Textbook of Tinnitus

Winfried Schlee • Berthold Langguth
Dirk De Ridder • Sven Vanneste
Tobias Kleinjung • Aage R. Møller
Editors

Textbook of Tinnitus

Second Edition

Springer

Editors
Winfried Schlee
Institute for Information and Process Management
Eastern Switzerland University of Applied Sciences
St. Gallen, Switzerland

Dirk De Ridder
Department of Surgical Sciences
University of Otago
Dunedin, New Zealand

Tobias Kleinjung
Department of Otorhinolaryngology – Head and Neck Surgery
University Hospital of Zurich, University of Zurich
Switzerland, Switzerland

Berthold Langguth
Department of Psychiatry and Psychotherapy
Interdisciplinary Tinnitus Clinic, University of Regensburg, Bezirksklinikum,
Regensburg, Germany

Sven Vanneste
School of Psychology
Global Brain Health Institute & Trinity College of Dublin Institute for Neuroscience
Dublin, Dublin, Ireland

Aage R. Møller
Neuroscience Program
University of Texas, Dallas School of Brain & Behavioral Sciences
Richardson, TX, USA

ISBN 978-3-031-35646-9 ISBN 978-3-031-35647-6 (eBook)
https://doi.org/10.1007/978-3-031-35647-6

This Springer imprint is published by the registered company Springer Nature Switzerland AG
The registered company address is: Gewerbestrasse 11, 6330 Cham, Switzerland

Foreword

I never thought I would survive with tinnitus for 15 years; I never thought that 15 years later the scientific community that knows so much more about tinnitus would have achieved so little in translating that knowledge into treatments.

These thoughts are also made more powerful when put in perspective with what the global scientific community has achieved in just the span of two full years of the COVID pandemic, in terms of identifying an unknown source of a new illness, discovering its mechanism of action of disease in the body and then the creation, testing, and worldwide distribution of a vaccine.

What lessons can be learned from a comparison between researching tinnitus, a disease that is not fatal but is the cause of suffering for at least a billion people and has been known for years, and research on COVID, a previously unknown illness?

When it comes to accomplishment in scientific discovery, numbers count, numbers of minds working on a problem. Not necessarily collectively but sheer numbers from the standpoint of building from ongoing literature created during the path of discovery. Sheer numbers and unlimited financial resources coming from a tremendous sense of urgency derived from what was seen immediately to be a deadly infectious disease crippling an entire world and its economy.

None of these is seen to be the case with tinnitus. Looking more closely we may find that when it comes to tinnitus simply throwing huge numbers of research manpower and unlimited financial resources at the problem might not produce results proportionally as expected.

What are the ingredients which make tinnitus still without a clear treatment? The point of difference may partially lie in the location of the pathology, namely the brain. Certainly COVID affects the brain, but the initial mechanism producing the pathology of COVID is not the workings of the brain but instead the immune system. Not that the immune system isn't immensely complex but certainly not to the extent of the human brain. And one needs only to think of the amount of research manpower and resources that has been targeted towards other brain disorders such as addiction, Alzheimer's disease, and depression to understand the complexity of the problem intrinsic to the brain.

The age old question is if the human brain is too complex for it to be able to understand itself.

Where does this leave us in terms of a strategy going forward? Does one continue with the same strategies with the idea that consistency is equivalent to persistence, a necessary quality for success or does one seek a different path? A basic principle underlying the strategy of discovering the treatment of a problem is to thoroughly understand the mechanism that has caused the problem and then with this alter the mechanism or alter the structure of the damage.

But this may not be a possible strategy for treatments of brain disorders given our level of basic science knowledge at this time.

So does that mean we must wait for basic science to catch up? No, not necessarily and there are examples in which treatments of neurological disorders have occurred even with an incomplete understanding of the mechanisms of the disorder. Transcranial Magnetic Stimulation and psychedelics for treatment of depression and cannabis for chronic pain and mood disorders are examples. These are treatments that have been discovered and integrated into practice before the underlying mechanisms have been completely known. This does not mean that research into the underlying causes of tinnitus should be abandoned but that lessons learned from other treatments of brain disorders can contribute to a possible different direction for treatment research.

Until more "firepower" is available we need less bureaucracy and a more bold approach including, for example, psychedelic drugs as a potential treatment. In the meantime we need to bring into clinical practice what we have already learned; acoustic stimulation being a prime example. Discovery without application is an empty endeavour and so being able to close this gap is a necessary achievement for the actual alleviation of suffering, which after all is our final goal.

Likewise there can also be benefit from examination of the very definition of the word treatment to include prevention. This is especially true for acoustic trauma and the various preventions of it yielding profound benefits at very low expenditures.

It all speaks to the issue of research strategy decision. But research itself does not exist in a vacuum but instead is the outcome of what produces it, namely a team. There must be motivation to drive integration and collaboration between teams to produce a research accomplishment. Results would naturally follow with the removal of redundancy and subsequent refocusing of resources on the core activities essential for research success.

It always seems impossible until it's done (Nelson Mandela)

Tinnitus Research Initiative
Monte Carlo, Monaco

Matteo de Nora

Preface

Highlights

- The book describes both the theoretical background of the different forms of tinnitus and detailed knowledge of state-of-the-art treatment of tinnitus.
- The book is written for clinicians and researchers by clinicians and researchers in tinnitus.
- It provides up-to-date information in forms that are suitable for those who diagnose and treat patients with tinnitus in their clinical praxis as clinical audiologists, dentists, neurologists, neurosurgeons, otolaryngologists, physical/manual therapists, psychiatrists, and psychologists.
- The book can also serve as a reference for clinicians who do not treat tinnitus patients routinely because of its organization and extensive subject index.
- The book is intended to serve as a reference for researchers interested in tinnitus who want to learn about basic principles and become familiar with the state of the art in tinnitus diagnosis and treatment.

Tinnitus (ringing in the ears) has many forms, and the severity of tinnitus ranges widely from being non-problematic to severely affecting a person's daily life. How loud the tinnitus is perceived does not directly relate to how much it distresses the patient. Thus, even tinnitus very close to the hearing threshold can be a disabling symptom. It can reduce the quality of life by generating anxiety and concentration problems, impairing the ability to do intellectual work, making it difficult to sleep, causing depression and sometimes even leading to suicide. Tinnitus can already occur at young age, but its prevalence steadily increases with the degree of age-related hearing loss and can reach 20% for people aged 65 and over. Moreover, tinnitus incidence is increasing dramatically with increased leisure noise, more work-related noise trauma, and longer lifespan.

Tinnitus is highly heterogeneous; it varies in its perceptual characteristics, its course, its co-morbidities, and its impact on the individual. Accordingly, there is also a high heterogeneity in tinnitus pathophysiology and in the response to specific treatments.

The different forms of tinnitus have similarities with different kinds of pain and can be considered phantom perceptions, i.e. the conscious awareness of a *percept* in the absence of an external stimulus. Moreover, there is no objective proof that someone has tinnitus or not. It remains a subjective perception, which can only be assessed in its characteristics and expression by the person concerned.

For a long time, it was believed that the anatomical location of the physiological abnormalities that caused the tinnitus was the ear, in particular the inner ear. However, it was later understood that most forms of tinnitus are caused by abnormalities in the central nervous system and that these abnormalities are often caused by expression of neural plasticity.

Many structures of the body, such as the ear, the auditory nervous system, the somatosensory system, other parts of the brain, and muscles of the head and the neck, are directly or indirectly involved in different forms of tinnitus. To treat and understand the pathology of tinnitus, therefore, requires involvement of many specialties of medicine, psychology, and neuroscience.

Tinnitus may occur after noise exposure and administration of pharmacological agents, but the cause of subjective tinnitus is often unknown. Severe tinnitus is often accompanied by symptoms such as hyperacusis (lowered tolerance to sound) and distortion of sounds. Affective disorders such as phonophobia (fear of sound) and depression often occur in individuals with severe tinnitus. With such differences in attributes, it is not reasonable to expect that a single cause can be responsible for severe tinnitus, again a factor that makes managing the tinnitus patient a challenge for health care professionals.

In 2006, the Tinnitus Research Initiative (TRI) was created as a foundation with the mission to find a cure for tinnitus by connecting researchers and clinicians from all over the world. In view of the complexity of tinnitus, TRI has facilitated interdisciplinary research efforts, and has put emphasis on neuroscience as most forms of tinnitus are disorders of the nervous system. The TRI wants to unite all researchers and clinicians globally in one front to fight the battle against this enigmatic symptom. It was also realized that only a few clinicians are specifically trained in tinnitus treatment, and there was a lack of suitable books that cover both basic research and clinical management of tinnitus.

This motivated us in 2010 to create a comprehensive textbook, the *Textbook of Tinnitus*. Special emphasis was placed on covering all relevant aspects of tinnitus and the perspective from many specialties of medicine, surgery, psychology, and neuroscience.

The fact that tinnitus is not a single disease but a group of diseases means that tinnitus cannot be effectively treated by a single approach, and several disciplines of health care must be involved in managing the patient with tinnitus. Treatment of the patient with severe tinnitus requires collaborations between clinicians in many different fields of medicine, audiology, and psychology. Accordingly, tinnitus research and treatment have been performed by a variety of disciplines, viewing the problem from various perspectives, focusing on different targets, and using diverse approaches. Therefore, the first edition of the *Textbook of Tinnitus* involved authors from diverse areas of expertise such as audiology, dentistry, clinical and experimental psychology, neurology, neuroscience, neurosurgery, otolaryngology, pharmacology, physical/manual therapy, psychiatry, data science, and software engineering.

Thus, the *Textbook of Tinnitus* has filled a void by providing a comprehensive overview of the different forms of tinnitus, their pathophysiology and their treatment. However, since the publication of the first edition of the *Textbook of Tinnitus* in 2010, tinnitus research has dramatically evolved. This development is evidenced by the pure amount of tinnitus-related research papers in PubMed which has doubled since 2010 (see Fig. 1).

This rapid development in Tinnitus Research made a new edition of the *Textbook of Tinnitus* urgently necessary. In view of the substantial increase in knowledge, we decided to modify the structure of the book and most chapters are newly written, and a few had major updates.

But the goal of the book remained the same. It is directed towards the clinician and aims to provide detailed information about diagnosis of the various different forms of tinnitus and their treatment. In addition, it provides an overview of what is known about the pathophysiology of different kinds of tinnitus and about new developments in the field.

The second edition brings together in a single book contributions from many different areas of basic science, clinical research, and health care to guide the management of the tinnitus patient.

The 60 chapters in this book express the independent views of the authors, some of which may diverge and some may complement one and another. With the experience from the first edition, that many readers only read single chapters and not the whole book, we tried to organize each chapter so that it contains all necessary information if read alone, which in turn resulted in some overlap across chapters.

The book has eight parts, I Basics About Tinnitus, II Neurobiology of Tinnitus, III Pathophysiological Models, IV Animal Research, V Diagnosis and Assessment, VI Management

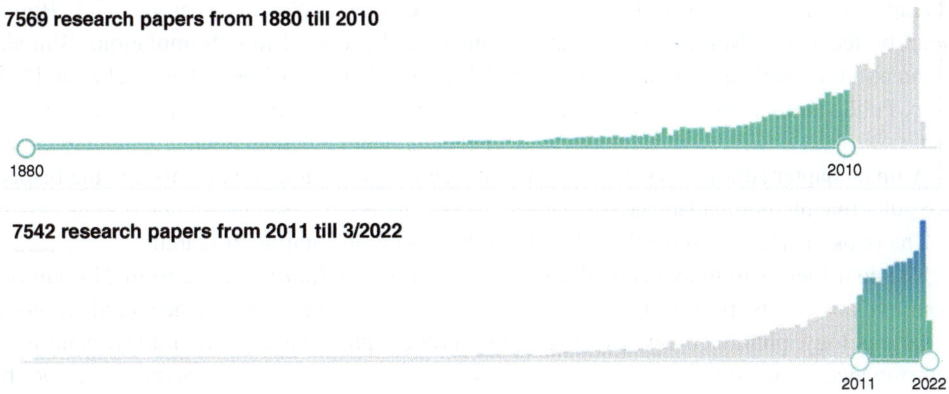

Fig. 1 Amount of research papers, found with the search term "Tinnitus" in pub-med

of Specific Forms of Tinnitus, VII Tinnitus Treatment, and VIII an Outlook about Future Directions.

The first part *Basics About Tinnitus* starts with a chapter about the history of tinnitus research, which is followed by two chapters dealing with the definition of tinnitus, tinnitus disorder, and other syndromes, which are characterized by hypersensitivity to sounds, such as hyperacusis and misophonia. The part also includes chapters on the epidemiology of tinnitus, the role of genetics in tinnitus, and risk factors for tinnitus. The last two chapters deal with the heterogeneity of tinnitus and the similarities between tinnitus and pain.

The second part *Neurobiology of Tinnitus* starts with a chapter about the anatomy and physiology of the auditory system. The next two chapters cover alterations of the cochlea after noise trauma and the molecular biology of the central nervous system in tinnitus. Further chapters deal with the interaction between the somatosensory and the auditory system, with auditory deprivation and with neural plasticity of the auditory system. The last two chapters of this part cover the knowledge about structural and functional alterations in patients with tinnitus detected by magnetic resonance imaging, electro- and magnetoencephalography.

In the third part various *Pathophysiological Models* of tinnitus are discussed. In detail, these are the Bayesian Model, the Neuronal Gain Model, the Noise Cancellation Model, the Neurophysiological Model, a Psychological Model, and a Neuroinflammatory Model of tinnitus.

The fourth part *Animal Research* includes a chapter on Animal Models of Hyperacusis and a chapter on the Translation of Animal Findings to Humans in Tinnitus Research.

The fifth part *Diagnosis and Assessment* starts with a chapter with the TRI flowchart for the diagnosis of tinnitus, followed by chapters on Tinnitus History Taking and Tinnitus Questionnaires. Further chapters deal with the otological and the audiological assessment of tinnitus, neuroradiological tests in the diagnosis of tinnitus, and the clinical assessment of the somatosensory system.

The sixth part deals with the *Management of Specific Forms of Tinnitus*. Separate chapters deal with various forms of tinnitus, which are characterized either by specific clinical or demographic features, pathophysiological patterns, or by specific co-morbidities. In detail, these are Conductive and Sensorineural Hearing Loss, Meniere's Disease and a Set of Rare Disorders with Tinnitus, Vestibular Schwannoma, Microvascular Compression of the Vestibulocochlear Nerve, Cerebrovascular Diseases, Somatosensory Tinnitus, Trauma-Associated Tinnitus, Tinnitus in Children and Adolescents, Tinnitus with Hyperacusis, and Tinnitus with Psychiatric Comorbidities.

The seventh part *Tinnitus Treatment* covers the various therapeutic approaches, which have been developed for the management of tinnitus. These include Tinnitus Counselling, Cognitive Behavioural Therapy, Mindfulness-Based Treatment, Auditory Treatments, Tinnitus Retraining

Therapy, Pharmacotherapy, Tinnitus Activity Treatment, Neural Therapy and Botox, Neurobiofeedback, Non-invasive Brain Stimulation, Invasive Brain Stimulation, Bimodal Stimulation, Complementary and Alternative Therapies, E-Health-Based Approaches and Self Help. Public and Patient Involvement as an important new development is also covered in this part.

A final chapter summarizes the current evidence for the various treatments and the respective guideline recommendations.

The book closes with some thoughts about the Future of Tinnitus Research.

The contributors to the second edition of the *Textbook of Tinnitus* come from 21 countries from five continents, from many different disciplines (audiology, data science, epidemiology, otolaryngology, pharmacology, psychiatry, psychology, physiotherapy, radiology, neurology, neuroscience, neurosurgery, software engineering), and also involve people affected by tinnitus. This multinational and multidisciplinary group evolved in the context of the "The Tinnitus Research Initiative" (TRI), which has promoted collaborative interdisciplinary research on tinnitus during the past 15 years. This book would not exist without Mr. Matteo de Nora, who founded and funded the Tinnitus Research Initiative and without him, also Tinnitus Research would not be where it is now.

We would also like to take this opportunity to remember all those who contributed to the *Textbook of Tinnitus* and who have since passed away. We mourn the loss of Hilde De Ridder-Symoens, Carlos Herraiz, Larry Roberts, David Baguley, and Aage Moller. All of them were passionate about advancing the treatment of tinnitus and alleviating the suffering of tinnitus sufferers. We will keep them and their achievements deep in our memory. This is especially true for Aage Moller, the spiritus rector of the *Textbook of Tinnitus*. As the *Textbook of Tinnitus* would not exist without Aage Moller and due to our special relationship with him, we have also added an obituary for the "father of tinnitus research".

Regensburg, Germany — Berthold Langguth
Zürich, Switzerland — Tobias Kleinjung
Regensburg, Germany — Winfried Schlee
Dublin, Ireland — Sven Vanneste
Dunedin, New Zealand — Dirk De Ridder

Aage Moller: A Father of Tinnitus Research

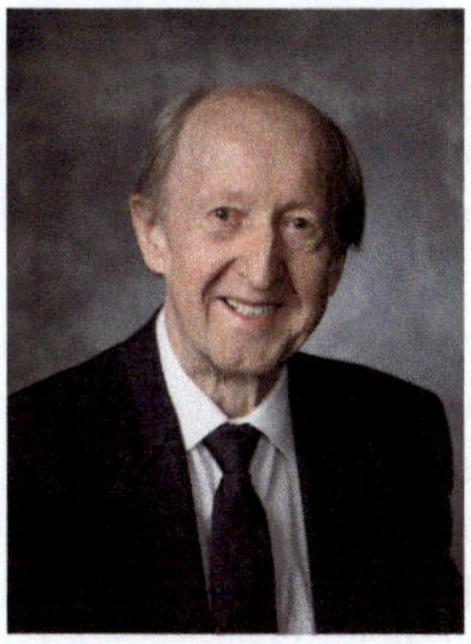

Aage Moller left us at the age of 90. Born in Denmark, trained at the Karolinska in Sweden, spent some research time in Kenya, and later had 2 academic careers, one in the neurosurgical operation theatre in Pittsburgh, and later, when most people retire, he joined the University of Texas at Dallas, where he was still actively teaching till a few months ago.

These facts are of little importance, as Aage will be remembered as a "Great Man", both in academia and as a human. His academic career needs no introduction, having published more than 200 scientific papers, more than 100 book chapters, more than 10 books, and edited among others the first *Textbook of Tinnitus*. But the way he did it is exemplary for his wonderful personality, kind yet firm, open-minded but no-nonsense, famous, yet humble, but above all, Aage was a man of dedication, dedication to the field of auditory neuroscience, dedicated to his students, not only in Dallas, but all over the world. This dedication also led to a second typical characteristic of Aage: courage. Scientifically he was unafraid to go beyond the trodden path. He studied audiology, neuroscience, pain, fear, autism, intraoperative neurophysiology, and pushed the concept of maladaptive plasticity as a cause for pain and tinnitus before that was en vogue. He was also one of first to endorse translational neuroscience, bridging the gap between basic neuroscience and clinicians. When he had trouble getting manuscripts accepted for publication because the journals were only interested in auditory research performed with pure tones, which had little translational value for clinicians, he founded a new journal in 1978, dedicated to translational approaches of hearing: *Hearing Research*. He was its chief editor for 27 years, read every single submission, and sometimes accepted manuscripts if one of his reviewers rejected it, if he saw merit in the manuscript. *Hearing Research* is now a standard in the field of auditory (neuro)science. He would accept research performed with complex noise as a stimulus, speech sounds, but the research had to be either basic or translational, not clinical audiology nor pure ENT. His journal had to fill a gap.

But Aage was more than a wonderful teacher, researcher, and journal editor. His interest in humanity led to motivating politicians in preventing work-related noise trauma in the 1970s, long before anybody became interested in it. He also published about the hidden dramas in the medical system, with the same goal: prevention of trauma, iatrogenic trauma.

Everybody who knew him has a story to tell, of how they met, and what Aage has meant for their career and how that resulted in life-long friendship. One of the co-authors, as a very young neurosurgeon interested in microvascular decompression surgery for hemifacial spasm and tinnitus asked Aage if he would be willing to become a co-promotor of my PhD thesis. I had never met him, he had never heard of me, as I hadn't published one single paper. Even though he was a famous scientist and I am Mr Nobody he answered my email immediately, writing that whether he would be willing to become co-promotor depended on my personality, as most neurosurgeons he knew were very arrogant, and he had no interest in spending time on educating an arrogant new specimen. He proposed to meet at 5:30 AM in the morning in Brussels the next month, when he was on one of his many lecturing tours, and had a 3 hour lay-over in Zaventem airport in Belgium. In the airport he took the time to listen to my proposal and gauge my behaviour and attitude. He suggested I get to writing a paper and send it to him. The first paper came back with 99% corrected in red, with only a few words still left in black fond. The second paper was a little better, with 85% in red, and progressively my success rate went up. Soon afterwards, he came to visit me in the operation theatre, because he wanted to see how my surgical nerve decompression technique was, most likely to verify whether the results of the manuscripts we would submit together were to be trusted. And I visited him in Pittsburgh and later in Dallas. Progressively the professor-student relationship turned into a friendship, by blurring the existing hierarchical boundaries under his instigation. And I am sure, many of us have had similar experiences. It demonstrates how Aage was not only a great scientist, but also a great human being.

Many readers will know him for his dedication to the tinnitus field, which he has helped to establish from a neglected research domain to a somewhat accepted scientific field. It was his inspirational guidance, his unselfish help, his organizational capacity, and never-ending support that brought many of us in the field. He can truly be called A Father of Tinnitus Research, not only because of the scientific work he has performed, but because he has been a father to an entire generation of young tinnitus researchers, and with Aage's death, the tinnitus field loses a pioneer, a teacher, an inspiration, and a friend for many.

Aage, you will be missed.

Contents

Part I Basics About Tinnitus

1 **History of Tinnitus** 3
Dirk De Ridder and Hilde De Ridder-Symoens

2 **Tinnitus, Tinnitus Disorder, and Other Phantom Perceptions** 17
Berthold Langguth and Dirk De Ridder

3 **Hypersensitivity to Sounds** 25
Laure Jacquemin, Martin Schecklmann, and David M. Baguley

4 **Epidemiology of Tinnitus: Frequency of the Condition** 35
Carlotta M. Jarach, Alessandra Lugo, Marco Scala, Christopher R. Cederroth, Werner J. D. Garavello, Winfried Schlee, Berthold Langguth, and Silvano Gallus

5 **Genetic Contribution to Tinnitus and Tinnitus Disorder** 49
Christopher R. Cederroth, Natalia Trpchevska, Sana Amanat, Alvaro Gallego-Martinez, and José Antonio Lopez-Escamez

6 **Environmental and Occupational Risk Factors for Tinnitus** 59
Deborah A. Hall and Roshni Biswas

7 **Tinnitus Heterogeneity, Different Types of Tinnitus, and Gender Aspects** 71
Berthold Langguth

8 **Similarities Between Tinnitus and Pain** 81
Dirk De Ridder and Aage R. Møller

Part II Neurobiology of Tinnitus

9 **Anatomy and Physiology of the Auditory System** 101
Gabriel Byczynski, Sven Vanneste, and Aage R. Møller

10 **Cochlear Changes After Noise Trauma** 115
María Eugenia Gómez-Casati and Ana Belén Elgoyhen

11 **Molecular Biology of the Central Auditory System and Tinnitus** 123
Rahilla Tarfa and Thanos Tzounopoulos

12 **Tinnitus and the Somatosensory System** 135
Aage R. Møller and Dirk De Ridder

13 **The Role of Auditory Deprivation** 145
Tobias Kleinjung and Aage R. Møller

14 **Neuroplasticity of the Auditory System** 149
Jos J. Eggermont

15 **Structural and Functional MRI-Based Neuroimaging in Tinnitus** 165
Katherine Adcock, Dirk De Ridder, and Sven Vanneste

16 **The Electrophysiological Explorations in Tinnitus Over the Decades Using EEG and MEG** 175
Anusha Yasoda-Mohan and Sven Vanneste

Part III Pathophysiological Models

17 **The Bayesian Brain and Tinnitus** 189
Dirk De Ridder, Sven Vanneste, William Sedley, and Karl Friston

18 **Central Gain Model for Tinnitus: A Review on Noise-Induced Plasticity or When Less at the Periphery Is More in the Center** 205
Vinay Parameshwarappa and Arnaud J. Norena

19 **The Frontostriatal Gating Model of Tinnitus** 221
Josef P. Rauschecker

20 **The Neurophysiological Model of Tinnitus and Decreased Sound Tolerance** 231
Pawel J. Jastreboff

21 **Psychological Models of Tinnitus** 251
Nicolas Dauman, Lise Hobeika, Soly Erlandsson, Rilana Cima, Laurence McKenna, Severine Samson, and Alain Londero

22 **Neuroinflammation Model of Tinnitus** 269
Weihua Wang and Shaowen Bao

Part IV Animal Research for Tinnitus

23 **Animal Models of Hyperacusis: Neural Hyperactivity in Auditory, Emotional, Arousal, Memory, and Motor Networks** 283
Richard Salvi, Guang-Di Chen, Xiaopeng Liu, Ben Auerbach, Dalian Ding, Yu-Chen Chen, and Senthilvelan Manohar

24 **Translating Animal Findings to Humans in Tinnitus Research** 301
Yiwen Zheng and Paul F. Smith

Part V Diagnosis and Assessment

25 **Diagnosis and Flowchart** 315
Berthold Langguth

26 **Tinnitus History Taking** 321
Berthold Langguth

27 **Tinnitus Questionnaires** 329
Berthold Langguth and Annick Gilles

28 **Clinical Otorhinolaryngological Assessment** 345
Tobias Kleinjung and Alain Londero

29 **Audiological Assessment for Tinnitus** 351
Giriraj S. Shekhawat, Karen Sparrow, and Lisa Callahan

30 **Clinical Neuroimaging in the Evaluation of Tinnitus** 363
Bernhard Schuknecht and Tobias Kleinjung

31 **Clinical Assessment of the Somatosensory System** 377
Tanit Ganz Sanchez and Sarah Michiels

Part VI Management of Specific Forms of Tinnitus

32 **Conductive and Sensorineural Hearing Loss** 385
Tobias Kleinjung and Alain Londero

33 **Meniere's Disease, a Set of Rare Disorders with Tinnitus** 399
Patricia Perez-Carpena, Lidia Frejo, and Jose Antonio Lopez-Escamez

34 **Tinnitus and Vestibular Schwannoma** 413
Dirk De Ridder and Tobias Kleinjung

35 **Microvascular Compression of the Vestibulocochlear Nerve** 423
Dirk De Ridder

36 **Tinnitus and Cerebrovascular Diseases** 439
Anna Piera, Alejandro Ponz, and Jose Miguel Láinez

37 **Cervical and Masticatory Somatosensory System** 447
Sarah Michiels and Tanit Ganz Sanchez

38 **Trauma-Associated Tinnitus** 457
Dirk De Ridder

39 **Tinnitus in Children and Adolescents** 465
Susanne S. Nemholt and David M. Baguley

40 **Pulsatile Tinnitus** 483
Jae-Jin Song and Dirk De Ridder

41 **Hyperacusis and Tinnitus** 501
Martin Schecklmann, Laure Jacquemin, and David M. Baguley

42 **Tinnitus and Psychiatric Comorbidities** 515
Berthold Langguth and Michael Landgrebe

Part VII Tinnitus Treatment

43 **Tinnitus Counselling and Psychoeducation** 529
Grant D. Searchfield, Martin Schecklmann, and Maria Kleinstaeuber

44 **CBT for Tinnitus** 545
Thomas Fuller and Derek J. Hoare

45 **Mindfulness and Tinnitus** 563
Laurence McKenna and Florian Vogt

46 **Auditory Treatments of Tinnitus** 575
Magdalena Sereda and Derek J. Hoare

47 **Tinnitus Retraining Therapy** 589
Pawel J. Jastreboff and Margaret M. Jastreboff

48 **Tinnitus Pharmacotherapy** 617
Ana Belén Elgoyhen and Berthold Langguth

49 **Tinnitus Activities Treatment** 631
Ann E. Perreau and Richard S. Tyler

50 **Neural Therapy, Botulinum Toxin** 645
Eberhard Biesinger, Jose Miguel Lainez, Marlene M. Speth, and Veronika Vielsmeier

51 **Neurofeedback** 653
Patrick Neff and Martin Meyer

52 **Noninvasive Brain Stimulation** 667
Sven Vanneste and Tobias Kleinjung

53 **Invasive Brain Stimulation** 679
Dirk De Ridder and Sven Vanneste

54 **Bimodal Stimulation for the Treatment of Tinnitus** 693
Sven Vanneste and Berthold Langguth

55 **Complementary and Alternative Therapies** 705
Alain Londero and Deborah A. Hall

56 **Public and Patient Involvement in Tinnitus Research** 717
Patrick K. A. Neff, Maryam Shabbir, Hazel Goedhart, Markku Vesala, Georgina Burns-O'Connell, and Deborah A. Hall

57 **Mobile Health Solutions for Tinnitus** 731
Muntazir Mehdi, Franz J. Hauck, Ruediger Pryss, and Winfried Schlee

58 **Autonomous Tinnitus Management (Self-Help for Tinnitus)** 739
Don J. McFerran and Nic Wray

59 **Tinnitus Treatment: Evidence and Guidelines** 763
Berthold Langguth, Tobias Kleinjung, Winfried Schlee, Sven Vanneste, and Dirk De Ridder

Part VIII Future Directions

60 **The Future of Tinnitus Research: "In Crazy We Believe, in Science We Trust"** 781
Dirk De Ridder, Sven Vanneste, Aage R. Møller, Tobias Kleinjung, Berthold Langguth, and Winfried Schlee

Index 787

Contributors

Katherine Adcock Global Brain Health Institute and Institute of Neuroscience, Trinity College Dublin, Dublin, Ireland

Lab for Clinical and Integrative Neuroscience, Trinity Institute for Neuroscience, School of Psychology, Trinity College Dublin, Dublin, Ireland

Sana Amanat Otology and Neurotology Group CTS495, Department of Genomic Medicine, GENYO-Centre for Genomics and Oncological Research Pfizer/University of Granada/Junta de Andalucía, PTS, Granada, Spain

Ben Auerbach Center for Hearing and Deafness, 137 Cary Hall, University at Buffalo, Buffalo, NY, USA

David M. Baguley NIHR Biomedical Research Centre, School of Medicine, University of Nottingham, Nottingham, UK

Mental Health and Clinical Neurosciences, School of Medicine, University of Nottingham, Nottingham, UK

Nottingham Audiology Services, Nottingham University Hospitals, Nottingham, UK

Nottingham Biomedical Research Centre, National Institute for Health Research, Ropewalk House, Nottingham, UK

Hearing Sciences, Mental Health and Clinical Neurosciences, School of Medicine, University of Nottingham, Nottingham, UK

Nottingham University Hospitals NHS Trust, Nottingham, UK

Shaowen Bao Department of Physiology, University of Arizona, Tucson, AZ, USA

Eberhard Biesinger Private Practice, Centre of Otorhinolaryngology, Lindenberg, Germany

Roshni Biswas Hearing Sciences Group, Division of Clinical Neuroscience, School of Medicine, University of Nottingham, Nottingham, UK

National Institute for Health Research (NIHR) Nottingham Biomedical Research Centre (BRC), Nottingham, UK

Georgina Burns-O'Connell British Tinnitus Association, Sheffield, UK

Gabriel Byczynski Lab for Clinical & Integrative Neuroscience, Trinity Institute for Neuroscience, School of Psychology, Trinity College Dublin, Dublin, Ireland

Lisa Callahan College of Education, Psychology, and Social Work, Flinders University, Adelaide, Australia

Christopher R. Cederroth Laboratory of Experimental Audiology, Department of Physiology and Pharmacology, Karolinska Institutet, Stockholm, Sweden

National Institute for Health Research Nottingham Biomedical Research Centre, Nottingham University Hospitals National Health Service Trust, Nottingham, UK

Division of Clinical Neuroscience, Hearing Sciences, School of Medicine, University of Nottingham, Nottingham, UK

Translational Hearing Research, Tübingen Hearing Research Center, Department of Otolaryngology, Head and Neck Surgery, University of Tübingen, Tübingen, Germany

Guang-Di Chen Center for Hearing and Deafness, 137 Cary Hall, University at Buffalo, Buffalo, NY, USA

Yu-Chen Chen Department of Radiology, Nanjing First Hospital, Nanjing Medical University, Nanjing, China

Rilana Cima Department of Clinical Psychological Science, Maastricht University, Maastricht, Netherlands

Adelante, Centre for Expertise in Rehabilitation and Audiology, Hoensbroek, Limburg, Netherlands

Nicolas Dauman Département de Psychologie, Université de Poitiers, Univ Rennes, Univ Angers, Univ Brest, RPPSY, Poitiers, France

Dirk De Ridder Section of Neurosurgery, Department of Surgical Sciences, University of Otago, Dunedin, New Zealand

Hilde De Ridder-Symoens Emeritus of Department of Medieval History, Free University of Amsterdam, Amsterdam, The Netherlands

Department of Early Modern History, University of Ghent, Gent, Belgium

Dalian Ding Center for Hearing and Deafness, 137 Cary Hall, University at Buffalo, Buffalo, NY, USA

Jos J. Eggermont University of Calgary, Calgary, AB, Canada

Ana Belén Elgoyhen Instituto de Investigaciones en Ingeniería Genética y Biología Molecular "Dr. Héctor N. Torres," Consejo Nacional de Investigaciones Científicas y Técnicas, Buenos Aires, Argentina

Soly Erlandsson Department of Social and Behavioural Science, University West, Trollhättan, Sweden

Lidia Frejo Otology and Neurotology Group CTS 495, Department of Genomic Medicine, Centro de Genómica e Investigación Oncológica (GENyO) Pfizer-Universidad de Granada-Junta de Andalucía, Granada, Spain

Sensorineural Pathology Programme, Centro de Investigación Biomédica en Red en Enfermedades Raras, Madrid, Spain

Karl Friston Wellcome Trust Centre for Neuroimaging, University College London, London, UK

Thomas Fuller Clinical Psychological Science, Faculty of Psychology and Neuroscience, Maastricht University, Maastricht, The Netherlands

Alvaro Gallego-Martinez Otology and Neurotology Group CTS495, Department of Genomic Medicine, GENYO-Centre for Genomics and Oncological Research Pfizer/University of Granada/Junta de Andalucía, PTS, Granada, Spain

Silvano Gallus Istituto di Ricerche Farmacologiche Mario Negri IRCCS, Department of Environmental Health Sciences, Milan, Italy

Werner J. D. Garavello School of Medicine and Surgery, University of Milan-Bicocca, Department of Otorhinolaryngology, Milan, Italy

Annick Gilles Faculty of Medicine and Health Sciences, Department of Translational Neuroscience, University of Antwerp, Wilrijk, Belgium

Department of Otorhinolaryngology and Head Neck Surgery, Antwerp University Hospital, Edegem, Belgium

Department of Education, Health and Social Work, University College Ghent, Ghent, Belgium

Hazel Goedhart Tinnitus Hub, London, UK

Tinnitus Hub, Amsterdam, The Netherlands

María Eugenia Gómez-Casati Instituto de Farmacología, Facultad de Medicina, Universidad de Buenos Aires, Buenos Aires, Argentina

Deborah A. Hall Hearing Sciences Group, Division of Clinical Neuroscience, School of Medicine, University of Nottingham, Nottingham, UK

National Institute for Health Research (NIHR) Nottingham Biomedical Research Centre (BRC), Nottingham, UK

Heriot-Watt University Malaysia, Putrajaya, Malaysia

Hearing Sciences, Mental Health and Clinical Neurosciences, School of Medicine, University of Nottingham, Nottingham, UK

Department of Psychology, School of Social Sciences, Heriot-Watt University Malaysia, Putrajaya, Malaysia

Franz J. Hauck Institute of Distributed Systems, Ulm University, Ulm, Germany

Derek J. Hoare NIHR Nottingham Biomedical Research Centre, Hearing Sciences, Mental Health and Clinical Neurosciences, School of Medicine, University of Nottingham, Nottingham, UK

Hearing Sciences, Mental Health and Clinical Neurosciences, School of Medicine, University of Nottingham, Nottingham, UK

NIHR Nottingham Biomedical Research Centre, Nottingham, UK

Lise Hobeika Univ. Lille, ULR 4072 - PSITEC - Psychologie: Interactions Temps Émotions Cognition, Lille, France

Institut du Cerveau et de la Moelle épinière–ICM, INSERM U 1127, CNRS UMR 7225, Sorbonne Université, Paris, France

Laure Jacquemin University Department of Otorhinolaryngology and Head and Neck Surgery, Antwerp University Hospital, Edegem, Belgium

Department of Translational Neurosciences, Faculty of Medicine and Health Sciences, University of Antwerp, Wilrijk, Belgium

Carlotta M. Jarach Istituto di Ricerche Farmacologiche Mario Negri IRCCS, Department of Environmental Health Sciences, Milan, Italy

Margaret M. Jastreboff JHDF, Inc., Guilford, CT, USA

Pawel J. Jastreboff Department Otolaryngology, School of Medicine, Emory University, Atlanta, GA, USA

JHDF, Inc., Ellicott City, MD, USA

JHDF, Inc., Guilford, CT, USA

Tobias Kleinjung Department of Otorhinolaryngology – Head and Neck Surgery, University Hospital of Zurich, University of Zurich, Zurich, Switzerland

Maria Kleinstaeuber Department of Psychology, Emma Eccles Jones College of Education and Human Services, Utah State University, Logan, UT, USA

Jose Miguel Lainez Department of Neurology, University Clinic Hospital, Catholic University of Valencia, Valencia, Spain

Michael Landgrebe Department of Psychiatry, Psychosomatics and Psychotherapy, kbo-Lech-Mangfall-Hosptial Agatharied, Hausham, Germany

Berthold Langguth Department of Psychiatry and Psychotherapy, Interdisciplinary Tinnitus Clinic, University of Regensburg, Regensburg, Germany

Xiaopeng Liu Center for Hearing and Deafness, 137 Cary Hall, University at Buffalo, Buffalo, NY, USA

Alain Londero Hôpital Européen Georges Pompidou, Assistance Publique - Hôpitaux de Paris, Paris, France

Faculté de Médecine Paris Descartes - Université de Paris, Paris, France

Service ORL et CCF, Hôpital Européen Georges Pompidou, Assistance Publique—Hôpitaux de Paris, Faculté de Médecine Paris Descartes—Université de Paris, Paris, France

Jose Antonio Lopez-Escamez Otology and Neurotology Group CTS 495, Department of Genomic Medicine, Centro de Genómica e Investigación Oncológica (GENyO) Pfizer-Universidad de Granada-Junta de Andalucía, Granada, Spain

Department of Otolaryngology, Hospital Universitario Virgen de las Nieves, Instituto de Investigación Biosanitaria, ibs.GRANADA, Granada, Spain

Sensorineural Pathology Programme, Centro de Investigación Biomédica en Red en Enfermedades Raras, Madrid, Spain

Division of Otolaryngology, Department of Surgery, Universidad de Granada, Granada, Spain

Meniere's Disease Neuroscience Research Program, Faculty of Medicine & Health, School of Medical Sciences, The Kolling Institute, University of Sydney, Sydney, New South Wales, Australia

Alessandra Lugo Istituto di Ricerche Farmacologiche Mario Negri IRCCS, Department of Environmental Health Sciences, Milan, Italy

Meniere's Disease Neuroscience Research Program, Faculty of Medicine & Health, School of Medical Sciences, The Kolling Institute, University of Sydney, Sydney, New South Wales, Australia

Senthilvelan Manohar Center for Hearing and Deafness, 137 Cary Hall, University at Buffalo, Buffalo, NY, USA

Don J. McFerran Tinnitus UK (Formerly the British Tinnitus Association), Sheffield, UK

Laurence McKenna Royal National ENT and Eastman Dental Throat Nose and Ear Hospitals, University College Hospitals, London, UK

Ear Institute, UCL, London, UK

Muntazir Mehdi Institute of Clinical Epidemiology and Biometry, University of Wuerzburg, Würzburg, Germany

Martin Meyer University Research Priority Program "Dynamics of Healthy Aging", University of Zurich, Zurich, Switzerland

Department of Comparative Language Science, University of Zurich, Zurich, Switzerland

Center for the Interdisciplinary Study of Language Evolution (ISLE), University of Zurich, Zurich, Switzerland

Cognitive Psychology Unit, Alpen-Adria University Klagenfurt, Klagenfurt am Wörthersee, Austria

Sarah Michiels Musculoskeletal Rehabilitation, REVAL Rehabilitation Research Center, Faculty of Rehabilitation Sciences and Physiotherapy, Hasselt University, Diepenbeek, Belgium

Anusha Yasoda-Mohan Global Brain Health Institute and Institute of Neuroscience, Trinity College Dublin, Dublin, Ireland

Lab for Clinical and Integrative Neuroscience, Trinity Institute for Neuroscience, School of Psychology, Trinity College Dublin, Dublin, Ireland

Aage R. Møller Neuroscience Program, School of Brain and Behavioral Sciences, University of Texas, Richardson, TX, USA

Neuroscience Program, University of Texas, Dallas School of Brain and Behavioral Sciences, Richardson, TX, USA

Patrick K. A. Neff Neuro-X Institute, École Polytechnique Fédérale de Lausanne (EPFL), Geneva, Switzerland

Department of Radiology and Medical Informatics, University of Geneva, Geneva, Switzerland

Department of Psychiatry and Psychotherapy, University of Regensburg, Regensburg, Germany

Centre for Cognitive Neuroscience and Department of Psychology, Paris-Lodron Universität Salzburg, Salzburg, Austria

Department of Otorhinolaryngology - Head and Neck Surgery, University Hospital of Zurich, University of Zurich, Zürich, Switzerland

Susanne S. Nemholt Kommunikationscentret, The Social Division in the Capital Region of Denmark, Hellerup, Denmark

Arnaud J. Norena UMR CNRS 7291, Aix-Marseille University, Marseille, France

Vinay Parameshwarappa UMR CNRS 7291, Aix-Marseille University, Marseille, France

Patricia Perez-Carpena Otology and Neurotology Group CTS 495, Department of Genomic Medicine, Centro de Genómica e Investigación Oncológica (GENyO) Pfizer-Universidad de Granada-Junta de Andalucía, Granada, Spain

Department of Otolaryngology, Hospital Universitario Virgen de las Nieves, Instituto de Investigación Biosanitaria, ibs.GRANADA, Granada, Spain

Sensorineural Pathology Programme, Centro de Investigación Biomédica en Red en Enfermedades Raras, Madrid, Spain

Ann E. Perreau Department of Communication Sciences and Disorders, Augustana College, Rock Island, IL, USA

Department of Otolaryngology—Head and Neck Surgery, University of Iowa, Iowa City, IA, USA

Anna Piera Department of Neurology, Hospital Clínico Universitario, Universidad Católica de Valencia, Valencia, Spain

Alejandro Ponz Department of Neurology, Hospital Clínico Universitario, Universidad Católica de Valencia, Valencia, Spain

Ruediger Pryss Institute of Clinical Epidemiology and Biometry, University of Wuerzburg, Würzburg, Germany

Josef P. Rauschecker Georgetown University Medical Center, Washington, DC, USA

Richard Salvi Center for Hearing and Deafness, 137 Cary Hall, University at Buffalo, Buffalo, NY, USA

Severine Samson Univ. Lille, ULR 4072 - PSITEC - Psychologie: Interactions Temps Émotions Cognition, Lille, France

Institut du Cerveau et de la Moelle épinière–ICM, INSERM U 1127, CNRS UMR 7225, Sorbonne Université, Paris, France

AP-HP, GH Pitié-Salpêtrière-Charles Foix, Unité d'Epileptologie, Paris, France

Tanit Ganz Sanchez Otolaryngology Department, University of São Paulo Medical School, São Paulo, Brazil

Marco Scala Istituto di Ricerche Farmacologiche Mario Negri IRCCS, Department of Environmental Health Sciences, Milan, Italy

Martin Schecklmann Department of Psychiatry and Psychotherapy, Interdisciplinary Tinnitus Clinic, University of Regensburg, Regensburg, Germany

Winfried Schlee Department of Psychiatry and Psychotherapy, Interdisciplinary Tinnitus Clinic, University of Regensburg, Regensburg, Germany

Institute for Information and Process Management, Eastern Switzerland University of Applied Sciences, St. Gallen, Switzerland

Bernhard Schuknecht Medical Radiological Institute, Zurich, Switzerland

Grant D. Searchfield Audiology Section, School of Population Health, Faculty of Medical and Health Sciences, The University of Auckland, Auckland, New Zealand

Eisdell Moore Centre, The University of Auckland, Auckland, New Zealand

Centre for Brain Research, The University of Auckland, Auckland, New Zealand

William Sedley Translational and Clinical Research Institute, Newcastle University, Newcastle upon Tyne, UK

Magdalena Sereda NIHR Nottingham Biomedical Research Centre, Nottingham, UK

Hearing Sciences, Mental Health and Clinical Neurosciences, School of Medicine, University of Nottingham, Nottingham, UK

Maryam Shabbir Hearing Sciences, Mental Health and Clinical Neurosciences, School of Medicine, University of Nottingham, Nottingham, UK

Giriraj S. Shekhawat College of Education, Psychology, and Social Work, Flinders University, Adelaide, Australia

Ear Institute, University College London, London, UK

Tinnitus Research Initiative, Regensburg, Germany

Paul F. Smith Department of Pharmacology and Toxicology, School of Biomedical Sciences, University of Otago, Dunedin, New Zealand

Brain Health Research Centre, University of Otago, Dunedin, New Zealand

Brain Research New Zealand, Christchurch, New Zealand

Eisdell Moore Centre for Hearing and Balance Research, University of Auckland, Auckland, New Zealand

Jae-Jin Song Department of Otorhinolaryngology-Head and Neck Surgery, Seoul National University Bundang Hospital, Seongnam, Republic of Korea

Karen Sparrow College of Education, Psychology, and Social Work, Flinders University, Adelaide, Australia

Marlene M. Speth Department of Otorhinolaryngology - Head and Neck Surgery, Kantonsspital Aarau, Aarau, Switzerland

Rahilla Tarfa School of Medicine, University of Pittsburgh, Pittsburgh, PA, USA

Natalia Trpchevska Laboratory of Experimental Audiology, Department of Physiology and Pharmacology, Karolinska Institutet, Stockholm, Sweden

Richard S. Tyler Department of Otolaryngology—Head and Neck Surgery, University of Iowa, Iowa City, IA, USA

Department of Communication Sciences and Disorders, University of Iowa, Iowa City, IA, USA

Thanos Tzounopoulos Department of Otolaryngology, University of Pittsburgh, Pittsburgh, PA, USA

Pittsburgh Hearing Research Center, University of Pittsburgh, Pittsburgh, PA, USA

Sven Vanneste Global Brain Health Institute, Trinity College Dublin, Dublin, Ireland

Trinity College Institute for Neuroscience, Trinity College Dublin, Dublin, Ireland

School of Psychology, Trinity College Dublin, Dublin, Ireland

Global Brain Health Institute and Institute of Neuroscience, Trinity College Dublin, Dublin, Ireland

Lab for Clinical and Integrative Neuroscience, Trinity Institute for Neuroscience, School of Psychology, Trinity College Dublin, Dublin, Ireland

School of Psychology, Global Brain Health Institute and Trinity College Institute for Neuroscience, Trinity College Dublin, Dublin, Ireland

Markku Vesala Tinnitus Hub, London, UK

Tinnitus Hub, Amsterdam, The Netherlands

Veronika Vielsmeier Department of Otorhinolaryngology, University of Regensburg, Regensburg, Germany

Florian Vogt Royal National ENT and Eastman Dental Hospital, University College Hospitals, London, UK

Weihua Wang Department of Physiology, University of Arizona, Tucson, AZ, USA

Nic Wray Tinnitus UK (Formerly the British Tinnitus Association), Sheffield, UK

Yiwen Zheng Department of Pharmacology and Toxicology, School of Biomedical Sciences, University of Otago, Dunedin, New Zealand

Brain Health Research Centre, University of Otago, Dunedin, New Zealand

Brain Research New Zealand, Christchurch, New Zealand

Eisdell Moore Centre for Hearing and Balance Research, University of Auckland, Auckland, New Zealand

Part I

Basics About Tinnitus

History of Tinnitus

1

Dirk De Ridder and Hilde De Ridder-Symoens

Abstract

Tinnitus is as old as humanity. The first written record of tinnitus as a medical condition comes from Mesopotamia in the seventh CBC. Tinnitus was still considered a punishment from the Gods and treatment consisted of charms. This changed with Hippocrates, in the fifth CBC who believed diseases were caused naturally and provided a brain-based explanation for tinnitus, as part of a constellation of symptoms, typical for infections. Several physicians and scientists proposed treatments, consisting of diet and herbal medicine, all of which seem to have an anti-inflammatory, anti-infectious effect and, being antioxidants, were neuroprotective. Later, sound therapy was added and opioids, targeting the tinnitus-associated suffering. After the advances made in the second century AD, the centre of medical science shifted to Byzantium, with Alexander de Tralles in the sixth century proposing tinnitus as the result of a raised irritability of the auditory sense. The Islamic golden age, between the eighth and fourteenth centuries, moves the centre of medicine to the Near East, North Africa, and Spain. Avicenna in the tenth century relates tinnitus to a hangover, trauma, or medication. Yet, treatments and explanations largely remained unchanged. The first cadaveric dissections in Italy during the Renaissance in the fifteenth and sixteenth centuries increased anatomical knowledge dramatically, yet, this detailed anatomical knowledge did not lead to novel insights nor treatments. In the Renaissance, Paracelsus claimed that not the illustrious ancients were to be followed, but nature itself. He was the first to describe that noise trauma like riffles or bells could generate tinnitus. His treatment added scarifications to the ear and venesection under the tongue. In the sixteenth century, the French physician Jean Fernel was the first to propose that deafness, tinnitus, and pain have a common origin, a very prescient insight. The scientific revolution in the seventeenth century with Descartes and Du Verney added a mechanistic auditory nerve and brain-centred explanation for tinnitus. In the early eighteenth century, Rivinus and Cotugno described tinnitus caused by convulsive contractions of the Eustachian muscle or stapedial muscle. The nineteenth century saw the birth of science as a profession, and Itard differentiated between true (objective) and false (subjective) tinnitus based on carotid compression. He further distinguished between idiopathic, based on noise trauma, and symptomatic false tinnitus, associated with other diseases. The German otologists classified tinnitus in detail and the first journal paper dedicated exclusively to tinnitus was published in 1841 in Germany. In the twentieth century, new audiological techniques permitted to describe frequency and loudness matching, as well as masking procedures, and in the twenty-first century novel brain imaging techniques identified many of the brain structures involved in the generation of tinnitus and its associated suffering. Yet, no treatment has emerged, based on this detailed knowledge, that can successfully treat tinnitus and tinnitus disorder.

D. De Ridder (✉)
Section of Neurosurgery, Department of Surgical Sciences, University of Otago, Dunedin, New Zealand
e-mail: dirk.deridder@otago.ac.nz

H. De Ridder-Symoens
Emeritus of Department of Medieval History, Free University of Amsterdam, Amsterdam, The Netherlands

Department of Early Modern History, University of Ghent, Gent, Belgium

W. Schlee et al. (eds.), *Textbook of Tinnitus*, https://doi.org/10.1007/978-3-031-35647-6_1

Graphical Abstract

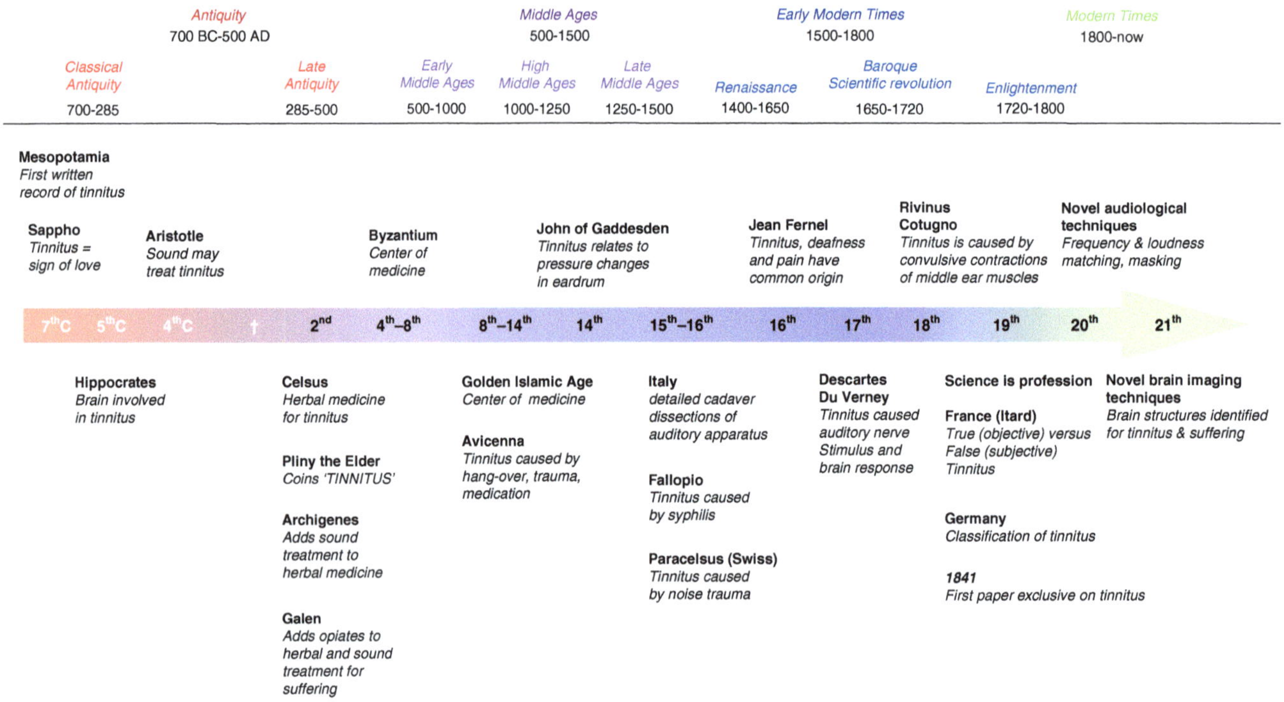

Highlights

- Seventh CBC: first written record of tinnitus in Mesopotamia, and Sappho describes tinnitus as a sign of rapturous love. Tinnitus was still considered a punishment from the Gods and treatment consisted of charms.
- Fifth CBC: Hippocrates, first brain-based explanation for tinnitus.
- Fourth CBC: Aristotle suggests tinnitus could be treated with sound therapy.
- Second century AD:
  - Celsus describes tinnitus treatment with diet and herbal medicine.
  - Pliny the Elder coins the word 'tinnitus'.
  - Archigenes adds sound treatment to the herbal medicines.
  - Galen adds opiates to the sound and herbal treatment targeting the tinnitus-associated suffering.
- Fourth–eighth century: centre of medical science shifts to Byzantium.
- Eighth–fourteenth century: during Islamic Golden Age centre of medicine to the Near East, North Africa, and Spain. Avicenna in the tenth century relates tinnitus to a hangover, trauma, or medication. Yet treatments and explanations largely remained unchanged.
- Fourteenth century of the middle ages John of Gaddesden suggests tinnitus may be related to pressure changes of the ear drum.
- Fifteenth–sixteenth century: first cadaveric dissections in Italy during the Renaissance increased anatomical knowledge dramatically, yet, this detailed anatomical knowledge did not lead to novel insights nor treatments.
  - Fallopio suggested that tinnitus was caused by the movement of Avicenna's vapours in the cavities of the ear or syphilis.
  - Paracelsus was first to describe that noise trauma could generate tinnitus.
- Sixteenth century: Jean Fernel was first to propose that deafness, tinnitus, and pain have a common origin.
- Seventeenth century Enlightenment triggers scientific revolution, with a mechanistic auditory nerve and brain-centred explanation for tinnitus,
- Eighteenth century: tinnitus is caused by convulsive contractions of the Eustachian muscle or stapedial muscle.
- Nineteenth century: science is a profession,

- France: Itard differentiates between true (objective) and false (subjective) tinnitus and subjective tinnitus can be idiopathic (noise trauma) or symptomatic (associated with other diseases).
- Germany: otologists classified tinnitus in detail and the first journal paper dedicated exclusively to tinnitus was published in 1841.
- England: psychological aspects of tinnitus recognized, as well as early treatment.

- Twentieth century: new audiological techniques to describe frequency and loudness matching, as well as masking procedures.
- Twenty-first century: novel brain imaging techniques identify many of the brain structures involved in the generation of tinnitus and its associated suffering.

Introduction

Tinnitus is an enigmatic symptom. Throughout most of history, with few exceptions, it has been considered an ear problem, whereas since the beginning of the third millennium it is generally considered a problem located within the brain, even if triggered in the brain.

The so-called earliest historic reference to tinnitus, dating back to the nineteenth CBC, in the Ebers papyrus, a 20 m long scroll written in hieratic characters, in which tinnitus was considered the consequence of a 'bewitched' ear [1], is controversial [2]. The ear is only mentioned seven times in the Ebers papyrus, and the reference to 'bewitched' comes from paragraph 768, which begins as "treatment for an ear which is strange, having conglomerated pus" [1]. The word strange is unclear: it may be translated as conspicuous, rather than strange [3].

Classical Antiquity (700 BC–285 AD)

The honour of the first citation of tinnitus may not be related to medicine, but to a female poet describing love. Sappho of Lesbos (600 BC) mentions tinnitus in one of her odes [4]. In the first century BC, the Roman poet Catullus, famous for his love poetry dedicated at his muse Lesbia, writes of tinnitus as a sign of rapturous love. His verses in poem 51 are an almost exact translation of one of Sappho, Plato's tenth muse, her odes [4]. Catullus version reads as:

> My tongue is paralyzed,
> A weak fire runs through my limbs,
> My ears are ringing with an inward sound,
> Night veils both my eyes [4]

And Sappho's original version reads as:

> My tongue fails and a subtle
> Fire races beneath my skin,
> I see nothing with my eyes
> And my ears hum [4]

Apart from the romantic idea that tinnitus's first description may be attributed to love, tinnitus in a medical context can be identified on the cuneiform clay tablets from Mesopotamia, from the Assyrian King Assurbanipal's (668–628 BC) extensive library [3, 5] in Nineveh, the capital of Assyria, in northern Mesopotamia. This library, the first library in world history, contained over 30,000 clay tablets. The Assyrians still considered diseases to be caused by Gods, ghosts, and spirits who were angry. Therefore, diseases were treated not only by products from nature, but also charms. From the many thousands of clay tablets, 600 deal with medicine, and of these about 20 refer to tinnitus, expressed as 'singing' ten times in these clay tablets [1, 5]. One clay tablet reads as "If the hand of a ghost seizes on a man, and his ears sing, myrrh, …" [1, 5]. It is unclear whether this refers to musical hallucinosis or tinnitus, but the advice is to install some mixtures in the ear and sign a charm each time. Twice a 'whispering' ear is mentioned, which is treated by a charm alone, and twice a 'speaking' ear is mentioned [3]. It is also unclear whether this refers to tinnitus or rather to verbal hallucinations in the setting of schizophrenia. The treatment for a 'speaking' ear is different and does not consist of singing a charm, but to drink mustard in beer. Considering that the treatments for a 'singing', 'whispering', and 'speaking' ear are different, it is speculative to think that these tablets refer to tinnitus, musical hallucinosis, and verbal hallucinations.

Western civilization started in Mesopotamia around 10.000 BC, as part of the fertile crescent, which also included the Nile valley in Egypt. Already in 3000 BC, Mesopotamia traded with both Egypt and the Indus Valley civilizations. It is unclear whether the oldest Mesopotamian civilization was the single cradle of all civilizations or whether the Indus valley civilization developed independently or under influence of Mesopotamia, as was the Egyptian, Greek, and the rest of Western civilization.

A competitor for the oldest reference is the Ayurveda dating back to 1500 BC from the Indus valley civilization in India. The Ayurveda is a multi-author compilation that evolved through centuries and is based on 3 early scripts, the Charaka Samhita, the Sushruta Samhita, and the Bhela Samhita. The current version, however, dates back to the first and second century AD. It contains 28 ear diseases and tinnitus is described as either 'buzzing' or 'ringing'. Tinnitus is accompanied by hearing loss. When the patient perceives dissonances or pleasant sound, this may be an ominous sign for "being carried off", i.e. for imminent hallucination or delirium [3].

Hippocrates, the father of Western medicine, lived in Greece from 460 to 377 BC, i.e. a contemporary of Plato and Pericles. He was the first physician to believe that diseases were caused naturally, not because of superstition and Gods [6]. As such, he separated medicine from religion: disease was not a punishment inflicted by the Gods, but rather the result of environmental factors, diet, and living habits [6]. His work is compiled in the *Corpus Hippocraticum*, which consists of 60 books, and it mentions tinnitus six times [7]. The entire corpus was translated in French by Littre in 1839 and 1861 [8], and in English by Adams in 1849 [6]. Hippocrates uses three different descriptions of tinnitus: *echos* (sound), *bombos* (humm, buzz), and *psophos* (gentle noise). Tinnitus can also be part of a constellation of symptoms and then should be considered an alarming symptom. Hippocrates describes tinnitus, associated with deafness and violent headache, likely referring to otogenic meningitis. He attempts to give a pathophysiological explanation, involving the brain: "There is impairment of hearing partly because of the internal noise and buzzing, and partly because of the swelling of the brain and the cerebral veins; the excess of warmth makes the brain fill the vacant space, which is there towards to ear, following this the air is no more present in the same quantity as before and does not give the same sound anymore". He continues by stating that "…if water or phlegm erupts through the nostrils or through the mouth, the patient will recover. If not, he will usually die at about the seventh day" [8].

Aristotle (384–322 BC), or one of his epigones of the peripatetic school, wrote in chapter 32 of the *Problemata Physica* about 13 problems, exclusively linked to the ear. Problem 9 addresses masking for the first time. It reads as follows: "Why is it that buzzing in the ear ceases if one makes a sound?" [1]. The answer is: "Is it because a greater sound drives out the less?" [3]. It is unclear whether this theoretical solution to the tinnitus problem was applied clinically as a treatment in Aristotle's time.

Lucretius (99–55 BC), the Roman Epicurean poet and philosopher from the first century BC, mentions tinnitus twice in his De Natura Rerum (About the Nature of Things). Like Hippocrates, he describes tinnitus in a constellation of symptoms, associated with fear and terror, accompanied by sweating, pallor, loss of speech, blurring of the eyes, and collapsing limbs [3].

The Greek Aulus Cornelius Celsus (c. 25 BC–c. 50 AD), living in the Roman empire, also known as the Cicero of medical writing, was not a physician, but a writer. Yet, he compiled everything known about medicine in multiple books, *De Medicina* (On Medicine) [1]. Celsus described a condition "in which the ears produce a ringing noise within themselves; and this also prevents them from perceiving sounds from without" [9], and called this 'sonare'. There were three different conditions in which sonare could emerge, each with a different prognosis [1]. " It is least serious when due to cold in the head; worse when occasioned by diseases or prolonged pains in the head; worst of all when it precedes the onset or serious maladies, especially epilepsy" [9]. This is reminiscent of Hippocrates' association of tinnitus, hearing loss and headaches as an ominous sign. Celsus describes different treatments to each of the 3 versions of sonare. For the cold-associated sonare, the ear should be cleaned and the breath held (=Valsalva manoever) until humor comes out of the ear. For the sonare associated with headaches, exercise, rubbing, affusion, and gargling should be added to a diet of food that make tin and a mixture of different ingredients dropped into the ear: radish juice, combined with rose oil, or with juice of wild cucumber. Another treatment was instilment of castoreum with vinegar and laurel oil, and the patient should abstain from wine, as long as the sonare is not gone. The same latter treatment is used for those cases in which the sonare was not associated with cold or headaches, but laurel could be replaced by iris oil. These mixtures may have been used as anti-inflammatory, antibacterial agents to treat ear infections as causes of tinnitus, and antioxidants as treatments for excitotoxicity as cause of tinnitus, and may have been neuroprotective. It is evident that these mixtures would have been discovered serendipitously, as medicine at that time was most likely unaware of the concepts of microbes, neuroprotection, and antioxidants. Radish has antibacterial activity against gram PLUS_SPI and gram-bacteria, as well as an antioxidant potential [10] and is neuroprotective [11]. Castoreum is a yellowish exudate, consisting of at least 24 compounds, and released from the castor sacs of mature beavers, used to scent mark their territory. Salicin, one of its compounds, is a precursor of aspirin and is analgesic and anti-inflammatory [12]. Furthermore, it has weak antibacterial characteristics [13]. Vinegar is both a good cleaning product and an antimicrobial (bacteria, viruses, and fungi) agent, accelerating wound healing [14] and considered the holy grail for infected wound management [15]. Furthermore, via its effect on monoamino-oxidase, an enzyme that breaks down dopamine, noradrenaline, and serotonin, it has a neuroprotective effect [16, 17]. Laurel oil has anti-inflammatory [18], antioxidant [18] and antibacterial [19] capacities as well. Rose oil promotes wound healing by modulating macrophage activity [20], reducing inflammation, and promoting skin barrier repair by topical application [21]. In addition to its anti-inflammatory properties, it also has analgesic, antioxidant, and neuroprotective effects [22]. Cucumber also has antioxidant, wound healing, and antimicrobial potential [23], as well as neuroprotective effects [24]. Iris oil also has antimicrobial (bacteria, plasmodium, fungi), anti-inflammatory, and antioxidant activity [25, 26], as well as neuroprotective properties [26].

The word 'tinnitus' can be attributed to Pliny the Elder (23/24–79 AD), a Roman military commander, naturalist, and complier of scientific knowledge [3]. Tinnitus is derived from tinnire, to ring, as can also be seen in tintinnabulum, a small bell mounted on a pole, placed in a Roman Catholic basilica to signify the church's link with the Pope. Pliny the Elder also used the word 'sonitus', the Latin for noise, so he made a distinction between what currently would be called pure tone tinnitus and noise-like tinnitus (sonitus). Pliny, like Celsus, also was not a physician, and he also lived in the first century AD, being a friend of the emperor Vespasianus. The Roman historian Suetonius (c. 69–122 AD) wrote that when the Vesuvius erupted in 79 AD, he was nearby, commanding part of the Roman fleet, and ordered to be put ashore to investigate the spectacle at close range, but was trapped and died, victim of his scientific curiosity. However, this version of Pliny's death is contested. He wrote the first encyclopaedia ever, the 37 volume *Naturalis Historia*, dedicated to the emperor Titus, covering all known branches of scientific discovery, including medicine, one book per topic. His treatments for tinnitus are reminiscent of Celsus and consist of pouring cumin, mixed with veal suet, or honey in the ears "when there are noises or ringing in them" [27]. Another mixture that can be applied in the ear consists of honey, rose oil and pomegranate, and juice of chard as well as styrax. Cumin is an antibacterial [28], antiviral [29] and antifungal [30] agent. It is beneficial in neutrophilic inflammatory diseases [31] and has anti-inflammatory, antioxidant, and neuroprotective properties [32]. Honey also has antimicrobial capacities and improves wound healing [33]. Furthermore, honey contains chrysin, which has anti-inflammatory, antioxidant, and neuroprotective properties [34]. Pomegranate also has antioxidant, anti-inflammatory, antimicrobial, and neuroprotective effects [35]. Benzoin resin, made from styrax shrubs, is sedative and relaxant, as well as disinfectant (against bacteria, fungi, and viruses), local anaesthetic, and seems to promote healing [36, 37].

Interestingly, in the Babylonian Talmud, the central text of Rabbinic Judaism, dating to the fifth century AD, tinnitus is called Titus' curse [38]. The Roman general Titus (39–81 AD), son of emperor Vespasianus and later on emperor himself, ended the Jewish Rebellion in 70 AD and destroyed the second (Herod's) temple in Jerusalem, for which he was cursed by God by giving him tinnitus [38]. He treated it by going to the blacksmith as he noted that the hammering silenced his tinnitus. Yet after 30 days, the effect of the sound therapy wore off [38].

Archigenes of Apamea was a Greco-Syrian physician who lived in Rome during Trajan's rule (98–117), a contemporary of Celsus and Pliny the Elder. His treatment for tinnitus consisted of a similar mixture Celsus described of castoreum and vinegar; this time with seeds of hemlock. Hemlock contains the toxin coniine, which has antibacterial [39] antispasmodic, and analgesic capacities. At low doses, hemlock activates muscles, peripheral, and autonomic nerves as well as the spinal cord, but at high doses it blocks these same nervous structures [40]. It acts as a nicotinic acetylcholine receptor [41] and GABAa inhibitor [42]. Coniine's most famous victim is Socrates who was sentenced to death by poison chalice containing poison hemlock in 399 BC [41, 43, 44]. Archigenes added sound to the tinnitus treatment, by shouting alternatingly with a shrill and deep voice through a tube to treat subjective head noises. He thus is the first to use sound treatment via an instrument [3], as well as the first to propose a multimodal approach.

Tinnitus is also mentioned in an Egyptian source, the *Fayyum Medical Book* from Crocodilopolis, written in demotic, which dates back to the second century AD, i.e. the Ptolemaic Roman period. In this book, Greek influences were incorporated in ancient Egyptian Medicine. It is assumed that it is based on earlier work dating back to second and third CBC [3].

In the same second century AD, a Greek physician born in Pergamon by the name of Claudius Galenus (129–199), better known as Galen, lived and worked in Athens, Alexandria, and Rome. He became the physician of the gladiators as well as of the emperor Marcus Aurelius. Galen's voluminous work would dominate Western medicine for nearly 1400 years. He mentions tinnitus ten times and proposes that tinnitus is due to vapours exhaled from the stomach [3]. This occurs in conditions of heat, coldness, with trauma or an upset stomach, following too much drinking of wine, after violent vomiting, or sometimes after medications applied in the ears [3]. Galen cites Archigenes, and likely also prescribed mixtures to pour into the ears, sound treatments, but on top of that he proposed the use of opium and mandragora (=nightshade), as to dull the sensibility of the brain [45], so that the tinnitus would be less annoying. Mandragora contains atropine and scopolamine, and apart from its anticholinergic effects, like hemlock, it also has sedative, analgesic, narcotic effects [46]. This suggests that Galen not only tried to treat the cause and loudness, but also the suffering component of the tinnitus, much alike current approaches.

Late Antiquity (285–500)

Classical antiquity ended with the Roman Empire's Crisis of the Third Century (235–284), when considerable social, cultural, and organizational changes occurred in the Roman Empire, starting with the reign of Diocletian in 285, who began the custom of splitting the Empire into Eastern Byzantine and Western portions ruled by multiple emperors simultaneously. Late Antiquity can thus be seen as a transitional period between classical antiquity and the early Muslim conquests (622–750), which are considered the start of the Middle Ages.

After the advances made by Celsus, Pliny the Elder, Archigenes, and Galen, the center of medical science shifted to Byzantium.

In the sixth century AD, Alexander of Tralles (ca. 525–ca. 605), whose brother designed the Hagia Sophia in Constantinople, was a well-known physician in the Byzantine Empire, who dedicated an entire book chapter to tinnitus. He proposed that tinnitus is the result of a raised irritability of the auditory sense. The tinnitus may be caused partly by gaseous thick air, partly by stagnation of humors, or by weakness after a general disease. His treatments consisted of instilling the well-known castoreum, vinegar, honey, hemlock seeds, and natron in the ear [3]. Natron, a mixture of sodium salts, was used in Egypt to clean the house and body, being an antiseptic, as well as used to treat infections caused by fungi and parasites [47].

One century later, Paulus of Aegina (c. 625–c. 690) prescribed similar treatments as Alexander of Tralles, ending the Greek-Alexandrian-Roman tradition of medicine, which was replaced by the developments occurring within the Islamic golden age between the eighth and fourteenth centuries (medieval period of Islam).

Early Middle Ages (500–1000)

The prophet Muhammad was also a military leader, conquering the entire Arabic Peninsula. After his death in 632, the caliphs (=successors) would continue the Muslim expansion culminating in a large Umayyad Caliphate that extended from the Arabic Peninsula to Persia, North Africa, and Spain.

The illiterate Muhammad had Allah's inspiration and revelations written down by his companions in the Quran, and his words and actions were recorded in the Hadith. These two most important Islamic works place values on education and emphasize the importance of acquiring knowledge, driving the Islamic caliphate to heavily sponsor scholars. These patrons initially requested translations of Greek texts of Hippocrates, Aristotle, Galen, Plato, Archimedes, and others into Arabic, as to acquire all knowledge available in the conquered territories, including Turkey, Persia, the entire Near East, North Africa, and Iberia. This translation movement from the eighth to tenth century AD involved many scholars from conquered areas, including scholars belonging to Nestorian (Christian) church of Mesopotamia. The assimilated scientific knowledge was collected in the House of Wisdom, the great library of Bagdad (destroyed by Mongols in 1258). In the West, Cordoba in the Caliphate of Córdoba (929–1031) and Toledo, both on the Iberian Peninsula, fulfilled the same function as centres of translation of ancient knowledge into Arabic. Already in the late seventh century, Christian Toledo became a main centre of literacy and writing and under the Moorish rule (711/712–1085), the translations continued. After its Reconquista in 1085, the Christians inherited vast libraries containing some of the leading scientific and philosophical books, not only of the ancient world, but of the Islamic East, the cutting edge of scientific knowledge, yet largely written in Arabic. Toledo continued the School of Translators where Arab, Jewish, and Christian scholars worked together and translated books of philosophy and science from Arabic, Jewish, and Greek into Latin and local Romance vernacular (Castilian), thus letting long-lost knowledge spread through Christian Europe again. Most translators were paid and personally supervised by the king, and the School of Translators declined after king Alfonso X the Wise was succeeded by his brother Sancho IV in 1284, losing its predominance as a bridge between different religions and cultures [48, 49]. Thanks to these translations, the polymath Aristotle (384–322 BC) became the greatest ancient scholar with absolute authority in medieval Europe. The comments of the Cordoba Muslim polymath Averroes (1126–1198), and the Dominican friar, philosopher, and Doctor of the Church Thomas Aquinas have reinforced this central position. It was only under the influence of the scientific revolution in the early modern period that the authority of Aristotle was overthrown.

The book production was facilitated by the large production of paper. Paper was invented in China, attributed to Cai Lun (50/62–121 AD). Even though paper already existed since three centuries, Cai Lun added tree bark and hemp ends to the production process of paper, which resulted in the large-scale manufacture and progressive worldwide spread of paper. In the Hadith, Muhammad instructed to seek knowledge, even in China [50]. In the eighth century, after the battle of Talas in 751, between the Islamic caliphate and China, papermaking was introduced via Chinese prisoners and spread to the Islamic world, replacing papyrus and parchment. The paper manufacturing process was refined, and machinery was designed for bulk manufacturing. This permitted Islamic assembly-line methods of hand-copying manuscripts to turn out editions far larger than any available in Europe for centuries.

The Persian and Arabian scholars and physicians of the caliphate developed their own schools and medical systems after the translation movement was finished. Rhazes (ca. 865–925) mentions tinnitus in the ninth century, as does Avicenna (980–1037) in the eleventh century, both from Persia. Avicenna developed a systematic classification of all known diseases, consisting of aetiology, symptomatology, and treatment for each disease. This was compiled in his Canon Medicinae [1, 3]. According to Avicenna, tinnitus is caused by vapours, trapped in ear cavities, that can give rise to different forms of tinnitus: *sonitus* (tone, sound, noise), *tinnitus* (ringing), and *sibilus* (hissing) [3]. Based on translations from Galen, Avicenna relates tinnitus to a hangover, trauma, or medication, i.e. he was the first to identify ototoxic tinnitus. Analogous to Galen, Avicenna proposes opium, henbane, and castoreum, instilment of almond oil in the ears, but also added vomiting, purging, and taking baths [3]. Henbane belongs to the same family as mandragora, proposed as tinnitus treatment by Galen. Almond oil acts as an antioxidant, is neuroprotective, and has dermatologic emollient and sclerosant properties [51].

Treatments for tinnitus still consisted of fumigations of the ears or instilment of heated urine of an ox mixed with vinegar and myrrh. Myrrh is a strong analgesic, antiseptic, antibacterial, antifungal, antioxidant, anti-inflammatory, and antiepileptic product from the bark of commiphora (cinnamon) trees [52].

In the sixth century, Benedict of Nursia, the patron saint of Europe, founded its first Benedictine Abbey in Monte Cassino (529 AD). This abbey was sacked and rebuilt to flourish in the eleventh and twelfth centuries. It maintained good relations with the Eastern Church, even receiving patronage from Byzantine emperors, becoming the most famous cultural, educational, and medical centre of Europe. The abbey housed a great library in Medicine and other sciences, attracting many physicians to come and gain medical and other knowledge. The earliest Institution of Higher Education in Europe started nevertheless in nearby Salerno (802 AD), a Mediterranean port, permitting books of Avicenna (980–1037) to arrive by sea. The Carthaginian physician, Constantine the African (d. before 1098/1099) came to Salerno and translated many texts from Arabic. This included works from Hippocrates, Galen, Razes, and Avicenna.

High Middle Ages (1000–1250)

The Carolingian Renaissance in the Carolingian Empire of Charlemagne and his successors which covered a territory of current France, Germany, and Northern Italy was followed by the Ottonian Byzantine Renaissance in the tenth century and the Renaissance of the twelfth century.

The Carolingian Renaissance of the eighth and ninth centuries in Northern Europe (France, Germany, Northern Italy) stimulated scientific and philosophical activities. Higher education took place for hundreds of years in cathedral schools or monastic schools, in which canons and monks taught classes. These cathedral schools evolved into the first universities which started operating in Bologna (1088), Paris (1150), Oxford (1167), Cambridge (1209), Salamanca (1218), and many more cities during the thirteenth century.

Similarly, Montpellier came to prominence in the twelfth century as a trading centre, and analogous to Salerno, with trading links across the Mediterranean world. Cultural life flourished because of tolerance of Muslims, Jews, and Cathars. In 1180, William VIII of Montpellier gave freedom for all to teach medicine in Montpellier, and in 1220, the faculty of medicine was established by a legate of Pope Honorius III. The medical faculty has, over the centuries, been one of the major and oldest continuous centres for medical teaching in Europe.

The English physician Gilbertus Anglicus (c. 1180–c. 1250), who trained in Salerno, wrote a treatise *Compendium Medicinae* [1], a comprehensive overview of the best practice in pharmacology, medicine, and surgery at the time. In it, he described four kinds of tinnitus, all with a different aetiology and different treatment [3]. One kind was a great windy matter moving up and down, with no specific treatment, tinnitus due to heat should be treated by almond oil in the ear, tinnitus due to cold by ear drops of castoreum or myrrh, or alternatively by juice of radish or leek, rose oil, or women's milk [3]. Leek, belonging to the onion family, in addition to its anti-inflammatory properties, has antioxidant, antibacterial, antiviral, and immune-enhancing properties [53]. The fourth kind of tinnitus was related to feebleness of the ears and was treated by juice of wormwood mixed with vinegar. Wormwood containing artemisia has antibacterial, antiviral, antihelmintic, and antifungal properties, as well as anti-inflammatory, antioxidant, analgesic, antidepressant, and neuroprotective effects [54, 55].

The Late Middle Ages (1250–1400)

The 'Waning of the Middle Ages', as the fourteenth and fifteenth centuries are described by the Dutch cultural historian Johan Huizinga (1872–1945), is also known as the Crisis of the Late Middle Ages with a series of demographic, political, and religious events that ended centuries of European stability [56]. The Great Famine of 1315–1317 and Black Death of 1347–1351 reduced the population by 20–50 million people, or between 1/3 and 2/3 of the entire European population, depending on the region. Popular revolts of peasants or town people against nobility and clergy resulted in constant wars within and between countries. Furthermore, the Western schism between 1378 and 1417 resulted in a revolt within the catholic church, in which bishops residing in Rome and Avignon both claimed to be the true Pope. In 1409, the Council of Pisa declared both Popes illegitimate and elected a third Pope, residing in Pisa. The solution came in 1417, at the Council of Constance, when the Popes of Rome and Pisa abdicated, the Pope of Avignon was excommunicated, and a new Pope residing in Rome was elected.

John of Gaddesden (1280–1361), also known as John Anglicus, his medical works, alongside those of Gilbertus Anglicus, "formed part of the core curriculum that underpinned the practice of medicine for the next 400 years" [57]. He proposed to suck pus out of the ear via a small tube, and this may also work for subjective tinnitus without a clear cause. This was the first proposal that pressure changes on the tympanum may modulate tinnitus [3].

The Renaissance (1400–1650)

Giorgio Vasari (1511–1574) who coined the term *Rinascita* (French: *Renaissance*) believed that after a period of decline during the Middle Ages, a new golden age had dawned, which was nothing less than a rebirth of the achievements of classical antiquity.

The Renaissance, starting in Florence with Petrarca (1304–1374) in the late fourteenth century, brought about dramatic changes in how the world was perceived and conceived, in comparison to the dogmatic and rigid feudal medieval scholastic approach. The demographic changes resulting from the massive death toll of the Great Famine and Black Death created a relative wealth in survivors who became interested in the world rather than heaven, focusing on worldly beauty and accepting innovation, as nothing was stable anymore, demographically, politically, and religiously. The medieval adage memento mori (remember to die) was replaced by carpe diem (seize the day). This secularization was clearly expressed in the arts and literature, by a realistic tendency rather than an idealistic base. But the mixture of individualism and secularization also permitted Nicolaus Copernicus (1473–1543) to state that the sun was the centre of the universe, and not the earth (1514). Furthermore, imminent death also triggered a self-centred focus: individualism was born, and individuals, not born in nobility, were capable of reaching unseen status in society, based on their artistic, scientific, or political aptness.

Secularization required another bacon to guide their lives, rather than religion, and Greek and Roman antiquity was chosen. Christopher Columbus (1451–1506) rediscovered the Greek concept, dating back to Pythagoras in the sixth CBC that the world was spherical. By the first CBC, Pliny the Elder wrote in his *Naturalis Historia* encyclopaedia that everybody agreed that the earth was spherical. By this renaissance idea, Columbus accidentally discovered America (1492). Martin Luther (1483–1546) protested against the abuse of selling indulgences and many other abuses in the Catholic church (1517), initiating the Protestant Reformation. All the new ideas could rapidly spread once the printing press was developed by the goldsmith Johannes Gutenberg (ca. 1400–1468) around 1440. The Renaissance concept of innovation, experiment, and empiricism, in contrast to blind dogmatic acceptance of religion and the ancient writers, was replaced by human dissection in the older and newly founded universities in Italy, France, Germany, England, and the Netherlands. Especially in Italy, the anatomist professors performed detailed anatomical dissections of the human body [58, 59]. This permitted Andreas Vesalius (1514–1564) to describe the malleus and incus, Giovanni Filippo Ingrassia (1510–1580) the stapes, Gabriele Fallopio (1523–1562) the facial canal, Bartolomeo Eustachi (ca. 1500/1510–1574) the tube bearing his name and the tensor tympani, and Giulio Casseri (1561–1616) detailed the stapedius [3]. Yet, this detailed anatomical knowledge did not lead to novel insights nor treatments. At the same time, Paracelsus (ca. 1493–1541) claimed that not the illustrious ancients were to be followed, but nature itself. He publicly burned books by Galen and Avicenna to make his point, at the start of his lectures [1]. He was also the first to teach and write in the vernacular, rather than Latin, whose usance would increase during the early modern period. He was the first to describe that noise trauma like riffles or bells could generate tinnitus [3]. His treatment was performed in stages. In the first stage, scarifications were applied to the ear, if that did not benefit, cupping behind the ear was proposed, followed by venesection under the tongue [45]. And if that doesn't work, Paracelsus stated that nothing else could be performed [3]. This last statement is what most medical doctors still claim, suggesting that indeed, tinnitus research has not advanced a lot, and truly missed a renaissance.

In the sixteenth century, the French physician Jean Fernel (1497–1558), physician to Catherine de Medici and King Henry II of France, was the first to coin the term physiology, to describe the study of the body's function. He also was the first to describe the spinal cord. In his work *Universa Medicina,* he was the first to propose that deafness, tinnitus, and pain have a common origin, a very prescient insight. It took nearly 500 years for Rodolfo Llinas to state the same, when he coined the term thalamocortical dysrhythmia, as a common pathophysiological mechanism underlying pain, tinnitus, and depression [60]. He added a fifth kind of tinnitus to Anglicus's four types, namely strepitus, which is the consequence of a noise trauma, yet he offers no new therapy [3].

In a similar fashion, Fallopio suggested that tinnitus was caused by the movement of Avicenna's vapours in the cavities of the ear, and this is based on Alexander de Tralles, who was influenced by Hippocrates and Galen. Yet, Fallopio also proposed something new, in that tinnitus could result from syphilis. Syphilis was first diagnosed in Naples, in 1494, after Columbus' return from the Americas, and is considered a New World disease.

The first to question whether mastoidectomy could potentially treat those trapped vapours was the early seventeenth century French anatomist Jean Riolan the Younger (1580–1657) [45], the personal physician to Marie de Medici; however, it is unclear whether he ever attempted this approach [3].

The Scientific Revolution (1650–1720) and Enlightenment (1720–1800)

As the cultural Renaissance came to an end in the middle of the seventeenth century, the scientific Renaissance triggered the Scientific Revolution, followed by an intellectual social movement, known as the Enlightenment. Science came to flourish, under influence of the development of the scientific method by Francis Bacon (1561–1626); the two main elements of the scientific method are the use of mathematics and measurement to give precise determinations of how the world and its parts work [61]. At the same time, the methodological doubt and mechanical philosophy were introduced by René Descartes (1596–1650), separating religion from science. The mechanization and mathematization of the world were best reflected by Sir Isaac Newton (1643–1727), the greatest physicist of all times, who developed the laws of motion, gravity, and co-invented calculus with Gottfried Wilhelm (von) Leibnitz (1646–1716). Whereas Newton was still an alchemist, Robert Boyle (1627–1691) separated chemistry from alchemy. New knowledge of chemistry superseded the theory that all things are made up of earth, air, fire, and water, and the old Aristotelian ideas began to be discarded. The mechanical philosophy combined with scientific experimentation and mathematization paved the way for the development of institutionalization of science, and in 1660, the first scientific society to be established was the Royal Society of London.

Francis Bacon, according to Voltaire, the father of the scientific method, experienced tinnitus after a noise exposure caused by a lyre, which disappeared 15 min later. He also expressed the fact that noise trauma could induce tinnitus, analogous to what Paracelsus and Fernel had claimed. [3]

Descartes proposed in 'The Passions of the Souls' (1649) that sound reaches the ends of nerves, which transmit the signal to the pineal gland, where it becomes conscious. His compatriot, anatomist and physiologist Joseph-Guichard Du Verney (1648–1730), further developed this concept and anticipated much of Hermann von Helmholtz's (1821–1894) theory of resonance. He states that there is no difference between external sounds exciting the auditory nerve and brain or a pathological activation of the auditory nerve [3]. This differs from a real internal sound, such as heart beat synchronous tinnitus, which according to Du Verney is related to a dilated artery. He calls these sounds that can often be heard by other people 'tintements'. Du Verney also distinguishes between 'tintements' caused by brain disorders and ear disorders [3].

Also in the seventeenth century, tinnitus is seen as part of a constellation of tinnitus, hemicrania, and vertigo, associated with hysterical convulsions by the Swiss Physician Johann Jakob Wepfer [1, 3]. Mechanistically, this was due to a blocked ear, whether by cerumen, secretion, or other causes, which prevents the circulation of free air. He distinguished between objective and subjective tinnitus by occluding the external meatus with a finger or drinking cup [1]; as treatment noise is applied, by banging two stones together, going back to Archigenes [3].

The eighteenth century, also known as the century of reason, was characterized by the British industrial revolution, as well as the American, French, and Haitian revolutions. Yet, in medicine, no great scientific advancements are made. In 1745, the Leyden jar was invented, an electrical component which stores a high-voltage electric charge, i.e. a forerunner of the electrical battery, invented by Volta in 1800. The first application of electricity to the treatment of tinnitus is attributed to Georg Daniel Wibel in 1768, in which he reported considerable success in the treatment of tinnitus and hearing loss with electrical stimulation, however, without describing details of the technique used. [1]

The German Lorenz Heister (1683–1758) proposed the use of a silver tube some 23 cm long which was introduced into the external meatus and used to create a negative pressure on the tympanic membrane [1], thereby recapitulating John of Gaddesden's suggestion made 400 years earlier.

In the same eighteenth century, the German professor August Rivinus, alias Bachmann (1652–1723), explained tinnitus by convulsive contractions of the middle ear muscles. But according to the Italian anatomist and professor of surgery at Naples' University, Domenico Cotugno (1736–1822), tinnitus is caused by convulsive contractions of the Eustachian muscle or stapedial muscle [3]. Based on meticulous dissections of the labyrinth and aqueducts, he postulated that contractions of the stapedial muscle would pull the stapes into the vestibulum, which would move intracochlear fluid activating the cochlear nerve, thereby generating tinnitus [3]. Thus, reasoning based on anatomical knowledge prevails, in keeping with the era.

Modern Times (1800-Now)

After the French Revolution in 1789, which created the fundamental principles of liberal democracy, based on the concepts of liberté (freedom), égalité (equality), and fraternité (brotherhood), Napoleon raise to power. Napoleon summarized his career as follows: "I closed the gulf of anarchy and brought order out of chaos. I rewarded merit regardless of birth or wealth, wherever I found it. I abolished feudalism and restored equality to all religion and before the law. I fought the decrepit monarchies of the Old Regime because the alternative was the destruction of all this. I purified the Revolution." [62]

The reward of merit regardless of birth or wealth in the nineteenth century permitted the birth of science as a profession. The term scientist was coined in 1833 by the polymath

William Whewell (1794–1866), replacing the old word 'natural philosopher' [63]. The first periodicals date from 1665, when the French *Journal des sçavans* and the English *Philosophical Transactions of the Royal Society* began to systematically publish research results. Yet, until the end of the eighteenth century, the usual way to circulate new medical insights was by means of books, lectures, and personal letters. Only in the early nineteenth century, publishing in scientific journals became more routine as a means of communication [64, 65].

This professionalism created a wealth of new discoveries. Charles Darwin(1809–1882) and Alfred Wallace (1823–1913) described evolution theory, Louis Pasteur (1822–1895) made the first vaccine against rabies, Dmitri Mendeleev (1834–1907) created the periodic table of elements, Michael Faraday (1791–1867) and James Clerk Maxwell (1831–1879) developed electromagnetism, Said Carnot (1796–1832), James Watt (1736–1819), and Ludwig Boltzman (1844–1906) described thermodynamics, and Carl Friedrich Gauss (1777–1855) became the prince of mathematics, calling it the queen of science. And with this advance of science, also otology was changed dramatically by a book of paramount importance *Traité des maladies de l'oreille et de l'audition* by Jean Marc Gaspard Itard (1774–1838), who became the leading figure in audiology and otology. His unorthodox approach may be explained by his unorthodox life. In an attempt to evade compulsory military service as a soldier during the French Revolution, his uncle the abbot Itard intervened for him and had him appointment as an assistant surgeon at the military hospital of Toulon, even though he worked at a bank and had no medical training [3]. He was later appointed deputy surgeon, and in 1799, a physician at the National Institute of the Deaf and Mutes. He trained with René Laennec (1781–1826), the inventor of the stethoscope, and who described tinnitus as an acoustic hallucination, because when he examined tinnitus with his invention, he could not hear the sound perceived by the patient. Apart from some medical inventions, such as the Itard catheter for insertion in the Eustachian tube, and his description of pneumothorax and Tourette's syndrome, Itard also described numbness of the tympanic membrane in otosclerosis. Yet, his claim to fame comes from two other events. He became known for his efforts to educate "Victor, le sauvage de l'Aveyron" [1], a Mowgli figure abandoned in the wilderness and found by hunters. He also treated the French philosopher and pedagogue Jean-Jacques Rousseau (1712–1778), who developed sudden hearing loss and tinnitus after a severe illness. Rousseau described his tinnitus in his "Confessions". Itard follows du Verney's approach to tinnitus and describes true and false tinnitus [1, 3]. True tinnitus is the result of vascular disorders or obstructions of auditory passages, in contrast to false tinnitus, which is not related to any existing noise [3]. To distinguish the two, Itard taught to compress the carotid arteries. If the tinnitus disappears it is true tinnitus, if not, false tinnitus. The same procedure also tells if the hearing loss is the consequence of the tinnitus, as most of his patients claimed. If the hearing improves on compressing the carotids, this confirms that the tinnitus causes the tinnitus [3]. False tinnitus is more common than true tinnitus and can be subdivided into symptomatic and idiopathic false tinnitus [3]. Idiopathic false tinnitus is due to violent excitation of the auditory nerve by loud noises such as explosions, guns and rifles, or loud machines [3]. Symptomatic false tinnitus is more common than idiopathic false tinnitus and occurs in sedentary life, hypochondriacs, hysterical women, in patients with worms, gastric disorders, menorrhagia, rheumatism, cachexia, and similar disorders [3]. False tinnitus can mimic all kinds of noises, including cries of animals, human voices, and can thus be likened to hallucinations. He also described a third form of tinnitus, 'fantastic tinnitus', auditory hallucinations, related to psychological disorders in which the treatment was that of the underlying disorder [1]. Treatment of true tinnitus consists of irritant foot baths and bleedings, by applying leaches to the neck or ears, or by venesection of the saphenous or jugular veins [3]. Treatment of false tinnitus involves antispasmodics, friction massage of the head, or warmth applications to the ears. Furthermore, Itard describes how to cover up the internal noise, whether real or false, by an external noise, at least equally loud. As an example, he provides a brisk open fire, especially when using green or slightly wet wood, riding a car on a bumpy road, listening to different musical instruments or living in a noisy neighbourhood. Itard thus translated Aristotle's masking concept, which was picked up by Archigenes and Galen and practiced by Titus into a treatment [3].

Another French physician, Jean-Antoine Saissy (1756–1822) reiterates Itard, but adds a treatment of his own, which consists of inhaling tobacco smoke and pressing it through the Eustachian tubes in the middle ears. The same approach was tested by the English otologist Joseph Toynbee (1815–1866), who suffered tinnitus himself. He investigated the application of chloroform and hydrocyanide via the same way, resulting in his premature death. When he was found death by his butler, a notebook was found with notes "on the effect of inhalation of chloroform on tinnitus, when pressed into the tympanum", together with an empty bottle of chloroform, and a half empty bottle of hydrocyanide, a constituent of tobacco smoke, and a third full bottle of ether [3].

Toynbee's nineteenth century compatriot, the Irish otologist William Robert Wilde (1815–1876), father of the English playwright Oscar Wilde, noted that the tinnitus is described in relation to their living conditions, social rank, or life style [3]. People from rural areas would describe their tinnitus as humming of bees, rushing of water, or singing of birds, whereas people from urban areas would describe it as hammering, sounds of steam machines, or rolling of carts. Furthermore, servants describe their tinnitus as ringing, and old women as the sound of tea kettles [3].

John Harrison Curtis (1778–1860) did recognize the psychological aspects of tinnitus and advocated psychological cures involving rest, spa treatment, and the like, which is still proposed currently. He also identified the importance of early treatment of the tinnitus, arguing that the long-term psychological consequences could be a change of the sound into auditory hallucinations [1]. Even though the transition from tinnitus to hallucinations has no scientific backup, it has been shown that early treatment of tinnitus carries a better prognosis than delayed treatments [66–68].

At the same time, in Germany, much energy was spent on classifying and detailing tinnitus. Eduard Schmalz (1801–1871), who as a physician worked at the institute for deaf-mutes in Dresden, describes 52 cases of tinnitus. For each case report, he details its location (left, right, bilateral, or in the head), its nature (continuous, fluctuating, pulsatile), its subjective loudness and pitch, and its association with hearing loss, hyperacusis, as well as diplacusis and vertigo [3].

The first article exclusively on tinnitus was published in 1841 in Casper's *Wochenschrift*, by Wilhelm Kramer (1801–1876). Its title was *Bemerkungen ober das Ohrenklingen*, and it detailed 707 cases of tinnitus out of 1000 cases of ear diseases.

The evolution of the understanding of tinnitus up to the twentieth century followed the Kuhnian principle that scientific evolution is essentially based on novel ideas, and that the most fitting idea survives, in a Darwinian way [69]. In contrast, Peter Galison proposed that scientific evolution is the consequence of the development of novel technology [70], and this philosophy was the main driver of understanding of tinnitus starting in the twentieth century.

In the first half of the twentieth century, Edmund Prince Fowler tested tinnitus in a rigorous way, using modern audiological equipment. He developed frequency and loudness matching, as well as masking procedures [3].

At the end of the twentieth century, the CT and MRI were invented, permitting unrivalled imaging possibilities of the structure and function of the brain; this resulted in attempts to identify brain-based pathophysiological mechanisms that can explain the development of tinnitus. This shift in pathophysiological thinking is actually a return to Hippocratic concepts, who already envisioned the involvement of the brain in the generation of tinnitus. In 1990, Pawel Jastreboff described tinnitus as a conditioned response to deafferentation, i.e. auditory deprivation, linking it to the known brain neurophysiology [71]. Yet this model was anatomically agnostic.

The turn of the twentieth to twenty-first century would trigger many neuroanatomy and neurophysiology-based approaches to explain the generation of tinnitus. This was based on novel functional brain imaging technology, such as magnetoencephalography (MEG), source localized EEG, and functional magnetic resonance imaging. Rodolfo Llinas, using MEG, developed the concept of thalamocortical dysrhythmia, linking specific oscillatory changes in the auditory cortex to tinnitus, as a consequence of auditory deprivation [60]. This model proposed a common mechanism for tinnitus, pain, Parkinson's disease, depression, and slow wave epilepsy [60], 500 years after Fernel had proposed this possibility. This model led to attempts to treat tinnitus by neuromodulation, i.e. magnetic and electrical stimulation of the auditory cortex [72], which has not entered mainstream treatment, because of contradictory meta-analytic evidence [73–75].

At the beginning of the twenty-first century, Winfried Schlee proposed that tinnitus was not a symptom resulting from phrenological overactivity of the auditory cortex, but an emergent property of network dysfunctioning [76, 77]. Based on this concept, multitarget brain stimulation has been proposed [78, 79], yet due to technological limitations of the neuromodulation devices, this approach has not been incorporated in clinical practice.

All these concepts were related to auditory deafferentation, i.e. a deprivation of auditory input. In 2010, Josef Rauschecker proposed a fundamentally different theory, in which the tinnitus percept would be related to a deficiency of a noise cancelling pathway [80], analogous to what had been suggested for chronic pain [81]. These two opposite models were subsequently unified in a tinnitus imbalance model, in which tinnitus is identified as the consequence of an imbalance between sound input and sound suppression [82], also based on similar pain models [81–83]. And most recently, this model has become integrated in a Bayesian brain model by Dirk De Ridder, in which the balance critically depends on the predictive capacities of the brain [82, 84, 85]. Tinnitus is thus seen as a prediction error, resulting from auditory deafferentation, and resulting in a memory-based filling-in of the missing auditory information, driving the suppression of the noise cancelling pathway [82, 86, 87]. Other models consider tinnitus to be the consequence of chronic neuroinflammation of the auditory system [88], analogous to what has been posited for chronic pain [89].

With each new pathophysiological model, novel treatment approaches were developed, yet, up to 2020, no pharmacological, nor auditory-based (hearing aids, masking devices), nor neuromodulation treatments (TMS, tDCS, etc.) has received FDA or CE approval or reimbursement. Itard's statement (1821) that treatment of tinnitus is generally unsuccessful and in most cases the physicians' orientation must be towards the relief of disturbing symptoms is "unfortunately" still largely true [1]. This furthermore also leads to an excess of quack treatments, who try to fill the medical gap with sometimes, but unfortunately not always, well-intentioned remedies. As such, all current treatments for tinnitus remain off-label, clearly demonstrating that further pathophysiological refinements are highly needed.

Exploring the past to understand the present and shape the future [90], reiterates Confucius, and this overview of tinnitus research can hopefully benefit researchers to apply the same philosophy and take up research where earlier researchers have stopped, due to a lack of knowledge, insight, or technology.

References

1. Stephens SD. The treatment of tinnitus--a historical perspective. J Laryngol Otol. 1984;98:963–72. https://doi.org/10.1017/s0022215100147802.
2. Dietrich S. Earliest historic reference of 'tinnitus' is controversial. J Laryngol Otol. 2004;118:487–8. https://doi.org/10.1258/0022215041615182.
3. Feldmann H. Tinnitus: diagnosis and treatment. In: Shulman A, et al, editors. Lea and Febiger, 1991. p. 3–37.
4. Freeman P. Searching for Sappho: the lost songs and world of the first woman poet. W.W. Norton; 2016.
5. Thompson RC. Assyrian praescriptions for diseases of the ears. J R Asiat Soc. 1931;1-25:1.
6. Adams F. The genuine works of Hippocrates. William Woods and Company; 1891.
7. Maltby MT. Ancient voices on tinnitus: the pathology and treatment of tinnitus in Celsus and the Hippocratic Corpus compared and contrasted. Int Tinnitus J. 2012;17:140–5. https://doi.org/10.5935/0946-5448.20120025.
8. Littre E. Oeuvres completes d'Hippocrate. Bailliere; 1840.
9. Spencer WG. Celsus De Medicina with an English translation. William Heinemann; 1961.
10. Iyda JH, et al. Chemical composition and bioactive properties of the wild edible plant Raphanus raphanistrum L. Food Res Int. 2019;121:714–22. https://doi.org/10.1016/j.foodres.2018.12.046.
11. Choi SJ, Park CK, Shin DH. Protective effects of radish extract against neurotoxicity in mice and PC12 cells. J Med Food. 2020;23:523–34. https://doi.org/10.1089/jmf.2019.4563.
12. Liu J, et al. Systems pharmacology analysis of synergy of TCM: an example using saffron formula. Sci Rep. 2018;8:380. https://doi.org/10.1038/s41598-017-18764-2.
13. Burdock GA. Safety assessment of castoreum extract as a food ingredient. Int J Toxicol. 2007;26:51–5. https://doi.org/10.1080/10915810601120145.
14. Zinn MK, Bockmuhl D. Did granny know best? Evaluating the antibacterial, antifungal and antiviral efficacy of acetic acid for home care procedures. BMC Microbiol. 2020;20:265. https://doi.org/10.1186/s12866-020-01948-8.
15. Agrawal KS, et al. Acetic acid dressings: finding the holy grail for infected wound management. Indian J Plast Surg. 2017;50:273–80. https://doi.org/10.4103/ijps.IJPS_245_16.
16. Tripathi S, Mazumder PM. Neuroprotective efficacy of apple cider vinegar on zinc-high fat diet-induced mono amine oxidase alteration in murine model of AD. J Am Coll Nutr. 2021;1-10:658. https://doi.org/10.1080/07315724.2021.1948933.
17. Tripathi S, Mitra Mazumder P. Comprehensive investigations for a potential natural prophylaxis-a cellular and murine model for apple cider vinegar against hydrogen peroxide and scopolamine induced oxidative stress. Drug Dev Res. 2021;83:105. https://doi.org/10.1002/ddr.21849.
18. Grenier A, et al. Antioxidant, anti-inflammatory, and anti-aging potential of a Kalmia angustifolia extract and identification of some major compounds. Antioxidants (Basel). 2021;10:1373. https://doi.org/10.3390/antiox10091373.
19. Frankova A, et al. Antibacterial activities of plant-derived compounds and essential oils toward Cronobacter sakazakii and Cronobacter malonaticus. Foodborne Pathog Dis. 2014;11:795–7. https://doi.org/10.1089/fpd.2014.1737.
20. Lei Z, et al. Rosehip oil promotes excisional wound healing by accelerating the phenotypic transition of macrophages. Planta Med. 2019;85:563–9. https://doi.org/10.1055/a-0725-8456.
21. Lin TK, Zhong L, Santiago JL. Anti-inflammatory and skin barrier repair effects of topical application of some plant oils. Int J Mol Sci. 2017;19:70. https://doi.org/10.3390/ijms19010070.
22. Ayati Z, et al. Phytochemistry, traditional uses and pharmacological profile of rose hip: a review. Curr Pharm Des. 2018;24:4101–24. https://doi.org/10.2174/1381612824666181010151849.
23. Khan A, et al. Biological and medicinal application of Cucumis sativus Linn. - review of current status with future possibilities. J Complement Integr Med. 2021;19:843. https://doi.org/10.1515/jcim-2020-0240.
24. Ibrahim DS. Neuroprotective effect of Cucumis melo Var. flexuosus leaf extract on the brains of rats with streptozotocin-induced diabetes. Metab Brain Dis. 2017;32:69–75. https://doi.org/10.1007/s11011-016-9886-y.
25. Mykhailenko O, et al. Qualitative and quantitative analysis of Ukrainian iris species: a fresh look on their antioxidant content and biological activities. Molecules. 2020;25:4588. https://doi.org/10.3390/molecules25194588.
26. Yousefsani BS, Boozari M, Shirani K, Jamshidi A, Dadmehr M. A review on phytochemical and therapeutic potential of Iris germanica. J Pharm Pharmacol. 2021;73:611–25. https://doi.org/10.1093/jpp/rgab008.
27. Jones IH, Knudsen VO. Certain aspects of tinnitus, particularly treatment. Laryngoscope. 1928;14:283–4.
28. Yabalak E, Ibrahim F, Erdogan Eliuz EA. Natural sanitizer potential of Cuminum cyminum and applicable approach for calculation of Kovats retention index of its compounds. Int J Environ Health Res. 2021;1-12:158. https://doi.org/10.1080/09603123.2021.2011159.
29. Yadav PK, Jaiswal A, Singh RK. In silico study on spice-derived antiviral phytochemicals against SARS-CoV-2 TMPRSS2 target. J Biomol Struct Dyn. 2021;40:1–11. https://doi.org/10.1080/07391102.2021.1965658.
30. Barashkova AS, Sadykova VS, Salo VA, Zavriev SK, Rogozhin EA. Nigellothionins from black cumin (Nigella sativa L.) seeds demonstrate strong antifungal and cytotoxic activity. Antibiotics (Basel). 2021;10:166. https://doi.org/10.3390/antibiotics10020166.
31. Korinek M, et al. Anti-inflammatory and antimicrobial volatile oils: fennel and cumin inhibit neutrophilic inflammation via regulating calcium and MAPKs. Front Pharmacol. 2021;12:674095. https://doi.org/10.3389/fphar.2021.674095.
32. Sarkar C, et al. Therapeutic perspectives of the black cumin component thymoquinone: a review. Food Funct. 2021;12:6167–213. https://doi.org/10.1039/d1fo00401h.
33. Tashkandi H. Honey in wound healing: an updated review. Open Life Sci. 2021;16:1091–100. https://doi.org/10.1515/biol-2021-0084.
34. Stompor-Goracy M, Bajek-Bil A, Machaczka M. Chrysin: perspectives on contemporary status and future possibilities as pro-health agent. Nutrients. 2021;13:2038. https://doi.org/10.3390/nu13062038.
35. Fahmy HA, Farag MA. Ongoing and potential novel trends of pomegranate fruit peel; a comprehensive review of its health ben-

efits and future perspectives as nutraceutical. J Food Biochem. 2021;46:e14024. https://doi.org/10.1111/jfbc.14024.
36. Mahfooz S, Itrat M, Uddin H, Khan TN. Unani medicinal herbs as potential air disinfectants: an evidence-based review. Rev Environ Health. 2021;37:155. https://doi.org/10.1515/reveh-2021-0087.
37. Sharif A, Nawaz H, Rehman R, Mushtaq A, Rashid U. A review on bioactive potential of benzoin resin. Int J Chem Biochem Sci. 2016;10:106–10.
38. Dan B. Titus's tinnitus. J Hist Neurosci. 2005;14:210–3.
39. Di Napoli M, et al. Anti-Pseudomonas aeruginosa activity of hemlock (Conium maculatum, Apiaceae) essential oil. Nat Prod Res. 2019;33:3436–40. https://doi.org/10.1080/14786419.2018.1477151.
40. Bowman WC, Sanghvi IS. Pharmacological actions of hemlock (Conium maculatum) alkaloids. J Pharm Pharmacol. 1963;15:1–25. https://doi.org/10.1111/j.2042-7158.1963.tb12738.x.
41. Hotti H, Rischer H. The killer of socrates: coniine and related alkaloids in the plant kingdom. Molecules. 2017;22(11):1962. https://doi.org/10.3390/molecules22111962.
42. Berger M, Chen Y, Bampali K, Ernst M, Maulide N. Expeditious synthesis of polyacetylenic water hemlock toxins and their effects on the major GABAA receptor isoform. Chem Commun (Camb). 2018;54:2008–11. https://doi.org/10.1039/c7cc09801d.
43. Arihan O, Boz M, Iskit AB, Ilhan M. Antinociceptive activity of coniine in mice. J Ethnopharmacol. 2009;125:274–8. https://doi.org/10.1016/j.jep.2009.06.032.
44. Dayan AD. What killed Socrates? Toxicological considerations and questions. Postgrad Med J. 2009;85:34–7. https://doi.org/10.1136/pgmj.2008.074922.
45. Politzer A. Geschichte der Ohrenheilkunde, vol. 1. Enke Verlag; 1907.
46. Fatur K. "Hexing Herbs" in ethnobotanical perspective: a historical review of the uses of anticholinergic solanaceae plants in Europe. Econ Bot. 2020;74:140–58.
47. Josset P. Therapeutic uses of natron in ancient Egypt and the Greco-Roman world. Rev Hist Pharm (Paris). 1996;44:385–96.
48. Burnett C. Vocabulary of teaching and research between middle ages and renaissance, vol. 8. In: Weijers O, editor. CIVICIMA; 1995.
49. Alverny M-T. Renaissance and renewal in the twelfth century. In: Benson RL, Constable G, editors. Harvard University Press; 1982.
50. Berkey J. Encyclopedia of islam and the muslim world. In: Martin CR, editor. MacMillan Reference; 2004.
51. Ouzir M, Bernoussi SE, Tabyaoui M, Taghzouti K. Almond oil: a comprehensive review of chemical composition, extraction methods, preservation conditions, potential health benefits, and safety. Compr Rev Food Sci Food Saf. 2021;20:3344–87. https://doi.org/10.1111/1541-4337.12752.
52. Latha S, Selvamani P, Prabha T. Pharmacological uses of the plants belonging to the genus commiphora. Cardiovasc Hematol Agents Med Chem. 2021;19:101–17. https://doi.org/10.2174/1871525718666200702125558.
53. Marefati N, et al. The effect of Allium cepa extract on lung oxidant, antioxidant, and immunological biomarkers in ovalbumin-sensitized rats. Med Princ Pract. 2018;27:122–8. https://doi.org/10.1159/000487885.
54. Ding J, et al. Artemisia scoparia: traditional uses, active constituents and pharmacological effects. J Ethnopharmacol. 2021;273:113960. https://doi.org/10.1016/j.jep.2021.113960.
55. Batiha GE, et al. Bioactive compounds, pharmacological actions, and pharmacokinetics of wormwood (Artemisia absinthium). Antibiotics (Basel). 2020;9:353. https://doi.org/10.3390/antibiotics9060353.
56. Goldsmith JL. The crises of the late middle ages: the case of France. Fr Hist. 1995;9:417–50.
57. Pearn J. Two medieval doctors: Gilbertus Anglicus (c1180–c1250) and John of Gaddesden (1280–1361). J Med Biogr. 2013;21:3–7.
58. Brockliss L. A history of the University in Europe Vol. 2: Universities in Early Modern Europe (1500–1800). In: De Ridder-Symoens H, editor. Cambridge University Press; 1992. p. 563–620; medicine p. 609–20.
59. Siraisi N. A history of the University in Europe Vol. 1: Universities in the Middle Ages. In: De Ridder-Symoens H, Cambridge University Press; 1992. p. 360–87.
60. Llinas RR, Ribary U, Jeanmonod D, Kronberg E, Mitra PP. Thalamocortical dysrhythmia: a neurological and neuropsychiatric syndrome characterized by magnetoencephalography. Proc Natl Acad Sci U S A. 1999;96:15222–7.
61. Henry J. The scientific revolution and the origins of modern science, chap. 3. Palgrave; 2002.
62. Currathers HA. Napoleon on campaign. Pen & Sword Books Limited; 2014.
63. Miller DP. The story of 'scientist: the story of a word'. Ann Sci. 2017;74:255–61. https://doi.org/10.1080/00033790.2017.1390155.
64. Fyfe A, McDougall-Waters J, Moxham N. 350 years of scientific periodicals. Notes Rec R Soc Lond. 2015;69:227–39. https://doi.org/10.1098/rsnr.2015.0036.
65. Kronick DA. A history of scientific & technical periodicals: the origins and development of the scientific and technical press, 1665–1790, 2nd ed. The Scarecrow Press; 1976.
66. Kleinjung T, et al. Which tinnitus patients benefit from transcranial magnetic stimulation? Otolaryngol Head Neck Surg. 2007;137:589–95. https://doi.org/10.1016/j.otohns.2006.12.007.
67. De Ridder D, Heijneman K, Haarman B, van der Loo E. Tinnitus in vascular conflict of the eighth cranial nerve: a surgical pathophysiological approach to ABR changes. Prog Brain Res. 2007;166:401–11. https://doi.org/10.1016/S0079-6123(07)66039-7.
68. De Ridder D, et al. Transcranial magnetic stimulation for tinnitus: influence of tinnitus duration on stimulation parameter choice and maximal tinnitus suppression. Otol Neurotol. 2005;26:616–9.
69. Kuhn T. The structure of scientific revolutions. 3rd ed. University of Chicago Press; 1962.
70. Galison P. Image and logic. University of Chicago Press; 1997.
71. Jastreboff PJ. Phantom auditory perception (tinnitus): mechanisms of generation and perception. Neurosci Res. 1990;8:221–54.
72. De Ridder D, et al. Magnetic and electrical stimulation of the auditory cortex for intractable tinnitus. Case report. J Neurosurg. 2004;100:560–4.
73. Dong C, et al. Low-frequency repetitive transcranial magnetic stimulation for the treatment of chronic tinnitus: a systematic review and meta-analysis of randomized controlled trials. Biomed Res Int. 2020;2020:3141278. https://doi.org/10.1155/2020/3141278.
74. Lefebvre-Demers M, Doyon N, Fecteau S. Non-invasive neuromodulation for tinnitus: a meta-analysis and modeling studies. Brain Stimul. 2020;14:113–28. https://doi.org/10.1016/j.brs.2020.11.014.
75. Liang Z, et al. Repetitive transcranial magnetic stimulation on chronic tinnitus: a systematic review and meta-analysis. BMC Psychiatry. 2020;20:547. https://doi.org/10.1186/s12888-020-02947-9.
76. Schlee W, Hartmann T, Langguth B, Weisz N. Abnormal resting-state cortical coupling in chronic tinnitus. BMC Neurosci. 2009;10:11. https://doi.org/10.1186/1471-2202-10-11.
77. Schlee W, Weisz N, Bertrand O, Hartmann T, Elbert T. Using auditory steady state responses to outline the functional connectivity in the tinnitus brain. PLoS One. 2008;3:e3720. https://doi.org/10.1371/journal.pone.0003720.
78. Kleinjung T, et al. Combined temporal and prefrontal transcranial magnetic stimulation for tinnitus treatment: a pilot study. Otolaryngol Head Neck Surg. 2008;138:497–501. https://doi.org/10.1016/j.otohns.2007.12.022.

79. De Ridder D, Vanneste S. Multitarget surgical neuromodulation: combined C2 and auditory cortex implantation for tinnitus. Neurosci Lett. 2015;591:202–6. https://doi.org/10.1016/j.neulet.2015.02.034.
80. Rauschecker JP, Leaver AM, Muhlau M. Tuning out the noise: limbic-auditory interactions in tinnitus. Neuron. 2010;66:819–26.
81. De Ridder D, Adhia D, Vanneste S. The anatomy of pain and suffering in the brain and its clinical implications. Neurosci Biobehav Rev. 2021;130:125–46. https://doi.org/10.1016/j.neubiorev.2021.08.013.
82. De Ridder D, Vanneste S. The Bayesian brain in imbalance: medial, lateral and descending pathways in tinnitus and pain: a perspective. Prog Brain Res. 2021;262:309–34. https://doi.org/10.1016/bs.pbr.2020.07.012.
83. Vanneste S, De Ridder D. Chronic pain as a brain imbalance between pain input and pain suppression. Brain Commun. 2021;3:fcab014. https://doi.org/10.1093/braincomms/fcab014.
84. De Ridder D, Joos K, Vanneste S. The enigma of the tinnitus-free dream state in a Bayesian world. Neural Plast. 2014;2014:612147. https://doi.org/10.1155/2014/612147.
85. De Ridder D, Vanneste S, Freeman W. The Bayesian brain: phantom percepts resolve sensory uncertainty. Neurosci Biobehav Rev. 2014;44C:4–15. https://doi.org/10.1016/j.neubiorev.2012.04.001.
86. Song JJ, et al. The balance between Bayesian inference and default mode determines the generation of tinnitus from decreased auditory input: a volume entropy-based study. Hum Brain Mapp. 2021;42:4059. https://doi.org/10.1002/hbm.25539.
87. Vanneste S, De Ridder D. Deafferentation-based pathophysiological differences in phantom sound: tinnitus with and without hearing loss. NeuroImage. 2016;129:80–94. https://doi.org/10.1016/j.neuroimage.2015.12.002.
88. Wang W, et al. Neuroinflammation mediates noise-induced synaptic imbalance and tinnitus in rodent models. PLoS Biol. 2019;17:e3000307. https://doi.org/10.1371/journal.pbio.3000307.
89. Ji RR, Xu ZZ, Gao YJ. Emerging targets in neuroinflammation-driven chronic pain. Nat Rev Drug Discov. 2014;13:533–48. https://doi.org/10.1038/nrd4334.
90. Grasek S. Explore the past to understand the present and shape the future. Soc Educ. 2008;72:367–70.

Tinnitus, Tinnitus Disorder, and Other Phantom Perceptions

2

Berthold Langguth and Dirk De Ridder

Abstract

Tinnitus is a phantom perception, analogous to hallucinations, visual snow, or some forms of chronic pain. These phantom perceptions can be associated with affective, cognitive, and behavioural symptoms, which are largely defining the related distress and the functional disability.

Accordingly, it has recently been proposed that tinnitus without and with suffering (or distress) should be differentiated by distinct terms: "tinnitus" for the former and "tinnitus disorder" for the latter. "Tinnitus" was defined as 'the conscious awareness of a tonal and/or noise sound for which there is no identifiable corresponding external acoustic source'. By contrast, "tinnitus disorder" was defined as 'tinnitus plus tinnitus-associated suffering with or without functional disability.' Tinnitus was further differentiated in objective and subjective, pulsatile and non-pulsatile, constant and intermittent, or acute and chronic.

Whereas tinnitus is a simple or elementary form of auditory phantom perception, musical hallucinosis and verbal hallucinations are more complex auditory phantom phenomena not only limited to sound perception, but also containing semantic content. Whereas verbal hallucinations are a typical feature of a psychiatric condition (i.e. psychosis or schizophrenia), musical hallucinosis commonly results from severe auditory deprivation, deafferentation, or deafness without altered consciousness.

Hallucinations can also occur in other sensory modalities—visual, olfactory, gustatory, tactile, proprioceptive, vestibular, nociceptive, thermoceptive, and chronoceptive. Hallucinations can be associated with sensory deprivation, drug use (particularly deliriants), sleep deprivation, psychosis, neurological disorders, and delirium tremens.

B. Langguth (✉)
Department of Psychiatry and Psychotherapy, University of Regensburg, Bezirksklinikum, Regensburg, Germany
e-mail: Berthold.Langguth@medbo.de

D. De Ridder
Section of Neurosurgery, Department of Surgical Sciences, University of Otago, Dunedin, New Zealand
e-mail: dirk.deridder@otago.ac.nz

W. Schlee et al. (eds.), *Textbook of Tinnitus*, https://doi.org/10.1007/978-3-031-35647-6_2

Graphical Abstract

Tinnitus and Tinnitus Disorder

Tinnitus is the conscious awareness of a tonal or composite noise for which there is no identifiable corresponding external sound source.

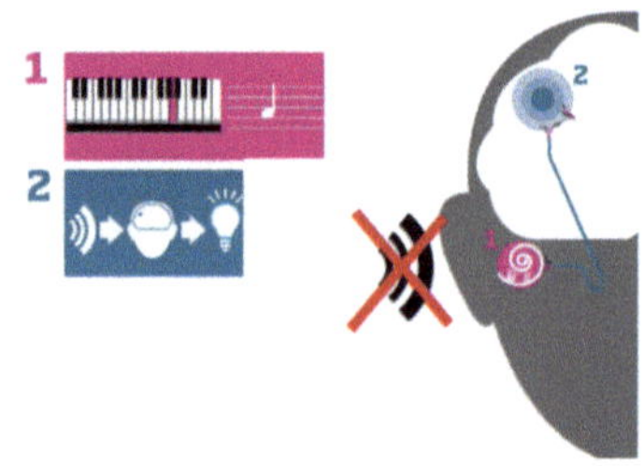

Tinnitus Disorder is the conscious awareness of a tonal or composite noise for which there is no identifiable corresponding external sound source, associated with emotional and/or cognitive dysfunction, and/or autonomic arousal, leading to behavioral changes and functional disability.

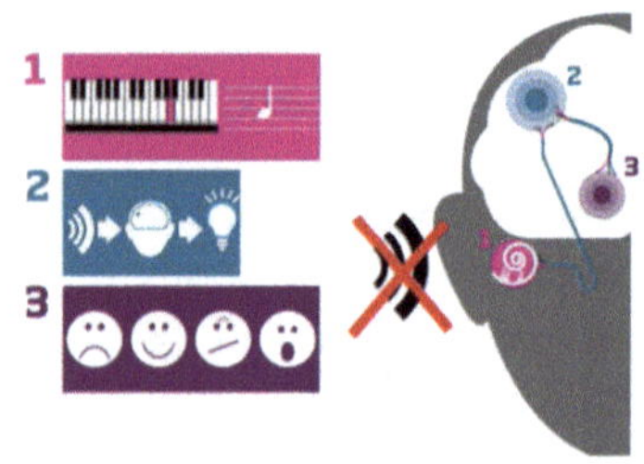

Highlights

- In a recent consensus article from an international and multidisciplinary group of tinnitus experts, it was proposed to differentiate "Tinnitus" from "Tinnitus disorder".
- "Tinnitus" was defined as 'the conscious awareness of a tonal and/or noise sound for which there is no identifiable corresponding external acoustic source'.
- "tinnitus disorder" was defined as 'tinnitus plus tinnitus-associated suffering with or without functional disability.'
- Operational diagnostic criteria were proposed in analogy to the diagnostic classification of chronic pain syndromes in ICD 11 and DSM V.

Introduction

An indispensable precondition for both clinical and scientific research is a clear and commonly accepted definition of a clinical term. Moreover, such a definition is essential for correct placement of a disorder within the existing classification systems such as the International Classification of Disorders (ICD) or the Diagnostic and Statistical Manual of Mental Disorders (DSM). A commonly accepted definition is a requirement for epidemiological research, for estimation of the global health and economic cost of tinnitus, as well as for health insurances and health care regulators. Moreover, commonly accepted definitions are important for the purposes of population and web-based surveys and for the purpose of identifying patient subgroups.

Traditionally, definitions of tinnitus did not differentiate between people who experience tinnitus and those who experience tinnitus together with tinnitus-associated emotional distress and functional disability.

However, for the purpose of clinical research, the degree of suffering is most relevant. In chronic pain, which is commonly considered the somatosensory analogue of chronic tinnitus [1–3], it has been shown that the perceived disability of the pain is only weakly ($R = 0.232$) correlated with pain intensity [4], but strongly ($R = 0.52$) with catastrophizing [5], i.e. the affective interpretation of pain, which determines the pain-associated suffering [6]. In the tinnitus field, it has also been shown that the quality of life is predicted by tinnitus catastrophizing and tinnitus-related fear, but not by psychophysical measures of tinnitus [7].

Many efforts have been made over the last decades to quantify the severity of tinnitus by assessing the related emotional distress and the tinnitus-associated handicap [8, 9] either by self-report questionnaires or by structured interviews. In spite of these efforts, a commonly accepted definition for tinnitus and its varying degree of emotional distress and functional disability is still lacking, and no diagnostic criteria have been established for the different forms of tinnitus.

Commonly Used Definitions, Diagnostic Criteria, and Diagnostic Classification

Multiple definitions of tinnitus have been published, from "ringing or buzzing in the ears" (Oxford Dictionary) to "the conscious experience of a sound that originates in the head of its owner" or "the conscious perception of an auditory sensation in the absence of a corresponding external stimulus" [10–13].

'Ringing in the ears' is clearly too simplistic – and frequently people perceive the origin of the phantom sound not in the ears, but in the head or even outside the head. Furthermore, tinnitus is not always described as 'ringing', but commonly also as hissing, cricket-like, or other sounds. Some definitions are more comprehensive descriptors of tinnitus, but are unhelpful because they include musical hallucinosis [14] or auditory hallucinations (e.g. the perception of voices in schizophrenia) and do not differentiate between etiologically different types of tinnitus, namely subjective and objective tinnitus. The term "objective tinnitus" (or its synonym "somatosound") is used to describe sounds that are generated by a sound source in the body, for example, by muscle contractions or blood flow. In this setting, the sound is present in the "internal environment" and heard by the auditory apparatus in contrast to subjective tinnitus, where no corresponding audible sound source can be found.

As with pain, tinnitus consists not only of a sensory discriminatory component, often expressed as tinnitus loudness and frequency or pitch, but also has an affective component, reflecting its unpleasantness [3], distress [15], or mood changes [16–18].

These tinnitus-associated symptoms can lead to comorbidities such as depression, anxiety, sleep disturbances, as well as cognitive problems such as concentration, attention, or memory problems [13, 19] (see also Chap. 21). In order to quantify the impact of tinnitus on quality of life, several self-report questionnaires have been developed and validated. These are used to stratify tinnitus patients according to the severity of their perceived tinnitus and also as outcome measurement for clinical trials [8, 9].

But tinnitus is not only heterogeneous with respect to its comorbidities, the associated emotional distress, or the associated functional disability. The pathophysiology of tinnitus can be heterogeneous, as tinnitus can be a symptom of specific pathologies, such as Meniere's disease, otosclerosis, or vestibular schwannoma. If such a specific etiology is not identified, the tinnitus is sometimes also called "idiopathic". The majority of subjects presenting with so-called "idiopathic" tinnitus have hearing loss measurable with conventional pure tone audiometry [10, 20, 21]. And even in tinnitus patients with normal standard pure tone audiometry, there may be some form of hearing loss [22–24].

With more sophisticated investigations, cochlear dysfunction can be detected even in the presence of a normal audiogram. These include high frequency audiometry [25, 26], distortion product otoacoustic emissions (DPOAE) [27], threshold equalizing in noise (TEN) testing [23], or auditory evoked potentials [22]. Recently, the term "hidden hearing loss" has been introduced to describe auditory symptoms such as tinnitus or poor speech discrimination in combination with a normal pure tone audiometry, a pattern that could be related to cochlear synaptopathy, evident in animal studies [28].

Finally, tinnitus is not adequately represented in current classification systems; in ICD 10, only as H93.1 as an otologic disorder without any consideration of the affective component, and in DSM IV and V, tinnitus is not yet represented at all.

Lack of Objective Tinnitus Biomarkers

Tinnitus is most often a subjective experience, currently without an objective measure, which has to be considered in the development of an operational definition of tinnitus. From an audiological perspective, it has been shown that weak or no correlation exists between changes in psychoacoustic measurements (matched tinnitus loudness or pitch) and changes in self-reported tinnitus suffering, and importantly, the changes in self-reported suffering, but not the change in psychoacoustic measurements, correlate with global subjective improvement [29, 30].

Currently, no objective biomarker has been established, neither for the existence of tinnitus, nor for the degree of suffering even if structural MRI brain scans [31] as well as electroencephalographic measurements [32] have shown some promise by discriminating people with tinnitus from those without tinnitus.

In the absence of an ability to objectively measure the sensory and affective components of the subjective tinnitus percept, an operational definition based on biomarkers is not possible. However, this does not mean that an operational definition of tinnitus cannot be put forward. For many disorders that are primarily characterized by their subjective experience, there exist established operational definitions in DSM or ICD.

Proposal for a Definition of Tinnitus and Tinnitus Disorder

Very recently, a group of international experts from different disciplines proposed in a consensus paper to differentiate between tinnitus and tinnitus disorder and proposed the following definitions [33]:

"Tinnitus" can be defined as 'the conscious awareness of a tonal and/or noise sound for which there is no identifiable corresponding external acoustic source'.

By contrast "tinnitus disorder" can best be defined as 'tinnitus plus tinnitus-associated emotional distress and functional disability.'

Tinnitus definitions include objective and subjective, pulsatile and non-pulsatile, constant and intermittent, and acute and chronic, but exclude more complex auditory phantom percepts such as musical hallucinosis and auditory or verbal hallucinations.

Proposal for Diagnostic Criteria

Based on the well-known analogy between chronic tinnitus and chronic pain, diagnostic criteria for tinnitus disorder could be similar to pain disorder criteria for Somatic Symptom Disorder in DSM-5.

The diagnostic criteria for Somatic Symptom Disorder noted in DSM 5 are:

1. One or more somatic symptoms that are distressing or result in significant disruption of daily life.
2. Excessive thoughts, feelings, or behaviours related to the somatic symptoms or associated health concerns as manifested by at least one of the following:
   (a) disproportionate and persistent thoughts about the seriousness of one's symptoms,
   (b) persistently high level of anxiety about health or symptoms,
   (c) excessive time and energy devoted to these symptoms or health concerns.
3. Although any one somatic symptom may not be continuously present, the state of being symptomatic is persistent (typically more than 6 months).

The somatic symptom disorder can be specified as "with predominant pain" (previously pain disorder) for individuals whose somatic symptoms predominantly involve pain.

Based on the pathophysiological, clinical, and treatment analogies between chronic pain and chronic tinnitus, it is proposed that tinnitus disorder falls under the somatic symptom disorder specified as "with predominant tinnitus". The other specifications could also be maintained:

Persistent: A persistent course is characterized by severe symptoms, marked impairment, and long duration (more than 6 months; Criterion C).

Mild: Only one of the symptoms specified in Criterion 2 is fulfilled.

Moderate: Two or more of the symptoms specified in Criterion 2 are fulfilled.

Severe: Two or more of the symptoms specified in Criterion 2 are fulfilled, plus there are multiple somatic complaints (or one very severe somatic symptom).

The severity of somatic symptom disorder is graded in the DSM-5 according to the number of the mentioned symptoms. As this procedure seems to be rather rough, it is recommended to complement it by using validated self-report instruments for assessing the individual tinnitus severity.

Tinnitus, Musical Hallucinosis, and Auditory Hallucinations

A stimulus produces an effect on the different sensory receptors, inducing sensation [3]. Perception in contrast has been defined as the act of interpreting and organizing a sensory stimulus to produce a meaningful experience of the world and of oneself [3]. Both sensation and perception can be conscious or unconscious [34]. Unconscious perception means that one responds to a stimulus even though one is not consciously aware of the stimulus, for example in priming [34]. Consciousness is a multifaceted concept that has two major components: awareness of environment and of self (i.e. the content of consciousness) and wakefulness (i.e. the level of consciousness). For tinnitus to be heard by a person, both wakefulness and awareness are required.

A first step in defining tinnitus relates to the acknowledgement that all patients with tinnitus are consciously aware of a sound that (even is transient) has no acoustic source, i.e. for which there is no identifiable corresponding sound source externally or from inside one's body. The sound percept of tinnitus can be tonal or noise -like, it can have a pattern, e.g. resemble the sounds of crickets or cicades, but it has no specific meaning cognitively. This is in contrast to other auditory phantom percepts such as musical hallucinations and verbal or auditory hallucinations. Hallucinations have been defined in DSM IV-TR as "A sensory perception that has the compelling sense of reality of a true perception but that occurs without external stimulation of the relevant sensory organ" [35]. Furthermore, hallucinations may be simple (i.e. unformed or "geometric") or complex (i.e. formed) [36]. Simple hallucinations by definition incorporate tinnitus, but a complex auditory or verbal hallucination differs by its semantic content from tinnitus.

Whereas musical hallucinosis are usually encountered in people with severe hearing loss, verbal hallucinations are typical for psychosis, as encountered in schizophrenia [37].

In the ICD-10, "organic hallucinosis" is defined as: "A disorder of persistent or recurrent hallucinations, usually visual or auditory, that occur in clear consciousness and may or may not be recognized by the subject as such. Delusional elaboration of the hallucinations may occur, but delusions do not dominate the clinical picture; insight may be preserved" [38]. In other words, hallucinosis is a constant state of hallucinations, but in a non-psychotic state. And they differ from delusions, which are not perceptual problems, but problems of belief.

DSM-5 defines a delusion as: "fixed beliefs that are not amenable to change in light of conflicting evidence" [39]. This is not applicable to tinnitus, as even though some tinnitus patients initially look for an external sound source explaining their tinnitus, they quickly realize the sound is generated inside their ears or head.

Hallucinations and hallucinosis should be excluded from the definition of tinnitus, even if transitions between tinnitus, musical hallucinosis, and verbal hallucinations are described in the literature [14, 40].

Thus, a preliminary definition could be that "tinnitus is the conscious awareness of a constant or intermittent sound that has no intrinsic meaning and for which there is no identifiable corresponding external sound source". As such, tinnitus is a sign of dysfunctional auditory sensation and perception.

Tinnitus is likened to chronic pain and visual snow. Whereas many manuscripts describe the analogy between chronic pain and tinnitus [1–3, 32, 41–52], very few have been detailed on the analogy between tinnitus and visual snow [53, 54]. Visual snow (VS) is described as constant, flickering static across the entire visual field. Diagnosis of visual snow syndrome requires the presence of visual snow for >3 months, alongside at least two of the following visual symptoms: palinopsia (=abnormal persistence or recurrence of an image in time), enhanced entoptic phenomena (= visual effects whose source is within the eye itself), photophobia, and impaired night vision (nyctalopia) [55].

Relevant Aspects for the Definition and Diagnostic Classification of Tinnitus

Objective and Subjective Tinnitus

Both definitions, tinnitus and tinnitus disorder, can be applied to objective and subjective tinnitus. It suffices that 'external' in the definition actually means 'external to the body', and as such 'tinnitus is the conscious awareness of a constant or intermittent sound that has no intrinsic meaning and for which there is no identifiable corresponding external (to the body) sound source.' Objective tinnitus is then described as tinnitus that can be attributed to an internal sound source, whereas subjective tinnitus is tinnitus with no reference to an internal sound source. As somatosounds, which lead to objective tinnitus, are generated within the body by muscular contraction or vascular bruits, this entity is included by the definition. In the same way, pulsatile tinnitus is captured by this definition.

This definition of objective tinnitus covers also all the cases in which the perceptual characteristics suggest an internal sound source even if the exact source cannot be identified. An example is pulse-synchronous tinnitus in which a vascular origin (hypertension, dehiscence, fistula, tumor, aneursym, stenosis, etc.) is expected, but is not identifiable by the respective diagnostic tests. Also in tinnitus with typical characteristics of muscular origin, it is sometimes difficult to retrieve the exact etiology (middle ear muscles, palatal muscles, etc.)

There are some criticisms about the terms "subjective tinnitus" and "objective tinnitus". The term "subjective tinnitus" is somewhat misleading, as there exist neuronal correlates of subjective tinnitus, which can be measured objectively by neuroimaging techniques, at least on the group level. Moreover, the term "subjective tinnitus" might suggest that the tinnitus exists only in the subjective experience of the individual or is even imagined by the patient. As alternative terms for "subjective tinnitus" and "objective tinnitus", the terms "primary tinnitus" (instead of subjective tinnitus) and "secondary tinnitus" (instead of objective tinnitus) were proposed. However, the terms subjective and objective tinnitus are much more common and widely used.

Acute and Chronic Tinnitus

For the differentiation between acute and chronic tinnitus, typically a duration of 3 or 6 months is chosen. However, there is no empirical evidence neither for 3 nor for 6 months.

It is generally accepted that the mechanisms involved in the generation of tinnitus differ from the mechanisms involved in the maintenance of tinnitus, but the temporal dynamics of this transition are still largely unclear. Moreover, neuroimaging research suggests that even after several years neurobiological changes still occur [56, 57].

From a clinical perspective, a differentiation between acute and chronic tinnitus could be guided by the chance of spontaneous recovery or by the efficacy of specific interventions for acute tinnitus, but also here there exist no convincing data.

Most guidelines use 6 months duration as criterion for chronic tinnitus. In a recent manuscript, 3 months were proposed as a cut-off for the transition from acute to chronic tinnitus in analogy with chronic pain, which is currently defined in ICD11 as pain extending beyond 3 months [58–60]. Similarly, 3 months is also a timeframe for defining chronic visual snow syndrome [55]. Thus, it seems reasonable to also use a duration of 3 months to differentiate between acute and chronic tinnitus.

Conclusion

A theoretical definition can be constructed that differentiates tinnitus without and with suffering. Whereas the first can be defined as 'tinnitus is the conscious awareness of a tonal and/or noise sound for which there is no identifiable corresponding external sound source', the latter can be defined as 'tinnitus disorder is the conscious awareness of a tonal and/or noise sound with associated suffering for which there is no identifiable corresponding external sound source.' These definitions include objective and pulsatile tinnitus, but exclude more complex auditory phantom percepts such as musical hallucinosis and auditory or verbal hallucinations.

An operational definition of "tinnitus" and some of its subforms is presented in Box 2.1. A definition of "tinnitus disorder" is proposed based on the current DSM 5 'somatic symptom disorder', analogous to pain, but then specified as tinnitus (see Box 2.2).

The subdivision between tinnitus as a sound percept without a corresponding external sound source and tinnitus disorder, which is tinnitus with its associated suffering, may be beneficial both for clinicians and researchers.

Box 2.1: Proposal for the Definition of Tinnitus and Tinnitus Disorder

Tinnitus is the conscious awareness of a tonal and/or noise sound for which there is no identifiable corresponding external sound source.

Tinnitus disorder is the conscious awareness of a tonal and/or noise sound with associated suffering and/or disability for which there is no identifiable corresponding external sound source.

Minimum time criterion: The tinnitus lasts at least 5 min and occurs on the majority of days.

Acute tinnitus: tinnitus with a duration of less than 3 months.

Chronic tinnitus: tinnitus with a duration of at least 3 months.

Objective tinnitus: tinnitus can be attributed to an internal sound source.

Subjective tinnitus: tinnitus without reference to an internal sound source.

Box 2.2: Proposal for Diagnostic Criteria for Tinnitus Disorder

According to the criteria for somatic symptom disorder specified as "with predominant tinnitus".

1. Tinnitus that is distressing or results in significant disruption of daily life.
2. Excessive thoughts, feelings, or behaviors related to tinnitus or associated health concerns (e.g. hyperacusis, insomnia, headache) as manifested by at least one of the following:
   (a) disproportionate and persistent thoughts about the seriousness of one's tinnitus,
   (b) persistently high level of anxiety about tinnitus.
   (c) excessive time and energy devoted to tinnitus.
3. Although the tinnitus sound may not be continuously present, the state of being symptomatic is persistent (typically more than 3 months).

Persistent: A persistent course is characterized by severe symptoms, marked impairment, and long duration (more than 3 months).

Mild: Only one of the symptoms specified in Criterion 2 is fulfilled.

Moderate: Two symptoms specified in Criterion 2 are fulfilled.

Severe: Two or more of the symptoms specified in Criterion 2 are fulfilled, plus there are multiple somatic complaints (or one very severe somatic symptom) (e.g. headache, insomnia, vertigo).

References

1. Moller AR. Similarities between severe tinnitus and chronic pain. J Am Acad Audiol. 2000;11:115–24.
2. Moller AR. Tinnitus and pain. Prog Brain Res. 2007;166:47–53.
3. De Ridder D, Elgoyhen AB, Romo R, Langguth B. Phantom percepts: tinnitus and pain as persisting aversive memory networks. Proc Natl Acad Sci U S A. 2011;108(20):8075–80.
4. Garbi Mde O, Hortense P, Gomez RR, da Silva TC, Castanho AC, Sousa FA. Pain intensity, disability and depression in individuals with chronic back pain. Rev Lat Am Enfermagem. 2014;22(4):569–75.

5. Kovacs FM, Seco J, Royuela A, Pena A, Muriel A, Spanish Back Pain Research Network. The correlation between pain, catastrophizing, and disability in subacute and chronic low back pain: a study in the routine clinical practice of the Spanish National Health Service. Spine. 2011;36(4):339–45.
6. Wade JB, Riddle DL, Price DD, Dumenci L. Role of pain catastrophizing during pain processing in a cohort of patients with chronic and severe arthritic knee pain. Pain. 2011;152(2):314–9.
7. Cima RF, Crombez G, Vlaeyen JW. Catastrophizing and fear of tinnitus predict quality of life in patients with chronic tinnitus. Ear Hear. 2011;32(5):634–41.
8. Langguth B, Goodey R, Azevedo A, Bjorne A, Cacace A, Crocetti A, et al. Consensus for tinnitus patient assessment and treatment outcome measurement: tinnitus research initiative meeting, Regensburg, July 2006. Prog Brain Res. 2007;166:525–36.
9. Hall DA, Haider H, Szczepek AJ, Lau P, Rabau S, Jones-Diette J, et al. Systematic review of outcome domains and instruments used in clinical trials of tinnitus treatments in adults. Trials. 2016;17(1):270.
10. Moller AR. Tinnitus: presence and future. Prog Brain Res. 2007;166:3–16.
11. Elgoyhen AB, Langguth B, De Ridder D, Vanneste S. Tinnitus: perspectives from human neuroimaging. Nat Rev Neurosci. 2015;16:632.
12. Langguth B, Kreuzer PM, Kleinjung T, De Ridder D. Tinnitus: causes and clinical management. Lancet Neurol. 2013;12(9):920–30.
13. Baguley D, McFerran D, Hall D. Tinnitus. Lancet. 2013;382(9904):1600–7.
14. Vanneste S, Song JJ, De Ridder D. Tinnitus and musical hallucinosis: the same but more. NeuroImage. 2013;82:373–83.
15. Vanneste S, Plazier M, van der Loo E, Van de Heyning P, Congedo M, De Ridder D. The neural correlates of tinnitus-related distress. NeuroImage. 2010;52(2):470–80.
16. Joos K, Vanneste S, De Ridder D. Disentangling depression and distress networks in the tinnitus brain. PLoS One. 2012;7(7):e40544.
17. Leaver AM, Renier L, Chevillet MA, Morgan S, Kim HJ, Rauschecker JP. Dysregulation of limbic and auditory networks in tinnitus. Neuron. 2011;69(1):33–43.
18. Langguth B, Landgrebe M, Kleinjung T, Sand GP, Hajak G. World J Biol Psychiatry. 2011;12(7):489–500.
19. Langguth B. A review of tinnitus symptoms beyond 'ringing in the ears': a call to action. Curr Med Res Opin. 2011;27(8):1635–43.
20. Norena A, Micheyl C, Chery-Croze S, Collet L. Psychoacoustic characterization of the tinnitus spectrum: implications for the underlying mechanisms of tinnitus. Audiol Neurootol. 2002;7(6):358–69.
21. Langguth B, Landgrebe M, Schlee W, Schecklmann M, Vielsmeier V, Steffens T, et al. Different patterns of hearing loss among tinnitus patients: a latent class analysis of a large sample. Front Neurol. 2017;8:46.
22. Schaette R, McAlpine D. Tinnitus with a normal audiogram: physiological evidence for hidden hearing loss and computational model. J Neurosci. 2011;31(38):13452–7.
23. Weisz N, Hartmann T, Dohrmann K, Schlee W, Norena A. High-frequency tinnitus without hearing loss does not mean absence of deafferentation. Hear Res. 2006;222(1–2):108–14.
24. Stouffer JL, Tyler RS. Characterization of tinnitus by tinnitus patients. J Speech Hear Disord. 1990;55(3):439–53.
25. Barnea G, Attias J, Gold S, Shahar A. Tinnitus with normal hearing sensitivity: extended high-frequency audiometry and auditory-nerve brain-stem-evoked responses. Audiology. 1990;29(1):36–45.
26. Vielsmeier V, Lehner A, Strutz J, Steffens T, Kreuzer PM, Schecklmann M, et al. The relevance of the high frequency audiometry in tinnitus patients with normal hearing in conventional pure-tone audiometry. Biomed Res Int. 2015;2015:302515.
27. Dadoo S, Sharma R, Sharma V. Oto-acoustic emissions and brainstem evoked response audiometry in patients of tinnitus with normal hearing. Int Tinnitus J. 2019;23(1):17–25.
28. Barbee CM, James JA, Park JH, Smith EM, Johnson CE, Clifton S, et al. Effectiveness of auditory measures for detecting hidden hearing loss and/or cochlear synaptopathy: a systematic review. Semin Hear. 2018;39(2):172–209.
29. Rabau S, Cox T, Punte AK, Waelkens B, Gilles A, Wouters K, et al. Changes over time of psychoacoustic outcome measurements are not a substitute for subjective outcome measurements in acute tinnitus. Eur Arch Otorhinolaryngol. 2015;272(3):573–81.
30. Hall DA, Mehta RL, Fackrell K. How to choose between measures of tinnitus loudness for clinical research? A report on the reliability and validity of an investigator-administered test and a patient-reported measure using baseline data collected in a phase IIa drug trial. Am J Audiol. 2017;26(3):338–46.
31. Boyen K, Langers DR, de Kleine E, van Dijk P. Gray matter in the brain: differences associated with tinnitus and hearing loss. Hear Res. 2013;295:67–78.
32. Vanneste S, To WT, De Ridder D. Tinnitus and neuropathic pain share a common neural substrate in the form of specific brain connectivity and microstate profiles. Prog Neuro-Psychopharmacol Biol Psychiatry. 2019;88:388–400.
33. De Ridder D, Schlee W, Vanneste S, Londero A, Weisz N, Kleinjung T, et al. Tinnitus and tinnitus disorder: theoretical and operational definitions (an international multidisciplinary proposal). Prog Brain Res. 2021;260:1–25.
34. Dehaene S, Naccache L, Le Clec HG, Koechlin E, Mueller M, Dehaene-Lambertz G, et al. Imaging unconscious semantic priming. Nature. 1998;395(6702):597–600.
35. Aleman A, de Haan EH. On redefining hallucination. Am J Orthopsychiatry. 1998;68(4):656–9.
36. Fraser CL, Lueck CJ. Illusions, hallucinations, and visual snow. Handb Clin Neurol. 2021;178:311–35.
37. Vanneste S, Song JJ, De Ridder D. Tinnitus and musical hallucinosis: the same but more. NeuroImage. 2013;82C:373–83.
38. World Health Organization. Organic hallucinosis. International Statistical Classification of Diseases and Related Health Problems. 10-R ed. Geneva: WHO; 1992.
39. Parnas J. Delusions, epistemology and phenophobia. World Psychiatry. 2015;14(2):174–5.
40. Marneros A, Beyenburg S, Berghaus A. Unilateral hallucinations and other psychotic symptoms due to otosclerosis. Psychopathology. 1997;30(2):89–92.
41. Arnold M, Bousser MG, Fahrni G, Fischer U, Georgiadis D, Gandjour J, et al. Vertebral artery dissection: presenting findings and predictors of outcome. Stroke. 2006;37(10):2499–503.
42. De Ridder D, De Mulder G, Menovsky T, Sunaert S, Kovacs S. Electrical stimulation of auditory and somatosensory cortices for treatment of tinnitus and pain. Prog Brain Res. 2007;166:377–88.
43. De Ridder D, Moller A. Similarities between treatments of tinnitus and central pain. In: Moller A, Langguth B, De Ridder D, Kleinjung T, editors. Textbook of tinnitus. New York: Springer; 2011. p. 753–62.
44. De Ridder D, Van de Heyning P. The Darwinian plasticity hypothesis for tinnitus and pain. Prog Brain Res. 2007;166:55–60.

45. De Ridder D, Vanneste S. The Bayesian brain in imbalance: medial, lateral and descending pathways in tinnitus and pain: a perspective. Prog Brain Res. 2021;262:309–34.
46. Kim YH, Park YG, Han KD, Vu D, Cho KH, Lee SY. Prevalence of tinnitus according to temporomandibular joint disorders and dental pain: the Korean National Population-based Study. J Oral Rehabil. 2018;45(3):198–203.
47. Langguth B, Hund V, Landgrebe M, Schecklmann M. Tinnitus patients with comorbid headaches: the influence of headache type and laterality on tinnitus characteristics. Front Neurol. 2017;8:440.
48. Llinas RR, Ribary U, Jeanmonod D, Kronberg E, Mitra PP. Thalamocortical dysrhythmia: a neurological and neuropsychiatric syndrome characterized by magnetoencephalography. Proc Natl Acad Sci U S A. 1999;96(26):15222–7.
49. Moller AR. Similarities between chronic pain and tinnitus. Am J Otol. 1997;18(5):577–85.
50. Rauschecker JP, May ES, Maudoux A, Ploner M. Frontostriatal gating of tinnitus and chronic pain. Trends Cogn Sci. 2015;19(10):567–78.
51. Tonndorf J. The analogy between tinnitus and pain: a suggestion for a physiological basis of chronic tinnitus. Hear Res. 1987;28(2–3):271–5.
52. Vanneste S, Song JJ, De Ridder D. Thalamocortical dysrhythmia detected by machine learning. Nat Commun. 2018;9(1):1103.
53. Lauschke JL, Plant GT, Fraser CL. Visual snow: a thalamocortical dysrhythmia of the visual pathway? J Clin Neurosci. 2016;28:123–7.
54. Renze M. Visual snow syndrome and its relationship to tinnitus. Int Tinnitus J. 2017;21(1):74–5.
55. Solly EJ, Clough M, Foletta P, White OB, Fielding J. The psychiatric symptomology of visual snow syndrome. Front Neurol. 2021;12:703006.
56. Schlee W, Hartmann T, Langguth B, Weisz N. Abnormal resting-state cortical coupling in chronic tinnitus. BMC Neurosci. 2009;10:11.
57. Schecklmann M, Landgrebe M, Poeppl TB, Kreuzer P, Manner P, Marienhagen J, et al. Neural correlates of tinnitus duration and distress: a positron emission tomography study. Hum Brain Mapp. 2013;34(1):233–40.
58. Scholz J, Finnerup NB, Attal N, Aziz Q, Baron R, Bennett MI, et al. The IASP classification of chronic pain for ICD-11: chronic neuropathic pain. Pain. 2019;160(1):53–9.
59. Treede RD, Rief W, Barke A, Aziz Q, Bennett MI, Benoliel R, et al. Chronic pain as a symptom or a disease: the IASP classification of chronic pain for the international classification of diseases (ICD-11). Pain. 2019;160(1):19–27.
60. Treede RD, Rief W, Barke A, Aziz Q, Bennett MI, Benoliel R, et al. A classification of chronic pain for ICD-11. Pain. 2015;156(6):1003–7.

Hypersensitivity to Sounds

3

Laure Jacquemin, Martin Schecklmann, and David M. Baguley

Abstract

The vocabulary and terminology used with regard to *hypersensitivity to sounds* are varied and imprecise. In this chapter, we explore and clarify understanding of hypersensitivity to sounds in adults, by identifying specific forms of decreased sound tolerance, such as recruitment, phonophobia, and misophonia. Due to the ill-defined terminology and insufficient literature, clear distinctions between diagnoses are hampered. These disorders of sound tolerance can be part of a more general medical disorder and, as such, have multiple comorbidities. Furthermore, they are complex and involve physiological and psychological aspects. As such, cognitive behavioural therapy and exposure therapy are often proposed for treatment, but evidence is lacking. Recently, there is a substantial and growing interest within both the clinical and research communities regarding decreased sound tolerance. Further progress can be made by reaching a consensus on the definition of loudness tolerance disorders and its subtypes, as well as investigating the treatment of these subtypes.

David Baguley has died before the publication of this book.

L. Jacquemin (✉)
University Department of Otorhinolaryngology and Head and Neck Surgery, Antwerp University Hospital, Edegem, Belgium

Department of Translational Neurosciences, Faculty of Medicine and Health Sciences, University of Antwerp, Wilrijk, Belgium
e-mail: laure.jacquemin@uza.be

M. Schecklmann
Department of Psychiatry and Psychotherapy, Interdisciplinary Tinnitus Clinic, University of Regensburg, Regensburg, Germany

D. M. Baguley (Deceased)
Nottingham Biomedical Research Centre, National Institute for Health Research, Nottingham, UK

Hearing Sciences, Mental Health and Clinical Neurosciences, School of Medicine, University of Nottingham, Nottingham, UK

Nottingham University Hospitals NHS Trust, Nottingham, UK

W. Schlee et al. (eds.), *Textbook of Tinnitus*, https://doi.org/10.1007/978-3-031-35647-6_3

Graphical Abstract

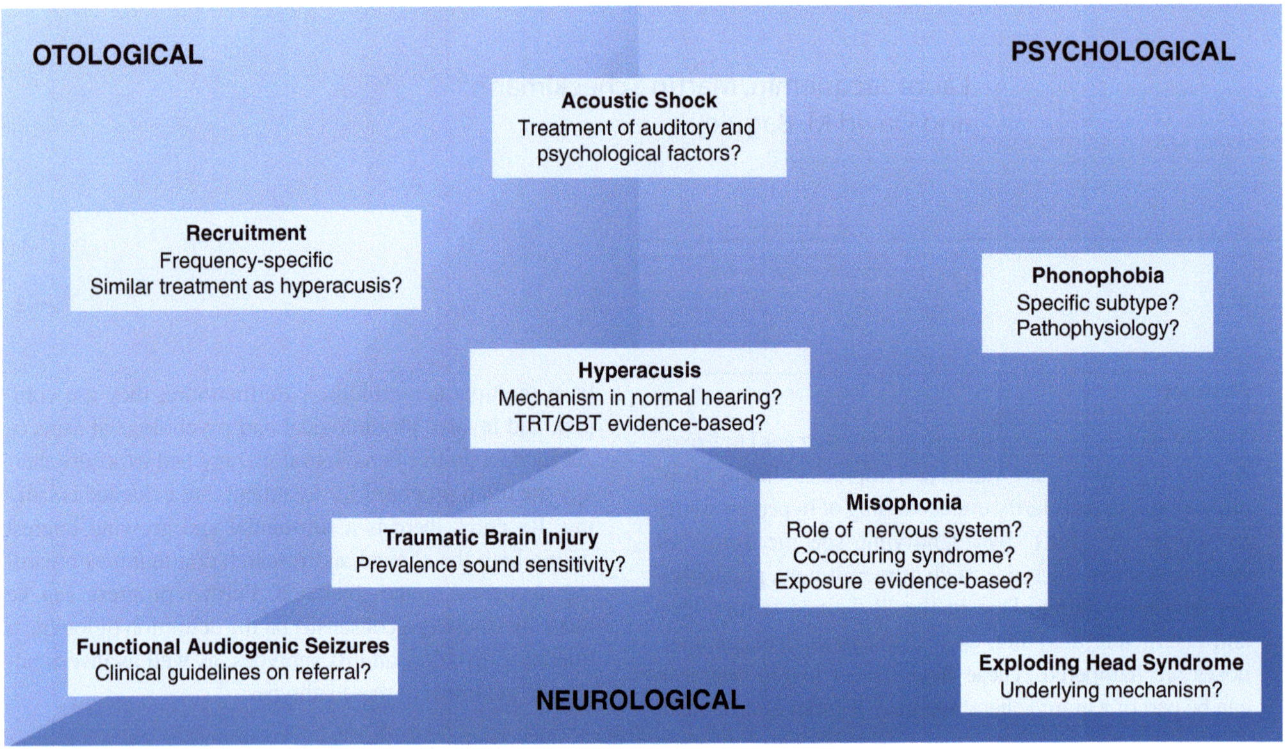

Highlights

- Consensus on the definition of loudness tolerance disorders and its subtypes potentially improves future epidemiological studies.
- There is insufficient literature supporting the subtyping of misophonia and phonophobia.
- CBT and exposure are most frequently proposed for treatment of different loudness tolerance disorders, but evidence is lacking.
- Hyperacusis and recruitment differ in trigger noises and might require different management options.
- Acoustic shock is a recently recognized condition, with occurrence of both auditory and psychological factors.
- Exploding head syndrome, traumatic brain injury, and functional audiogenic seizures involve the auditory pathway in some manner, but potentially need referral.

General Oversensitivity

Audiologists, Otologists, and Auditory Neuroscientists have generally concerned themselves with disorders of reduced hearing—but there are some patients who complain that their hearing is oversensitive. The vocabulary and terminology used in this regard are varied and imprecise, including reduced, decreased, or collapsed sound tolerance, hyperacusis, and loudness tolerance disorders. Furthermore, these symptoms can be part of a more general medical disorder and, as such, have multiple comorbidities. More specifically, persons with an *environmental intolerance* (EI) attribute several idiopathic, multisystem symptoms (e.g. cognitive problems, affected well-being) to a specific environmental exposure (e.g. odorous chemicals, electromagnetic fields, everyday sounds) [1]. A central pathophysiology has been suggested to explain the overlap of these symptoms [2]. In this chapter, we seek to explore and clarify understanding of hypersensitivity to sounds and to lead the reader into an understanding of current knowledge in this regard. To achieve that, we will focus on 'what is hyperacusis?', but also 'what is not hyperacusis?' by identifying specific forms of decreased sound tolerance and patient's experiences, and to then consider areas of overlap, and to identify unanswered research questions. In each case, we shall consider definitions, epidemiology, mechanisms, and treatments. The focus of this chapter will be on adults.

Hyperacusis

Hyperacusis literally means *excessive hearing*. The term has been in use in the medical literature for over 80 years, but there has been given minimal attention to it. A clinician Delphi survey by Adams and colleagues (2020) reached consensus on a definition for hyperacusis, namely "reduced tolerance to sounds that are perceived as normal to the majority of the population or were perceived as normal to the person before" [3]. This contrasts with the 'normal' preferences most people have regarding specific sounds or sound levels without affecting their everyday lives and social interactions. The framework proposed by Tyler and colleagues (discussed below) was the first to recognize pain hyperacusis as a separate entity [4]. The pathophysiology behind this experience of sound-evoked pain will be discussed further in this chapter.

Prevalence numbers of hyperacusis vary from 3.2% to 17.2% in the general adult population [3]. This variability can be explained by the subjective nature of this symptom, and as such, the results of epidemiological research are highly dependent on the formulated question. The consensus on the definition reached in 2020 can improve future epidemiological studies.

Common complaints of patients with hyperacusis are discomfort, headache, concentration difficulties, fatigue, and anxiety [3]. As these experiences vary between patients, the framework of Tyler and colleagues suggests subtypes of hyperacusis based on its defining feature: annoyance, loudness, fear, or pain [4]. Many patients with hyperacusis experience two or more of these aspects and data indicate that the hyperacusis experience can be very complex [5].

Besides the well-known comorbidity with tinnitus, other medical conditions also often co-occur with hyperacusis (see Table 3.1 for a full overview). With regard to psychiatric comorbidities, there seems to be an overrepresentation of anxiety disorders and anxiety-related personality traits, such as neuroticism [12]. It is important to bear in mind that hyperacusis can also be part of a more general perception disorder (including visual and somatosensory stimuli) [3]. It was shown that hyperacusis in tinnitus is associated with general hypersensitivity as indicated by increased subjective pain-related problems, increased vertigo, and by an overestimation of tinnitus pitch and hearing problems [22].

Table 3.1 Exemplary comorbidities in hyperacusis

Developmental Disorder
Autism spectrum disorder [6]
Neurological Disorder
Tay-Sachs disease [7]
Chronic fatigue syndrome [8]
Fibromyalgia/chronic pain [9]
Migraine [10]
Psychiatric Disorder
Depression [11]
Post-traumatic stress disorder [12]
Anxiety disorder (e.g. social phobia, generalized anxiety disorder, agoraphobia) [12]
Infectious Disease
Lyme disease [13]
Otologic Disorder
Meniere's disease [14]
Superior semicircular canal syndrome [15, 16]
Acoustic Shock [17]
Perilymph fistula [18]
Genetic Disorder
Williams syndrome [19, 20]
Cri du chat syndrome [21]

As the research field of hyperacusis is emergent, parallels can be drawn from the understanding of these comorbidities. For example, the association with migraine made Abouzari and colleagues investigate the effect of migraine therapy on hyperacusis [23]. Similarly, it might be noteworthy to look at the rich field of chronic pain. Also, in pain disorders, hypersensitivity problems can be found—hyperalgesia. In chronic pain, perceptual experiences are distorted in many different sensory modalities, including the auditory perception [24]. Especially, the phenomenon of 'pain hyperacusis' might be better understood by investigating the associations with chronic and/or neuropathic pain. Future research might benefit from learning from chronic pain research, similar as tinnitus research has profit from it.

While increased auditory input can lead to a decrease in central auditory excitability (e.g. after prolonged exposure to moderate-level sounds) [25], the central auditory system can become more excitable due to reduced auditory input (e.g. hearing impairment) [26]. These gain adaptations might be an attempt to optimally use the full input range. These changes can lead to tinnitus, when there is an increase in auditory spontaneous rates, and hyperacusis, when there is an increase in sound-evoked rates [27]. According to this so-called homeostatic model, not all types and degrees of hearing loss lead to these auditory symptoms (e.g. depending on the damage to inner or outer hair cells). But this model seems to fail in explaining why tinnitus and hyperacusis also occur in normal hearing subjects. However, there might be more subtle deafferentation without audiometric thresholds shifts, as demonstrated by cochlear dead regions testing and speech-in-noise recognition tests [28, 29]. The model using increased gain for explanation of tinnitus and hyperacusis is well recognized, but other models are also discussed and proposed [30–32] (please also see Chap. 18 on Neural gain). Importantly, activation at the level of the auditory cortex is more closely related to the perception of the stimuli rather than its physical characteristics [33, 34]. It was also speculated that recruitment is a risk factor for developing hyperacusis due to progressive avoidance behaviour (please see also the subchapter on recruitment below).

Literature on sound-evoked pain draws attention to a poorly understood experience, explained by a population of fibres in the cochlear nerve involved in pain perception (i.e. type II unmyelinated fibres) [35–37]. More specifically, there seems to be an alternative neuronal pathway from cochlea to brainstem that is activated by tissue-damaging noise. This involves a novel sensory modality, as the nervous system detects stimuli that can damage this tissue, further triggering sensations of pain or nausea for example [36].

In the chapter on *hyperacusis in tinnitus*, the management options available are discussed with psychoeducation and counselling in different forms being the most applied treatments (i.e. cognitive behavioural therapy (CBT), tinnitus retraining therapy (TRT) with sound therapy). However, evidence on this topic is limited with only a handful of studies focusing on hyperacusis as a primary complaint [38]. While some more innovative approaches have been suggested (multi-modal migraine prophylaxis therapy [23], round and oval window reinforcement [39]), stepwise reduction of avoidance behaviour and lowering the perceived distress by applying TRT or CBT principles is the recommended approach for now (please see also Chap. 41 on the management of hyperacusis and tinnitus).

Recruitment

The fact that hearing loss causes problems in the detection of lower intensity sounds is obvious, but it often results also in moderately intense sounds to be perceived as very loud. This phenomenon is called 'recruitment'. The dynamic range is smaller at some frequencies, leaving only a small range of levels that are audible and comfortable [40]. In contrast, every-day sounds (independent of the frequency) become intolerable (and even painful sometimes) in hyperacusis.

Recruitment refers to an abnormally large loudness at an elevated threshold (i.e. missing loudness compensation) [41]. This takes place for sounds and frequencies of sounds for which sensorineural hearing loss is evident. A typical phenomenon is that due to damage of the outer hair cells (which dampen intense sounds and amplify quiet sounds), people will ask others to speak louder, but when speech is louder ask the others not to speak so loudly. Thus, sensorineural hearing loss leads to a reduced auditory dynamic range (i.e. the difference between the loudest undistorted and the quietest discernible sound).

As damage to the outer hair cells cannot yet be cured, symptomatic treatment is necessary. First, hearing aids may help compensate for hearing loss and for reduced auditory dynamic range with sophisticated hearing aid fitting. Prescription algorithms using compression can match device output to the user's dynamic range and preferentially amplify soft speech sounds. Second, sound therapy can be another treatment option in order to increase the reduced auditory dynamic range [42]. These therapies can be part of a structured counselling approach, which can also include psychoeducation on recruitment and related avoidance strategies. However, research on the similarities and divergences of recruitment and hyperacusis is lacking, which leaves the question open if these two conditions should be treated similarly or require a different approach.

Misophonia

Misophonia (i.e. literally meaning *hatred of sound*) is defined as a disorder of decreased tolerance to specific sounds or stimuli associated with these sounds [43], for example a dislike of chewing, sniffing, or slurping sounds [44], and this set of triggers differs across patients [45]. Reactions to sound depend on the history, the evaluation of that sound, and the psychological profile for a given subject, as well as the context in which the sound is presented. An important characteristic of misophonia is that this sound tolerance problem does not depend on the physical characteristics, such as frequency and intensity [46]. Another aspect is that the sounds are related to other people. Historically, there were different definitions of misophonia such as hatred of sound [47] or an abnormal reaction to a sound with a specific meaning for the patient [48]. Commonly, misophonia describes a "disproportionate level of hate, anger, rage, and disgust toward a person producing sounds associated with eating (e.g. chewing and swallowing) or breathing" [47]. A variant of misophonia relates to adverse reactions to repetitive movements of another person in proximity. This phenomenon is called *misokinesia* [49]. The relationships between misophonia and misokinesia are as yet obscure.

The first model to explain this phenomenon was described by the Jastreboff's [46], suggesting that misophonia is developed and maintained through associative learning mechanisms that are activated in certain contexts. Hence, neurophysiological systems responsible for emotion, memory, and learning play an important role in the pathophysiology. Researchers have explored objective measures for this phenomenon. A study by Edelstein and colleagues suggested that misophonic responses can be measured through skin conductance responses (representing autonomic nervous system activity), but stated that this relationship might be mediated by other clinical conditions present [45]. A candidate for a neurophysiological marker for misophonia might be the N1 event-related potential (ERP) component according to Schröder and colleagues with N1 being often associated with auditory attention [50]. With regard to the location of these maladaptive brain processes, functional magnetic resonance imaging (fMRI) research indicated a potential role of the anterior insular cortex (AIC) [51]. This so-called 'core hub of the salience network' detects personally important stimuli in the environment and directs attention to it [52]. The discussed studies have one major limitation in common: causal relationships between the neurological measure and misophonia could not be proven. Nevertheless, the discussed peripheral and central nervous systems play a role, and as such, should be further investigated. Misophonia may be more related to psychological/brain causes—instead of somatic/hearing causes—compared to other conditions such as temporomandibular joint disorder or superior canal dehiscence, in which one's own body sounds are perceived and not filtered out by neuronal filter mechanisms. These reactions to one's own body sounds are more similar to tinnitus than to misophonia (hatred) or phonophobia (anxiety) (please see also the subchapter on phonophobia below).

Prevalence numbers of misophonia in a general population are lacking, yet a small number of studies provide some insight. For example, Naylor and colleagues administered the Amsterdam Misophonia scale (A-Miso-S) in a UK undergraduate medical student population. Surprisingly, a total of 49.1% of the students demonstrated clinically significant misophonic symptoms: 37% mild symptoms, 12% moderate symptoms, and 0.3% severe symptoms [53]. No extreme cases were indicated. A similar study in Chinese undergraduates demonstrated an overall prevalence of 20%, with 6% of the participants showing severe or extreme symptoms [54]. When focussing on a subpopulation of inpatients with depression, Siepsiak and colleagues found a prevalence of 11.7% according to the MisoQuest questionnaire [55]. The lower rates of misophonia in patients with depression compared to a general student population are unexpected and can be explained by the use of different questionnaires in these studies or affirm the role of higher cortical emotion-processing areas. Hence, there is a need for further investigation of assessment tools for misophonia.

Clinical interviews can be conducted to check if the patient meets the criteria and questionnaires can provide information about the severity of the complaints (e.g. MisoQuest, Amsterdam Misophonia Scale, Misophonia Questionnaire) [56–58]. A psychoacoustic test was lacking until 2021, when Enzler and colleagues published a test that could assess misophonia reliably and quickly. The test quantifies aversion towards different sources or events, such as mouth, breathing, nasal, throat sounds, and repetitive sounds [59].

An online study in 300 patients with misophonia reported that the symptoms start in childhood or early teenage years for most of the participants, with an increase in severity over time [60]. The impact on a persons' life with misophonia can be immense as it can lead to angry feelings, social isolation, and considerable psychological distress [52].

Publications on misophonia start in the early 2000s [46], raising attention to this phenomenon in various disciplines (e.g. audiology, neuroscience, psychiatry, psychology). The most common comorbid psychological disorders are obsessive-compulsive disorder (OCD), obsessive-compulsive personality disorder, and post-traumatic stress disorder (PTSD) [58]. This latter disorder seems also related to the severity of the misophonic symptoms [60]. Brout and colleagues pointed out: "It is unclear whether misophonia is a unique constellation of symptoms or a trandiagnostically co-occurring syndrome found across other disorders" [52].

As higher cortical brain structures are proposed to be involved in misophonia, the Jastreboff's suggested to 'retrain' the brain through repeated exposure to the misophonic triggers with new and positive conditioned responses following the exposure [46]. However, randomized controlled trials to investigate the effectiveness of this therapy are lacking. Furthermore, CBT for misophonia has been investigated by Schröder and colleagues in an open trial with eight bi-weekly group CBT sessions compared to a waiting list [61]. This study showed significant reductions in misophonia symptoms in 48% of the participants. Effectiveness of pharmacological treatments, on the other hand, is unknown [52].

Phonophobia

Phonophobia (i.e. literally meaning *fear of sound*) is defined as an anxiety disorder that is characterized as a persistent, abnormal, and unwarranted fear of sound (often everyday sounds) shaped by an emotional meaning [46]. Typical examples are children's voices for teachers or telephone ringing for office workers [62]. Based on the concepts of Jastreboff's (conditioning of sounds with physiological reactions as an etiological model), it is considerable that phonophobia is a specific subtype of misophonia. However, if it is a real subtype or rather a variation of sound tolerance disorders, it is the topic of current discussions. All of these conditions have emotional, cognitive, physiological, and behavioural reactions to specific sounds in common and are more or less associated with somatic and/or hearing complaints. It is important to note that misophonia and phonophobia are related to specific sounds or in more detail sounds with a specific meaning to the patient or sounds which are associated with negative learning experience in contrast to recruitment or hyperacusis.

It is important to differentiate phonophobia's different meanings, including the sound intolerances during migraine headaches described in neurological literature [63]. For example, when searching for manuscript titles with 'phonophobia' on PubMed, half of the publications cover migraine-related phonophobia.

Prevalence numbers are hard to find in literature, as most studies focus on patients with a secondary complaint of phonophobia and, for example, a primary complaint of tinnitus. These patients often find it hard to separate the different symptoms (e.g. hyperacusis, phonophobia, insomnia) they experience when filling out a questionnaire [62].

It is possible that over time the triggering stimuli become generalized and, as such, a broad spectrum of sounds become phobic. In other words, what started as phonophobia for a certain sound might evolve into a general hypersensitivity to noise.

Little is known about the pathophysiology of phonophobia. The peripheral and central auditory pathways are often intact. It is assumed that certain learning or conditioning processes are at the core. As it is assumed that the phonophobic reactions are exaggerated, these reactions should be treated. Thus, CBT is often suggested as a treatment to deal with these maladaptive reactions. However, there is little literature to support this. As a first step, its pathophysiology should be better understood. What is the role of the auditory system? Or should we focus on psychological models to explain this condition? These questions should be answered before exploring management options. Moreover, it is unclear how many adults suffer from this condition and how heterogeneous this population is. In other words, we have a name for a defined condition without knowing how many people suffer from it, why they suffer from it, and how we can decrease suffering. On the other hand, one may take it easy and categorize phonophobia as only one of the numerous possible phobias. By doing this, the mechanism and treatment are rather clear (i.e. learning processes and CBT).

Exploding Head Syndrome

The rather lurid term Exploding Head Syndrome (EHS) refers to a benign condition wherein an individual perceives a sudden, transient, and intense noise at the onset of sleep [64]. The term EHS was first used by Pearce [65]. This can be accompanied by the perception of a flash of light, and/or jerking of the body. These experiences can be frequent and may be highly alarming or distressing for the individual. By definition, therefore, EHS falls into the category of a parasomnia, though it has rarely been considered in that context. Other terminology that has been used for EHS includes 'snapping of the brain' and 'episodic cranial shock'—these in an early report from 1920 [66], and 'sensory discharges' [64].

The literature regarding epidemiological features of EHS is sparse, and what there is consists mainly of case reports or ill-defined case series. As such, definitive information on prevalence and incidence is not available. Trends in the literature include more reports of ENS in women than men (potentially due to the greater likelihood of women consulting their doctor than men [67]) and an onset of EHS in middle age. Associations with excessive smoking and stress have been proposed. Minimal information regarding natural history or longitudinal data is available.

The mechanisms of EHS are unclear, but there appear to be no associations with hearing loss, tinnitus, or hyperacusis. As such, it appears not to have an otological nor audiological basis, though the noise percept must involve the auditory pathway in some manner. Frese and colleagues reported neurological and structural neuroimaging in a series of six adults with EHS: all investigations were normal [68]. Studies to image the EHS activity, either with functional neuroimaging or MEG, have not been undertaken to date, and the unpredictable and very transient nature of EHS in individuals who by definition are either at the cusp of sleep or actually asleep would represent substantial challenges. An attempt at polysomnography has been inconclusive [69]. The reported coupling of EHS with a visual percept, and/or a motor experience might indicate cortical involvement, but this would be speculative at present.

There are no clinical trials for treatment of EHS in the literature. The benign nature of EHS, which though unpleasant is not associated with harm, has led several authors to advocate reassurance as a treatment [70, 71], though where stress and/or anxiety has been indicated as association or cause, common sense dictates that these may be addressed also.

Acoustic Shock

Acoustic Shock is a relatively recently recognized condition [17, 72] wherein patients experience a variable combination/clusters of the following symptoms [73]: otalgia, hyperacusis, tinnitus, cochlear hearing loss, anxiety and fear, hypervigilance, and sleep disturbance. It is instigated by exposure to an abrupt, sudden, and unexpected sound, such as a transient noise through the headphones used by call-centre workers, or an alarm in proximity. The index sound exposure is often intense though this is not always the case: the unexpected nature of the sound and proximity to the ear appear as if not more important than loudness [74]. The presence and extent of cochlear hearing loss is variable, indicating that this is a phenomenon distinct from both traditional noise-induced hearing loss and acoustic trauma, though in the case of combat blast injury these may overlap. Acoustic shock was first identified in call-centre workers, who on cold calling may experience retaliation to a perceived incursion by an individual screaming down their telephone or striking the microphone with keys or some other object. Data regarding the prevalence and incidence of acoustic shock are not yet available.

A number of potential mechanisms for acoustic shock have been proposed. These include cochlear injury, tonic contraction of the tensor tympani middle ear muscle [75], and psychological mechanisms, either in conjunction with auditory involvement [74] or in isolation [76]. Following a case report of acoustic shock where there was no indication of cochlear hearing loss [77], a 'integrative' model has been proposed, involving the tensor tympani muscle, the trigeminal nerve, and the trigeminal cervical complex [78]: at the time of writing, this has not been independently corroborated or validated. An additional possibility is that the otalgia component of acoustic shock, which is the most consistent symptom experienced [17], may involve potentiation and/or activation of the nociceptive cochlear nerve fibres discussed above [36].

No clinical controlled trials of treatments for acoustic shock have been reported to date, and the pragmatic use of existing strategies for the symptom components of hyperacusis and tinnitus occurs. Given the observed occurrence of both auditory and psychological factors as described, the investigation of the efficacy of treatment protocols that addressed each and all of the components is indicated.

Decreased Sound Tolerance Associated with Traumatic Brain Injury

Head injury may lead to hearing problems in a number of different ways. Direct trauma to the temporal bone, which may involve temporal bone fracture, can lead to cochlear hearing loss, tinnitus, and in very severe cases avulsion of the cochlear nerve may occur [79]. Other cases of traumatic brain injury (TBI) may be indirect, including blast injuries, and the audio-vestibular consequences may be less clear, as the neurological impact may involve widespread challenges to central auditory structures and pathways [80].

TBI is a prevalent condition with a report of 2.5 million emergency department episodes per year in the USA [81]. In some populations, such as armed forces engaged in active combat, exposure to TBI may be repeated [82]. Within the population there are experiences of confusion and memory loss, and these may be long standing. The prevalence of audiovestibular problems following TBI is well known, but has not been robustly determined, and the natural history is unknown. The issues may include hearing loss, auditory-processing disorders, tinnitus, hyperacusis, and imbalance, and the combination of such challenges with cognitive issues may be additive and debilitating. Regarding specific issues with sound tolerance following TBI, reports exhibit the problems with definitions seen elsewhere. Up to 32% of adults experiencing TBI reported that they were 'bothered by noise' up to 12 months post injury [83], but this is a non-standard question for hyperacusis (and decreased sound tolerance) and it may reflect emotional disinhibition (which is common in the TBI population) as well as sound tolerance challenges.

TBI can adversely affect each and every part of the auditory pathway, from cochlea, to brainstem, to midbrain, to cortex. Additionally, systems of memory, cognition, and emotional regulation may also be impacted, and these issues may increase the burden of managing decreased sound tolerance, tinnitus, and hearing loss. Papesh and colleagues (2018) advocate for comprehensive auditory evaluation in the TBI population, and a battery including assessment of speech understanding in noise, temporal processing, dichotic listening, and the use of long latency auditory-evoked potentials [80]. This is a standard to which many clinical services might aspire but fail to achieve. While there are undoubted challenges in this regard, involving clinic resources and the limited attention span, patience, and concentration abilities of the TBI patient population, more diligent assessment of such patients is undoubtedly indicated. It should be noted though that there is exceeding sparse validation data for auditory assessments in the TBI population.

Theodoroff and colleagues (2019) state that several questions remain unanswered concerning the underlying mechanisms of noise sensitivity following TBI, which impedes the development of effective interventions for this specific type of decreased sound tolerance. More specifically, it might not be modality-specific, but rather related to impaired sensory gating. Hence, the need for an audiologist, psychologist, or neurologist to be involved is unknown [84].

Functional Audiogenic Seizures

In the Audiology and Otolaryngology communities, the term 'functional' or "dissociative", when applied to hearing loss, has traditionally carried a strong implication of malingering or deliberate falsehood. In the Neurology community, however, there is a very different perspective: the idea that a symptom may not have a detectable physiological cause or lesion, but may genuinely arise from emotional or psychological challenges [85]. The term functional neurological disorders (FND) is used. An analogy can be made between symptoms that derive from *hardware* problems (e.g. cochlear hearing loss, or auditory dyschrony) and those from *software* problems within the central nervous system (including the auditory system). Such symptoms can include the entire spectrum of neurological disorders and have been estimated to account for 16% of neurological consultations, rendering FND the second most common diagnosis in outpatient neurology [86].

There are a small, but important, population of individuals who experience a seizure when hearing an abrupt and unexpected sound. Such audiogenic seizures can be debilitating and limiting to everyday activities. There may be extreme reliance on hearing protection. The literature in this regard is sparse and emergent. In some situations there can be a potentiation or disinhibition of startle reflexes, such as in cerebral palsy (Baguley, clinical experience), but in other cases there may be a functional aspect to the situation [87].

The epidemiology of functional audiogenic seizure is unknown. It is rare, but potentially each clinician working with patients with decreased sound tolerance may see one or two patients in a career, and hence it is worthy of consideration.

The mechanisms of functional audiogenic seizure are clearly complex and potentially specific to each individual patient. The role of the Audiologist and Otologist in such situations is to be aware of the possibility of such a clinical presentation, and then to refer to specialist Neurology clinicians, who if active in FND will be supported by Psychology and Physiotherapy colleagues.

The role of ear-related clinicians in treatment may be limited, but the introduction of the need for referral needs to be sensitive and based in compassion. Once within an FND treatment programme, patients with functional audiogenic seizure may require some audiological input to support the gradual reduction of use of hearing protection, and this may involve the use of ear level sound generators.

Closing Remarks

Disorders of sound tolerance are complex and involve physiological and psychological aspects. The terminology used in this area is ill-defined, and in an individual patient it may not be possible to make clear distinctions between diagnoses. What is encouraging, however, is that there is substantial and growing interest within both the clinical and research communities regarding decreased sound tolerance, which bodes well for future progress.

Acknowledgement David Baguley is supported by the UK National Institute of Health Research (NIHR), but his views are his own and do not represent those of NIHR nor the UK Department of Health and Social Care.

References

1. Palmquist E, Claeson AS, Neely G, Stenberg B, Nordin S. Overlap in prevalence between various types of environmental intolerance. Int J Hyg Environ Health. 2014;217(4–5):427–34.
2. Viziano A, Micarelli A, Alessandrini M. Noise sensitivity and hyperacusis in patients affected by multiple chemical sensitivity. Int Arch Occup Environ Health. 2017;90(2):189–96.
3. Adams B, Sereda M, Casey A, Byrom P, Stockdale D, Hoare DJ. A Delphi survey to determine a definition and description of hyperacusis by clinician consensus. Int J Audiol. 2020;1-7:607.
4. Tyler RS, Pienkowski M, Roncancio ER, Jun HJ, Brozoski T, Dauman N, et al. A review of hyperacusis and future directions: part I. Definitions and manifestations. Am J Audiol. 2014;23(4):402–19.
5. Ke J, Du Y, Tyler RS, Perreau A, Mancini PC. Complaints of people with Hyperacusis. J Am Acad Audiol. 2020;31(08):553–8.
6. Danesh AA, Lang D, Kaf W, Andreassen WD, Scott J, Eshraghi AA. Tinnitus and hyperacusis in autism spectrum disorders with emphasis on high functioning individuals diagnosed with Asperger's syndrome. Int J Pediatr Otorhinolaryngol. 2015;79(10):1683–8.
7. Karimzadeh P, Jafari N, Nejad Biglari H, Jabbeh Dari S, Ahmad Abadi F, Alaee MR, et al. GM2-Gangliosidosis (Sandhoff and Tay Sachs disease): diagnosis and neuroimaging findings (an Iranian pediatric case series). Iranian J Child Neurol. 2014;8(3):55–60.
8. Jason LA, Taylor RR, Kennedy CL. Chronic fatigue syndrome, fibromyalgia, and multiple chemical sensitivities in a community-based sample of persons with chronic fatigue syndrome-like symptoms. Psychosom Med. 2000;62(5):655–63.
9. Geisser ME, Glass JM, Rajcevska LD, Clauw DJ, Williams DA, Kileny PR, et al. A psychophysical study of auditory and pressure sensitivity in patients with fibromyalgia and healthy controls. J Pain. 2008;9(5):417–22.
10. Kelman L, Tanis D. The relationship between migraine pain and other associated symptoms. Cephalalgia. 2006;26(5):548–53.
11. Paulin J, Andersson L, Nordin S. Characteristics of hyperacusis in the general population. Noise Health. 2016;18(83):178–84.
12. Jüris L, Andersson G, Larsen HC, Ekselius L. Psychiatric comorbidity and personality traits in patients with hyperacusis. Int J Audiol. 2013;52(4):230–5.
13. Nields JA, Fallon BA, Jastreboff PJ. Carbamazepine in the treatment of Lyme disease-induced hyperacusis. J Neuropsychiatry Clin Neurosci. 1999;11(1):97–9.
14. Brandy WT, Lynn JM. Audiologic findings in hyperacusic and non-hyperacusic subjects. Am J Audiol. 1995;4(1):46–51.
15. Ward BK, Carey JP, Minor LB. Superior canal dehiscence syndrome: lessons from the first 20 years. Front Neurol. 2017;8:177.
16. Nikkar-Esfahani A, Whelan D, Banerjee A. Occlusion of the round window: a novel way to treat hyperacusis symptoms in superior semicircular canal dehiscence syndrome. J Laryngol Otol. 2013;127(7):705–7.
17. McFerran DJ, Baguley DM. Acoustic shock. J Laryngol Otol. 2007;121(4):301–5.
18. Fukaya T, Nomura Y. Audiological aspects of idiopathic perilymphatic fistula. Acta Otolaryngol Suppl. 1988;456:68–73.
19. Klein AJ, Armstrong BL, Greer MK, Brown FR 3rd. Hyperacusis and otitis media in individuals with Williams syndrome. J Speech Hear Disord. 1990;55(2):339–44.
20. Gothelf D, Farber N, Raveh E, Apter A, Attias J. Hyperacusis in Williams syndrome: characteristics and associated neuroaudiologic abnormalities. Neurology. 2006;66(3):390–5.
21. Espirito Santo LD, Moreira LM, Riegel M. Cri-Du-chat syndrome: clinical profile and chromosomal microarray analysis in six patients. Biomed Res Int. 2016;2016:5467083.

22. Schecklmann M, Landgrebe M, Langguth B, T. R. I. Database Study Group. Phenotypic characteristics of hyperacusis in tinnitus. PLoS One. 2014;9(1):e86944.
23. Abouzari M, Tan D, Sarna B, Ghavami Y, Goshtasbi K, Parker EM, et al. Efficacy of multi-modal migraine prophylaxis therapy on hyperacusis patients. Ann Otol Rhinol Laryngol. 2020;129(5):421–7.
24. Suhnan AP, Finch PM, Drummond PD. Hyperacusis in chronic pain: neural interactions between the auditory and nociceptive systems. Int J Audiol. 2017;56(11):801–9.
25. Pienkowski M, Eggermont JJ. Long-term, partially-reversible reorganization of frequency tuning in mature cat primary auditory cortex can be induced by passive exposure to moderate-level sounds. Hear Res. 2009;257(1–2):24–40.
26. Kotak VC, Fujisawa S, Lee FA, Karthikeyan O, Aoki C, Sanes DH. Hearing loss raises excitability in the auditory cortex. J Neurosci Off J Soc Neurosci. 2005;25(15):3908–18.
27. Pienkowski M, Tyler RS, Roncancio ER, Jun HJ, Brozoski T, Dauman N, et al. A review of hyperacusis and future directions: part II. Measurement, mechanisms, and treatment. Am J Audiol. 2014;23(4):420–36.
28. Weisz N, Hartmann T, Dohrmann K, Schlee W, Norena A. High-frequency tinnitus without hearing loss does not mean absence of deafferentation. Hear Res. 2006;222(1–2):108–14.
29. Gilles A, Schlee W, Rabau S, Wouters K, Fransen E, Van de Heyning P. Decreased speech-in-noise understanding in young adults with tinnitus. Front Neurosci. 2016;10:288.
30. Sedley W. Tinnitus: does gain explain? Neuroscience. 2019;407:213–28.
31. Zeng FG. Tinnitus and hyperacusis: central noise, gain and variance. Curr Opin Physio. 2020;18:123–9.
32. Eggermont JJ. Separate auditory pathways for the induction and maintenance of tinnitus and hyperacusis? Prog Brain Res. 2021;260:101–27.
33. Langers DR, van Dijk P, Schoenmaker ES, Backes WH. fMRI activation in relation to sound intensity and loudness. NeuroImage. 2007;35(2):709–18.
34. Röhl M, Uppenkamp S. Neural coding of sound intensity and loudness in the human auditory system. J Assoc Res Otolaryngol. 2012;13(3):369–79.
35. Hickox AE, Liberman MC. Is noise-induced cochlear neuropathy key to the generation of hyperacusis or tinnitus? J Neurophysiol. 2014;111(3):552–64.
36. Flores EN, Duggan A, Madathany T, Hogan AK, Márquez FG, Kumar G, et al. A non-canonical pathway from cochlea to brain signals tissue-damaging noise. Curr Biol. 2015;25(5):606–12.
37. Liu C, Glowatzki E, Fuchs PA. Unmyelinated type II afferent neurons report cochlear damage. Proc Natl Acad Sci U S A. 2015;112(47):14723–7.
38. Fackrell K, Potgieter I, Shekhawat GS, Baguley DM, Sereda M, Hoare DJ. Clinical interventions for hyperacusis in adults: a scoping review to assess the current position and determine priorities for research. Biomed Res Int. 2017;2017:2723715.
39. Silverstein H, Wu YH, Hagan S. Round and oval window reinforcement for the treatment of hyperacusis. Am J Otolaryngol. 2015;36(2):158–62.
40. Lesica NA. Why do hearing aids fail to restore normal auditory perception? Trends Neurosci. 2018;41(4):174–85.
41. Buus S, Florentine M. Growth of loudness in listeners with cochlear hearing losses: recruitment reconsidered. J Assoc Res Otolaryngol. 2002;3(2):120–39.
42. Formby C, Hawley ML, Sherlock LP, Gold S, Payne J, Brooks R, et al. A sound therapy-based intervention to expand the auditory dynamic range for loudness among persons with sensorineural hearing losses: a randomized placebo-controlled clinical trial. Semin Hear. 2015;36(2):77–110.
43. Swedo S, Baguley DM, Denys D, Dixon LJ, Erfanian M, Fioretti A, et al. A Consensus definition of misophonia: using a delphi process to reach expert agreement. medRxiv. 2021:2021.04.05.21254951.
44. Aazh H, Landgrebe M, Danesh AA, Moore BC. Cognitive behavioral therapy for alleviating the distress caused by tinnitus, Hyperacusis and Misophonia: current perspectives. Psychol Res Behav Manag. 2019;12:991–1002.
45. Edelstein M, Brang D, Rouw R, Ramachandran V. Misophonia: physiological investigations and case descriptions. Front Hum Neurosci. 2013;7:296.
46. Jastreboff M, Jastreboff P. Decreased sound tolerance and tinnitus retraining therapy (TRT). Aust N Z J Audiol. 2002;24:74–84.
47. Potgieter I, MacDonald C, Partridge L, Cima R, Sheldrake J, Hoare DJ. Misophonia: a scoping review of research. J Clin Psychol. 2019;75(7):1203–18.
48. Jastreboff PJ, Jastreboff MM. Treatments for decreased sound tolerance (Hyperacusis and Misophonia). Semin Hear. 2014;35(02):105–20.
49. Jaswal SM, De Bleser AKF, Handy TC. Misokinesia is a sensitivity to seeing others fidget that is prevalent in the general population. Sci Rep. 2021;11(1):17204.
50. Schroder A, van Diepen R, Mazaheri A, Petropoulos-Petalas D, Soto de Amesti V, Vulink N, et al. Diminished n1 auditory evoked potentials to oddball stimuli in misophonia patients. Front. Behav Neurosci. 2014;8:123.
51. Kumar S, Tansley-Hancock O, Sedley W, Winston JS, Callaghan MF, Allen M, et al. The brain basis for Misophonia. Curr Biol. 2017;27(4):527–33.
52. Brout JJ, Edelstein M, Erfanian M, Mannino M, Miller LJ, Rouw R, et al. Investigating misophonia: a review of the empirical literature, clinical implications, and a research. Agenda. 2018;12:36.
53. Naylor J, Caimino C, Scutt P, Hoare DJ, Baguley DM. The prevalence and severity of misophonia in a UK undergraduate medical student population and validation of the Amsterdam Misophonia scale. Psychiatry Q. 2021;92(2):609–19.
54. Zhou X, Wu MS, Storch EA. Misophonia symptoms among Chinese university students: incidence, associated impairment, and clinical correlates. J Obsessive-Compuls Relat Disord. 2017;14:7–12.
55. Siepsiak M, Sobczak AM, Bohaterewicz B, Cichocki Ł, Dragan WŁ. Prevalence of misophonia and correlates of its symptoms among inpatients with depression. Int J Environ Res Public Health. 2020;17(15):5464.
56. Siepsiak M, Sliwerski A, Lukasz Dragan W. Development and psychometric properties of MisoQuest-A new self-report questionnaire for misophonia. Int J Environ Res Public Health. 2020;17(5):1797.
57. Wu MS, Lewin AB, Murphy TK, Storch EA. Misophonia: incidence, phenomenology, and clinical correlates in an undergraduate student sample. J Clin Psychol. 2014;70(10):994–1007.
58. Schroder A, Vulink N, Denys D. Misophonia: diagnostic criteria for a new psychiatric disorder. PLoS One. 2013;8(1):e54706.
59. Enzler F, Loriot C, Fournier P, Noreña AJ. A psychoacoustic test for misophonia assessment. Sci Rep. 2021;11(1):11044.
60. Rouw R, Erfanian M. A large-scale study of Misophonia. J Clin Psychol. 2018;74(3):453–79.
61. Schröder AE, Vulink NC, van Loon AJ, Denys DA. Cognitive behavioral therapy is effective in misophonia: an open trial. J Affect Disord. 2017;217:289–94.
62. Schaaf H, Klofat B, Hesse G. Hyperacusis, phonophobia, and recruitment. Abnormal deviations of hearing associated with hypersensitivity to sound. HNO. 2003;51(12):1005–11.
63. Kalita J, Misra UK, Bansal R. Phonophobia and brainstem excitability in migraine. Eur J Neurosci. 2021;53(6):1988–97.
64. Sharpless BA. Exploding head syndrome. Sleep Med Rev. 2014;18(6):489–93.
65. Pearce JM. Exploding head syndrome. Lancet (London, England). 1988;2(8605):270–1.

66. Armstrong-Jones R. Snapping of the brain. Lancet. 1920;196(5066):720.
67. Campbell SM, Roland MO. Why do people consult the doctor? Fam Pract. 1996;13(1):75–83.
68. Frese A, Summ O, Evers S. Exploding head syndrome: six new cases and review of the literature. Cephalalgia. 2014;34(10):823–7.
69. Sachs C, Svanborg E. The exploding head syndrome: polysomnographic recordings and therapeutic suggestions. Sleep. 1991;14(3):263–6.
70. Evans RW, Pearce JM. Exploding head syndrome. Headache. 2001;41(6):602–3.
71. Feketeova E, Buskova J, Skorvanek M, Mudra J, Gdovinova Z. Exploding head syndrome--a rare parasomnia or a dissociative episode? Sleep Med. 2014;15(6):728–30.
72. Parker WAE, Parker VL, Parker G, Parker AJ. Acoustic shock: an update review. J Laryngol Otol. 2020:1–6.
73. Milhinch JC. Acoustic shock injury: real or imaginary? 2002. Available from: https://www.audiologyonline.com/articles/acoustic-shock-injury-real-or-1172
74. Baguley DM, Cope TE, McFerran DJ. Functional auditory disorders. Handb Clin Neurol. 2016;139:367–78.
75. Westcott M. Acoustic shock injury (ASI). Acta Otolaryngol Suppl. 2006;556:54–8.
76. Hooper RE. Acoustic shock controversies. J Laryngol Otol. 2014;128(Suppl 2):S2–9.
77. Londero A, Charpentier N, Ponsot D, Fournier P, Pezard L, Noreña AJ. A case of acoustic shock with post-trauma trigeminal-autonomic activation. Front Neurol. 2017;8:420.
78. Noreña AJ, Fournier P, Londero A, Ponsot D, Charpentier N. An integrative model accounting for the symptom cluster triggered after an acoustic shock. Trends Hear. 2018;22:2331216518801725.
79. Merchant SN, Nadol JB, Schuknecht HF. Schuknecht's pathology of the ear. Shelton, CT: People's Medical Pub. House-USA; 2010.
80. Papesh MA, Theodoroff SM, Gallun FJ. Traumatic brain injury injury and auditory processing. In: Fagelson M, Baguley DM, editors. Hyperacusis and disorders of sound intolerance. San Diego: Plural Publishers; 2018. p. 149–66.
81. Centers for Disease Control and Prevention. Report to congress on traumatic brain injury in the united states: epidemiology and rehabilitation. Atlanta, GA: National Center for Injury Prevention and Control; Division of Unintentional Injury Prevention; 2015.
82. Agimi Y, Earyes L, Deressa T, Stout K. Estimating repeat traumatic brain injury in the U.S. military, 2015–2017. Mil Med. 2021;187:e360.
83. Dikmen S, Machamer J, Fann JR, Temkin NR. Rates of symptom reporting following traumatic brain injury. J Int Neuropsychol Soc. 2010;16(3):401–11.
84. Theodoroff SM, Reavis KM, Griest SE, Carlson KF, Hammill TL, Henry JA. Decreased sound tolerance associated with blast exposure. Sci Rep. 2019;9(1):10204.
85. Carson A, Lehn A. Epidemiology. In: Hallet M, Stone J, Carson A, editors. Functional neurologic disorders. 139: handbook of clinical neurology; 2016. p. 47–60.
86. Stone J, Carson A, Duncan R, Roberts R, Warlow C, Hibberd C, et al. Who is referred to neurology clinics?—the diagnoses made in 3781 new patients. Clin Neurol Neurosurg. 2010;112(9):747–51.
87. Baguley DM. Functional audiogenic seizure. In: Fagelson M, Kimball SH, editors. Tinnitus and hyperacusis casebook. New York: Thieme Medical Publishers; 2021.

Epidemiology of Tinnitus: Frequency of the Condition

4

Carlotta M. Jarach, Alessandra Lugo, Marco Scala, Christopher R. Cederroth, Werner J. D. Garavello, Winfried Schlee, Berthold Langguth, and Silvano Gallus

Abstract

We conducted an umbrella review of the scientific literature followed by a systematic review to comprehensively collect existing evidence on global prevalence from national or regional representative samples of tinnitus. The present chapter shows selected results from a comprehensive recently published systematic review and meta-analysis (Jarach et al., 2022; *JAMA Neurol.* 2022;79(9):888–900).

Out of 767 publications retrieved in November 2021, we identified 113 eligible publications and extracted prevalence estimates from 89 articles included in the meta-analyses. We present here results from 81 articles with available information on any or severe tinnitus. Overall, prevalence of any tinnitus was 14.4% in adults and 13.6% in children; prevalence of severe tinnitus was 2.3% in adults and 2.7% in children.

Prevalence estimates did not significantly differ by sex, while tinnitus prevalence increased with increasing age: any tinnitus was reported by 9.7% of young adults, 13.7% of middle-aged adults, and 23.6% of older adults. Corresponding estimates for severe tinnitus were 0.4% in young adults, 2.7% in middle aged, and 6.9% among older adults, respectively.

Our results indicate that globally tinnitus affects more than 740 million people and is felt as a major problem by more than 120 million subjects, mostly aged 65 years or more.

C. M. Jarach · A. Lugo · M. Scala · S. Gallus (✉)
Istituto di Ricerche Farmacologiche Mario Negri IRCCS, Department of Environmental Health Sciences, Milan, Italy
e-mail: silvano.gallus@marionegri.it

C. R. Cederroth
Laboratory of Experimental Audiology, Department of Physiology and Pharmacology, Karolinska Institutet, Stockholm, Sweden

National Institute for Health Research Nottingham Biomedical Research Centre, Nottingham University Hospitals National Health Service Trust, Nottingham, UK

Division of Clinical Neuroscience, Hearing Sciences, School of Medicine, University of Nottingham, Nottingham, UK

W. J. D. Garavello
School of Medicine and Surgery, University of Milan-Bicocca, Department of Otorhinolaryngology, Milan, Italy

W. Schlee
Department of Psychiatry and Psychotherapy, Interdisciplinary Tinnitus Clinic, University of Regensburg, Regensburg, Germany

B. Langguth
Klinik und Poliklinik für Psychiatrie, Psychosomatik und Psychotherapie, Universität Regensburg Bezirksklinikum, Regensburg, Germany

W. Schlee et al. (eds.), *Textbook of Tinnitus*, https://doi.org/10.1007/978-3-031-35647-6_4

Graphical Abstract

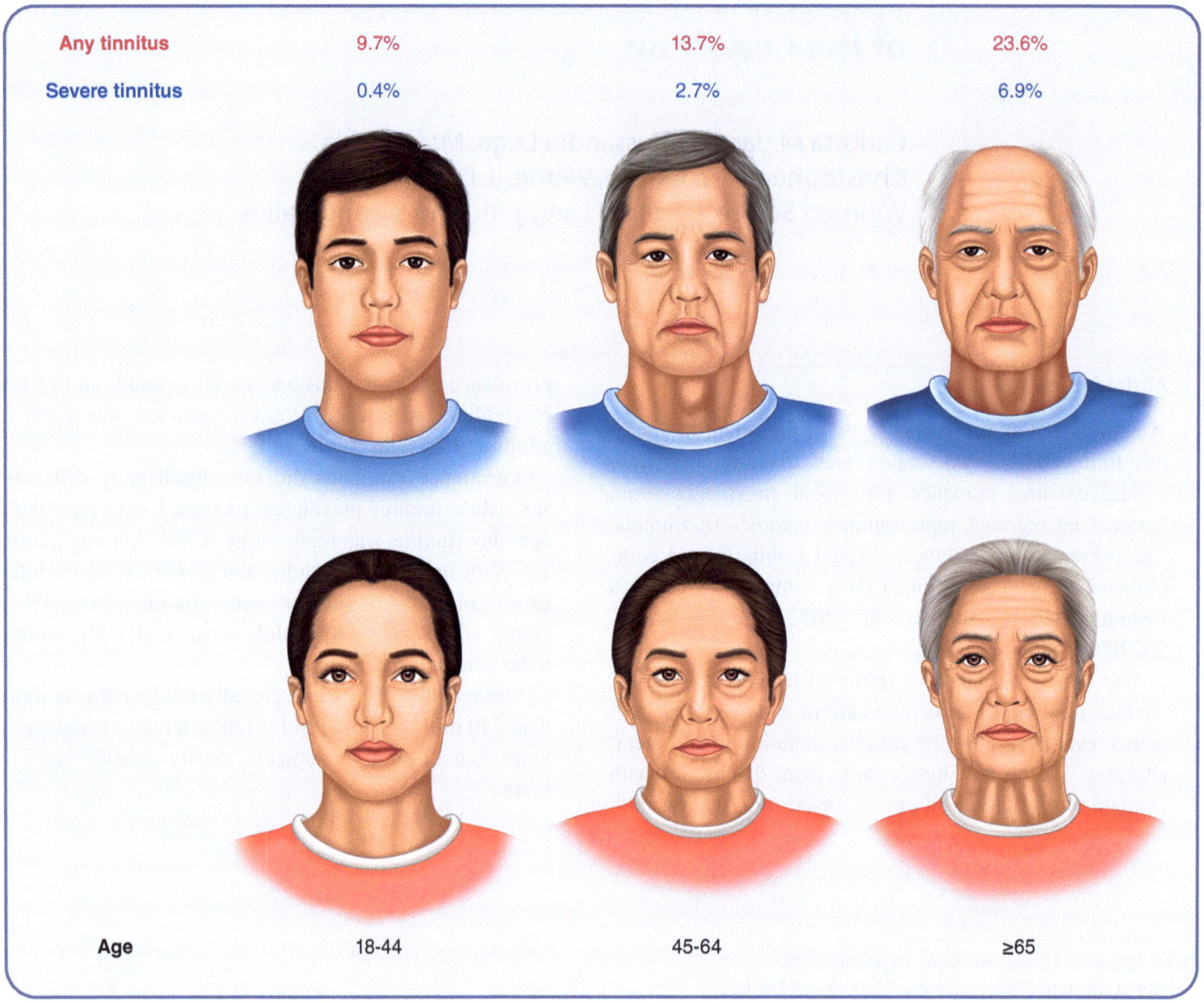

Highlights

- This chapter is based on a comprehensive systematic review of over a 100 epidemiological studies on tinnitus published in JAMA Neurology;
- Based on this review 14.4% of the adult population report tinnitus, with 2.3% of the adult population suffering from severe tinnitus;
- Pooled tinnitus prevalence in children was 13.6% with high variations depending on the question used to assess the symptom;
- Tinnitus prevalence is similar among sexes and increases with increasing age.

Introduction

Available data on the frequency (i.e., prevalence and incidence) of tinnitus in the general population are highly variable [1]. The reasons behind this variability are to be found not only in tinnitus multifactorial etiology, its associated disorders, and the various characteristics, but also in the subjective nature of tinnitus and the lack of diagnostic standards [2, 3]. While multiple studies have shown an increase in tinnitus prevalence and its severity as a function of age, no clear consensus exists concerning the relationship with sex [4].

The few longitudinal studies on tinnitus make it difficult to estimate the incidence of this symptom. Moreover, the prevalence of tinnitus, which is estimated as either point prevalence, period prevalence, or lifetime prevalence [4], ranges widely [1]. A systematic review which tried to identify and collect data about the global prevalence of tinnitus was published in 2016 by McCormack and colleagues [1]. According to the authors, due to the diversity of available data, it was not possible to perform a meta-analysis, nor was it possible to compare prevalence rates across studies. Location bias, inconsistency in the definition used, and reporting by different age bands were mainly responsible for such impossibility [1].

As the literature on tinnitus has grown substantially in the last few years, we decided to provide an update of the evidence, which also would consider pediatric tinnitus [5], which we published elsewhere [6]. This chapter will provide the main results on any and severe tinnitus estimates, but we invite to consult our publication for more details, especially regarding incidence estimates.

Methods

The present systematic review on prevalence of tinnitus is based on a systematic review of meta-analyses, pooled analyses, and systematic reviews (umbrella review) providing data complemented by a traditional review of all original articles on prevalence of tinnitus.

We conducted an umbrella review to systematically collect existing evidence on the prevalence of tinnitus. For this review, the Preferred Reporting Items for Systematic review and Meta-Analyses (PRISMA) guidelines [7] were followed. The review is based on literature research in PubMed and Embase from November 2021. Details can be seen elsewhere [6].

Pooled prevalence of any tinnitus and severe tinnitus was estimated, for children and adults, and separately by tinnitus definition (see [6]). For any tinnitus (AT), we identified six possible classes of definitions (A1–A6), while for severe tinnitus (ST) five possible classes (S1-S5).

We used forest plots to picture outcomes. We quantified the heterogeneity using the I^2 statistic, which expresses the percentage of the total observed variability due to heterogeneity (0–40%: little heterogeneity; 30–60%: moderate heterogeneity; 50–90%: substantial heterogeneity; 75–100%: considerable heterogeneity, according to the Cochrane Collaboration). I^2 can be calculated from Cochran's Q according to the formula: I^2 = 100% X (Cochran's Q – degrees of freedom). All statistical analyses will be performed using the software RStudio-software version 1.4.1717.

Results

Details on country, age group, and tinnitus definition of the 81 eligible articles [2, 8–87] on any and severe tinnitus included in meta-analyses are summarized in Jarach et al. [6].

Prevalence of Any Tinnitus in Adults

The pooled prevalence estimate of any tinnitus in adults was 14.4% (95% CI 12.6–16.5; 55 studies; I^2: 100%). Among all studies, the estimates ranged from 4.1% (95% CI 3.7–4.4) to 37.2% (95% CI 34.6–39.9). Prevalence of any tinnitus did not differ according to tinnitus classes of definitions (p-value among strata 0.130): the prevalence of those who were asked "have you experienced tinnitus?" (A1) was 17.5% (95% CI 14.0–21.8; 12 studies; I^2: 100%), that for those who were asked "for more than 5 minutes?" (A2) was 13.7% (95% CI 10.7–17.4; 9 studies; I^2: 100%), for "have you experienced tinnitus during the last months?" (A3) was 14.2% (95% CI 10.0–19.8; 7 studies; I^2: 100%), for "during the last months, have you experienced tinnitus which lasts for more than 5 minutes?" (A4) was 16.0 (95% CI 13.1–19.4; 18 studies; I^2: 99%), for those assessing tinnitus through a specific scale (A5) was 9.3% (95% CI 3.2–24.1; 3 studies; I^2: 100%), and for those who were asked other tinnitus definitions (A6) was 9.6% (95% CI 6.3–14.3; 6 studies; I^2: 100%).

Prevalence of Any Tinnitus in Children

The pooled prevalence estimate of any tinnitus in children was 13.6% (95% CI 8.5–21.0; 27 studies; I^2: 100%). Among all studies, this estimate ranged from 0.7% (95% CI 0.6–0.8) to 66.9% (95% CI 62.6–71.0). Prevalence of any tinnitus in children was heterogeneous in strata of tinnitus definition classes (*p*-value among strata 0.013): where the word "tinnitus" was not present in the question (AN) the prevalence was 20.4% (95% CI 14.4–28.0; 18 studies; I^2: 99%), and for those where it was present (AT) it was 5.6% (95% CI 2.0–14.8; 9 studies; I^2: 100%).

Tinnitus Prevalence According to Age Groups

Pooled prevalence estimate of any tinnitus was 9.7% (95% CI 7.4–12.5; 22 studies; I^2: 100%) in young adults, 13.7% (95% CI 11.0–17.0; 30 studies; I^2: 100%) in middle aged adults, and 23.6% (95% CI 19.4–28.5; 31 studies; I^2: 99%) among the older adults.

Tinnitus Prevalence According to Sex and World Regions

The pooled prevalent estimate for any tinnitus in adults was 14.1% (95% CI 11.6–17.0; 31 studies; I^2: 100%) in men and 13.1% (95% CI 10.5–16.2; 30 studies; I^2: 100%) in women (*p*-value among strata 0.620). Any tinnitus in adults was significantly different among continents ranging from 5.2% (95% CI 4.7–5.7; 1 study) in Africa to 21.9% (95% CI 20.2–23.8; 1 study) in South America (*p*-value among strata <0.001). Presence of tinnitus was not differing among Gross Domestic Product (GDP) per capita tertiles (*p*-value among strata 0.750), but it differed according to latitude (*p*-value among strata 0.025). Figures 4.1, 4.2, and 4.3 show the estimates according to the different continent, latitude, and GDP.

Prevalence of Severe Tinnitus in Adults

The pooled prevalence estimate of severe tinnitus in adults was 2.3% (95% CI 1.7–3.4; 34 studies; I^2: 99%). Among all studies, the estimates ranged from 0.5% (95% CI 0.3–0.7) to 12.6% (95% CI 11.1–14.1). Severity in adults was different according to tinnitus definition classes (*p*-value among strata <0.001): for those who were asked "are you bothered by your tinnitus?" (S1) the pooled prevalence of severe tinnitus was 6.4% (95% CI 4.2–9.6; 7 studies; I^2: 100%), for "how much are you bothered by your tinnitus?" (S2) was 1.3% (95% CI 1.1–1.7; 21 studies; I^2: 93%), for "does your tinnitus interfere with sleep and concentration?" (S3) (one study only) identified a prevalence of 3.0% (95% CI 2.5–3.6), for tinnitus severity assessed through a validated scale (S4) was 2.9% (95% CI 0.9–9.2; 3 studies; I^2: 99%), and for other tinnitus severity definitions (S5) was 7.3% (95% CI 5.4–9.9; 2 studies; I^2: 100%).

Prevalence of Severe Tinnitus in Different Age Groups and According to Sex and World Regions

The pooled prevalence estimate of severe tinnitus in children was 2.7% (95% CI 0.8–8.4; 10 studies; I^2: 99%). Among adults, it was 0.4% (95% CI: 0.3–0.7; 2 studies) for young adults, 2.7% (95% CI: 1.6–4.7; 3 studies; I^2: 97%) for middle-aged adults, and 6.9% (95% CI: 2.6–17.4; 4 studies; I^2: 99%) for the older adults. It was 2.3% (95% CI 1.1–4.6; 8 studies; I^2: 100%) in men and 2.7% (95% CI 1.7–4.3; 7 studies; I^2: 99%) in women (*p*-value among strata 0.660). Tinnitus severity in adults was significantly different among continents ranging from 0.8% (95% CI 0.6–1.0; 1 study) in Africa to 12.6% (95% CI 11.1–14.1; 1 study) in South America (*p*-value among strata <0.001). The prevalence of severe tinnitus did not differ significantly by GDP per capita tertiles, nor by latitude. Figures 4.4, 4.5, and 4.6 show the pooled estimates.

Any tinnitus per continent	#	s. size	%	[95% CI]
Africa				
Khedr, 2010 (EG) [45]	439	8484	5.2	[4.7; 5.7]
Asia				
Fujii, 2011 (JP) [27]	2312	14423	16.0	[15.4; 16.6]
Jalessi, 2013 (IR) [42]	146	3194	4.6	[3.9; 5.4]
Kim, 2015 (KR) [47]	4234	20500	20.7	[20.1; 21.2]
Park, 2014b (KR) [70]	4950	25100	19.7	[19.2; 20.2]
Sugiura, 2008 (JP) [81]	743	2193	33.9	[31.9; 35.9]
Xu, 2011 (CN) [87]	918	6333	14.5	[13.6; 15.4]
Yang, 2018 (CN) [88]	387	3705	10.4	[9.5; 11.5]
Pooled estimate		**75448**	**15.2**	**[9.8; 22.9]**
Heterogeneity: $I^2 = 99\%$, $p < 0.01$				
Europe				
Axelsson, 1989 (SE) [10]	337	2378	14.2	[12.8; 15.6]
Baigi, 2011 (SE) [11]	2024	12166	16.6	[16.0; 17.3]
Bernhardt, 2011 (DE) [12]	393	4308	9.1	[8.3; 10.0]
Biswas, 2022 (BG) [14]	285	1007	28.3	[25.5; 31.2]
Biswas, 2022 (DE) [14]	108	911	11.9	[9.8; 14.1]
Biswas, 2022 (ES) [14]	155	1000	15.5	[13.3; 17.9]
Biswas, 2022 (FR) [14]	137	971	14.1	[12.0; 16.5]
Biswas, 2022 (GR) [14]	152	945	16.1	[13.8; 18.6]
Biswas, 2022 (IE) [14]	82	941	8.7	[7.0; 10.7]
Biswas, 2022 (IT) [14]	134	979	13.7	[11.6; 16.0]
Biswas, 2022 (LV) [14]	194	957	20.3	[17.8; 23.0]
Biswas, 2022 (PL) [14]	126	762	16.5	[14.0; 19.4]
Biswas, 2022 (PT) [14]	155	958	16.2	[13.9; 18.7]
Biswas, 2022 (RO) [14]	208	984	21.1	[18.6; 23.8]
Biswas, 2022 (UK) [14]	154	1007	15.3	[13.1; 17.7]
Coles, 1984 (UK) [19]	888	8069	11.0	[10.3; 11.7]
Coles, 1984b (UK) [19]	810	7645	10.6	[9.9; 11.3]
Davis, 1989, (UK) [21]	3533	35330	10.0	[9.7; 10.3]
Davis, 1989b, (UK) [21]	765	10778	7.1	[6.6; 7.6]
Dorner, 2010, (AT) [23]	74	686	10.8	[8.6; 13.4]
Engdahl, 2012, (NO) [24]	7049	49948	14.1	[13.8; 14.4]
Gallus, 2015 (IT) [28]	183	2952	6.2	[5.4; 7.1]
Hannaford, 2005 (UK) [33]	2684	15140	17.7	[17.1; 18.3]
Hasson, 2010 (SE) [35]	2989	11213	26.7	[25.8; 27.5]
Herr, 2016 (DE) [36]	207	1489	13.9	[12.2; 15.8]
Johansson, 2003 (SE) [43]	76	575	13.2	[10.6; 16.3]
Krog, 2010 (NO) [48]	9579	51574	18.6	[18.2; 18.9]
Kuttila, 2005 (FI) [49]	259	1721	15.0	[13.4; 16.8]
Lugo, 2019 (SE) [53]	16066	71542	22.5	[22.2; 22.8]
Oosterloo, 2021 (NL) [67]	1304	6098	21.4	[20.4; 22.4]
Palmer, 2002 (UK) [68]	527	12907	4.1	[3.7; 4.4]
Parving, 1993 (DK) [71]	576	3387	17.0	[15.8; 18.3]
Quaranta, 1996 (IT) [73]	315	2170	14.5	[13.1; 16.1]
Rademaker, 2021 (NL) [74]	254	932	27.3	[24.4; 30.2]
Schubert, 2021 (NL) [78]	39625	124651	31.8	[31.5; 32.0]
Pooled estimate		**449081**	**14.7**	**[12.7; 16.9]**
Heterogeneity: $I^2 = 100\%$, $p = 0$				
North America				
Choi, 2020 (US) [17]	605	3669	16.5	[15.3; 17.7]
Cooper, 1994 (US) [20]	945	6342	14.9	[14.0; 15.8]
House, 2018 (US) [40]	388	1314	29.5	[27.1; 32.1]
Masterson, 2016 (US) [56]	2243	23393	9.6	[9.2; 10.0]
Nondahl, 2002 (US) [63]	308	3737	8.2	[7.4; 9.2]
Nondahl, 2010 (US) [64]	308	3737	8.2	[7.4; 9.2]
Nondahl, 2011 (US) [65]	345	3267	10.6	[9.5; 11.7]
Shargorodsky, 2010 (US) [79]	3587	14178	25.3	[24.6; 26.0]
Weiss, 1972 (US) [83]	622	6672	9.3	[8.6; 10.0]
Pooled estimate		**66309**	**13.4**	**[9.8; 18.1]**
Heterogeneity: $I^2 = 100\%$, $p = 0$				
Oceania				
Gopinath, 2010 (AU) [32]	481	1292	37.2	[34.6; 39.9]
Wu, 2015 (NZ) [86]	4771	79976	6.0	[5.8; 6.1]
Pooled estimate		**81268**	**16.2**	**[4.0; 47.7]**
Heterogeneity: $I^2 = 100\%$, $p < 0.01$				
South America				
Oiticica, 2015 (BR) [66]	430	1960	21.9	[20.1; 23.8]
Pooled estimate		**682550**	**14.4**	**[12.6; 16.5]**
Heterogeneity: $I^2 = 100\%$, $p = 0$				
Test for subgroup differences: $\chi^2_5 = 523.96$, df = 5 ($p < 0.01$)				

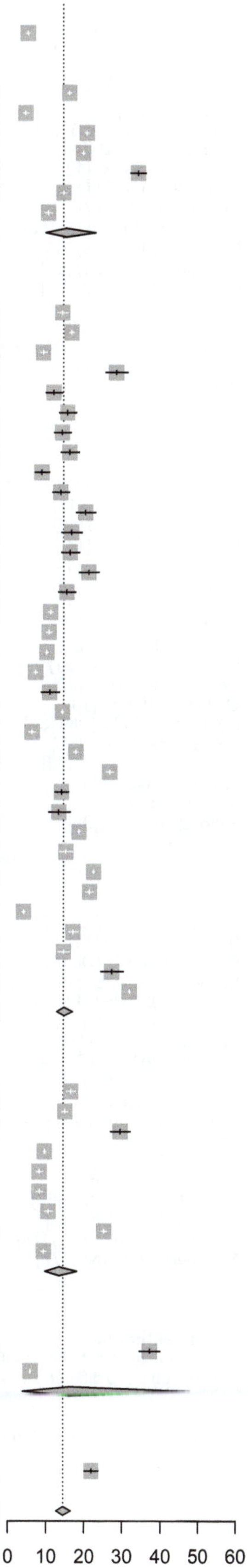

Fig. 4.1 Forest plot of any tinnitus prevalence in adults, by continent. CI, confidence interval. In brackets, country codes follow ISO 3166-1 alpha-2 codes

Any tinnitus per equator tert	#	s. size	%	[95% CI]
40°				
Biswas, 2022 (GR) [14]	152	945	16.1	[13.8; 18.6]
Biswas, 2022 (PT) [14]	155	958	16.2	[13.9; 18.7]
Choi, 2020 (US) [17]	605	3669	16.5	[15.3; 17.7]
Cooper, 1994 (US) [20]	945	6342	14.9	[14.0; 15.8]
Fujii, 2011 (JP) [27]	2312	14423	16.0	[15.4; 16.6]
Gopinath, 2010 (AU) [32]	481	1292	37.2	[34.6; 39.9]
House, 2018 (US) [40]	388	1314	29.5	[27.1; 32.1]
Jalessi, 2013 (IR) [42]	146	3194	4.6	[3.9; 5.4]
Khedr, 2010 (EG) [45]	439	8484	5.2	[4.7; 5.7]
Kim, 2015 (KR) [47]	4234	20500	20.7	[20.1; 21.2]
Masterson, 2016 (US) [56]	2243	23393	9.6	[9.2; 10.0]
Nondahl, 2002 (US) [63]	308	3737	8.2	[7.4; 9.2]
Nondahl, 2010 (US) [64]	308	3737	8.2	[7.4; 9.2]
Nondahl, 2011 (US) [65]	345	3267	10.6	[9.5; 11.7]
Oiticica, 2015 (BR) [66]	430	1960	21.9	[20.1; 23.8]
Park, 2014b (KR) [70]	4950	25100	19.7	[19.2; 20.2]
Shargorodsky, 2010 (US) [79]	3587	14178	25.3	[24.6; 26.0]
Sugiura, 2008 (JP) [81]	743	2193	33.9	[31.9; 35.9]
Weiss, 1972 (US) [83]	622	6672	9.3	[8.6; 10.0]
Pooled estimate		**145358**	**15.0**	**[11.5; 19.4]**
Heterogeneity: I^2 = 100%, p = 0				
40°−51°				
Biswas, 2022 (BG) [14]	285	1007	28.3	[25.5; 31.2]
Biswas, 2022 (ES) [14]	155	1000	15.5	[13.3; 17.9]
Biswas, 2022 (FR) [14]	137	971	14.1	[12.0; 16.5]
Biswas, 2022 (IT) [14]	134	979	13.7	[11.6; 16.0]
Biswas, 2022 (RO) [14]	208	984	21.1	[18.6; 23.8]
Biswas, 2022 (UK) [14]	154	1007	15.3	[13.1; 17.7]
Coles, 1984 (UK) [19]	888	8069	11.0	[10.3; 11.7]
Coles, 1984b (UK) [19]	810	7645	10.6	[9.9; 11.3]
Davis, 1989, (UK) [21]	3533	35330	10.0	[9.7; 10.3]
Davis, 1989b, (UK) [21]	765	10778	7.1	[6.6; 7.6]
Dorner, 2010, (AT) [23]	74	686	10.8	[8.6; 13.4]
Gallus, 2015 (IT) [28]	183	2952	6.2	[5.4; 7.1]
Hannaford, 2005 (UK) [33]	2684	15140	17.7	[17.1; 18.3]
Palmer, 2002 (UK) [68]	527	12907	4.1	[3.7; 4.4]
Quaranta, 1996 (IT) [73]	315	2170	14.5	[13.1; 16.1]
Wu, 2015 (NZ) [86]	4771	79976	6.0	[5.8; 6.1]
Xu, 2011 (CN) [87]	918	6333	14.5	[13.6; 15.4]
Yang, 2018 (CN) [88]	387	3705	10.4	[9.5; 11.5]
Pooled estimate		**191639**	**11.7**	**[9.4; 14.5]**
Heterogeneity: I^2 = 100%, p = 0				
=52°				
Axelsson, 1989 (SE) [10]	337	2378	14.2	[12.8; 15.6]
Baigi, 2011 (SE) [11]	2024	12166	16.6	[16.0; 17.3]
Bernhardt, 2011 (DE) [12]	393	4308	9.1	[8.3; 10.0]
Biswas, 2022 (DE) [14]	108	911	11.9	[9.8; 14.1]
Biswas, 2022 (IE) [14]	82	941	8.7	[7.0; 10.7]
Biswas, 2022 (LV) [14]	194	957	20.3	[17.8; 23.0]
Biswas, 2022 (PL) [14]	126	762	16.5	[14.0; 19.4]
Engdahl, 2012, (NO) [24]	7049	49948	14.1	[13.8; 14.4]
Hasson, 2010 (SE) [35]	2989	11213	26.7	[25.8; 27.5]
Herr, 2016 (DE) [36]	207	1489	13.9	[12.2; 15.8]
Johansson, 2003 (SE) [43]	76	575	13.2	[10.6; 16.3]
Krog, 2010 (NO) [48]	9579	51574	18.6	[18.2; 18.9]
Kuttila, 2005 (FI) [49]	259	1721	15.0	[13.4; 16.8]
Lugo, 2019 (SE) [53]	16066	71542	22.5	[22.2; 22.8]
Oosterloo, 2021 (NL) [67]	1304	6098	21.4	[20.4; 22.4]
Parving, 1993 (DK) [71]	576	3387	17.0	[15.8; 18.3]
Rademaker, 2021 (NL) [74]	254	932	27.3	[24.4; 30.2]
Schubert, 2021 (NL) [78]	39625	124651	31.8	[31.5; 32.0]
Pooled estimate		**345553**	**17.0**	**[14.4; 19.9]**
Heterogeneity: I^2 = 100%, p = 0				
Pooled estimate		**682550**	**14.4**	**[12.6; 16.5]**
Heterogeneity: I^2 = 100%, p = 0				
Test for subgroup differences: χ^2_2 = 7.32, df = 2 (p = 0.03)				

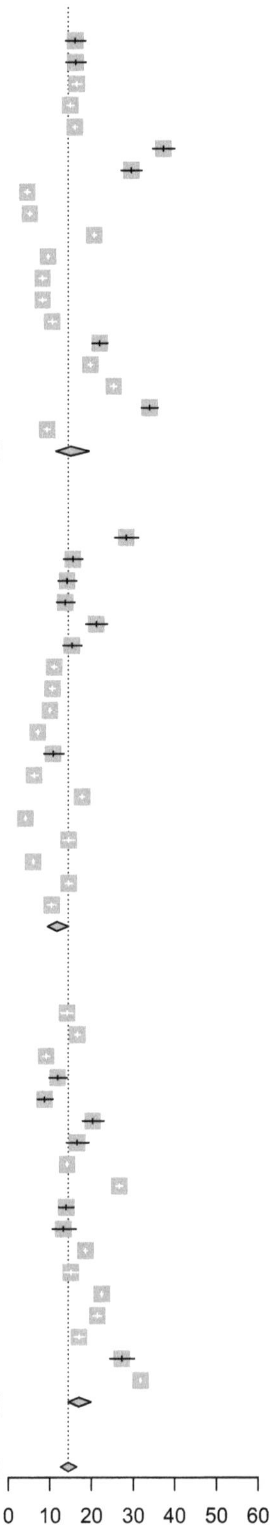

Fig. 4.2 Forest plot of any tinnitus prevalence in adults, by latitude. CI, confidence interval. In brackets, country codes follow ISO 3166-1 alpha-2 codes

Any tinnitus per GDP tert	#	s. size	%	[95% CI]
<4100$				
Biswas, 2022 (BG) [14]	285	1007	28.3	[25.5; 31.2]
Biswas, 2022 (ES) [14]	155	1000	15.5	[13.3; 17.9]
Biswas, 2022 (FR) [14]	137	971	14.1	[12.0; 16.5]
Biswas, 2022 (GR) [14]	152	945	16.1	[13.8; 18.6]
Biswas, 2022 (IT) [14]	134	979	13.7	[11.6; 16.0]
Biswas, 2022 (LV) [14]	194	957	20.3	[17.8; 23.0]
Biswas, 2022 (PL) [14]	126	762	16.5	[14.0; 19.4]
Biswas, 2022 (PT) [14]	155	958	16.2	[13.9; 18.7]
Biswas, 2022 (RO) [14]	208	984	21.1	[18.6; 23.8]
Gallus, 2015 (IT) [28]	183	2952	6.2	[5.4; 7.1]
Jalessi, 2013 (IR) [42]	146	3194	4.6	[3.9; 5.4]
Khedr, 2010 (EG) [45]	439	8484	5.2	[4.7; 5.7]
Kim, 2015 (KR) [47]	4234	20500	20.7	[20.1; 21.2]
Oiticica, 2015 (BR) [66]	430	1960	21.9	[20.1; 23.8]
Park, 2014b (KR) [70]	4950	25100	19.7	[19.2; 20.2]
Quaranta, 1996 (IT) [73]	315	2170	14.5	[13.1; 16.1]
Xu, 2011 (CN) [87]	918	6333	14.5	[13.6; 15.4]
Yang, 2018 (CN) [88]	387	3705	10.4	[9.5; 11.5]
Pooled estimate		**82961**	**14.3**	**[11.4; 17.7]**
Heterogeneity: $I^2 = 99\%$, $p = 0$				
4100–5200$				
Axelsson, 1989 (SE) [10]	337	2378	14.2	[12.8; 15.6]
Baigi, 2011 (SE) [11]	2024	12166	16.6	[16.0; 17.3]
Bernhardt, 2011 (DE) [12]	393	4308	9.1	[8.3; 10.0]
Biswas, 2022 (DE) [14]	108	911	11.9	[9.8; 14.1]
Biswas, 2022 (UK) [14]	154	1007	15.3	[13.1; 17.7]
Coles, 1984 (UK) [19]	888	8069	11.0	[10.3; 11.7]
Coles, 1984b (UK) [19]	810	7645	10.6	[9.9; 11.3]
Davis, 1989, (UK) [21]	3533	35330	10.0	[9.7; 10.3]
Davis, 1989b, (UK) [21]	765	10778	7.1	[6.6; 7.6]
Dorner, 2010, (AT) [23]	74	686	10.8	[8.6; 13.4]
Fujii, 2011 (JP) [27]	2312	14423	16.0	[15.4; 16.6]
Gopinath, 2010 (AU) [32]	481	1292	37.2	[34.6; 39.9]
Hannaford, 2005 (UK) [33]	2684	15140	17.7	[17.1; 18.3]
Hasson, 2010 (SE) [35]	2989	11213	26.7	[25.8; 27.5]
Herr, 2016 (DE) [36]	207	1489	13.9	[12.2; 15.8]
Johansson, 2003 (SE) [43]	76	575	13.2	[10.6; 16.3]
Kuttila, 2005 (FI) [49]	259	1721	15.0	[13.4; 16.8]
Lugo, 2019 (SE) [53]	16066	71542	22.5	[22.2; 22.8]
Palmer, 2002 (UK) [68]	527	12907	4.1	[3.7; 4.4]
Sugiura, 2008 (JP) [81]	743	2193	33.9	[31.9; 35.9]
Wu, 2015 (NZ) [86]	4771	79976	6.0	[5.8; 6.1]
Pooled estimate		**295749**	**13.8**	**[10.9; 17.2]**
Heterogeneity: $I^2 = 100\%$, $p = 0$				
>5200$				
Biswas, 2022 (IE) [14]	82	941	8.7	[7.0; 10.7]
Choi, 2020 (US) [17]	605	3669	16.5	[15.3; 17.7]
Cooper, 1994 (US) [20]	945	6342	14.9	[14.0; 15.8]
Engdahl, 2012, (NO) [24]	7049	49948	14.1	[13.8; 14.4]
House, 2018 (US) [40]	388	1314	29.5	[27.1; 32.1]
Krog, 2010 (NO) [48]	9579	51574	18.6	[18.2; 18.9]
Masterson, 2016 (US) [56]	2243	23393	9.6	[9.2; 10.0]
Nondahl, 2002 (US) [63]	308	3737	8.2	[7.4; 9.2]
Nondahl, 2010 (US) [64]	308	3737	8.2	[7.4; 9.2]
Nondahl, 2011 (US) [65]	345	3267	10.6	[9.5; 11.7]
Oosterloo, 2021 (NL) [67]	1304	6098	21.4	[20.4; 22.4]
Parving, 1993 (DK) [71]	576	3387	17.0	[15.8; 18.3]
Rademaker, 2021 (NL) [74]	254	932	27.3	[24.4; 30.2]
Schubert, 2021 (NL) [78]	39625	124651	31.8	[31.5; 32.0]
Shargorodsky, 2010 (US) [79]	3587	14178	25.3	[24.6; 26.0]
Weiss, 1972 (US) [83]	622	6672	9.3	[8.6; 10.0]
Pooled estimate		**303840**	**15.6**	**[12.3; 19.5]**
Heterogeneity: $I^2 = 100\%$, $p = 0$				
Pooled estimate		**682550**	**14.4**	**[12.6; 16.5]**

Heterogeneity: $I^2 = 100\%$, $p = 0$
Test for subgroup differences: $\chi^2_2 = 0.59$, df = 2 ($p = 0.75$)

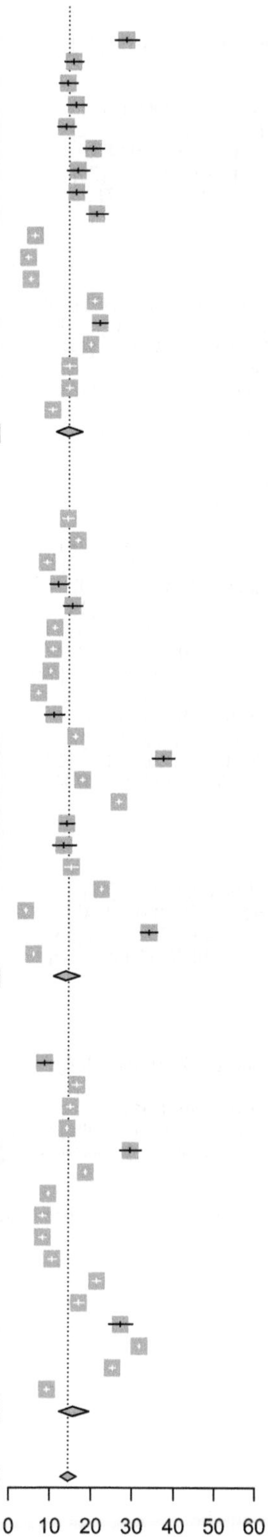

Fig. 4.3 Forest plot of any tinnitus prevalence in adults, by Gross Domestic Product (GDP). CI, confidence interval. In brackets, country codes follow ISO 3166-1 alpha-2 codes

Severe tinnitus per continent	#	s. size	%	[95% CI]
Africa				
Khedr, 2010 (EG) [45]	67	8484	0.8	[0.6; 1.0]
Asia				
Fujii, 2011 (JP) [27]	360	14423	2.5	[2.2; 2.8]
Jalessi, 2013 (IR) [42]	92	3207	2.9	[2.3; 3.5]
Kim, 2015 (KR) [47]	146	19290	0.8	[0.6; 0.9]
Park, 2014b (KR) [70]	1466	25100	5.8	[5.6; 6.1]
Xu, 2011 (CN) [87]	31	6333	0.5	[0.3; 0.7]
Pooled estimate		**68353**	**1.8**	**[0.8; 3.9]**
Heterogeneity: I^2 = 100%, p < 0.01				
Europe				
Axelsson, 1989 (SE) [10]	58	2378	2.4	[1.9; 3.1]
Biswas, 2022 (BG) [14]	20	1007	2.0	[1.2; 3.1]
Biswas, 2022 (DE) [14]	9	912	1.0	[0.5; 1.9]
Biswas, 2022 (ES) [14]	17	1000	1.7	[1.0; 2.7]
Biswas, 2022 (FR) [14]	10	971	1.0	[0.5; 1.9]
Biswas, 2022 (GR) [14]	18	945	1.9	[1.1; 3.0]
Biswas, 2022 (IE) [14]	6	941	0.6	[0.2; 1.4]
Biswas, 2022 (IT) [14]	8	979	0.8	[0.4; 1.6]
Biswas, 2022 (LV) [14]	13	957	1.4	[0.7; 2.3]
Biswas, 2022 (PL) [14]	8	761	1.1	[0.5; 2.1]
Biswas, 2022 (PT) [14]	14	958	1.5	[0.8; 2.4]
Biswas, 2022 (RO) [14]	41	984	4.2	[3.0; 5.6]
Biswas, 2022 (UK) [14]	9	1007	0.9	[0.4; 1.7]
Coles, 1984 (UK) [19]	654	8069	8.1	[7.5; 8.7]
Coles, 1984b (UK) [19]	665	7645	8.7	[8.1; 9.4]
Davis, 1989, (UK) [21]	565	35330	1.6	[1.5; 1.7]
Gallus, 2015 (IT) [28]	36	2952	1.2	[0.9; 1.7]
Hannaford, 2005 (UK) [33]	333	15140	2.2	[2.0; 2.4]
Hasson, 2010 (SE) [35]	943	11213	8.4	[7.9; 8.9]
Krog, 2010 (NO) [48]	4699	51574	9.1	[8.9; 9.4]
Lugo, 2019 (SE) [53]	1995	71542	2.8	[2.7; 2.9]
Oosterloo, 2021 (NL) [67]	160	6098	2.6	[2.2; 3.1]
Parving, 1993 (DK) [71]	102	3387	3.0	[2.5; 3.6]
Pooled estimate		**226750**	**2.2**	**[1.6; 3.1]**
Heterogeneity: I^2 = 99%, p = 0				
North America				
Choi, 2020 (US) [17]	40	3669	1.1	[0.8; 1.5]
House, 2018 (US) [40]	134	1314	10.2	[8.6; 12.0]
Nondahl, 2002 (US) [63]	285	3737	7.6	[6.8; 8.5]
Nondahl, 2011 (US) [65]	43	3267	1.3	[1.0; 1.8]
Pooled estimate		**11987**	**3.3**	**[1.2; 8.8]**
Heterogeneity: I^2 = 99%, p < 0.01				
South America				
Oiticica, 2015 (BR) [66]	246	1960	12.6	[11.1; 14.1]
Pooled estimate		**317534**	**2.3**	**[1.7; 3.1]**
Heterogeneity: I^2 = 99%, p = 0				
Test for subgroup differences: χ^2_4 = 476.55, df = 4 (p < 0.01)				

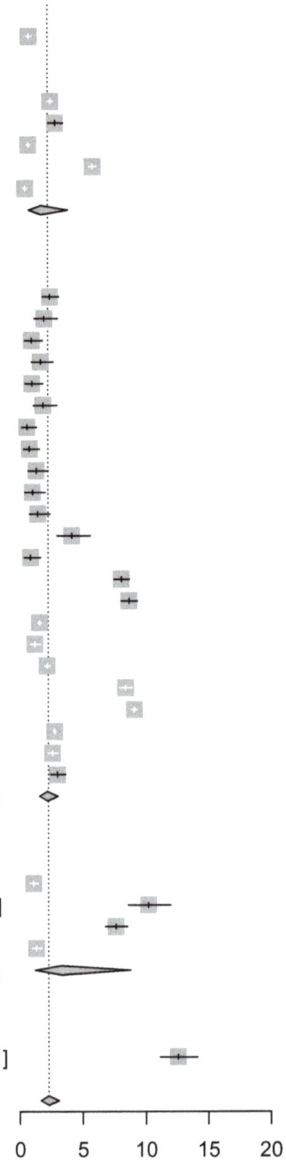

Fig. 4.4 Forest plot of severe tinnitus prevalence in adults, by continent. CI, confidence interval. In brackets, country codes follow ISO 3166-1 alpha-2 codes

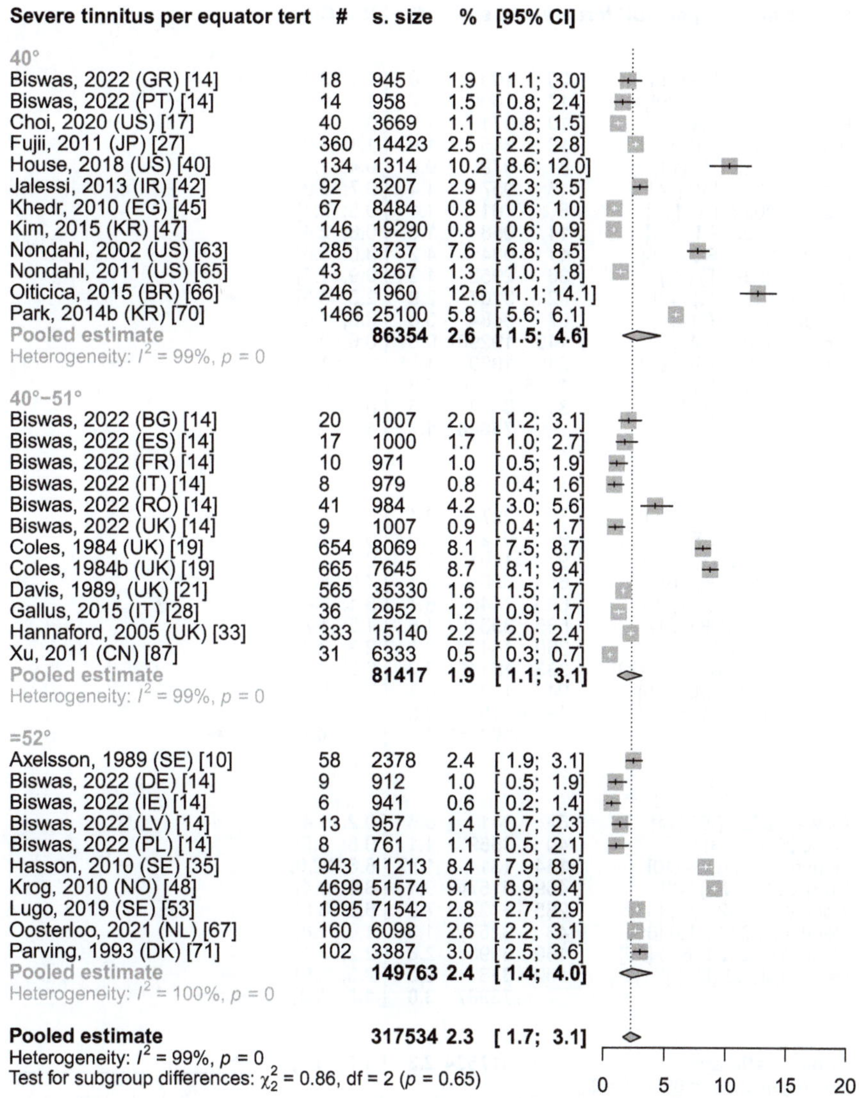

Fig. 4.5 Forest plot of severe tinnitus prevalence in adults, by latitude. CI, confidence interval. In brackets, country codes follow ISO 3166-1 alpha-2 codes

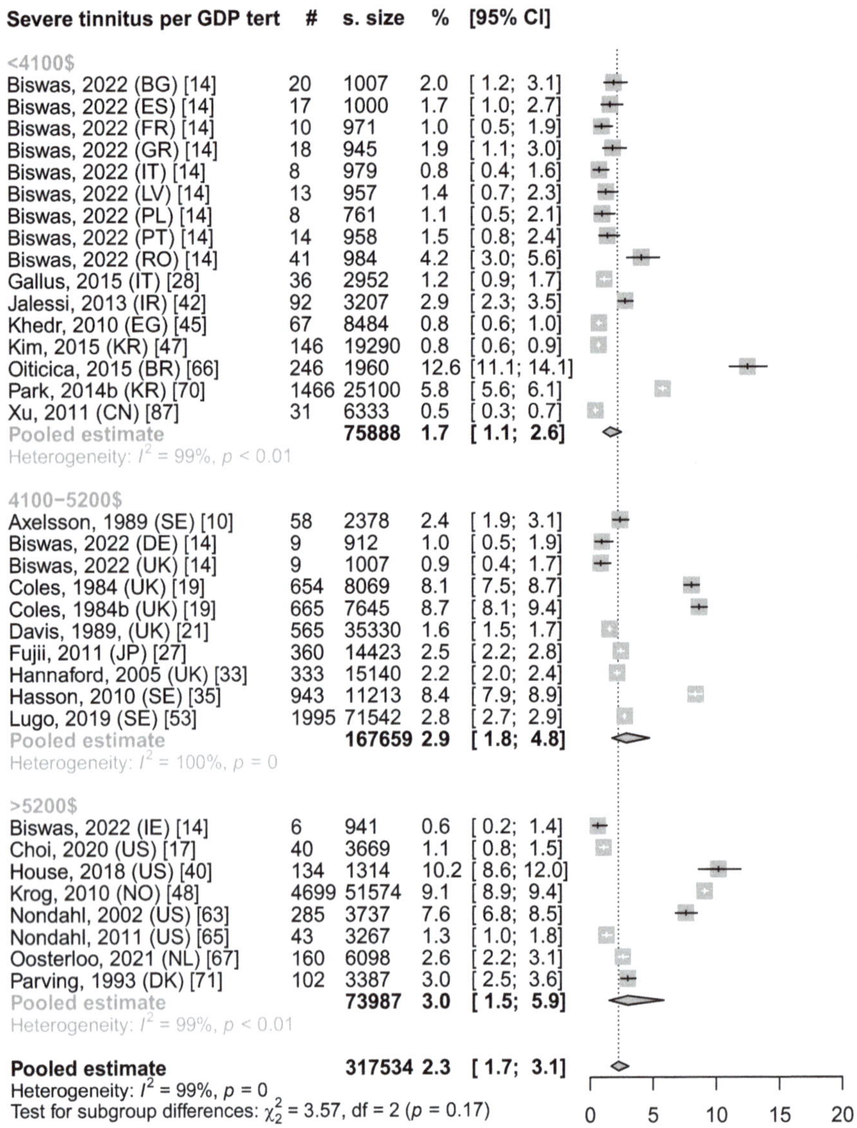

Fig. 4.6 Forest plot of severe tinnitus prevalence in adults, by Gross Domestic Product (GDP). CI, confidence interval. In brackets, country codes follow ISO 3166-1 alpha-2 codes

Conclusions

In this chapter we reported the main results of a systematic review on the prevalence of tinnitus worldwide that we published elsewhere [6], summarizing estimates from 81 original studies from 1972 to 2021. According to our estimates, about 15% of the adult population have tinnitus and approximately every sixth person with tinnitus (2% of the whole adult population) suffers from a severe form of tinnitus. Tinnitus prevalence is similar among sexes and increases with increasing age.

The review reveals a high variability of assessment methodologies across studies [1, 88, 89]. Therefore, the questions used for any tinnitus assessment were grouped in 6 different classes and for severe tinnitus in 5 different classes. Despite the substantial heterogeneity of estimates within any tinnitus definition classes, we did not find significant differences across classes. This suggests that not all the variability of the prevalence estimates is explained by the variability of the used definitions. At the same time, in our results we observed that children are more susceptible to the interpretation of the question addressed to assess tinnitus: a possible reason behind this lies in the fact that children are more frequently asked "do you hear a noise inside your head/ears?", without mentioning the name of the symptom. This leads us to agree with some researchers, who suggest that children are prone to report tinnitus to please the interviewers [90], a phenomenon which would explain the much higher estimates of any and particularly severe tinnitus prevalence in children rather than young adults. Furthermore, the prevalence estimates in children can also be influenced by a sampling bias. In all the studies with children, the parents have to agree that their children are interviewed, and it is possible that those parents who suffer from tinnitus themselves are more likely to allow a study participation of their children. Given the genetic heritability of tinnitus, this could inflate the prevalence estimates in children [91]. Nevertheless, in spite of the increasing number of research on the subject, tinnitus still remains an insufficient and unrecognized problem in the pediatric population [92] (see also Chap. 39).

In accordance with previous studies, prevalence of tinnitus increases with increasing age [2, 4, 41, 69]. In severe tinnitus this increase is even more pronounced. Whereas the prevalence of any tinnitus in the older adults is 2.5 times that of middle-aged adults, the prevalence of severe tinnitus is 20 times that of young adults.

Concerning the association between sex and tinnitus, the literature is not unanimous [2, 93]. In the current analysis, neither any nor severe tinnitus was related to the sex of the participants.

As addressed [4], scanty information is available on the differences among countries, and we were only partially able to fill the gap; in fact, Africa and South America are not well-represented. We found only 2 studies on any tinnitus prevalence and 2 studies on severe tinnitus prevalence from those two continents.

An association between socio-economic status and tinnitus has been theorized [34, 94]. However, although with all the limitations of an ecological analysis [95, 96], here we did not find a relationship between per-capita GDP and tinnitus prevalence.

It has been suggested that tinnitus may follow a seasonal pattern with worsening in the winter relative to the summer [97]. Thus, the hours of sun per day or temperatures might play a role for tinnitus severity or onset. Here we found that those countries having their main city at an intermediate level of latitude (40–51°) had the lowest prevalence of tinnitus. Future analytical studies should address this issue more in details.

Importantly, we included only studies based on samples representative of the general population, excluding ad hoc populations exposed to selected risk factors, such as veterans and musicians. In these two peculiar populations, the prevalence of tinnitus was reported with a point estimate of 31% [98] in veterans and 26% in musicians [99], thus much higher than in the general adult population.

Generalizing our estimates to the whole global population, more than 740 million people experience tinnitus, and over 120 million people worldwide suffer from a severe form of it. Such estimates give tinnitus the same order of magnitude of the global leading causes of years lived with disability, namely low back pain, migraine, and other hearing loss [100]. Health politicians should consider this impressive prevalence, playing a leading role in conveying funding, ultimately to boost research on tinnitus and hence improving the care and the lives of patients suffering from tinnitus.

Acknowledgements We are grateful to the support of Cavalier Savani, President of A. I. T. ONLUS Associazione Italiana Tinnitus.

Funding Unification of Treatments and Interventions for Tinnitus Patients—UNITI project, which has received funding from the European Union's Horizon 2020 Research and Innovation Programme, Grant Agreement Number 848261; Tinnitus Genetic and Environmental Risks—Tiger project, which has received funding from the European Union's Horizon 2020 Research and Innovation Programme, Grant Agreement Number GNP-182.

References

1. McCormack A, Edmondson-Jones M, Somerset S, et al. A systematic review of the reporting of tinnitus prevalence and severity. Hear Res. 2016;337:70–9.
2. Gallus S, Lugo A, Garavello W, et al. Prevalence and determinants of tinnitus in the Italian adult population. Neuroepidemiology. 2015;45(1):12–9.
3. McFerran DJ, Stockdale D, Holme R, et al. Why is there no cure for tinnitus? Front Neurosci. 2019;13:802.
4. Biswas R, Hall DA. Prevalence, incidence, and risk factors for tinnitus. Curr Top Behav Neurosci. 2020;51:3–28.
5. Lugo A, Bosetti C, Peveri G, et al. Dose-response relationship between cigarette smoking and site-specific cancer risk: protocol for a systematic review with an original design combining umbrella and traditional reviews. BMJ Open. 2017;7(10):e018930.
6. Jarach CM, Lugo A, Scala M, et al. Global prevalence and incidence of tinnitus: a systematic review and meta-analysis. JAMA Neurol. 2022;79(9):888–900.
7. Moher D, Liberati A, Tetzlaff J, et al. Preferred reporting items for systematic reviews and meta-analyses: the PRISMA statement. PLoS Med. 2009;6(7):e1000097.
8. Akhter R, Morita M, Ekuni D, et al. Self-reported aural symptoms, headache and temporomandibular disorders in Japanese young adults. BMC Musculoskelet Disord. 2013;14:58.
9. Aksoy S, Akdogan O, Gedikli Y, et al. The extent and levels of tinnitus in children of Central Ankara. Int J Pediatr Otorhinolaryngol. 2007;71(2):263–8.
10. Axelsson A, Ringdahl A. Tinnitus--a study of its prevalence and characteristics. Br J Audiol. 1989;23(1):53–62.
11. Baigi A, Oden A, Almlid-Larsen V, et al. Tinnitus in the general population with a focus on noise and stress: a public health study. Ear Hear. 2011;32(6):787–9.
12. Bernhardt O, Mundt T, Welk A, et al. Signs and symptoms of temporomandibular disorders and the incidence of tinnitus. J Oral Rehabil. 2011;38(12):891–901.
13. Bhatt JM, Lin HW, Bhattacharyya N. Prevalence, severity, exposures, and treatment patterns of tinnitus in the United States. JAMA Otolaryngol Head Neck Surg. 2016;142(10):959–65.

14. Biswas R, Lugo A, Akeroyd MA, et al. Tinnitus prevalence in Europe: a multi-country cross-sectional population study. Lancet Reg Health Eur. 2022;12:100250.
15. Bogo R, Farah A, Karlsson KK, et al. Prevalence, incidence proportion, and heritability for tinnitus: a longitudinal twin study. Ear Hear. 2017;38(3):292–300.
16. Brunnberg E, Linden-Bostrom M, Berglund M. Tinnitus and hearing loss in 15-16-year-old students: mental health symptoms, substance use, and exposure in school. Int J Audiol. 2008;47(11):688–94.
17. Choi JS, Yu AJ, Voelker CCJ, et al. Prevalence of tinnitus and associated factors among Asian Americans: results from a national sample. Laryngoscope. 2020;130(12):E933–e940.
18. Coelho CB, Sanchez TG, Tyler RS. Tinnitus in children and associated risk factors. Prog Brain Res. 2007;166:179–91.
19. Coles RR. Epidemiology of tinnitus: (1) prevalence. J Laryngol Otol Suppl. 1984;9:7–15.
20. Cooper JC Jr. Health and Nutrition Examination Survey of 1971-75: part II. Tinnitus, subjective hearing loss, and Well-being. J Am Acad Audiol. 1994;5(1):37–43.
21. Davis AC. The prevalence of hearing impairment and reported hearing disability among adults in Great Britain. Int J Epidemiol. 1989;18(4):911–7.
22. Demeester K, van Wieringen A, Hendrickx JJ, et al. Prevalence of tinnitus and audiometric shape. B-ENT. 2007;3(Suppl 7):37–49.
23. Dorner TE, Stronegger WJ, Rebhandl E, et al. The relationship between various psychosocial factors and physical symptoms reported during primary-care health examinations. Wien Klin Wochenschr. 2010;122(3–4):103–9.
24. Engdahl B, Krog NH, Kvestad E, et al. Occupation and the risk of bothersome tinnitus: results from a prospective cohort study (HUNT). BMJ Open. 2012;2(1):e000512.
25. Folmer RL, McMillan GP, Austin DF, et al. Audiometric thresholds and prevalence of tinnitus among male veterans in the United States: data from the National Health and Nutrition Examination Survey, 1999–2006. J Rehabil Res Dev. 2011;48:503–15.
26. Frei P, Mohler E, Braun-Fahrlander C, et al. Cohort study on the effects of everyday life radio frequency electromagnetic field exposure on non-specific symptoms and tinnitus. Environ Int. 2012;38:29–36.
27. Fujii K, Nagata C, Nakamura K, et al. Prevalence of tinnitus in community-dwelling Japanese adults. J Epidemiol. 2011;21(4):299–304.
28. Gates GA, Cooper JC Jr, Kannel WB, et al. Hearing in the elderly: the Framingham cohort, 1983-1985. Part I. Basic audiometric test results. Ear Hear. 1990;11(4):247–56.
29. Gibrin PC, Melo JJ, Marchiori LL. Prevalence of tinnitus complaints and probable association with hearing loss, diabetes mellitus and hypertension in elderly. Codas. 2013;25(2):176–80.
30. Gilles A, Van Hal G, De Ridder D, et al. Epidemiology of noise-induced tinnitus and the attitudes and beliefs towards noise and hearing protection in adolescents. PLoS One. 2013;8(7):e70297.
31. Gopinath B, McMahon CM, Rochtchina E, et al. Incidence, persistence, and progression of tinnitus symptoms in older adults: the Blue Mountains Hearing Study. Ear Hear. 2010;31(3):407–12.
32. Hannaford PC, Simpson JA, Bisset AF, et al. The prevalence of ear, nose and throat problems in the community: results from a national cross-sectional postal survey in Scotland. Fam Pract. 2005;22(3):227–33.
33. Hannula S, Bloigu R, Majamaa K, et al. Self-reported hearing problems among older adults: prevalence and comparison to measured hearing impairment. J Am Acad Audiol. 2011;22(8):550–9.
34. Hasson D, Theorell T, Westerlund H, et al. Prevalence and characteristics of hearing problems in a working and non-working Swedish population. J Epidemiol Community Health. 2010;64(5):453–60.
35. Herr RM, Loerbroks A, Bosch JA, et al. Associations of organizational justice with tinnitus and the mediating role of depressive symptoms and burnout-findings from a cross-sectional study. Int J Behav Med. 2016;23(2):190–7.
36. Holgers KM. Tinnitus in 7-year-old children. Eur J Pediatr. 2003;162(4):276–8.
37. Holgers KM, Pettersson B. Noise exposure and subjective hearing symptoms among school children in Sweden. Noise Health. 2005;7(27):27–37.
38. Holgers KM, Juul J. The suffering of tinnitus in childhood and adolescence. Int J Audiol. 2006;45(5):267–72.
39. House L, Bishop CE, Spankovich C, et al. Tinnitus and its risk factors in african americans: the Jackson Heart Study. Laryngoscope. 2018;128(7):1668–75.
40. Humphriss R, Hall AJ, Baguley DM. Prevalence and characteristics of spontaneous tinnitus in 11-year-old children. Int J Audiol. 2016;55(3):142–8.
41. Jalessi M, Farhadi M, Asghari A, et al. Tinnitus: an epidemiologic study in Iranian population. Acta Med Iran. 2013;51(12):886–91.
42. Johansson MS, Arlinger SD. Prevalence of hearing impairment in a population in Sweden. Int J Audiol. 2003;42(1):18–28.
43. Juul J, Barrenas ML, Holgers KM. Tinnitus and hearing in 7-year-old children. Arch Dis Child. 2012;97(1):28–30.
44. Khedr EM, Ahmed MA, Shawky OA, et al. Epidemiological study of chronic tinnitus in Assiut, Egypt. Neuroepidemiology. 2010;35(1):45–52.
45. Kim YH, Jung HJ, Kang SI, et al. Tinnitus in children: association with stress and trait anxiety. Laryngoscope. 2012;122(10):2279–84.
46. Kim HJ, Lee HJ, An SY, et al. Analysis of the prevalence and associated risk factors of tinnitus in adults. PLoS One. 2015;10(5):e0127578.
47. Krog NH, Engdahl B, Tambs K. The association between tinnitus and mental health in a general population sample: results from the HUNT study. J Psychosom Res. 2010;69(3):289–98.
48. Kuttila S, Kuttila M, Le Bell Y, et al. Recurrent tinnitus and associated ear symptoms in adults. Int J Audiol. 2005;44(3):164–70.
49. Landalv D, Malmstrom L, Widen SE. Adolescents' reported hearing symptoms and attitudes toward loud music. Noise Health. 2013;15(66):347–54.
50. Lasisi AO, Abiona T, Gureje O. Tinnitus in the elderly: profile, correlates, and impact in the Nigerian Study of Ageing. Otolaryngol Head Neck Surg. 2010;143(4):510–5.
51. Loprinzi PD, Lee H, Gilham B, et al. Association between accelerometer-assessed physical activity and tinnitus, NHANES 2005-2006. Res Q Exerc Sport. 2013;84(2):177–85.
52. Lugo A, Trpchevska N, Liu X, et al. Sex-specific association of tinnitus with suicide attempts. JAMA Otolaryngol Head Neck Surg. 2019;145(7):685–7.
53. Mahboubi H, Oliaei S, Kiumehr S, et al. The prevalence and characteristics of tinnitus in the youth population of the United States. Laryngoscope. 2013;123(8):2001–8.
54. Marmut Z, Belojevic G, Backovic D, et al. Tinnitus among Serbian secondary school students in relation to their behavior and habits. Noise Health. 2014;16(69):73–8.
55. Masterson EA, Themann CL, Luckhaupt SE, et al. Hearing difficulty and tinnitus among U.S. workers and non-workers in 2007. Am J Ind Med. 2016;59(4):290–300.
56. McCormack A, Edmondson-Jones M, Fortnum H, et al. The prevalence of tinnitus and the relationship with neuroticism in a middle-aged UK population. J Psychosom Res. 2014;76(1):56–60.
57. Melo JJ, Meneses CL, Marchiori LL. Prevalence of tinnitus in elderly individuals with and without history of occupational noise exposure. Int Arch Otorhinolaryngol. 2012;16(2):222–5.
58. Michikawa T, Nishiwaki Y, Kikuchi Y, et al. Prevalence and factors associated with tinnitus: a community-based study of Japanese elders. J Epidemiol. 2010;20(4):271–6.

59. Mills RP, Albert DM, Brain CE. Tinnitus in childhood. Clin Otolaryngol Allied Sci. 1986;11(6):431–4.
60. Nemholt S, Schmidt JH, Wedderkopp N, et al. A cross-sectional study of the prevalence and factors associated with tinnitus and/or hyperacusis in children. Ear Hear. 2020;41(2):344–55.
61. Nodar RH. Tinnitus aurium in school age children: a survey. J Audiol Res. 1972;12:133–5.
62. Nondahl DM, Cruickshanks KJ, Wiley TL, et al. Prevalence and 5-year incidence of tinnitus among older adults: the epidemiology of hearing loss study. J Am Acad Audiol. 2002;13(6):323–31.
63. Nondahl DM, Cruickshanks KJ, Wiley TL, et al. The ten-year incidence of tinnitus among older adults. Int J Audiol. 2010;49(8):580–5.
64. Nondahl DM, Cruickshanks KJ, Huang GH, et al. Tinnitus and its risk factors in the Beaver Dam offspring study. Int J Audiol. 2011;50(5):313–20.
65. Oiticica J, Bittar RS. Tinnitus prevalence in the city of Sao Paulo. Braz J Otorhinolaryngol. 2015;81(2):167–76.
66. Oosterloo BC, Croll PH, de Jong RJB, et al. Prevalence of tinnitus in an aging population and its relation to age and hearing loss. Otolaryngol Head Neck Surg. 2021;164(4):859–68.
67. Palmer KT, Griffin MJ, Syddall HE, et al. Occupational exposure to noise and the attributable burden of hearing difficulties in Great Britain. Occup Environ Med. 2002;59(9):634–9.
68. Park B, Choi HG, Lee HJ, et al. Analysis of the prevalence of and risk factors for tinnitus in a young population. Otol Neurotol. 2014;35(7):1218–22.
69. Park KH, Lee SH, Koo JW, et al. Prevalence and associated factors of tinnitus: data from the Korean National Health and Nutrition Examination Survey 2009-2011. J Epidemiol. 2014;24(5):417–26.
70. Parving A, Hein HO, Suadicani P, et al. Epidemiology of hearing disorders. Some factors affecting hearing. The Copenhagen Male Study. Scand Audiol. 1993;22(2):101–7.
71. Piotrowska A, Raj-Koziak D, Lorens A, et al. Tinnitus reported by children aged 7 and 12 years. Int J Pediatr Otorhinolaryngol. 2015;79(8):1346–50.
72. Quaranta A, Assennato G, Sallustio V. Epidemiology of hearing problems among adults in Italy. Scand Audiol Suppl. 1996;42:9–13.
73. Rademaker MM, Smit AL, Brabers AEM, et al. Using different cutoffs to define tinnitus and assess its prevalence-a survey in the Dutch general population. Front Neurol. 2021;12:690192.
74. Raj-Koziak D, Gos E, Swierniak W, et al. Prevalence of tinnitus in a sample of 43,064 children in Warsaw, Poland. Int J Audiol. 2020;60:1–7.
75. Rhee J, Lee D, Suh MW, et al. Prevalence, associated factors, and comorbidities of tinnitus in adolescents. PLoS One. 2020;15(7):e0236723.
76. Salonen J, Johansson R, Joukamaa M. Alexithymia, depression and tinnitus in elderly people. Gen Hosp Psychiatry. 2007;29(5):431–5.
77. Schubert NMA, Rosmalen JGM, van Dijk P, et al. A retrospective cross-sectional study on tinnitus prevalence and disease associations in the Dutch population-based cohort lifelines. Hear Res. 2021;411:108355.
78. Shargorodsky J, Curhan GC, Farwell WR. Prevalence and characteristics of tinnitus among US adults. Am J Med. 2010;123(8):711–8.
79. Stouffer JL, Tyler RS. Characterization of tinnitus by tinnitus patients. J Speech Hear Disord. 1990;55(3):439–53.
80. Sugiura S, Uchida Y, Nakashima T, et al. Tinnitus and brain MRI findings in Japanese elderly. Acta Otolaryngol. 2008;128(5):525–9.
81. Tan HE, Lan NSR, Knuiman MW, et al. Associations between cardiovascular disease and its risk factors with hearing loss-A cross-sectional analysis. Clin Otolaryngol. 2018;43(1):172–81.
82. Weiss NS. Relation of high blood pressure to headache, epistaxis, and selected other symptoms. The United States Health Examination Survey of Adults. N Engl J Med. 1972;287(13):631–3.
83. Welch D, Dawes PJ. Personality and perception of tinnitus. Ear Hear. 2008;29(5):684–92.
84. Widen SE, Erlandsson SI. Self-reported tinnitus and noise sensitivity among adolescents in Sweden. Noise Health. 2004;7(25):29–40.
85. Wu BP, Searchfield G, Exeter DJ, et al. Tinnitus prevalence in New Zealand. N Z Med J. 2015;128(1423):24–34.
86. Xu X, Bu X, Zhou L, et al. An epidemiologic study of tinnitus in a population in Jiangsu province, China. J Am Acad Audiol. 2011;22(9):578–85.
87. Yang H, Cai Y, Guo H, et al. Prevalence and factors associated with tinnitus: data from adult residents in Guangdong province, South of China. Int J Audiol. 2018;57(12):892–9.
88. Biswas R, Lugo A, Genitsaridi E, et al. Modifiable lifestyle-related risk factors for tinnitus in the general population: an overview of smoking, alcohol, body mass index and caffeine intake. In: Langguth B, Kleinjung T, De Ridder D, et al., editors. Tinnitus-an interdisciplinary approach towards individualized treatment. London: Elsevier; 2021. p. 1–24.
89. Biswas R, Lugo A, Gallus S, et al. Standardized questions in English for estimating tinnitus prevalence and severity, hearing difficulty and usage of healthcare resources, and their translation into 11 European languages. Hear Res. 2019;377:330–8.
90. Baguley DM, McFerran DJ. Tinnitus in childhood. Int J Pediatr Otorhinolaryngol. 1999;49(2):99–105.
91. Maas IL, Bruggemann P, Requena T, et al. Genetic susceptibility to bilateral tinnitus in a Swedish twin cohort. Genet Med. 2017;19(9):1007–12.
92. Savastano M, Marioni G, de Filippis C. Tinnitus in children without hearing impairment. Int J Pediatr Otorhinolaryngol. 2009;73(Suppl 1):S13–5.
93. Park RJ, Moon JD. Prevalence and risk factors of tinnitus: the Korean National Health and Nutrition Examination Survey 2010-2011, a cross-sectional study. Clin Otolaryngol. 2014;39(2):89–94.
94. Martinez C, Wallenhorst C, McFerran D, et al. Incidence rates of clinically significant tinnitus: 10-year trend from a cohort study in England. Ear Hear. 2015;36(3):e69–75.
95. Neumark Y. What can ecological studies tell us about death? Isr J Health Policy Res. 2017;6(1):52.
96. Morgenstern H. Uses of ecologic analysis in epidemiologic research. Am J Public Health. 1982;72(12):1336–44.
97. Plante DT, Ingram DG. Seasonal trends in tinnitus symptomatology: evidence from internet search engine query data. Eur Arch Otorhinolaryngol. 2015;272(10):2807–13.
98. Theodoroff SM, Lewis MS, Folmer RL, et al. Hearing impairment and tinnitus: prevalence, risk factors, and outcomes in US service members and veterans deployed to the Iraq and Afghanistan wars. Epidemiol Rev. 2015;37:71–85.
99. Di Stadio A, Dipietro L, Ricci G, et al. Hearing loss, tinnitus, hyperacusis, and diplacusis in professional musicians: a systematic review. Int J Environ Res Public Health. 2018;15(10):2120.
100. Disease GBD, Injury I, Prevalence C. Global, regional, and national incidence, prevalence, and years lived with disability for 328 diseases and injuries for 195 countries, 1990-2016: a systematic analysis for the Global Burden of Disease Study 2016. Lancet. 2017;390(10100):1211–59.

Genetic Contribution to Tinnitus and Tinnitus Disorder

5

Christopher R. Cederroth, Natalia Trpchevska, Sana Amanat, Alvaro Gallego-Martinez, and José Antonio Lopez-Escamez

Abstract

Tinnitus is a subjective perception of sound reported in almost 15% of the global population. Tinnitus can be found associated with hearing loss, hyperacusis, noise exposure, and several comorbidities such as anxiety or headache. Several environmental factors may trigger this symptomatology, though genetic variation may modulate and facilitate the development of a chronic or severe tinnitus phenotype. Currently, a strong genetic heritability has been observed in studies with twins and adoptees. Also, sex differences and familial aggregation have been observed in tinnitus, suggesting a relevant genetic background. Genome-wide association studies and exome/genome sequencing can decipher the contribution of common and rare genetic variations in the genome to the different phenotypes observed in tinnitus patients. A burden of rare missense variants in several synaptic genes, including *ANK2, AKAP9,* and *TSC2,* was found in Spanish individuals with MD and tinnitus extreme phenotype and replicated in Swedish patients with severe tinnitus. However, several of these new candidate variants are pending confirmation, and replication in an independent cohort and functional validation is needed before their clinical translation. High-throughput sequencing may elucidate the genetic structure of severe tinnitus combining genetic and clinical data in early personalized diagnosis and genetic therapy.

C. R. Cederroth (✉)
Laboratory of Experimental Audiology, Department of Physiology and Pharmacology, Karolinska Institutet, Stockholm, Sweden

National Institute for Health Research (NIHR) Nottingham Biomedical Research Centre, Nottingham University Hospitals NHS Trust, Nottingham, UK

Translational Hearing Research, Tübingen Hearing Research Center, Department of Otolaryngology, Head and Neck Surgery, University of Tübingen, Tübingen, Germany
e-mail: christopher.cederroth@ki.se

N. Trpchevska
Laboratory of Experimental Audiology, Department of Physiology and Pharmacology, Karolinska Institutet, Stockholm, Sweden
e-mail: natalia.trpchevska@ki.se

S. Amanat · A. Gallego-Martinez
Otology and Neurotology Group CTS495, Department of Genomic Medicine, GENYO-Centre for Genomics and Oncological Research Pfizer/University of Granada/Junta de Andalucía, PTS, Granada, Spain
e-mail: sa30@sanger.ac.uk; alvaro.gallego@genyo.es

J. A. Lopez-Escamez (✉)
Otology and Neurotology Group CTS495, Department of Genomic Medicine, GENYO-Centre for Genomics and Oncological ResearchPfizer/University of Granada/Junta de Andalucía, PTS, Granada, Spain

Meniere's Disease Neuroscience Research Program, Faculty of Medicine & Health, School of Medical Sciences, The Kolling Institute, The University of Sydney, Sydney, New South Wales, Australia

Department of Surgery, Division of Otolaryngology, University of Granada, Granada, Spain
e-mail: jalopezescamez@ugr.es; Jose.lopezescamez@sydney.edu.au

W. Schlee et al. (eds.), *Textbook of Tinnitus*, https://doi.org/10.1007/978-3-031-35647-6_5

Graphical Abstract

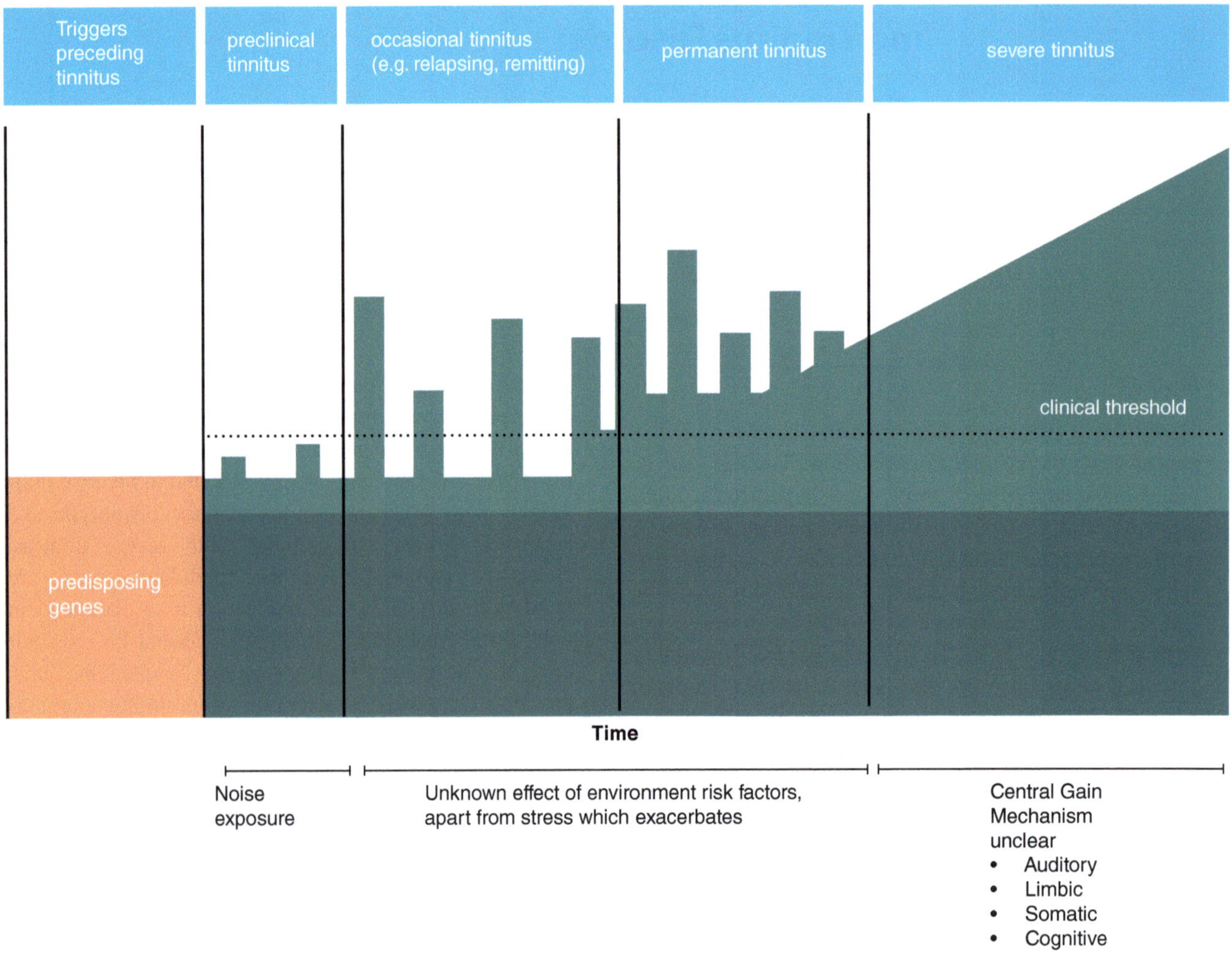

Hypothetical Sketch of the Development of Tinnitus Over Time: Several factors that predispose to tinnitus are at play during the subclinical phase of the disease, before clinically recognizable symptoms are present. The light blue area represents the progression of tinnitus severity, and bars denote events that alter plasticity along the auditory pathway, some of which such as mild noise overexposure do not reach a clinical threshold (e.g., THI > 58). Indeed, lifestyle and environmental factors that predispose an individual to tinnitus (like environmental noise exposure) might act years before clinical onset, complicating epidemiological studies. Arrows denote episodes of acute damage to the auditory system (e.g., overexposure to noise). Eventually, most individuals with occasional tinnitus enter a permanent phase. It is critical to obtain detailed understanding on mechanisms that allow tinnitus to develop and sustain, preferably via studies that combine genetic risk factors with lifestyle and environmental factors.

Highlights

- Scientific evidence pinpoints the relevance of genetic risk factors along with environmental factors in the development of tinnitus and its severity.
- Differences in the age of onset, familial aggregation, and sex-predominant diagnosis found in patients with tinnitus may derive from an important genetic background.
- Genome-wide association analysis has been an important step in the discovery of genetic markers related to tinnitus in large populations. However, whole-genome sequencing methodologies are needed to understand the complex genetic architecture of tinnitus.
- Research in the genetic background of tinnitus is still in its first steps, with new omic-based technologies being the main scientific resources to elucidate the complexity of tinnitus across different genetic populations.

Textbox

- Genotyping: methodology for determining genetic markers of an individual by biological assay and comparing with another individual or reference sequence. This methodology allows to determine the genetic difference between individuals in the form of alleles.
- Allele: Gene variant form.
- WGS: Whole-Genome Sequencing. Methodology based in the determination of the entire DNA sequence of an organism.
- WES: Whole-Exome Sequencing. Methodology based in the determination of the exome, or coding sequence, of an organism. Exome only covers around 1–2% of the entire genome of an individual.
- GWAS: Genome-Wide Association Analysis. Statistical methodology of association between common variants or genetic markers and complex traits by comparing a large set of genotyped individuals.
- Indels: Insertion and Deletions. Short alterations in the DNA as a variant between 1 and 10,000 base pairs in length. Insertion variants are the addition of one or more nucleotide base pairs into a DNA sequence, while a deletion is a loss of certain nucleotides in the DNA.
- SNP: Single Nucleotide Polymorphism, a point alteration of genetic aberration where a reference nucleotide changes for a less frequent nucleotide, probably altering the resulted amino-acid or protein (missense variants) or not (synonymous variants).
- Phenotype: Set of observable traits and characteristics that define an organism covering its morphology, its physiology, as well as developmental processes and behavior.
- Missense variants: Genomic variants that have an impact on the coded amino-acid. Missense variants are generally more damaging on the final protein form than synonymous variants, which have no consequence on the resulting amino-acid.
- MAF: Minor allele frequency. Frequency of the less common allele in a defined locus in a given population. MAF can also be defined as the frequency of the second common allele in the case of several alleles in a specific locus.
- CADD: Combined Annotation-Dependent Depletion score. It is a score to estimate the pathogenicity of a rare variant.
- Synaptic genes: Genes coding for proteins related to the synapse; the structure that allows the signaling between the neurons in the nervous system by electrical or chemical signals.
- OR: Odds ratio. Statistic value that quantifies the strength of association between two frequencies.

Introduction

Research into the etiology of tinnitus has never been as interesting and provocative as in the past 5 years [1, 2]. There has been progress on several fronts, but in particular with regard to the molecular genetics of this disorder of the ear and brain [3]. Still, a number of critically important and unresolved issues remain to establish the validity of the results. The recent progress in this historically difficult area of research does not seem to be widely appreciated, which is why this chapter aims to provide a high-level review of progress, its limitations, and the implications for clinical and research practice.

Tinnitus is a multifactorial condition, whose pathophysiological mechanisms remain poorly known. As for most psychiatric conditions, tinnitus cannot be objectively diagnosed and self-reports translate into a kaleidoscope of signs and symptoms that vary in frequency, percepts, duration, and severity [4, 5]. Indeed, the lack of such objective measures or pathological features of high sensitivity and specificity preempts an accurate diagnosis [6]. Severe tinnitus, for which often individuals seek medical help, represents a small proportion of the population (~2%, please see also Chap. 4 on the epidemiology of tinnitus). The contrastingly high prevalence of self-reported tinnitus (ranging from 15% to 25% of the population) may be ground to tinnitus being considered a symptom rather than a disorder or a disease. Moreover, in ENT clinics, tinnitus often comes as secondary to primary auditory complaints and idiopathic tinnitus, often non-explained by an accompanying hearing loss, remains enigmatic.

The onset of tinnitus is most often sporadic, being perceived intermittently, and then increases in frequency and occurrence until becoming constant. As tinnitus becomes more frequent or constant [7], a resulting impact on life quality is observed, with accompanying stress, anxiety, and depression [8]. While tinnitus has a large impact on societal costs and public health [9–11], its contribution to years lived with disability remains uncovered, likely due to the lack of nation-wide surveys with standardized definitions of clinical relevance. While a full picture of the societal, familial, and personal impacts is lacking, individuals with severe tinnitus have elevated risk of suicide attempts [12, 13], which underscores the pressing need for more effective preventive, diagnostic, and treatment strategies (Table 5.1).

Table 5.1 Characteristics of tinnitus. Lambda (λs) refers to the sibling recurrence risk ratio

Features	Associated details	Reference
Prevalence		[14]
Any tinnitus	17%	
Unilateral	6.68%	
Bilateral	8.49%	
Constant	7.38%	
Severe	2.55%	
Significant tinnitus (SigT)	2.77%	
Suicide attempts	4.4%	[12, 13]
Yearly cost		[9–11]
Medical (per person per year)	GB£750 million	
Total per year (societal and medical)	€6.8 billion	
Heritability		
Twins (Uni- or bilateral tinnitus)	27–68%	[15, 16]
Adoptees (SigT)	31%	[17]
Familial aggregation (severe)	λs = 5.03–10.25	[14]
Replicated candidate genes associated with tinnitus		
Genes with common variants	*COL11A1*, *GRK6*, *MFHAS1*, *MSRA*, *XKR6*, *C8orf12*, AF131215.5, and *BLK*	[18]
Genes with rare variants	*ANK2*, *AKAP9* and *TSC2*	[19]

Major efforts in the tinnitus community, aided by exceptional advances in technology and genomic knowledge, have propelled the field and identified robust and replicable findings. We believe it timely to provide an update on the genetics of tinnitus, along with considerations of its implications.

Tinnitus as a Disorder

Due to the lack of operational or standardized definition of tinnitus, the diagnostic criteria for tinnitus have not been established so far. In the world health organization's ICD11 catalogue, tinnitus has been defined as a nonspecific symptom associated with hearing disorders rather a clinical entity. Recently, a group of tinnitus experts has proposed new definitions of tinnitus in order to classify it either as a symptom or as a disorder. Tinnitus as a symptom is defined as the conscious awareness of a tonal or composite noise for which there is no identifiable corresponding external sound source. In contrast, tinnitus is defined as a disorder when it is associated with emotional distress, cognitive dysfunction, and/or autonomic arousal ultimately leading towards behavioral changes and functional disability [20] (please see also Chap. 2 on the definition of tinnitus and tinnitus disorder).

Evidence to Support Heritability in Tinnitus Disorder

In literature, the evidence to support a genetic contribution to tinnitus is limited to a few epidemiological and genetic studies showing conflicting results, and most of the largest studies were conducted in Sweden. Studies in twins, adoptees, and familial aggregation have been widely used to depict the relative contributions of genetics and environmental components to the risk of a specific trait. Although there are many assumptions and methodological issues with these "old genetics" approaches, when applied to optimized tinnitus definitions, these have yielded remarkably consistent findings. In spite of a large number of studies evaluating the relationship between tinnitus and other environmental factors (cross-sectional studies), a handful of studies were published in either case-controls or longitudinal designs to determine risk factors for tinnitus (Fig. 5.1). This reveals major gaps in knowledge such as the impact of perinatal and childhood events, maternal stress, and viral infections. In the last decade, however, several genetic epidemiological studies have suggested that specific tinnitus subtypes may be differentially impacted by genetic or environmental factors. The large number of definitions used for tinnitus in these studies account for the lack of replication, with heritability ranging from 2% to 68% depending on the definition (Table 5.1). To summarize this literature briefly, both adoption and twin studies indicate that this familial transmission is mainly due to genetic effects and suggest negligible shared environment effects, which thus excludes perinatal origins as a contributor to tinnitus. Thus, tinnitus should be viewed as a complex trait resulting from both genetic and environmental interactions (please see also Chap. 6 on environmental and occupational risk factors).

Twins Studies

One of the largest twin studies conducted on tinnitus subjects was performed using data from the Swedish Twin Registry, in which authors reported a high concordance between monozygotic twins with bilateral tinnitus and a high heritability of 0.62 in young women with bilateral tinnitus [15].

Adoptees-Based Studies

Another study in Sweden was performed to determine whether the above findings were potentially confounded by shared environmental factors. For this purpose, the study used national registry data and identified adoptees, biological parents, and adoptive parents with or without clinically

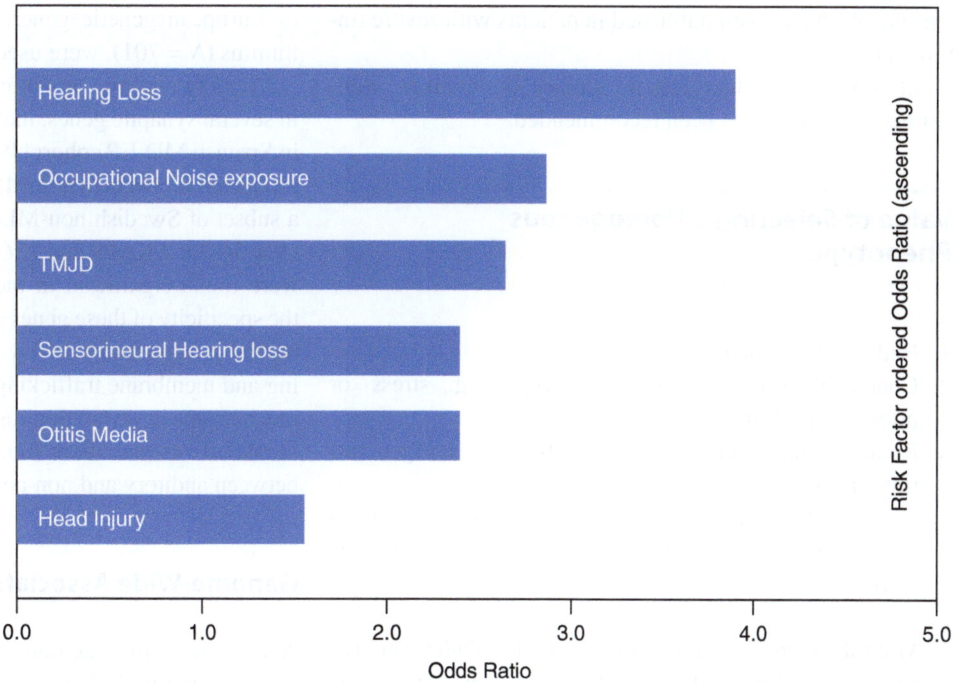

Fig. 5.1 Comparisons of a selected set of risk factors for tinnitus from longitudinal and/or case/control studies. Hearing loss [21], occupational noise exposure [22], temporomandibular joint disorders [23], sensorineural hearing loss [24], otitis media [24], head injury [21]

reported tinnitus (ICD_{10}: 93.1). The results showed that the familial transmission of tinnitus was due in part to genetics, but was not influenced by shared environmental effects [17]. However, since the study covered two generations whose diagnostic criteria may have changed over time, it is likely that the observed heritability of 0.32 was underestimated.

Familial Aggregation

Since the genetics of tinnitus appeared to be differentially affected depending on tinnitus subtypes, a familial aggregation study was conducted to determine the recurrence risk of various forms of tinnitus among siblings. This study has found that the recurrence risk ratio is significantly higher for severe tinnitus than for constant tinnitus or lateralized tinnitus [14]. This liability for severe tinnitus was twofold greater in females than in males. Overall, this report highlighted the relevance of stratifying tinnitus by severity and sex in future studies.

Overall, severe tinnitus can be described as distressing disorder in 1% of population affecting quality of life. It aggregates strongly within families with ninefold risk for a sibling to develop tinnitus if the other has severe tinnitus [14], which is in the range of what has been described for schizophrenia. As these findings have not been replicated elsewhere, more clinical and genetics work is required to assess the transmission of severe tinnitus within families and in sporadic cases, something which has never been commonly practiced in ENT clinics.

Genetic Approaches behind the Tinnitus Riddle

Methods to assess the genome have become increasingly complete and cost-effective, and large-scale genome projects have driven the advances in genotyping, sequencing, and bioinformatic analysis. Large consortia have been critical in gaining statistical power. Despite these advances, progress in the genetic quest of tinnitus has been disappointingly slow [25, 26], likely due to the disbelief that tinnitus is no more than a mere symptom of hearing loss. A large number of studies failed in identifying genetic variants through candidate gene approaches, likely due to small sample size and poor/inappropriate tinnitus phenotype, self-reported tinnitus, lack of the utilization of standardized tools to measure tinnitus severity, and those that found positive results were never replicated in independent cohorts [25, 26]—a crucial step in the external validity of genetic findings.

Genomic Studies for Tinnitus

Genome and Exome Studies

Improvements in technologies have enabled the evaluation of most of the protein-coding regions of the genome (the "exome") via high-throughput sequencing. This is an area of high interest because the confident identification of rare variants of strong effect could be valuable since they would pinpoint a single key gene likely amenable to molecular biology. Only a small exome sequencing study with a replication cohort has been published in patients with severe tinnitus [19].

In order to conduct genetic studies on tinnitus, well-defined phenotype has been recommended.

Value of Selecting a Homogenous Phenotype

1. Reduction in genetic noise
2. Characterization of tinnitus phenotype (e.g., stress- or noise-induced tinnitus)
3. Reduced selection bias of individuals with heterogeneous tinnitus phenotype
4. Controlled biasness on tinnitus-related biasness induced by comorbidities (i.e., hearing loss, headache, anxiety, insomnia).

Multiple approaches have been applied to understand the genetic basis of tinnitus [27, 28]. Emerging data support the role for rare and common variants in increasing its risk. However, only two studies as of yet report robust and replicable genomic findings for tinnitus. Interestingly, the genetic basis of tinnitus has multiple points of convergence with anxiety and insomnia. It is possible that with further work, the results will lead to revisions in the classification of tinnitus subtypes.

Exome-Based Extreme Phenotype (EP) Study

Variations in phenotype for quantitative traits can be represented by a bell-shaped graph as mild, intermediate, and severe phenotypes, where mild and severe phenotypes are located at the tails of the distribution, and most of the subjects show an intermediate phenotype (center part of the distribution) [29]. EP covers both extreme ends of a phenotype distributions, i.e., mild and severe. However, Amanat et al. covered only one extreme, i.e., severe phenotype [19]. This severe phenotype occurs in extreme cases that could exhibit an excess of rare variants.

To conduct this study, exome sequencing of Spanish Meniere disease patients ($N = 59$) with severe tinnitus was performed and this group was further divided into two subgroups of MD-extreme phenotype (EP) and MD- almost extreme phenotype (AEP) based on tinnitus handicap inventory (THI) scores. Two validation cohorts, genomes of Non-MD Swedish tinnitus individuals ($N = 97$) and exomes of European genetic generalized epilepsy patients without tinnitus ($N = 701$), were used.

Authors reported an enrichment of rare missense variants in several synaptic genes, including *ANK2, AKAP9,* and *TSC2* in Spanish MD-EP cohort [19]. This enrichment in *ANK2* was replicated in Swedish non-MD tinnitus individuals and also in a subset of Swedish non-MD individuals with severe tinnitus ($N = 34$) for AKAP9 and *TSC2*. However, none of these genes were found significant in the epilepsy cohort demonstrating the specificity of these genes with tinnitus. The significant biological process and pathways were cytoskeletal protein binding and membrane trafficking in neurons. Thus, the proposed mechanisms in severe tinnitus involve axon initial segment, an increased axonal branching, and enhanced connectivity between auditory and non-auditory brain regions.

Genome-Wide Association Study

A small-scale pilot genome-wide association study (GWAS) on 167 tinnitus individuals from Belgium was conducted. Unfortunately, none of the SNPs could pass the significant threshold of 3.4e–7. But gene set enrichment analysis evidenced metabolic pathways associated with serotonin reception-mediated signaling, endoplasmatic reticulum stress, and oxidative stress [30].

Recently, a large GWAS conducted in >200,000 individuals with self-reported tinnitus from the UK Biobank and replicated in the US Million Veteran Program (MVP) cohort has reported 3 loci in noncoding region (rs143424888, rs553448379, rs11249981) with small effect size that explained approximately 6% of the heritability [18]. MVP cohort was not controlled for noise exposure, but was known for tinnitus risk factors. Eight candidate genes were predicted (*COL11A1, GRK6, MFHAS1, MSRA, XKR6, C8orf12,* AF131215.5, and *BLK*). However, the broad phenotype that was selected to define tinnitus - being occasionally and constantly perceived with a prevalence of near 30% - may have accounted for a rather low number of associated loci, when compared to age-related hearing loss [31]. This GWAS is a pioneering contribution to define the genetic architecture of noise-induced hearing loss and tinnitus, but their findings cannot be extended to any tinnitus phenotype.

A recent GWAS comprising 91,424 individuals from UK biobank was conducted to understand the molecular mechanisms of tinnitus. Three variants in *RCOR1* gene including chr14:103042287, rs4900545, and rs4906228 were found significant, but these findings were not replicated in a second, independent cohort [32] (Table 5.2).

Table 5.2 Summary of significant GWAS findings on different tinnitus cohorts. Replicated variants in different studies are marked in bold. Details for each study are referenced in last column

Locus	Description	OMIM	Cytogenetic band	Variant	*p*-value	Reference
ZNF318	ZINC FINGER PROTEIN 318	617,512	6p21.1	**rs553448379**	2.10E-08	[18]
COL11A1	COLLAGEN, TYPE XI, ALPHA-1	120,280	1p21.1	**rs143424888**	8.50E-09	[18]
MSRA	PEPTIDE METHIONINE SULFOXIDE REDUCTASE	601,250	8p23.1	**rs11249981**	4.60E-08	[18]
BANK1	B-CELL SCAFFOLD PROTEIN WITH ANKYRIN REPEATS 1	610,292	4q24	rs17249745	1.30–09	[18]
SORCS3	SORTILIN-RELATED VPS10 DOMAIN-CONTAINING RECEPTOR 3	606,285	10q25.1	rs72815660	9.70E-09	[18]
MON2	REGULATOR OF ENDOSOME-TO-GOLGI TRAFFICKING	616,822	12q14.1	rs11174489	3.80E-09	[18]
RCOR1	REST COREPRESSOR	607,675	14q32.31-q32.32	rs4906228	1.70E-08	[32]
RCOR1	REST COREPRESSOR	607,675	14q32.31-q32.32	rs4900545	1.80E-08	[32]
RCOR1	REST COREPRESSOR	607,675	14q32.31-q32.32	14:103042287_CT_C	3.50E-08	[32]
UBAC2	LIPOCALIN-INTERACTING MEMBRANE RECEPTOR	610,007	12q13.12	rs7336872	5.94E-08	[32]
ARID5B	AT-RICH INTERACTION DOMAIN-CONTAINING PROTEIN 5B	608,538	10q21.2	rs118053011	9.89E-08	[32]
WDPCP	WD REPEAT-CONTAINING PLANAR CELL POLARITY EFFECTOR	613,580	2p15	rs61734468	3.96E-10	[33]

Deciphering the Genetic Structure of Tinnitus and Tinnitus Disorder

Tinnitus is a common trait, and it probably results in the interaction of common variants with a small effect size with environmental factors such as noise exposure that induce epigenetic changes across life span. GWAS have identified and replicated few common variants in patients reporting tinnitus with noise-induced hearing loss, particularly in the loci of *COL11A1*, *SLC29A1,* and *TNKS* genes [18]; however, the observed values for the OR and their etiological fractions are very low and these common variants should be considered as modifiers of the susceptibility to develop tinnitus (Fig. 5.2).

Tinnitus disorder defined as the condition associated with emotional, cognitive, or behavioral changes is considered a more "rare disease" (<1% of the general population) compared with tinnitus defined as a symptom. It is probably the result of the combined effect of multiple common and rare variants with a high effect size that may lead to a severe phenotype. Rare variants in *ANK2* and *TCS2* genes have been identified and replicated in few individuals with an extreme tinnitus phenotype in Spanish and Swedish individuals, showing higher OR and etiological fraction values. These should be considered as variants increasing the risk to develop severe tinnitus, or tinnitus disorder [20] (Fig. 5.2).

All these variants associated with tinnitus or tinnitus disorder are single nucleotide variants, and the genetic architecture of tinnitus probably involves additional types of variants including small structural variants (insertion, deletions) and copy number variants, as it has been found in other brain disorders [34]. However, this remains to be investigated in the context of tinnitus.

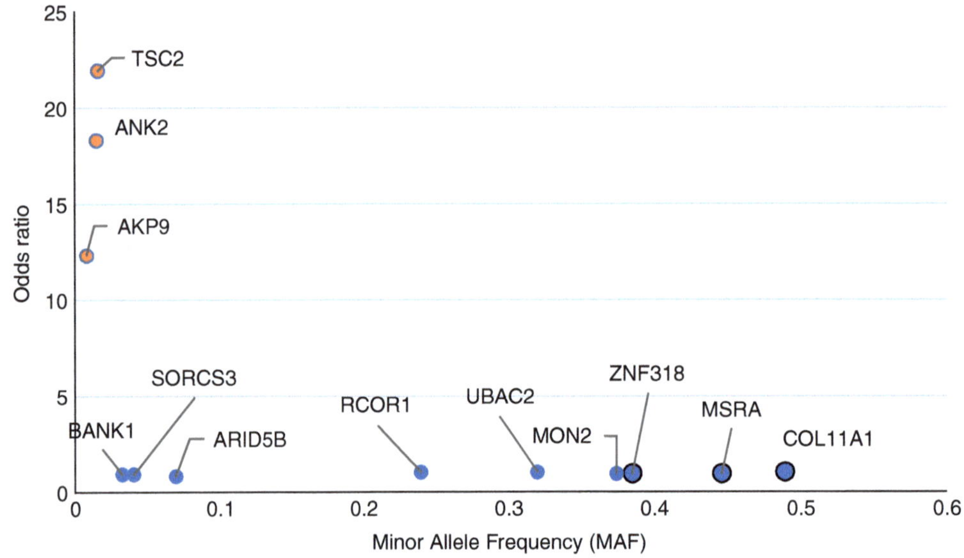

Fig. 5.2 The genetic landscape of tinnitus. The effect of the variants associated with tinnitus as a function of their allelic frequency observed in different tinnitus genomic studies. Rare variants (with frequencies <1%) with a large effect size are found in a low number of individuals, while common variants (with frequencies >1%) with a small effect size are reported in a larger number of individuals. Orange dots represent OR for genes enriched in rare missense variants in exome sequencing studies selecting individual with tinnitus extreme phenotype. Blue dots represent OR for common variants associated to self-reported tinnitus in genome-wide association studies (GWAS). Odds ratio from GWAS studies was calculated from beta values from their respective studies. Note: This could not be done for WDPCP; neither OR nor Beta was provided to calculate OR. MAF used in representation is the aggregated MAF for each rare missense variant found for each gene. Variants included in candidate genes observed in exome analysis and their respective MAF are: 4:114262911:A>G—0; 4:114277102:T>G—0; 4:114294509:G>C—0; 4:114294537:G>A—0.0039 for ANK2 gene; 7:91622303:G>C—0.003; 7:91631849:A>G—0; 7:91643610:G>A—0.0004; 7:91670121:G>A—0.0001; 7:91700267:T>C—0.0038; 7:91732039:G>C—0.0038 for AKAP9 gene; and 16:2110765:C>T—0.0009; 16:2129140:C>T—0; 16:2133726:C>T—0.00007; 16:2138096:C>T—0.0003 for TSC2 gene

Limitations and Perspectives

One of the limitations emerging from past genetic research in tinnitus has been the very limited sample size often yielding unpowered studies in absence of replication in independent cohorts. Indeed, there is only a handful of replicated studies that have been able to identify variants associated with defined tinnitus subtypes. However, it appears that there are limited tinnitus definitions in large biobanks (or a lack of appropriate tinnitus phenotyping at recruitment), which calls for a larger involvement of ENT clinics in collecting biosamples for genetic research [35, 36]. This would require the uniformization of the clinical assessment of tinnitus, since even throughout Europe, there is a large heterogeneity on how this is assessed by physicians [37]. For instance, this could involve the standard use of tinnitus questionnaires such as the THI or the TFI, with predefined EU cut-offs for different scales of severity.

The emerging genetic data suggest that the more severe the tinnitus, the greater its genetic liability. It is thus possible that in the future, a new classification of severe tinnitus as a neurological disorder (in opposition to, for instance, occasional tinnitus as a symptom) may provide new guidance not only in fundamental research, but also in clinical research, ultimately leading to improved therapeutic interventions. Moreover, the identification of sex and gender as important biological variables (SABV) in tinnitus research may lead to the identification of sex-targeted treatments with greater success in treatment outcomes. Such are the ambitions from several EU projects such as TIGER (https://tiger.tinnitusresearch.net/) and UNITI (https://uniti.tinnitusresearch.net/), which are pioneering biobanking with in-depth phenotyping within large clinical trials.

Acknowledgments This study has been partially funded by H2020 MSCA-ITN-2016-722046 [38], the H2020-SC1-2019-848261 [39], and the GNP-182 GENDER-Net Co-Plus Fund (JALE and CRC). The project leading to these results has received funding from "la Caixa" Foundation (ID 100010434), under agreement LCF/PR/DE18/52010002 (JALE). This project is a part of European School of Interdisciplinary Tinnitus (ESIT) research and Sana Amanat was a PhD student in Biomedicine Program at the University of Granada. CRC received additional funding from Forschung Für Leben, Svenska Läkaresällskapet (SLS-779681), Hörselforskningsfonden (503). The data handling for STOP and SweGen cohorts was enabled by resources provided by the Swedish National Infrastructure for Computing (SNIC) at UPPMAX partially funded by the Swedish Research Council through grant agreement no. 2018-05973.

References

1. Shore SE, Roberts LE, Langguth B. Maladaptive plasticity in tinnitus--triggers, mechanisms and treatment. Nat Rev Neurol. 2016;12(3):150–60. https://doi.org/10.1038/nrneurol.2016.12.
2. Elgoyhen AB, Langguth B, De Ridder D, Vanneste S. Tinnitus: perspectives from human neuroimaging. Nat Rev Neurosci. 2015;16(10):632–42. https://doi.org/10.1038/nrn4003.
3. Cederroth CR, Trpchevska N, Langguth B. A new buzz for tinnitus-it's in the genes! JAMA Otolaryngol Head Neck Surg. 2020;146(11):1025–6. https://doi.org/10.1001/jamaoto.2020.2919.
4. BaguleyD,McFerranD,HallD.Tinnitus.Lancet.2013;382(9904):1600–7. https://doi.org/10.1016/S0140-6736(13)60142-7.
5. Langguth B, Kreuzer PM, Kleinjung T, De Ridder D. Tinnitus: causes and clinical management. Lancet Neurol. 2013;12(9):920–30. https://doi.org/10.1016/S1474-4422(13)70160-1.
6. Jackson R, Vijendren A, Phillips J. Objective measures of tinnitus: a systematic review. Otol Neurotol. 2019;40(2):154–63. https://doi.org/10.1097/MAO.0000000000002116.
7. Edvall NK, Mehraei G, Claeson M, Lazar A, Bulla J, Leineweber C, Uhlén I, Canlon B, Cederroth CR. Alterations in auditory brain stem response distinguish occasional and constant tinnitus. J Clin Invest. 2022;132(5):e155094. https://doi.org/10.1172/JCI155094.
8. Schlee W, Hall DA, Edvall NK, Langguth B, Canlon B, Cederroth CR. Visualization of global disease burden for the optimization of patient management and treatment. Front Med (Lausanne). 2017;4:86. https://doi.org/10.3389/fmed.2017.00086.
9. Stockdale D, McFerran D, Brazier P, Pritchard C, Kay T, Dowrick C, et al. An economic evaluation of the healthcare cost of tinnitus management in the UK. BMC Health Serv Res. 2017;17(1):577. https://doi.org/10.1186/s12913-017-2527-2.
10. Maes IH, Cima RF, Vlaeyen JW, Anteunis LJ, Joore MA. Tinnitus: a cost study. Ear Hear. 2013;34(4):508–14. https://doi.org/10.1097/AUD.0b013e31827d113a.
11. Goldstein E, Ho CX, Hanna R, Elinger C, Yaremchuk KL, Seidman MD, et al. Cost of care for subjective tinnitus in relation to patient satisfaction. Otolaryngol Head Neck Surg. 2015;152(3):518–23. https://doi.org/10.1177/0194599814566179.
12. Seo JH, Kang JM, Hwang SH, Han KD, Joo YH. Relationship between tinnitus and suicidal behaviour in Korean men and women: a cross-sectional study. Clin Otolaryngol. 2016;41(3):222–7. https://doi.org/10.1111/coa.12500.
13. Lugo A, Trpchevska N, Liu X, Biswas R, Magnusson C, Gallus S, et al. Sex-specific association of tinnitus with suicide attempts. JAMA Otolaryngol Head Neck Surg. 2019;145(7):685–7. https://doi.org/10.1001/jamaoto.2019.0566.
14. Trpchevska N, Bulla J, Prada Hellberg M, Edvall NK, Lazar A, Mehraei G, et al. Sex-dependent aggregation of tinnitus in Swedish families. J Clin Med. 2020;9(12):3812. https://doi.org/10.3390/jcm9123812.
15. Maas IL, Bruggemann P, Requena T, Bulla J, Edvall NK, Hjelmborg JVB, et al. Genetic susceptibility to bilateral tinnitus in a Swedish twin cohort. Genet Med. 2017;19(9):1007–12. https://doi.org/10.1038/gim.2017.4.
16. Bogo R, Farah A, Karlsson KK, Pedersen NL, Svartengren M, Skjonsberg A. Prevalence, incidence proportion, and heritability for tinnitus: a longitudinal twin study. Ear Hear. 2016;38:292. https://doi.org/10.1097/AUD.0000000000000397.
17. Cederroth CR, PirouziFard M, Trpchevska N, Idrizbegovic E, Canlon B, Sundquist J, et al. Association of Genetic vs environmental factors in Swedish adoptees with clinically significant tinnitus. JAMA Otolaryngol Head Neck Surg. 2019;145:222. https://doi.org/10.1001/jamaoto.2018.3852.
18. Clifford RE, Maihofer AX, Stein MB, Ryan AF, Nievergelt CM. Novel risk loci in tinnitus and causal inference with neuropsychiatric disorders among adults of European ancestry. JAMA Otolaryngol Head Neck Surg. 2020;146:1015. https://doi.org/10.1001/jamaoto.2020.2920.
19. Amanat S, Gallego-Martinez A, Sollini J, Perez-Carpena P, Espinosa-Sanchez JM, Aran I, et al. Burden of rare variants in synaptic genes in patients with severe tinnitus: an exome based extreme phenotype study. EBioMedicine. 2021;66:103309. https://doi.org/10.1016/j.ebiom.2021.103309.
20. De Ridder D, Schlee W, Vanneste S, Londero A, Weisz N, Kleinjung T, et al. Tinnitus and tinnitus disorder: theoretical and operational definitions (an international multidisciplinary proposal). Prog Brain Res. 2021;260:1–25. https://doi.org/10.1016/bs.pbr.2020.12.002.
21. Nondahl DM, Cruickshanks KJ, Wiley TL, Klein R, Klein BE, Tweed TS. Prevalence and 5-year incidence of tinnitus among older adults: the epidemiology of hearing loss study. J Am Acad Audiol. 2002;13(6):323–31.
22. Dougherty AL, MacGregor AJ, Han PP, Viirre E, Heltemes KJ, Galarneau MR. Blast-related ear injuries among U.S. military personnel. J Rehabil Res Dev. 2013;50(6):893–904. https://doi.org/10.1682/JRRD.2012.02.0024.
23. Bernhardt O, Mundt T, Welk A, Koppl N, Kocher T, Meyer G, et al. Signs and symptoms of temporomandibular disorders and the incidence of tinnitus. J Oral Rehabil. 2011;38(12):891–901. https://doi.org/10.1111/j.1365-2842.2011.02224.x.
24. Aarhus L, Engdahl B, Tambs K, Kvestad E, Hoffman HJ. Association between childhood hearing disorders and tinnitus in adulthood. JAMA Otolaryngol Head Neck Surg. 2015;141(11):983–9. https://doi.org/10.1001/jamaoto.2015.2378.
25. Vona B, Nanda I, Shehata-Dieler W, Haaf T. Genetics of tinnitus: still in its infancy. Front Neurosci. 2017;11:236. https://doi.org/10.3389/fnins.2017.00236.
26. Lopez-Escamez JA, Bibas T, Cima RF, Van de Heyning P, Knipper M, Mazurek B, et al. Genetics of tinnitus: an emerging area for molecular diagnosis and drug development. Front Neurosci. 2016;10:377. https://doi.org/10.3389/fnins.2016.00377.
27. Lopez-Escamez JA, Amanat S. Heritability and genetics contribution to tinnitus. Otolaryngol Clin N Am. 2020;53(4):501–13. https://doi.org/10.1016/j.otc.2020.03.003.
28. Amanat S, Gallego-Martinez A, Lopez-Escamez JA. Genetic inheritance and its contribution to tinnitus. Curr Top Behav Neurosci. 2021;51:29–47. https://doi.org/10.1007/7854_2020_155.
29. Amanat S, Requena T, Lopez-Escamez JA. A systematic review of extreme phenotype strategies to search for rare variants in genetic studies of complex disorders. Genes. 2020;11(9):987. https://doi.org/10.3390/genes11090987.
30. Gilles A, Van Camp G, Van de Heyning P, Fransen E. A pilot Genome-wide Association Study identifies potential metabolic pathways involved in tinnitus. Front Neurosci. 2017;11:71.
31. Trpchevska N, Freidin MB, Broer L, Oosterloo BC, Yao S, Zhou Y, et al. Genome-wide association meta-analysis identifies 48 risk variants and highlights the role of the stria vascularis in hearing loss. Am J Hum Genet. 2022;109(6):1077–91. https://doi.org/10.1016/j.ajhg.2022.04.010. Epub 2022 May 16.
32. Wells HRR, Abidin FNZ, Freidin MB, Williams FMK, Dawson SJ. Genome-wide association study suggests that variation at the RCOR1 locus is associated with tinnitus in UK biobank. Sci Rep. 2021;11(1):6470. https://doi.org/10.1038/s41598-021-85871-6.
33. Urbanek ME, Zuo J. Genetic predisposition to tinnitus in the UK biobank population. Sci Rep. 2021;11(1):18150. https://doi.org/10.1038/s41598-021-97350-z.
34. Kaminsky EB, Kaul V, Paschall J, Church DM, Bunke B, Kunig D, et al. An evidence-based approach to establish the functional and clinical significance of copy number variants in intellectual and developmental disabilities. Genet Med. 2011;13(9):777–84. https://doi.org/10.1097/GIM.0b013e31822c79f9.

35. Szczepek AJ, Frejo L, Vona B, Trpchevska N, Cederroth CR, Caria H, et al. Recommendations on collecting and storing samples for genetic studies in hearing and tinnitus research. Ear Hear. 2019;40(2):219–26. https://doi.org/10.1097/AUD.0000000000000614.
36. Cederroth CR, Kähler A, Sullivan PF, Lopez-Escamez JA. Genetics of tinnitus: time to biobank phantom sounds. Front Genet. 2017;8:110.
37. Fuller TE, Haider HF, Kikidis D, Lapira A, Mazurek B, Norena A, et al. Different teams, same conclusions? A systematic review of existing clinical guidelines for the assessment and treatment of tinnitus in adults. Front Psychol. 2017;8:206. https://doi.org/10.3389/fpsyg.2017.00206.
38. Schlee W, Hall DA, Canlon B, Cima RFF, de Kleine E, Hauck F, et al. Innovations in doctoral training and research on tinnitus: the European School on Interdisciplinary Tinnitus Research (ESIT) perspective. Front Aging Neurosci. 2017;9:447. https://doi.org/10.3389/fnagi.2017.00447.
39. Schlee W, Schoisswohl S, Staudinger S, Schiller A, Lehner A, Langguth B, et al. Towards a unification of treatments and interventions for tinnitus patients: the EU research and innovation action UNITI. Prog Brain Res. 2021;260:441–51. https://doi.org/10.1016/bs.pbr.2020.12.005.

Environmental and Occupational Risk Factors for Tinnitus

6

Deborah A. Hall and Roshni Biswas

Abstract

Many people may not realise that they use epidemiologic information to make daily decisions affecting their health. From reading nutritional information on food packaging to walking 10,000 steps every day-these health behaviours are underpinned by epidemiologists' assessment of risk. Generally speaking, environmental risks to health are defined as all the external physical, chemical, biological, and work-related factors that affect a person's health. This chapter summarises current debates about environmental and work-related risk factors for tinnitus. Topics span genetic, physiological, behavioural and environmental domains, demography, and lifestyle.

D. A. Hall (✉)
Hearing Sciences Group, Division of Clinical Neuroscience, School of Medicine, University of Nottingham, Nottingham, UK

National Institute for Health Research (NIHR) Nottingham Biomedical Research Centre (BRC), Nottingham, UK

Heriot-Watt University Malaysia, Putrajaya, Malaysia
e-mail: deborah.hall@hw.ac.uk

R. Biswas
Hearing Sciences Group, Division of Clinical Neuroscience, School of Medicine, University of Nottingham, Nottingham, UK

National Institute for Health Research (NIHR) Nottingham Biomedical Research Centre (BRC), Nottingham, UK

W. Schlee et al. (eds.), *Textbook of Tinnitus*, https://doi.org/10.1007/978-3-031-35647-6_6

Graphical Abstract

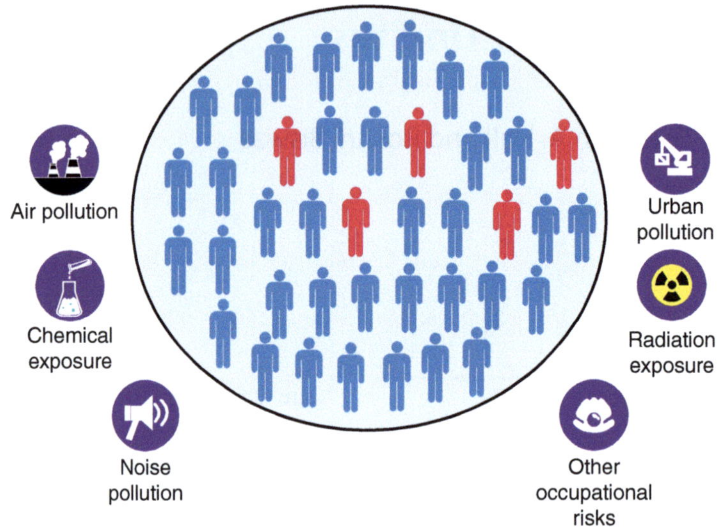

Highlights

- In this chapter, we bring together research studies and debates that are rather scattered across the literature.
- The World Health Organization is committed to reducing exposure to hazardous environmental and occupational risks.
- Noise-induced hearing-related problems are widely recognised as one of the most prominent occupational diseases, but they can also result from leisure noise exposure.
- There is a reasonable body of evidence that chemical exposures increase the risk of hearing loss and/or tinnitus, but perhaps mostly at higher concentrations of exposure.
- A small number of recently published studies point to job stress as a risk factor for tinnitus.
- Key features of urban design play a role in encouraging physical activity which might play a protective role in reducing the risk.
- There appears to be no evidence for an association between tinnitus and exposure to poor air quality or to radio-frequency electromagnetic fields.

Introduction

Many people may not realise that they use epidemiologic information to make daily decisions affecting their health. For example, whenever someone decides to put on a face mask when travelling on public transport, wear ear plugs when going to a live rock music gig, or climb the stairs rather than take an escalator, they may be influenced, consciously or subconsciously, by epidemiologists' assessment of risk [1]. Generally speaking, environmental risks to health are defined as all the external physical, chemical, biological, and work-related factors that affect a person's health [2]. They include pollution, radiation, noise, land use patterns, work environment, and climate change. Many of these were recently proposed by the World Health Organization (WHO) [3] to be major areas of environmental action needed in order to prevent common non-communicable diseases such as cancers, depression, and cardiovascular, respiratory, and musculo-skeletal diseases.

Tinnitus refers to a health condition that is characterised by a phantom sound perceived in the head or ears. It is often treated in the scientific literature as if it was a single phenomenon, but in reality there are likely to be many different causes, many different physiological and psychological mechanisms involved, and hence many different subtypes. This can make the study of tinnitus rather challenging at times. Susceptibility to different risk factors may help to shed light on some of these mechanisms and subtypes. Therefore, debates about tinnitus have considered a range of factors that can potentially increase risk; notably genetic, physiological, behavioural and environmental domains, demography, and lifestyle. As a non-communicable disease, the impact of environmental and occupational risk factors on tinnitus is now being explored. The purpose of this chapter is to introduce the reader to some of these debates since research studies and supporting evidence are relatively scarce and fairly scattered across the literature.

Levels of Evidence

The most reliable source of evidence on risk comes from longitudinal studies that follow study participants forward over time, and interventional studies. Due to the ethical and feasibility constraints involved if manipulating environmental risks as part of an interventional study design, longitudinal studies form the mainstay of evidence. Longitudinal studies are useful for assessing incidence and establishing causal hypothesis.

Incidence is a measure of the number of new cases of tinnitus (i.e. the probability of developing tinnitus) obtained by following up tinnitus-free individuals over a specified observation period. Measures of incidence count new tinnitus cases in the numerator. The denominator is the number of tinnitus-free people in the population at the start of the observation period. Because all of new tinnitus cases (numerator) are also represented in the denominator, incidence is a *proportional* value.

Various measures of effect are used to quantify the strength of association between the exposure and the outcome, i.e. tinnitus. Either the ratio or the difference in the frequency measures between the exposed and unexposed individuals is utilised to calculate measures of effect. Relative risk (RR), Odds ratio (OR), and Hazards ratio (HR) are some commonly used measures of effect. RR is calculated by the ratio of the probability of the outcome occurring in the exposed group compared to the probability of the outcome occurring in the non-exposed group. An RR of 1.0 means that tinnitus is equally likely in both exposed and non-exposed groups. Values greater than 1.0 indicate that the exposure leads to an increased risk, while values lower than 1.0 indicate a decreased risk, but only if the 95% confidence interval (CI) for the RR estimate does not span the value of 1.0. OR reflects the degree of association between tinnitus given a known exposure. It is calculated by the ratio of the odds of an exposure between the tinnitus cases and controls in a case-control study. An OR greater or lesser than 1.0 and not overlapping with 1.0 indicates that the exposure differs between groups. HR is another measure used for dichotomous variables and is calculated as the hazard in the exposed groups divided by the hazard in the unexposed groups. In longitudinal studies, a single estimate of HR summarises the experience from the entire follow-up period. Estimates of HR are interpreted in the same way as RR [4].

Without evidence that observes cases over time or compares cases and controls, the risk cannot be deemed as causal for tinnitus. Instead, it might only be correlational in nature. Unfortunately, for many tinnitus risk factors, much of the high-level evidence is not yet there to present a compelling message.

Environmental and Occupational Risk Factors for Tinnitus

The underlying pathophysiology of tinnitus is unclear. The most widely reported risk factor for tinnitus is hearing loss/hearing difficulty with tinnitus seen as a potential consequence of compensatory neuroplastic events in the central auditory pathway [5]. But even so, a multinational prevalence survey conducted on 11,427 adults in Europe reported that 6.5% people with no hearing difficulty experience tinnitus, and approximately 30% with severe hearing difficulty do not experience tinnitus [6] This relationship is also predisposed to confounding by factors such as age, noise exposure, and ototoxic medications which are additional known risk factors for both hearing problems and tinnitus [7]. Some of these factors are environmental, but many are not. These complexities make it challenging to tease apart the inter-relationships between tinnitus, hearing problems, and other risks such as environmental risks.

The WHO 2017 [3] report on preventing non-communicable diseases by reducing environmental risk factors focuses on the reduction of exposure to hazardous environmental and occupational risks. It is interesting to note that, according to WHO, current estimates of the disease burden from non-communicable diseases due to environmental risks are likely to be underestimated. This is because of the challenges in assessing associations with long lag times, multiple toxic exposures, complex pathways, or difficulties in assessing exposures.

Air Pollution

To our knowledge, there are no specific studies examining the association between tinnitus and exposure to poor air quality. However, we found one interesting cross-sectional study exploring the association between hearing loss and exposure to poor air quality. This study assessed auditory brainstem response (ABR) in participants living in the Metropolitan Mexico City area compared with matched controls living in clean air regions. The findings indicate that living in a polluted region significantly disrupted the ABR wave delay and inter-wave intervals which the authors interpret as preliminary evidence for the harmful effect of air pollution causing neuroinflammation and cochlear synaptopathy, leading to compensatory neuroplasticity and increased auditory gain [8]. In a retrospective cohort study using a Taiwanese health insurance database, there was increased risk of clinically diagnosed sensorineural hearing loss following increased exposure to air pollutants, namely carbon monoxide and nitrogen dioxide. Nitrogen dioxide is a reactive nitrogen species that can induce inflammation by oxidative stress thereby damaging hair cells. Carbon monoxide causes toxicity by impairing oxygen carrying capacity of blood, but there are no reports explaining its association with hearing loss [9]. Although these results are preliminary, given the pathophysiological links between hearing loss and tinnitus, it would not be unreasonable to extrapolate these predictions to tinnitus.

Chemical Exposures

A recent article gives us a succinct yet scholarly overview of the common chemical pollutants that cause damage to the peripheral auditory system [10]. The authors explain that environmental or occupational exposure to organic solvents and heavy metals are major causes of ototoxicity. Given that such exposures often occur at the same time, synergistic interactions may potentiate hearing damage in susceptible individuals. However, this is not supported by observations in at least one case-control study which showed that relative risk of tinnitus increases linearly as a function of the numbers of daily ototoxic exposures [11].

Many of the ototoxic organic solvents target the mid-frequency region of the cochlea leading to hearing problems, while others, such as styrene, are known to induce cochlear oxidative stress. The degree of hearing loss associated with exposure to these compounds depends on the type of organic solvent and its concentration level. Of further concern is that exposure to organic solvents may have a synergistic effect with exposure to noise. This enhances the damage to outer hair cells and increases the risk of noise-induced hearing loss. The authors raised particular concerns over benzene, ethyl benzene, toluene, and xylene since these make up around 60% of all non-methane volatile organic compounds in the urban atmosphere and they are highly ototoxic. These compounds originate from crude oil and petroleum products and are primarily released into the environment through vehicles in heavy traffic urban areas.

A longitudinal study on a US-based population has demonstrated associations between exposures of organic solvents and prevalence of high-frequency hearing loss for benzene (OR = 1.43, 95% CI = 1.15–1.78), ethylbenzene (OR = 1.24, 95% CI = 1.02–1.50), and toluene (OR = 1.27, 95% CI = 1.06–1.52) [12]. However, this was true only for the higher concentrations of exposure and none of the ORs in the multiple multivariate logistic regression analyses remained statistically significant ($p \geq 0.05$) between organic solvents and self-reported tinnitus after adjusting for covariates. The authors are cautious to point out that there is potential for information bias in the measurement of tinnitus, noise, and other covariates as study participants may incorrectly remember events from the past. They therefore called for further research to validate their findings.

Heavy metals such as cadmium, lead, cobalt, arsenic, and mercury are also ototoxic. For example, exposure to cadmium and lead damages the cochlear hair cells and induces oxidative stress, and cumulative exposures can therefore cause hearing problems. Cadmium is common in the ambient air in industrialised urban areas because it is released into the atmosphere when burning fossil fuels or incinerating municipal waste. It is also found in contaminated food such as shellfish and vegetables. Lead is common in batteries, solder, pipes, pottery, roofing materials, and in some cosmetics and paints.

Tobacco smoking is the most important single source of cadmium exposure in the general population. Exposure to secondhand smoke is recognised as an environmental and occupational risk factor. This can arise from a range of home, work, or social settings. Secondhand smoke contains the same toxic chemicals that are inhaled by smokers, including nicotine, carbon monoxide, benzene, formaldehyde, and cyanide. To our knowledge, there is only one study directly examining the association between tinnitus and secondhand smoke, and this was cross-sectional in design. From a sample of US high school and college students, a significant main effect of noise exposure on tinnitus occurrence and an interaction of second-hand smoke exposure and noise were revealed, but the regression analysis showed no main effect of secondhand smoke on tinnitus [13]. The motivation for this study may have come from an earlier study by one of the same authors which suggested harmful effects on central auditory processing. Specifically, that study found evidence of toxic effects of secondhand smoke exposure by evoked potentials with decreased ABR wave V/I amplitude ratio and longer (delayed) latency of the auditory middle latency Pb response in the exposed group compared to unexposed matched controls [14].

There is a much larger body of evidence on the risks of personal smoking for developing tinnitus. For example, results from a systematic review and meta-analysis of 20 such original studies give confidence in the claim that smoking significantly is associated with tinnitus [15]. In that study, no matter how smoking was defined it was found to increase the risk of developing tinnitus: current smoking (OR = 1.21, 95%CI = 1.09–1.35); former smoking (OR = 1.13, 95%CI = 1.01–1.26); and ever smoking (OR = 1.20, 95%CI = 1.11–1.30). This finding perhaps implies that even people who quit smoking might not reverse the risk. However, the authors are clear to point out that their result does not necessarily mean that smoking directly causes tinnitus. Importantly, smokers are known to differ from non-smokers in a number of relevant health behaviours which might also predispose to developing tinnitus. For example, smokers are more likely to be exposed to occupational or leisure noise and less likely to wear hearing protection in those noisy places. As such, tinnitus could instead be seen as the consequence of combined risky behaviours, and those risky behaviours might prevail even after the person has quit smoking.

At least one study has investigated the combined effects of multiple chemical exposures [11]. In this case-control study, cases were Australian military personnel deployed in international operations to East Timor and Bougainville in Southeast Asia, while controls were serving members not deployed to those regions. The authors paid particular attention to the impact of daily exposure to multiple potential ototoxic factors during deployment. The results of univariate logistic regression with self-reported moderate/severe tinnitus as the dependent variable showed increased risks from self-reported daily exposure to solvents and degreasing agents (OR = 2.02, 95% CI = 1.42–2.87), heavy metals (OR = 3.28, 95% CI = 2.01–5.37), engine exhaust causing eye irritation (OR = 3.08, 95% CI = 2.15–4.43), and intense smoke such as from fires (OR = 2.46, 95% CI = 1.30–4.67), as well as tobacco smoking (OR = 1.39, 95% CI = 1.06–1.82). A multivariable logistic regression to consider the potential impact of multiple concurrent exposures demonstrated that daily exposure to four or more ototoxic factors was associated with up to a four-fold increase in the risk of moderate/severe tinnitus (OR = 3.98, 95% CI = 2.25–7.05).

Noise Pollution

The WHO has recognised that noise (i.e. 'unwanted sounds') is a leading environmental nuisance in the European region, and the public complains about excessive noise more and more often [16]. In fact, noise exposure has been described as 'the new secondhand smoke' [17]. The most common environmental sources of noise pollution originate from: transportation (road traffic, railway, and aircraft), wind turbines, leisure activities (live music, use of personal listening devices, sporting events, etc.), and workplace settings.

Leisure activities represent a considerable source of excessive noise; especially for the younger generation. In 2008, the Scientific Committee on Emerging and Newly Identified Hazards and Risk (SCENIHR) [18] expressed the opinion that prolonged exposure to sounds from personal listening devices can result in temporary and permanent hearing threshold shifts and tinnitus. However, the scientific data available at the time on tinnitus were inadequate to draw firm conclusions. There are some compelling indicators from cross-sectional studies. For example, an internet-based population study found that high exposure to leisure music (OR = 1.39, 95% CI = 1.24–1.55), workplace noise (OR = 2.05, 95% CI = 1.48–2.82), hearing difficulty, and age were all independently associated with increased tinnitus [19]. However, even 10 years on from the SCENIHR report, new data are still inconclusive. For example, a systematic review published in 2017 on behalf of WHO concluded from the findings of five studies that there was no association between prolonged listening to loud music through personal listening devices and tinnitus, or the results were contradictory and all of the evidence was of low quality [20]. The same review failed to find any published studies assessing the association between noise from road traffic, railways, aircraft, and wind turbines on hearing loss or tinnitus.

Regarding occupational risks, noise-induced hearing loss is recognised by the European Union as one of the most prominent occupational diseases across the member states. In many commercial sectors, noise levels regularly exceed regulatory limits. In 2005, the European Agency for Health and Safety at Work [21] identified sectors with the highest levels of ambient noise; namely agriculture, construction, engineering, woodworking, foundries and the foods and drinks, and entertainment industries. Unsurprisingly therefore, these are the sectors with a high prevalence of hearing loss in the workforce (i.e. agriculture, forestry and fishing, mining and quarrying, extraction, energy and water supply, manufacturing, and construction). The report suggested that employees with full-time non-permanent contracts were most exposed to loud noise. This group often has less information available relating to health and safety issues, less training, and less formal supervision and control in the workplace. The report also identified a worrying trend towards exposure to loud noise affecting increasing numbers of younger workers, perhaps in combination with the risks posed by unsafe music listening behaviours.

The effect of noise pollution on tinnitus is somewhat expected given that noise-induced hearing loss is a well-known risk factor for hearing. The pathophysiology of tinnitus is often explained as a maladaptive neuroplastic response within the central auditory pathways to sensory deprivation due to hearing loss. There are several potential mechanisms. One is the proposal that hyper-excitability within the central auditory system occurs through the downregulation of inhibitory cortical processes following damage to the cochlea or to auditory projection pathways [22]. Another is temporal synchrony in spontaneous firing patterns of neurons in the auditory cortex [23].

Other Occupational Risks

Of the occupational risks described in Table 6.1, arguably the most relevant for tinnitus is that of stress. Stress is the body's reaction to harmful situations (whether real or perceived) and it's generally accepted that the long-term effects of stress are damaging to physical and psychological health. Stress triggers the release of stress hormones; cortisol and adrenaline. Cortisol mediates the endocrine stress response and is secreted by the adrenal gland (kidney) as the end product of the hypothalamic-pituitary-adrenal (HPA) axis which involves structures in the central nervous and endocrine systems [24] (see Fig. 6.1a). Cortisol increases sugars (glucose) in the bloodstream, alters immune system responses, and suppresses the digestive system. Adrenaline increases heart rate, elevates blood pressure, and boosts energy supplies. Long-term activation of the stress-response system and the overexposure to cortisol and other stress hormones can disrupt almost all of the body's processes. In this way, stress can be either a triggering or aggravating factor for many diseases and pathological conditions (please see also the role of stress in animal models as discussed in Chap. 23). It is suggested that chronic tinnitus may already lead to a long-term dysregulation of the HPA axis via the connectivity between the auditory system and HPA axis via the limbic system [24] (see Fig. 6.1b). This misbalances the negative feedback that is responsible for maintaining homeostasis under normal conditions. Work-related stress, as well as other stressors, can push this further off balance.

Table 6.1 Environmental and occupational risk factors defined by WHO (2017) [3]

Risk	Description/examples
Air pollution	Transport emissions, energy generation and industrial emissions, and domestic lighting and heating
Chemical exposure	Organic solvents, heavy metals, pesticides, asbestos, formaldehyde, and second-hand tobacco smoke
Noise pollution	Leisure noise (e.g. prolonged exposure to loud music), occupational noise (e.g. industrial noise, military, musicians), and transportation noise (e.g. vehicles and aircraft)
Other occupational risks	Ergonomic factors and injuries (e.g. poor work postures, prolonged sitting, prolonged computer use), working conditions (e.g. sedentary life style), occupational stress, and work-life imbalance
Radiation exposure	Exposures to ionizing (e.g. radon) and ultra-violet radiation
Urban planning	Transport infrastructure facilitating walking and cycling, and favourable land-use patterns

A search of 'occupational stress' AND 'tinnitus' revealed a small number of recently published cross-sectional studies indicating stress as a risk factor. One survey of bus drivers in Bangkok, Thailand, found that job strain as measured by the ratio between demand and control was significantly associated with self-reported tinnitus (OR = 1.55, CI 95% = 1.17–2.05) [24]. Similarly, a perceived imbalance between effort and reward reported by hospital nurses in Urumqi, Northwest China, was predictive of self-reported tinnitus (OR = 1.49, CI 95% = 1.11–2.00) [25]. Both sets of findings came from a logistic regression model which adjusted for age, marital status, education, smoking, alcohol consumption, physical exercise, and occupational noise exposure. Another observational study surveyed workers in a deep gold mine in Jilin province, Northeast China [26]. Common adverse effects for the 179 respondents were tinnitus (47%), hearing loss (44%), and being easily tired (31%). Multivariate analyses showed that reporting more than one adverse effect in the deep-underground and continuously spending more than 8 hours in this environment were significant predictors of psychological problems as measured by the Symptom Checklist-90-Revised (SCL-90-R).

In a cross-sectional study on call-centre operators in Taiwan, a multivariate logistic regression analysis showed female gender (OR = 1.67, 95% CI = 1.15–2.43) and perceived high level of stress (OR = 1.24, 95% CI = 1.43–3.51) to be strongly associated with tinnitus, with a significant interaction between gender and stress level (OR = 3.27, 95% CI = 1.40–7.66) [27]. Occupational stress was also associated with other physical discomforts and health complaints such as eye strain, hoarse throat, chronic cough, peptic ulcer, chest tightness, frequent urination, and musculoskeletal discomfort.

Radiation Exposure

Radiation refers to energy and is ubiquitous in our everyday lives, from visible light to radiowaves and X-rays. The properties of the energy include oscillating electric and magnetic fields, and so it's often referred to by its other name 'electromagnetic waves' (Fig. 6.2). The electromagnetic spectrum covers electromagnetic waves with frequencies from below 1 Hz to above 10^{25} Hz, corresponding to wavelengths from thousands of kilometres to the fraction of the size of an atom.

The greatest risk of exposure to human health is from 'ionising radiation' which includes energy in the high ultraviolet radiation range, X-rays and gamma rays (Fig. 6.2). Exposure to radiation in this range is sufficient to cause chemical reactions in living organisms. Nevertheless, normal everyday exposure to ionising radia-

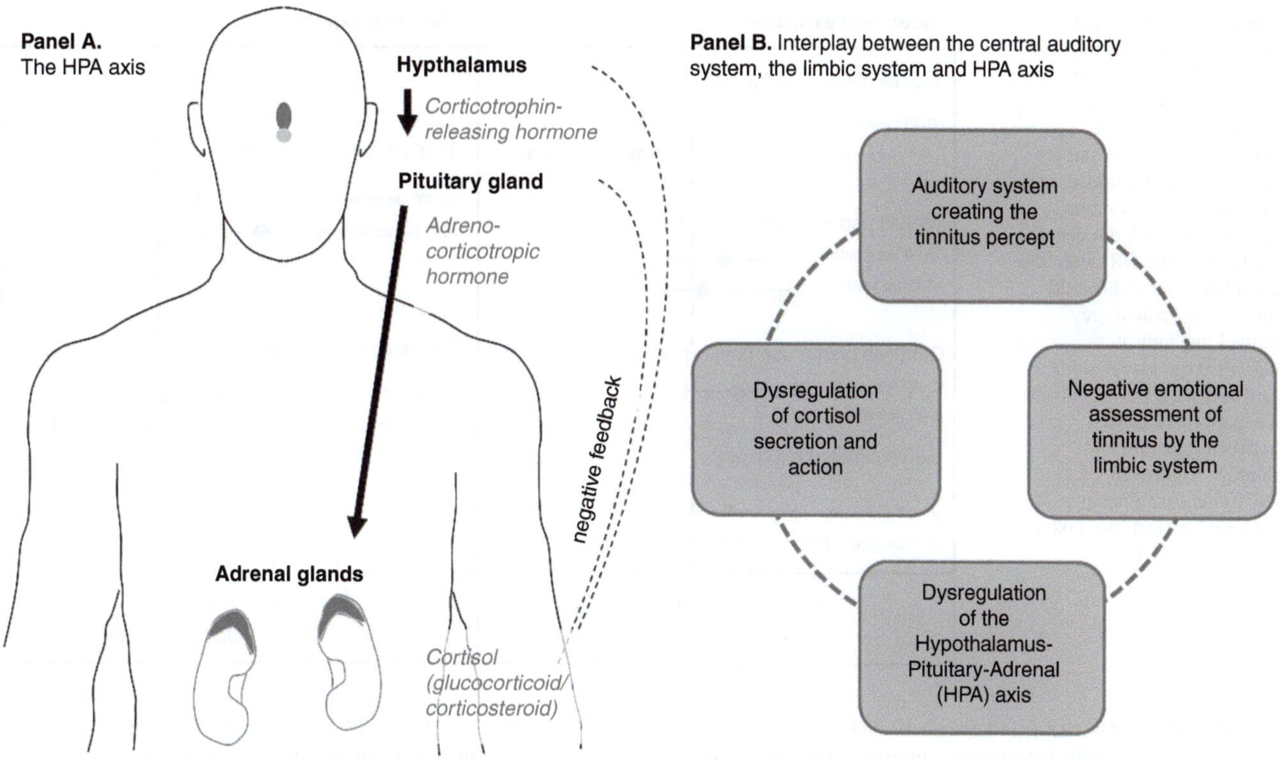

Fig. 6.1 Panel (**a**) illustrates the hypothalamic-pituitary-adrenal (HPA) axis which involves structures in the central nervous and endocrine systems that determine the control of cortisol release as part of the human stress response. Panel (**b**) illustrates the interplay between this HPA axis, and the central auditory system, and limbic system in the context of tinnitus. Panel B is derived from de Kloet and Szczepek [24]

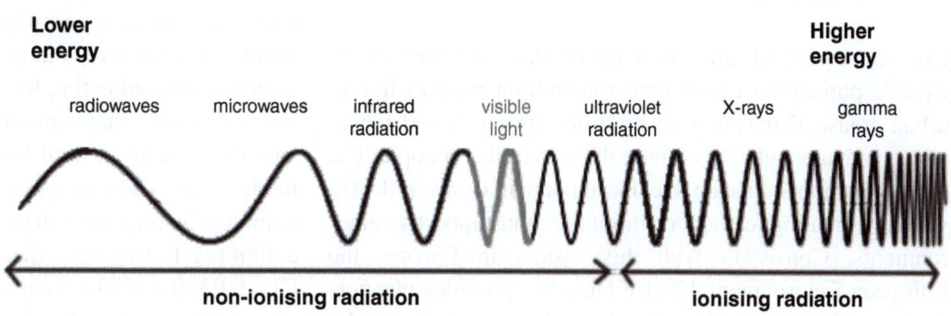

Fig. 6.2 The electromagnetic spectrum

tion is low. Instead, the greatest public opinion shows a general concern about chronic exposure to non-ionising radiation, particularly radio-frequency waves (Fig. 6.2) such as those produced by mobile phones and cordless phones (near-field personal exposure) or broadcast transmitters (far-field residential exposure). The risk to tinnitus from these sources has been assessed in at least one cohort study [28]. Here the authors surveyed the Basel population in Switzerland at baseline and one-year follow-up to assess the association between exposure level and tinnitus. Two levels of exposures were classified as 50–90th percentile and >90th percentile, compared to the <50th percentile as reference. Modelling was adjusted for other major environmental risk factors including degree of urbanity, physical activity, occupational risk factors such as stress and nightshift work, demographics, and lifestyle. Results showed no evidence that exposure to radio-frequency electromagnetic fields in everyday life puts people at risk of developing tinnitus (Fig. 6.3). However, the authors do caveat these findings by saying that absolute magnitude of exposures was substantially below the national legislative standard limits.

Certain individuals claim to experience electromagnetic hypersensitivity because they react to the presence of radiofrequencies at extremely low intensities. A recent review of this literature suggests that many hypersensitive individuals appear to have impaired detoxification systems that become overloaded by excessive oxidative stress [29]. As we saw in section "Chemical Exposures", this can have direct negative physiological effects on the central auditory system. Whether

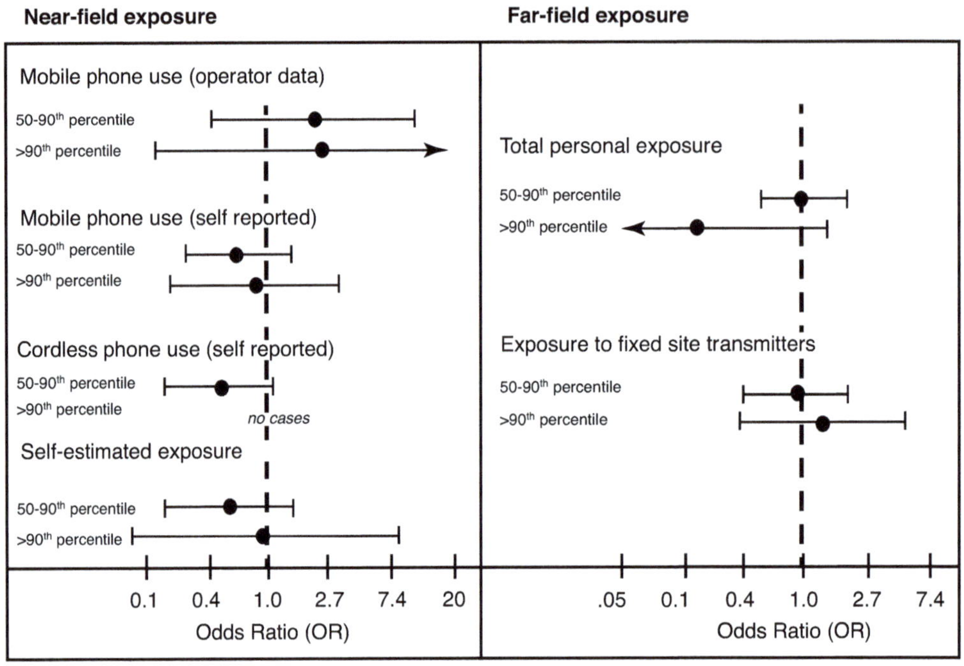

Fig. 6.3 Results of the logistic regression analyses for the cohort ($n = 455$) showing the association between the different exposure surrogates and the development of tinnitus over the one-year observation period. The black dot denotes the value of the OR, with 95% confidence intervals (solid lines). The vertical grey dashed line indicates OR = 1.0 (no association). Leftward ORs (<1.0) indicate a negative association between exposure and tinnitus. Rightward ORs (>1.0) indicate a positive association. (Data are taken from Frei et al. [28])

or not hypersensitivity predisposes to a risk of tinnitus from exposure to radio-frequency energy remains to be determined.

Urban Planning

Growing industrialisation now means that over 50% of the world's population (more than four billion people) live in urban areas, increasingly in high density cities and mega-cities, with a population of more than ten million people. The United Nation's Sustainable Development Goals reflect a vision of creating resilient communities and supportive environments. Consistent with this vision, in Europe, the European Environmental Noise Directive provides planners in all member states with a legislative framework for implementing specialised 'smart' tools that inform noise management action plans and ensure that European cities are intelligently developed (Fig. 6.4).

The evidence for noise pollution as a risk factor for tinnitus has been presented in section "Noise Pollution". Yet, the urban environment has a much broader impact on the risk of non-communicable disease with respect to the degree to which it promotes a sedentary lifestyle and obesity and discourages physical activity. Transport infrastructure such as footpaths and cycle routes that facilitate walking and cycling and favourable land-use patterns such as parks and pavements are associated with protection against a range of non-communicable diseases and obesity.

Many studies have confirmed that good urban design qualities can play a role in encouraging physical activity [31]. Physical activity can therefore be seen as a proxy measure for the urban environment. Protection against the risk of tinnitus has been examined in at least one cohort study. The National Health and Nutrition Examination Survey (NHANES) in the US, led by the Centers for Disease Control and Prevention, has collected data using accelerometer-assessed physical activity and self-reported tinnitus at least over the period 2005–2006 [32]. For adolescents, after adjusting for gender, systolic blood pressure, poverty status, race/ethnicity, cotinine, body mass index, and age, results showed that every one-minute increase in moderate-to-vigorous physical activity reduced the risk of a tinnitus lasting more than 3 months by 4% compared with a tinnitus lasting less than 3 months (OR = 0.96, 95% CI = 0.93–0.99). For older adults with hypertension, results showed that every 60-minute increase in light-intensity physical activity reduced the risk of tinnitus by 21% compared with no tinnitus (OR = 0.79, 95% CI = 0.65–0.96). Indirect benefits to tinnitus from physical activity could be that it generally promotes good cardiovascular health and improves health-related quality of life. The clinical implications of these findings are that hearing healthcare professionals are encouraged to promote physical activity to help prevent or treat tinnitus. At least one cross-sectional study also reported that higher levels of physical activity were significantly associated with lower levels of tinnitus severity, as well as improved health-related quality of life [33]. This is positive corroborating evidence from an independent US sample and with self-reported data using the Godin Leisure-Time Exercise Question, even if direct causality cannot be established.

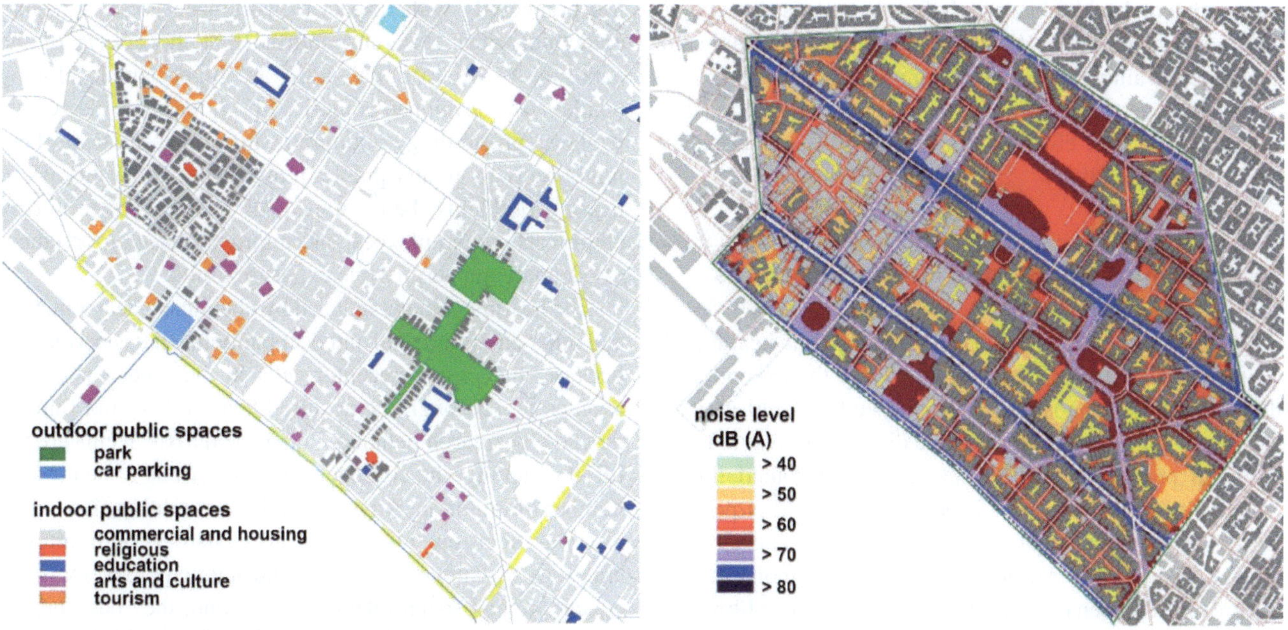

Fig. 6.4 Strategic maps of Thessaloniki city centre, Greece. The left hand map shows the predominant uses of the public spaces and buildings, while the right hand map shows ambient noise levels. Noise levels are averaged over a 24-h period and include all sound sources such as road, railway, and industry. (Adapted from Vogiatzis and Remy (Figs. 12 and 14) [30])

Physical activity also protects against obesity which strains the body's circulatory system leading to higher blood pressure, lower circulation, and poor oxygenation of cells, including hair cells in the inner ear. NHANES data collection for the period 2007–2010 included data on obesity, self-reported physical activity, and hearing loss [34]. The questionnaire that was used asked about time spend during sedentary activity (i.e. inactivity), while hearing loss was assessed by full audiometric examination. The multivariate analysis adjusted for age, sex, race/ethnicity, obesity, poverty income ratio, ear infections, loud noise exposure, and smoking. Results for hearing showed that obese adolescents had a greater risk of high-frequency hearing loss (defined as ≥15 dB HL in either ear for the average 3–6 kHz) compared to the normal weight adolescents (OR = 1.95, 95% CI = 1.19–3.21), and this association remained even when the hours of sedentary activity were added as co-variate in the model. Tinnitus was not assessed in this study.

Preventive Strategies

The United Nations argues that it's essential to tackle non-communicable disease through the reduction of exposure to hazardous environmental and occupational risks in order to achieve its Sustainable Development Goals, particularly goal 3 which encourages healthy lives and promotes well-being for all the world's citizens, across the lifespan.

Excessive noise exposure has been identified as a global health hazard. In the US, the National Institute for Occupational Safety and Health (NIOSH) recommends that workers should not be exposed to noise at a level that exceeds 85 decibels (dBA) 8-h time-weighted average [34]. In other countries, similar legislative directives define standards for employers to ensure that occupational noise exposure is limited in the workplace. Employers are required to conduct risk assessment, and where noise levels exceed, the legal limit protection measures must be provided such as use of personal hearing protective devices and regular hearing screening using audiometric testing [35–37].

While preventive strategies for hearing provide protection against damaging noise levels, other forms of protection are required if the workplace has exposures to non-acoustic occupational risks. One article set out the scientific rationale for using hearing conservation strategies in noisy workplaces where workers are exposed to ototoxic chemicals, even when those ambient noise levels fall within the regulatory limits [38]. The concern here is that noise exposure may potentiate or interact synergistically with numerous toxic substances. The combination often results in hearing loss that can be temporary or permanent, depending on the level of noise, the type and dose of the chemical, and the duration of the exposure.

In the US, the Occupational Safety and Health Administration has set standards for employers to maintain exposures below the permissible noise exposure limit, where there is chemical exposure as well [39]. Even in workers exposed to ototoxic substances below the permissible chemical exposure limit, employers should provide relevant health and safety training, use engineering controls such as isolation, enclosures, and ventilation, offer personal protective equipment, and/or eliminate unnecessary tasks that expose their workforce [39].

Concluding Remarks and Future Directions

There is a strong geopolitical diversity in public health policies and in healthcare systems and, with the exception of European Union, most are country-specific. Multi-national studies of some non-communicable diseases have noted variation in prevalence estimates and have attributed this to country-specific differences in economic prosperity/poverty, access to medicines and health care, climatic and environmental factors, and racial composition. Common diseases where this has been observed include breast cancer [40], type 1 diabetes [41], and type 2 diabetes [42]. A global systematic review reported a positive correlation between country-level affluence and the incidence of childhood type 1 diabetes [41], and a positive correlation between the relative change in Gross Domestic Product (GDP) per capita and the relative change in the disease over between the periods 1975–1999 and 2000–2017. Although genetic susceptibility is known to differ across ethnic groups, these country-specific differences cannot fully explain the global variability and the increase in incidence observed over these five decades. In the case of breast cancer, the more affluent EU countries report a higher incidence of breast cancer, attributable to the longer established Western lifestyle [39]. But at the same time, these countries also show a higher survival rate, attributable to the higher availability of effective treatments. Generally speaking, countries with a higher GDP per capita are known to allocate more resources to health and safety [43]. However, for tinnitus, the patterns of risk and survival (recovery) might not necessarily be the same because there are no available effective treatments for hearing loss and tinnitus.

A country's economic affluence is commonly measured by the Purchasing Power Parity or GDP per capita. For hearing loss and tinnitus, there is no real evidence on the association between a country's economic status and the risk of developing hearing-related problems. Perhaps the lack of multi-national studies has prevented such data explorations. Nevertheless, on an individual level, personal wealth has been associated with a greater likelihood of experiencing a clinically significant tinnitus [44]. Interestingly, this association has been explained by other (non-economic) factors associated with higher socioeconomic status such as less exposure to noisy industrial workplace, greater uptake of hearing protection, greater expectations about good health, and expecting or insisting upon onward medical referral. More generally with respect to workplace noise exposure, epidemiological research confirms that the effects of the exposure to occupational noise are higher in developing compared to developed countries [45] (please see also Chap. 4 on the epidemiology of tinnitus). Preventive strategies here might reply to greater public of awareness about the risk to hearing problems, better uptake of hearing protection by employers and employees, and improved legal enforcement of occupational permissible exposure limits.

The hearing damage induced by chemicals, heavy metals, and other environmental and occupational risks is permanent because the sensory receptor cells in the inner ear cannot regenerate. Although the acquired hearing loss and tinnitus induced by environmental pollutants and toxic agents are not life-threatening, the consequences are serious to health in a number of important ways. First, these conditions have devastating effects on children (see also Chap. 39 on tinnitus in children) by impairing speech and language development, education, and social integration. Second, they have broad-ranging and negative effects on quality of life. Third, they are linked to social isolation, cognitive decline, dementia, depression, and even suicide. Fourth, they impose a huge economic burden through loss of productivity at work, unemployment, and disability claims. As the prevalence of hearing loss and tinnitus worldwide is estimated to rise, there is a critical need to identify emerging risk factors that pollute the environment and discover effective prevention and treatment strategies.

Generally speaking, studies assessing risks for developing tinnitus tend to focus on individual-level characteristics, such as age, gender, hearing status, comorbidities, and lifestyle. It certainly makes sense to identify high-risk individuals and focus on personalised assessment and management techniques, especially given the high degree of tinnitus heterogeneity. Nonetheless, ignoring environmental and occupational risks at a population level, or group level, perhaps detracts from considering tinnitus as a public health problem.

The authors of the studies presented in this chapter have sometimes taken the opportunity to identify unanswered questions to define the research agenda. With respect to the risk of noise exposure through leisure activities, Śliwińska-Kowalska and Zaborowski [20] suggest that further evidence is needed to understand the consequence of long-term exposures to leisure music on hearing and to provide practical guidance for personal listening device users.

Oftentimes, the authors of systematic reviews comment on the low quality of included studies which prevents them from drawing firm conclusions or recommendations. For example, Śliwińska-Kowalska and Zaborowski [20] excluded 33 out of 38 potentially relevant articles because there was either a lack of data on any audiometric assessment which prevented them from determining the risk of noise exposure through using personal listening devices, or a lack of information about the noise levels that people exposed themselves to. More generally, the WHO Guideline Development Group has written about the challenge in conducting a long-term objective exposure assessment for assessing the risk of hearing loss due to environmental exposure to noise. Specifically, the group highlighted a need for research to develop a comprehensive methodology as an alternative to the equal energy principle outlined in the ISO standard [46].

A deeper understanding of modifiable risk and protective factors is imperative for the prevention of disease and injury, through public health campaigns and government legislation. For example, smoke-free legislation is a good example of how nations can respond to encourage positive health behaviours. Smoking bans protect non-smokers from the dangers of passive smoking and encourage smokers to quit or to reduce consumption. Adopting socio-ecological perspectives of health encourages us to assess how multiple levels of influence, such as those related to behavioural and environmental factors, affect health and disease among populations, and how these contexts are interrelated. The dynamic interplay among behavioural and environmental factors adds to the complexity of addressing public health problems, requiring interdisciplinary collaborations to develop innovative, multi-pronged solutions. We hope that by synthesizing the disparate evidence on environmental and occupational risk factors for tinnitus within a single chapter, we can inspire and motivate others to rise to find relevant strategies for reducing tinnitus risk.

References

1. Centers for Disease Control and Prevention (CDC). Principles of epidemiology in public health practice. An introduction to applied epidemiology and biostatistics. 3rd ed. Atlanta: US Department of Health and Human Services; 2012.
2. Prüss-Ustün A, van Deventer E, Mudu P, Campbell-Lendrum D, Vickers C, Ivanov I, Forastiere F, Gumy S, Dora C, Adair-Rohani H, Neira M. Environmental risks and non-communicable diseases. BMJ. 2019;364:l265. https://doi.org/10.1136/bmj.l265.
3. World Health Organization. Preventing non-communicable diseases (NCDs) by reducing environmental risk factors. Geneva: World Health Organization; 2017. Accessed 19 January 2021.
4. Biswas R, Hall DA. Prevalence, incidence, and risk factors for tinnitus. In: Current topics in behavioral neurosciences. Berlin, Heidelberg: Springer; 2020. https://doi.org/10.1007/7854_2020_154.
5. Baguley D, McFerran D, Hall DA. Tinnitus. Lancet. 2013;382(9904):1600–7. https://doi.org/10.1016/S0140-6736(13)60142-7.
6. Biswas R, Lugo A, Akeroyd MA, Schlee W, Gallus S, Hall DA. Tinnitus prevalence in Europe: a multi-country cross-sectional population study. The Lancet Regional Health-Europe. 2022;12:100250.
7. Eggermont JJ. Tinnitus and neural plasticity (Tonndorf lecture at the XIth International Tinnitus Seminar, Berlin, 2014). Hear Res. 2015;319:1–11. https://doi.org/10.1016/j.heares.2014.10.002.
8. Calderón-Garcidueñas L, Kulesza RJ, Mansour Y, et al. Increased gain in the auditory pathway, Alzheimer's disease continuum, and air pollution: peripheral and central auditory system dysfunction evolves across pediatric and adult urbanites. J Alzheimers Dis. 2019;70(4):1275–86. https://doi.org/10.3233/jad-190405.
9. Chang KH, Tsai SC, Lee CY, Chou RH, Fan HC, Lin FC, Lin CL, Hsu YC. Increased risk of sensorineural hearing loss as a result of exposure to air pollution. Int J Environ Res Public Health. 2020;17(6):1969. https://doi.org/10.3390/ijerph17061969.
10. Rosati R, Jamesdaniel S. Environmental exposures and hearing loss. Int J Environ Res Public Health. 2020;17(13):4879. https://doi.org/10.3390/ijerph17134879.
11. Kirk KM, McGuire A, Nielsen L, Cosgrove T, McClintock C, Nasveld PE, Treloar SA. Self-reported tinnitus and ototoxic exposures among deployed Australian Defence Force personnel. Mil Med. 2011;176(4):461–7. https://doi.org/10.7205/milmed-d-10-00353.
12. Staudt AM, Whitworth KW, Chien LC, Whitehead LW, Ruiz G, de Porras D. Association of organic solvents and occupational noise on hearing loss and tinnitus among adults in the U.S., 1999-2004. Int Arch Occup Environ Health. 2019;92(3):403–13. https://doi.org/10.1007/s00420-019-01419-2.
13. Money LE, Ramkissoon I. Effects of secondhand smoke exposure and noise exposure on tinnitus occurrence in college students and adolescents. J Am Acad Audiol. 2020;31(4):286–91. https://doi.org/10.3766/jaaa.19032.
14. Ramkissoon I, Batavia M. Effects of secondhand smoke exposure on hearing and auditory evoked potentials, ABR and AMLR in young adults. J Am Acad Audiol. 2018;29(8):685–95. https://doi.org/10.3766/jaaa.16161.
15. Veile A, Zimmermann H, Lorenz E, Becher H. Is smoking a risk factor for tinnitus? A systematic review, meta-analysis and estimation of the population attributable risk in Germany. BMJ Open. 2018;8(2):e016589. https://doi.org/10.1136/bmjopen-2017-016589.
16. World Health Organisation (WHO). 2021. https://www.euro.who.int/en/health-topics/environment-and-health/noise/data-and-statistics Accessed 10 Jan 2021.
17. Van Dort P, Schöner G. Noise exposure 'the new secondhand smoke' - how is it addressed in building certification schemes. IOP Conf Ser: Earth Environ Sci. 2020;588:032063. https://doi.org/10.1088/1755-1315/588/3/032063.
18. Scientific Committee on Emerging and Newly Identified Health Risks (SCENIHR). Potential health risks of exposure to noise from personal music players and mobile phones including a music playing function. Brussels: European Commission; 2008.
19. Moore DR, Zobay O, Mackinnon RC, Whitmer WM, Akeroyd MA. Lifetime leisure music exposure associated with increased frequency of tinnitus. Hear Res. 2017;347:18–27. https://doi.org/10.1016/j.heares.2016.10.030.
20. Śliwińska-Kowalska M, Zaborowski K. WHO environmental noise guidelines for the European region: a systematic review on environmental noise and permanent hearing loss and tinnitus. Int J Environ Res Public Health. 2017;14(10):E1139.
21. European Agency for Health and Safety at Work. Risk observatory: thematic report. Noise in figures. Luxembourg: Office for Official Publications of the European Communities; 2005. Accessed 19 January 2021.
22. Eggermont JJ, Roberts LE. The neuroscience of tinnitus. Trends Neurosci. 2004;27(11):676–82. https://doi.org/10.1016/j.tins.2004.08.010.
23. Noreña AJ, Eggermont JJ. Changes in spontaneous neural activity immediately after an acoustic trauma: implications for neural correlates of tinnitus. Hear Res. 2003;183(1–2):137–53. https://doi.org/10.1016/s0378-5955(03)00225-9.

24. de Kloet ER, Szczepek AJ. Stress and glucocorticoid action in the brain and ear: implications for tinnitus. In: Szczepek AJ, Mazurek B, editors. Tinnitus and stress: an interdisciplinary companion for healthcare professionals. Cham: Springer; 2017. p. 7–35. https://doi.org/10.1007/978-3-319-58397-6_2.
25. Li J, Kaewboonchoo O, Jiang Y, Naknoi S, Loerbroks A. A stressful work environment is associated with tinnitus: initial evidence from Asia. Gen Hosp Psychiatry. 2017;47:A1–3. https://doi.org/10.1016/j.genhosppsych.2017.04.010.
26. Liu J, Liu Y, Ma T, Gao M, Zhang R, Wu J, Zou J, Liu S, Xie H. Subjective perceptions and psychological distress associated with the deep underground: a cross-sectional study in a deep gold mine in China. Medicine (Baltimore). 2019;98(22):e15571. https://doi.org/10.1097/MD.0000000000015571.
27. Lin Y-H, Chen C-Y, Lu S-Yi. Physical discomfort and psychosocial job stress among male and female operators at telecommunication call centers in Taiwan. Appl Ergon. 2009;40(4):561–8. https://doi.org/10.1016/j.apergo.2008.02.024.
28. Frei P, Mohler E, Braun-Fahrländer C, Fröhlich J, Neubauer G, Röösli M, the QUALIFEX-team. Cohort study on the effects of everyday life radio frequency electromagnetic field exposure on non-specific symptoms and tinnitus. Environ Int. 2012;38:29–36. https://doi.org/10.1016/j.envint.2011.08.002.
29. Stein Y, Udasin IG. Electromagnetic hypersensitivity (EHS, microwave syndrome) – review of mechanisms. Environ Res. 2020;186:109445. https://doi.org/10.1016/j.envres.2020.109445.
30. Vogiatzis K, Remy N. Environmental noise mapping as a smart urban tool development. In: Bobek V, editor. Smart Urban development. IntechOpen; 2019. https://doi.org/10.5772/intechopen.88449.
31. Sivam A, Karuppannan S, Koohsari MJ, Sivam A. Does urban design influence physical activity in the reduction of obesity? A review of evidence. The Open Urban Stud J. 2012;2012(5):14–21. https://doi.org/10.2174/1874942901205010014.
32. Loprinzi PD, Lee H, Gilham B, Cardinal BJ. Association between accelerometer-assessed physical activity and tinnitus, NHANES 2005–2006. Res Q Exerc Sport. 2013;84(2):177–85. https://doi.org/10.1080/02701367.2013.784840.
33. Carpenter-Thompson JR, McAuley E, Husain FT. Physical activity, tinnitus severity, and improved quality of life. Ear Hear. 2015;36(5):574–81. https://doi.org/10.1097/AUD.0000000000000169.
34. Scinicariello F, Carroll Y, Eichwald J, et al. Association of obesity with hearing impairment in adolescents. Sci Rep. 2019;9:1877. https://doi.org/10.1038/s41598-018-37739-5.
35. US Department of Health and Human Services. Preventing occupational hearing loss. A practical guide. 1996. https://www.cdc.gov/niosh/docs/96-110/pdfs/96-110.pdf?id=10.26616/NIOSHPUB96110. Accessed 19 Jan 2021.
36. EU Directive 2003/10/EC. 2003. https://eur-lex.europa.eu/legal-content/EN/TXT/?uri=CELEX%3A02003L0010-20190726. Accessed 20 Jan 2021.
37. Safe Work Australia. Australian work health and safety strategy 2012–2022. 2017. https://www.safeworkaustralia.gov.au/system/files/documents/1902/australian-work-health-safety-strategy-2012-2022v2.pdf. Accessed 19 Jan 2021.
38. Morata TC. Promoting hearing health and the combined risk of noise-induced hearing loss and ototoxicity. Audiol Med. 2007;5(1):33–40. https://doi.org/10.1080/16513860601159018.
39. US Department of Labor. Occupational Safety and Health Agency. Preventing hearing loss caused by chemical (ototoxicity) and noise exposure. 2018. https://www.osha.gov/dts/shib/shib030818.html. Accessed 19 Jan 2021.
40. Dafni U, Tsourti Z, Alatsathianos I. Breast cancer statistics in the European Union: incidence and survival across European countries. Breast Care (Basel). 2019;14(6):344–53. https://doi.org/10.1159/000503219.
41. Gomez-Lopera N, Pineda-Trujillo N, Diaz-Valencia PA. Correlating the global increase in type 1 diabetes incidence across age groups with national economic prosperity: a systematic review. World J Diabetes. 2019;10(12):560–80. https://doi.org/10.4239/wjd.v10.i12.560.
42. Haynes-Maslow L, Leone LA. Examining the relationship between the food environment and adult diabetes prevalence by county economic and racial composition: an ecological study. BMC Public Health. 2017;17:648. https://doi.org/10.1186/s12889-017-4658-0.
43. World Health Organization. 2016. Global Health Observatory data repository. https://apps.who.int/gho/data/view.main.GHEDCHEGDPSHA2011WBv?lang=en. Accessed 19 Jan 2021.
44. Martinez C, Wallenhorst C, McFerran D, Hall DA. Incidence rates of clinically significant tinnitus: 10-year trend from a cohort study in England. Ear Hear. 2015;36(3):e69–75. https://doi.org/10.1097/AUD.0000000000000121.
45. Nandi SS, Dhatrak SV. Occupational noise-induced hearing loss in India. Indian J Occupat Environ Med. 2008;12(2):53–6. https://doi.org/10.4103/0019-5278.43260.
46. World Health Organization (WHO). Environmental noise guidelines for the European Region. Copenhagen: World Health Organization; 2018. https://www.euro.who.int/__data/assets/pdf_file/0008/383921/noise-guidelines-eng.pdf.

Tinnitus Heterogeneity, Different Types of Tinnitus, and Gender Aspects

7

Berthold Langguth

Abstract

Tinnitus is a highly heterogeneous condition with respect to its perceptual characteristics, its etiology, its comorbidities, and its burden. Different forms of tinnitus also differ in their pathophysiology and presumably in their response to specific treatments. Thus, tinnitus heterogeneity is a major challenge in the identification of efficient tinnitus treatments.

Several strategies have been applied to identify more homogeneous tinnitus subtypes. In particular, it has been tried to identify subtypes from large databases. These approaches suggest that the majority of tinnitus patients cannot be categorized in clearly delineated (i.e. distinct) subtypes. Instead, the heterogeneity is better explained by patient characteristics falling along various continua.

This has important implications for both clinical management and research.

In order to optimize treatment for the individual patient, a personalized treatment plan should be developed, considering the tinnitus profile, the comorbidities, the psychological distress, the gender, and the previous treatment experiences of the patient. Moreover, it is essential to consider tinnitus heterogeneity in research designs.

B. Langguth (✉)
Department of Psychiatry and Psychotherapy, University of Regensburg, Bezirksklinikum, Regensburg, Germany
e-mail: Berthold.Langguth@medbo.de

W. Schlee et al. (eds.), *Textbook of Tinnitus*, https://doi.org/10.1007/978-3-031-35647-6_7

Graphical Abstract

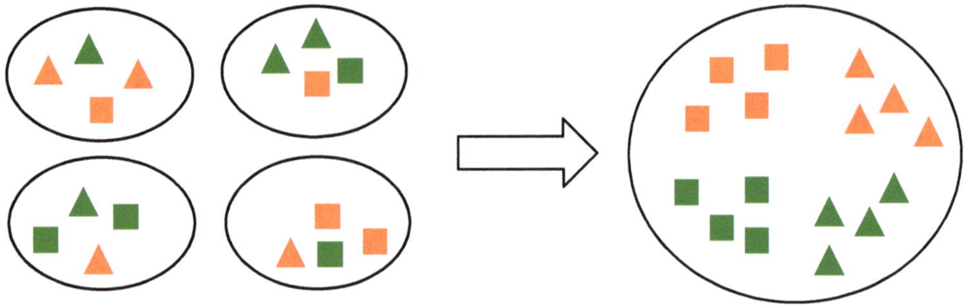

Tinnitus is a heterogeneous condition:
• investigation of small samples results in incongruent results
• one possibility to address this heterogeneity is the pooling of these samples in order to identify homogeneous subgroups

One strategy to better understand the heterogeneity is the creation of large patient databases based on standardized clinical assessm e n t

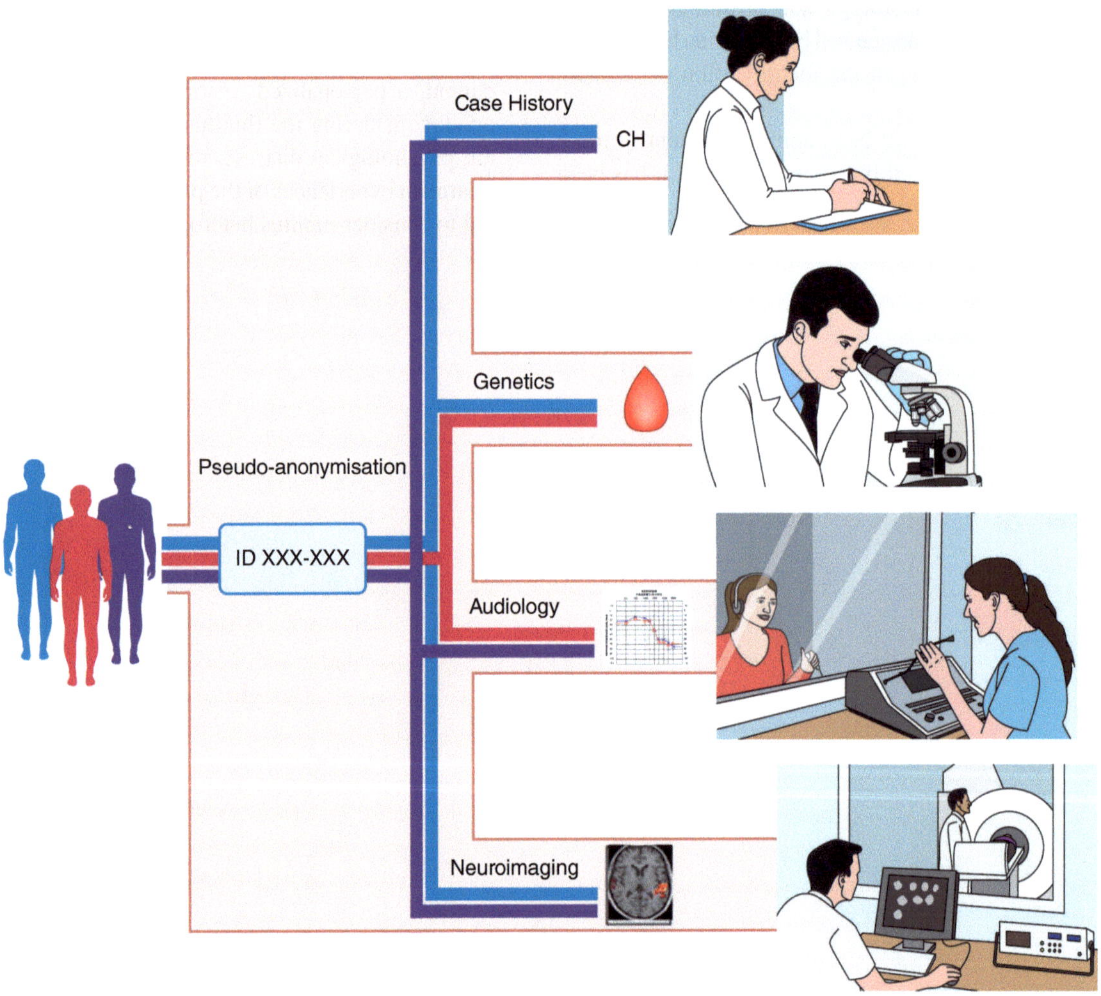

Highlights

- Tinnitus with its numerous pathophysiological mechanisms and clinical manifestations is a highly heterogeneous condition.
- Tinnitus in males and females differs in prevalence, appearance, and response to treatment.
- Tinnitus heterogeneity has hampered both fundamental and clinical research.
- Tinnitus heterogeneity should be considered in research by using appropriate research designs and in clinical management by personalized treatment.

Tinnitus Heterogeneity

Tinnitus studies are characterized by a large variability in the results. This variability is observed both in treatment studies and in studies that address the pathophysiology of tinnitus, e.g. by using neuroimaging methods. This variability in results suggests that tinnitus is a heterogenous condition and this heterogeneity in turn might explain that tinnitus remains a scientific and clinical enigma, despite a substantial increase in research efforts in the recent years.In general, "heterogeneity" describes the fact that there is a non-uniform appearance of a substance, organism, or disease. Whenever there is a non-uniformity in at least one quality, we can call it "heterogeneous." Tinnitus patients differ on at least six dimensions: First, tinnitus patients may present diverse clinical profiles with respect to the *perception of tinnitus* (e.g., laterality of tinnitus, tinnitus pitch, ringing, buzzing, hissing, or cricket sounds). Additionally, tinnitus can be occasional or permanent, acute or chronic, pulsatile or non-pulsatile, intermittent, or constant. Second, tinnitus can be associated with multiple *etiologies*—hearing loss, temporomandibular joint disorder, psychological conditions, and aging being among the most common ones. Third, there are numerous related *comorbidities* that add to the complex clinical picture of tinnitus (e.g., hyperacusis, anxiety, depression, sleep disorders, headache, concentration problems). A fourth dimension is the inter-individual variability of the *interference* of tinnitus with sounds, orofacial maneuvers, or pharmacological interventions such as lidocaine. The fifth dimension is the associated tinnitus distress. The psychological impact of the ongoing tinnitus perception differs largely among patients and within patients over time. Sixth, there is a large variation of responses to the various investigated treatments [1, 2].The heterogeneity in these six dimensions is highly relevant both for research and for clinical management. The current interpretation of this observed heterogeneity is that several different tinnitus subtypes may exist and that these different subtypes may have different etiologies and different clinical profiles. Presumably, these subtypes differ in their pathophysiology and in their responses to specific treatments. The assumption of the existence of distinct subtypes resembles the situation with headaches, which is another heterogeneous disorder. The International Headache Society identifies more than 150 different types of headaches [3]. This subtypisation was essential for the development of effective therapies. Triptans for example are effective for migraine [4], but not for other headache forms. However, in contrast to headache, in tinnitus so far, the diagnostic criteria to identify the potentially existing tinnitus subtypes are not known.In this chapter, the various dimensions of tinnitus heterogeneity and their relevance for research and clinical management will be discussed.

Perceptual Heterogeneity

Tinnitus can have various perceptual characteristics. It can be perceived on one side, on both sides, and within the head. The sound character can be ringing, buzzing, hissing, or cricket sounds. It can have a tone-like or a noise-like character or a combination of various tones and noises. The tinnitus pitch can vary from a low frequency sound to a high frequency sound. Some patients also report that they perceive multiple distinguishable sounds. Further variable characteristics concern the time course. It can be acute or chronic, intermittent or constant, occasional or permanent, it can fluctuate and finally it can have a pulsatile character. Some of these characteristics point to specific etiologies or specific pathophysiological aspects. As an example, a pulsatile tinnitus, which is synchronous to the heartbeat, has probably a vascular origin (see also Chap. 40).

Etiologic Heterogeneity

Several etiologic factors can contribute to tinnitus. The most important risk factor for tinnitus development is hearing loss. Further relevant etiologic factors include temporomandibular disorder, neck muscle strains, and emotional factors, such as distress or emotional trauma. In many cases, there is a combination of several etiologic factors, which play a role for the emergence of tinnitus. The relevance of the different etiologic factors might vary from individual to individual. For patient management the identification of the relevant etiologic factors is important, as they represent potential targets for treatment.

Heterogeneity in Comorbidities

Tinnitus is frequently accompanied by comorbidities. The increased co-occurrence suggests that tinnitus and the comorbidity are mutually dependent either by sharing common pathophysiologic mechanisms or etiologic factors or by causing each other. Moreover, it has been shown that patients differ in their tinnitus characteristics depending on their comorbidities [5–7]. Typical comorbidities include hyperacusis, speech comprehension difficulties, insomnia, anxiety, depression, or headache. Comorbidities can precede the tinnitus, they can begin together with the tinnitus, or they can develop after the tinnitus. Comorbidities play a major role for the impact of tinnitus on quality of life. Moreover, they are relevant for the clinical management as an individual treatment plan should include treatment of comorbidities.

Heterogeneity in Interference with Tinnitus

Typically, tinnitus interferes with external sounds. External sounds typically mask tinnitus, but in some individuals, they can also increase tinnitus loudness. External sounds can also induce a reduction of tinnitus loudness, which outlasts the external sound by a short period. This phenomenon is called "residual inhibition". However, the extent of residual inhibition and the optimal sound to induce residual inhibition varies among people with tinnitus. It is assumed that this variability reflects differences in the neuronal activity in central auditory pathways across individuals.

About 60% of all people with tinnitus can modulate their tinnitus by movements of the head, face, or the neck [8]. Presumably, this clinical phenomenon reflects the interaction between the trigeminal nerve and C2 afferents with the auditory pathway on the level of the dorsal cochlear nucleus [9] and is a characteristic of "somatic tinnitus" [10] (see also Chaps. 12, 31, and 37).

Another example of the variability of interference is the variable effect of lidocaine on tinnitus. Whereas most people with tinnitus perceive a reduction of their tinnitus after intravenous lidocaine application, tinnitus remains unchanged or gets louder in others. Presumably, these groups differ in their pathophysiological mechanisms.

Heterogeneity in Tinnitus Severity

The subjectively perceived severity of tinnitus can vary from no impairment to most severe impairment in almost all aspects of life. Perceptual characteristics of the tinnitus can only explain a small part of this variability [11]. More important factors are personality traits and comorbidities [12, 13]. The tinnitus severity is an essential aspect of an individual's tinnitus, as it determines tinnitus-related disability and tinnitus-related handicap. The tinnitus severity is relevant for the diagnostic and therapeutic management of the individual patient (see Chap. 25) and is the most frequently used primary outcome of therapeutic interventions.

Heterogeneity in Response to Treatment

Many different pharmacological and non-pharmacological treatments have been investigated in tinnitus [14, 15]. Most treatment studies did not reveal a significant difference between the intervention group and the control group and were therefore considered negative. However, in most of these studies the response to treatment was highly heterogeneous. This means that some study participants responded to the intervention, even if most others did not show a response. It is obvious that it would be highly desirable to identify criteria that can predict the outcome to a given intervention. A first step in this direction has been made by the analysis of self-reported effects of various therapeutic interventions in a large sample. This study has shown that response to certain treatments has an impact on the outcome of other treatments [2]. This result indicates that response to treatment might be a useful criterion for subtyping patients.

Gender Aspects

Many epidemiological studies have revealed higher prevalence and intensity of tinnitus in the male population [16, 17]. This is somewhat surprising, as other stress-related disorders such as chronic pain syndromes, anxiety, or depression are all more frequent in women. At least to some extent, the increased prevalence of tinnitus in men can be explained by a higher degree of hearing loss in men. The higher risk for hearing loss in men is probably related to both biological and environmental factors. Men have a higher biological susceptibility for the acquisition of hearing loss [18], and presumably a higher exposition to occupational noise. Moreover, there exist sex-related differences in auditory function, in the neuronal pattern underlying tinnitus and probably also in the response to specific therapeutic methods. All these aspects will be discussed in the following paragraphs.

Sex Differences in Sound Processing

Sex differences have been found for morphology and function of the auditory system both in animals and humans [19].

One explanation for these differences are the influence of sex hormones on the development and the function of the auditory system, with estrogen playing a crucial role. Both animal and human studies suggest that estrogens have a beneficial effect on hearing function and that females are protected against hearing loss because of estrogen and its signaling pathways [20, 21]. Several clinical reports have observed that the level of estrogen and its derivatives positively influence amplitudes of optoacoustic emissions and latencies of the auditory brain stem response [22–25]. In a large study of postmenopausal women, the serum estradiol level was associated with hearing loss [26]. These observations are consistent with hearing ailments identified in Turner syndrome, where estrogen deficiency is reported to provoke a hearing loss similar to presbycusis [27].

Higher testosterone levels result in a decrease in OAE amplitudes [28] and an increase of nerve cell thresholds at the level of the midbrain [29]. In animals, this effect depends on the frequency and the type of stimulus and its importance in mating [29, 30].

Taken together, testosterone has rather a detrimental effect on hearing sensitivity, whereas estrogen has a protective influence on the peripheric auditory structures [31, 32].

Sex hormones, therefore, play an important role in regulating sensitivity and selectivity of hearing, starting already at the periphery, where females are given the advantage of better preservation of cochlear structures with reported higher reactiveness to the acoustic environment.

This might not only protect from the development of tinnitus, but could also influence the responsiveness of female tinnitus patients to acoustic stimulation.

Sex Differences in Higher Order Auditory Processing

Sex differences exist also at higher levels of the auditory pathway in language and music processing [19]. Women are better in performing speech-related tasks, whereas men have advantages in the processing of pitch and melody [33, 34]. In line with these findings, women have advantages in the processing of fast-changing auditory input [35], imminent to linguistic features. In contrast, men have better pitch and loudness discrimination [34].

At the level of auditory cortices, women demonstrate larger bilateral cortical volume and a reduction of left side asymmetry related to lateral specialization in verbal processing [36, 37], a phenomenon also observable in patterns of activation in BOLD signal, which indicates more diffuse processing of phonological tasks in women [38]. Analogical findings are reported in men, who also reveal more distributed activity when processing pitch [33].

Sex differences in neural patterns characteristic for auditory paradigms also emerge for higher-level cognitive functions like working memory and top-down perception [39, 40]. For instance, in auditory oddball tasks, women exhibit faster reactions for deviant, infrequent stimuli, while men were reported to reveal an increased mismatch-negativity wave corresponding to a stronger neural response to novelty [40]. Moreover, repetition suppression, i.e., less pronounced neural auditory response to repeated stimuli, is observed to a lesser extent in women suggesting that women are less prone to the effect of habituation.

According to the Bayesian brain model (see also Chap. 17), top-down predictions or expectations are an inherent ingredient of conscious perception [41]. In this context, the bias toward novelty in men, as well as faster reactions to oddball stimuli and decreased habituation in women, suggests that women may reveal a more dynamic update of predictions [42].

Sex differences in neural activity in tinnitus and in response to specific treatments.

Imaging and treatment studies provide some support for sex-related differences in the neuronal mechanisms of tinnitus.

In a recent case series, thirteen postmenopausal women with tinnitus reported tinnitus improvement after treatment with estrogens [43].

Significant differences between males and females were also found in patterns of oscillatory brain activity in tinnitus patients [44, 45]. These differences at the neural level may play a role for differences in outcome of various therapeutic interventions: Vascular decompression of the auditory nerve results in a significant improvement (decrease in tinnitus loudness) in 54% of women compared to 29% of men [46]. In a study using bilateral transcranial direct current stimulation (tDCS), the reduction of tinnitus intensity and distress was more pronounced in women [47].

More favourable therapy outcomes in females were also reported in studies using repetitive transcranial magnetic stimulation (rTMS) [48] and auditory stimulation [49, 50]. In a recent large study, in which gender effects on various therapeutic approaches were investigated, females had better outcomes with tDCS and orofacial treatment, whereas men benefited more from a combination of Tinnitus retraining therapy and cognitive behavioural therapy [51].

Even if these results suggest a general tendency towards more favourable outcomes in females, these data should be interpreted with caution, as all these analyses were post-hoc analysis and not analyses according to a predefined statistical analysis plan with correction for multiple comparisons.

Approaches to Address Heterogeneity

The large variability in clinical and perceptual characteristics of tinnitus, the variable response to most therapeutic interventions, and the impact of gender, all point to a considerable pathophysiological heterogeneity of tinnitus. There is consensus in the research community that a deeper understanding of this heterogeneity is key for advances in the understanding of the neuronal mechanisms of the different forms of tinnitus and for the development of more efficient treatment interventions [1]. Several strategies have been proposed to address this heterogeneity:

Clinical Identification of Tinnitus Subtypes

One strategy consists in the identification of distinct clinical subtypes with a clearly delineated etiology and pathophysiology. An example for such a subtype is the so-called "typewriter tinnitus", which is characterized by paroxysmal attacks of unilateral staccato tinnitus and a good response to the anticonvulsant carbamazepine, based on the pathophysiologic assumption of an underlying neurovascular conflict [52]. However, unfortunately only very few such subtypes could be identified and most of these subtypes refer to objective tinnitus. Thus, only very few tinnitus patients can be categorized in such clearly delineated subtypes.

Tinnitus Patient Databases for the Identification of Subtyping Criteria

In the quest for the identification of subtypes, databases have been created, in which various patient characteristics have been collected to enable data-driven and hypothesis-driven subtyping analysis [53–55]. Analysis of these databases revealed that etiologic aspects such as pattern of hearing loss [56] or onset related to trauma [57] represent relevant criteria for subtyping. Similarly comorbidities such as temporomandibular joint disorder [7], headache [5], or hyperacusis [6] have bene identified as relevant criteria.

However, even if patients with and without a given characteristic (e.g. patients with TMJ disorders versus patients without TMJ disorders) differed in many other aspects of tinnitus, these analyses did not reveal clearly distinguishable subtypes, as the characteristics of the two groups largely overlapped. In addition, data-driven analyses revealed only subtypes with largely overlapping clusters.

These findings suggest that the heterogeneity is better explained by patient characteristics falling along various continua which can contribute towards a profile across multiple domains [58–60]. Given this distinction, the 'subtyping' approach (identification of subgroups as distinct categories of tinnitus) for addressing tinnitus heterogeneity has to be complemented by a 'profiling' approach to characterize individual patients based on the distribution pattern of symptoms along a continuum or multiple continua.

Identification of Tinnitus Subtypes by Treatment Response

The identification of tinnitus subgroups is primarily motivated by the expectation that this will help to identify more efficient treatments for tinnitus patients. It is assumed that pathophysiologically more homogeneous patient samples will reduce the variability in the outcome of therapeutic trials and increase the chances, to identify efficient treatment options for specific subtypes. Thus, the envisaged strategy would be as follows:

1. Identify a tinnitus subtype, which represents a clinical entity with characteristic clinical and pathophysiological criteria
2. Identify a treatment, which specifically targets the pathophysiological abnormalities of this subtype
3. Evaluate this treatment with a clinical trial in patients with this specific tinnitus subtype

Even if this strategy sounds reasonable, it has not yet been proven successful for the majority of tinnitus patients, as already the identification of subtypes represents a major challenge, which has not yet been successfully solved.

Therefore, an alternative strategic approach has been proposed. In this alternative approach, the delineation of subtypes is based on the response to specific treatments and can be illustrated as follows:

1. A specific treatment is tested in a large and heterogeneous sample of clinically and pathophysiologically well-characterized patients
2. Responders and non-responders are compared in post-hoc comparisons, whether they differ in their clinical and/or pathophysiological characteristics
3. A confirmatory study in which only patients with responder characteristics are includeds

A first proof of principle for this approach comes from a recent study, in which a large sample of patients reported about their experiences with various treatments. This study revealed that the response to one treatment is a significant predictor for the response to another treatment [2].

However, a major shortcoming of this approach is the need for confirmatory studies, as post-hoc analyses of clinical trials always bear the risk that positive results emerge by randomness. With increasing numbers of post-hoc analyses, significant findings for subgroups will emerge, even if there is no real effect. It is possible to control for this risk by defining a priori a limited number of hypotheses-driven subgroup analyses and by correcting accordingly for multiple comparisons, but this in turn limits the chances to detect unexpected associations between specific criteria and treatment response.

Genetic Heterogeneity

Subtypisation according to genetic variants is a commonly used approach for the identification of biologically distinct disease entities. Even if recent research revealed first hints for the relevance of genetic factors in tinnitus [61], the overall knowledge about genetic and epigenetic risk factors for tinnitus is still limited. Moreover, the available data suggest that in tinnitus—similar like in other frequent disorders such as depression, diabetes, or hypertension—there exist a larger number of relevant gene variants, which interact with each other and with environmental factors in a complex way, which makes it very difficult to identify subtypes based on genetic variants.

On the other hand, genetic research has helped to identify relevant clinical characteristics for delineating subtypes. This can be illustrated by the example of tinnitus laterality. Genetic research has underscored that bilateral and unilateral tinnitus represent different disease entities, as genetic variants, which are relevant for the development of bilateral tinnitus, play no role for the development of unilateral tinnitus [62].

Implications of Tinnitus Heterogeneity on Clinical Management

The heterogeneity of tinnitus has also important implications for the clinical management, as it requires a personalized approach. Even if there exist no established evidence-based approaches for specific tinnitus subgroups, it is possible to develop personalized treatment plans for individual patients.

First, the individually relevant etiologic factors should be identified and treated (e.g. hearing loss or temporomandibular joint dysfunction). Second, the individually most relevant aspect of tinnitus should be the primary focus of treatment (e.g. insomnia or fear from worsening of the tinnitus). Third, comorbidities should be considered in the treatment plan (e.g. headaches, depression, hyperacousis), and fourth, modulation of tinnitus by specific interventions should guide the choice of treatments (e.g. tinnitus reduction by sound or neck movements suggests a potential efficacy of sound therapy or physiotherapy, respectively).

Conclusion

This heterogeneity of tinnitus is a major obstacle for the identification of efficient tinnitus treatments [14, 15].

Several strategies have been applied to identify more homogeneous tinnitus subtypes. In particular, it has been tried to identify subtypes from large databases, either according to clinical hypotheses or purely data-driven. These approaches suggest that the majority of tinnitus patients cannot be categorized in clearly delineated (i.e. distinct) subtypes. Instead, the heterogeneity is better explained by patient characteristics falling along various continua which can contribute towards a profile across multiple domains [58]. Given this distinction, the 'subtyping' approach (identification of subgroups as distinct categories of tinnitus) for addressing tinnitus heterogeneity has to be complemented by a 'profiling' approach to characterize individual patients based on the distribution pattern of symptoms along a continuum or multiple continua.

This has important implications for both clinical management and research.

In order to optimize treatment for the individual patient, a personalized treatment plan should be developed, considering the tinnitus profile, the comorbidities, the psychological distress, the gender, and the previous treatment experiences of the patient.

Moreover, it is essential to consider tinnitus heterogeneity in research designs, e.g. by a stepwise approach, where in a first step response characteristics are identified before the efficacy of a given intervention is tested in the appropriate patient group.

References

1. Cederroth CR, Gallus S, Hall DA, Kleinjung T, Langguth B, Maruotti A, et al. Editorial: towards an understanding of tinnitus heterogeneity. Front Aging Neurosci. 2019;11:53.
2. Simoes J, Neff P, Schoisswohl S, Bulla J, Schecklmann M, Harrison S, et al. Toward personalized tinnitus treatment: an exploratory study based on internet crowdsensing. Front Public Health. 2019;7:157.
3. Headache Classification Committee of the International Headache Society (IHS) the international classification of headache disorders, 3rd edition. Cephalalgia. 2018;38(1):1–211.
4. Cameron C, Kelly S, Hsieh SC, Murphy M, Chen L, Kotb A, et al. Triptans in the acute treatment of migraine: a systematic review and network meta-analysis. Headache. 2015;55(Suppl 4):221–35.
5. Langguth B, Hund V, Landgrebe M, Schecklmann M. Tinnitus patients with comorbid headaches: the influence of headache type and laterality on tinnitus characteristics. Front Neurol. 2017;8:440.
6. Schecklmann M, Landgrebe M, Langguth B, TRI Database Study Group. Phenotypic characteristics of hyperacusis in tinnitus. PLoS One. 2014;9(1):e86944.
7. Vielsmeier V, Kleinjung T, Strutz J, Burgers R, Kreuzer PM, Langguth B. Tinnitus with temporomandibular joint disorders: a specific entity of tinnitus patients? Otolaryngol Head Neck Surg. 2011;145:748.
8. Sanchez TG, da Silva LA, Brandao AL, Lorenzi MC, Bento RF. Somatic modulation of tinnitus: test reliability and results after repetitive muscle contraction training. Ann Otol Rhinol Laryngol. 2007;116(1):30–5.
9. Shore SE, Roberts LE, Langguth B. Maladaptive plasticity in tinnitus--triggers, mechanisms and treatment. Nat Rev Neurol. 2016;12(3):150–60.
10. Michiels S, Ganz Sanchez T, Oron Y, Gilles A, Haider HF, Erlandsson S, et al. Diagnostic criteria for somatosensory tinnitus: a Delphi process and face-to-face meeting to establish consensus. Trends Hear. 2018;22:2331216518796403.
11. Hiller W, Goebel G. Factors influencing tinnitus loudness and annoyance. Arch Otolaryngol Head Neck Surg. 2006;132(12):1323–30.
12. Milerova J, Anders M, Dvorak T, Sand PG, Koniger S, Langguth B. The influence of psychological factors on tinnitus severity. Gen Hosp Psychiatry. 2013;35(4):412–6.

13. Langguth B, Kleinjung T, Fischer B, Hajak G, Eichhammer P, Sand PG. Tinnitus severity, depression, and the big five personality traits. Prog Brain Res. 2007;166:221–5.
14. Elgoyhen AB, Langguth B. Pharmacological approaches to the treatment of tinnitus. Drug Discov Today. 2010;15(7–8):300–5.
15. Langguth B, Kreuzer PM, Kleinjung T, De Ridder D. Tinnitus: causes and clinical management. Lancet Neurol. 2013;12(9):920–30.
16. Shargorodsky J, Curhan GC, Farwell WR. Prevalence and characteristics of tinnitus among US adults. Am J Med. 2010;123(8):711–8.
17. Gallus S, Lugo A, Garavello W, Bosetti C, Santoro E, Colombo P, et al. Prevalence and determinants of tinnitus in the Italian adult population. Neuroepidemiology. 2015;45(1):12–9.
18. Lien KH, Yang CH. Sex differences in the triad of acquired sensorineural hearing loss. Int J Mol Sci. 2021;22(15):8111.
19. Nolan LS. Age-related hearing loss: why we need to think about sex as a biological variable. J Neurosci Res. 2020;98(9):1705–20.
20. Shuster BZ, Depireux DA, Mong JA, Hertzano R. Sex differences in hearing: probing the role of estrogen signaling. J Acoust Soc Am. 2019;145(6):3656.
21. Fetoni AR, Picciotti PM, Paludetti G, Troiani D. Pathogenesis of presbycusis in animal models: a review. Exp Gerontol. 2011;46(6):413–25.
22. Delhez A, Lefebvre P, Pequeux C, Malgrange B, Delacroix L. Auditory function and dysfunction: estrogen makes a difference. Cell Mol Life Sci. 2020;77(4):619–35.
23. Dehan CP, Jerger J. Analysis of gender differences in the auditory brainstem response. Laryngoscope. 1990;100(1):18–24.
24. Snihur AW, Hampson E. Sex and ear differences in spontaneous and click-evoked otoacoustic emissions in young adults. Brain Cogn. 2011;77(1):40–7.
25. Adriztina I, Adnan A, Adenin I, Haryuna SH, Sarumpaet S. Influence of hormonal changes on audiologic examination in normal ovarian cycle females: an analytic study. Int Arch Otorhinolaryngol. 2016;20(4):294–9.
26. Kim SH, Kang BM, Chae HD, Kim CH. The association between serum estradiol level and hearing sensitivity in postmenopausal women. Obstet Gynecol. 2002;99(5 Pt 1):726–30.
27. Hederstierna C, Hultcrantz M, Rosenhall U. Estrogen and hearing from a clinical point of view; characteristics of auditory function in women with turner syndrome. Hear Res. 2009;252(1–2):3–8.
28. McFadden D, Champlin CA. Comparison of auditory evoked potentials in heterosexual, homosexual, and bisexual males and females. J Assoc Res Otolaryngol. 2000;1(1):89–99.
29. Miranda JA, Wilczynski W. Sex differences and androgen influences on midbrain auditory thresholds in the green treefrog, Hyla cinerea. Hear Res. 2009;252(1–2):79–88.
30. Arch VS, Narins PM. Sexual hearing: the influence of sex hormones on acoustic communication in frogs. Hear Res. 2009;252(1–2):15–20.
31. Caras ML. Estrogenic modulation of auditory processing: a vertebrate comparison. Front Neuroendocrinol. 2013;34(4):285–99.
32. McCullar JS, Oesterle EC. Cellular targets of estrogen signaling in regeneration of inner ear sensory epithelia. Hear Res. 2009;252(1–2):61–70.
33. Gaab N, Keenan JP, Schlaug G. The effects of gender on the neural substrates of pitch memory. J Cogn Neurosci. 2003;15(6):810–20.
34. Rammsayer TH, Troche SJ. On sex-related differences in auditory and visual sensory functioning. Arch Sex Behav. 2012;41(3):583–90.
35. Jerger J, Hall J. Effects of age and sex on auditory brainstem response. Arch Otolaryngol. 1980;106(7):387–91.
36. Kulynych JJ, Vladar K, Jones DW, Weinberger DR. Gender differences in the normal lateralization of the supratemporal cortex: MRI surface-rendering morphometry of Heschl's gyrus and the planum temporale. Cereb Cortex. 1994;4(2):107–18.
37. Rademacher J, Morosan P, Schleicher A, Freund HJ, Zilles K. Human primary auditory cortex in women and men. Neuroreport. 2001;12(8):1561–5.
38. Shaywitz BA, Shaywitz SE, Pugh KR, Constable RT, Skudlarski P, Fulbright RK, et al. Sex differences in the functional organization of the brain for language. Nature. 1995;373(6515):607–9.
39. Chorlian DB, Rangaswamy M, Manz N, Kamarajan C, Pandey AK, Edenberg H, et al. Gender modulates the development of theta event related oscillations in adolescents and young adults. Behav Brain Res. 2015;292:342–52.
40. Nagy E, Potts GF, Loveland KA. Sex-related ERP differences in deviance detection. Int J Psychophysiol. 2003;48(3):285–92.
41. Friston K. A theory of cortical responses. Philos Trans R Soc Lond Ser B Biol Sci. 2005;360(1456):815–36.
42. Auksztulewicz R, Friston K. Repetition suppression and its contextual determinants in predictive coding. Cortex. 2016;80:125–40.
43. Lai JT, Liu CL, Liu TC. Hormone replacement therapy for chronic tinnitus in menopausal women: our experience with 13 cases. Clin Otolaryngol. 2017;42(6):1366–9.
44. Weiler EW, Brill K, Tachiki KH, Wiegand R. Electroencephalography correlates in tinnitus. Int Tinnitus J. 2000;6(1):21–4.
45. Vanneste S, Joos K, De RD. Prefrontal cortex based sex differences in tinnitus perception: same tinnitus intensity, same tinnitus distress, different mood. PLoS One. 2012;7(2):e31182.
46. Moller MB, Moller AR, Jannetta PJ, Jho HD. Vascular decompression surgery for severe tinnitus: selection criteria and results. Laryngoscope. 1993;103(4 Pt 1):421–7.
47. Frank E, Schecklmann M, Landgrebe M, Burger J, Kreuzer P, Poeppl TB, et al. Treatment of chronic tinnitus with repeated sessions of prefrontal transcranial direct current stimulation: outcomes from an open-label pilot study. J Neurol. 2012;259(2):327–33.
48. De Ridder D, De Mulder G, Verstraeten E, Seidman M, Elisevich K, Sunaert S, et al. Auditory cortex stimulation for tinnitus. Acta Neurochir Suppl. 2007;97(Pt 2):451–62.
49. Partyka M, Neff P, Bacri T, Michels J, Weisz N, Schlee W. Gender differentiates effects of acoustic stimulation in patients with tinnitus. Prog Brain Res. 2021;263:25–57.
50. Neff PKA, Schoisswohl S, Simoes J, Staudinger S, Langguth B, Schecklmann M, et al. Prolonged tinnitus suppression after short-term acoustic stimulation. Prog Brain Res. 2021;262:159–74.
51. Van der Wal A, Luyten T, Cardon E, Jacquemin L, Vanderveken OM, Topsakal V, et al. Sex differences in the response to different tinnitus treatment. Front Neurosci. 2020;14:422.
52. Mardini MK. Ear-clicking "tinnitus" responding to carbamazepine. N Engl J Med. 1987;317(24):1542.
53. Meikle MB. Electronic access to tinnitus data: the Oregon Tinnitus Data Archive. Otolaryngol Head Neck Surg. 1997;117(6):698–700.
54. Witsell DL, Schulz KA, Moore K, Tucci DL. Implementation and testing of research infrastructure for practice-based research in hearing and communication disorders. Otolaryngol Head Neck Surg. 2011;145(4):565–71.
55. Landgrebe M, Zeman F, Koller M, Eberl Y, Mohr M, Reiter J, et al. The Tinnitus Research Initiative (TRI) database: a new approach for delineation of tinnitus subtypes and generation of predictors for treatment outcome. BMC Med Inform Decis Mak. 2010;10:42.
56. Langguth B, Landgrebe M, Schlee W, Schecklmann M, Vielsmeier V, Steffens T, et al. Different patterns of hearing loss among tinnitus patients: a latent class analysis of a large sample. Front Neurol. 2017;8:46.
57. Kreuzer PM, Landgrebe M, Schecklmann M, Staudinger S, Langguth B. Trauma-associated tinnitus: audiological, demographic and clinical characteristics. PLoS One. 2012;7(9):e45599.
58. van den Berge MJC, Free RH, Arnold R, de Kleine E, Hofman R, van Dijk JMC, et al. Cluster analysis to identify possible subgroups in tinnitus patients. Front Neurol. 2017;8:115.
59. Schlee W, Hall DA, Canlon B, Cima RFF, de Kleine E, Hauck F, et al. Innovations in doctoral training and research on tinnitus: the European school on interdisciplinary tinnitus research (ESIT) perspective. Front Aging Neurosci. 2017;9:447.

60. Genitsaridi E, Partyka M, Gallus S, Lopez-Escamez JA, Schecklmann M, Mielczarek M, et al. Standardised profiling for tinnitus research: the European School for Interdisciplinary Tinnitus Research Screening Questionnaire (ESIT-SQ). Hear Res. 2019;377:353–9.
61. Cederroth CR, Trpchevska N, Langguth B. A new buzz for tinnitus-It's in the genes! JAMA Otolaryngol Head Neck Surg. 2020;146(11):1025–6.
62. Maas IL, Bruggemann P, Requena T, Bulla J, Edvall NK, Hjelmborg JVB, et al. Genetic susceptibility to bilateral tinnitus in a Swedish twin cohort. Genet Med. 2017;19(9):1007–12.

Similarities Between Tinnitus and Pain

8

Dirk De Ridder and Aage R. Møller

Abstract

Chronic pain and tinnitus share analogous anatomical and pathophysiological mechanisms leading to similarities in clinical presentation and resulting in common treatment approaches.

Yet, there is an important difference as well. Acute pain is the result of activation of specific dedicated pain pathways, for which there is no tinnitus counterpart.

Chronic pain is slightly more prevalent than tinnitus, 25% vs. 15%, and both symptoms are on the rise, also being comorbid.

Clinically, both are entirely subjective symptoms that can be associated with suffering in 20% of patients. Chronic pain can be associated with allodynia and hyperpathia, and tinnitus with hyperacusis and misophonia. Both can have a wind-up phenomenon.

Both share electrophysiological similarities in that alpha oscillatory resting state activity is replaced by theta-gamma cross-frequency coupling in the respective sensory cortex. The presence of pain and tinnitus results from an imbalance between two pain and tinnitus provoking pathways and one descending pain and noise cancelling pathway, respectively.

The thalamocortical dysrhythmic activity present in the lateral pathway is embedded in the triple cognitive network, essential for conscious perception and related to pain or tinnitus-related suffering.

The transition from acute to chronic pain and tinnitus is related to maladaptive learning via conditioning, based on abnormal connectivity between the nucleus accumbens and the descending pain and noise canceling pathway, respectively. The persistence of chronic pain and tinnitus may be linked to neuroinflammation, which is the result of genetic and epigenetic factors, combined with altered microbiome.

Aage R. Møller has died before the publication of this book.

D. De Ridder (✉)
Section of Neurosurgery, Department of Surgical Sciences, University of Otago, Dunedin, New Zealand
e-mail: dirk.deridder@otago.ac.nz

A. R. Møller (Deceased)
Neuroscience Program, School of Brain & Behavioral Sciences, University of Texas, Richardson, TX, USA

W. Schlee et al. (eds.), *Textbook of Tinnitus*, https://doi.org/10.1007/978-3-031-35647-6_8

Graphical Abstract

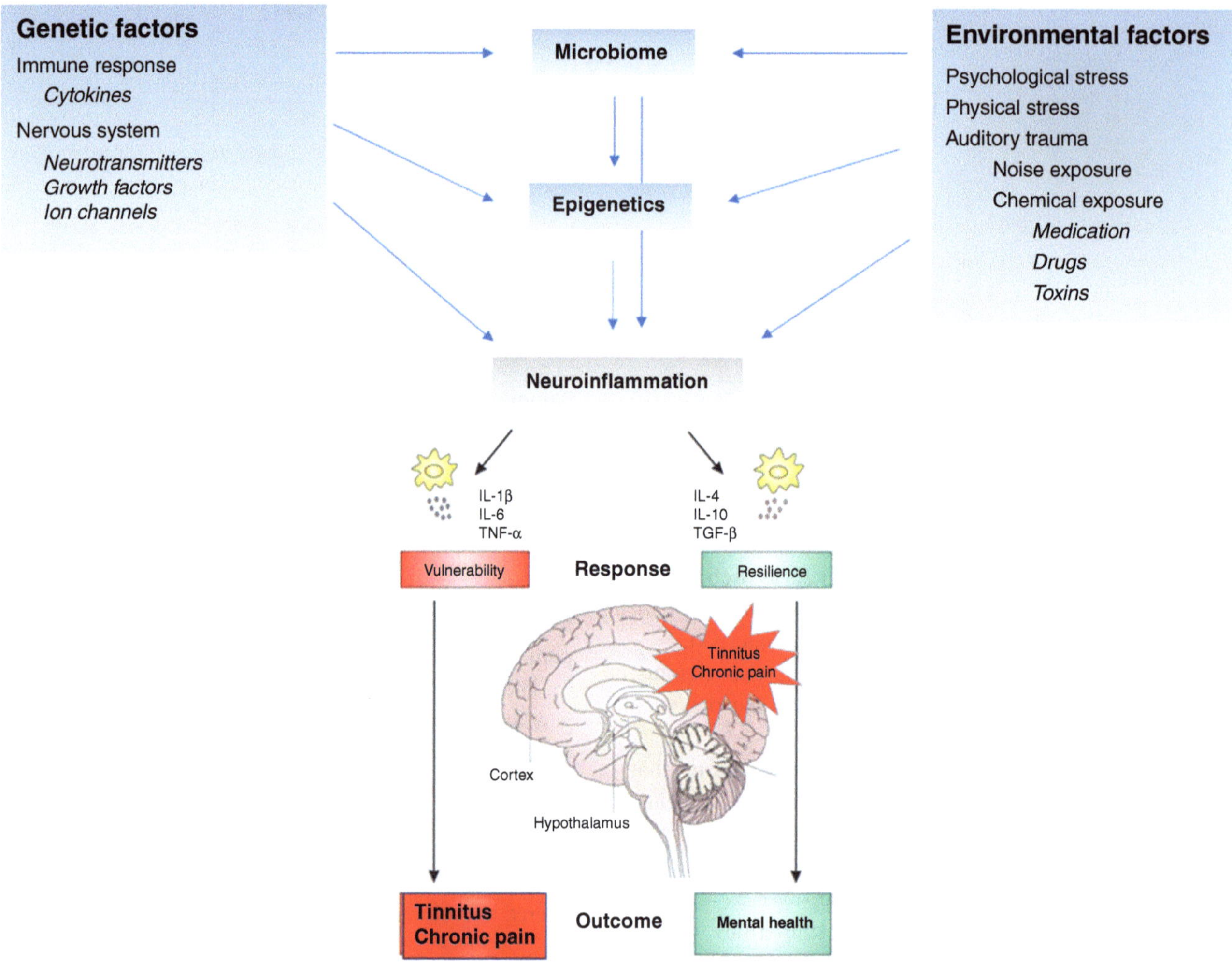

Highlights

- Chronic pain and tinnitus share analogous anatomical and pathophysiological mechanisms
- The common pathophysiology leads to similarities in clinical presentation
- The similar clinical presentation results in common treatment approaches
- There is an important difference: acute pain is the result of activation of specific dedicated pain pathways, for which there is no tinnitus counterpart
- Chronic pain is slightly more prevalent than tinnitus, 25% vs. 15%
- Both symptoms have an increasing incidence
- Chronic pain and tinnitus are comorbid
- Clinically, both are entire subjective symptoms that can be associated with suffering in 20% of patients
- Both chronic pain and tinnitus fill in missing sensory information
- Chronic pain can be associated with allodynia and hyperpathia, and tinnitus with hyperacusis and misophonia
- Both can have a wind-up phenomenon
- Both share electrophysiological similarities in that alpha oscillatory resting state activity is replaced by theta-gamma cross-frequency coupling in the respective sensory cortex
- The presence of pain and tinnitus results from an imbalance between two pain and tinnitus provoking pathways and one descending pain and noise cancelling pathway, respectively
- The thalamocortical dysrhythmic activity present in the lateral pathway is embedded in the triple cognitive network, essential for conscious perception and related to pain or tinnitus-related suffering
- The transition from acute to chronic pain and tinnitus is related to maladaptive learning via condition-

ing, based on abnormal connectivity between the nucleus accumbens and the descending pain and noise canceling pathway, respectively
- The persistence of chronic pain and tinnitus may be linked to neuroinflammation, which is the result of genetic and epigenetic factors, combined with altered microbiome
- Based on the similar clinical picture and similar pathophysiology, analogous treatments have been developed for both symptoms, consisting of pharmacological, neuromodulatory, and psychological approaches

Introduction

Chronic pain and tinnitus share analogous anatomical and pathophysiological mechanisms leading to similarities in clinical presentation and resulting in common treatment approaches.

The clinical similarities between tinnitus and pain have been described since the 1980s [1–4]. Both symptoms are subjective and may fluctuate in character and quality. Both symptoms compensate for deafferented sensory information: the tinnitus pitch reflects the individual's frequency spectrum of the hearing loss [5], and neuropathic pain is felt as coming from the area that was initially innervated by the injured neural structure [6]. For example, phantom pain is perceived in the missing body part [6, 7]. Both symptoms are associated with perceptual changes. For example, touching the area of neuropathic pain can create a painful sensation (allodynia) and tinnitus patients frequently perceive specific sounds as unpleasant (misophonia). A noxious stimulus in neuropathic pain patients often generates an explosive and prolonged feeling of pain (hyperpathia), like hyperacusis seen in some tinnitus patients, in which a sound is being perceived as too loud or painful. Many individuals with chronic pain experience a worsening of their pain from repeated stimulation (the "wind-up" phenomenon) [2]. This is similar to the increasingly unpleasant feeling from repetitive sounds that many individuals with severe tinnitus experience [2].

Furthermore, both phantom pain and tinnitus can result in or are associated with stress, anxiety, and depression, which can lead to sleep disturbances and fatigue, a decrease in quality of life, and disability, associated with concentration and memory problems, and sometimes even lead to suicide in both clinical conditions [3].

However, there is also an important difference between pain and tinnitus [8]. Whereas physiological pain exists, i.e. pain resulting from nociceptive receptor activation and transmitted via existing pain pathways, no obvious physiological tinnitus exists.

Neuropathic pain generation has been explained by the pathophysiological gate theory of pain [9] and was incorporated in a Darwinian plasticity model [10], suggesting that the brain will look for missing information in the environment. The pathophysiological similarities have been studied anatomically and electrophysiologically. Anatomically, tinnitus and pain have been likened to an aversive memory-like mechanism [8], involving the parahippocampus, insula, anterior cingulate, and respective sensory cortex. Electrophysiologically, both symptoms have been associated with a reduction of resting state alpha activity in thalamus and cortex and emergence of cross-frequency coupled theta-gamma activity, also known as thalamocortical dysrhythmia [11–16]. These anatomical and electrophysiological explanations have been incorporated in a Bayesian brain model for tinnitus and pain [17, 18]. This model states that the brain predicts sensory input, based on a generative model of the self in the world, and if the brain is deprived of sensory input, it will pull the missing information from memory [17, 18]. This Bayesian brain model has been further extended into the triple network model both for tinnitus and pain, explaining the paradoxical salience attached to the phantom percept, as well as the cognitive and emotional aspects of the pain and sound [19, 20].

Prevalence of Chronic Neuropathic Pain and Chronic Tinnitus

One of the problems in getting consistent epidemiologic data is similar for pain and tinnitus, namely that there is no generally accepted definition to use in these epidemiological studies [21]. This not only includes what pain and tinnitus are, but also how much of the time the symptom is present, and at what time one can speak of 'chronic' pain and tinnitus. Chronic pain was used to be defined as pain that persists beyond the point of healing, but now is simplified to any pain that persists after 3 months [22]. Chronic pain has been subdivided in multiple entities, a feature that has not been succesfully applied to tinnitus [21, 22].

The prevalence of chronic pain has been estimated at 20% of the population of Europe [23] and USA [24], and even higher, up to 30% in China [25] and the developing world [26]. For tinnitus, a meta-analysis has identified a prevalence of about 15% in Europe and worldwide [27, 28]. About 1000 people out of 100,000 get tinnitus every year [28], and the incidence is increasing in time [29]. For chronic pain, the incidence is 10× higher (10%), and on the rise as well [30]. One reason may be that the prevalence of chronic pain [24] and chronic tinnitus [27, 28] increases with age. Furthermore, tinnitus and chronic pain are comorbid [31, 32], not only for headache [33], neck pain [34], and TMJ [35] pain, but also multisite [31] and joint [36] pain.

There are many causes or risk factors that are related to tinnitus and chronic pain.

Common Risk Factors for Chronic Pain and Tinnitus

Individuals with head injuries are prone to develop chronic pain and tinnitus [37].

Childhood adversity is a risk factor for the development of chronic pain [38, 39] and possibly tinnitus [40–43] in adulthood. Furthermore, childhood adversity is related to many other risk factors for tinnitus and chronic pain, such as asthma, arthritis, obesity, insomnia, diabetes, hypertension, infections, cancer, and other diseases [44]. Indeed, asthma [45, 46], arthritis [45, 46], obesity [46, 47], insomnia [48, 49], diabetes [46, 50], and hypertension [50, 51] are risk factors for tinnitus [44, 45, 47, 48, 50] and chronic pain [46, 49, 51].

Meta-analyses have shown that anxiety and depression are present in about 20% of pain [52] and tinnitus [28] patients. Whether anxiety and depression are resultant from tinnitus and cause tinnitus or associated via common risk factors has not yet been fully elucidated. Yet, for both tinnitus [53] and chronic pain [52], higher severity of the symptom correlates with increased anxiety and depression and psychiatric distress [36], suggesting there is a clear correlation between the physical and psychological components of chronic pain and tinnitus.

Tinnitus and Pain Definitions: Tinnitus and Pain, Tinnitus Disorder, and Pain Disorder

Pain has been defined by the IASP and WHO in ICD11 as 'an unpleasant sensory and emotional experience associated with, or resembling that associated with, actual or potential tissue damage' [54]. Pain thus consists of a sensory and an emotional component. As with pain, tinnitus also consists not only of a sensory component, characterized by a specific intensity or loudness, and by a specific frequency or pitch, but also an affective-motivational component, reflecting its unpleasantness [8] and its related distress [55]. Tinnitus-associated distress involves an autonomic, sympathetic component [56] and should be differentiated from mood changes, such as anxiety and depression, which are associated with different neural correlates [57]. Suffering is the result of a dysfunctional cognitive, emotional, and autonomic response [58–60]. For example, this could include depression, and anxiety, as well as sleep disturbances, concentration, attention, and memory problems [61, 62], common to both tinnitus and pain [36, 63] (Figs. 8.1 and 8.2).

Pain can exist without suffering, especially if the numeric rating scale is below 5, but also with suffering and disability [64]. Similarly, tinnitus can exist with and without suffering

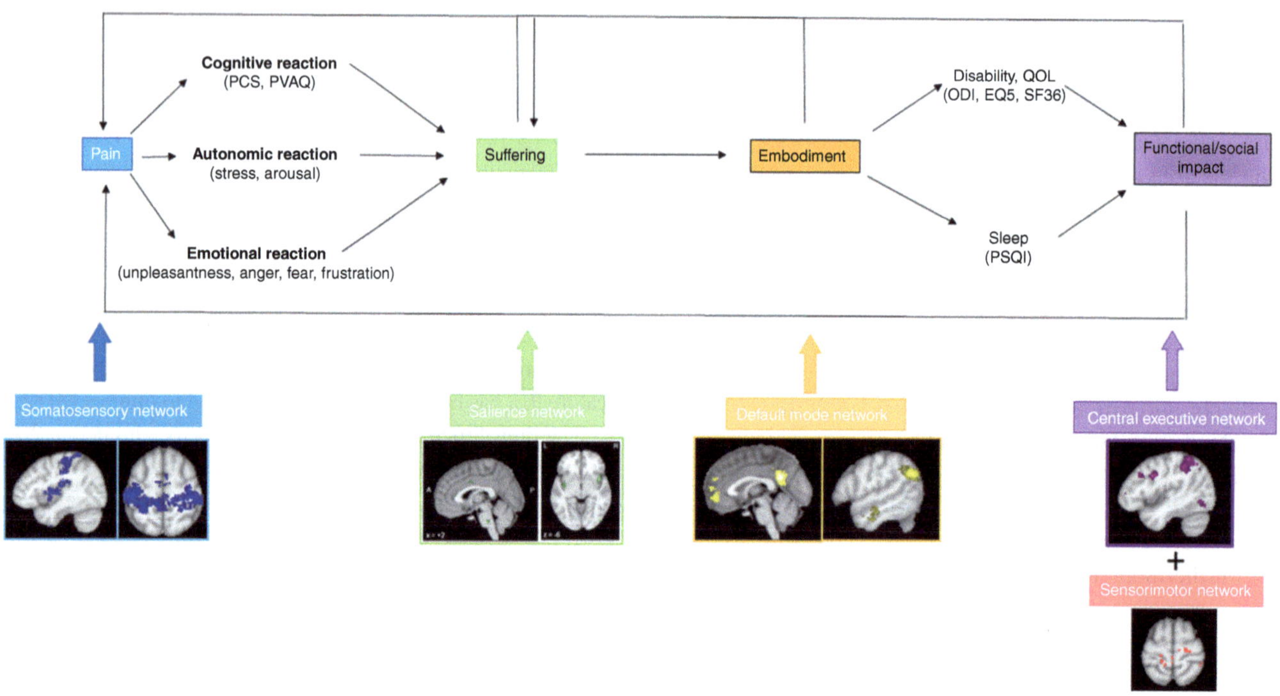

Fig. 8.1 Mechanism of pain and suffering

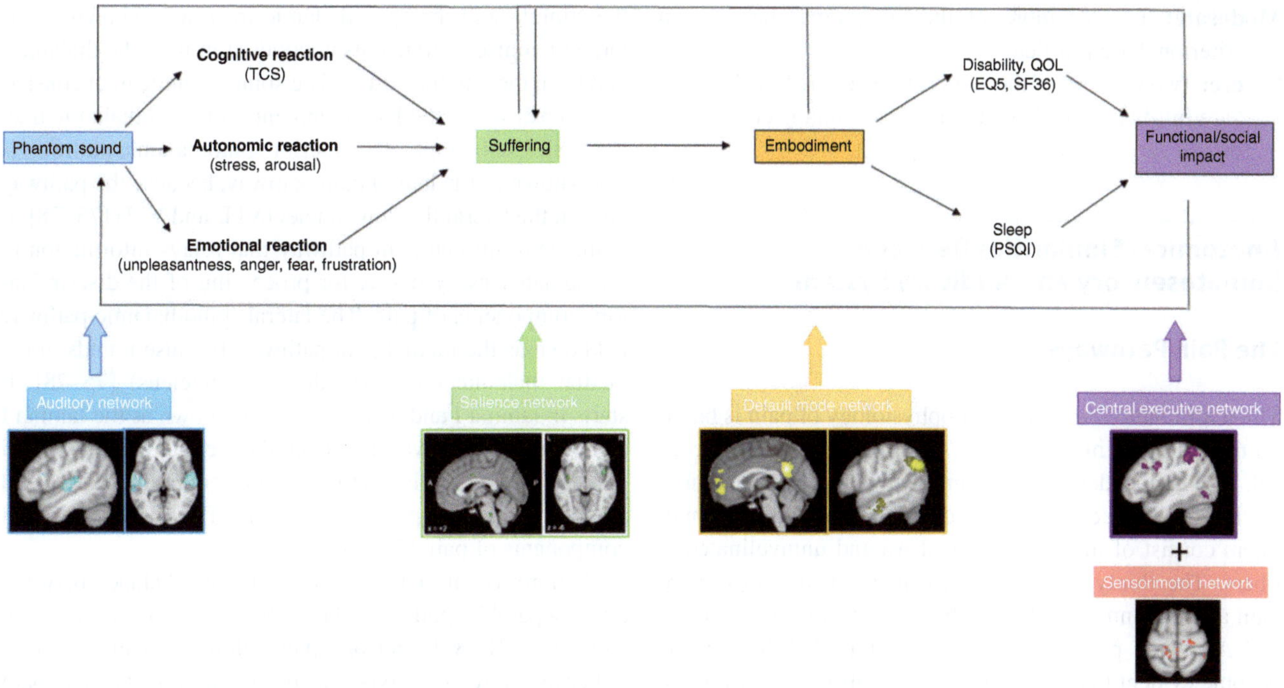

Fig. 8.2 Mechanism of tinnitus and suffering

[21]. Hence, tinnitus has been defined as the conscious awareness of a tonal or composite noise for which there is no identifiable corresponding external acoustic source. Tinnitus Disorder, on the other hand, has been defined "as tinnitus that is associated with emotional distress, cognitive dysfunction, and/or autonomic arousal, leading to behavioral changes and functional disability" [21]. In other words: "Tinnitus" describes the auditory or sensory component, whereas "Tinnitus Disorder" reflects the auditory component and the associated suffering [21].

WHO ICD-11 Definition

When aligning the definition of tinnitus with the ICD11 definition of pain, the tinnitus ICD11 definition proposal would be 'Tinnitus is the conscious awareness of a tonal or composite noise for which there is no identifiable corresponding external acoustic source, which when associated with emotional distress, cognitive dysfunction, and/or autonomic arousal, leading to behavioral changes and functional disability becomes a disorder'.

Disorder in DSM-5

The American Psychiatric Association publishes the Diagnostic and Statistical Manual of Mental Disorders. The diagnostic criteria for Somatic Symptom Disorder are noted in DSM 5, its most recent version are the following:

1. One or more somatic symptoms that are distressing or result in significant disruption of daily life.
2. Excessive thoughts, feelings, or behaviors related to the somatic symptoms or associated health concerns as manifested by at least one of the following:
   - disproportionate and persistent thoughts about the seriousness of one's symptoms,
   - persistently high level of anxiety about health or symptoms,
   - excessive time and energy devoted to these symptoms or health concerns.
3. Although any one somatic symptom may not be continuously present, the state of being symptomatic is persistent (typically more than 6 months).

The somatic symptom disorder can be specified as "with predominant pain" (previously pain disorder) for individuals whose somatic symptoms predominantly involve pain.

Based on the pathophysiological, clinical, and treatment analogies between chronic pain and chronic tinnitus, it is proposed that tinnitus disorder falls under the somatic symptom disorder specified as "with predominant tinnitus". The other specifications could also be maintained:

Persistent: A persistent course is characterized by severe symptoms, marked impairment, and long duration (more than 6 months; Criterion 3). It would make sense to change this into 3 months (see above).

Mild: Only one of the symptoms specified in Criterion 2 is fulfilled.

Moderate: Two or more of the symptoms specified in Criterion 2 are fulfilled.

Severe: Two or more of the symptoms specified in Criterion 2 are fulfilled, plus there are multiple somatic complaints (or one very severe somatic symptom).

Anatomical Similarities Between Somatosensory and Auditory System

The Pain Pathways

The traditional view on the pathophysiology of pain is based on the pain gate model of pain, localized in the spinal cord [9]. Pain is considered a problem of imbalance between large thickly myelinated Aβ fibers and small fibers [9]. The small fibers consist of thinly myelinated Aδ and unmyelinated C fibers. The thinly myelinated Aδ fibers encode fast sharp pain and the unmyelinated C fibers result in slow dull pain, and Aβ fibers process touch information [65]. Yet, it has become evident that this simple but beautiful concept is not tenable, as all fiber types exist in low and high threshold versions [66–68]. Aδ fibers are proposed to detect change, as they have the lowest threshold, transmit information at low velocity, are activated by stimulus on/offset, and have large receptive fields, responding to any hair movement [67]. Aβ fibers transmit the content of change that is detected by the Aδ fibers. They also have low thresholds, but transmit at high velocity, meaning they carry the highest information content and respond to specific hair cells. Aβ fibers are activated by on/offset and persists during stimulation [68]. C fibers encode whether the stimulus is beneficial or detrimental, which phenomenologically is expressed as pleasantness or unpleasantness of the stimulus [69]. All these fiber types have their cell bodies in the dorsal root ganglion. In the dorsal root ganglion, C fibers make up 70% of all fibers, Aδ about 3%, and Aβ 27% [70]. From the dorsal root ganglion, the different fiber types continue to the dorsal horn of the spinal cord to end in different layers of the spinal cord. Low threshold C fibers end in layer II, low threshold Aδ fibers in layer III, and low threshold Aβ fibers in layer IV [71]. High threshold C fibers end in layer I and II, high threshold Aδ fibers end in layer I and V, and high threshold Aβ fibers end in layers I to V [72, 73].

From the dorsal horn, at least four pathways relay the information to the brain, three ipsilaterally and one pathway crosses at the level of the entry in the spinal cord. The ipsilateral pathways include the postsynaptic dorsal column, the spinocerebellar and the spinocervical pathways [74]. The anterolateral system crosses to the contralateral side and divides in three pathways. The spinoreticular tract is involved in processing alertness and arousal in response to painful stimuli, the spinotectal tract orients eyes and head towards the stimuli, and the spinothalamic tract, also known as the lateral lemniscus, transmits nocuous stimuli to the thalamus, and from there to the cortex. The spinothalamic tract consists of two pathways, the lateral and anterior spinothalamic tract [75–78]. Confusingly, the anterior spinothalamic pathway is also known as the lateral pain pathway, because the pathway ends in the lateral thalamic nuclei (VPL and VPI) [75–78]. It is the conventional pain pathway that relays information to the somatosensory cortex for processing of the discriminatory components of pain. The lateral spinothalamic pathway is known as the medial pain pathway, because it ends in the medial thalamic nuclei (mediodorsal nucleus) [75–78]. It starts in lamina I and is therefore also known as the lamina I spinothalamic pathway, and from the medial thalamic nuclei the information is relayed to the anterior cingulate cortex and anterior insula, for processing of the affective-motivational components of pain [75–78].

A more recent view envisions pain as a balance between three separable pathways [17, 79, 80], two pain-evoking pathways [81, 82], and one pain inhibitory pathway [83], rather than three fiber types, as proposed in the original pain gate model [9]. The lateral pain pathway, as described above, encodes the discriminatory sensory [82] component, i.e. how painful a stimulus is, the characteristics of the pain (burning, throbbing, …) and the location of the pain. It is a pain-specific pathway, in contrast to the medial pain pathway, which is nonspecific, and encodes suffering [79]. Indeed, the medial pathway encodes the motivational/affective component of pain [75, 82, 84, 85], i.e., the unpleasantness via the rostral anterior cingulate cortex [84] and catastrophizing via the anterior insula [86]. When combined, this explains suffering [59], as demonstrated clinically and by functional imaging meta-analysis [79]. The medial pathway also encodes distress, an autonomic arousal state [56], and consequentially drives the attention to the pain, as confirmed by cingulotomies, which decrease not only the affective component of pain but also attention paid to pain [87]. The medial pathway is nonspecific, in that it overlaps with suffering or distress-experienced tinnitus [88], but also symptoms such as breathlessness (air hunger) [89–92], hunger [93], thirst [94–96], social exclusion [97], and others. It is fundamentally a salience pathway [98] that attaches a behavioral relevance to the pain and tinnitus and maintains the pain into consciousness [99, 100].

The descending pain modulating pathway runs from the dorsolateral prefrontal cortex to the pregenual anterior cingulate cortex to the reticular nucleus of the thalamus, periaqueductal grey, and is relayed from there to the rostroventral medulla oblongata and spinal cord [75, 83, 101]. It also involves the (para)hippocampal area [101], which links the pain percept to context [102, 103].

The pain inhibitory pathway suppresses ongoing pain in a state-dependent manner [83] and determines the presence

[104, 105], i.e. most likely the duration of chronic neuropathic pain during the day, analogous to what is known in tinnitus [106]. The medial and lateral pain pathways process noxious stimuli in parallel [107] and can be individually modulated without affecting the other pathway [82], as evidenced by both cingulotomies/lobotomies [108], mood changes, and distraction [82]. In lobotomies, the unpleasantness is removed from the pain, but the intensity remains the same, and mood influences the unpleasantness but not the intensity of the pain [82, 109]. But in contrast, distraction reduces pain intensity without decreasing unpleasantness [82].

Pain is context-dependent [110], as evident in soldiers evacuated from the battle front [111]. Observations made in wounded soldiers evacuated from the frontline clearly documented that there is no relationship between the extent of the injury and the presence or intensity of the experienced pain, in contrast to civilian trauma [111]. In the frontline of a battlefield, surviving is more behaviorally relevant, i.e., more salient, than perceiving pain, as pain could lead to immobilization, and thus prevent appropriate measures (fight or flight response) essential for staying alive. In Beecher's words, who studied the soldiers coming from the battle front: "The intensity of suffering is largely determined by what the pain means to the patient" [111]. Thus, the intensity of the suffering is largely determined by the salience of the pain in a specific context. In sado-masochism, pain can be perceived as pleasant, the opposite of suffering. However, the noxious stimulus is only perceived as pleasurable in the very specific erotic context [112]. When a sadomasochist hits his finger with a hammer in a nonerotic context, the pain will feel equally unpleasant and causes the same amount of suffering as for a non-sadomasochist [112]. Pleasant pain is mediated via activation of the descending pain inhibitory pathway, whereas unpleasant pain is processed via the medial pain system [84, 113].

Another example of context dependent pain is placebo analgesia [110], in which the combination of expectation, affect, and social context results in pain suppression in the absence of an active treatment [114].

Pain can lead to perceived disability, which is predominantly related to the suffering or catastrophizing [115], and less so to the painfulness [116]. Forty percent of the total effect of pain severity on functional disability is mediated by pain catastrophizing [117]. Yet, there may be an indirect effect of painfulness. A cluster analysis in patients seen at a neurosurgical clinic for back and leg pain demonstrated that visual analogue scores (VAS) for painfulness of 5 or less are associated with normal catastrophizing (suffering) scores, normal quality of life, and normal disability scores. VAS painfulness scores of 6 and higher are associated with suffering but no disability, whereas VAS painfulness >7 are associated with suffering and disability [64]. This suggests that some threshold exists (VAS 5) above which painfulness results in suffering, and another threshold (VAS 7) above which painfulness becomes associated with suffering plus disability [64].

The Auditory Pathways

The auditory system is organized in way that is analogous to the somatosensory system.

When evaluating tinnitus, the separation between the medial and lateral pathway is less obvious than for pain. The auditory cortex, part of the lateral sensory pathway, is also involved in affective processing [118], and the anterior cingulate cortex and insula, part of the affective pathway, are also involved in loudness processing [119]. A possible explanation may be that tinnitus loudness and tinnitus distress correlate [120–123]. Therefore, loudness and distress may obviously correlate with the same brain areas. Yet, it cannot be excluded that tinnitus loudness and distress encoding areas truly overlap. The lobotomy data do suggest that one may change the affective suffering component without altering the loudness component [124, 125], and that the medial and lateral pathways are thus truly separable.

The medial auditory pathway appears to be very similar to the medial pain pathway [17]. Indeed, the medial 'salience' system is activated by sounds as well [126–128], and the pathways largely overlap [129] with the medial pain pathways. This also explains why the dorsal anterior cingulate cortex is involved in both pain and tinnitus, as demonstrated by a machine learning approach looking at the commonalities between pain and tinnitus [14].

Transcranial magnetic stimulation [130], transcranial direct current stimulation [131], and implants [132] of the dorsal anterior cingulate cortex all modulate both the tinnitus loudness perception and the affective component, in keeping with the functional imaging literature.

The descending auditory inhibitory pathways, also known as the noise cancelling pathways, can be reconstructed based on the published literature. Analogous to the descending pain inhibitory pathways, the pre-to-subgenual anterior cingulate cortex is involved [133–135]. It has been hypothesized that this connects to the reticular nucleus of the thalamus [133, 134]. The pgACC may also connect to the ventral tectal longitudinal column [136–138], which lies between the somatosensory periaqueductal gray and visual dorsal tectal longitudinal column [139], and is involved in sound suppression [136–138]. The ventral tectal longitudinal column connects to the olive in the brainstem [140], from where the olivocochlear bundle transmits inhibitory information to the cochlea [141, 142].

In summary, based on the existing literature about the anatomy and physiology of the auditory pathways, it can be proposed that the somatosensory system and auditory system are very similar in structure and function.

Pain and Tinnitus as an Intracranial Balance Problem

Pain can be regarded as a balance between pain input and pain suppression [80, 85, 143]. When pain input equals suppression no pain is perceived, but when input is increased and/or suppression is decreased, pain ensues. This has been well described as the pain gate at the level of the spinal cord [54] and can be conceptualized at the level of the brain as well [23, 80, 85, 143].

When a patient calls on a healthcare professional to treat his or her pain, the patient will tell he or she "is in pain". What the patient actually conveys is that she has a certain amount of painfulness associated with a certain amount of suffering, present during a certain amount of time [79]. Each of these three aspects of pain can be related to one of the three abovementioned pathways: the lateral painfulness pathway, the medial suffering pathway, and the descending perceptual pathway which can be visualized by functional magnetic resonance imaging (fMRI). A neurosynth meta-analysis of 420 fMRI studies (www.neurosynth.org) confirms that in chronic pain all three pathways are involved.

Similarly, when a patient with tinnitus calls on a healthcare professional to treat his or her tinnitus, the patient will tell he or she has tinnitus. This means that the patient perceives the phantom sound with a certain amount of loudness associated with a certain amount of suffering, present during the day during a certain amount of time. Also, each of these three components can be related to one of the three abovementioned pathways: the lateral loudness pathway, the medial suffering pathway, and the descending perceptual pathway.

In pain, using EEG, one can compute a balance between the three pathways by selecting one area as main hub for each pathway: the somatosensory cortex (SSC) activity as a proxy for the lateral pain-specific ascending pathway, the dorsal anterior cingulate cortex (dACC) activity as a proxy for the medial suffering pathway, and the pregenual anterior cingulate cortex (pgACC) activity as a proxy for the descending pain inhibitory pathway [80, 144]. Using source localization with sLORETA [145], the current density, i.e. the amount of current in a voxel, can be computed in the pregenual anterior cingulate cortex, the dorsal anterior cingulate cortex, and the somatosensory cortex, and the balance between the areas can be calculated using the formula 'pain = current density (dACC + SSC)/2× current density pgACC', which reflects the balance of the activity between the two pain evoking pathways and the one pain suppressing pathway [80, 85]. This balance indeed correlates with the presence and intensity of the pain [80].

A balance can only be maintained when these three areas communicate. This can be visualized by computing functional and effective connectivity. Functional connectivity, as expressed by lagged phase synchronization between the pgACC, dACC, and SSC, is reduced in chronic (neuropathic) pain in comparison to healthy controls without pain [80]. Thus, the pain input and pain suppression become uncoupled, leading to an imbalance, i.e. pain [79]. But functional connectivity does not explain from where to where in the brain the information flows. Effective connectivity shows the direction of the functional connectivity. In healthy controls without pain, the pgACC sends information to the dACC and SSC. This suggests that the pgACC inhibits activity in the dACC and SSC, preventing or suppressing pain by maintaining a balance between pain input (dACC+SSC) and pain suppression (pgACC). In contrast, in chronic pain, the effective connectivity is disturbed, with reversed information flow from the dACC to the pgACC, likely reducing the inhibitory capacity of the pgACC [80]. This assumes that both the pgACC and dACC effective connectivities are inhibitory, which is possible as both these areas have GABA receptors [146].

Considering the analogy between the somatosensory and auditory system described above, it can be hypothesized that in tinnitus a similar mechanism is at work, in which tinnitus is the result of an imbalance between the dACC, auditory cortex (AC), and pgACC. This is in keeping with a previously proposed model [88], which attempted to reconcile the noise cancelling deficiency model of tinnitus [133, 134] and the deafferentation-based models of tinnitus [16, 88]. However, it has been shown that in tinnitus there are likely 2 different pathophysiological mechanisms, one for tinnitus with hearing loss, and one for tinnitus without hearing loss [18, 147, 148]. This is reminiscent of the difference between neuropathic pain and fibromyalgia. Neuropathic pain is related to sensory deafferentation, whereas in fibromyalgia pain suppression, mediated via the pgACC, is deficient [143, 149, 150]. Whereas tinnitus without hearing loss involves the pgACC, tinnitus with little hearing loss involves the auditory cortex, and tinnitus with more severe hearing loss involves the parahippocampus [18, 147, 148], the main hub of auditory memory [151–153]. Thus, the imbalance may be based on different triggers in patients with tinnitus with and without hearing loss.

What Controls the Imbalance in Pain and Tinnitus?

The balance between pain input and suppression is likely controlled by the reward/dysreward system [17, 79]. The reward system can be simplified as a balance between positive and negative reward prediction errors, computed by the nucleus accumbens and habenula, respectively [154]. The habenula is also connected to the ventral tegmental area, as well as periaqueductal gray, dorsal anterior cingulate cortex and insula, thalamus and somatosensory cortex, all involved in pain processing [155, 156]. Furthermore, it receives input from the nucleus accumbens [155, 156], permitting a balance function between nucleus accumbens, ventral tegmental area, and habenula. Consequently, the ventral tegmental area may be arbitrating between the reward and dysreward system and compute the final balance.

The chronification of pain has been linked to the emergence of both increased functional [157] and structural connectivity [158] between the nucleus accumbens and the pregenual anterior cingulate cortex. This could be explained as a paradoxical reward associated with the pain.

In tinnitus, the same pathological functional connectivity has been demonstrated between the nucleus accumbens and the pregenual anterior cingulate cortex as well as between the nucleus accumbens and the auditory cortex [159], suggesting a similar mechanism may be at play. However, in this study no correlation was made with tinnitus chronification, albeit that all patients had chronic tinnitus. Yet, it does suggest that a paradoxical reward may underlie chronic tinnitus as well.

Integrating the Bayesian Brain with Imbalance

Based on Helmholtz's active inference concept for vision, also known as the predictive brain, a new model for brain functioning has been proposed, called the Bayesian brain [18, 160–164], which is basically the predictive brain model with added updating via sensorimotor exploration of the environment [162, 164, 165]. Bayesian inference can therefore be conceptualized as the use of sensorimotor and social information from the environment to update memory-based prior representations or models of the world (held before acquiring new inputs) to produce posterior representations (that emerge after acquiring those sensory or social inputs) and which integrate action-relevant information [166]. The Bayesian brain model has also been applied to tinnitus [18, 147, 148, 167, 168] (see Chap. 17). In summary, brains are prediction machines, essential in navigation/movement, using information from previous experiences (memory), to predict future events (intelligence), based on current context, in relation to the self, to reduce uncertainty, important for natural and sexual selection.

The brain can make multiple predictions in parallel [160, 169] and the prediction that best fits the sensory sampling survives and becomes the next percept [169]. If in doubt, the percept will switch between predictions, as readily noted in the Rubin vase and the Necker cube illusions. The reliability of the current behavioral strategy is encoded by ventral medial prefrontal cortex and pregenual anterior cingulate cortex [160], while the reliability of alternative behavioral strategies is encoded by lateral frontopolar cortex. When the reliability of the current strategy decreases, the behavioral strategy switches to the alternative. This switching is encoded by rostral to dorsal anterior cingulate cortex, and the rejection of the current strategy is encoded by ventrolateral prefrontal cortex, while the confirmation of new behavioral strategy as actor is encoded by ventral striatum, i.e. nucleus accumbens [160]. Translating this to chronic pain, it can be proposed that in chronic pain the dorsal anterior cingulate cortex switches the current pain-free state to a painful state (via the habenula). The accumbens confirms the painful state as beneficial, i.e. as the new reference state. The pregenual anterior cingulate cortex confirms the painful state as reliable and the functional connectivity between the nucleus accumbens and pregenual anterior cingulate cortex maintains the painful state. Indeed, chronification of acute to chronic pain involves the presence of both functional [157] and structural connectivity [158] between the nucleus accumbens and the pregenual anterior cingulate cortex [157, 158]. This concept can also be translated to chronic tinnitus. In chronic tinnitus, the dorsal anterior cingulate cortex switches the current tinnitus-free state to a tinnitus state (via the habenula). The accumbens confirms the tinnitus state as beneficial, i.e. as the new reference state. The pregenual anterior cingulate cortex confirms the tinnitus state as reliable and the functional connectivity between the nucleus accumbens and pregenual anterior cingulate cortex maintains the tinnitus state. This can also explain the functional connectivity between the nucleus accumbens and the pregenual anterior cingulate cortex as well as the functional connectivity between the nucleus accumbens and the auditory cortex [159]. In tinnitus patients with high distress, i.e. suffering, the connectivity extends to other areas and also involves connections between the habenula and dorsal anterior cingulate cortex, ventral tegmental area and parahippocampal area, nucleus accumbens and dorsal anterior cingulate cortex, and between the nucleus accumbens and parahippocampal area [159], incorporating both the contextual and the affective component of tinnitus in the reference state network.

Neuroinflammation in Chronic Pain and Tinnitus

Neuroinflammation, i.e. a local inflammation of tissue within the PNS and CNS, is characterized by infiltration of immune cells, activation of glial cells, and production of inflammatory mediators, such as chemokines and cytokines, as well as neuroactive substances [170]. Neuroinflammation plays an important role in the transition from acute to chronic pain, as well as in the persistence of chronic pain [171–176].

Whenever tissue damage occurs, a local inflammation ensues in the area of the tissue damage. Neuroinflammation could be induced by altered, i.e. prolonged increased C fiber activity, aka neurogenic neuroinflammation [170, 177]. Chronic pain is associated with a long-lasting and sometimes even permanent central sensitization that persists after acute inflammation has been resolved [178]. This inflammatory response in the peripheral tissue triggers an inflammation in the dorsal root ganglion, resulting in peripheral sensitization, clinically expressed as pain hypersensitivity [179]. The neuroinflammation in the DRG subsequently causes an inflammatory response in the dorsal horn of the spinal cord [179], resulting in central sensitization, clinically expressed as allodynia [179]. From the dorsal horn, the inflammation is further relayed to the brain [179]. When the medial pathway is involved, this leads to alterations in the affective component of pain; when the lateral pathway is inflamed, the sensory discriminatory component of pain, i.e. painfulness, worsens. Indeed, in chronic pain the frequency of painfulness is associated with a neuroinflammation of the lateral pathways [180] and the suffering is related to neuroinflammation of the medial pathways [181].

Similarly, tinnitus has been linked to neuroinflammation [182–184], starting with a peripheral inflammation at the level of the cochlea, spreading to cochlear nucleus, extending to the inferior colliculus, medial geniculate body, and ultimately to the primary and secondary auditory cortex [184].

The sympathetic and parasympathetic nervous systems are involved in inflammation. The sympathetic system can be both pro-inflammatory and anti-inflammatory [185, 186], whereas the parasympathetic nervous system is generally considered anti-inflammatory [187, 188]. Consequently, it is unsurprising that both the sympathetic and parasympathetic nervous systems are involved in the pathophysiology of chronic pain and tinnitus.

Role of the Autonomic Nervous System in Chronic Pain and Tinnitus

The autonomic nervous system consists of the sympathetic (SNS), parasympathetic (PNS), and enteric nervous system [189]. The sympathetic nervous system releases noradrenaline at its target organs where it activates alpha and beta receptors. Activation of the SNS leads to a state of overall elevated activity and attention: a fight or flight response [189]. This is characterized by increased sensory perception with pupil dilation, increased visual and auditory sensory detection, as well as increased energy generation and delivery to muscles via blood pressure and heart rate elevation, increased respiratory rate, and glycogenolysis as to prepare for the fight or flight reaction. This increased cardiac and muscular energy delivery is combined with reduced energy delivery at the gastrointestinal tract, leading to gastrointestinal peristalsis. The SNS also activates the adrenal gland to secrete adrenaline and noradrenaline and influences the immune system. The parasympathetic system, on the other hand, releases acetylcholine that acts on muscarinic receptors at its target organs inducing a rest, digest, and restore response [189]. The activity of the sympathetic and parasympathetic nervous systems is tightly balanced, most commonly antagonistic in direction, thereby creating an inverted-U curve profile of target activation.

The Sympathetic Nervous System (SNS)

The SNS is involved in pain perception via different mechanisms at different levels, from the periphery to the brain [190]. Sympathetically driven noradrenaline release enhances afferent skin sensitivity, as well as increases sensitivity of the vasculature [190]. Furthermore, the number of nociceptors is increased, as are the number of sympathetic fibers that contact the dorsal root ganglion leading to peripheral sensitization [190]. The sympathetic nervous system is also involved in the inflammatory response in the dorsal horn and brain, leading to central sensitization, clinically expressed as allodynia [190].

The involvement of the sympathetic nervous system in pain is most clearly evidenced in complex regional pain syndrome (CRPS) [191], sympathetically mediated pain [192], and autonomic headaches [193]. Furthermore, sympathetic nerve blocks and sympathectomies can relieve some of these pain syndromes, albeit that there is no meta-analytic scientific evidence for it [194].

The SNS is also involved in tinnitus [20, 56, 195–197] at multiple levels, from cochlea [198] to cortex [21, 56, 196]. Sympathetic hyperactivity is a risk factor [199] for stress-induced tinnitus [198], but also a consequence of tinnitus, leading to a vicious circle of stress and tinnitus. Stress may be involved in tinnitus via the hypothalamus-pituitary-adrenal axis (HPA axis), the sympathetic-adreno-medullar (SAM) axis, and the immune axis [198]. Sympathetic blocks may be beneficial for the treatment of tinnitus [200], especially tinnitus in the setting of Meniere's disease [201, 202], as could be sympathectomies [203].

Parasympathetic Nervous System (PNS)

Meta-analytic evidence shows that the parasympathetic system is suppressed in chronic pain [204], in keeping with activation of the PNS when no danger is present, to generate a rest and digest state. Vagus nerve stimulation can reduce sympathetic activity and increase parasympathetic activity [205]. Activating the suppressed vagus nerve by transcutaneous stimulation improves pain, especially in headaches, more specifically in cluster headache [206] and migraine [206], but also more generally after surgery [207], as evidenced by meta-analytic data.

Tinnitus is also associated with sympathetic dominance and non-invasive vagus nerve stimulation reduces this sympathetic preponderance in tinnitus patients [197]. This is associated with a small improvement in tinnitus loudness [208], albeit not in all studies [209]. A systematic review on invasive and non-invasive vagus nerve stimulation confirmed the small benefit on distress and loudness [210]. Whether vagus nerve stimulation is paired to acoustic stimulation or not does not seem to matter [208, 210–212].

The Microbiome in Chronic Pain and Tinnitus

The microbiome comprises a complex collection of microorganisms, with their genes and metabolites, colonizing different parts of the body [213]. The microbiome communicates in a bidirectional way with its host via immunological, hormonal, and neural pathways [214]. The neural pathways involve both spinal and vagal communication channels [215]. The signals generated by gut microbes can alter brain structure and function, while autonomic nervous system activity can affect the microbiome by modulating the intestinal environment and by directly regulating microbial behavior [216]. The microbiome assists in the bioconversion of nutrients and detoxification, supporting immunity, protecting against pathogenic microbes, and maintaining health [213], including mental health [215]. The microbiome is formed by the age of 3 and can be influenced by many factors, including genetics, the way of childbirth, diet, age, stress, toxins, and drugs [217]. The disruption of this balance, which is called dysbiosis, is associated with a plethora of diseases, including chronic pain [214, 218–220] and possibly tinnitus [221].

Treatment of Chronic Neuropathic Pain and Chronic Tinnitus

Treatment analogies exist between chronic pain and tinnitus, as do differences [222]. The main difference between the treatment of chronic pain and tinnitus is that there are specific physiological pain pathways, which can be addressed by 'pain killers' such as anti-inflammatory products and opioids [8]. There is no such analogy for tinnitus.

The pathophysiological and electrophysiological similarities between chronic pain and tinnitus have resulted in similar therapeutic approaches, involving pharmacology, neuromodulation, and psychological treatment proposals.

Even though there is no pharmacological treatment for tinnitus that is approved by the FDA and CE, many medications have been tested that are also used in some forms of chronic pain [223]. Pharmacologically, lidocaine or lidocaine-like drugs were tested both in pain and tinnitus [224], as are antiepileptics [225, 226], and antidepressants, even though meta-analytic evidence does not support their use in tinnitus [225, 226]. But also neuromodulation treatments consisting of noninvasive and invasive stimulation of the somatosensory cortex and auditory cortex were developed [222, 227, 228]. Other common therapy modalities that have been studied include cognitive behavior therapy [229, 230], as well as acupuncture [231, 232] and low level laser therapy [233, 234]. The similarities in treatment approaches might be related not only to anatomical and pathophysiological analogies, but also to the cross-modal interaction between senses, as electrical stimulation of the somatosensory system (trigeminal nerve) system could change the perception of tinnitus [235].

Similarly, psychological treatments have been used, especially cognitive behavioral therapy, for both chronic pain [230] and tinnitus [229]. These treatments attempt to improve the suffering associated with chronic pain and tinnitus.

Also, noninvasive and invasive neuromodulation have been used as a treatment for chronic pain and tinnitus [236]. Noninvasive treatments consist of transcranial magnetic stimulation, transcranial electrical stimulation, and neurofeedback [237]. Transcranial electrical stimulation comes in three forms, transcranial direct current stimulation, transcranial random noise stimulation, and transcranial alternating current stimulation [237]. Invasive neuromodulation comes under the form of implanted electrodes, for chronic pain especially at the level of the spinal cord, but also peripherally and intracranially [136]. For tinnitus, these implants remain predominantly experimental. For details of these treatments, the reader is referred to the specific chapters.

Conclusion: Common Etiopathology in Chronic Pain and Tinnitus

Chronic pain and tinnitus may share a common pathophysiology leading to a shared electrophysiology (Figs. 8.3 and 8.4).

Both symptoms are related to genetic factors, which include genetic polymorphisms that influence immune and

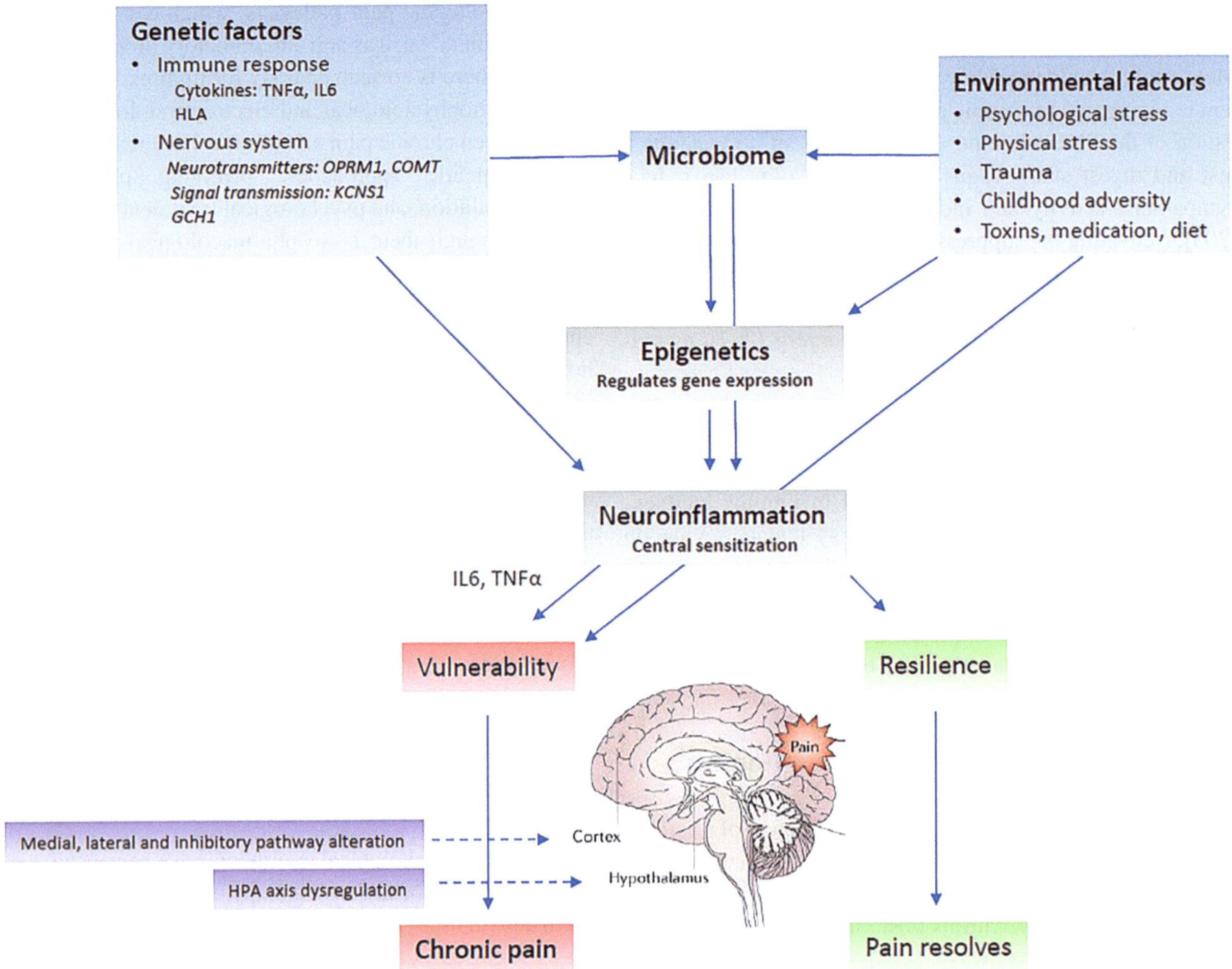

Fig. 8.3 Pathophysiology of chronic pain

nervous system functioning [19, 20, 79]. The expression of these risk genes is triggered by environmental factors, which include psychological and physical stress, trauma and toxins, medication, or diet [19, 20, 79]. For chronic pain, there exists a strong correlation with childhood adversity [38, 39], which has been suggested for tinnitus as well [40, 41], but not unequivocally demonstrated. These environmental factors exert their influence via alterations in the microbiome as well as by epigenetic modifications of genes involved in neural and/or immunological processing. This leads to a final common pathway of neuroinflammation. The neuroinflammation has been hypothesized to alter the tinnitus [183, 184, 238] and pain [171, 173, 180] network and its integration into the triple network and emotional network [19, 20, 79]. A shared pathological electrophysiology then ensues, consisting of pathological cross-frequency coupling, known as thalamocortical dysrhythmia [12, 14, 16], which becomes embedded in the triple network, required for conscious processing of the pain and tinnitus percept, as well as the suffering in pain disorder and tinnitus disorder [19–21, 79].

Based on the similar clinical picture and similar pathophysiology, analogous treatments have been developed for both symptoms, consisting of pharmacological, neuromodulatory, and psychological approaches.

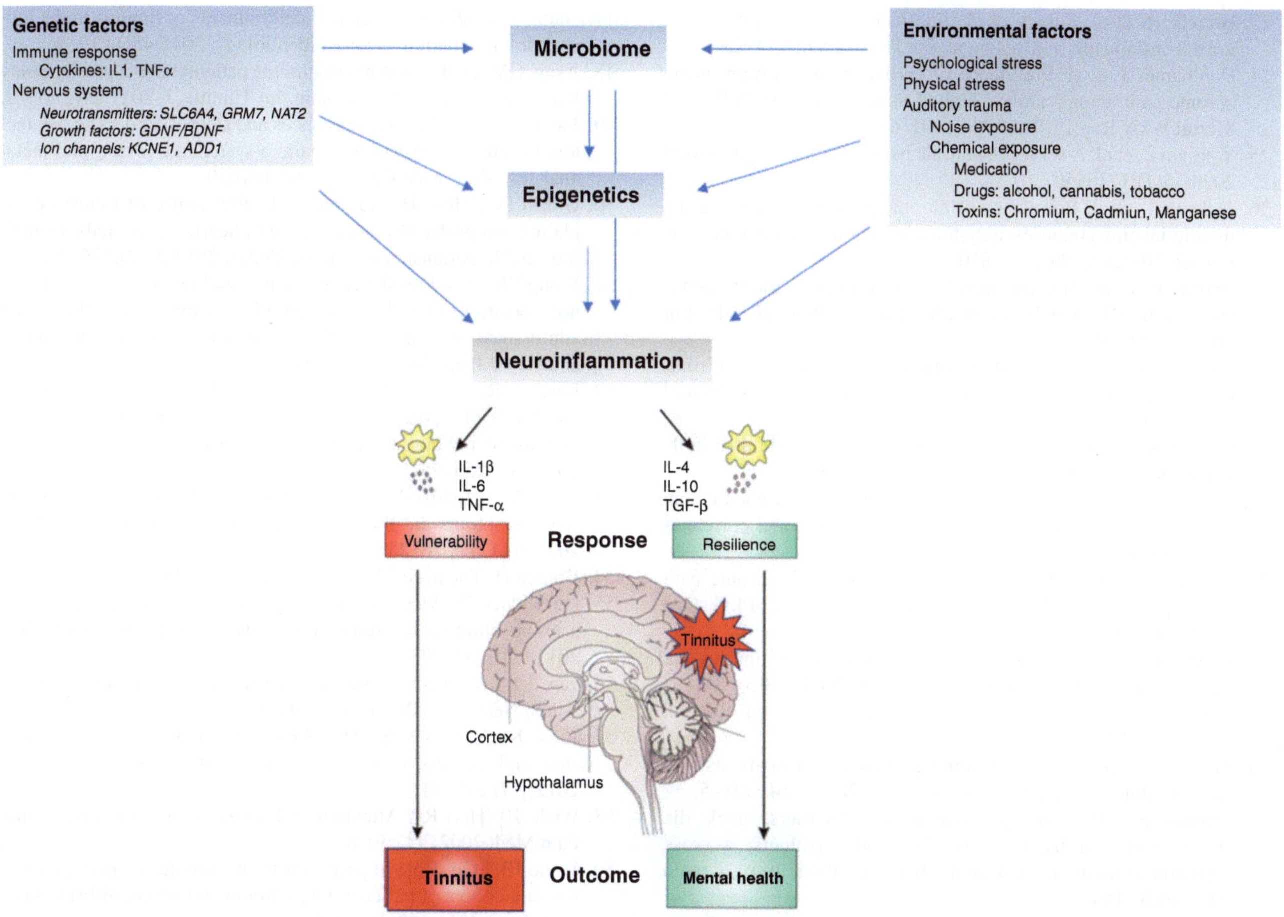

Fig. 8.4 Pathophysiology of tinnitus

References

1. Tonndorf J. The analogy between tinnitus and pain: a suggestion for a physiological basis of chronic tinnitus. Hear Res. 1987;28(2–3):271–5.
2. Moller AR. Similarities between severe tinnitus and chronic pain. J Am Acad Audiol. 2000;11(3):115–24.
3. Moller AR. Similarities between chronic pain and tinnitus. Am J Otol. 1997;18(5):577–85.
4. Moller AR. Tinnitus and pain. Prog Brain Res. 2007;166:47–53.
5. Norena A, et al. Psychoacoustic characterization of the tinnitus spectrum: implications for the underlying mechanisms of tinnitus. Audiol Neurootol. 2002;7(6):358–69.
6. Flor H, Nikolajsen L, Staehelin Jensen T. Phantom limb pain: a case of maladaptive CNS plasticity? Nat Rev Neurosci. 2006;7(11):873–81.
7. Ramachandran VS, Hirstein W. The perception of phantom limbs. The D O Hebb lecture. Brain. 1998;121(Pt 9):1603–30.
8. De Ridder D, et al. Phantom percepts: tinnitus and pain as persisting aversive memory networks. Proc Natl Acad Sci U S A. 2011;108(20):8075–80.
9. Melzack R, Wall PD. Pain mechanisms: a new theory. Science. 1965;150(699):971–9.
10. De Ridder D, Van de Heyning P. The Darwinian plasticity hypothesis for tinnitus and pain. Prog Brain Res. 2007;166:55–60.
11. De Ridder D, et al. Theta-gamma dysrhythmia and auditory phantom perception. J Neurosurg. 2011;114(4):912–21.
12. De Ridder D, et al. Thalamocortical dysrhythmia: a theoretical update in tinnitus. Front Neurol. 2015;6:124.
13. To WT, et al. Thalamocortical dysrhythmia underpin the log-dynamics in phantom sounds. Prog Brain Res. 2021;262:511–26.
14. Vanneste S, Song JJ, De Ridder D. Thalamocortical dysrhythmia detected by machine learning. Nat Commun. 2018;9(1):1103.
15. Jeanmonod D, et al. Neuropsychiatric thalamocortical dysrhythmia: surgical implications. Neurosurg Clin N Am. 2003;14(2):251–65.
16. Llinas RR, et al. Thalamocortical dysrhythmia: a neurological and neuropsychiatric syndrome characterized by magnetoencephalography. Proc Natl Acad Sci U S A. 1999;96(26):15222–7.
17. De Ridder D, Vanneste S. The Bayesian brain in imbalance: medial, lateral and descending pathways in tinnitus and pain: a perspective. Prog Brain Res. 2021;262:309–34.
18. De Ridder D, Vanneste S, Freeman W. The Bayesian brain: phantom percepts resolve sensory uncertainty. Neurosci Biobehav Rev. 2014;44C:4–15.
19. De Ridder D, et al. Pain and the triple network model. Front Neurol. 2022;13:757241.
20. De Ridder D, et al. Tinnitus and the triple network model: a perspective. Clin Exp Otorhinolaryngol. 2022;15:205.
21. De Ridder D, et al. Tinnitus and tinnitus disorder: theoretical and operational definitions (an international multidisciplinary proposal). Prog Brain Res. 2021;260:1–25.
22. Treede RD, et al. Chronic pain as a symptom or a disease: the IASP Classification of Chronic Pain for the International Classification of Diseases (ICD-11). Pain. 2019;160(1):19–27.

23. Breivik H, et al. Survey of chronic pain in Europe: prevalence, impact on daily life, and treatment. Eur J Pain. 2006;10(4):287–333.
24. Dahlhamer J, et al. Prevalence of chronic pain and high-impact chronic pain among adults - United States, 2016. MMWR Morb Mortal Wkly Rep. 2018;67(36):1001–6.
25. Yongjun Z, et al. A survey of chronic pain in China. Libyan J Med. 2020;15(1):1730550.
26. Jackson T, et al. Prevalence of chronic pain in low-income and middle-income countries: a systematic review and meta-analysis. Lancet. 2015;385(Suppl 2):S10.
27. Biswas R, et al. Tinnitus prevalence in Europe: a multi-country cross-sectional population study. Lancet Reg Health Eur. 2022;12:100250.
28. Jarach CM, et al. Global prevalence and incidence of tinnitus: a systematic review and meta-analysis. JAMA Neurol. 2022;79(9):888–900.
29. Stohler NA, et al. A study on the epidemiology of tinnitus in the United Kingdom. Clin Epidemiol. 2019;11:855–71.
30. Zajacova A, Grol-Prokopczyk H, Zimmer Z. Pain trends among american adults, 2002-2018: patterns, disparities, and correlates. Demography. 2021;58(2):711–38.
31. Ausland JH, et al. Tinnitus and associations with chronic pain: the population-based Tromso Study (2015-2016). PloS One. 2021;16(3):e0247880.
32. Isaacson JE, et al. Clinical associations between tinnitus and chronic pain. Otolaryngol Head Neck Surg. 2003;128(5):706–10.
33. Langguth B, et al. Tinnitus and headache. Biomed Res Int. 2015;2015:797416.
34. Michiels S, et al. Cervical spine dysfunctions in patients with chronic subjective tinnitus. Otol Neurotol. 2015;36(4):741–5.
35. Cimino R, et al. Temporomandibular disorders, neck disability, and oral parafunctions in tinnitus patients: a cross-sectional epidemiological study from Southern Italy. Cranio. 2022;40(6):485–93.
36. Park E, et al. Psychiatric distress as a common risk factor for tinnitus and joint pain: a national population-based survey. Clin Exp Otorhinolaryngol. 2020;13(3):234–40.
37. Kreuzer PM, et al. Trauma-associated tinnitus. J Head Trauma Rehabil. 2014;29(5):432–42.
38. Pierce J, et al. Characterizing pain and generalized sensory sensitivity according to trauma history among patients with knee osteoarthritis. Ann Behav Med. 2021;55:853.
39. You DS, Meagher MW. Childhood adversity and pain facilitation. Psychosom Med. 2018;80(9):869–79.
40. Aazh H, Danesh AA, Moore BCJ. Parental mental health in childhood as a risk factor for anxiety and depression among people seeking help for tinnitus and hyperacusis. J Am Acad Audiol. 2019;30(9):772–80.
41. Aazh H, Landgrebe M, Danesh AA. Parental mental illness in childhood as a risk factor for suicidal and self-harm ideations in adults seeking help for tinnitus and/or hyperacusis. Am J Audiol. 2019;28(3):527–33.
42. Aazh H, Langguth B, Danesh AA. Parental separation and parental mental health in childhood and tinnitus and hyperacusis disability in adulthood: a retrospective exploratory analysis. Int J Audiol. 2018;57(12):941–6.
43. Aazh H, Puri BK, Moore BCJ. Parental separation and parental mental health in childhood and risk of insomnia in adulthood among patients with tinnitus. J Am Acad Audiol. 2020;31(3):217–23.
44. Nelson CA, et al. Adversity in childhood is linked to mental and physical health throughout life. BMJ. 2020;371:m3048.
45. Kim HJ, et al. Analysis of the prevalence and associated risk factors of tinnitus in adults. PloS One. 2015;10(5):e0127578.
46. Guh DP, et al. The incidence of co-morbidities related to obesity and overweight: a systematic review and meta-analysis. BMC Public Health. 2009;9:88.
47. Gallus S, et al. Prevalence and determinants of tinnitus in the italian adult population. Neuroepidemiology. 2015;45(1):12–9.
48. Asnis GM, et al. Insomnia in tinnitus patients: a prospective study finding a significant relationship. Int Tinnitus J. 2021;24(2):65–9.
49. Varallo G, et al. Sleep disturbances and sleep disorders as risk factors for chronic postsurgical pain: a systematic review and meta-analysis. Sleep Med Rev. 2022;63:101630.
50. Gibrin PC, Melo JJ, Marchiori LL. Prevalence of tinnitus complaints and probable association with hearing loss, diabetes mellitus and hypertension in elderly. Codas. 2013;25(2):176–80.
51. Wong CK, et al. Prevalence, incidence, and factors associated with non-specific chronic low back pain in community-dwelling older adults aged 60 years and older: a systematic review and meta-analysis. J Pain. 2022;23(4):509–34.
52. Fonseca-Rodrigues D, et al. Correlation between pain severity and levels of anxiety and depression in osteoarthritis patients: a systematic review and meta-analysis. Rheumatology (Oxford). 2021;61(1):53–75.
53. Park M, et al. Association between tinnitus and depressive symptoms in the South Korean population. PloS One. 2021;16(12):e0261257.
54. Bonica JJ. The need of a taxonomy. Pain. 1979;6(3):247–8.
55. De Ridder D, Vanneste S, Congedo M. The distressed brain: a group blind source separation analysis on tinnitus. PloS One. 2011;6(10):e24273.
56. van der Loo E, et al. Insular lateralization in tinnitus distress. Auton Neurosci. 2011;165(2):191–4.
57. Joos K, Vanneste S, De Ridder D. Disentangling depression and distress networks in the tinnitus brain. PLoS One. 2012;7(7):e40544.
58. Wade JB, Hart RP. Attention and the stages of pain processing. Pain Med. 2002;3(1):30–8.
59. Wade JB, et al. Role of pain catastrophizing during pain processing in a cohort of patients with chronic and severe arthritic knee pain. Pain. 2011;152(2):314–9.
60. Craig AD. A new view of pain as a homeostatic emotion. Trends Neurosci. 2003;26(6):303–7.
61. Baguley D, McFerran D, Hall D. Tinnitus. Lancet. 2013;382(9904):1600–7.
62. Langguth B. A review of tinnitus symptoms beyond 'ringing in the ears': a call to action. Curr Med Res Opin. 2011;27(8):1635–43.
63. Lerman SF, et al. Longitudinal associations between depression, anxiety, pain, and pain-related disability in chronic pain patients. Psychosom Med. 2015;77(3):333–41.
64. Raymaekers V, et al. Real world data collection and cluster analysis in patients with sciatica due to lumbar disc herniation. Clin Neurol Neurosurg. 2022;217:107246.
65. Julius D, Basbaum AI. Molecular mechanisms of nociception. Nature. 2001;413(6852):203–10.
66. Djouhri L. Electrophysiological evidence for the existence of a rare population of C-fiber low threshold mechanoreceptive (C-LTM) neurons in glabrous skin of the rat hindpaw. Neurosci Lett. 2016;613:25–9.
67. Djouhri L. Adelta-fiber low threshold mechanoreceptors innervating mammalian hairy skin: a review of their receptive, electrophysiological and cytochemical properties in relation to Adelta-fiber high threshold mechanoreceptors. Neurosci Biobehav Rev. 2016;61:225–38.
68. Djouhri L, Lawson SN. Abeta-fiber nociceptive primary afferent neurons: a review of incidence and properties in relation to other afferent A-fiber neurons in mammals. Brain Res Brain Res Rev. 2004;46(2):131–45.
69. Olausson H, et al. The neurophysiology of unmyelinated tactile afferents. Neurosci Biobehav Rev. 2010;34(2):185–91.
70. Lawson SN, Fang X, Djouhri L. Nociceptor subtypes and their incidence in rat lumbar dorsal root ganglia (DRGs): focussing

on C-polymodal nociceptors, Abeta-nociceptors, moderate pressure receptors and their receptive field depths. Curr Opin Physiol. 2019;11:125–46.

71. Li L, et al. The functional organization of cutaneous low-threshold mechanosensory neurons. Cell. 2011;147(7):1615–27.
72. Comitato A, Bardoni R. Presynaptic inhibition of pain and touch in the spinal cord: from receptors to circuits. Int J Mol Sci. 2021;22(1):414.
73. Woodbury CJ, et al. Identity of myelinated cutaneous sensory neurons projecting to nocireceptive laminae following nerve injury in adult mice. J Comp Neurol. 2008;508(3):500–9.
74. Peirs C, Dallel R, Todd AJ. Recent advances in our understanding of the organization of dorsal horn neuron populations and their contribution to cutaneous mechanical allodynia. J Neural Transm (Vienna). 2020;127(4):505–25.
75. Craig AD. How do you feel? Interoception: the sense of the physiological condition of the body. Nat Rev Neurosci. 2002;3(8):655–66.
76. Craig AD, Dostrovsky J. Medulla to thalamus. In: Wall P, Melzack R, editors. Textbook of pain. Edingburgh: Churchill-Livingstone; 1999. p. 183–214.
77. Craig AD, Zhang ET, Blomqvist A. Association of spinothalamic lamina I neurons and their ascending axons with calbindin-immunoreactivity in monkey and human. Pain. 2002;97(1-2):105–15.
78. Dostrovsky JO. Role of thalamus in pain. Prog Brain Res. 2000;129:245–57.
79. De Ridder D, Adhia D, Vanneste S. The anatomy of pain and suffering in the brain and its clinical implications. Neurosci Biobehav Rev. 2021;130:125–46.
80. Vanneste S, De Ridder D. Chronic pain as a brain imbalance between pain input and pain suppression. Brain Commun. 2021;3(1):fcab014.
81. Price DD. Psychological and neural mechanisms of the affective dimension of pain. Science. 2000;288(5472):1769–72.
82. Bushnell MC, Ceko M, Low LA. Cognitive and emotional control of pain and its disruption in chronic pain. Nat Rev Neurosci. 2013;14(7):502–11.
83. Fields H. State-dependent opioid control of pain. Nat Rev Neurosci. 2004;5(7):565–75.
84. Rainville P, et al. Pain affect encoded in human anterior cingulate but not somatosensory cortex. Science. 1997;277(5328):968–71.
85. De Ridder D, Vanneste S. Burst and tonic spinal cord stimulation: different and common brain mechanisms. Neuromodulation. 2016;19(1):47–59.
86. Mathur VA, et al. High frequency migraine is associated with lower acute pain sensitivity and abnormal insula activity related to migraine pain intensity, attack frequency, and pain catastrophizing. Front Hum Neurosci. 2016;10:489.
87. Cohen RA, et al. Impairments of attention after cingulotomy. Neurology. 1999;53(4):819–24.
88. De Ridder D, et al. An integrative model of auditory phantom perception: tinnitus as a unified percept of interacting separable subnetworks. Neurosci Biobehav Rev. 2014;44:16–32.
89. von Leupoldt A, et al. Dyspnea and pain share emotion-related brain network. Neuroimage. 2009;48(1):200–6.
90. Liotti M, et al. Brain responses associated with consciousness of breathlessness (air hunger). Proc Natl Acad Sci U S A. 2001;98(4):2035–40.
91. Brannan S, et al. Neuroimaging of cerebral activations and deactivations associated with hypercapnia and hunger for air. Proc Natl Acad Sci U S A. 2001;98(4):2029–34.
92. Parsons LM, et al. Neuroimaging evidence implicating cerebellum in the experience of hypercapnia and hunger for air. Proc Natl Acad Sci U S A. 2001;98(4):2041–6.
93. Tataranni PA, et al. Neuroanatomical correlates of hunger and satiation in humans using positron emission tomography. Proc Natl Acad Sci U S A. 1999;96(8):4569–74.
94. Denton D, et al. Correlation of regional cerebral blood flow and change of plasma sodium concentration during genesis and satiation of thirst. Proc Natl Acad Sci U S A. 1999;96(5):2532–7.
95. Denton D, et al. Neuroimaging of genesis and satiation of thirst and an interoceptor-driven theory of origins of primary consciousness. Proc Natl Acad Sci U S A. 1999;96(9):5304–9.
96. Farrell MJ, et al. Effect of aging on regional cerebral blood flow responses associated with osmotic thirst and its satiation by water drinking: a PET study. Proc Natl Acad Sci U S A. 2008;105(1):382–7.
97. Eisenberger NI. The pain of social disconnection: examining the shared neural underpinnings of physical and social pain. Nat Rev Neurosci. 2012;13(6):421–34.
98. Seeley WW, et al. Dissociable intrinsic connectivity networks for salience processing and executive control. J Neurosci. 2007;27(9):2349–56.
99. Boly M, et al. Baseline brain activity fluctuations predict somatosensory perception in humans. Proc Natl Acad Sci U S A. 2007;104(29):12187–92.
100. Sadaghiani S, Hesselmann G, Kleinschmidt A. Distributed and antagonistic contributions of ongoing activity fluctuations to auditory stimulus detection. J Neurosci. 2009;29(42):13410–7.
101. Kong J, et al. Exploring the brain in pain: activations, deactivations and their relation. Pain. 2010;148(2):257–67.
102. Aminoff E, Gronau N, Bar M. The parahippocampal cortex mediates spatial and nonspatial associations. Cereb Cortex. 2007;17(7):1493–503.
103. Aminoff EM, Kveraga K, Bar M. The role of the parahippocampal cortex in cognition. Trends Cogn Sci. 2013;17(8):379–90.
104. Moens M, et al. Spinal cord stimulation modulates cerebral function: an fMRI study. Neuroradiology. 2012;54(12):1399–407.
105. Watanabe K, et al. Altered cerebral blood flow in the anterior cingulate cortex is associated with neuropathic pain. J Neurol Neurosurg Psychiatry. 2018;89(10):1082–7.
106. Song JJ. Dysfunctional noise cancelling of the rostral anterior cingulate cortex in tinnitus patients. PloS One. 2015;10(4):e0123538.
107. Frot M, et al. Parallel processing of nociceptive A-delta inputs in SII and midcingulate cortex in humans. J Neurosci. 2008;28(4):944–52.
108. Freeman W, Watts JW. Psychosurgery. 2nd ed. Springfield: Charles C Thomas; 1950.
109. Villemure C, Bushnell MC. Mood influences supraspinal pain processing separately from attention. J Neurosci. 2009;29(3):705–15.
110. Carlino E, Frisaldi E, Benedetti F. Pain and the context. Nat Rev Rheumatol. 2014;10(6):348–55.
111. Beecher HK. Relationship of significance of wound to pain experienced. JAMA. 1956;161(17):1609–13.
112. Kamping S, et al. Contextual modulation of pain in masochists: involvement of the parietal operculum and insula. Pain. 2016;157(2):445–55.
113. Leknes S, et al. The importance of context: when relative relief renders pain pleasant. Pain. 2013;154(3):402–10.
114. Atlas LY. A social affective neuroscience lens on placebo analgesia. Trends Cogn Sci. 2021;25(11):992–1005.
115. Kovacs FM, et al. The correlation between pain, catastrophizing, and disability in subacute and chronic low back pain: a study in the routine clinical practice of the Spanish National Health Service. Spine (Phila Pa 1976). 2011;36(4):339–45.
116. Garbi Mde O, et al. Pain intensity, disability and depression in individuals with chronic back pain. Rev Lat Am Enfermagem. 2014;22(4):569–75.

117. Besen E, et al. The role of pain catastrophizing as a mediator in the work disability process following acute low back pain. J Appl Biobehav Res. 2017;22(1):e12085.
118. Schecklmann M, et al. Auditory cortex is implicated in tinnitus distress: a voxel-based morphometry study. Brain Struct Funct. 2013;218(4):1061–70.
119. De Ridder D, Congedo M, Vanneste S. The neural correlates of subjectively perceived and passively matched loudness perception in auditory phantom perception. Brain Behav. 2015;5:e00331.
120. Wallhausser-Franke E, et al. Tinnitus: distinguishing between subjectively perceived loudness and tinnitus-related distress. PloS One. 2012;7(4):e34583.
121. Probst T, et al. Emotion dynamics and tinnitus: daily life data from the "TrackYourTinnitus" application. Sci Rep. 2016;6:31166.
122. Hiller W, Goebel G. Factors influencing tinnitus loudness and annoyance. Arch Otolaryngol Head Neck Surg. 2006;132(12):1323–30.
123. Bruggemann P, et al. Impact of multiple factors on the degree of tinnitus distress. Front Hum Neurosci. 2016;10:341.
124. Beard AW. Results of leucotomy operations for tinnitus. J Psychosom Res. 1965;9(1):29–32.
125. Elithorn A. Prefrontal leucotomy in the treatment of tinnitus. Proc R Soc Med. 1953;46(10):832–3.
126. Iannetti GD, Mouraux A. From the neuromatrix to the pain matrix (and back). Exp Brain Res. 2010;205(1):1–12.
127. Legrain V, et al. The pain matrix reloaded: a salience detection system for the body. Prog Neurobiol. 2011;93(1):111–24.
128. Mouraux A, et al. A multisensory investigation of the functional significance of the "pain matrix". Neuroimage. 2011;54(3):2237–49.
129. Langers D, Melcher JR. Hearing without listening: functional connectivity reveals the engagement of multiple nonauditory networks during basic sound processing. Brain Connect. 2011;1(3):233–44.
130. Vanneste S, et al. Repetitive transcranial magnetic stimulation frequency dependent tinnitus improvement by double cone coil prefrontal stimulation. J Neurol Neurosurg Psychiatry. 2011;82(10):1160–4.
131. Vanneste S, De Ridder D. Bifrontal transcranial direct current stimulation modulates tinnitus intensity and tinnitus-distress-related brain activity. Eur J Neurosci. 2011;34(4):605–14.
132. De Ridder D, Joos K, Vanneste S. Anterior cingulate implants for tinnitus: report of 2 cases. J Neurosurg. 2016;124(4):893–901.
133. Leaver AM, et al. Dysregulation of limbic and auditory networks in tinnitus. Neuron. 2011;69(1):33–43.
134. Rauschecker JP, Leaver AM, Muhlau M. Tuning out the noise: limbic-auditory interactions in tinnitus. Neuron. 2010;66(6):819–26.
135. Seydell-Greenwald A, et al. Functional MRI evidence for a role of ventral prefrontal cortex in tinnitus. Brain Res. 2012;1485:22–39.
136. De Ridder D, et al. Surgical brain modulation for tinnitus: the past, present and future. J Neurosurg Sci. 2012;56(4):323–40.
137. Marshall AF, et al. Auditory response properties of neurons in the tectal longitudinal column of the rat. Hear Res. 2008;244(1-2):35–44.
138. Saldana E, et al. The TLC: a novel auditory nucleus of the mammalian brain. J Neurosci. 2007;27(48):13108–16.
139. Aparicio MA, Saldana E. The dorsal tectal longitudinal column (TLCd): a second longitudinal column in the paramedian region of the midbrain tectum. Brain Struct Funct. 2014;219(2):607–30.
140. Vinuela A, et al. Connections of the superior paraolivary nucleus of the rat: II. Reciprocal connections with the tectal longitudinal column. Front Neuroanat. 2011;5:1.
141. Attanasio G, et al. Protective effect of the cochlear efferent system during noise exposure. Ann N Y Acad Sci. 1999;884:361–7.
142. Moore JK, Simmons DD, Guan Y. The human olivocochlear system: organization and development. Audiol Neurootol. 1999;4(6):311–25.
143. De Ridder D, Vanneste S. Occipital nerve field transcranial direct current stimulation normalizes imbalance between pain detecting and pain inhibitory pathways in fibromyalgia. Neurotherapeutics. 2017;14(2):484–501.
144. De Ridder D, et al. All bursts are equal, but some are more equal (to burst firing): burstDR stimulation versus Boston burst stimulation. Expert Rev Med Devices. 2020;17(4):289–95.
145. Pascual-Marqui RD. Standardized low-resolution brain electromagnetic tomography (sLORETA): technical details. Methods Find Exp Clin Pharmacol. 2002;24(Suppl D):5–12.
146. Palomero-Gallagher N, et al. Cytology and receptor architecture of human anterior cingulate cortex. J Comp Neurol. 2008;508(6):906–26.
147. Vanneste S, De Ridder D. Deafferentation-based pathophysiological differences in phantom sound: tinnitus with and without hearing loss. Neuroimage. 2016;129:80–94.
148. Vanneste S, Alsalman O, De Ridder D. Top-down and bottom-up regulated auditory phantom perception. J Neurosci. 2019;39(2):364–78.
149. Jensen KB, et al. Overlapping structural and functional brain changes in patients with long-term exposure to fibromyalgia pain. Arthritis Rheum. 2013;65(12):3293–303.
150. Robinson ME, et al. Gray matter volumes of pain-related brain areas are decreased in fibromyalgia syndrome. J Pain. 2011;12(4):436–43.
151. De Ridder D, et al. Amygdalohippocampal involvement in tinnitus and auditory memory. Acta Otolaryngol Suppl. 2006;556:50–3.
152. De Ridder D, Vanneste S. Targeting the parahippocampal area by auditory cortex stimulation in tinnitus. Brain Stimul. 2014;7:709.
153. Laureano MR, et al. Memory networks in tinnitus: a functional brain image study. PloS One. 2014;9(2):e87839.
154. Garrison J, Erdeniz B, Done J. Prediction error in reinforcement learning: a meta-analysis of neuroimaging studies. Neurosci Biobehav Rev. 2013;37(7):1297–310.
155. Shelton L, Becerra L, Borsook D. Unmasking the mysteries of the habenula in pain and analgesia. Prog Neurobiol. 2012;96(2):208–19.
156. Shelton L, et al. Mapping pain activation and connectivity of the human habenula. J Neurophysiol. 2012;107(10):2633–48.
157. Baliki MN, et al. Corticostriatal functional connectivity predicts transition to chronic back pain. Nat Neurosci. 2012;15(8):1117–9.
158. Mansour AR, et al. Brain white matter structural properties predict transition to chronic pain. Pain. 2013;154(10):2160–8.
159. Hullfish J, et al. Functional connectivity analysis of fMRI data collected from human subjects with chronic tinnitus and varying levels of tinnitus-related distress. Data Brief. 2018;21:779–89.
160. Donoso M, Collins AG, Koechlin E, Human cognition. Foundations of human reasoning in the prefrontal cortex. Science. 2014;344(6191):1481–6.
161. Friston K, Kilner J, Harrison L. A free energy principle for the brain. J Physiol Paris. 2006;100(1-3):70–87.
162. Knill DC, Pouget A. The Bayesian brain: the role of uncertainty in neural coding and computation. Trends Neurosci. 2004;27(12):712–9.
163. Kording K. Decision theory: what "should" the nervous system do? Science. 2007;318(5850):606–10.
164. Friston K. The free-energy principle: a unified brain theory? Nat Rev Neurosci. 2010;11(2):127–38.
165. De Ridder D, Vanneste S, Freeman W. The Bayesian brain: phantom percepts resolve sensory uncertainty. Neurosci Biobehav Rev. 2012;44:4.

166. Jackson JH. Remarks on evolution and dissolution of the nervous system. Br J Psychiatry. 1887;33(141):25–48.
167. De Ridder D, Joos K, Vanneste S. The enigma of the tinnitus-free dream state in a Bayesian world. Neural Plast. 2014;2014:612147.
168. Lee SY, et al. No auditory experience, no tinnitus: lessons from subjects with congenital- and acquired single-sided deafness. Hear Res. 2017;354:9–15.
169. De Ridder D, Verplaetse J, Vanneste S. The predictive brain and the "free will" illusion. Front Psychol. 2013;4:131.
170. Xanthos DN, Sandkuhler J. Neurogenic neuroinflammation: inflammatory CNS reactions in response to neuronal activity. Nat Rev Neurosci. 2014;15(1):43–53.
171. Ji RR, Xu ZZ, Gao YJ. Emerging targets in neuroinflammation-driven chronic pain. Nat Rev Drug Discov. 2014;13(7):533–48.
172. White FA, Bhangoo SK, Miller RJ. Chemokines: integrators of pain and inflammation. Nat Rev Drug Discov. 2005;4(10):834–44.
173. Ellis A, Bennett DL. Neuroinflammation and the generation of neuropathic pain. Br J Anaesth. 2013;111(1):26–37.
174. Gao YJ, Ji RR. Chemokines, neuronal-glial interactions, and central processing of neuropathic pain. Pharmacol Ther. 2010;126(1):56–68.
175. Kawasaki Y, et al. Cytokine mechanisms of central sensitization: distinct and overlapping role of interleukin-1beta, interleukin-6, and tumor necrosis factor-alpha in regulating synaptic and neuronal activity in the superficial spinal cord. J Neurosci. 2008;28(20):5189–94.
176. Ho IHT, et al. Spinal microglia-neuron interactions in chronic pain. J Leukoc Biol. 2020;108:1575.
177. Hathway GJ, et al. Brief, low frequency stimulation of rat peripheral C-fibres evokes prolonged microglial-induced central sensitization in adults but not in neonates. Pain. 2009;144(1-2):110–8.
178. Christianson CA, et al. Spinal TLR4 mediates the transition to a persistent mechanical hypersensitivity after the resolution of inflammation in serum-transferred arthritis. Pain. 2011;152(12):2881–91.
179. Goncalves Dos Santos G, et al. Neuraxial cytokines in pain states. Front Immunol. 2019;10:3061.
180. Albrecht DS, et al. The neuroinflammatory component of negative affect in patients with chronic pain. Mol Psychiatry. 2019;26:864.
181. Albrecht DS, et al. Imaging of neuroinflammation in migraine with aura: a [(11)C]PBR28 PET/MRI study. Neurology. 2019;92(17):e2038–50.
182. Hwang JH, et al. Expression of tumor necrosis factor-alpha and interleukin-1beta genes in the cochlea and inferior colliculus in salicylate-induced tinnitus. J Neuroinflammation. 2011;8:30.
183. Wang W, et al. Neuroinflammation mediates noise-induced synaptic imbalance and tinnitus in rodent models. PLoS Biol. 2019;17(6):e3000307.
184. Mennink LM, et al. The role of inflammation in tinnitus: a systematic review and meta-analysis. J Clin Med. 2022;11(4):1000.
185. Pongratz G, Straub RH. The sympathetic nervous response in inflammation. Arthritis Res Ther. 2014;16(6):504.
186. Carr L, et al. Neural mechanisms of empathy in humans: a relay from neural systems for imitation to limbic areas. Proc Natl Acad Sci U S A. 2003;100(9):5497–502.
187. Czura CJ, Friedman SG, Tracey KJ. Neural inhibition of inflammation: the cholinergic anti-inflammatory pathway. J Endotoxin Res. 2003;9(6):409–13.
188. Pereira MR, Leite PE. The involvement of parasympathetic and sympathetic nerve in the inflammatory reflex. J Cell Physiol. 2016;231(9):1862–9.
189. Waxenbaum JA, Reddy V, Varacallo M. Anatomy, autonomic nervous system. Treasure Island: StatPearls; 2021.
190. Crockett A, Panickar A. Role of the sympathetic nervous system in pain. Anaesth Intens Care Med. 2011;12(2):50–4.
191. Knudsen LF, et al. Complex regional pain syndrome: a focus on the autonomic nervous system. Clin Auton Res. 2019;29(4):457–67.
192. Chen SS, Zhang JM. Progress in sympathetically mediated pathological pain. J Anesth Perioper Med. 2015;2(4):216–25.
193. Matharu MS, Goadsby PJ. Trigeminal autonomic cephalgias. J Neurol Neurosurg Psychiatry. 2002;72(Suppl 2):ii19–26.
194. O'Connell NE, et al. Local anaesthetic sympathetic blockade for complex regional pain syndrome. Cochrane Database Syst Rev. 2016;7:CD004598.
195. Datzov E, et al. Tinnitus, heart rate variability, and some biochemical indicators. Int Tinnitus J. 1999;5(1):20–3.
196. Vanneste S, De Ridder D. Brain areas controlling heart rate variability in tinnitus and tinnitus-related distress. PloS One. 2013;8(3):e59728.
197. Ylikoski J, et al. Non-invasive vagus nerve stimulation reduces sympathetic preponderance in patients with tinnitus. Acta Otolaryngol. 2017;137(4):426–31.
198. Szczepek AJ, Mazurek B. Neurobiology of stress-induced tinnitus. Curr Top Behav Neurosci. 2021;51:327–47.
199. Lee W, et al. Objective multidisciplinary measurements of sleep disturbance and autonomic dysfunction as risk factors for chronic subjective tinnitus. J Formos Med Assoc. 2023;122:470.
200. Koning HM, Dyrbye BA, van Hemert FJ. Percutaneous radiofrequency lesion of the superior cervical sympathetic ganglion in patients with tinnitus. Pain Pract. 2016;16(8):994–1000.
201. Adlington P, Warrick J. Stellate ganglion block in the management of tinnitus. J Laryngol Otol. 1971;85(2):159–68.
202. Warrick JW. Stellate ganglion block in the treatment of Meniere's disease and in the symptomatic relief of tinnitus. Br J Anaesth. 1969;41(8):699–702.
203. Passe ER. Sympathectomy in relation to Meniere's disease, nerve deafness and tinnitus; a report on 110 cases. Acta Otolaryngol. 1952;42(1-2):133–51.
204. Tracy LM, et al. Meta-analytic evidence for decreased heart rate variability in chronic pain implicating parasympathetic nervous system dysregulation. Pain. 2016;157(1):7–29.
205. Clancy JA, et al. Non-invasive vagus nerve stimulation in healthy humans reduces sympathetic nerve activity. Brain Stimul. 2014;7(6):871–7.
206. Lai YH, et al. Cervical noninvasive vagus nerve stimulation for migraine and cluster headache: a systematic review and meta-analysis. Neuromodulation. 2020;23(6):721–31.
207. Patel ABU, et al. Trans-auricular vagus nerve stimulation to reduce perioperative pain and morbidity: protocol for a single-blind analyser-masked randomised controlled trial. BJA Open. 2022;2:None.
208. De Ridder D, Langguth B, Vanneste S. Vagus nerve stimulation for tinnitus: a review and perspective. Prog Brain Res. 2021;262:451–67.
209. Raj-Koziak D, et al. Effectiveness of transcutaneous vagus nerve stimulation for the treatment of tinnitus: an interventional prospective controlled study. Int J Audiol. 2023:1–10.
210. Stegeman I, et al. Tinnitus treatment by vagus nerve stimulation: a systematic review. PloS One. 2021;16(3):e0247221.
211. De Ridder D, et al. Placebo-controlled vagus nerve stimulation paired with tones in a patient with refractory tinnitus: a case report. Otol Neurotol. 2015;36(4):575–80.
212. De Ridder D, et al. Safety and efficacy of vagus nerve stimulation paired with tones for the treatment of tinnitus: a case series. Neuromodulation. 2014;17(2):170–9.
213. Scotti E, et al. Exploring the microbiome in health and disease: implications for toxicology. Toxicol Res Appl. 2017;1:1–37.
214. Ustianowska K, et al. The role of the human microbiome in the pathogenesis of pain. Int J Mol Sci. 2022;23(21):13267.
215. Mayer EA. Gut feelings: the emerging biology of gut-brain communication. Nat Rev Neurosci. 2011;12(8):453–66.

216. Osadchiy V, Martin CR, Mayer EA. The gut-brain axis and the microbiome: mechanisms and clinical implications. Clin Gastroenterol Hepatol. 2019;17(2):322–32.
217. Bar-Yosef Mayer DE, Vandermeersch B, Bar-Yosef O. Shells and ochre in Middle Paleolithic Qafzeh Cave, Israel: indications for modern behavior. J Hum Evol. 2009;56(3):307–14.
218. Guo R, et al. Pain regulation by gut microbiota: molecular mechanisms and therapeutic potential. Br J Anaesth. 2019;123(5):637–54.
219. Li S, et al. The role of bacteria and its derived metabolites in chronic pain and depression: recent findings and research progress. Int J Neuropsychopharmacol. 2020;23(1):26–41.
220. Nijs J, et al. Nutritional intervention in chronic pain: an innovative way of targeting central nervous system sensitization? Expert Opin Ther Targets. 2020;24(8):793–803.
221. Megantara I, et al. The role of gut dysbiosis in the pathophysiology of tinnitus: a literature review. Int Tinnitus J. 2022;26(1):27–41.
222. De Ridder D, Moller A. Similarities between treatments of tinnitus and central pain. In: Moller A, et al., editors. Textbook of tinnitus. New York: Springer; 2011. p. 753–62.
223. Szczepek AJ. Clinical pharmacology of tinnitus: design and evaluation. In: Hock FJ, Gralinski MR, editors. Drug discovery and evaluation: methods in clinical pharmacology. Switzerland: Springer Nature; 2020. p. 209–21.
224. Shea JJ, Emmett JR. The medical treatment of tinnitus. J Laryngol Otol Suppl. 1981;4:130–8.
225. Hoekstra CE, et al. Anticonvulsants for tinnitus. Cochrane Database Syst Rev. 2011;(7):CD007960.
226. Baldo P, et al. Antidepressants for patients with tinnitus. Cochrane Database Syst Rev. 2012;(9):CD003853.
227. De Ridder D, et al. Electrical stimulation of auditory and somatosensory cortices for treatment of tinnitus and pain. Prog Brain Res. 2007;166:377–88.
228. De Ridder D, Perera S, Vanneste S. State of the art: novel applications for cortical stimulation. Neuromodulation. 2017;20(3):206–14.
229. Fuller T, et al. Cognitive behavioural therapy for tinnitus. Cochrane Database Syst Rev. 2020;1:CD012614.
230. Morley S, Eccleston C, Williams A. Systematic review and meta-analysis of randomized controlled trials of cognitive behaviour therapy and behaviour therapy for chronic pain in adults, excluding headache. Pain. 1999;80(1–2):1–13.
231. Huang K, et al. Acupuncture for tinnitus: a systematic review and meta-analysis of randomized controlled trials. Acupunct Med. 2021;39:264.
232. Feng Z, et al. Acupuncture for neuropathic pain: a meta-analysis of randomized control trials. Front Neurol. 2022;13:1076993.
233. Chen CH, et al. Efficacy of low-level laser therapy for tinnitus: a systematic review with meta-analysis and trial sequential analysis. Brain Sci. 2020;10(12):931.
234. Glazov G, Yelland M, Emery J. Low-level laser therapy for chronic non-specific low back pain: a meta-analysis of randomised controlled trials. Acupunct Med. 2016;34(5):328–41.
235. Shulman A. External electrical stimulation in tinnitus control. Am J Otol. 1985;6(1):110–5.
236. Vanneste S, De Ridder D. Noninvasive and invasive neuromodulation for the treatment of tinnitus: an overview. Neuromodulation. 2012;15:350.
237. De Ridder D, Adhia D, Langguth B. Tinnitus and brain stimulation. Curr Top Behav Neurosci. 2021;51:249.
238. Shulman A, et al. Neuroinflammation and tinnitus. Curr Top Behav Neurosci. 2021;51:161–74.

Part II

Neurobiology of Tinnitus

Anatomy and Physiology of the Auditory System

9

Gabriel Byczynski, Sven Vanneste, and Aage R. Møller

Abstract

To provide context for the anatomical and functional aspects of tinnitus and its manifestation, this chapter discusses the anatomy and physiology of the auditory system. The approach begins at the ear, moving through the process of transduction, to peripheral nervous system components, and ending at the central nervous system regions of the auditory system. There is emphasis on the ascending and descending auditory systems, and their contributions to the development and etiology of tinnitus. In addition to anatomy, this section also discusses functional aspects of the auditory nervous system including a background of animal studies of auditory function, frequency selectivity, and neural connectivity. The chapter concludes with a discussion of how tinnitus may arise through the anatomical layout of the auditory nervous system. Diseases that arise from phantom sensations, the contribution of hidden hearing loss, and brain regions relating to tinnitus are discussed. This chapter fundamentally aims to provide sufficient anatomical and physiological of the auditory system background to allow the reader to better understand the structures and functions underlying tinnitus and its manifestation.

Aage R. Møller has died before the publication of this book.

G. Byczynski
Lab for Clinical & Integrative Neuroscience, Trinity Institute for Neuroscience, School of Psychology, Trinity College Dublin, Dublin, Ireland

S. Vanneste (✉)
Global Brain Health Institute, Trinity College Dublin, Dublin, Ireland

Trinity College Institute for Neuroscience, Trinity College Dublin, Dublin, Ireland

School of Psychology, Trinity College Dublin, Dublin, Ireland
e-mail: sven.vanneste@tcd.ie

A. R. Møller (Deceased)
Neuroscience Program, School of Brain & Behavioral Sciences, University of Texas, Richardson, TX, USA

Highlights

- The auditory system is divided into central and peripheral, ascending and descending systems, and the classical and nonclassical pathways.
- Tinnitus may arise via neural circuitry connectedness that overlaps and arises into perception via frontal and parietal regions.
- Hidden hearing loss may contribute to tinnitus by causing network hyperexcitability and sensitivity.

Introduction

This chapter reviews the anatomy and physiology of the auditory system, emphasizing structures and functions often involved in tinnitus. It is therefore not an extensive overview of auditory anatomy and function, but rather, it is more focused on pertinent anatomy and physiology relating to tinnitus.

The mammalian auditory system consists generally of four main components: (1) the ear, which conducts sounds to; (2) the cochlea, where the sounds are separated based on frequency, and which is also the point of sensory transduction through hair cells; (3) the auditory nerve; and (4) the central auditory nervous system. Within the central auditory nervous system, there is further anatomical and functional division, including regional population of neurons divided into layers within the auditory cortices [1]. There are also numerous associated regions, for example, Wernicke's area and the angular gyrus. The angular gyrus specifically has been posited as playing a role in tinnitus perception [1, 2].

This chapter will follow the path of sound through the ear, cochlea, auditory nerve, and auditory cortices, with details of the classical and nonclassical pathways of the auditory system, ascending and descending systems, frequency selectivity, and ending with a discussion of phantom sensations and their associated neural networks. Through emphasizing

W. Schlee et al. (eds.), *Textbook of Tinnitus*, https://doi.org/10.1007/978-3-031-35647-6_9

structural and functional anatomy relating to tinnitus, this chapter aims to have provided relevant and current information on the neurobiological underpinnings of tinnitus.

The Ear

The first point for sound entering the auditory system is the ear. Anatomically, sound first travels through the outer, middle, and inner sections of the ear and ear canal, the conductive regions, and lastly, the cochlea where they are transduced into neural code. The conductive bones, or ossicles, have very little importance to tinnitus and therefore are scarcely covered here. Instead, we will begin with the cochlea.

The cochlea is a complex structure, and its basilar membrane is the point where sound is spectrally divided (see Fig. 9.1) The membrane is also where transduction occurs, specifically at the sensory cells which line it. The two types of sensory cells, inner hair cells and outer hair cells, are morphologically similar, but have functional differences. Inner hair cells transduce sound into neural code using mechanoelectrical transducer channels [5]. The hair cells are the fundamental auditory receptor cells and control discharges in the main group of auditory nerve fibers. The outer hair cells amplify the motion of the basilar membrane, and in doing so, act as a cochlear amplifier. The elongations and shortening of the outer hair cells is most pronounced for low sound intensity, adding approximately 50 dB of sensitivity [6]. In fact, the nonlinearity of the outer hair cells can be used in clinical diagnosis using otoacoustic emission tests. An example of this nonlinearity is shown in a guinea pig in Fig. 9.2.

The active role of outer hair cells also causes the cochlea to generate sound, called otoacoustic emissions. These emissions can be recorded using a microphone placed in the ear canal and are divided into a few variations including spontaneous otoacoustic emission (SOAE), transient-evoked otoacoustic emission (TEOAE), and distortion product otoacoustic emission (DPOAE) (see Fig. 9.3). SOAEs are often associated with normal cochlear function; however, they may also be associated with hearing loss or pathology at high frequencies [10]. TEOAEs, on the other hand, often carry clinical potential to detect hearing loss risk relating to outer hair-cell dysfunction [11]. Similarly, DPOAEs are also an effective tool for clinical diagnostic purposes, indicating cochlear development and hair cell integrity [12].

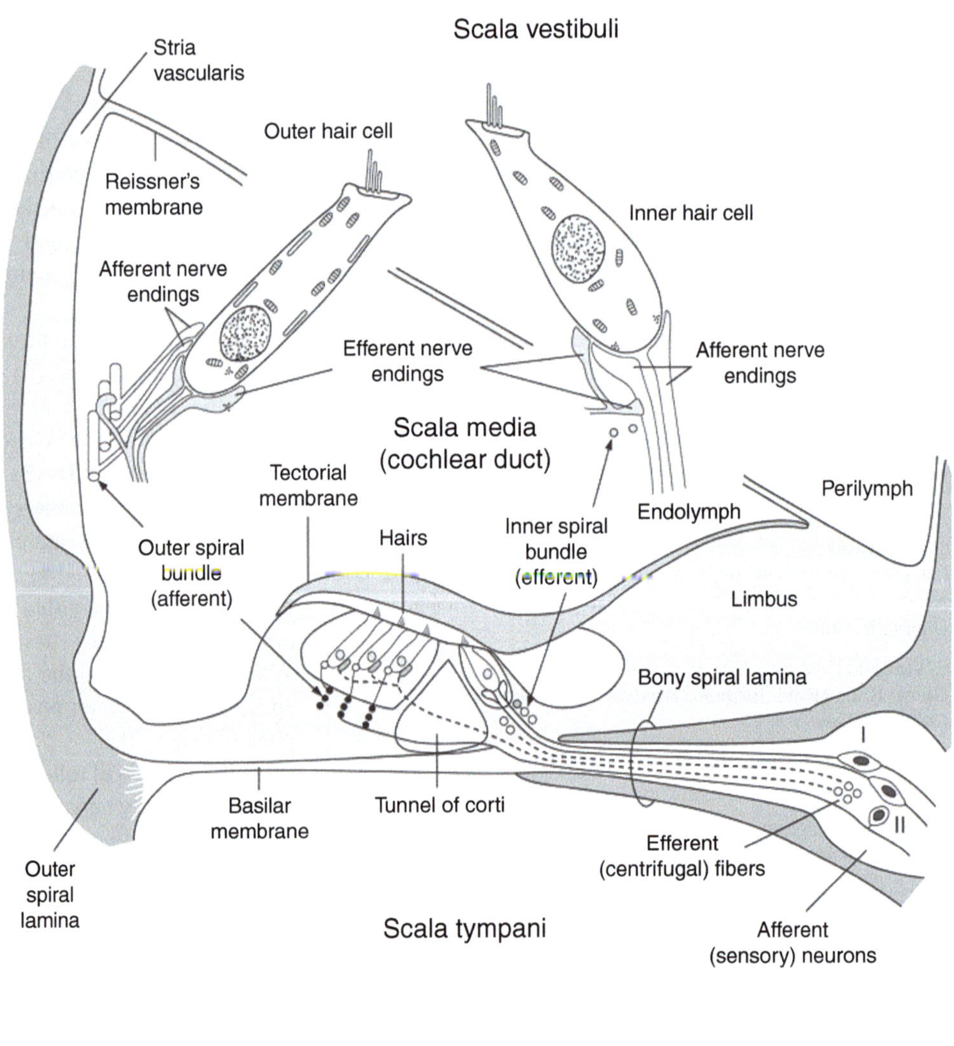

Fig. 9.1 Schematic drawing of a cross-section of the cochlea showing the organ of Corti. Outer and inner hair cells are shown as inserts [3, 4]

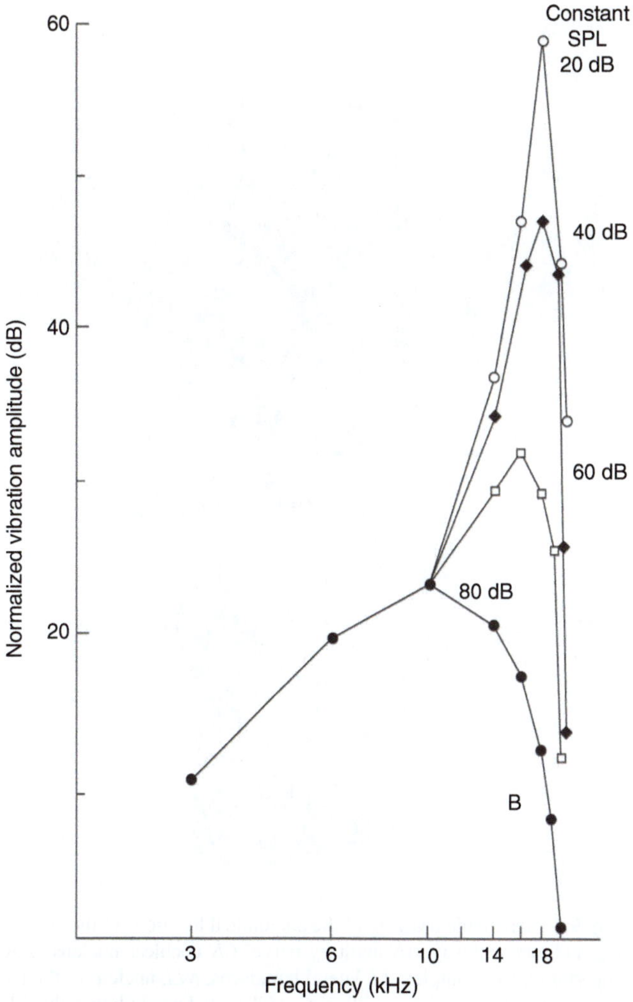

Fig. 9.2 Vibration amplitude at a single point of the basilar membrane of a guinea pig obtained using pure tones as test sounds at four different intensities. The amplitude scale is normalized, and the individual curves would have coincided if the basilar membrane motion had been linear [7, 8]

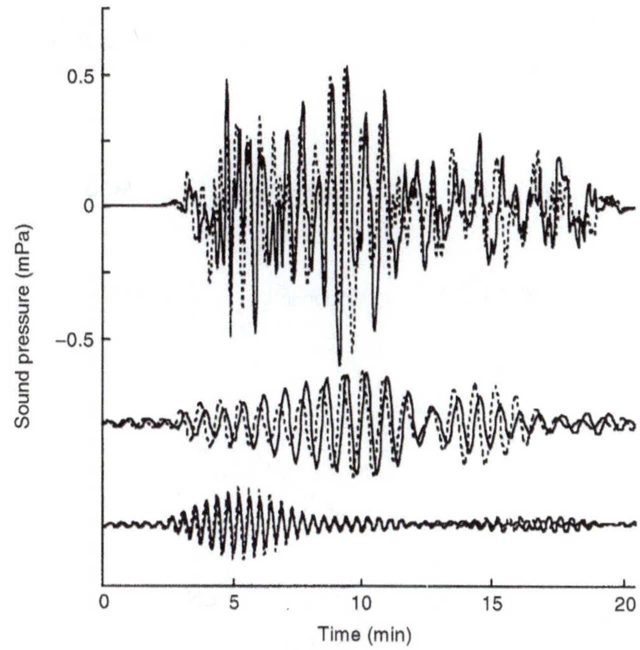

Fig. 9.3 Click evoked otoacoustic emission (TEOAE). The solid and the dashed lines are the response in two different body positions [3, 9]

Anatomy of the Auditory Nervous System

After transduction, the neural code then passes to the auditory nervous system, consisting of two parallel ascending pathways and two reciprocal descending pathways. The ascending pathways each project to the auditory cortices through the cochlear nuclei (CN), lateral lemniscus (LL), inferior colliculus (IC), and medial geniculate body (MG). The descending pathways intuitively begin at the cerebral cortex and project down to the cochlea (see Figs. 9.4 and 9.5 for visual representations).

The sensory cells in the cochlea are innervated by the auditory nerve, which conducts signals to the CN, the first nucleus of the ascending pathway. The CN itself is divided into the anterior ventral cochlear nuclei (AVCN), the posterior ventral cochlear nuclei (PVCN), and the dorsal cochlear nuclei (DCN) (Figs. 9.4 and 9.5). Each fiber of the auditory nerve bifurcates, and one of the branches divides again, making it possible for each nerve fiber to connect to neurons in each of the three divisions of cochlear nucleus (Fig. 9.6). This represents an example of parallel processing allowing the same information to be processed in different nerve cell populations. The cells in the three divisions project to the nucleus of the inferior colliculus through the dorsal (stria of Monaco), the medial (stria of Held), and ventral stria (trapezoidal body). The fibers give off collateral to the nuclei of the SOC [15].

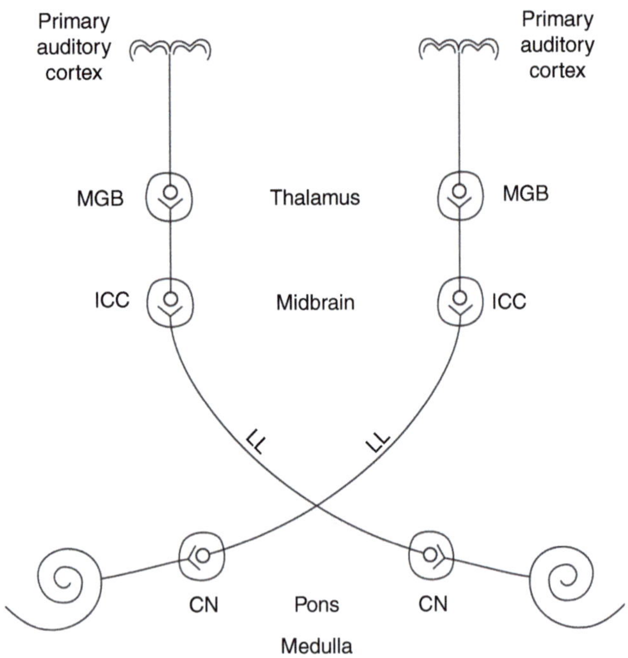

Fig. 9.4 Schematic drawing of the anatomical locations of the ascending auditory pathway. *AN* auditory nerve, *CN* cochlear nucleus, *SOC* superior olivary complex, *LL* lateral lemniscus, *NLL* nucleus of the lateral lemniscus, *IC* inferior colliculus, *MG* medial geniculate body [13]

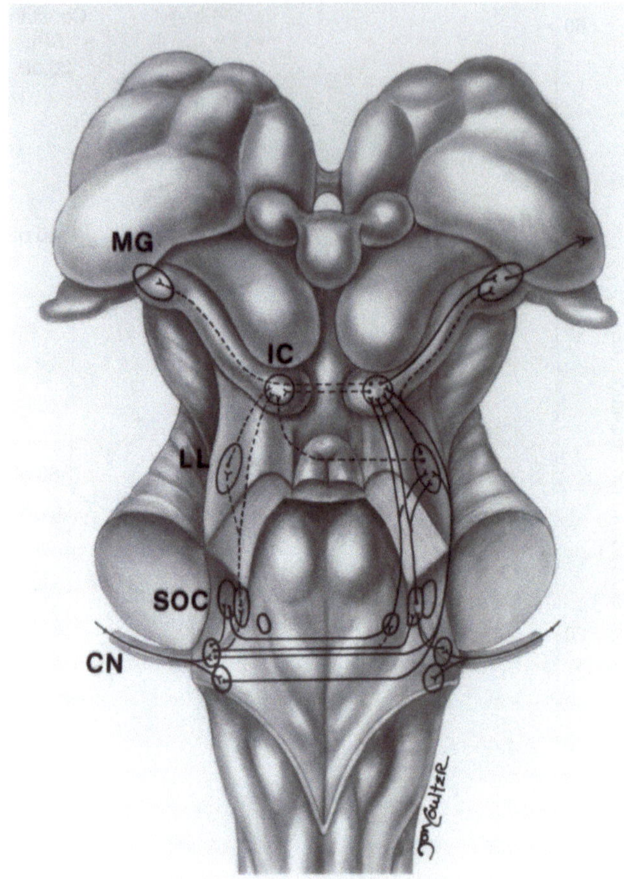

Fig. 9.5 Schematic drawing of the anatomical locations of the ascending auditory pathway. *AN* auditory nerve, *CN* cochlear nucleus, *SOC* superior olivary complex, *LL* lateral lemniscus, *NLL* nucleus of the lateral lemniscus, *IC* inferior colliculus, *MG* medial geniculate body [14]

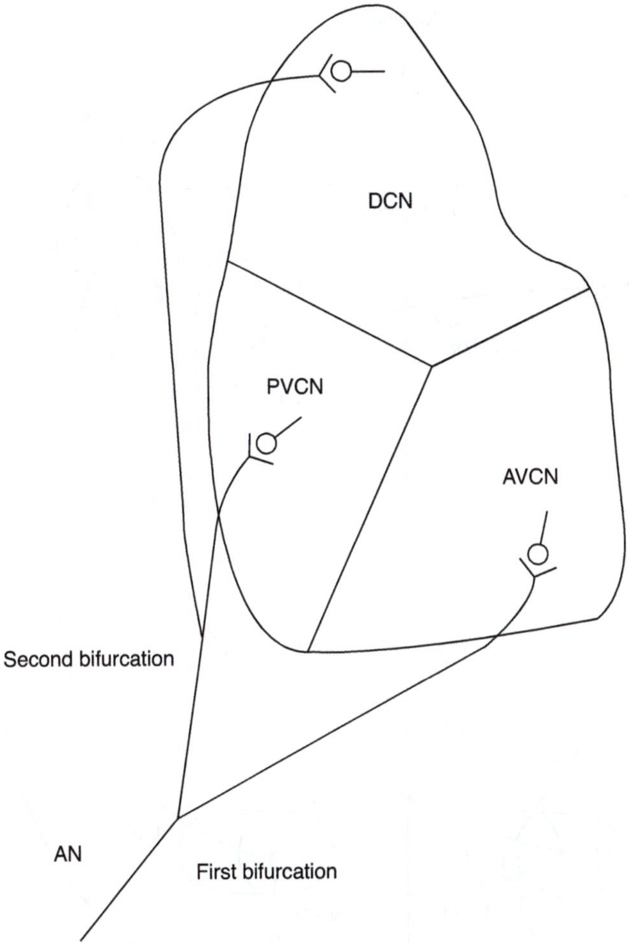

Fig. 9.6 Schematic drawing of the cochlear nucleus shows the auditory nerve's connections with the three main divisions and the cochlear nucleus. *DCN* dorsal cochlear nucleus, *PVCN* posterior ventral cochlear nucleus, *AVCN* anterior ventral cochlear nucleus [3]

Ascending Systems

Pertaining to the ascending pathways of the auditory system, two sensory pathways are identified: the classical pathways and the nonclassical pathways. The classical pathways are known as the lemniscal system, or the 'specific' system, while the nonclassical pathways are referred to as the extralemniscal system, or 'unspecific' system. These systems may also be referred to as the 'slow and accurate' and 'fast and dirty' pathways, respectively. Both the classical and nonclassical pathways make essential connections to the lateral nucleus of the amygdala through either the high route or the low route [16] (see Figs. 9.7 and 9.10).

The low route uses subcortical connections from the lateral and medial thalamus and is not normally active in adults with tinnitus; however, there are indications that the nonclassical auditory pathways are active in children [18]. Some forms of tinnitus may involve the extra lemniscal pathways, meaning that subcortical connections to the amygdala are active in some individuals (and children) with tinnitus or other disorders, including autism [19–22].

The high route uses a long chain of neurons in the primary and secondary auditory cortices, followed by neurons in several associate cortices. The cells of the ICC project to the ventral part of the thalamic auditory nucleus. Cells in the medial geniculate body (MGB) project to the primary auditory cortex, secondary cortex, anterior and posterior auditory fields, and other auditory divisions [23] (Fig. 9.8). In the nonclassical pathways, the thalamic nuclei project to secondary auditory cortex and associate cortices, skipping the primary auditory cortex. The dorsal and medial thalamus additionally route to several subcortical structures including the amygdala and hypothalamus (Fig. 9.9).

The extralemniscal system begins at the midbrain with connections from the ICC to the IC, external nucleus (ICX), and dorsal cortex of the IC (DC) [25]. The ICX receives projections from the trigeminal ganglion [26, 27], the spinal part of the fifth nerve nucleus [28], and the dorsal part of the spinal cord [29]. The organization of the system therefore allows input from the somatosensory system to the auditory pathways [30].

There is comparatively less known facts about the functional role of the nonclassical pathways, since cells in the nonclassical pathways respond less distinctly to stimulation, and to a generally broader range of stimuli. They also integrate information on a broader spatial scale, with some neurons in the nonclassical pathways responding to nonauditory modalities. There is, however, no sign of cross-modal interaction in typical adults, the exception being individuals with tinnitus and autism; suggesting that nonclassical pathways are not normally active in adults. Figure 9.10 shows a depiction of connections between the classical and nonclassical routes.

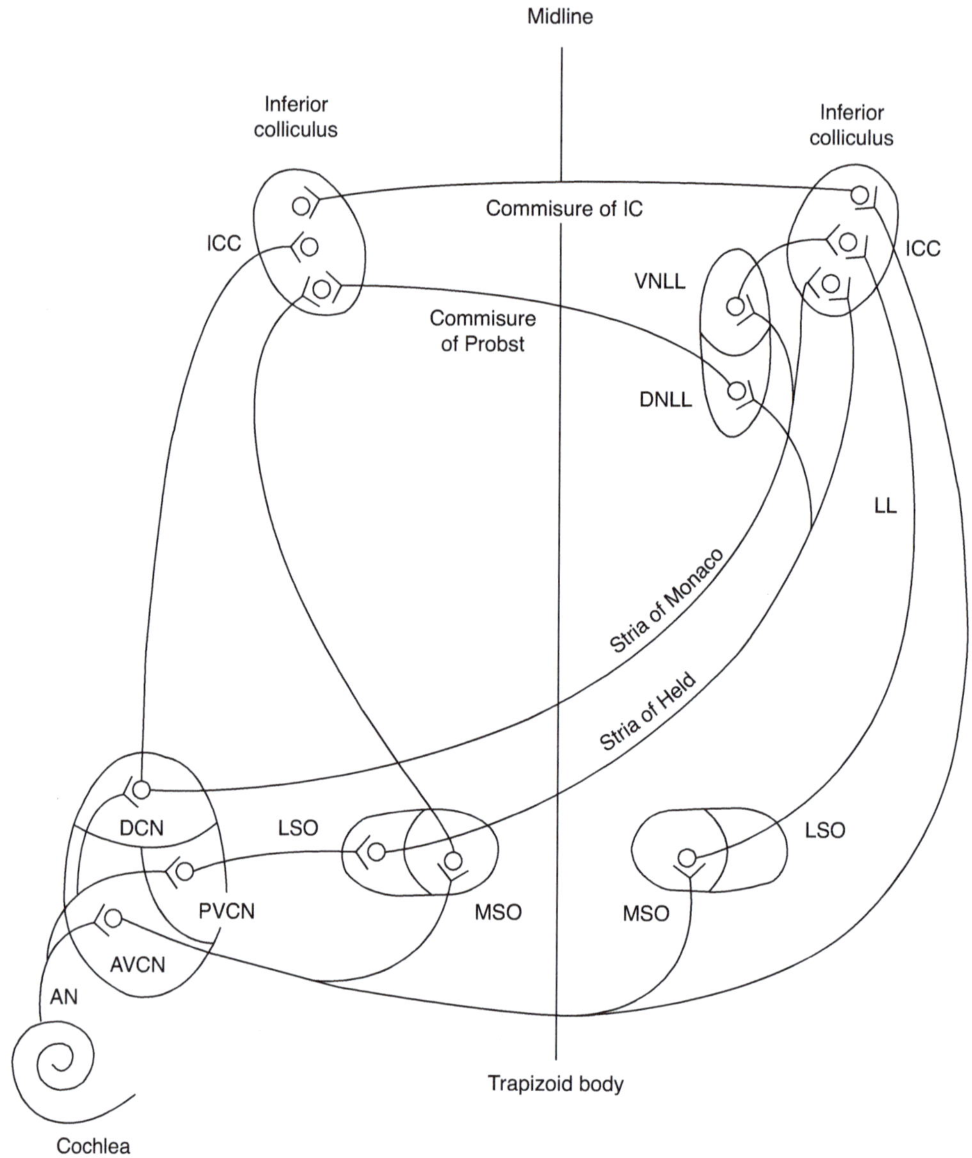

Fig. 9.7 More detailed drawing of the ascending auditory pathways from the ear to the central nucleus of the inferior colliculus (ICC). *AVCN* anterior ventral cochlear nucleus, *PVCN* posterior ventral cochlear nucleus, *DCN* dorsal cochlear nucleus, *LSO* lateral superior olive, *NTB* nucleus of the trapezoidal body, *MSO* medial superior olive, *SH* stria of Held (intermediate stria), *SM* stria of Monakow (dorsal stria), *LL* nucleus of the lateral lemniscus, *DNLL* dorsal nucleus of the lateral lemniscus, *VNLL* ventral nucleus of the lateral lemniscus, *ICC* central nucleus of the inferior colliculus [3]

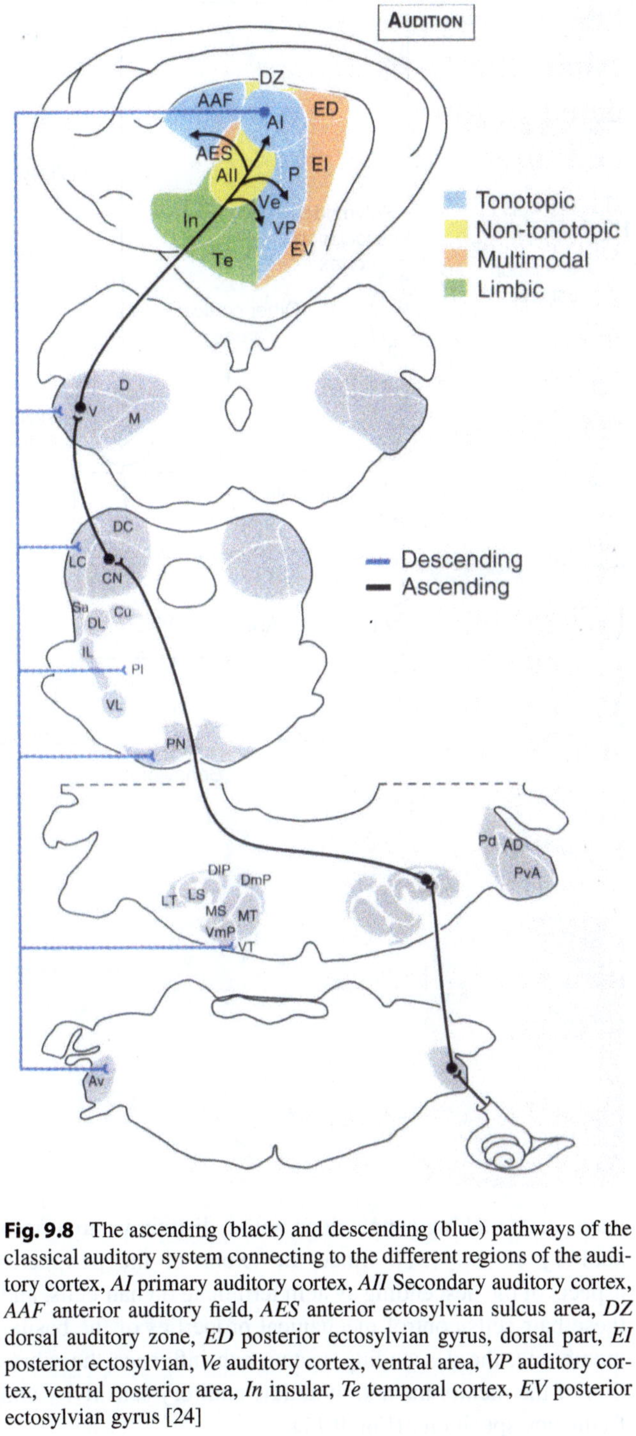

Fig. 9.8 The ascending (black) and descending (blue) pathways of the classical auditory system connecting to the different regions of the auditory cortex, *AI* primary auditory cortex, *AII* Secondary auditory cortex, *AAF* anterior auditory field, *AES* anterior ectosylvian sulcus area, *DZ* dorsal auditory zone, *ED* posterior ectosylvian gyrus, dorsal part, *EI* posterior ectosylvian, *Ve* auditory cortex, ventral area, *VP* auditory cortex, ventral posterior area, *In* insular, *Te* temporal cortex, *EV* posterior ectosylvian gyrus [24]

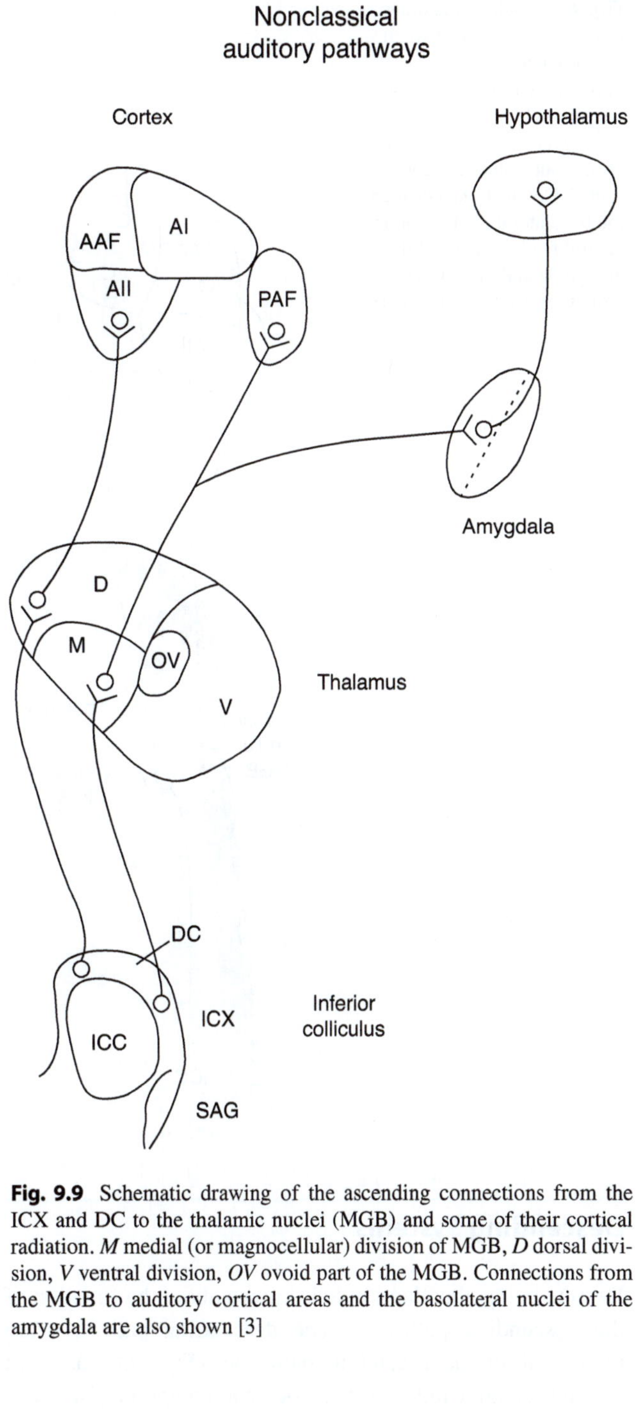

Fig. 9.9 Schematic drawing of the ascending connections from the ICX and DC to the thalamic nuclei (MGB) and some of their cortical radiation. *M* medial (or magnocellular) division of MGB, *D* dorsal division, *V* ventral division, *OV* ovoid part of the MGB. Connections from the MGB to auditory cortical areas and the basolateral nuclei of the amygdala are also shown [3]

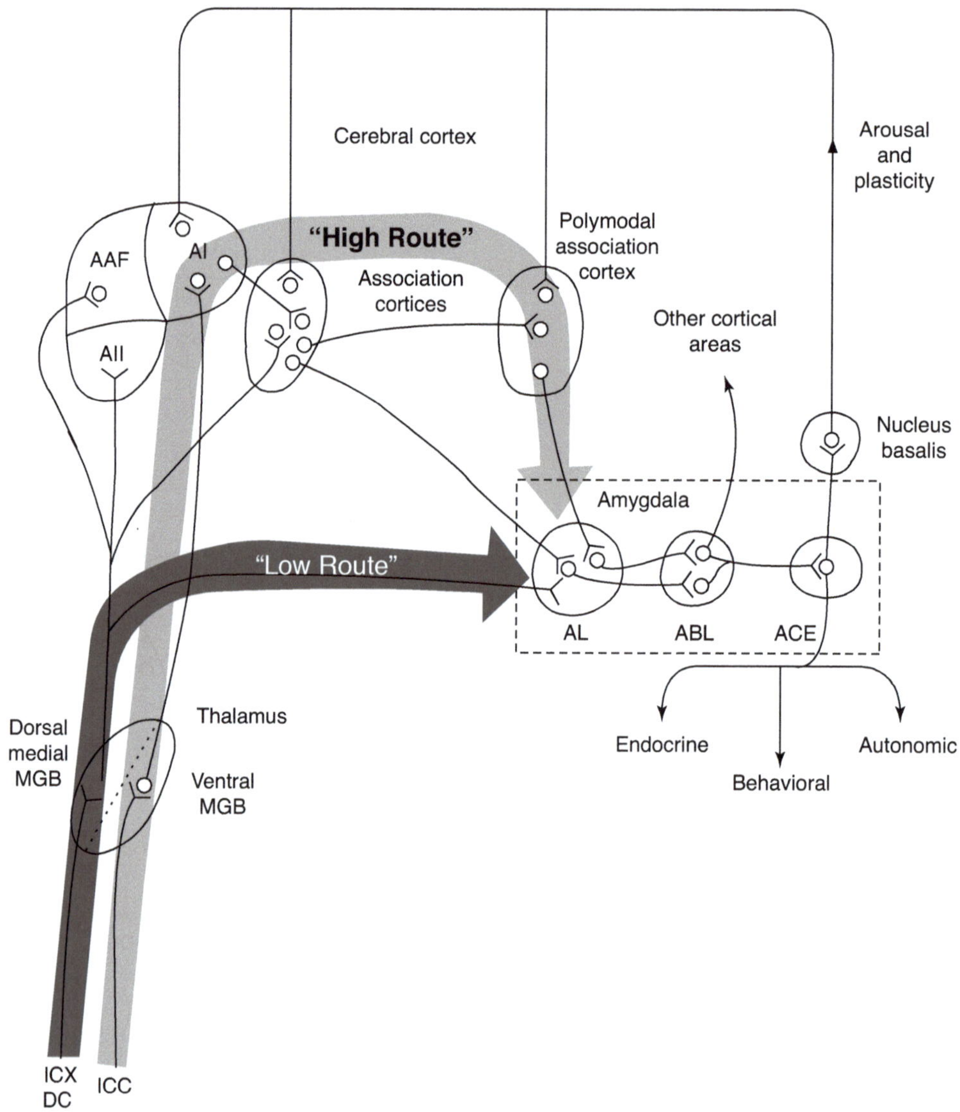

Fig. 9.10 Schematic drawing of the connections between the classical and the non-classical routes and the lateral nucleus of the amygdala (AL), showing the "high route" and the "low route." Connections between the basolateral (ABL) and the central nuclei (ACE) of the amygdala and other CNS structures are also shown [16, 17]

Descending Systems

Despite being abundant, little is known about the function of the descending pathways. The descending pathways are reciprocal to the ascending pathways (Fig. 9.8) and are located as far caudal as the cochlear receptors [24]. The descending system is often described as having three pathways, each making connections with a distinctive area from auditory centers [31]. Since the axons of the peripheral aspects of the descending system terminate on hair cells, and these hair cells control mechanical properties of the basilar membrane, the descending system can influence the vibration of the membrane and modulate auditory sensitivity and frequency specificity (Fig. 9.11).

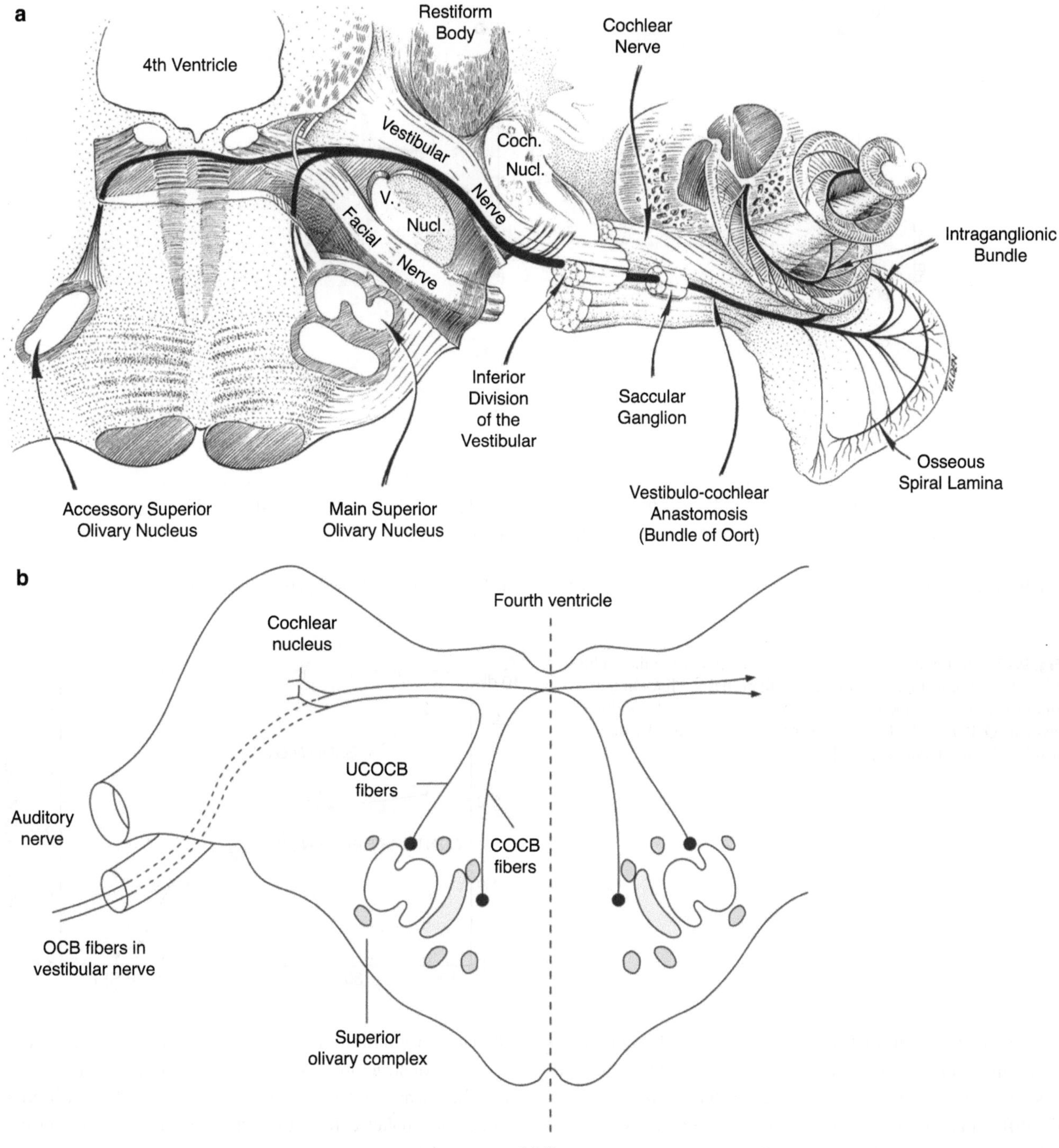

Fig. 9.11 (**a**) Origin of efferent supply to the cochlea [32]. (**b**) Olivocochlear system in the cat. The uncrossed olivocochlear bundle (UCOCB) and the crossed olivocochlear bundle (COCB) are shown [33]

Frequency Selectivity in the Auditory Nervous System

Nerve cells and axons in the auditory system are tuned to a spectrum of sounds resulting from the frequency selectivity of the basilar membrane. The frequency selectivity manifests through influence of the descending system, as well as the anatomical composition of the membrane. Figure 9.12 shows a family of tuning curves in a cat's auditory nerve, illustrating sharpness of the tuning of the auditory nerve changing with its tuned frequency. Figure 9.13 also gives an example of how auditory fiber tuning varies with stimulus intensity.

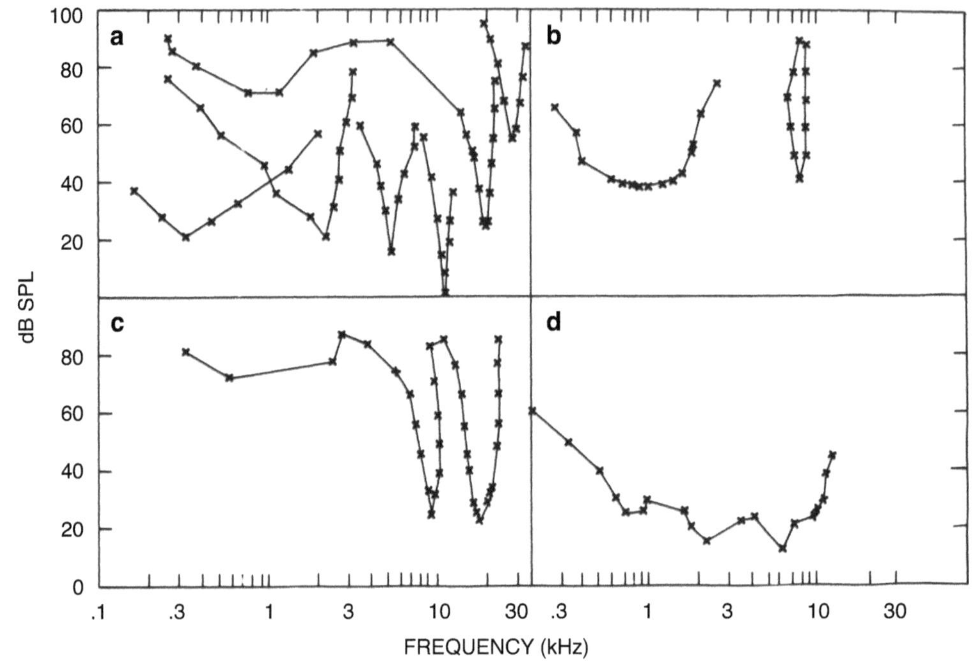

Fig. 9.12 Examples of frequency tuning curves with different shapes obtained from neurons of the superior olivary complex of the cat [34]

Fig. 9.13 Shift in the center frequency (solid lines) and the width of the tuning of a single auditory nerve fiber (dashed line) in the auditory nerve as a function of the stimulus intensity. The width is given a "Q10dB," which is the center frequency divided by the width at 10 dB above the peak [35]

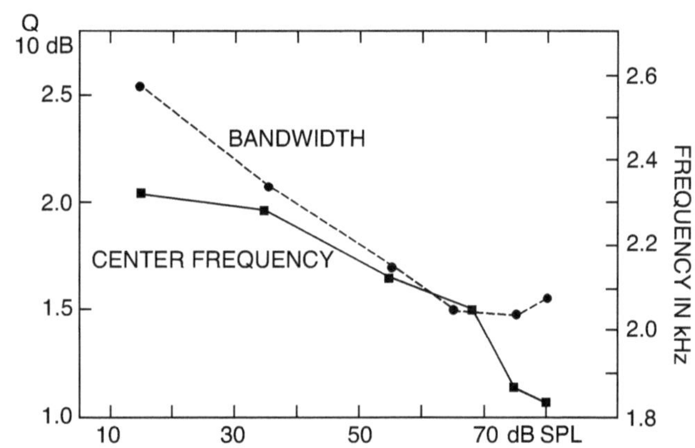

Frequency tuning that results from the cochlear processes is modified in neural processes within the auditory nervous system. This is particularly important as the tuning of cells in the different ascending auditory pathway structures varies significantly. For example, tuning differs in sharpness between the auditory nerve fiber and the cells of CN, where the CN has much sharper tuning. In fact, the CN tuning depends on the number of nerve fibers converging on the cell, and furthermore, their excitatory or inhibitory characteristics. Here we see that lateral inhibition becomes relevant in shaping the tuning curves of structures. Where lateral inhibition sharpens tuning, the convergence of nerve fibers tuned to different frequencies makes cells in the structures of the ascending system more broadly tuned compared to the auditory nerve fibers. The number of functional connections that a cell receives in fact determines the width and center frequency of the tuning of many cells in the ascending system and is furthermore dependent on the synaptic efficacy of the connections.

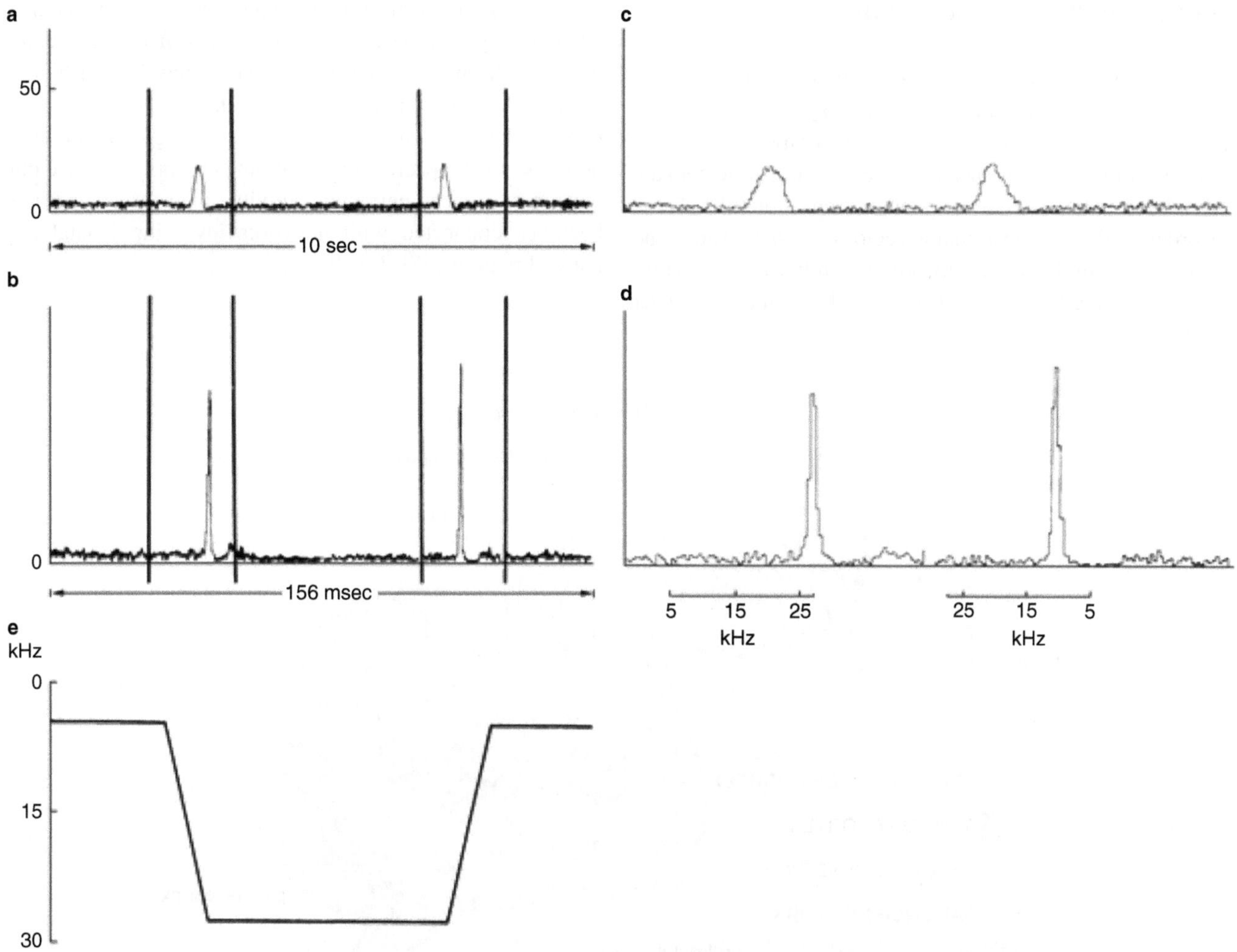

Fig. 9.14 Period histograms of a cell in the cochlear nucleus of a rat in response to tones, the frequency of which varied between 5 and 25 kHz at different rates. (**a**) and (**c**): Slow rate, (**b**) and (**d**): Fast rate. The top histograms (**a** and **c**, slow rate) show the responses obtained when the duration of a complete cycle was 10 s, and the lower histograms (**b** and **d**, fast rates) show the responses obtained when the duration of a complete cycle was 156 ms. The change in the frequency of the stimulus tone was accomplished by having a trapezoidal waveform control of the frequency of the sound generator (**e**). The two left-hand graphs (**a** and **b**) are histograms of a full modulation cycle, and the right-hand graphs (**c** and **d**) show the details between the vertical lines in the left-hand graphs [36]

Importantly, given the relationship between synaptic efficacy and synaptic plasticity, the tuning of these cells is dynamic. Activation of the cerebral cortex can be altered through neural plasticity, and neuroplastic changes alter not only the anatomical area of the activated cortex, but its associate cell tuning. Generally, studies are concerned with the response to a steady frequency (i.e., simple tones); however, it is shown that with rapid frequency variation, studies show sharper tuning compared to single, static frequency (Fig. 9.14).

Using more complex sounds, as opposed to single tone presentation, response patterns become more complex, as shown in cells of the CN. The response patterns become largely dependent on the rate of tonal change, meaning that complex sound responses cannot simply be interpolated from the results of their component simple pure tones. The nonlinear behavior is more pronounced in responses of cells in higher-order nuclei of the auditory nuclei including the cerebral cortices.

Disease of Phantom Sensation

Thus far, this chapter has covered the fundamental anatomy and function of the auditory nervous system required to understand how tinnitus may manifest. Many forms of tinnitus and other diseases such as those of neuropathic pain are considered to be disorders of phantom sensation [37]. These disorders often involve many regions of the brain, and changes in neural connectivity are often related to the symptoms and manifestations of neuropathic pain and sever tinnitus.

Many brain structures including the subgenual and dorsal anterior cingulate cortices, precuneus, and frontal cortex are involved in phantom sensations, and it may indeed be that tinnitus, like other phantom sensation-based disorders, are perceived as the consequence of overlapping dynamic brain networks [37]. Specifically, phantom percepts may arise into awareness when neuronal activity in sensory cortices becomes connected with networks involving frontal and parietal regions [37] (Fig. 9.15).

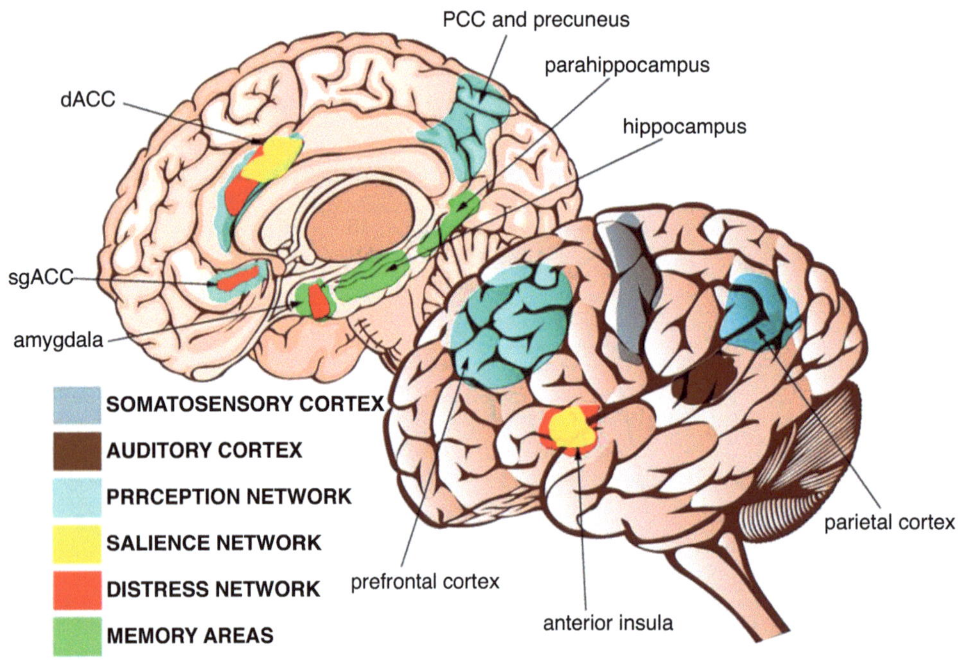

Fig. 9.15 Brain networks involved in phantom perception. Sensory deafferentation causes neuroplastic changes resulting in increased activation of the primary sensory cortex: somatosensory cortex (gray) in the case of phantom pain and auditory cortex (brown) in the case of tinnitus. Awareness of the stimulus arises when this activity is connected to a larger coactivated awareness or perceptual network. This perceptual network involves subgenual (sgACC) and dorsal anterior cingulate cortex (dACC) and posterior cingulate cortex (PCC), precuneus, parietal cortex, and frontal cortex (blue). Salience to the phantom percept is reflected by activating the dACC and the anterior insula (yellow). Because of a constant learning process, the phantom percept becomes associated with distress, which is reflected by a nonspecific distress network consisting of the anterior cingulate cortex (sgACC and dACC), anterior insula, and amygdala (red). The persistence of the phantom percept is due to memory mechanisms involving the parahippocampal area, amygdala, and hippocampus (green) [37]

Hidden Hearing Loss

In addition to network-related alterations which may indeed be a factor influencing the perception of phantom perceptions which may be the case for tinnitus, other theories returned to the more traditional target of a cochlear role. Traditional theories of tinnitus implicated the possibility that cochlear damage triggered tinnitus sensations. This claim was met with contradictory results showing that tinnitus patients often present with normal audiograms [38]. There is still a role for the cochlea in tinnitus, however, in the realm of so-called "hidden hearing loss". Using auditory brainstem response (ABR) data, research has shown that reduced ABR wave I amplitudes and ABR wave V latency in tinnitus patents reflect deficits in cochlear processing, despite a normal audiogram [38]. In the presence of activity deprivation, excitatory synapses become exaggerated, with inhibitory synapses being decreased. It is believed that this combination of compensations to reduced cochlear processing results in hyperexcitation of networks amplifying spontaneous activity. The role of higher-level brain networks playing a role in phantom perception is then easily connected with excitation resulting from input deprivation, ultimately producing the phantom sensation.

Conclusions

This chapter discusses what we regard to be the relevant neurobiological and anatomical aspects of tinnitus. The brain as a whole is a highly complex and interconnected organ, and therefore, it must be acknowledged that the limits to which neuroanatomy plays a role in tinnitus are not reached in this section.

References

1. Flint PW, Haughey BH, Lund VJ, Robbins KT, Thomas JR, Francis HW, Lesperance MM. Cummings otolaryngology: head and neck surgery. Amsterdam: Elsevier; 2020.
2. Song J-J, De Ridder D, Van de Heyning P, Vanneste S. Mapping tinnitus-related brain activation: an activation-likelihood estimation Metaanalysis of PET studies. J Nucl Med. 2012;53(10):1550–7. https://doi.org/10.2967/jnumed.112.102939.
3. Moller AR. Sensory systems: anatomy, physiology and pathophysiology. Houston: Gulf Professional Publishing; 2003.
4. Shepherd G. Neurobiology. New York: Oxford University Press; 1994.
5. Fettiplace R. Hair cell transduction, tuning, and synaptic transmission in the mammalian cochlea. Compr Physiol. 2017;7(4):1197–227. https://doi.org/10.1002/cphy.c160049.
6. Stebbins WC, Hawkins JE Jr, Johnson LG, Moody DB. Hearing thresholds with outer and inner hair cell loss. Am J Otolaryngol. 1979;1(1):15–27. https://doi.org/10.1016/s0196-0709(79)80004-6.
7. Johnstone BM, Patuzzi R, Yates GK. Basilar membrane measurements and the travelling wave. Hear Res. 1986;22:147–53. https://doi.org/10.1016/0378-5955(86)90090-0.
8. Sellick P, Patuzzi R, Johnstone B. Measurement of basilar membrane motion in the Guinea pig using the Mössbauer technique. J Acoust Soc Am. 1982;72(1):131–41.
9. Büki B, Avan P, Ribari O. The effect of body position on transient otoacoustic emission. In: Intracranial and intralabyrinthine fluids. Berlin: Springer; 1996. p. 175–81.
10. Baiduc RR, Lee J, Dhar S. Spontaneous otoacoustic emissions, threshold microstructure, and psychophysical tuning over a wide frequency range in humans. J Acoust Soc Am. 2014;135(1):300–14. https://doi.org/10.1121/1.4840775.
11. Keefe DH, Feeney MP, Hunter LL, Fitzpatrick DF, Blankenship CM, Garinis AC, et al. High frequency transient-evoked otoacoustic emission measurements using chirp and click stimuli. Hear Res. 2019;371:117–39. https://doi.org/10.1016/j.heares.2018.09.010.
12. Abdala C, Visser-Dumont L. Distortion product Otoacoustic emissions: a tool for hearing assessment and scientific study. Volta Rev. 2001;103(4):281–302.
13. Møller AR. Monitoring auditory evoked potentials. In: Intraoperative neurophysiological monitoring. Totowa, NJ: Humana Press; 2006. pp. 85-124. https://doi.org/10.1007/978-1-59745-018-8_6.
14. Møller AR. Evoked potentials in intraoperative monitoring. Williams & Wilkins; 1988.
15. Walton JP, Burkard R. 40 - neurophysiological manifestations of aging in the peripheral and central auditory nervous system. In: Hof PR, Mobbs CV, editors. Functional neurobiology of aging. San Diego: Academic Press; 2001. p. 581–95.
16. LeDoux JE. Brain mechanisms of emotion and emotional learning. Curr Opin Neurobiol. 1992;2(2):191–7.
17. Møller AR. Neural plasticity and disorders of the nervous system. Cambridge: Cambridge University Press; 2006.
18. Moller AR, Rollins PR. The non-classical auditory pathways are involved in hearing in children but not in adults. Neurosci Lett. 2002;319(1):41–4.
19. Møller AR. Neurophysiologic abnormalities in autism. New autism research developments. 2007;137–58.
20. Møller AR. Neural plasticity: for good and bad. Prog Theor Phys Suppl. 2008;173:48–65.
21. Møller AR, Kern JK, Grannemann B. Are the non-classical auditory pathways involved in autism and PDD? Neurol Res. 2005;27(6):625–9.
22. Møller AR, Møller MB, Yokota M. Some forms of tinnitus may involve the extralemniscal auditory pathway. Laryngoscope. 1992;102(10):1165–71.
23. Chen L, Wang X, Ge S, Xiong Q. Medial geniculate body and primary auditory cortex differentially contribute to striatal sound representations. Nat Commun. 2019;10(1):418. https://doi.org/10.1038/s41467-019-08350-7.
24. Winer JA, Lee CC. The distributed auditory cortex. Hear Res. 2007;229(1–2):3–13.
25. Aitkin L. The auditory midbrain: structure and function in the central auditory pathway. Berlin: Springer; 1986.
26. Jain R, Shore S. External inferior colliculus integrates trigeminal and acoustic information: unit responses to trigeminal nucleus and acoustic stimulation in the Guinea pig. Neurosci Lett. 2006;395(1):71–5.
27. Wiberg M, Westman J, Blomqvist A. Somatosensory projection to the mesencephalon: an anatomical study in the monkey. J Comp Neurol. 1987;264(1):92–117.
28. Zhou J, Shore S. Convergence of spinal trigeminal and cochlear nucleus projections in the inferior colliculus of the Guinea pig. J Comp Neurol. 2006;495(1):100–12.

29. Aitkin L, Dickhaus H, Schult W, Zimmermann M. External nucleus of inferior colliculus: auditory and spinal somatosensory afferents and their interactions. J Neurophysiol. 1978;41(4):837–47.
30. Aitkin L, Kenyon C, Philpott P. The representation of the auditory and somatosensory systems in the external nucleus of the cat inferior colliculus. J Comp Neurol. 1981;196(1):25–40.
31. Huffman RF, Henson OW Jr. The descending auditory pathway and acousticomotor systems: connections with the inferior colliculus. Brain Res Brain Res Rev. 1990;15(3):295–323. https://doi.org/10.1016/0165-0173(90)90005-9.
32. Schuknecht HF. Pathology of the ear. Cambridge: Harvard University Press; 1974.
33. Møller AR. Hearing: anatomy, physiology, and disorders of the auditory system. San Diego: Plural Publishing; 2012.
34. Guinan JJ, Norris BE, Guinan SS. Single auditory units in the superior olivary complex: II: locations of unit categories and tonotopic organization. Int J Neurosci. 1972;4(4):147–66. https://doi.org/10.3109/00207457209164756.
35. Møller AR. Frequency selectivity of single auditory-nerve fibers in response to broadband noise stimuli. J Acoust Soc Am. 1977;62(1):135–42.
36. Møller AR. Coding of sounds with rapidly varying spectrum in the cochlear nucleus. J Acoust Soc Am. 1974;55(3):631–40.
37. De Ridder D, Elgoyhen AB, Romo R, Langguth B. Phantom percepts: tinnitus and pain as persisting aversive memory networks. Proc Natl Acad Sci. 2011;108(20):8075–80. https://doi.org/10.1073/pnas.1018466108.
38. Schaette R, McAlpine D. Tinnitus with a normal audiogram: physiological evidence for hidden hearing loss and computational model. J Neurosci. 2011;31(38):13452–7. https://doi.org/10.1523/jneurosci.2156-11.2011.

Cochlear Changes After Noise Trauma

10

María Eugenia Gómez-Casati and Ana Belén Elgoyhen

Abstract

- Tinnitus, sound perception without an external source, occurs in 15% of the population and is the most reported disability for soldiers after combat. Noise overexposure is the single most important known factor leading to tinnitus.
- In addition, single exposures to blasts or acute harming sounds, but also chronic expositions to moderate noise can lead to long-term consequences to hearing, such us permanent hearing threshold shifts as well as poor speech discrimination in noisy environments. Almost half a billion people in the world have disabling hearing loss and 1.1 billion young people (aged between 12 and 35 years old) are at risk of losing their hearing due to recreational noise.
- Thus, exposure to excessive noise is the most common preventable cause leading to hearing loss and tinnitus.
- Noise overexposure leads to damage of mechanosensory hair cells and/or their stereocilia, synaptic ribbon reduction, and auditory nerve deterioration.
- The clinical significance of noise-induced hearing loss (NIHL) and noise-induced tinnitus has driven efforts to understand the underlying molecular, physiological, and biochemical mechanisms in order to search for therapeutic agents that act as otoprotectants.

M. E. Gómez-Casati (✉)
Instituto de Farmacología, Facultad de Medicina, Universidad de Buenos Aires, Buenos Aires, Argentina

A. B. Elgoyhen
Instituto de Investigaciones en Ingeniería Genética y Biología Molecular "Dr. Héctor N. Torres," Consejo Nacional de Investigaciones Científicas y Técnicas, Buenos Aires, Argentina

W. Schlee et al. (eds.), *Textbook of Tinnitus*, https://doi.org/10.1007/978-3-031-35647-6_10

Graphical Abstract

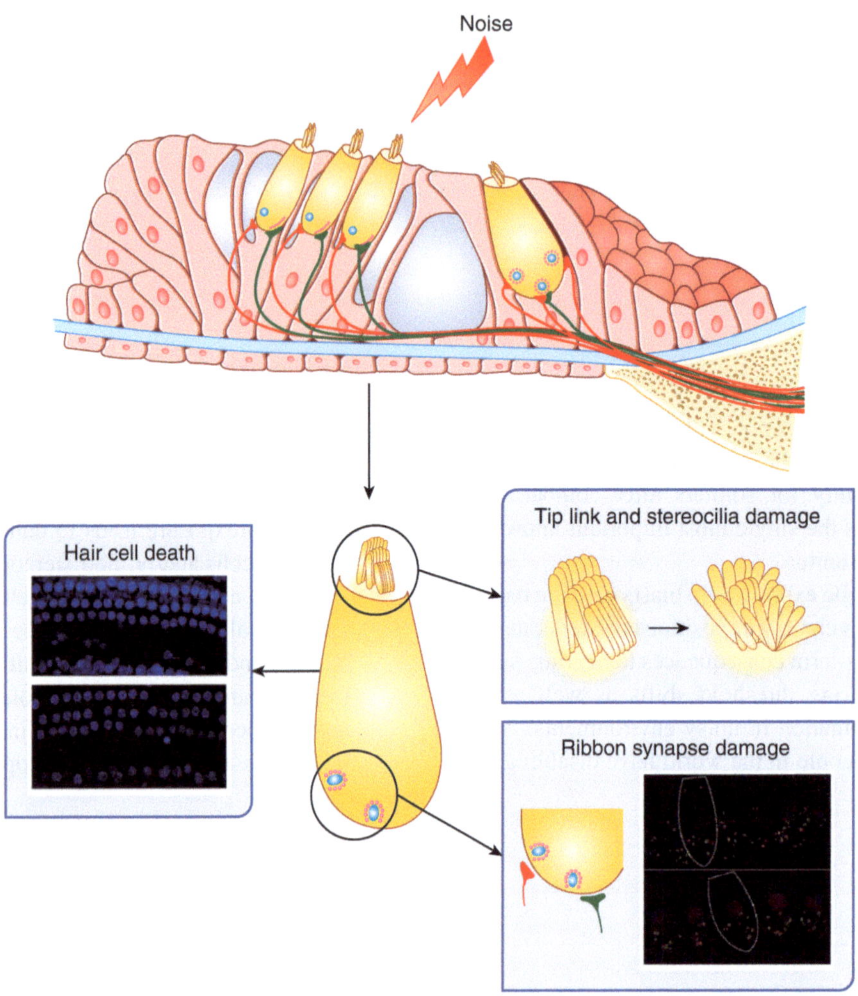

An overview of cochlear changes after noise trauma:

- Hair cells' tip links and stereocilia can be damaged
- Ribbon synapses can be lost due to exposure to loud noise or prolonged exposure to milder noise, even in absence of permanent hearing threshold shift. Right: immunolabeling of CTBP2 (a component of ribbon synapses, red puncta) and GluA2 (AMPA receptor, expressed at the auditory nerve terminal) at the base of hair cells
- Hair cell death. Left: whole mount of organ Corti stained with the nuclear dye Draq5 (blue) to visualize the sites of missing hair cells

Introduction

Tinnitus is frequently accompanied by hearing loss and the frequency spectrum of the perceived tinnitus sound correlates to the frequency range of the hearing loss [1]. In fact, in most cases auditory deprivation is the initial step in the generation of tinnitus. Peripheral deafferentation due to cochlear damage leads to increased spontaneous neuronal activity at various auditory pathway relays (except in the auditory nerve) all the way to the auditory cortex [2]. However, nearly 25% of all patients with tinnitus have normal hearing thresholds according to the conventional audiogram (125 Hz–8 kHz range) [3]. In spite of this, hearing abnormalities might still accompany tinnitus in patients with normal thresholds. Thus, patients with apparently normal audiograms might have hearing loss at higher frequencies not covered by standard clinical practice. An additional important number of patients might have hidden hearing loss, which is undetectable by conventional audiometry [4]. Therefore, cochlear changes which are at the onset of hearing loss likely trigger the ignition of most tinnitus cases. In this regard, within the environmental preventable factors that contribute the most to hearing loss is the exposure to loud noise, which can be of occupational, recreational, or environmental origin [5–7]. Moreover, prolonged noise and/or blast exposures are the most common known factors leading to tinnitus [8]. In fact, exposure to loud sound is the way to generate an animal model to study tinnitus [9]. Therefore, the cochlear pathophysiological consequences of exposure to loud sounds are most likely at the onset of tinnitus.

Exposure to overly loud sounds leading to noise-induced hearing loss (NIHL) and tinnitus is a worldwide concern that leads to considerable communication and affective problems for affected individuals and presents a significant socioeconomic factor [10]. Despite several identified details about its etiology, the underlying mechanisms that induce NIHL have been only partially identified. Research on animal models and on autopsy tissue samples from humans has shown that overexposure to noise can cause damage to several structures in the middle and inner ear. Depending on the kind of noise exposure, duration, and intensity, temporary or permanent auditory threshold shifts can occur. Noise of very high sound pressure levels, such as bomb blasts or jet engine at takeoff (~140 dB SPL), can break the eardrum and lift the entire sensory epithelium from its cellular anchorage [11, 12]. Chronic exposures to high to moderate sound pressure levels, like those present in a noisy industrial unit, do not cause an apparent damage to the middle ear; rather, there is an ongoing degeneration of the sensory epithelium in the inner ear [13]. It has been described that traumatizing acoustical stimuli of octave-band noise produces damage to the cochlea at the regions half an octave above the noise band and in more basal regions [14–17]. The anatomical consequences of noise exposure in the inner ear are varied and have been studied over decades, establishing several important ones such as damage to mechanosensory hair cells and/or their stereocilia, auditory neurons, and other specialized cells in the inner ear [14, 15, 18, 19]. The degree of damage, as well as the identity of the injured structures, depends on the intensity and the duration of the noise exposure.

Hair cell loss is particularly detrimental because they are the sensory cells in the inner ear, responsible for the detection and transduction of acoustic signals. Out of the two types of hair cells that coexist in mammalian inner ears, outer hair cells (OHCs) have shown the highest sensitivity to noise exposure, especially at the basal, high-frequency, cochlear turn [15, 18, 19]. Provided that hair cells in mammals do not regenerate [20], cell death represents a predictor of deficit in hearing capacity throughout the individual's life. While intense noise exposure leads to hair cell death, more moderate exposures that spare the cells still produce damage to structures such as the stereocilia of both OHCs and inner hair cells (IHCs) [15, 21, 22]. For example, overstimulation of the hair bundle can disrupt or break the tip links, uncoupling the mechanotransduction channel complex from mechanical stimuli and leading to hair cell dysfunction [23, 24]. Intracellularly, hair cells also show evidence of susceptibility to noise such as vacuolation of endoplasmic reticulum and swollen mitochondria, suggesting that metabolic stress is an important issue [25]. Another well-described consequence of overexposure to low to moderate noise is the degeneration of synapses between IHCs and auditory nerve fibers connecting the auditory periphery with the brain, i.e., the so-called ribbon synapses [16]. A massive swelling of auditory nerve terminals has been described, which can increase several fold in size [18, 26]. This swelling appears minutes after the acoustic trauma, and initial studies showed that it could be reverted within days, paving the way to the concept that this synaptic aspect of the noise exposure is only temporary. However, a series of recent studies drastically changed this view, showing that a low to moderate noise exposure, which produces only a transient loss of hearing sensitivity, actually generates long-term changes to neurons in the inner ear [16]. A permanent reduction in the number of ribbon synapses was noted, together with a delayed reduction in the number of somas corresponding to auditory neurons occurring in the following few weeks or even months postexposure [16]. Neuronal loss is an important factor contributing to the degree of sensory impairment in cases of inner ear pathology. Furthermore, the degree of neuronal survival following hair cell loss is an important determinant for the success of prostheses such as cochlear implants designed to directly stimulate the fibers of the VIIIth nerve.

The clinical burden of acoustic trauma due to exposure to loud sounds has driven efforts to understand the underlying molecular, physiological, and biochemical mechanisms in order to develop targeted therapeutics to prevent and/or protect the hearing of noise-exposed individuals. Moreover, it highlights the urgent need to promote improved noise exposure policies for hearing protection together with more efficient standards of NIHL and noise-induced tinnitus risk assessments.

Noise-Induced Hearing Loss Measurements

The most common functional measurement to analyze the degree of NIHL is the auditory threshold. In humans, this is evaluated by an audiometric screening: a measure of the lowest pure-tone sound pressure level across the speech spectrum (500–4000 Hz) to elicit an auditory perception [27]. Auditory brainstem responses (ABRs) and distortion product otoacoustic emissions (DPOAEs) are the two minimally invasive physiological measurements typically used in animal work on NIHL. The ABR is an evoked potential recorded from subdermal electrodes in the scalp by averaging the electrical response to many identical acoustic stimuli punctate in time. It represents synchronized activity of several classes of neurons in the ascending auditory pathway [28]. In response to very short tone pips at different frequencies delivered to the eardrum, the summed activity of cochlear nerve fibers can be recorded and the threshold for ABR can be estimated as the lowest stimulus level required to produce a response. The first peak of the ABR represents the summed activity of cochlear nerve fibers synapsing on IHCs [29, 30]. Cochlear thresholds can also be measured via DPOAEs, which are mechanical distortions created by nonlinearities in OHC transduction when the cochlea is stimulated simultaneously by two close pure-tone frequencies. DPOAEs can be detected as an objective sound by a sensitive microphone placed in the external ear canal [31, 32]. Therefore, these two complementary techniques for assessing cochlear function enable to analyze the degree of noise-induced threshold shift and to perform a differential diagnosis of OHC versus IHC/auditory nerve dysfunction throughout the cochlea, from low-frequency apical turn to the high-frequency basal tip [16].

Noise-Induced Hair Cell Loss

Exposure to a very high sound pressure level for a short time as well as long-term exposures to moderate noise can lead to a permanent damage to hair cells causing permanent auditory threshold elevation. In animal models of NIHL, permanent threshold shifts at a given frequency test can be correlated by the pattern of hair cell loss or damage as a function of the cochlear region [21]. The cytocochleogram is used to quantify hair cell damage or death along the whole length of the cochlea from base to apex and it can be expressed as fractional hair cell loss versus frequency [33]. As stated above, OHCs at the basal cochlear region are more vulnerable to noise [14]. Above a specific intensity level, OHCs show signs of metabolic exhaustion with the accumulation of reactive oxygen and nitrogen species (ROS and RNS, respectively) [34]. Another consequence of noise exposure is an increase of free Ca^{2+} in OHCs immediately after acoustic overstimulation, to which both entry through ion channels and release from intracellular stores might contribute [35–37]. Augmented intracellular Ca^{2+} concentration after exposure to high-intensity levels can be assumed from an increase in the Ca^{2+}-binding protein calmodulin (CaM), a key mediator of calcium signaling [38]. Since OHCs have the fundamental capacity to amplify low-intensity stimuli to make them detectable [39], the loss of functional OHCs (either by cell death or by sterereocilia damage) can elevate auditory thresholds by as much as 50 dB SPL at high-frequency regions [40, 41]. It has been described that noise-induced OHC loss in guinea pigs is associated with the apoptotic cell-death pathway [42]. Cochlear perfusion with a cell permeable peptide that blocks a key enzyme within the apoptosis pathway prevents the noise-induced OHCs loss [43]. Among the possible strategies to prevent hair cell death, the use of antioxidants to neutralize ROS and/or RNS and caspase or cell death inhibitors could have a potential pharmacotherapeutic value for hair cells' functional and morphological integrity.

Noise-Induced Stereocilia Damage

The intense hair bundle stimulation that occurs during prolonged and/or intense noise exposures can raise the force on tip links and cause their disruption [44]. Tip links are essential for coupling mechanical stimuli to the opening of the mechanotransduction channels [24]. Within 24 h, tip links can be regenerated after *in vitro* breakage, followed by a recovery of the hair bundle and restoration of mechanotransduction [45, 46]. However, more work is needed to characterize tip link regeneration *in vivo*. It has been proposed that tip links' breakage and repair contribute to the temporary auditory threshold shift seen after noise trauma [47]. Electron microscopy studies have also shown stereocilia core damage following acoustic trauma. Changes in stereocilia F-actin cores have been described including: actin depolymerization, loss of F-actin crosslinkers, rootlet breakage, and stereocilia fusion [48–51]. After acoustic trauma, a reduction in the number of stereocilia, height and width, was visualized by gaps in fluorescent phalloidin staining, which might decrease bundle stiffness and sensitivity [52]. A replacement of the entire hair bundle has been described after nonlethal insults in frogs and chickens [44, 53]. Evidence of hair bundle replacement in mammalian organs of Corti is limited: damaged hair cells can survive for a prolonged time and regrow their stereocilia in cultured embryonic and in neonatal rat utricles after laser lesioning [54] and gentamicin treatment *in vitro* [55], respectively.

Noise-Induced Synapse Damage

Auditory nerve fibers transmit electrical signals from the periphery to the cochlear nucleus in the brainstem. Each unmyelinated auditory nerve terminal receives signals from a single IHC via a sole ribbon synapse [56, 57], but each IHC is innervated by around 10–20 auditory nerve fibers, depending on the cochlear frequency region and species [58–60]. Synapses between IHCs and spiral ganglion neurons are also sensitive to low or moderate sound overexposure. Dramatic swelling of auditory nerve terminals in the synaptic zone at the contact point with IHCs has been shown to occur early after exposure, followed by a partial recovery within days [18, 26]. This swelling is prevented with the application of specific glutamate receptor antagonists during the noise protocol and mimicked by acute cochlear perfusion of agonists in the absence of sound, suggesting a type of glutamate excitotoxicity, since glutamate is the neurotransmitter at the IHC-synapses [61–65].

With the development of immunostaining techniques to quantify the synaptic contacts between IHCs and auditory nerve terminals with a confocal microscope [66, 67], synapses in normal ears and those exposed to traumatic noise were evaluated [16]. This technique used one antibody against a major protein in the presynaptic ribbon, located on the hair cell side of each synapse, and a second antibody against a subtype of glutamate receptor, located in the auditory nerve terminal [67]. By using this fast method for quantifying synapses in fixed tissue, Kujawa and Liberman [16] have shown that moderate noise exposures that preserve hair cells and hearing thresholds reduce supra-threshold responses through immediate elimination of roughly 40% of IHC-auditory nerve fibers' synapses. This is followed by delayed loss of spiral ganglion cells. This reduction in cochlear synapses correlates with a reduction in ABR peak 1 amplitude at suprathreshold intensities (e.g., at 80 dB SPL), without changes in ABR thresholds [16, 68, 69]. Once the synapse has been damaged, the affected neuron is functionally disconnected from the IHC and incapable of sending sensory information to the central nervous system. This cochlear synaptopathy that occurs in the absence of hair cell loss and without changes in threshold sensitivity has been called hidden hearing loss, because the dysfunction is not visible by a standard audiometric test [4]. The mechanism underlying hidden hearing loss has been analyzed through single fiber recordings in guinea pigs after exposure to noise [70]. Auditory nerve fibers contacting each IHC differ in sensitivity to sound and spontaneous discharge rate (SR), i.e., the spike rate without an external sound source [71]. They are classified into three groups according to the correlation between thresholds and SR: low-SR, medium-SR, and high-SR [72]. These three subtypes can innervate the same IHC at different positions along the basolateral surface of the cell and project to different cell types of the cochlear nucleus [57]. Low and medium-SR fibers have thinner axons, fewer mitochondria, make synaptic contacts on the modiolar side of the IHC, and activate at high sound intensity levels. In contrast, high-SR fibers have thicker axons, more mitochondria, tend to synapse on the pillar side, and respond at low sound intensity levels [57]. It has been proposed that such diversity of auditory nerve fibers allows the wide dynamic range of sound intensities encoded by the cochlea and signal coding in noisy backgrounds [73–75]. By recording from large populations of single auditory nerve fibers in guinea pigs, Furman et al. (2013) have reported that after noise exposure there is a selective loss of the low-SR, high threshold fibers and that surviving fibers show normal responses [70]. Although the loss of low SR fibers does not lead to changes in auditory thresholds, it might contribute to hearing difficulties in noisy environments [76]. A more recent work performed in mice where sound-evoked and spontaneous activity from single auditory nerve fibers recordings were performed after acoustic trauma have shown no selective loss of low-SR fibers. Instead, loss of both SR fibers, together with a recovery in single-fiber thresholds to pre-exposure levels, and an increase in the strength of tone-burst responses in the presence of continuous masking noise were observed [77]. This study suggests that noise-induced cochlear synaptopathy varies across different species and that, in mouse, the noise-induced hyperexcitability seen in central auditory circuits is also observed at the level of the auditory nerve [77]. The inability to understand speech-in-noise is one of the main complaints hearing care professionals receive from both young and aged patients with normal audiograms [78]. Standard hearing tests in quiet provides a good measure of the state of the sensory cells in the inner ear after noise-induced hearing loss. However, the most vulnerable elements are the synapses between IHCs and auditory nerve fibers. Speech-in-noise tests or performance on other complex auditory tasks may be a useful measure of noise-induced neuropathy.

Noise-Induced Cochlear Molecular Changes

High-throughput analysis of gene expression by RNA-sequencing (RNA-seq) is emerging as a valuable tool for comprehensive analyses of global gene expression patterns [79]. A widespread molecular understanding of noise-induced changes in the inner ear is required in order to design targeted pharmacological therapeutics to prevent hearing loss and tinnitus. A recent work identified the inner ear cell-type-specific molecular landscape after acoustic trauma by using RiboTag and single-cell RNA sequencing [80]. After exposure to loud noise, there is an induction of the transcription factors STAT3 and IRF7 and immune-related genes across all inner ear cell types [80]. Indeed, inhibiting the JAK2/STAT3-signaling pathway reduces the degeneration of OHCs and prevents both ABR and DPOAEs threshold elevation following acoustic overstimulation [81]. The transcription factor IRF7 plays a role in the Toll-like receptor-signaling pathway, thought to be part of the innate immune response to stress [80]. The expression level of IRF7 is rapidly upregulated 1 day post-noise exposure, implicating the Toll-like receptor-signaling pathway in the molecular response of the inner ear cells to acoustic trauma [82]. The transcriptional changes of immune-related genes in the cochlea suggest that specific inflammatory mechanisms are involved in post-noise processes [80]. In the lateral wall compartment, important for generating and maintaining the endocochlear potential, there is a downregulation in the expression of potassium transport genes after acoustic trauma [80]. At the auditory nerve level, activation of the ATF3/4 stress response pathway, which is known as the integrated stress response pathway, is observed only in high-SR fibers (i.e., the noise-resistant fibers that activate at low sound intensity levels) [80]. It has been suggested that the gene expression program activated by this pathway optimizes the cellular response to stress and is dependent on the nature and intensity of the stimuli. Although the integrated stress response pathway is primarily a pro-survival, homeostatic program, exposure to severe stress can drive signaling toward cell death [83]. High-SR fibers also exhibit a reduction in the expression of genes involved in synaptic transmission, suggesting that they might protect the neurons from glutamatergic excitotoxicity due to sustained exposure to loud noise [80]. In fact, neuronal damage due to excitotoxicity is prevented with the application of glutamate receptor antagonists during noise exposure [61–65]. Following acoustic trauma, there is a downregulation of genes that function in mRNA metabolic processes (e.g.,

Sfpq, Hnrnpu, and Snrrnp48) in OHCs [80]. However, in supporting cells, genes that function in nerve impulse transmission (e.g., Grm3, Asic2, and Cacna1e) are specifically repressed and genes encoding structural proteins involved in cell adhesion and migration (e.g., Podxl and Itgb1) are induced [80]. Knowing which signaling pathways across inner ear cell types are activated in response to noise will help to identify noise-induced changes with the final goal to discover candidate therapeutics to prevent and/ or treat noise-induced hearing loss and tinnitus.

Conclusions

Exposure to loud noise is the most common preventable cause leading to hearing loss and tinnitus. Unless action is taken, it is likely that the number of people with disabling hearing loss and tinnitus will grow over the coming years. Despite the clinical concern, there are currently no registered treatments that protect and/or restore hearing. During the last 15 years, a lot of progress has been made in understanding the underlying molecular, physiological, and biochemical mechanisms involved in hair cell and nerve damage after noise overexposure. Together with several experimental studies in animal models of noise-induced hearing loss, some therapies are becoming available which can be used in humans. Because no treatment is now available to reverse cochlear damage, implementation of preventative strategies and awareness of hearing health is essential. Prevention activities should comprise those affecting young people, improvement of noise legislation, and encouragement of use of hearing protectors.

Acknowledgments Agencia Nacional de Promoción Científica y Tecnológica (Argentina) to M.E.G-C and A.B.E, Pew Charitable Trust (USA) to M.E.G-C, National Organization for Hearing Research (USA) to M.E.G-C, NIH Grant R01 DC001508 (USA) (Paul A. Fuchs and A.B.E) and Scientific Grand Prize from the Fondation Pour L'Audition (France) to A.B.E.

References

1. Norena A, Micheyl C, Chéry-Croze S, Collet L. Psychoacoustic characterization of the tinnitus spectrum: implications for the underlying mechanisms of tinnitus. Audiol Neurootol. 2002;7:358–69.
2. Elgoyhen AB, Langguth B, De Ridder D, Vanneste S, De Ridder D, Vanneste S. Tinnitus: perspectives from human neuroimaging. Nat Rev Neurosci. 2015;16:632. https://doi.org/10.1038/nrn4003.
3. Tang J, Ji B, Liu L. [Study of hearing loss in 200 patients with subjective tinnitus]. Lin Chung Er Bi Yan Hou Tou Jing Wai Ke Za Zhi. 2011;16:726–9.
4. Schaette R, McAlpine D. Tinnitus with a normal audiogram: physiological evidence for hidden hearing loss and computational model. J Neurosci. 2011;31:13452–7.
5. Concha-Barrientos M, Campbell-Lendrum D, Steenland K. Occupational noise: assessing the burden of disease from work-related hearing impairment at national and local levels/Marisol Concha-Barrientos, Diarmid Campbell-Lendrum, Kyle Steenland. Geneva: World Health Organisation (WHO Environment Burd. Dis. Ser. No 9). 2004. https://apps.who.int/iris/handle/10665/43001.
6. Lie A, Skogstad M, Johannessen HA, Tynes T, Mehlum IS, Nordby KC, Engdahl B, Tambs K. Occupational noise exposure and hearing: a systematic review. Int Arch Occup Environ Health. 2016;89:351–72.
7. Śliwińska-Kowalska M, Zaborowski K. WHO environmental noise guidelines for the European region: a systematic review on environmental noise and permanent hearing loss and tinnitus. Int J Environ Res Public Health. 2017;14:1139. https://doi.org/10.3390/ijerph14101139.
8. Henry JA, Dennis KC, Schechter MA. General review of tinnitus: prevalence, mechanisms, effects, and management. J Speech Lang Hear Res. 2005;48:1204–35.
9. Galazyuk A, Brozoski TJ. Animal models of tinnitus: a review. Otolaryngol Clin N Am. 2020;53:469–80.
10. WHO. World Health Organisation. 2018. https://www.who.int/pbd/deafness/estimates/en/.
11. Kerr AG, Byrne JE. Concussive effects of bomb blast on the ear. J Laryngol Otol. 1975;89:131–44.
12. Hamernik RP, Turrentine G, Roberto M, Salvi R, Henderson D. Anatomical correlates of impulse noise-induced mechanical damage in the cochlea. Hear Res. 1984;13:229–47.
13. Clark WW, Bohne BA, Boettcher FA. Effect of periodic rest on hearing loss and cochlear damage following exposure to noise. J Acoust Soc Am. 1987;82:1253–64.
14. Liberman MC, Kiang NY. Acoustic trauma in cats. Cochlear pathology and auditory-nerve activity. Acta Otolaryngol Suppl. 1978;358:1–63.
15. Robertson D, Johnstone B, McGill T. Effects of loud tones on the inner ear: a combined electrophysiological and ultrastructural study. Hear Res. 1980;2:39–53.
16. Kujawa SG, Liberman MC. Adding insult to injury: cochlear nerve degeneration after "temporary" noise-induced hearing loss. J Neurosci. 2009;29:14077–85.
17. Kim KX, Payne S, Yang-Hood A, Li SZ, Davis B, Carlquist J, Ghaffari BV, Gantz JA, Kallogjeri D, Fitzpatrick JAJ, Ohlemiller KK, Hirose K, Rutherford MA. Vesicular glutamatergic transmission in noise-induced loss and repair of Cochlear ribbon synapses. J Neurosci. 2019;39:4434–47.
18. Spoendlin H. Primary structural changes in the organ of Corti after acoustic overstimulation. Acta Otolaryngol. 1971;71:166–76.
19. Wang Y, Hirose K, Liberman MC. Dynamics of noise-induced cellular injury and repair in the mouse cochlea. J Assoc Res Otolaryngol. 2002;3:248–68.
20. Edge AS, Chen ZY. Hair cell regeneration. Curr Opin Neurobiol. 2008;18:377–82.
21. Liberman MC, Dodds LW. Single-neuron labeling and chronic cochlear pathology. III. Stereocilia damage and alterations of threshold tuning curves. Hear Res. 1984;16:55–74.
22. Saunders JC, Dear SP, Schneider ME. The anatomical consequences of acoustic injury: a review and tutorial. J Acoust Soc Am. 1985;78:833–60.
23. Pickles JO, Osborne MP, Comis SD. Vulnerability of tip links between stereocilia to acoustic trauma in the Guinea pig. Hear Res. 1987;25:173–83.
24. Assad JA, Shepherd GMG, Corey DP. Tip-link integrity and mechanical transduction in vertebrate hair cells. Neuron. 1991;7:985–94.
25. Wong ACY, Ryan AF. Mechanisms of sensorineural cell damage, death and survival in the cochlea. Front Aging Neurosci. 2015;0:58.

26. Robertson D. Functional significance of dendritic swelling after loud sounds in the Guinea pig cochlea. Hear Res. 1983;9:263–78.
27. Le TN, Straatman LV, Lea J, Westerberg B. Current insights in noise-induced hearing loss: a literature review of the underlying mechanism, pathophysiology, asymmetry, and management options. J Otolaryngol. 2017;46:46–1.
28. Melcher J, Kiang NY. Generators of the brainstem auditory evoked potential in cat. III: identified cell populations. Hear Res. 1996;93:52–71.
29. Buchwald JS, Huang CM. Far-field acoustic response: origins in the cat. Science. 1975;189:382–4.
30. Antoli-Candela F, Jr, Kiang NYS. Unit activity underlying the N1 potential. In: Naunton RF, Fernandez C, editors. Evoked Electrical Activity in the Auditory Nervous System. Academic Press; New York: 1978. pp. 165–91.
31. Shera CA, Guinan JJ Jr. Evoked otoacoustic emissions arise by two fundamentally different mechanisms: a taxonomy for mammalian OAEs. J Acoust Soc Am. 1999;105:782–98.
32. Robles L, Ruggero MA. Mechanics of the mammalian cochlea. Physiol Rev. 2001;81:1305–52.
33. Liberman MC. Advances in experimental medicine and biology, vol. 875. New York: Springer; 2016. p. 1–7. https://link.springer.com/chapter/10.1007/978-1-4939-2981-8_1.
34. Lynch ED, Gu R, Pierce C, Kil J. Ebselen-mediated protection from single and repeated noise exposure in rat. Laryngoscope. 2004;114:333–7.
35. Maurer J, Heinrich UR, Mann W. Morphologic damage and changes of intracellular calcium-binding sites after acute noise trauma in the organ of corti of the Guinea pig. ORL J Otorhinolaryngol Relat Spec. 1993;55:7–12.
36. Fridberger A, Åke Flock M, Ulfendahl BF. Acoustic overstimulation increases outer hair cell Ca2+ concentrations and causes dynamic contractions of the hearing organ. Proc Natl Acad Sci U S A. 1998;95:7127.
37. Oliver D, Ludwig J, Reisinger E, Zoellner W, Ruppersberg JP, Fakler B. Memantine inhibits efferent cholinergic transmission in the cochlea by blocking nicotinic acetylcholine receptors of outer hair cells. Mol Pharmacol. 2001;60:183–9.
38. Zuo H, Cui B, She X, Wu M. Changes in Guinea pig cochlear hair cells after sound conditioning and noise exposure. J Occup Health. 2008;50:373–9.
39. Dallos P. Cochlear amplification, outer hair cells and prestin. Curr Opin Neurobiol. 2008;18:370–6.
40. Dallos P, Harris D. Properties of auditory nerve responses in absence of outer hair cells. J Neurophysiol. 1978;41:365–83.
41. Saunders J, Cohen Y, Szymko Y. The structural and functional consequences of acoustic injury in the cochlea and peripheral auditory system: a five year update. J Acoust Soc Am. 1991;90:136–46.
42. Hu B, Guo W, Wang P, Henderson S, Jiang S. Intense noise-induced apoptosis in hair cells of Guinea pig cochleae. Acta Otolaryngol. 2000;120:19–24.
43. Wang J, Van De Water TR, Bonny C, de Ribaupierre F, Puel JL, Zine A. A peptide inhibitor of c-Jun N-terminal kinase protects against both aminoglycoside and acoustic trauma-induced auditory hair cell death and hearing loss. J Neurosci. 2003;23:8596–607.
44. Wagner EL, Shin J-BB. Mechanisms of hair cell damage and repair. Trends Neurosci. 2019;42:414–24.
45. Jia S, Yang S, Guo W, He D. Fate of mammalian cochlear hair cells and stereocilia after loss of the stereocilia. J Neurosci. 2009;29:15277–85.
46. Indzhykulian A, Stepanyan R, Nelina A, Spinelli K, Ahmed Z, Belyantseva I, Friedman T, Barr-Gillespie P, Frolenkov G. Molecular remodeling of tip links underlies mechanosensory regeneration in auditory hair cells. PLoS Biol. 2013;11:e1001583. https://doi.org/10.1371/JOURNAL.PBIO.1001583.
47. Zhao Y, Yamoah EN, Gillespie PG. Regeneration of broken tip links and restoration of mechanical transduction in hair cells. Proc Natl Acad Sci U S A. 1996;93:15469.
48. Tilney L, Saunders J, Egelman E, DeRosier D. Changes in the organization of actin filaments in the stereocilia of noise-damaged lizard cochleae. Hear Res. 1982;7:181–97.
49. Engström B, Flock A, Borg E. Ultrastructural studies of stereocilia in noise-exposed rabbits. Hear Res. 1983;12:251–64.
50. Liberman M. Chronic ultrastructural changes in acoustic trauma: serial-section reconstruction of stereocilia and cuticular plates. Hear Res. 1987;26:65–88.
51. Liberman MC, Dodds LW. Acute ultrastructural changes in acoustic trauma: serial-section reconstruction of stereocilia and cuticular plates. Hear Res. 1987;26:45–64.
52. Avinash G, Nuttall A, Raphael Y. 3-D analysis of F-actin in stereocilia of cochlear hair cells after loud noise exposure. Hear Res. 1993;67:139–46.
53. Gale JE, Meyers JR, Periasamy A, Corwin JT. Survival of bundleless hair cells and subsequent bundle replacement in the bullfrog's saccule. J Neurobiol. 2002;50:81–92.
54. Sobkowicz HM, August BK, Slapnick SM. Cellular interactions as a response to injury in the organ of corti in culture. Int J Dev Neurosci. 1997;15:463–85.
55. Zheng JL, Keller G, Gao W-QQW. Immunocytochemical and morphological evidence for intracellular self-repair as an important contributor to mammalian hair cell recovery. J Neurosci. 1999;19:2161–70.
56. Liberman MC. Morphological differences among radial afferent fibers in the cat cochlea: an electron-microscopic study of serial sections. Hear Res. 1980;3:45–63.
57. Liberman MC. Single-neuron labeling in the cat auditory nerve. Science. 1982;216:1239–41.
58. Liberman MC, Dodds LW, Pierce S. Afferent and efferent innervation of the cat cochlea: quantitative analysis with light and electron microscopy. J Comp Neurol. 1990;301:443–60.
59. Bohne BA, Kenworthy A, Carr CD. Density of myelinated nerve fibers in the chinchilla cochlea. J Acoust Soc Am. 1982;72:102–7.
60. Stamataki S, Francis HW, Lehar M, May BJ, Ryugo DK. Synaptic alterations at inner hair cells precede spiral ganglion cell loss in aging C57BL/6J mice. Hear Res. 2006;221:104–18.
61. Pujol R, Puel JL. Excitotoxicity, synaptic repair, and functional recovery in the mammalian cochlea: a review of recent findings. Ann N Y Acad Sci. 1999;884:249–54.
62. Puel J, Pujol R, Ladrech S, Eybalin M. Alpha-amino-3-hydroxy-5-methyl-4-isoxazole propionic acid electrophysiological and neurotoxic effects in the Guinea-pig cochlea. Neuroscience. 1991;45:63–72.
63. Puel JL, Ruel J, Gervais d'Aldin C, Pujol R. Excitotoxicity and repair of cochlear synapses after noise-trauma induced hearing loss. Neuroreport. 1998;9:2109–14.
64. Ruel J, Bobbin R, Vidal D, Pujol R, Puel J. The selective AMPA receptor antagonist GYKI 53784 blocks action potential generation and excitotoxicity in the Guinea pig cochlea. Neuropharmacology. 2000;39:1959–73.
65. Ruel J, Wang J, Rebillard G, Eybalin M, Lloyd R, Pujol R, Puel JL. Physiology, pharmacology and plasticity at the inner hair cell synaptic complex. Hear Res. 2007;227:19–27.
66. Khimich D, Nouvian R, Pujol R, Tom Dieck S, Egner A, Gundelfinger ED, Moser T. Hair cell synaptic ribbons are essential for synchronous auditory signalling. Nature. 2005;434:889–94.
67. Liberman LD, Wang H, Liberman MC. Opposing gradients of ribbon size and AMPA receptor expression underlie sensitivity differences among cochlear-nerve/hair-cell synapses. J Neurosci. 2011;31:801–8.

68. Boero LE, Castagna VC, Di Guilmi MN, Goutman JD, Elgoyhen AB, Gomez-Casati ME, Elgoyhen AB, Gómez-Casati ME. Enhancement of the medial olivocochlear system prevents hidden hearing loss. J Neurosci. 2018;38:7440–51.
69. Liberman LD, Liberman MC. Dynamics of cochlear synaptopathy after acoustic overexposure. J Assoc Res Otolaryngol. 2015;16:205–19.
70. Furman AC, Kujawa SG, Liberman MC. Noise-induced cochlear neuropathy is selective for fibers with low spontaneous rates. J Neurophysiol. 2013;110:577–86.
71. Kiang N, Watanabe T, Thomas E, Clark L. Discharge patterns of single fibers in the cat's auditory nerve. Cambridge: MIT Press; 1965.
72. Liberman MC. Auditory-nerve response from cats raised in a low-noise chamber. J Acoust Soc Am. 1978;63:442–55.
73. Costalupes JA. Representation of tones in noise in the responses of auditory nerve fibers in cats. I. Comparison with detection thresholds. J Neurosci. 1985;5:3261–9.
74. Liberman MC. Noise-induced and age-related hearing loss: new perspectives and potential therapies. F1000Research. 2017;6:1–11.
75. Young ED, Barta PE. Rate responses of auditory nerve fibers to tones in noise near masked threshold. J Acoust Soc Am. 1986;79:426–42.
76. Bharadwaj HM, Verhulst S, Shaheen L, Liberman MC, Shinn-cunningham BG. Cochlear neuropathy and the coding of supra-threshold sound. Front Sci Neurosci. 2014;8:1–18.
77. Suthakar K, Liberman MC. Auditory-nerve responses in mice with noise-induced cochlear synaptopathy. J Neurophysiol. 2021;126:2027. https://doi.org/10.1152/JN.00342.2021.
78. Frisina DR, Frisina RD. Speech recognition in noise and presbycusis: relations to possible neural mechanisms. Hear Res. 1997;106:95–104.
79. Mortazavi A, Williams BA, McCue K, Schaeffer L, Wold B. Mapping and quantifying mammalian transcriptomes by RNA-Seq. Nat Methods. 2008;5:621–8.
80. Milon B, Shulman ED, So KS, Cederroth CR, Lipford EL, Sperber M, Sellon JB, Sarlus H, Pregernig G, Shuster B, Song Y, Mitra S, Orvis J, Margulies Z, Ogawa Y, Shults C, Depireux DA, Palermo AT, Canlon B, Burns J, Elkon R, Hertzano R. A cell-type-specific atlas of the inner ear transcriptional response to acoustic trauma. Cell Rep. 2021;36:109758.
81. Wilson T, Omelchenko I, Foster S, Zhang Y, Shi X, Nuttall A. JAK2/STAT3 inhibition attenuates noise-induced hearing loss. PLoS One. 2014;9:e108276.
82. Cai Q, Vethanayagam R, Yang S, Bard J, Jamison J, Cartwright D, Dong Y, Hu B. Molecular profile of cochlear immunity in the resident cells of the organ of Corti. J Neuroinflammation. 2014;11:173.
83. Pakos-Zebrucka K, Koryga I, Mnich K, Ljujic M, Samali A, Gorman A. The integrated stress response. EMBO Rep. 2016;17:1374–95.

Molecular Biology of the Central Auditory System and Tinnitus

11

Rahilla Tarfa and Thanos Tzounopoulos

Abstract

Tinnitus is an auditory precept without any external input. In most cases, initial damage to the cochlea results in a change in peripheral auditory input that, in turn, triggers a change in central auditory mechanisms to compensate for this loss. This compensation, a combination of homeostatic and synaptic plasticity, results in an increased 'gain' in central auditory structures that may underlie the initiation of tinnitus. Changes at the molecular, cellular, and synaptic level in both auditory and nonauditory areas have been noted in animal models of tinnitus. Current research efforts to cure or clinically target to alleviate the tinnitus symptoms are focused on these areas and target these changes, including ion channel activators. Future studies should focus on unraveling the mechanisms of tinnitus precept induction and circuitry distribution for better treatment options.

Highlights

- Initial damage to the cochlear and a combination of resultant homeostatic and synaptic plasticity changes drive the maladaptive brain changes that induce tinnitus.
- A number of changes at the molecular, cellular, and synaptic levels in auditory and nonauditory structures underlie the induction and maintenance of tinnitus.
- The neuronal changes that are necessary and sufficient for the initiation and maintenance of tinnitus take place within these networks, but more work on how brain circuity changes to distribute and maintain the tinnitus precept is needed to drive therapeutic innovation.

R. Tarfa
School of Medicine, University of Pittsburgh, Pittsburgh, PA, USA
e-mail: rtarfa@uw.edu

T. Tzounopoulos (✉)
Department of Otolaryngology, University of Pittsburgh, Pittsburgh, PA, USA

Pittsburgh Hearing Research Center, University of Pittsburgh, Pittsburgh, PA, USA
e-mail: thanos@pitt.edu

Basics About Tinnitus

Definition

A common misconception of brain sensory processing is the basic premise that information is processed on an input-output operation. However, this negates and ignores the fact that the brain has a baseline of continuous ongoing computations that integrate internal information and external signals. As such, for hearing to occur, sound waves from the external environment are received via the ear and peripheral auditory system, and then integrated into the central auditory system, to not only facilitate the sense of audition but also our cognizance and perception of the new input. Tinnitus violates this design by presenting as an aberration in sound perception which manifests as the involuntary perception of phantom sounds in the absence of any external auditory input. The term 'tinnitus' itself is derived from the Latin root verb *tinnire*, meaning "to ring" [1], with records demonstrating attempts to define and treat tinnitus dating as far back to ancient Egypt [2]. It is differentiated from the auditory hallucinations well associated with psychotic disorders in that the sounds in tinnitus are indistinct [1] (see also Chap. 2).

Classification and Etiology

Tinnitus presents heterogeneously. Most patients report a hissing, sizzling, or ringing sound. It can be classified based

W. Schlee et al. (eds.), *Textbook of Tinnitus*, https://doi.org/10.1007/978-3-031-35647-6_11

on who perceives the sound—subjective vs. objective. Ninety-nine percent of patients perceive the sound alone, but on the rare occasion, 1% of the time, the sound can also heard by another person within inches of the patient (objective) [3]. It should be noted that the definition of 'objective tinnitus' deviates from the classic definition of tinnitus, as it has an identifiable cause. For reference, 'subjective tinnitus' is what most auditory neuroscientists study in the basic neuroscience literature.

Tinnitus can also be classified as pulsatile vs. nonpulsatile. The sound in pulsatile tinnitus is often in tune with the patient's heartbeat and is secondary to a vascular pathology such as: atherosclerotic disease, intracranial hypertension, vascular anatomic variants, or vascular tumors at the skull base [4]. Nonpulsatile tinnitus, on the other hand, is continuous [5]. Moreover, tinnitus can have a sudden onset, and patients report variability in how long it lasts, some reporting acute vs. chronic tinnitus (lasting >3 months) [5] (see also Chap. 2). This variability in classification remains one of the challenges in constructing an objective measurement tool that can be used to assess and diagnose tinnitus.

Neurobiology of the Auditory System and Pathophysiology Models of Tinnitus

The sense of audition begins with the peripheral auditory system, which handles the conduction and propagation of sound from the outer ear, up to the different portions of the brain to be processed and interpreted by the central auditory system. At the cellular level, altered spontaneous activity, in the form of hyperactivity, in various auditory nuclei of the auditory system following sensory damage is believed to be the most robust correlate of tinnitus [6]. Here, we discuss the anatomy and physiology of the different auditory and nonauditory nuclei that play key roles in auditory processing and the changes seen in the pathophysiology of tinnitus.

Anatomy and Physiology of the Peripheral Auditory Nervous System

The peripheral auditory system comprises the outer and middle ear, cochlea, and auditory nerve. Sounds are transmitted sequentially from the outer—>middle—>inner ear and then transferred to the neural pathways of both the peripheral and central auditory nervous system. The outer ear enables sound collection, localization, and direction to the external auditory meatus which directs the transmission to the tympanic membrane. The middle ear is air-filled and resides within the temporal bone. Overall, the middle ear serves to amplify the collected sound to the cochlear, thus overcoming the impedance mismatch between the outer ear and cochlea—which occurs due to a combination of the configuration of sound transduction and mechanics between the tympanic membrane and the lever action of the three small bones [7].

Cochlea

The cochlea is at the center of transducing acoustic sound into the electrical impulses that the brain can integrate, transmit, and interpret. The organ of corti, considered the hearing end organ, is comprised of an array of both outer and inner hair cells (OHCs and IHCs) and is positioned on top of the basilar membrane. Both hair cells change vibratory energy to electrical energy and are responsible for the transduction process. The auditory nerve, a component of the eight cranial nerve, is the final component of the peripheral nervous system and carries impulses from the cochlea to the brainstem.

In general, tinnitus is thought to be triggered by a set of abnormal events in the cochlea. Damage to the hair cells of the cochlea and/or fibers of the auditory nerve, due to presbycusis, noxious acoustic exposure, or ototoxic drugs, has been found to be the most common insult leading to tinnitus. Some of the earlier arguments in the field purported that tinnitus arose from overactivity in the cochlear nerve, while the rest of the central auditory nervous system involvement was thought to be minuscule [8]. However, this idea was refuted for two major reasons—cochlear damage resulted in decreased spontaneous and evoked firing activity, and surgical denervation of the cochlea did not result in the alleviation of tinnitus [8]. It is now known and appreciated that initial insult in the cochlea leads to a reduction in the transmission of neural activity from the cochlea to the central auditory system [9]. In addition, it is the loss of this input to the central auditory system that leads to compensatory mechanisms, which lead to the initiation and maintenance of tinnitus (more discussed below) (see also Chap. 2).

From recent studies, we now know that noxious acoustic exposure can cause significant but temporary threshold shifts (TTS) in hearing that lead to rapid loss of synapses (up to 50%) between the cochlear neurons and IHCs [10, 11]. OHCs are most vulnerable to noxious acoustic exposure, while IHCs are additionally sensitive due to presbycusis, although at much earlier timelines [10]. This synaptic loss, referred to as cochlear synaptopathy, has been shown to lead to axonal pruning, new axonal growth, synaptogenesis, excessive glutamate release, and tonotopic changes [12]. The combination of these sets of changes following the noxious insult is referred to as cochlear synaptopathy [11]; however, whether cochlear synaptopathy itself leads to tinnitus remains unclear.

It is important to note that while damage to the auditory nerves and/or cochlea is an initiating insult for tinnitus, many patients with tinnitus (10–15%) present with normal audiograms in the low frequency range below 8 kHz [13]. The converse is also true, wherein many patients present with peripheral auditory hearing dysfunction due to either high frequency hearing loss (where tinnitus occurs) or synaptopathy and, yet, do not have tinnitus. The current understanding is that tinnitus without any shifts in auditory thresholds may occur in patients who had some type of neuropathic damage to the cochlea as a result of either noxious acoustic exposure or presbycusis that doesn't unveil itself unless high frequency hearing is tested [14, 15]. In fact, the IHCs seem to be more susceptible to this type of damage as compared to the OHCs, especially in cells that are tuned to high frequencies or have a high depolarization threshold [14]. This "hidden hearing loss" [16] in tinnitus is supported by the reduction of the auditory brainstem response (ABR) Wave I in response to suprathreshold sounds in tinnitus patients as compared to normal hearing patients; however, Wave V (in the midbrain) is at high/normal levels, thus supporting the idea of "central gain" [13, 17] (see also Chap. 18; more discussed below).

Anatomy and Physiology of the Central Auditory Nervous System

The central auditory system is made up of the cochlear nucleus, superior olivary complex, lateral lemniscus, interior colliculus, medial geniculate body, and auditory cortex.

Dorsal Cochlear Nucleus (DCN)

Located in the pons is the cochlear nucleus, the first nuclei that comprises the central auditory nervous system. It consists of the dorsal cochlear nucleus (DCN), the posterior ventral cochlear nucleus, and the anterior ventral cochlear nucleus. The cochlear nucleus is also the first site of multisensory integration, receiving input from the auditory nerve fibers and somatosensory afferents [18]. Additionally, the output neurons of the DCN, the fusiform neurons, receive inputs from the trigeminal and dorsal column pathways. This somatosensory information is relayed via the granule cells' axons to the fusiform neurons and interneurons of the DCN [18].

Most notably, the fusiform cells, the output cells of the DCN, have been demonstrated to display hyperactive spontaneous activity in animal models of tinnitus. However, whether this is simply a sign of tinnitus or the initiating spark that causes tinnitus remains a subject of debate. The current prevailing and favored mechanism underlying tinnitus is the idea that a gain in the central auditory system compensates for sensory deprivation in peripheral auditory system, thereby altering neuronal sensitivity [8]. Studies show that a decrease in peripheral inputs resulting from cochlear damage results in increased activity in the central auditory nervous system [6]. One school of thought proposes that this increase in activity occurs to maintain neural coding efficiency at a ***set point*** in reaction to auditory deprivation [8]. As a result, a combination of plasticity mechanisms including homeostatic and synaptic plasticity mechanisms is employed in the central auditory structures, a "central gain" so to speak, that regulates both the sensitivity and adaptation of central neurons to the new distribution of sensory input following acoustic damage [6, 19]. This adaptation serves to ensure that the average central nervous system activity, more specifically in the DCN, is maintained at a set-point, and that the range of activity corresponds to the new modified, albeit decreased, range of cochlear inputs. *The result of this compensation is what is thought to be a crucial component in triggering tinnitus.*

Homeostatic Intrinsic Plasticity in the DCN

In the last few years, a fair amount of work has been done to investigate the hyperexcitability and long-term homeostatic plasticity changes in DCN neurons following tinnitus at the cellular level. These studies utilized tinnitus animal models of mice that allowed for the behavioral stratification of mice after noise exposure. Whole cell patch-clamp electrophysiology recordings from DCN neurons revealed decreased potassium currents from KCNQ2/3 channels [20], which belong to the family of subthreshold non-inactivating potassium channels, KCNQ1–5. More specifically, this change was noted only in the DCN regions that represent high frequency sounds. Moreover, the fusiform neurons in this DCN area had a decrease in KCNQ2/3 currents, consistent with the tinnitus-specific hyperactivity also observed in previous studies [20, 21].

These previous experiments utilizing animal models of tinnitus demonstrated that not all animals that are exposed to noise develop tinnitus. This question of why some mice are seemingly resilient to tinnitus was examined at the cellular level to see if there were any elements of homeostatic plasticity at play. Using the gap-startle animal model in mice to behaviorally sort animals based on whether they have tinnitus or not, they found that KNCQ2/3 displayed a bidirectional plasticity that determined whether mice were vulnerable or resilient to tinnitus [22]. In the mice vulnerable to tinnitus, the KCNQ2/3 channels underwent a leftward shift in their voltage of half-activation, thus less channels were available for activation, leading to the increased hyperexcitability or spontaneous firing rates noted in the fusiform cells of the DCNs in tinnitus animals [20, 22]. On the other hand, a recovery of the KCNC2/3 channels underlies the development of resilience to tinnitus [22]. Accordingly, the administration of retigabine, the pan-KCNQ2–5 activator, 4 days after noxious noise exposure, significantly reduced the portion of mice that developed tinnitus [22].

Interestingly, other currents also contribute to the homeostatic plasticity that provides tinnitus resilience. The fusiform neurons in the DCN nucleus of non-tinnitus mice were found to be biophysically distinct with reduced resting membrane potentials [22]. This was found to be due to a reduction in the hyperpolarization-activated cationic nucleotide-gated channels (HCN). More importantly, this HCN plasticity was found to temporally occur following KCNQ plasticity as demonstrated by the recovery of the channels. Additionally, with the intraperitoneal injection of retigabine to mice, these mice not only demonstrated an increased resilience to tinnitus and decreased hyperexcitability in their fusiform cells, but their fusiform cells also demonstrated decreased HCN currents. Thus, KCNQ plasticity, as demonstrated by KCNQ channel recovery, followed by HCN plasticity, as demonstrated by HCN reduction, are key determinants in driving the tinnitus resilience pathway.

Given that the modulation of KCNQ2/3 channels presents a key intervention point for eliciting resilience to tinnitus, a few studies have examined the suitability of KCNQ activators for clinical use, starting with preclinical studies. While the pan-KCNQ activator, retigabine, demonstrated therapeutic promise in behavioral studies by significantly reducing the number of mice that develop tinnitus in an animal model [22], its clinical use is not feasible. Following FDA approval for the treatment of partial seizures, retigabine was withdrawn from the market in 2017 due to severe side effects, including urinary retention, blue skin discoloration, and retinal dyspigmentation [23]. These side effects stemmed from a combination of two factors: i) poor selectivity of retigabine among KCNQ2–5 channels, and ii) binding of retigabine metabolites and their dimerization in melanin-containing layers which resulted in dyspigmentation [24, 25]. As a result, derivatives from retigabine have been chemically synthesized over the years, with the goal of arriving at therapeutically feasible compounds that can be funneled through preclinical development for eventual clinical use and cure of tinnitus. The most promising of these therapeutics is RL-81 from the second generation of KCNQ activators derived from retigabine [23, 26]. Not only is this the most potent KCNQ2/3 activator till date, but it is also the most specific for KCNQ2/3 over KCNQ4 and KCNQ5 [23, 27]. Lastly, in a modified SBAD operant animal model of tinnitus, a Marinos et al. showed that the administration of RL-81 only a week after noxious noise exposure significantly reduces the percentage of mice with behavioral evidence of tinnitus up to 2 weeks following noise exposure [26].

Homeostatic Synaptic Plasticity in the DCN

In addition to homeostatic plasticity, there is surmounting evidence to indicate that a combination of inhibitory and excitatory synaptic changes results in cumulative maladaptive plasticity processes in the DCN. A study examining sound-exposed rats that underwent tinnitus induction using 1 h of 17 kHz octave noise (116 dB SPL) demonstrated that rats with chronic high frequency tinnitus had significant reduction in their glycinergic receptor (GlyR) α_1 protein levels as well as GlyR binding sites [28]. Consistent with this, another study demonstrated that the application of vigabatrin, an inhibitor of GABA transaminase, resulted in a reduction in the number of rats that displayed tinnitus behavior [29]. Together, these data show that the downregulation of inhibitory synaptic transmission through reduction in glycinergic signaling contributes in part to the hyperactivity of DCN fusiform neurons observed in animal models of tinnitus.

Concurrent with changes in inhibitory synaptic plasticity, there is also evidence of changes that occur in glutamatergic synaptic neurotransmission in tinnitus animal models. Taking advantage of retrograde and anterograde transportation to projections of the DCN using labeled fluorescent conjugated dextran amine, following acoustic overexposure of 15 kHZ, 110 dB SPL for 6 h, there was an increased expression of vesicular glutamate transporters (VGLUT-2) in the DCN terminals [30]. Additional evidence of an increase in glutamatergic synaptic neurotransmission was found in animals displaying tinnitus behavior, reflected as an upregulation of VGLUT2 [31]. Moreover, this increase is thought to be due to increased somatosensory inputs and redistribution to the DCN in the weeks following acoustic trauma [32].

Another form of plasticity, spike-timing-dependent plasticity (STDP), contributes to the integration of multisensory input in the DCN. STDP occurs based on the temporal order of pre- and postsynaptic activity, with contributing modulation via NMDA and cholinergic receptors [33]. In normal hearing animals, STDP occurs between the parallel-fiber synapses and fusiform cells of the DCN [33]. When parallel fibers are presynaptically activated before fusiform cells, Hebbian plasticity or long-term potentiation (LTP) occurs [34]. When this order is reversed, long-term depression (LTD) or non-Hebbian plasticity, wherein synaptic strength is weakened, is noted instead [18]. STDP can be induced in DCN fusiform neurons by pairing auditory and transcutaneous stimulation activating the trigeminal and dorsal column afferents [18]. Furthermore, in GPIAS animal models of tinnitus, fusiform neurons displayed altered STDP reflected as increased LTP, while animals that did not develop tinnitus showed increased LTD [34, 35].

Further studies have examined whether STDP can be exploited to reduce tinnitus symptoms or behavior, especially since non-Hebbian plasticity or LTD results in the weakening of synapses.

LTD induction protocols using bimodal stimulation of the auditory and somatosensory pathways were explored as a means of reducing tinnitus behavior. Human GPIAS studies were conducted in which 20 min of auditory-somatosensory LTD bimodal stimulation of the DCN resulted in a reduction in physiological correlates and behavioral evidence of tinnitus [35]. Yet, another study aimed at reversing the tinnitus-induced plasticity utilized the pairing of auditory tones with brief vagal nerve stimulation in rats [36]. The idea is that increasing the number of cortical neurons tuned to another frequency other than the tinnitus frequency will overcome or reduce the overrepresented tinnitus frequency. Their study demonstrated that vagal nerve stimulation paired with multiple tones can reverse the increased cortical synchrony in rats and the number of animals with behavioral evidence of tinnitus [36]. Using bimodal stimulation to reverse or overcome the maladaptive plasticity in tinnitus remains an active area of research, with a recent study even combining bimodal auditory and lingual stimulation in human tinnitus patients over a 12-week period, which showed significant reduction in tinnitus symptoms, up to 1 year following treatment [37].

Inferior Colliculus (IC)

The inferior colliculus (IC) is a major nucleus structure in the afferent central auditory pathways, located in the posterior midbrain where all the ascending fibers from the lower brainstem auditory pathway converge. Here, there is a well-organized tonotopic organization with low to high frequencies represented from the dorsolateral to ventromedial location, ranging from sharpness to broad and multipeaks represented. This is the first location with the set of neurons that not only encode intensity, but also sound duration, and thus can sense gap detection in sound. Hence, the IC is thought to be a reasonable temporal processor of sound, although its phase locking is not as good as the neurons in the brainstem which are part of the lower levels in the central auditory pathway. Additionally, the IC contains different set of neurons that respond to either contralateral, ipsilateral, or binaural auditory inputs, thus demonstrating its role in both sound localization and lateralization.

Unlike the DCN, there is a lack of consensus on the pathological changes in the IC following tinnitus. While some studies demonstrated an increase in spontaneous firing in the IC, similar to the DCN in tinnitus mice [38, 39], other studies demonstrate this activity following noise exposure regardless of tinnitus behavior [40, 41]. Even more dissonant are the studies that show no change in spontaneous firing rate at all in the IC following noise exposure in rats screened for tinnitus using GPIAS [42]. Concern with regards to the inconsistencies stem from the variability in experimental design, induction protocols, animal models, and species widely used across these studies [33]. Another idea for this variability could be that there likely exists a microcircuit heterogeneity in the IC that remains unexplored [33]. As such subpopulation(s) within the IC may actually encode for tinnitus, and by studying a random sampling across various experiments, it is difficult to arrive at a unanimous conclusion on the plastic changes in the IC following tinnitus induction [33].

Among the studies that demonstrate IC hyperactivity following acoustic trauma, there is electrophysiological and molecular evidence. Increased activity in the IC is thought to depend on the activity in the DCN; however, studies have differed on this as one study showed abolishment of increased activity in IC following DCN ablation and another showed the opposite [43]. And yet, another study showed that IC is unlikely to maintain increased hyperactivity in the setting of cochlear ablation, within a window of up to 6 weeks [44]. Moreover, another study showed a marked reduction in IC hyperactivity in the setting of DCN ablation [45]. The findings from this study are consistent with studies that show loss of glycinergic inhibition within the DCN and reduction in evoked release of radioactively labelled glycine from the DCN following cochlear ablation [21, 46]. Consistent with these findings, another study showed decreased levels of glutamic acid decarboxylase (GAD) in synaptic clefts and γ-aminobutyric acid (GABA) release from the IC [43]. Altogether, the studies showing the persistence of tonotopic mapping and consistency of timing in the IC mirror the DCN following acoustic damage [43] likely point to the fact that tinnitus-related changes in the DCN are transmitted to the IC and beyond.

Thalamus

The medial geniculate body (MGB), located in the thalamus, is the next major component of the ascending central auditory pathway. The neurons in this region are not only highly variable anatomically, but also functionally. There are *on* neurons, which respond at the beginning of a short and quick stimulus, *off* neurons which respond when a stimulus is shut off, *sustained* neurons which are on for the duration of an input, the *late* neurons which are delayed to onset of the input, and lastly the *suppressive* neurons, which function as inhibitory neurons. The MCB is like the IC in terms of coding intensity and lateralization and localization of sound; however, it appears that these functions are more defined in the ventral portion of the MBG as compared to the dorsal or medial portion. The major output of the MBG is to the auditory cortex [47], with the medial portion receiving a lot of somatosensory input and sending projections to the ventral striatum and the amygdala [48, 49]. The thalamus being a key target of cortical modulation, in addition to its projection pathways vital for cognitive and emotional processing relevant to tinnitus, makes it an important integrative center in the pathophysiology of the disease.

Thalamic neurons are heavily modulated by inhibitory neurotransmission, which is essential for integrating incoming and outgoing neural stimuli, frequency tuning, and processing temporal information while gating information transmission to the auditory cortex. Single-unit recordings from the MGB in awake rats displaying tinnitus behavior were found to display increased spontaneous and burst firing when exposed to broadband noise and tones at the unit's characteristic frequency [50]. Further work has shown that the activation of extrasynaptic $GABA_A$ receptors [51] changes thalamic firing from tonic to burst firing mode. This change in firing activity results in a change in physiologic function that has been implicated in tinnitus. The thalamocortical dysrhythmia model is a proposed hypothesis thought to underlie tinnitus and chronic pain. In the case of tinnitus, increased inhibition acting via extrasynaptic $GABA_AR$ leads to a deactivation of T-type calcium channels which underlies a switch to burst firing in thalamic neurons and resultant low frequency oscillations in the delta or theta range [52–54]. These slow oscillations then reach the cortex and lead to gamma oscillations in the auditory cortex [53]. The gamma cortical oscillations are believed to correlate with the precept of tinnitus. In vitro animal experiments aimed at testing the thalamocortical dysrhythmia model found that stimulating extrasynaptic $GABA_AR$ in sound-exposed rats that displayed tinnitus behavior showed an increase in burst firing and $GABA_AR$ currents up to 3 months after a tinnitus-induced acoustic event [55].

Overall, while the thalamocortical dysrhythmia model is a favored model for explaining the tinnitus precept, the underlying mechanisms that lead to T-type calcium channel deactivation and hyperpolarization remain to be unanswered.

Auditory Cortex

The highest order auditory neurons are in the auditory cortex and subcortex. The auditory cortex, like the rest of the brain cortices, is comprised of six layers with distinct cell types labelled I–VI. Tonotopic organization of the primary auditory cortex shows that frequencies, low to high, are represented from rostro lateral to the caudomedial locations. The auditory cortex is involved in speech perception. Furthermore, ablation studies have given more insight into its overall role in auditory processing, as such animals have difficulty with pattern perception and temporal discrimination.

One of the best ways to examine the properties of the auditory cortex in tinnitus is via simultaneously recording from many neurons both before and after acoustic trauma. Over the years, both in vivo recordings from awake animals and imaging techniques like magnetoencephalography (MEG) and functional magnetic resonance imaging (fMRI) have been used to study tinnitus. Studies investigating the neurophysiological underpinnings of tinnitus in the auditory cortices have demonstrated the emergence and duration of both spontaneous and burst activity in the auditory cortex. Both types of firing activity were found to emerge over chronic time periods rather than acute time periods, with the frequency of burst activity significantly increased [56]. More importantly, the significance of this burst activity is related to increased synaptic reliability and thus synaptic plasticity [8, 57]. It is thought that a shift towards overrepresentation is noted in the preferred tuning frequencies of neurons in the hearing loss region in the auditory cortex, after noise overexposure. This resulted in these frequencies having an overrepresentation in the cortical tonotopic map [58, 59].

Neural synchrony is another major change noted to occur in the auditory cortex of animals with tinnitus following acoustic trauma. Multielectrode array recordings in anesthetized cats that had been exposed to noxious acoustic sound levels (5–6 kHz at 1225–120 dB SPL for 1 h) showed a shift in tuning curves to lower characteristic frequencies and a time-dependent increase in spontaneous firing rates in the auditory cortex [60]. Moreover, neural synchrony was also immediately observed following acoustic trauma, which aligns with the timeline of tinnitus immediately developing following noxious noise exposure, thus neural synchrony is thought to be a neural correlative for tinnitus [60, 61]. Consistent with this, following noise exposure (narrow-band, 12 kHz, 120 dB SPL, 1 h) in rats, there was an increase in local field potentials (LFP) and gap-startle reaction in awake rats [62].

In addition to observing acute changes in the auditory cortex in response to acoustic trauma, a few studies have also examined chronic changes in response to acoustic trauma. Cats were exposed for 2–4 h at ~120 dB SPL, 5 kHz and recorded from 7 to 16 weeks later [63, 64]. There was evident reorganization of tonotopic maps in the auditory cortex, and the spontaneous firing rates were higher in the reorganized areas, thought to be due to disinhibition in the tinnitus region. Moreover, there was also increased interneural synchrony that is thought to be due to chronic tinnitus reflected as high-frequency hearing loss due to noxious acoustic sounds.

MEG studies in human subjects with tinnitus demonstrated decreased alpha-band power with an increase in delta-band power as compared to controls [65]. This decrease is thought to be related to the tinnitus percept itself [66]. Additionally, gamma oscillations in tinnitus were also observed in patients with tinnitus [67]. Moreover, lateralization of gamma waves correlated with lateralization of perceived tinnitus [66].

Nonauditory Nuclei and Tinnitus

Interestingly, aside from the structures involved in the auditory pathway, nonauditory inputs are thought to be important following tinnitus induction. Evidence for this idea stems from previous work that showed modulation of the perception of tinnitus loudness from thalamic stimulation, abnormal activity in the somatosensory system, and contraction of head and neck musculature [68–70]. More recent studies in human utilizing neuroimaging and neural connectivity studies have demonstrated tinnitus-induced functional changes in the prefrontal, parietal and cingulate cortices, the limbic system, thalamus, and cerebellum [16], thus shedding light on the involvement of nonauditory structures in the maintenance of tinnitus. More importantly, the central gain enhancement has been noted in limbic areas such as the amygdala, adding to the observation that many patients with tinnitus report negative emotions including anxiety, depression, and sleep aberrations [71].

A functional magnetic resonance imaging (fMRI) study examining connectivity in tinnitus vs. non-tinnitus patients demonstrated distinct connectivity patterns with the auditory cortex-insula network present in tinnitus patients [72]. Additionally, increased functional connectivity was observed between the auditory cortex and the parahippocampal region. A noted increase of connectivity was also observed in nonauditory regions such as the brainstem, basal ganglia, nucleus accumbens, and cerebellum. As such, not only did this study imply a role for nonauditory regions in the pathophysiology of tinnitus, but also denotes a shift in these areas that normally function for attention, memory, and emotion, all areas that are related to the distress associated with chronic tinnitus.

Amygdala

Emotional salient information is processed in the amygdala and has been implicated in tinnitus. The lateral (LA) portion of the amygdala is most important for processing sound as it received input from a myriad of sensory systems including directly from the MGN and other secondary auditory association areas [71]. Both molecular and electrophysiological studies have provided evidence for the role of the amygdala in tinnitus. Following a 10 kHz noise exposure at 125–127 dB SPL in the left ear for 4 h, there was a noted increase in *c-fos* immunoreactivity in the LA, basolateral (BLA), and central (CeA) portions of the amygdala [73]. *C-fos* is a marker or neuronal activity and is a gene that is transiently activated and translated in response to a range of stimuli, including sensory stimuli, thus playing a role in neuronal plasticity [71]. In a follow-up study, *c-fos* was noted to be upregulated following traumatic noise exposure up to 7 h later, but only in the CeA [74], while another study found higher levels in the LA as compared to the CeA 3 h following traumatic noise exposure including tinnitus [75]. Additionally, multielectrode electrophysiological experiments were conducted in the BLA following a 10 kHz tone at 105 dB SPL for 3 h in both tinnitus and non-tinnitus rats sorted based on the gap startle reflex model [76]. The authors found significantly higher spontaneous firing rates in the BLA in rats with behavioral evidence of tinnitus at up to 6 weeks following noise exposure. They also noted increased neural synchrony in the BLA of tinnitus-behaving rats. Notably, activation using an NMDA partial agonist injected 15 min prior to traumatic sound exposure prevented the prior noted plastic changes in the amygdala, notably the expression of another molecular marker, Arc [77]. Lastly, fMRI studies involving the amygdala show that brain regions that connected the amygdala contribute the most to noted differences between tinnitus and control patients [78]. In another fMRI study, brain activation induced by emotional sounds has been investigated. In this study, patients with tinnitus showed a reduced amygdala activation as compared to healthy controls [79]. A similar finding of reduced amygdala activation in tinnitus patients was obtained in another fMRI study, in which the neural responses to emotionally expressive and neutral faces were investigated [80].

Hippocampus

The hippocampus has been well established as the brain region for learning and memory formation including spatial memory. Recent studies have established that hearing loss affects not only synaptic integrity, but also noxious sound exposure decreased hippocampal neurogenesis [71]. Moreover, the hippocampus receives both direct and indirect inputs from various auditory association cortices and the auditory cortex to help in the formation of long-term auditory memories. Evidence of the involvement of the hippocampus in tinnitus stems from a combination of behavioral, molecular, and electrophysiology experiments. Acoustic noise exposure of 4 kHz at 104 dB SPL for 30 mins to freely moving rats demonstrated a change in both the firing properties and place field positions [81], which persisted for 24 h following acoustic trauma. As such, this study provided evidence for the rapid induction of plastic changes following noxious noise exposure that leads to chronic changes in the hippocampus. Additionally, the effect of acoustic trauma on hippocampal neurogenesis was also investigated. Following exposure to a 12 kHz tone at 125 dB SPL for 2 h in a rat model of tinnitus, doublecortin, a microtubule-associated protein expressed in neuronal precursor cells and a marker of neurogenesis, was found to be downregulated in rats that displayed tinnitus behavior [82]. Additionally, evidence from in vitro experiments demonstrated an increase in the firing of the CA1 pyramidal neurons, as well as a decrease in long-term potentiation following acoustic trauma reflected as an increase in post-burst hyperpolarization due to a decrease in the hyperpolarization-activated cationic nucleotide-gated current (H-current) [83]. Moreover, at the synaptic level, there is an increase in inhibitory GABAergic transmission within the CA1 following noxious sound exposure [84].

Cingulate Cortex

Cingulate cortex is another limbic structure; however, it has been the least characterized with regard to its role in inducing the maladaptive plasticity noted in tinnitus [71]. A molecular study examining molecular makers following bilateral acoustic trauma of 132–142 dB SPL demonstrated that 1 h following noise trauma, there was a significant decrease in *c-fos* in the anterior cingulate cortex (ACC) [74]. There is recent evidence from human EEG studies to indicate that the functional connectivity within the cingulate cortex is changed as reflected in their alpha and beta frequency bands in response to the distress state in a tinnitus patient [85]. This study implicates the cingulate cortex as being part of the processing of tinnitus-related distress. Another study examined the age of onset of tinnitus-related distress neural substrates, examining the cingulate cortex and parahippocampus, and found that the cingulate cortex was more activated in late-onset tinnitus patients as compared to early-onset tinnitus, as reflected in their beta and gamma frequency bands [86]. There remains a large gap to be filled in specifying the exact role that the cingulate cortex plays in maintaining the maladaptive plasticity of tinnitus.

Future Perspectives

Much remains to be uncovered with regard to the mechanism of action and pathophysiology of tinnitus. While studies on the neurobiology of tinnitus have highlighted the site of initiation of tinnitus as well as the neuroplastic changes that follow to maintain tinnitus, much is yet to be uncovered on how these changes become distributed from auditory brain regions to nonauditory areas. More studies are needed on the early circuitry neuronal changes that initiate tinnitus and the changes that result in the tinnitus precept. Perhaps, real-time in vivo experiments that enable wide field two-photon calcium imaging shortly following acoustic changes in key auditory and nonauditory nuclei can provide insight into the critical window for such changes before the precept is developed.

The origin of the tinnitus precept remains unknown. What is clear is that there are insufficient studies designed to temporally capture the progression of tinnitus circuity changes as they occur and what we have are snapshots instead. Additionally, we lack the tools for simultaneous monitoring brain changes at small enough resolution that can unveil the concurrent neuroplastic changes in response to tinnitus. Even so, the difficulty of translating these animal model findings to human studies remains an obstacle (see Chap. 24).

Within a single brain nucleus, it is also unknown how the surrounding neuronal circuitry is affected by the homeostatic changes that have taken place in the neuronal correlates found to be sensitive due to tinnitus. For example, many studies have focused on the fusiform cells of the DCN demonstrating excitability, with little attention paid on the surrounding cells and nuclei and how the homeostatic changes in the DCN affect vertical transmission and synaptic plasticity of the other cells within the cochlear nucleus, and the role this may play in initiating and maintaining chronic tinnitus.

References

1. Baguley D, McFerran D, Hall D. Tinnitus. Lancet. 2013;382(9904):1600–7.
2. Heller AJ. Classification and epidemiology of tinnitus. Otolaryngol Clin N Am. 2003;36(2):239–48.
3. Understanding the facts [Internet]. 2015 [cited 2020 Oct 1]. https://www.ata.org/understanding-facts.
4. Miller TR, Serulle Y, Gandhi D. Arterial abnormalities leading to tinnitus. Neuroimaging Clin N Am. 2016;26(2):227–36.

5. Holmes S, Padgham ND. Review paper: more than ringing in the ears: a review of tinnitus and its psychosocial impact. J Clin Nurs. 2009;18(21):2927–37.
6. Galazyuk AV, Wenstrup JJ, Hamid MA. Tinnitus and underlying brain mechanisms. Curr Opin Otolaryngol Head Neck Surg. 2012 [cited 2020 Nov 11];20(5). https://www.ncbi.nlm.nih.gov/pmc/articles/PMC3886369/.
7. Musiek FE, Baran JA. The auditory system: anatomy, physiology, and clinical correlates. 2nd ed. San Diego: Plural Publishing; 2018. 513p.
8. Noreña AJ, Farley BJ. Tinnitus-related neural activity: theories of generation, propagation, and centralization. Hear Res. 2013;295:161–71.
9. Ruel J, Chabbert C, Nouvian R, Bendris R, Eybalin M, Leger CL, et al. Salicylate enables cochlear arachidonic-acid-sensitive NMDA receptor responses. J Neurosci. 2008;28(29):7313–23.
10. Fernandez KA, Guo D, Micucci S, De Gruttola V, Liberman MC, Kujawa SG. Noise-induced cochlear synaptopathy with and without sensory cell loss. Neuroscience. 2020;427:43–57.
11. Kujawa SG, Liberman MC. Adding insult to injury: Cochlear nerve degeneration after "temporary" noise-induced hearing loss. J Neurosci. 2009;29(45):14077–85.
12. Saunders JC. The role of central nervous system plasticity in tinnitus. J Commun Disord. 2007;40(4):313–34.
13. Schaette R, McAlpine D. Tinnitus with a normal audiogram: physiological evidence for hidden hearing loss and computational model. J Neurosci. 2011;31(38):13452–7.
14. Kujawa SG, Liberman MC. Synaptopathy in the noise-exposed and aging cochlea: primary neural degeneration in acquired sensorineural hearing loss. Hear Res. 2015;330(Pt B):191–9.
15. Furman AC, Kujawa SG, Liberman MC. Noise-induced cochlear neuropathy is selective for fibers with low spontaneous rates. J Neurophysiol. 2013;110(3):577–86.
16. Shore SE, Roberts LE, Langguth B. Maladaptive plasticity in tinnitus--triggers, mechanisms and treatment. Nat Rev Neurol. 2016;12(3):150–60.
17. Gu JW, Herrmann BS, Levine RA, Melcher JR. Brainstem auditory evoked potentials suggest a role for the ventral Cochlear nucleus in tinnitus. J Assoc Res Otolaryngol. 2012;13(6):819–33.
18. Wu C, Martel DT, Shore SE. Transcutaneous induction of stimulus-timing-dependent plasticity in dorsal cochlear nucleus. Front Syst Neurosci. 2015;9:116.
19. Cai S, Ma W-L, Young ED. Encoding intensity in ventral cochlear nucleus following acoustic trauma: implications for loudness recruitment. SpringerLink. [cited 2020]. https://link.springer.com/article/10.1007/s10162-008-0142-y.
20. Li S, Choi V, Tzounopoulos T. Pathogenic plasticity of Kv7.2/3 channel activity is essential for the induction of tinnitus. Proc Natl Acad Sci. 2013;110(24):9980–5.
21. Brozoski TJ, Bauer CA, Caspary DM. Elevated fusiform cell activity in the dorsal cochlear nucleus of chinchillas with psychophysical evidence of tinnitus. J Neurosci. 2002;22(6):2383–90.
22. Li S, Kalappa BI, Tzounopoulos T. Noise-induced plasticity of KCNQ2/3 and HCN channels underlies vulnerability and resilience to tinnitus. Elife. 2015;4:e07242.
23. Kumar M, Reed N, Liu R, Aizenman E, Wipf P, Tzounopoulos T. Synthesis and evaluation of potent KCNQ2/3-specific channel activators. Mol Pharmacol. 2016;89(6):667–77.
24. Groseclose MR, Castellino S. An investigation into Retigabine (Ezogabine) associated dyspigmentation in rat eyes by MALDI imaging mass spectrometry. Chem Res Toxicol. 2019;32(2):294–303.
25. Eskioglou E, Perrenoud MP, Ryvlin P, Novy J. Novel treatment and new drugs in epilepsy treatment. Curr Pharm Des. 2017;23(42):6389–98.
26. Marinos L, Kouvaros S, Bizup B, Hambach B, Wipf P, Tzounopoulos T. Transient delivery of a KCNQ2/3-specific channel activator 1 week after noise trauma mitigates noise-induced tinnitus. J Assoc Res Otolaryngol. 2021;22(2):127–39.
27. Liu R, Tzounopoulos T, Wipf P. Synthesis and optimization of Kv7 (KCNQ) potassium channel agonists: the role of fluorines in potency and selectivity. ACS Med Chem Lett. 2019;10(6):929–35.
28. Wang H, Brozoski TJ, Turner JG, Ling L, Parrish JL, Hughes LF, et al. Plasticity at glycinergic synapses in dorsal cochlear nucleus of rats with behavioral evidence of tinnitus. Neuroscience. 2009;164(2):747–59.
29. Yang S, Weiner BD, Zhang LS, Cho S-J, Bao S. Homeostatic plasticity drives tinnitus perception in an animal model. Proc Natl Acad Sci U S A. 2011;108(36):14974–9.
30. Barker M, Solinski HJ, Hashimoto H, Tagoe T, Pilati N, Hamann M. Acoustic overexposure increases the expression of VGLUT-2 mediated projections from the lateral vestibular nucleus to the dorsal Cochlear nucleus. PLoS One. 2012;7(5):e35955.
31. Heeringa AN, Wu C, Chung C, West M, Martel D, Liberman L, et al. Glutamatergic projections to the cochlear nucleus are redistributed in tinnitus. Neuroscience. 2018;391:91–103.
32. Zeng C, Yang Z, Shreve L, Bledsoe S, Shore S. Somatosensory projections to cochlear nucleus are upregulated after unilateral deafness. J Neurosci. 2012;32(45):15791–801.
33. Shore SE, Wu C. Mechanisms of noise-induced tinnitus: insights from cellular studies. Neuron. 2019;103(1):8–20.
34. Koehler SD, Shore SE. Stimulus timing-dependent plasticity in dorsal cochlear nucleus is altered in tinnitus. J Neurosci. 2013;33(50):19647–56.
35. Marks KL, Martel DT, Wu C, Basura GJ, Roberts LE, Schvartz-Leyzac KC, et al. Auditory-somatosensory bimodal stimulation desynchronizes brain circuitry to reduce tinnitus in guinea pigs and humans. Sci Transl Med. 2018 [cited 2021 Mar 29];10(422). https://stm.sciencemag.org/content/10/422/eaal3175.
36. Engineer ND, Riley JR, Seale JD, Vrana WA, Shetake JA, Sudanagunta SP, et al. Reversing pathological neural activity using targeted plasticity. Nature. 2011;470(7332):101–4.
37. Conlon B, Langguth B, Hamilton C, Hughes S, Meade E, Connor CO, et al. Bimodal neuromodulation combining sound and tongue stimulation reduces tinnitus symptoms in a large randomized clinical study. Sci Transl Med. 2020;12(564):eabb2830.
38. Bauer CA, Turner JG, Caspary DM, Myers KS, Brozoski TJ. Tinnitus and inferior colliculus activity in chinchillas related to three distinct patterns of cochlear trauma. J Neurosci Res. 2008;86(11):2564–78.
39. Longenecker RJ, Galazyuk AV. Development of tinnitus in CBA/CaJ mice following sound exposure. J Assoc Res Otolaryngol. 2011;12(5):647.
40. Berger JI, Coomber B, Wells TT, Wallace MN, Palmer AR. Changes in the response properties of inferior colliculus neurons relating to tinnitus. Front Neurol. 2014;5:203.
41. Longenecker RJ, Galazyuk AV. Variable effects of acoustic trauma on behavioral and neural correlates of tinnitus in individual animals. Front Behav Neurosci. 2016 [cited 2020 Sep 25];10. https://www.frontiersin.org/articles/10.3389/fnbeh.2016.00207/full.
42. Ropp T-JF, Tiedemann KL, Young ED, May BJ. Effects of unilateral acoustic trauma on tinnitus-related spontaneous activity in the inferior colliculus. J Assoc Res Otolaryngol. 2014;15(6):1007–22.

43. Berger JI, Coomber B. Tinnitus-related changes in the inferior colliculus. Front Neurol. 2015 [cited 2020 Nov 13];6. https://www.frontiersin.org/articles/10.3389/fneur.2015.00061/full.
44. Mulders WHAM, Ding D, Salvi R, Robertson D. Relationship between auditory thresholds, central spontaneous activity, and hair cell loss after acoustic trauma. J Comp Neurol. 2011;519(13):2637–47.
45. Manzoor NF, Licari FG, Klapchar M, Elkin RL, Gao Y, Chen G, et al. Noise-induced hyperactivity in the inferior colliculus: its relationship with hyperactivity in the dorsal cochlear nucleus. J Neurophysiol. 2012;108(4):976–88.
46. Potashner SJ, Suneja SK, Benson CG. Altered glycinergic synaptic activities in Guinea pig brain stem auditory nuclei after unilateral cochlear ablation. Hear Res. 2000;147(1–2):125–36.
47. Aitkin LM, Webster WR. Medial geniculate body of the cat: organization and responses to tonal stimuli of neurons in ventral division. J Neurophysiol. 1972;35(3):365–80.
48. Bordi F, LeDoux JE. Response properties of single units in areas of rat auditory thalamus that project to the amygdala. II. Cells receiving convergent auditory and somatosensory inputs and cells antidromically activated by amygdala stimulation. Exp Brain Res. 1994;98(2):275–86.
49. Bordi F, LeDoux JE. Response properties of single units in areas of rat auditory thalamus that project to the amygdala. I. Acoustic discharge patterns and frequency receptive fields. Exp Brain Res. 1994;98(2):261–74.
50. Kalappa BI, Brozoski TJ, Turner JG, Caspary DM. Single unit hyperactivity and bursting in the auditory thalamus of awake rats directly correlates with behavioural evidence of tinnitus. J Physiol. 2014;592(Pt 22):5065–78.
51. Cope DW, Hughes SW, Crunelli V. GABAA receptor-mediated tonic inhibition in thalamic neurons. J Neurosci. 2005;25(50):11553–63.
52. Llinás R, Urbano FJ, Leznik E, Ramírez RR, van Marle HJF. Rhythmic and dysrhythmic thalamocortical dynamics: GABA systems and the edge effect. Trends Neurosci. 2005;28(6):325–33.
53. Llinás RR, Ribary U, Jeanmonod D, Kronberg E, Mitra PP. Thalamocortical dysrhythmia: a neurological and neuropsychiatric syndrome characterized by magnetoencephalography. Proc Natl Acad Sci U S A. 1999;96(26):15222–7.
54. Llinás RR, Steriade M. Bursting of thalamic neurons and states of vigilance. J Neurophysiol. 2006;95(6):3297–308.
55. Sametsky EA, Turner JG, Larsen D, Ling L, Caspary DM. Enhanced GABAA-mediated tonic inhibition in auditory thalamus of rats with behavioral evidence of tinnitus. J Neurosci. 2015;35(25):9369–80.
56. Roberts LE. Neural plasticity and its initiating conditions in tinnitus. HNO. 2018;66(3):172–8.
57. Luo H, Pace E, Zhang J. Blast-induced tinnitus and hyperactivity in the auditory cortex of rats. Neuroscience. 2017;340:515–20.
58. Noreña AJ, Tomita M, Eggermont JJ. Neural changes in cat auditory cortex after a transient pure-tone trauma. J Neurophysiol. 2003;90(4):2387–401.
59. Robertson D, Irvine DRF. Plasticity of frequency organization in auditory cortex of Guinea pigs with partial unilateral deafness. J Comp Neurol. 1989;282(3):456–71.
60. Noreña AJ, Eggermont JJ. Changes in spontaneous neural activity immediately after an acoustic trauma: implications for neural correlates of tinnitus. Hear Res. 2003;183(1–2):137–53.
61. Pienkowski M, Eggermont JJ. Long-term, partially-reversible reorganization of frequency tuning in mature cat primary auditory cortex can be induced by passive exposure to moderate-level sounds. Hear Res. 2009;257(1–2):24–40.
62. Sun W, Deng A, Jayaram A, Gibson B. Noise exposure enhances auditory cortex responses related to hyperacusis behavior. Brain Res. 2012;1485:108–16.
63. Noreña AJ, Eggermont JJ. Enriched acoustic environment after noise trauma reduces hearing loss and prevents cortical map reorganization. J Neurosci. 2005;25(3):699–705.
64. Noreña AJ, Eggermont JJ. Enriched acoustic environment after noise trauma abolishes neural signs of tinnitus. Neuroreport. 2006;17(6):559–63.
65. Adjamian P, Sereda M, Zobay O, Hall DA, Palmer AR. Neuromagnetic indicators of tinnitus and tinnitus masking in patients with and without hearing loss. J Assoc Res Otolaryngol. 2012;13(5):715–31.
66. Weisz N, Moratti S, Meinzer M, Dohrmann K, Elbert T. Tinnitus perception and distress is related to abnormal spontaneous brain activity as measured by magnetoencephalography. PLoS Med. 2005;2(6):e153.
67. Weisz N, Müller S, Schlee W, Dohrmann K, Hartmann T, Elbert T. The neural code of auditory phantom perception. J Neurosci. 2007;27(6):1479–84.
68. Shi Y, Burchiel KJ, Anderson VC, Martin WH. Deep brain stimulation effects in patients with tinnitus: otolaryngol neck surg [Internet]. 2009 [cited 2020 Nov 18]. https://journals.sagepub.com/doi/10.1016/j.otohns.2009.05.020?url_ver=Z39.88-2003&rfr_id=ori%3Arid%3Acrossref.org&rfr_dat=cr_pub++0pubmed.
69. Møller AR, Møller MB, Yokota M. Some forms of tinnitus may involve the extralemniscal auditory pathway. Laryngoscope. 1992;102(10):1165–71.
70. Levine RA. Somatic (craniocervical) tinnitus and the dorsal cochlear nucleus hypothesis. Am J Otolaryngol. 1999;20(6):351–62.
71. Kapolowicz MR, Thompson LT. Plasticity in limbic regions at early time points in experimental models of tinnitus. Front Syst Neurosci. 2020 [cited 2021 Mar 14];13. https://www.frontiersin.org/articles/10.3389/fnsys.2019.00088/full.
72. Maudoux A, Lefebvre P, Cabay J-E, Demertzi A, Vanhaudenhuyse A, Laureys S, et al. Connectivity graph analysis of the auditory resting state network in tinnitus. Brain Res. 2012;1485:10–21.
73. Zhang JS, Kaltenbach JA, Wang J, Kim SA. Fos-like immunoreactivity in auditory and nonauditory brain structures of hamsters previously exposed to intense sound. Exp Brain Res. 2003;153(4):655–60.
74. Wallhäusser-Franke E, Mahlke C, Oliva R, Braun S, Wenz G, Langner G. Expression of c-fos in auditory and non-auditory brain regions of the gerbil after manipulations that induce tinnitus. Exp Brain Res. 2003;153(4):649–54.
75. Mahlke C, Wallhäusser-Franke E. Evidence for tinnitus-related plasticity in the auditory and limbic system, demonstrated by arg3.1 and c-fos immunocytochemistry. Hear Res. 2004;195(1–2):17–34.
76. Zhang J, Luo H, Pace E, Li L, Liu B. Psychophysical and neural correlates of noised-induced tinnitus in animals: intra- and inter-auditory and non-auditory brain structure studies. Hear Res. 2016;334:7–19.
77. Kapolowicz MR, Thompson LT. Acute high-intensity noise induces rapid Arc protein expression but fails to rapidly change GAD expression in amygdala and hippocampus of rats: effects of treatment with D-cycloserine. Hear Res. 2016;342:69–79.
78. Zimmerman BJ, Abraham I, Schmidt SA, Baryshnikov Y, Husain FT. Dissociating tinnitus patients from healthy controls using resting-state cyclicity analysis and clustering. Netw Neurosci. 2019;3(1):67–89.
79. Davies JE, Gander PE, Hall DA. Does chronic tinnitus alter the emotional response function of the amygdala?: a sound-evoked fMRI study. Front Aging Neurosci. 2017;9:31.
80. Rosengarth K, Kleinjung T, Langguth B, Landgrebe M, Lohaus F, Greenlee MW, et al. Chapter 9 - Altered brain responses to emotional facial expressions in tinnitus patients. In: Langguth B, Kleinjung T, De Ridder D, Schlee W, Vanneste S, editors. Progress

in brain research. Amsterdam: Elsevier; 2021 [cited 2022 Mar 27]. p. 189–207. (Tinnitus - An Interdisciplinary Approach Towards Individualized Treatment: Towards understanding the complexity of tinnitus; vol. 262). https://www.sciencedirect.com/science/article/pii/S0079612321000261.

81. Goble TJ, Møller AR, Thompson LT. Acute high-intensity sound exposure alters responses of place cells in hippocampus. Hear Res. 2009;253(1–2):52–9.
82. Kraus KS, Mitra S, Jimenez Z, Hinduja S, Ding D, Jiang H, et al. Noise trauma impairs neurogenesis in the rat hippocampus. Neuroscience. 2010;167(4):1216–26.
83. Cunha AOS, de Oliveira JAC, Almeida SS, Garcia-Cairasco N, Leão RM. Inhibition of long-term potentiation in the schaffer-CA1 pathway by repetitive high-intensity sound stimulation. Neuroscience. 2015 Dec;3(310):114–27.
84. Cunha AOS, de Deus JL, Ceballos CC, Leão RM. Increased hippocampal GABAergic inhibition after long-term high-intensity sound exposure. PLoS One. 2019;14(5):e0210451.
85. Vanneste S, De Ridder D. Stress-related functional connectivity changes between auditory cortex and cingulate in tinnitus. Brain Connect. 2015;5(6):371–83.
86. Song J-J, Vanneste S, Schlee W, Van de Heyning P, De Ridder D. Onset-related differences in neural substrates of tinnitus-related distress: the anterior cingulate cortex in late-onset tinnitus, and the frontal cortex in early-onset tinnitus. Brain Struct Funct. 2015;220(1):571–84.

Tinnitus and the Somatosensory System

12

Aage R. Møller and Dirk De Ridder

Abstract

Auditory-somatosensory interactions are characteristic of brain functioning and important for multisensory integration, speech, and suppression of self-generated sounds.

The auditory system is a distributed network of the lemniscal pathway and the extralemniscal pathway. The extralemniscal pathway connects to other sensory systems, as well as the limbic system. Under deafferentation, the extralemniscal system compensates for a degeneration of the lemniscal pathway. Consequently, the auditory system starts 'listening' to somatosensory system input, which may generate somatic (=somatosensory) tinnitus, in which changes in the somatosensory system influence tinnitus. This may also be reflected by the fact that tinnitus is associated with different forms of pain.

The mechanism has been partially elucidated and involves connections between the somatosensory and auditory system at all levels of the ascending pathways.

These connections can therapeutically be targeted by physical therapy, botulinum toxin injections, electrical somatosensory stimulation, and bimodal stimulation.

Aage R. Møller has died before the publication of this book.

A. R. Møller (Deceased)
Neuroscience Program, School of Brain & Behavioral Sciences, University of Texas, Richardson, TX, USA

D. De Ridder (✉)
Section of Neurosurgery, Department of Surgical Sciences, University of Otago, Dunedin, New Zealand
e-mail: Dirk.deridder@otago.ac.nz

Highlights

- Auditory-somatosensory interactions are common, a physiological part of multisensory integration.
- Auditory system is distributed and consists of lemniscal and extralemniscal systems.
- Lemniscal system processes auditory discriminatory components.
- Extralemniscal system connects to other senses and limbic system.
- Upon auditory deafferentation, the lemniscal system degenerates and extralemniscal compensates.
- Upon auditory deafferentation, the auditory system starts 'listening' to somatosensory (and visual) input.
- This cross-modal activation can result into somatic (=somatosensory) tinnitus.
- Somatic tinnitus comes in two forms, non-pulsatile and pulsatile.
- Somatic tinnitus may be treated by physical therapy, botulinum toxin injections, somatosensory stimulation, or bimodal stimulation.

Introduction

Formerly, it was regarded as an axiom that the information from the different sense organs was processed in specific and separate parts of the brain [1, 2]. This modular concept has gradually been eroded, and it has become evident that there is considerable interaction between systems that once were regarded as separate [1, 3]. As such, the brain can be regarded as a hierarchical modular network [4–6], in which topographic sensory maps are embedded within higher order non-topographic networks that process the sensory or memory-related information in social, cognitive, and emotional ways [7].

This fits with the concept of the brain as a complex adaptive system [8–10], in which nonlinear dynamics rule, and

W. Schlee et al. (eds.), *Textbook of Tinnitus*, https://doi.org/10.1007/978-3-031-35647-6_12

that can be studied by network science. The nervous system is highly adaptive, with reorganization of synaptic connections and strength in response to changes in afferent drive [11–13]. The dynamic changes of connections in the brain reflect the brain's response to changes in the environment, i.e., they are adaptive, yet may sometimes be maladaptive [14, 15].

It has been proposed that many brain disorders are connectivity disorders [9, 16], also known as dysconnectivity [17, 18] or dysconnection [19] disorders. In other words, many brain disorders are the consequence of altered connections within or between brain networks or brain circuits (= circuitopathy) [20], rather than mere activity problems, in which hypo- or hyperactivity of a hub in the brain is the main culprit of the brain disorder [21]. But ultimately, brain disorders might result from a combination of abnormal activity and connectivity [22], rather than a pure activity disorder [21].

Whereas initially tinnitus was regarded as the consequence of hyperactivity in the auditory cortex, as evidenced by fMRI [23], PET scan [24, 25], EEG [26], and MEG [27], it is now widely accepted that it is an emergent property of dynamically changing, overlapping, auditory, and non-auditory networks in the brain [28–56].

Some individuals with tinnitus [57] have signs of abnormal activation of the subcortical connections to the amygdala through the non-classical pathways (formerly named the extralemniscal pathways), which could result in associating the tinnitus sound to emotional responses. Thus, the non-classical pathway may link the auditory lateral, sound discriminating pathway, to the medial, suffering pathway [31], analogous to what has been described for pain [7]. This is in keeping with a new definition of tinnitus [58]. The proposed definition is: "Tinnitus is the conscious awareness of a tonal or composite noise for which there is no identifiable corresponding external acoustic source", which becomes Tinnitus Disorder "when associated with emotional distress, cognitive dysfunction, and/or autonomic arousal, leading to behavioral changes and functional disability." In other words, "Tinnitus" describes the auditory or sensory component, whereas "Tinnitus Disorder" reflects the auditory component and the associated suffering with or without disability.

It has been proposed that when functional connections develop between tinnitus sound processing pathways and pathways involved in suffering, that tinnitus evolves in tinnitus disorder [31].

Physiological Interaction Between the Auditory and the Somatosensory System

Athletes, musicians, and dancers combine visual, auditory, and somatosensory information to coordinate their movements [59]. Yet, somatosensory signals can interfere with hearing through the rich connections between different systems in the brain, and that is facilitated when the non-classical auditory pathways are active, such as in some individuals with tinnitus [60]. These interactions also exist between the auditory and the visual system, evident in, for example, lip-reading, the McGurk effect, and ventriloquism. The McGurk illusion occurs when the auditory component of one sound is paired with the visual component of another sound, leading to the perception of a third sound [61, 62].

In the same way somatosensory-auditory interactions can generate the skin parchment illusion [63], in which subjects rub their hands together while the sound of rubbing is recorded. When played back, the subjects report the skin on their hands turning dry as parchment [63]. The somatosensory-auditory interaction may also be involved in suppressing self-generated sounds, e.g., in chewing [64] and in permitting normal speech [65, 66].

Multisensory integration allows for more precise environmental representations than possible with a single sensory system, by enhancing coincident features from each sense [11, 67], in keeping with abductive reasoning, as described by the duck test: "When I see a bird that walks like a duck and swims like a duck and quacks like a duck, I call that bird a duck" [68].

This is in agreement with the recent concept of the organization of the auditory cortex as a distributed system [3, 69].

Cross-modal interaction may occur through activation of the non-classical auditory pathways, aka the extralemniscal system [60], a phylogenetically old, non-topographic multimodal system [70], a second auditory ascending pathway, along the phylogenetically more recent, topographic unimodal lemniscal system [70] (Table 12.1). The lemniscal, or core thalamocortical projection, carries tonotopically organized and auditory-specific information and is the same as the lateral auditory system [31], whereas the extralemniscal thalamocortical pathway forms part of an integrative system that plays an important role in multisensory integration, temporal pattern recognition, and certain forms of learning [107]. The extralemniscal nuclei send and receive feedforward and feedback projections among a wide constellation of midbrain, cortical, and limbic-related sites, i.e., the medial system, which support potential conduits for auditory information flow to higher auditory cortical areas, mediators for transitioning among arousal states, and synchronizers of activity across widely distributed cortical territories [108]. Cross-modal interaction between the somatosensory system and the auditory system may be more prevalent in young children than adults [109].

The multisensory interactions may occur by convergence of somatosensory and auditory pathways on different structures at every level of the ascending auditory pathway: the cochlear nucleus, inferior colliculus, medial geniculate body, and the auditory cortex [11, 110]. Cross-modal compensa-

Table 12.1 Overview of differences between the extralemniscal and lemniscal auditory pathways

Extralemniscal system—non-classical system	Lemniscal system—classical system
Nonspecific system	Specific system
Phylogenetically old [71, 72]	Phylogenetically recent [71, 72]
Unconscious reflexes [73, 74]	Conscious perception [73, 74]
To secondary cortex [75–78]	To primary sensory area [75–78]
Less tonotopic [75, 79–81]	Tonotopic [75, 79–81]
Slow spontaneous firing rate [82, 83]	Higher spontaneous firing rate [84–88]
Variable latency response [80, 89, 90]	Short latency response [80, 89, 90]
Rapid habituation to repetitive stimuli [79, 80, 90]	Slower habituation to repetitive stimuli [79, 80, 90]
Fires predominantly in burst mode [81, 91]	Fires in tonic mode [81, 91]
Stimulus detector [92, 93]	Feature detector [92, 93]
Non-linear [93–95]	Linear [93–95]
Overrides tonic mode [93–95]	Weaker than burst mode [93–95]
Processes changes in auditory environment [93, 96]	Processes the content of change in the auditory environment [93, 96]
Calbindin positive [75, 78, 97]	Parvalbumin positive [75, 78, 97]
Calbindin increases after deafferentation [98–101]	Parvalbumin decreases after deafferentation [102]
Multimodal [79, 103–106]	Unimodal [104]

tion, in which one sensory system replaces another following loss of input, is one facet of multisensory integration [12, 13] that may be of relevance for tinnitus. This may be mediated via the extralemniscal auditory system, as auditory deafferentation results in degeneration of the parvalbumin-rich lemniscal system [102] and an increase of the calbindin rich extralemniscal system [98–101], which is involved in multimodal compensation. This cross-modal compensation has been demonstrated in vitro, in vivo, and from a systems level perspective across all levels of the nervous system [11]. It has been studied intensively at the level of the cortex, in which early studies showed that when one sense is deprived of input, that sensory deprived cortex becomes invaded by input from other senses [12]; in other words, the deprived cortex starts 'listening' to other senses. This cross-modal plasticity also occurs in adults with mild-moderate hearing loss. In these people, activation of auditory cortical regions occurs in response to somatosensory stimulation, in contrast to people with normal hearing [111]. However, the cross-modal plasticity that occurs after loss of sensory input can significantly interfere with recovery from brain damage and mitigation of maladaptive effects is critical to maximizing the potential for recovery [112].

The cochlear nucleus (CN) is the first central nervous system station in the auditory system that integrates multisensory information [11] (Fig. 12.1). It receives input from the auditory nerve, auditory midbrain, auditory cortex, trigeminal and cervical ganglia, spinal trigeminal nucleus, and dorsal column nuclei [110, 113, 114]. Auditory pathways begin in the ventral and dorsal cochlear nucleus (VCN and DCN). The granule cell domain receives the majority of inputs from the somatosensory system. Somatosensory input terminates on the apical dendrites of fusiform cells in the dorsal cochlear nucleus, whereas auditory input terminates on the basal dendrites of the same fusiform cells [115]. Fusiform cells are, therefore, ideally placed for multisensory integration [115].

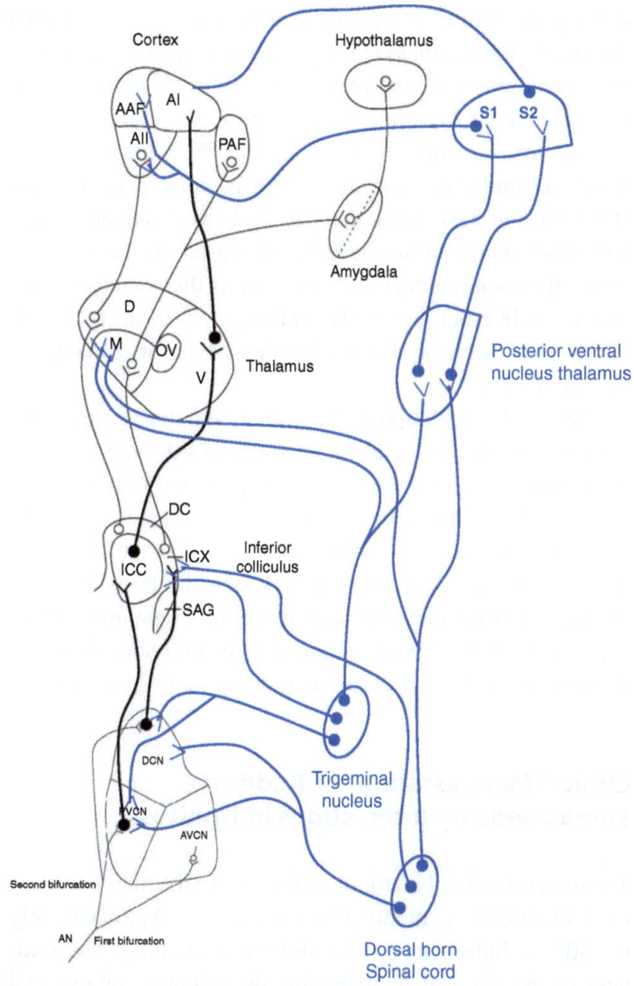

Fig. 12.1 Interactions between auditory (black) and somatosensory (blue) system in tinnitus

Vesicular glutamate transporters (VGLUTS) are transporter proteins that pack glutamate into vesicles prior to synaptic release. In the cochlear nucleus, VGLUT1 is predominantly associated with auditory nerve fiber terminals, whereas VGLUT2 is associated with somatosensory nuclei and their brainstem projections to the cochlear nucleus [116].

Following unilateral deafferentation of the cochlea, ipsilateral VGLUT1 expression in the cochlear nucleus is significantly decreased, and in contrast, ipsilateral VGLUT2 expression is significantly increased [117]. Thus, the somatosensory projections to the cochlear nucleus are upregulated after unilateral deafness [115], and the enhanced glutamatergic somatosensory input in the cochlear nucleus may cause the spontaneous hyperactivity associated with tinnitus [118]. Similar mechanisms are mimicked in the auditory cortex [119]. A similar mechanism is seen in noise overexposure [120]. In summary, noise damage leads to diminished auditory drive, which in turn leads to increased excitatory input from other non-auditory regions such as the somatosensory system, or in other words, the auditory system starts 'listening' to somatosensory input when deprived of its usual auditory input [11].

Electrical stimulation of the skin around the ear can modulate activity in the dorsal cochlear nucleus through both the direct pathways via the trigeminal system and indirect pathways via the dorsal raphe and the locus coeruleus [121, 122]. These findings are signs that the non-classical pathways are involved, as the classical pathways lack the basis for such interaction. It is mainly somatic receptors in the upper body that can modulate activity elicited by sound stimulation in the neurons of the non-classical auditory pathways [123].

Clinical Manifestations of Auditory-Somatosensory Interactions in Tinnitus

The temporomandibular joint and neck are the major sources of somatosensory modulation of tinnitus. Approximately 60–80% of individuals with tinnitus can modulate the loudness or the pitch of their tinnitus by voluntary or external manipulations of the jaw, movements of the eyes, or pressure applied to head and neck regions, including the temporomandibular joint [124–130], indicating a strong relationship between some forms of tinnitus and the somatosensory system [115]. The following findings indicate the presence of somatosensory influence: (1) neck or jaw pain that simultaneously appears with tinnitus, (2) neck/jaw symptoms that are simultaneously aggravated with tinnitus, (3) head or neck trauma preceding tinnitus, (4) varying pitch, loudness, and/or location, and (5) discrepancies in audiogram and unilateral tinnitus [131]. Somatic modulation does not occur in patients after previous noise exposure, and in patients with narrow band noise tinnitus maneuver-induced modulation is more common than in pure-tone tinnitus [127].

The simultaneous onset or increase and decrease of tinnitus with neck or jaw pain and the influence of certain postures are simple questions that most reliably diagnose somatic tinnitus [132].

A rare form of pulsatile tinnitus has been coined somatosensory pulsatile tinnitus syndrome [133, 134], with intermittent or constant heartbeat synchronous subjective tinnitus, but in whom the pulsatile tinnitus can not be objectively detected by the health care provider. In 90% of these patients, the pulsations can be suppressed with head and neck intense muscle contractions [134]. This is also believed to be due to somatosensory-auditory interactions. Three mechanisms have been proposed: (1) somatosensory afferents causing dysfunction of the CNS mechanisms that normally suppress self-generated cardiac and vascular sounds, (2) cardiac synchronous disinhibition of the auditory CNS by somatosensory afferents, and (3) a combination of 1 and 2 [134].

Treatments Based on Auditory-Somatosensory Interactions

1. Physical therapy.

   When treating the TMJ problem in tinnitus patients, 35% of the observed decrease in tinnitus severity can be attributed to a reduction in TMJ pain [135]. Especially younger female patients with a shorter duration of tinnitus and a higher initial score on the TQ somatic subscale have the best prognosis after multimodal orofacial therapy for somatic tinnitus [136].

   Similarly, in patients with cervicogenic somatic tinnitus, cervical physical therapy can have a positive effect on subjective tinnitus [137]. Especially those patients with covarying (increasing or decreasing simultaneously) tinnitus and neck complaints and a combination of low-pitched tinnitus and increasing tinnitus during inadequate cervical spine postures benefit from cervical physical therapy [138].
2. Botulinum toxin injections.

   Botox injections are routinely used for objective tinnitus in palatal myoclonus [139]. Botox is also given in the C2 and trigeminal dermatomas, as standard of practice for migraine, with or without comorbid depression [140, 141]. Considering that migraine and depression are well-known comorbidities of tinnitus [142, 143], one study followed up migraine patients with tinnitus comorbidity, and of the five patients with preexisting tinnitus, botox completely abolished the tinnitus in two, including one whose tinnitus of 10 years' duration resolved permanently with one treatment. The tinnitus loudness of the other four was attenuated between 70 and 100% for about 3 months, which paralleled their headaches response [144]. It has been proposed that botox acts on tinnitus via a reduction of peripheral inputs from cervical, temporal, frontal, and periauricular muscles [145], but considering that it inhibits the release of nociceptive mediators such as glutamate, substance P, and calcitonin gene-related peptide (CGRP) from nociceptive fibers [146], this may also be mediated via a somatosensory-auditory direct interaction.

3. Electrical stimulation of the C2 and trigeminal area.

   Furthermore, skin stimulation on face regions close to the ear [147] can affect a person's tinnitus [148, 149]. In addition, there is an increased prevalence of somatoform disorders in individuals with tinnitus [150] and reports of tinnitus occurring after dental pulpalgia that resolved after endodontic therapy [151]. Similarly, tinnitus occurs more frequently in individuals with craniocervical mandibular disorders such as temporomandibular joint syndrome [152–154]. Changes in tinnitus may even occur with stimulation of the median nerve on the wrist [60, 155, 156], all leading to the term "somatic tinnitus" [126].

   In the same way, electrical stimulation via TENS [157] or via implanted electrodes [158, 159] of the C2 dermatoma may also modulate tinnitus in a subset of patients. TENS can improve the quality of life in tinnitus patients [160], but can also modulate the loudness and character of tinnitus in some individuals [60]. In a group of 240 patients in whom tinnitus could be modulated by somatosensory events (e.g., tinnitus change with rotation, retro-, and antiflexion of neck) or modulated by pressure on head or face, real and sham TENS treatment was applied at the C2 dermatoma for 30 min (10 min of 6 Hz, followed by 10 min of 40 Hz and 10 min of sham), resulting in a significant tinnitus suppression [157]. Only 17.9% ($N = 43$) of the patients with tinnitus responded to C2 TENS. They had an improvement of 42.92%, and only 6 patients had a reduction of 100%, who were later implanted with a subcutaneous electrode for permanent tinnitus suppression [159].
4. Bimodal stimulation: electrical stimulation of C2 or trigeminal area plus sound presentation.

   In view of the low success rate of unimodal somatosensory stimulation for tinnitus, bimodal C2 and auditory stimulation [161], as well as bimodal trigeminal and auditory stimulation has been developed [162]. Whereas C2 plus auditory stimulation seems to yield a transient effect on both loudness and distress [161], the trigeminal plus auditory stimulation only exerts a benefit on the distress and not the loudness [162]. Whether long term benefits may result is currently unknown.

Conclusion

In conclusion, when the auditory input is altered because of hearing loss or overexposure to noise, the cochlear nucleus and other parts of the auditory pathways respond by starting to 'listen' to somatosensory input rather than auditory input. This is mediated via the extralemniscal system and results in hyperactivity of the auditory system, clinically expressed as somatosensory tinnitus. Treatment can consist of modulating the somatosensory input, by physical therapy, botox injections, electrical stimulation, or by reversing the maladaptive plasticity via bimodal stimulation.

References

1. Teichert M, Bolz J. How senses work together: cross-modal interactions between primary sensory cortices. Neural Plast. 2018;2018:5380921.
2. Moller A. New developments in neuroscience. J Integr Creative Stud. 2015;10:1–23.
3. Moller A. New developments in neuroscience. A review. Arch Neurol Neurosurg. 2019;2:48–58.
4. Fuster JM. The cognit: a network model of cortical representation. Int J Psychophysiol. 2006;60(2):125–32.
5. Meunier D, Lambiotte R, Bullmore ET. Modular and hierarchically modular organization of brain networks. Front Neurosci. 2010;4:200.
6. Stam CJ. Modern network science of neurological disorders. Nat Rev Neurosci. 2014;15(10):683–95.
7. De Ridder D, Adhia D, Vanneste S. The anatomy of pain and suffering in the brain and its clinical implications. Neurosci Biobehav Rev. 2021;130:125–46.
8. De Ridder D, Maciaczyk J, Vanneste S. The future of neuromodulation: smart neuromodulation. Expert Rev Med Devices. 2021;18(4):307–17.
9. Fornito A, Zalesky A, Breakspear M. The connectomics of brain disorders. Nat Rev Neurosci. 2015;16(3):159–72.
10. Freeman WJ, Kozma R, Werbos PJ. Biocomplexity: adaptive behavior in complex stochastic dynamical systems. Biosystems. 2001;59(2):109–23.
11. Wu C, Stefanescu RA, Martel DT, Shore SE. Listening to another sense: somatosensory integration in the auditory system. Cell Tissue Res. 2015;361(1):233–50.
12. Bavelier D, Neville HJ. Cross-modal plasticity: where and how? Nat Rev Neurosci. 2002;3(6):443–52.
13. Neville H, Bavelier D. Human brain plasticity: evidence from sensory deprivation and altered language experience. Prog Brain Res. 2002;138:177–88.
14. Moller A. Neuroplasticity and its dark sides: disorders of the nervous system. Dallas: Aage Moller Publishing; 2018.
15. Kucyi A, Davis KD. The dynamic pain connectome. Trends Neurosci. 2015;38(2):86–95.
16. Fornito A, Bullmore ET. Connectomics: a new paradigm for understanding brain disease. Eur Neuropsychopharmacol. 2014;25:733.
17. van den Heuvel MP, Sporns O. A cross-disorder connectome landscape of brain dysconnectivity. Nat Rev Neurosci. 2019;20(7):435–46.
18. Uhlhaas PJ. Dysconnectivity, large-scale networks and neuronal dynamics in schizophrenia. Curr Opin Neurobiol. 2013;23(2):283–90.
19. Diwadkar VA, Bakshi N, Gupta G, Pruitt P, White R, Eickhoff SB. Dysfunction and dysconnection in cortical-striatal networks during sustained attention: genetic risk for schizophrenia or bipolar disorder and its impact on brain network function. Front Psych. 2014;5:50.
20. Hannan AJ. Synaptopathy, circuitopathy and the computational biology of Huntington's disease. BMC Biol. 2018;16(1):71.
21. Crossley NA, Mechelli A, Scott J, et al. The hubs of the human connectome are generally implicated in the anatomy of brain disorders. Brain. 2014;137(Pt 8):2382–95.

22. Fu Z, Iraji A, Turner JA, et al. Dynamic state with covarying brain activity-connectivity: on the pathophysiology of schizophrenia. NeuroImage. 2020;224:117385.
23. Smits M, Kovacs S, de Ridder D, Peeters RR, van Hecke P, Sunaert S. Lateralization of functional magnetic resonance imaging (fMRI) activation in the auditory pathway of patients with lateralized tinnitus. Neuroradiology. 2007;49(8):669–79.
24. Andersson G, Lyttkens L, Hirvela C, Furmark T, Tillfors M, Fredrikson M. Regional cerebral blood flow during tinnitus: a PET case study with lidocaine and auditory stimulation. Acta Otolaryngol. 2000;120(8):967–72.
25. Eichhammer P, Hajak G, Kleinjung T, Landgrebe M, Langguth B. Functional imaging of chronic tinnitus: the use of positron emission tomography. Prog Brain Res. 2007;166:83–8.
26. van der Loo E, Gais S, Congedo M, et al. Tinnitus intensity dependent gamma oscillations of the contralateral auditory cortex. PLoS One. 2009;4(10):e7396.
27. Weisz N, Muller S, Schlee W, Dohrmann K, Hartmann T, Elbert T. The neural code of auditory phantom perception. J Neurosci. 2007;27(6):1479–84.
28. Burton H, Wineland A, Bhattacharya M, Nicklaus J, Garcia KS, Piccirillo JF. Altered networks in bothersome tinnitus: a functional connectivity study. BMC Neurosci. 2012;13:3.
29. Chen YC, Zhang H, Kong Y, et al. Alterations of the default mode network and cognitive impairment in patients with unilateral chronic tinnitus. Quant Imaging Med Surg. 2018;8(10):1020–9.
30. De Ridder D, Vanneste S. Targeting the parahippocampal area by auditory cortex stimulation in tinnitus. Brain Stimul. 2014;7:709.
31. De Ridder D, Vanneste S. The Bayesian brain in imbalance: medial, lateral and descending pathways in tinnitus and pain: a perspective. Prog Brain Res. 2021;262:309–34.
32. De Ridder D, Vanneste S, Weisz N, et al. An integrative model of auditory phantom perception: tinnitus as a unified percept of interacting separable subnetworks. Neurosci Biobehav Rev. 2014;44:16–32.
33. Eggermont JJ. Separate auditory pathways for the induction and maintenance of tinnitus and hyperacusis? Prog Brain Res. 2021;260:101–27.
34. Henderson-Sabes J, Shang Y, Perez PL, et al. Corticostriatal functional connectivity of bothersome tinnitus in single-sided deafness. Sci Rep. 2019;9(1):19552.
35. Hu J, Cui J, Xu JJ, Yin X, Wu Y, Qi J. The neural mechanisms of tinnitus: a perspective from functional magnetic resonance imaging. Front Neurosci. 2021;15:621145.
36. Hullfish J, Abenes I, Kovacs S, Sunaert S, De Ridder D, Vanneste S. Functional connectivity analysis of fMRI data collected from human subjects with chronic tinnitus and varying levels of tinnitus-related distress. Data Brief. 2018;21:779–89.
37. Hullfish J, Abenes I, Yoo HB, De Ridder D, Vanneste S. Frontostriatal network dysfunction as a domain-general mechanism underlying phantom perception. Hum Brain Mapp. 2019;40(7):2241–51.
38. Kim JY, Kim YH, Lee S, et al. Alteration of functional connectivity in tinnitus brain revealed by resting-state fMRI? A pilot study. Int J Audiol. 2012;51(5):413–7.
39. Lee MH, Solowski N, Wineland A, et al. Functional connectivity during modulation of tinnitus with orofacial maneuvers. Otolaryngol Head Neck Surg. 2012;147:757.
40. Maudoux A, Lefebvre P, Cabay JE, et al. Connectivity graph analysis of the auditory resting state network in tinnitus. Brain Res. 2012;1485:10.
41. Maudoux A, Lefebvre P, Cabay JE, et al. Auditory resting-state network connectivity in tinnitus: a functional MRI study. PLoS One. 2012;7(5):e36222.
42. Mohan A, Alexandra SJ, Johnson CV, De Ridder D, Vanneste S. Effect of distress on transient network dynamics and topological equilibrium in phantom sound perception. Prog Neuro-Psychopharmacol Biol Psychiatry. 2018;84(Pt A):79–92.
43. Mohan A, Davidson C, De Ridder D, Vanneste S. Effective connectivity analysis of inter- and intramodular hubs in phantom sound perception - identifying the core distress network. Brain Imaging Behav. 2020;14(1):289–307.
44. Mohan A, De Ridder D, Idiculla R, DSouza C, Vanneste S. Distress-dependent temporal variability of regions encoding domain-specific and domain-general behavioral manifestations of phantom percepts. Eur J Neurosci. 2018;48(2):1743–64.
45. Mohan A, De Ridder D, Vanneste S. Graph theoretical analysis of brain connectivity in phantom sound perception. Sci Rep. 2016;6:19683.
46. Mohan A, De Ridder D, Vanneste S. Emerging hubs in phantom perception connectomics. Neuroimage Clin. 2016;11:181–94.
47. Mohan A, Moreno N, Song JJ, De Ridder D, Vanneste S. Evidence for behaviorally segregated, spatiotemporally overlapping subnetworks in phantom sound perception. Brain Connect. 2017;7(3):197–210.
48. Schlee W, Mueller N, Hartmann T, Keil J, Lorenz I, Weisz N. Mapping cortical hubs in tinnitus. BMC Biol. 2009;7:80.
49. Schlee W, Weisz N, Bertrand O, Hartmann T, Elbert T. Using auditory steady state responses to outline the functional connectivity in the tinnitus brain. PLoS One. 2008;3(11):e3720.
50. To WT, De Ridder D, Hart J Jr, Vanneste S. Changing brain networks through non-invasive neuromodulation. Front Hum Neurosci. 2018;12:128.
51. Vanneste S, De Ridder D. Stress-related functional connectivity changes between auditory cortex and cingulate in tinnitus. Brain Connect. 2015;5:371.
52. Vanneste S, De Ridder D. Deafferentation-based pathophysiological differences in phantom sound: tinnitus with and without hearing loss. NeuroImage. 2016;129:80–94.
53. Vanneste S, Focquaert F, Van de Heyning P, De Ridder D. Different resting state brain activity and functional connectivity in patients who respond and not respond to bifrontal tDCS for tinnitus suppression. Exp Brain Res. 2011;210(2):217–27.
54. Vanneste S, Joos K, Ost J, De Ridder D. Influencing connectivity and cross-frequency coupling by real-time source localized neurofeedback of the posterior cingulate cortex reduces tinnitus related distress. Neurobiol Stress. 2018;8:211–24.
55. Vanneste S, To WT, De Ridder D. Tinnitus and neuropathic pain share a common neural substrate in the form of specific brain connectivity and microstate profiles. Prog Neuro-Psychopharmacol Biol Psychiatry. 2019;88:388–400.
56. Wineland AM, Burton H, Piccirillo J. Functional connectivity networks in nonbothersome tinnitus. Otolaryngol Head Neck Surg. 2012;147:900.
57. Crippa A, Lanting CP, van Dijk P, Roerdink JB. A diffusion tensor imaging study on the auditory system and tinnitus. Open Neuroimaging J. 2010;4:16–25.
58. De Ridder D, Schlee W, Vanneste S, et al. Tinnitus and tinnitus disorder: theoretical and operational definitions (an international multidisciplinary proposal). Prog Brain Res. 2021;260:1–25.
59. Sperdin HF, Cappe C, Murray MM. The behavioral relevance of multisensory neural response interactions. Front Neurosci. 2010;4:9.
60. Moller AR, Moller MB, Yokota M. Some forms of tinnitus may involve the extralemniscal auditory pathway. Laryngoscope. 1992;102(10):1165–71.
61. Kaiser J, Hertrich I, Ackermann H, Mathiak K, Lutzenberger W. Hearing lips: gamma-band activity during audiovisual speech perception. Cereb Cortex. 2005;15(5):646–53.
62. Kanaya S, Yokosawa K. Perceptual congruency of audio-visual speech affects ventriloquism with bilateral visual stimuli. Psychon Bull Rev. 2011;18(1):123–8.

63. Jousmaki V, Hari R. Parchment-skin illusion: sound-biased touch. Curr Biol. 1998;8(6):R190.
64. Shore SE, Zhou J. Somatosensory influence on the cochlear nucleus and beyond. Hear Res. 2006;216–217:90–9.
65. Trudeau-Fisette P, Ito T, Menard L. Auditory and somatosensory interaction in speech perception in children and adults. Front Hum Neurosci. 2019;13:344.
66. Ohashi H, Ito T. Recalibration of auditory perception of speech due to orofacial somatosensory inputs during speech motor adaptation. J Neurophysiol. 2019;122(5):2076–84.
67. Meredith MA. On the neuronal basis for multisensory convergence: a brief overview. Brain Res Cogn Brain Res. 2002;14(1):31–40.
68. Riley JW. Poems & prose sketches. Portable poetry; 2017.
69. Winer JA, Lee CC. The distributed auditory cortex. Hear Res. 2007;229(1–2):3–13.
70. De Ridder D. A heuristic pathophysiological model of tinnitus. In: Moller A, Langguth B, De Ridder D, Kleinjung T, editors. Textbook of tinnitus. New York: Springer; 2011. p. 171–98.
71. Strominger NL, Nelson LR, Dougherty WJ. Second order auditory pathways in the chimpanzee. J Comp Neurol. 1977;172(2):349–65.
72. Parvizi J, Damasio AR. Differential distribution of calbindin D28k and parvalbumin among functionally distinctive sets of structures in the macaque brainstem. J Comp Neurol. 2003;462(2):153–67.
73. Tennigkeit F, Schwarz DW, Puil E. Mechanisms for signal transformation in lemniscal auditory thalamus. J Neurophysiol. 1996;76(6):3597–608.
74. McCormick DA, Feeser HR. Functional implications of burst firing and single spike activity in lateral geniculate relay neurons. Neuroscience. 1990;39(1):103–13.
75. Jones EG. The thalamic matrix and thalamocortical synchrony. Trends Neurosci. 2001;24(10):595–601.
76. Jones EG. Viewpoint: the core and matrix of thalamic organization. Neuroscience. 1998;85(2):331–45.
77. Jones EG. Chemically defined parallel pathways in the monkey auditory system. Ann N Y Acad Sci. 2003;999:218–33.
78. Chiry O, Tardif E, Magistretti PJ, Clarke S. Patterns of calcium-binding proteins support parallel and hierarchical organization of human auditory areas. Eur J Neurosci. 2003;17(2):397–410.
79. Bordi F, LeDoux JE. Response properties of single units in areas of rat auditory thalamus that project to the amygdala. I. Acoustic discharge patterns and frequency receptive fields. Exp Brain Res. 1994;98(2):261–74.
80. Calford MB. The parcellation of the medial geniculate body of the cat defined by the auditory response properties of single units. J Neurosci. 1983;3(11):2350–64.
81. Hu B, Senatorov V, Mooney D. Lemniscal and non-lemniscal synaptic transmission in rat auditory thalamus. J Physiol. 1994;479(Pt 2):217–31.
82. Sherman SM, Koch C. The synaptic organization of the brain. Oxford: Oxford University Press; 1998.
83. Disterhoft JF, Olds J. Differential development of conditioned unit changes in thalamus and cortex of rat. J Neurophysiol. 1972;35(5):665–79.
84. Kawaguchi Y, Kubota Y. Correlation of physiological subgroupings of nonpyramidal cells with parvalbumin- and calbindinD28k-immunoreactive neurons in layer V of rat frontal cortex. J Neurophysiol. 1993;70(1):387–96.
85. Kawaguchi Y. Distinct firing patterns of neuronal subtypes in cortical synchronized activities. J Neurosci. 2001;21(18):7261–72.
86. Solbach S, Celio MR. Ontogeny of the calcium binding protein parvalbumin in the rat nervous system. Anat Embryol (Berl). 1991;184(2):103–24.
87. Baimbridge KG, Celio MR, Rogers JH. Calcium-binding proteins in the nervous system. Trends Neurosci. 1992;15(8):303–8.
88. Caillard O, Moreno H, Schwaller B, Llano I, Celio MR, Marty A. Role of the calcium-binding protein parvalbumin in short-term synaptic plasticity. Proc Natl Acad Sci U S A. 2000;97(24):13372–7.
89. Bordi F, LeDoux J, Clugnet MC, Pavlides C. Single-unit activity in the lateral nucleus of the amygdala and overlying areas of the striatum in freely behaving rats: rates, discharge patterns, and responses to acoustic stimuli. Behav Neurosci. 1993;107(5):757–69.
90. Bartlett EL, Smith PH. Anatomic, intrinsic, and synaptic properties of dorsal and ventral division neurons in rat medial geniculate body. J Neurophysiol. 1999;81(5):1999–2016.
91. He J, Hu B. Differential distribution of burst and single-spike responses in auditory thalamus. J Neurophysiol. 2002;88(4):2152–6.
92. Mooney DM, Zhang L, Basile C, et al. Distinct forms of cholinergic modulation in parallel thalamic sensory pathways. Proc Natl Acad Sci U S A. 2004;101(1):320–4.
93. Sherman SM. A wake-up call from the thalamus. Nat Neurosci. 2001;4(4):344–6.
94. Sherman SM. Tonic and burst firing: dual modes of thalamocortical relay. Trends Neurosci. 2001;24(2):122–6.
95. Swadlow HA, Gusev AG. The impact of 'bursting' thalamic impulses at a neocortical synapse. Nat Neurosci. 2001;4(4):402–8.
96. Ramcharan EJ, Cox CL, Zhan XJ, Sherman SM, Gnadt JW. Cellular mechanisms underlying activity patterns in the monkey thalamus during visual behavior. J Neurophysiol. 2000;84(4):1982–7.
97. Tardif E, Chiry O, Probst A, Magistretti PJ, Clarke S. Patterns of calcium-binding proteins in human inferior colliculus: identification of subdivisions and evidence for putative parallel systems. Neuroscience. 2003;116(4):1111–21.
98. Syka J. Plastic changes in the central auditory system after hearing loss, restoration of function, and during learning. Physiol Rev. 2002;82(3):601–36.
99. Forster CR, Illing RB. Plasticity of the auditory brainstem: cochleotomy-induced changes of calbindin-D28k expression in the rat. J Comp Neurol. 2000;416(2):173–87.
100. Caicedo A, d'Aldin C, Eybalin M, Puel JL. Temporary sensory deprivation changes calcium-binding proteins levels in the auditory brainstem. J Comp Neurol. 1997;378(1):1–15.
101. Garcia MM, Edward R, Brennan GB, Harlan RE. Deafferentation-induced changes in protein kinase C expression in the rat cochlear nucleus. Hear Res. 2000;147(1–2):113–24.
102. Rausell E, Cusick CG, Taub E, Jones EG. Chronic deafferentation in monkeys differentially affects nociceptive and nonnociceptive pathways distinguished by specific calcium-binding proteins and down-regulates gamma-aminobutyric acid type a receptors at thalamic levels. Proc Natl Acad Sci U S A. 1992;89(7):2571–5.
103. Itoh K, Kamiya H, Mitani A, Yasui Y, Takada M, Mizuno N. Direct projections from the dorsal column nuclei and the spinal trigeminal nuclei to the cochlear nuclei in the cat. Brain Res. 1987;400(1):145–50.
104. Moller AR. Hearing : its physiology and pathophysiology. 1st ed. San Diego: Academic Press; 2000.
105. Szczepaniak WS, Moller AR. Interaction between auditory and somatosensory systems: a study of evoked potentials in the inferior colliculus. Electroencephalogr Clin Neurophysiol. 1993;88(6):508–15.
106. Leinonen L, Hyvarinen J, Sovijarvi AR. Functional properties of neurons in the temporo-parietal association cortex of awake monkey. Exp Brain Res. 1980;39(2):203–15.
107. Hu B. Functional organization of lemniscal and nonlemniscal auditory thalamus. Exp Brain Res. 2003;153(4):543–9.
108. Lee CC. Exploring functions for the non-lemniscal auditory thalamus. Front Neural Circuits. 2015;9:69.
109. Moller AR, Rollins PR. The non-classical auditory pathways are involved in hearing in children but not in adults. Neurosci Lett. 2002;319(1):41–4.

110. Zhou J, Shore S. Convergence of spinal trigeminal and cochlear nucleus projections in the inferior colliculus of the Guinea pig. J Comp Neurol. 2006;495(1):100–12.
111. Cardon G, Sharma A. Somatosensory cross-modal reorganization in adults with age-related, early-stage hearing loss. Front Hum Neurosci. 2018;12:172.
112. Mao YT, Pallas SL. Compromise of auditory cortical tuning and topography after cross-modal invasion by visual inputs. J Neurosci. 2012;32(30):10338–51.
113. Li H, Mizuno N. Single neurons in the spinal trigeminal and dorsal column nuclei project to both the cochlear nucleus and the inferior colliculus by way of axon collaterals: a fluorescent retrograde double-labeling study in the rat. Neurosci Res. 1997;29(2):135–42.
114. Schofield BR, Coomes DL. Auditory cortical projections to the cochlear nucleus in Guinea pigs. Hear Res. 2005;199(1–2):89–102.
115. Shore SE, Roberts LE, Langguth B. Maladaptive plasticity in tinnitus--triggers, mechanisms and treatment. Nat Rev Neurol. 2016;12(3):150–60.
116. Zhou J, Nannapaneni N, Shore S. Vessicular glutamate transporters 1 and 2 are differentially associated with auditory nerve and spinal trigeminal inputs to the cochlear nucleus. J Comp Neurol. 2007;500(4):777–87.
117. Zeng C, Nannapaneni N, Zhou J, Hughes LF, Shore S. Cochlear damage changes the distribution of vesicular glutamate transporters associated with auditory and nonauditory inputs to the cochlear nucleus. J Neurosci. 2009;29(13):4210–7.
118. Zeng C, Yang Z, Shreve L, Bledsoe S, Shore S. Somatosensory projections to cochlear nucleus are upregulated after unilateral deafness. J Neurosci. 2012;32(45):15791–801.
119. Basura GJ, Koehler SD, Shore SE. Multi-sensory integration in brainstem and auditory cortex. Brain Res. 2012;1485:95–107.
120. Dehmel S, Pradhan S, Koehler S, Bledsoe S, Shore S. Noise overexposure alters long-term somatosensory-auditory processing in the dorsal cochlear nucleus--possible basis for tinnitus-related hyperactivity? J Neurosci. 2012;32(5):1660–71.
121. Zhang J, Guan Z. Pathways involved in somatosensory electrical modulation of dorsal cochlear nucleus activity. Brain Res. 2007;1184:121–31.
122. Kanold PO, Young ED. Proprioceptive information from the pinna provides somatosensory input to cat dorsal cochlear nucleus. J Neurosci. 2001;21(19):7848–58.
123. Aitkin LM. The auditory midbrain, structure, and function in the central auditory pathway. Clifton: Humana Press; 1986.
124. Rubinstein B, Axelsson A, Carlsson GE. Prevalence of signs and symptoms of craniomandibular disorders in tinnitus patients. J Craniomandib Disord. 1990;4(3):186–92.
125. Pinchoff RJ, Burkard RF, Salvi RJ, Coad ML, Lockwood AH. Modulation of tinnitus by voluntary jaw movements. Am J Otol. 1998;19(6):785–9.
126. Levine RA. Somatic (craniocervical) tinnitus and the dorsal cochlear nucleus hypothesis. Am J Otolaryngol. 1999;20(6):351–62.
127. Lee HY, Kim SJ, Choi JY. Somatic modulation in tinnitus: clinical characteristics and treatment outcomes. J Int Adv Otol. 2020;16(2):213–7.
128. Ralli M, Greco A, Turchetta R, Altissimi G, de Vincentiis M, Cianfrone G. Somatosensory tinnitus: current evidence and future perspectives. J Int Med Res. 2017;45(3):933–47.
129. Sanchez TG, Guerra GC, Lorenzi MC, Brandao AL, Bento RF. The influence of voluntary muscle contractions upon the onset and modulation of tinnitus. Audiol Neurootol. 2002;7(6):370–5.
130. Won JY, Yoo S, Lee SK, et al. Prevalence and factors associated with neck and jaw muscle modulation of tinnitus. Audiol Neurootol. 2013;18(4):261–73.
131. Michiels S, Ganz Sanchez T, Oron Y, et al. Diagnostic criteria for somatosensory tinnitus: a Delphi process and face-to-face meeting to establish consensus. Trends Hear. 2018;22:2331216518796403.
132. Michiels S, Cardon E, Gilles A, Goedhart H, Vesala M, Schlee W. Somatosensory tinnitus diagnosis: diagnostic value of existing criteria. Ear Hear. 2021;43(1):143–9.
133. Levine RA, Nam EC, Melcher J. Somatosensory pulsatile tinnitus syndrome: somatic testing identifies a pulsatile tinnitus subtype that implicates the somatosensory system. Trends Amplif. 2008;12(3):242–53.
134. Levine RA. Somatosensory pulsatile tinnitus syndrome (SSPT) revisited. Int Tinnitus J. 2021;25(1):39–45.
135. van der Wal A, Michiels S, Van de Heyning P, et al. Reduction of somatic tinnitus severity is mediated by improvement of temporomandibular disorders. Otol Neurotol. 2022;43(3):e309–15.
136. van der Wal A, Van de Heyning P, Gilles A, et al. Prognostic indicators for positive treatment outcome after multidisciplinary orofacial treatment in patients with somatosensory tinnitus. Front Neurosci. 2020;14:561038.
137. Michiels S, Van de Heyning P, Truijen S, Hallemans A, De Hertogh W. Does multi-modal cervical physical therapy improve tinnitus in patients with cervicogenic somatic tinnitus? Man Ther. 2016;26:125–31.
138. Michiels S, Van de Heyning P, Truijen S, Hallemans A, De Hertogh W. Prognostic indicators for decrease in tinnitus severity after cervical physical therapy in patients with cervicogenic somatic tinnitus. Musculoskelet Sci Pract. 2017;29:33–7.
139. Park JM, Kim WJ, Han JS, Park SY, Park SN. Management of palatal myoclonic tinnitus based on clinical characteristics: a large case series study. Acta Otolaryngol. 2020;140(7):553–7.
140. Herd CP, Tomlinson CL, Rick C, et al. Cochrane systematic review and meta-analysis of botulinum toxin for the prevention of migraine. BMJ Open. 2019;9(7):e027953.
141. Affatato O, Moulin TC, Pisanu C, et al. High efficacy of onabotulinumtoxinA treatment in patients with comorbid migraine and depression: a meta-analysis. J Transl Med. 2021;19(1):133.
142. Langguth B, Hund V, Landgrebe M, Schecklmann M. Tinnitus patients with comorbid headaches: the influence of headache type and laterality on tinnitus characteristics. Front Neurol. 2017;8:440.
143. Nowaczewska M, Wicinski M, Straburzynski M, Kazmierczak W. The prevalence of different types of headache in patients with subjective tinnitus and its influence on tinnitus parameters: a prospective clinical study. Brain Sci. 2020;10(11):776.
144. Ranoux D, Levine RA. Botulinum toxin can abolish and/or quiet tinnitus associated with chronic migraine: Serendipidous observations. Int Tinnitus J. 2022;25(2):133–6.
145. Lainez MJ, Piera A. Botulinum toxin for the treatment of somatic tinnitus. Prog Brain Res. 2007;166:335–8.
146. Dolly O. Synaptic transmission: inhibition of neurotransmitter release by botulinum toxins. Headache. 2003;43(Suppl 1):S16–24.
147. Herraiz C, Toledano A, Diges I. Trans-electrical nerve stimulation (TENS) for somatic tinnitus. Prog Brain Res. 2007;166:389–94.
148. Shulman A. External electrical tinnitus suppression: a review. Am J Otol. 1987;8(6):479–84.
149. Shulman A, Tonndorf J, Goldstein B. Electrical tinnitus control. Acta Otolaryngol. 1985;99(3–4):318–25.
150. Hiller W, Janca A, Burke KC. Association between tinnitus and somatoform disorders. J Psychosom Res. 1997;43(6):613–24.

151. Wright EF, Gullickson DC. Dental pulpalgia contributing to bilateral preauricular pain and tinnitus. J Orofac Pain. 1996;10(2):166–8.
152. Chole RA, Parker WS. Tinnitus and vertigo in patients with temporomandibular disorder. Arch Otolaryngol Head Neck Surg. 1992;118(8):817–21.
153. Morgan DH. Tinnitus of TMJ origin: a preliminary report. Cranio. 1992;10(2):124–9.
154. Gelb H, Gelb ML, Wagner ML. The relationship of tinnitus to craniocervical mandibular disorders. Cranio. 1997;15(2):136–43.
155. Cacace AT, Cousins JP, Parnes SM, et al. Cutaneous-evoked tinnitus. II. Review of neuroanatomical, physiological and functional imaging studies. Audiol Neurootol. 1999;4(5):258–68.
156. Cacace AT, Cousins JP, Parnes SM, et al. Cutaneous-evoked tinnitus. I. Phenomenology, psychophysics and functional imaging. Audiol Neurootol. 1999;4(5):247–57.
157. Vanneste S, Plazier M, Van de Heyning P, De Ridder D. Transcutaneous electrical nerve stimulation (TENS) of upper cervical nerve (C2) for the treatment of somatic tinnitus. Exp Brain Res. 2010;204(2):283–7.
158. De Ridder D, Vanneste S. Multitarget surgical neuromodulation: combined C2 and auditory cortex implantation for tinnitus. Neurosci Lett. 2015;591:202–6.
159. De Ridder D, Vanneste S, Menovsky T, Langguth B. Surgical brain modulation for tinnitus: the past, present and future. J Neurosurg Sci. 2012;56(4):323–40.
160. Aydemir G, Tezer MS, Borman P, Bodur H, Unal A. Treatment of tinnitus with transcutaneous electrical nerve stimulation improves patients' quality of life. J Laryngol Otol. 2006;120(6):442–5.
161. Marks KL, Martel DT, Wu C, et al. Auditory-somatosensory bimodal stimulation desynchronizes brain circuitry to reduce tinnitus in guinea pigs and humans. Sci Transl Med. 2018;10(422):eaal3175.
162. Conlon B, Langguth B, Hamilton C, et al. Bimodal neuromodulation combining sound and tongue stimulation reduces tinnitus symptoms in a large randomized clinical study. Sci Transl Med. 2020;12(564):eabb2830.

The Role of Auditory Deprivation

13

Tobias Kleinjung and Aage R. Møller

Abstract

Hearing loss is the most important factor in the development of tinnitus. This chapter describes the changes that occur in the central auditory system as a consequence of hearing loss. Deprivation of input to the auditory system can cause two types of functional changes: it can alter the balance between inhibition and excitation, and it can activate neuronal plasticity. Any type of hearing loss, such as conductive or sensorineural hearing loss, results in decreased input to the central auditory nervous system. Noise-induced hearing loss is an example of auditory deprivation and overuse, which in turn can activate neural plasticity. An altered balance between inhibition and excitation can change the gain in the central auditory system. If the gain is increased, this can lead to hyperactivity in the form of tinnitus. The effects on the balance between inhibition and excitation may subside when normal input to the auditory system occurs. However, activation of neuronal plasticity that may occur as a result of sensory stimulation may persist even after normal sensory stimulation is restored. Plastic changes may become permanent, and reversal of neuronal plasticity may require special measures.

Aage R. Møller has died before the publication of this book.

T. Kleinjung (✉)
Department of Otorhinolaryngology – Head and Neck Surgery, University Hospital of Zurich, University of Zurich, Zurich, Switzerland
e-mail: tobias.kleinjung@usz.ch

A. R. Møller (Deceased)
Neuroscience Program, School of Brain & Behavioral Sciences, University of Texas, Richardson, TX, USA

Highlights

- Deprivation of input to the auditory system can cause two kinds of change in function: It can alter the balance between inhibition and excitation and can activate neural plasticity.
- Hearing loss of any kind, such as conductive hearing loss or cochlear hearing loss, causes decreased input to the auditory nervous system.
- Noise-induced hearing loss is an example of deprivation of auditory stimulation and overexposure, which in itself may activate neural plasticity.
- Altered balance between inhibition and excitation can change the gain in the auditory system. If the gain is increased, it may cause hyperactivity in the form of tinnitus.
- The effect on the balance between inhibition and excitation may abate when normal input to the auditory system is established.
- Activation of neural plasticity, which may occur because of sensory stimulation, may last after restoring normal sensory stimulation.
- Plastic changes may become permanent, and reversal of neural plasticity may require special actions.

Introduction

The effect on the nervous system of sensory deprivation can be profound and is different when it occurs at birth or shortly thereafter, compared with occurring during adult life. The anatomical and functional development of the nervous system depends on sensory stimulation. Therefore, sound deprivation can have a stronger effect on young individuals than on adults [1]. The fact that there are indications that the non-classical pathways are normally active in children [2, 3] while not normally active in adults may influence the way children react to deprivation of sound compared with adults.

W. Schlee et al. (eds.), *Textbook of Tinnitus*, https://doi.org/10.1007/978-3-031-35647-6_13

Deprivation of input to the auditory system can mainly cause two different kinds of change in the function of the auditory nervous system, both of which can cause tinnitus: (1) It can decrease or shift the balance between excitation and inhibition and thereby increase the gain in the auditory nervous system and (2) deprivation of sensory stimulation can activate neural plasticity involving change in synaptic efficacy and sprouting of axons [4]. The effect of sound deprivation may not be easily observed because children do not complain of tinnitus in the same way as adults (see Chap. 39).

There are many ways that the auditory nervous system can be deprived of normal stimulation. Any form of hearing loss can cause some degree of sensory deprivation; whether it occurs through obstruction of the ear canal, disorders of the middle ear, or from disorders of the cochlea (see Chap. 32), it may have the same effect on the nervous system.

Tinnitus is common after noise-induced hearing loss (see Chaps. 32 and 38). Reduced hearing may activate neural plasticity, causing the form of tinnitus that occurs after exposure to loud sounds; however, overexposure in itself may also activate neural plasticity and thereby cause tinnitus. The tinnitus that occurs after exposure to noise, which causes hearing loss, or after a brief period of deprivation of sound often disappears after some time. In some instances, however, exposure to loud noise, especially impulsive or high-frequency sounds such as fire alarms, can cause permanent tinnitus.

It was earlier believed that increased neural firing was the cause of tinnitus, but more recent studies seem to indicate that temporal and spatial coherence of activity is more important for eliciting a sensation of the presence of sound including tinnitus [5, 6]. Noreña and Eggermont [7] showed a slight increase in spontaneous firing in cells in the auditory cortex after acoustic trauma.

Many different parts of the nervous system have been implicated in tinnitus. Some investigators have found evidence of altered spontaneous activity that is different at different levels of the auditory system [8]. There is evidence that tinnitus may be associated with less neural excitation in the periphery of the ascending auditory pathway, but greater activity in more central structures. Some have hypothesized that increased synchrony of neural firing can cause tinnitus. Other investigators have hypothesized that temporal coherence of firing in large groups of nerve cells is the cause of some forms of tinnitus [5, 9].

The frequency tuning in the cochlea is the basis for the tuning of nerve cells throughout the auditory nervous system. The acuity of tuning to sounds depends on the intensity of the sound; the higher the intensity, the broader the tuning [10, 11]. Increased temporal coherence of firing in many nerve cells may be caused by the broadening of the cochlea's tuning that occurs at higher sound intensities, thus causing a greater degree of overlap of different cells' response areas in the cortex. Unmasking of dormant synapses of interneurons, which often occur as a result of activation of neural plasticity, may also cause increased coherence of neural firing [4]. Changes in the relation between excitation and inhibition may likewise cause increased coherence and increased spontaneous firing. Both such changes may therefore be caused by reduced sensory stimulation.

Change in Balance Between Inhibition and Excitation

Single auditory nerve fibers have both excitatory and inhibitory response areas that mainly surround the excitatory areas [12]. The inhibition that is present in the response of single auditory nerve fibers is not caused by synaptic inhibition, but it is instead a form of suppression that is a result of cochlear nonlinearities [9]. Similar arrangement of suppression and excitation is present throughout the auditory nervous system, where the suppression is caused by synaptic inhibition. This means that a sound such as a tone will activate both inhibition and excitation. This suppression or inhibition is similar to what is in the visual system known as lateral inhibition. If pathologies of the cochlea result in a greater reduction of inhibition than excitation in a population of neurons, they may become sufficiently active to produce awareness of sound without sound reaching the ear, thus tinnitus. Tinnitus can be suppressed by proper arrangement of sound stimulation. Thus, sound in certain frequency regions can suppress some forms of tinnitus, and that may occur because such sounds contribute more to inhibition than excitation of specific populations of nerve cells. There are some indications that high-frequency sounds elicit stronger inhibitory influence on neurons in the cochlear nucleus more than low frequencies. This means that high-frequency hearing loss, which is common, may cause tinnitus because it reduces normally occurring inhibition. This can also explain why high-frequency stimulation can be effective in reducing some forms of tinnitus.

There is an interaction between inhibition and excitation along the ascending pathways including the cerebral cortices [13]. Lateral inhibition is especially prevalent in the inferior colliculus where interaction between excitation and inhibition is especially prevalent. It has been shown that selective damage to sensory cells (acoustic trauma) in the cochlea that reduces the evoked potentials recorded from the auditory nerve, in fact, increases the discharge rate of many neurons in the inferior colliculus [14], indicating that the deprivation stimulation caused by cochlear trauma has decreased inhibition in these third-order neurons of the ascending auditory pathways. The observed changes suggest that these cells receive inhibitory input from high-frequency regions of their response areas and this inhibition has been reduced by deprivation of stimulation caused by cochlear trauma.

Josef Syka and his collaborators have shown that acoustic trauma causes increased activity in central auditory structures [15, 16]. This means many investigators agree that neural activity in the auditory periphery is decreased by acoustic trauma, while it is increased at central levels such as the inferior colliculus and the cerebral cortex. Also, the edge effect [17] may be a consequence of lateral inhibition. The fact that tinnitus is more prevalent in elderly individuals may be explained by the reduction in inhibition that normally occurs with age [18], thereby shifting the balance between excitation and inhibition toward excitation.

Studies of temporal integration in the inferior colliculus of rats have shown decreased signs of GABAergic inhibitory activity in the cochlear nucleus after acoustic trauma [19]; administration of GABA A receptor agonists (benzodiazepines) reversed these changes [20].

Experience from treatment of people with tinnitus has also supported the hypothesis that deprivation of auditory stimulation decreases inhibition in the auditory nervous system.

Watanabe et al. [21] in a study of 600 individuals with tinnitus found that therapy with narrow band noise could suppress tinnitus in 66% of individuals, more so in individuals with presbycusis than sudden deafness. Souliere et al. [22] studied the effect of cochlear implants on loudness, annoyance, daily duration, location, and residual inhibition of tinnitus in 33 postlingual deafened individuals. Eighty-five percent of these individuals had tinnitus. The study showed a significant reduction in both loudness and annoyance. Fifty-four percent of the individuals who had tinnitus before implantation had a loudness decrease of 30% or more; 43% had a decrease in annoyance of 30% or more. The duration of the tinnitus decreased 30% or more in 48% of the individuals who had tinnitus before implantation. The fact that many of the participants in these studies experienced contralateral residual inhibition and tinnitus suppression suggests that a central mechanism contributed to their tinnitus.

Using a computational model of a lateral inhibition neural network, Kral and Majernik [23] showed evidence that lateral inhibition might be involved in some forms of tinnitus. These investigators suggested that the spontaneous activity in the auditory nerve, when subjected to lateral inhibition, could cause phantom perceptions in the absence of auditory stimulation that many individuals experience when placed in silence, such as in an acoustically shielded chamber used for audiologic testing. Kral and Majernik [23] suggested that neural noise normally generated in neural networks is generally masked by a sound stimuli or ambient broadband acoustic noise. Inhibition may balance excitation in response to broadband noise, but the spectrum of other kinds of noise determines to what extent the response will be suppressed by inhibition or whether excitation dominates.

Rubinstein et al. [24] have shown that stimulation with electrical impulses at a high rate applied to the cochlea can reduce tinnitus in some individuals. The fact that especially high-frequency electrical stimulation of the cochlea has a beneficial effect on tinnitus in both deaf individuals [22, 24] and individuals who do not have much hearing loss (see also Chap. 46) [22] supports these hypotheses. Other investigators [25–27] found that electrical stimulation of the cochlea can reduce some forms of tinnitus by counteracting the effect of reduced activation of the auditory nervous system.

Activation of Neural Plasticity

It is now generally accepted that the brain is a distributed system where many functions involve different parts of the brain. For example, it is well-known that many brain functions can be changed by activation of neuroplasticity, whereas functions such as long-term memory, sexual preference, and handedness seem to be "hard-wired" [28]. Many studies have confirmed that maladaptive plasticity plays an essential role in many common diseases, including some forms of tinnitus [29–31]. That activation of neuroplasticity plays a significant role in chronic neuropathic pain, spasticity, and probably diseases such as fibromyalgia is a well-established knowledge [32–34]. The strongest promoter of neural plasticity is deprivation of sensory stimulation [5, 35]. The effect of activation of neural plasticity can be changes in the function of the nervous system that occur with a short delay and last for just a short period for a long time.

It is assumed that acoustic trauma causes deprivation of input to the auditory nervous system because of the hearing loss it causes. There is, however, also the possibility that overstimulation may activate neural plasticity, which in turn can cause changes in the function of the nervous system that may result in tinnitus.

Studies in animals have shown evidence that auditory deprivation can cause cortical map modifications, and such cortical plasticity is associated with decreased inhibition [13, 36]. There are several ways that deprivation of sensory stimulation can immediately affect functions of the auditory nervous system. These matters are discussed in Chap. 14.

References

1. Persic D, et al. Regulation of auditory plasticity during critical periods and following hearing loss. Hear Res. 2020;397:107976.
2. Møller AR. Hearing: anatomy, physiology, and disorders of the auditory system. 2nd ed. Amsterdam: Academic Press; 2006.

3. Moller AR, Rollins PR. The non-classical auditory pathways are involved in hearing in children but not in adults. Neurosci Lett. 2002;319(1):41–4.
4. Møller AR. Neural plasticity and disorders of the nervous system. New York: Cambridge University Press; 2006.
5. Eggermont JJ, Roberts LE. The neuroscience of tinnitus. Trends Neurosci. 2004;27(11):676–82.
6. Møller AR. Pathophysiology of tinnitus. Otolaryngol Clin North Am. 2003;36:249–66.
7. Norena AJ, Eggermont JJ. Changes in spontaneous neural activity immediately after an acoustic trauma: implications for neural correlates of tinnitus. Hear Res. 2003;183(1–2):137–53.
8. Syka J. Plastic changes in the central auditory system after hearing loss, restoration of function, and during learning. Physiol Rev. 2002;82(3):601–36.
9. Ruggero MA. Responses to sound of the basilar membrane of the mammalian cochlea. Curr Opin Neurobiol. 1992;2:449–56.
10. Johnstone BM, Patuzzi R, Yates GK. Basilar membrane measurements and the traveling wave. Hear Res. 1986;22:147–53.
11. Møller AR. Frequency selectivity of the basilar membrane revealed from discharges in auditory nerve fibers. In: Evans EF, Wilson JP, editors. Psychophysics and physiology of hearing. London: Academic Press; 1977. p. 197–205.
12. Sachs MB, Kiang NYS. Two tone inhibition in auditory nerve fibers. J Acoust Soc Am. 1968;43:1120–8.
13. Eggermont JJ. Acquired hearing loss and brain plasticity. Hear Res. 2017;343:176–90.
14. Wang J, Ding D, Salvi RJ. Functional reorganization in chinchilla inferior colliculus associated with chronic and acute cochlear damage. Hear Res. 2002;168:238–49.
15. Syka J, Rybalko N, Popelar J. Enhancement of the auditory cortex evoked responses in awake Guinea pigs after noise exposure. Hear Res. 1994;78:158–68.
16. Syka J, Popelar J. Noise impairment in the Guinea pig. I. Changes in electrical evoked activity along the auditory pathway. Hear Res. 1982;8:263–72.
17. Gerken GM. Central tinnitus and lateral inhibition: an auditory brainstem model. Hear Res. 1996;97(1–2):75–83.
18. Caspary DM, et al. Immunocytochemical and neurochemical evidence for age-related loss of GABA in the inferior colliculus: implications for neural presbycusis. J Neurosci. 1990;10:2363–72.
19. Szczepaniak WS, Møller AR. Evidence of decreased GABAergic influence on temporal integration in the inferior colliculus following acute noise exposure: a study of evoked potentials in the rat. Neurosci Lett. 1995;196:77–80.
20. Szczepaniak WS, Møller AR. Effects of (-)-baclofen, clonazepam, and diazepam on tone exposure-induced hyperexcitability of the inferior colliculus in the rat: possible therapeutic implications for pharmacological management of tinnitus and hyperacusis. Hear Res. 1996;97:46–53.
21. Watanabe K, et al. [Suppression of tinnitus by band noise masker--a study of 600 cases]. Nihon Jibiinkoka Gakkai Kaiho. 1997;100(9):920–6.
22. Souliere CR Jr, et al. Tinnitus suppression following cochlear implantation. A multifactorial investigation. Arch Otolaryngol Head Neck Surg. 1992;118(12):1291–7.
23. Kral A, Majernik V. On lateral inhibition in the auditory system. Gen Physiol Biophys. 1996;15(2):109–27.
24. Rubinstein JT, et al. Electrical suppression of tinnitus with high-rate pulse trains. Otol Neurotol. 2003;24:478–85.
25. Portmann M, et al. Temporary. Tinnitus suppression in many through electrical stimulation of the cochlea. Acta Otolaryngol. 1979;87:249–99.
26. Cazals Y, Negrevergne M, Aran JM. Electrical stimulation of the cochlea in man: hearing induction and tinnitus suppression. J Am Audiol Soc. 1978;3:209–13.
27. Aran JM, Cazals I. Electrical suppression of tinnitus. In: Ciba Foundation symposium 85. London: Pitman Books; 1981. p. 217–25.
28. Moller A. The malleable brain: benefits and harm from plasticity of the brain. New York: Nova Science; 2009. p. 247.
29. Wang K, et al. Auditory neural plasticity in tinnitus mechanisms and management. Neural Plast. 2020;2020:7438461.
30. Roberts LE. Neural plasticity and its initiating conditions in tinnitus. HNO. 2018;66(3):172–8.
31. Shore SE, Roberts LE, Langguth B. Maladaptive plasticity in tinnitus--triggers, mechanisms and treatment. Nat Rev Neurol. 2016;12(3):150–60.
32. Bak MS, Park H, Kim SK. Neural plasticity in the brain during neuropathic pain. Biomedicine. 2021;9(6):624.
33. Henry DE, Chiodo AE, Yang W. Central nervous system reorganization in a variety of chronic pain states: a review. PM R. 2011;3(12):1116–25.
34. Li S. Spasticity, motor recovery, and neural plasticity after stroke. Front Neurol. 2017;8:120.
35. Moller AR. The role of neural plasticity in tinnitus. Prog Brain Res. 2007;166:37–45.
36. Rajan R. Plasticity of excitation and inhibition in the receptive field of primary auditory cortical neurons after limited receptor organ damage. Cereb Cortex. 2001;11(2):171–82.

Neuroplasticity of the Auditory System

14

Jos J. Eggermont

Abstract

Plasticity occurs at various time scales. In addition to neuronal spike-firing adaptation at a relatively short time scale, central neural responses can be decreased over much longer time periods, e.g., as in habituation. In particular, spectrotemporal receptive fields might have slower timescales of adaptation on the order of minutes to hours. A common hypothesis is that tinnitus results from a maladaptive imbalance between excitation and inhibition as a result of downregulation of inhibitory amino acid neurotransmission in the central auditory pathway. However, the effects of neural plasticity underlying noise exposure do not need to be maladaptive because the chronic tinnitus percept may be the result of experience-dependent plasticity with a percept engrained in memory as a result of continuous attention to it. Plastic changes in the adult auditory system do occur following noise exposure, from traumatic to environmental, causing permanent hearing loss, temporary loss, or no audiometric hearing loss. Tonotopic map changes are not required for tinnitus to occur; however, tonotopic maps in people with hearing loss without tinnitus were significantly different from those with normal hearing, whereas the maps of people with hearing loss and tinnitus were not. These results corroborate that map reorganization is a characteristic of hearing loss, not of tinnitus. It further raises the possibility that the spontaneous activity underlying tinnitus may prevent cortical map changes.

J. J. Eggermont (✉)
University of Calgary, Calgary, AB, Canada
e-mail: eggermon@ucalgary.ca

Highlights

- Discusses short-term to long-term plasticity
- Compares homeostatic and Hebbian plasticity
- Describes effects of critical period and cross-modal plasticity
- Plasticity from noise exposure; from environmental to traumatic
- Plasticity reflected in changing spontaneous firing rates and neural synchrony
- Neural synchrony changes are underlying network connectivity
- Tonotopic map changes are an epiphenomenon
- Does tinnitus result from maladaptive plasticity?

Introduction

Adjustment in auditory processing to physical changes during development or changing sound experiences is an aspect of neuroplasticity. Among others, neuroplasticity may allow coping with hearing loss resulting from noise exposure, disease, or aging. Plastic changes can be homeostatic, adjusting the frequency-specific gain in processing sound, and consequently leading to reorganization of tonotopic maps in thalamo-cortical areas. Changes may also occur in the connectivity between auditory structures and also between the auditory and other sensory systems, the latter called cross-modal plasticity. Tinnitus has been attributed to such plastic changes, hence called maladaptive plasticity.

Neuroplasticity can be distinguished in short-term and long-term forms. Short-term synaptic depression is reflected in the decrease of excitatory and inhibitory postsynaptic potentials or currents with repetitive stimulation. Similar to adaptation of spike firing [1, 2], short-term depression occurs and recovers on the time scale of milliseconds to seconds and reflects the decrease in presynaptic transmitter release followed by replenishment. As input rate increases, the size of

W. Schlee et al. (eds.), *Textbook of Tinnitus*, https://doi.org/10.1007/978-3-031-35647-6_14

synaptic responses is decreased, leading to an output rate that increases more slowly than the input rate. Thus, short-term depression regulates central gain. In contrast to decrease in synaptic strength, characteristic of depression, increased synaptic strength underlies facilitation, augmentation, and potentiation [3].

In addition to neuronal adaptation at a relatively short time scale, central neural responses can be decreased over much longer time periods, e.g., as in habituation. Other forms of synaptic plasticity on this time scale are long-term potentiation (LTP), long-term depression (LTD), and spike-timing-dependent plasticity (STDP), and also play important roles in determining neural responses. In particular, spectro-temporal receptive fields (STRFs) might have slower timescales of adaptation on the order of minutes to hours [4], and long-term synaptic modifications might set the neuronal response patterns to behaviorally important stimuli such as vocalizations [3].

Tonotopic Map Plasticity

Short-Term Plasticity

Sensory deafferentation results in rapid shifts in the receptive fields of cortical neurons. The rapidity of these shifts has led to the suggestion that subthreshold inputs may be unmasked by a selective loss of inhibition [5]. However, Scholl and Wehr [6] found "that acute acoustic trauma disrupted the balance of excitation and inhibition by selectively increasing and reducing the strength of inhibition at different positions within the receptive field in primary auditory cortex (A1). Inhibition was abolished for frequencies far below the trauma-tone frequency but was markedly enhanced near the edges of the region of elevated peripheral threshold." The changes occurred only for relatively high-level tones (Fig. 14.1). These changes in inhibition led to an expansion of receptive fields, but not by unmasking. Far below the trauma-tone frequency, decreased inhibition combined with prolonged excitation led to increased responses. Near the edges of the region of hearing loss, increased inhibition delayed rather than abolished responses. Thus, "rapid receptive field shifts caused by acoustic trauma are caused by distinct mechanisms at different positions within the receptive field, which depend on differential disruption of excitation and inhibition" [6].

Long-Term Plasticity

Short-term adaptation (up to 100 ms) reflects mostly synaptic suppression mechanisms after response to a stimulus. Long-term adaptation (up to a few seconds) is reflected in the habituation of neuronal responses to constant stimuli. Very long-term adaptation (several weeks) can lead to plastic changes in the cortex, most often facilitated during early development, by stimulus relevance or by behavioral states such as attention. Gourévitch and Eggermont [4] showed that long-term adaptation with a time course of tens of minutes may be detected in anesthetized adult cat A1 after a few minutes of listening to random-frequency tone pips. After the initial post-onset suppression, a slow recovery of the neuronal response strength to tones at or near their best frequency was observed for low-rate random sounds (four pips per octave per second) during stimulation. The firing rate at the end of stimulation (15 min) reached levels close to that observed during the initial onset response. The effect, clear for spikes and to a smaller extent also for local field potentials (LFPs), decreased with increasing spectro-temporal density of the sound and may therefore be of particular relevance in cortical processing (Fig. 14.2). In contrast to pure tone presentation, the multifrequency stimulus does not favor any frequency in particular. Thus, only the spectro-temporal sound density determines the recovery and further increase in firing rate during stimulation at the neurons' best frequency over time, which may be a crucial parameter for relevance of the sound in A1 [4].

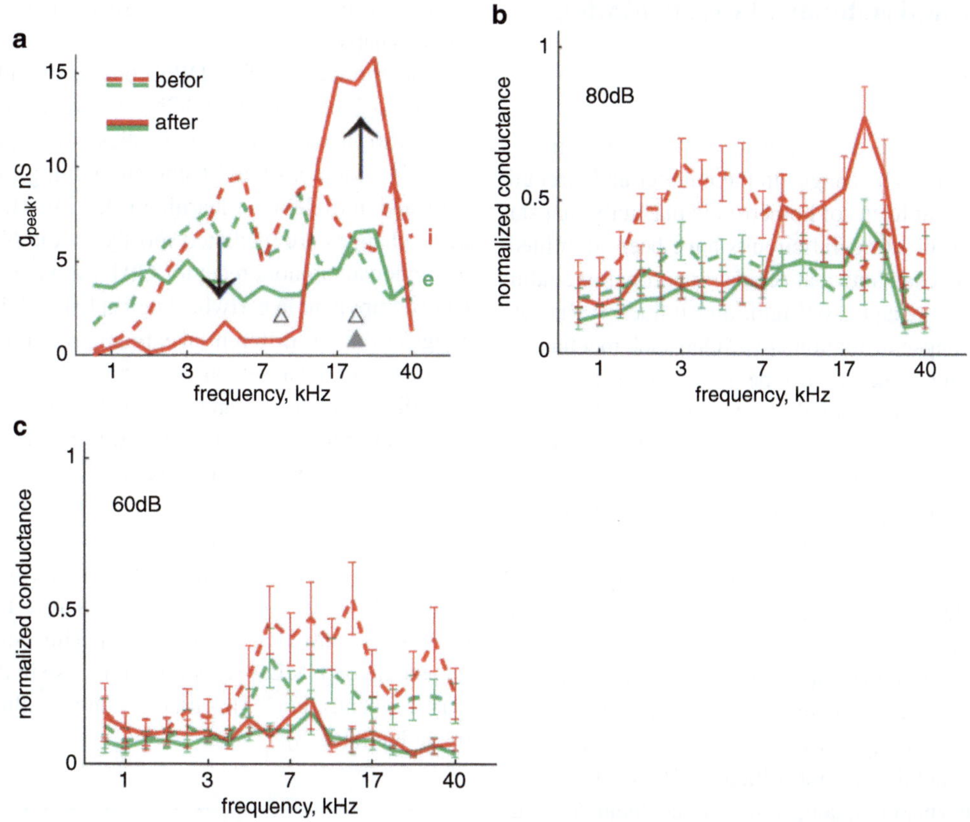

Fig. 14.1 After noise trauma, the balance of excitation and inhibition is disrupted in opposing directions at low and high frequencies. (**a**) Peak synaptic conductances as a function of tone frequency. Before acoustic trauma (dashed lines), inhibitory (red) and excitatory (green) conductances were approximately balanced throughout the receptive field. After trauma (solid lines), inhibition was abolished for frequencies <10 kHz (downward arrow), but was greatly enhanced for higher frequencies (upward arrow). Tone level = 80 dB SPL. Characteristic frequency for this cell was 26 kHz. (**b**) Peak synaptic conductances (normalized to peak inhibition for each cell) before (dashed lines) and after (solid lines) acoustic trauma for the population (n = 12 cells in 12 animals). Trauma-tone was 20 kHz, 10 min, 110–120 dB SPL for all cells. Tone level = 80 dB SPL. Inhibition (red) was consistently abolished at low frequencies and enhanced at high frequencies. Excitation (green) was affected to a lesser extent. (**c**) normalized peak synaptic conductances (as in **b**) for tone levels of 60 dB SPL. Both excitation and inhibition were reduced across all frequencies. (From Scholl and Wehr [6]. Disruption of balanced cortical excitation and inhibition by acoustic trauma. J. Neurophysiol. 100(2), 646–656. Free Access)

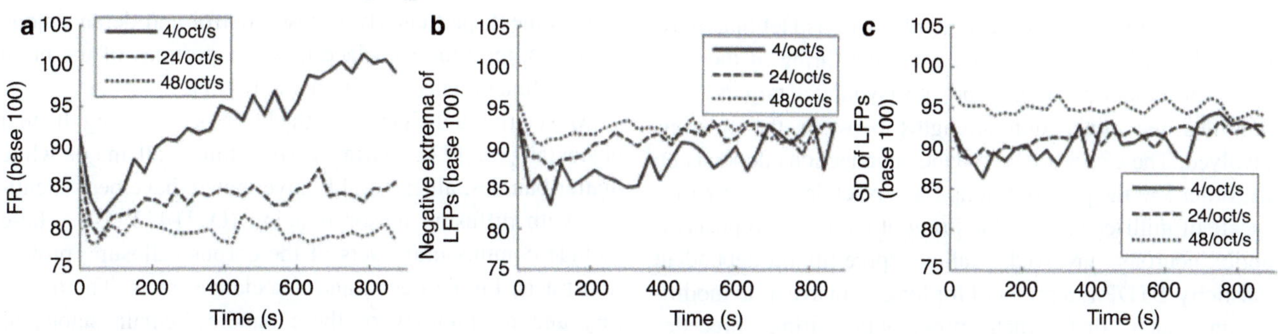

Fig. 14.2 Long-term average of (**a**) the firing rate (FR), (**b**) the negative extrema of the local field potential (LFP), and (**c**) the standard deviation (SD) of the LFP in the 100 ms following the presentation of best frequency tone pips, as a function of the density of the multifrequency tone pip presentation. The vertical scale is the same for (**a**, **b** and **c**). Base 100 is the FR (**a**) or the negative extrema (**b**) or SD (**c**). The time bin is 30 s: a point at time t shows the average value between time t and time $t+30$ s. (From Gourévitch and Eggermont [4] Spectrotemporal sound density-dependent long-term adaptation in cat primary auditory cortex. Eur J Neurosci 27: 3310–3321. Own copyright)

Homeostatic and Hebbian Plasticity Models

Homeostatic

"During learning and development, neural circuitry is refined, in part, through changes in the number and strength of synapses. Several forms of homeostatic plasticity that stabilize the properties of neural circuits have been identified. These include mechanisms that regulate neuronal excitability, stabilize total synaptic strength, and influence the rate and extent of synapse formation" [7]. "One such mechanism is synaptic scaling, which allows neurons to detect changes in their own firing rates through a set of calcium-dependent sensors that then regulate receptor trafficking to increase or decrease the accumulation of glutamate receptors at synaptic sites. Additional homeostatic mechanisms may allow local changes in synaptic activation to generate local synaptic adaptations, and network-wide changes in activity to generate network-wide adjustments in the balance between excitation and inhibition" [8, 9].

In accord with homeostatic plasticity, hyperacusis is likely an increased central gain resulting from hearing loss, which manifest itself, e.g., as steeper input-output functions of LFPs in the chinchilla inferior colliculus [10]. Furthermore, age-related presynaptic changes in the cochlear nucleus include reduced glycine levels, while in the auditory midbrain and cortex, GABA synthesis and release are altered [11]. Often increased gain is considered a functional equivalent to reduced inhibition, and vice versa. In broad terms, gain control is a major part of achieving homeostasis, i.e., the maintenance of a dynamic system within a preferred and relatively stable range of states [12].

Hebbian

The opposite type to homeostatic plasticity is Hebbian plasticity [13], which relies on the correlated firing of the neuron's presynaptic inputs and postsynaptic targets, and modifies the connection strengths between the neurons involved. The effect on the synaptic connections depends on the order and the precise timing (i.e., exact delay over a timescale of milliseconds) of the firing of the pre- and postsynaptic neurons involved, called spike-timing-dependent plasticity. STDP is a protocol for long-term synaptic modification, such that when presynaptic firing precedes postsynaptic spiking by <50 ms, LTP is induced, but when the postsynaptic cell routinely fires first, LTD is induced. With STDP, repeated presynaptic spike arrival a few milliseconds before postsynaptic action potentials leads in many synapse types to LTP of the synapses, whereas repeated spike arrival after postsynaptic spikes leads to LTD of the same synapse.

The application of STDP to plasticity and tinnitus in the dorsal cochlear nucleus (DCN) was reviewed by Wu et al. [14] who stated: "In vitro studies investigating STDP in DCN [15] demonstrated Hebbian learning rules in fusiform cells and anti-Hebbian learning rules cartwheel cells. While these changes are mediated mostly by the NMDA receptor, the endocannabinoid receptor CB1 was shown to control the LTD component in cartwheel cells [16]. Additional evidence suggests that the differential expression of this receptor at the parallel fiber synapses on fusiform and cartwheel cells, and thus the selective engagement of the endocannabinoid system, may partially explain the difference in the types of learning rules observed in these cells [16]. Furthermore, M1/M3 muscarinic acetylcholine receptors were shown to interact with the endocannabinoid system to control the size and sign of the associative long-term synaptic plasticity in fusiform cells by converting the postsynaptic Hebbian LTP to presynaptic anti-Hebbian LTD [17]. This conversion is also dependent on NMDA receptors and a rise in the postsynaptic Ca^{2+} concentration." This conversion was altered after tinnitus induction [18].

Developmental Plasticity

Structural and Connectivity Changes

One of the more dramatic changes in the brain—synaptic pruning—takes place throughout the first 20 years of life [19], and particularly in late childhood and adolescence, and may result in decreased local connectivity measures. Conversely, increased myelination throughout childhood and adolescence facilitates increased long-range functional correlations [20]. Increases in functional connectivity during development, particularly in task control and default-mode networks, tend to take place between portions of the brain that are functionally related in adults [21].

Most structural changes in the brain occur during the first postnatal year [22]. During early infancy, all major white matter bundles, albeit weakly myelinated, have been identified with diffusion tensor imaging (DTI) [23, 24]. These include commissural tracts of the corpus callosum, projection tracts, limbic tracts, and associative tracts. The trajectory and morphology of these bundles remain stable, as revealed by a longitudinal study, between birth and 2 years of age [25]. Short-range connections can also be visualized in the infant brain by MRI [26]. At the whole-brain level, an increase in global efficiency and integration and a decrease in segregation are observed in the structural networks during the first 2 postnatal years. Dubois et al. [22] emphasized that the auditory network is already functional in utero; in contrast, the visual network develops mainly after birth. Fransson et al. [27] reported that in the infant brain (mean age = 39 weeks gestational age) large parts of the auditory cortex were found to be bilaterally functional. He and Parikh [28] also found strong interhemispheric connectivity in the auditory network from early gestational age with minimal changes until term. However, at 52 weeks, the connections were significantly stronger than at 39 weeks corrected age. This early maturation may explain why topographical functional connectivity exists in the majority of congenitally, prelingually deaf [29].

Cross-Modal Plasticity

Cross-modal plasticity refers to the ability of an intact sensory modality (e.g., vision) to recruit cortical brain regions from a deprived sensory modality (e.g., audition) to carry out sensory processing. Following postnatal deafness, both somatosensory and visual modalities participate in cross-modal reinnervation of the AAF, consistent with the growing literature that documents deafness-induced cross-modal plasticity outside A1 [30]. Recordings in the auditory field of the anterior ectosylvian sulcus (FAES) of early-deafened adults revealed robust responses to visual stimulation as well as receptive fields that collectively represented the contralateral visual field. A second group of early-deafened cats was trained to localize visual targets in a perimetry array. In these animals, cooling loops were surgically placed on the FAES to reversibly deactivate the region, which resulted in substantial contralateral visual orienting deficits [31]. These results demonstrate that cross-modal plasticity can substitute one sensory modality for another while maintaining the functional repertoire of the reorganized region. Animal research in the congenitally deaf white cat has found limited evidence for reorganization in the connectivity of A1 [32].

In human studies, evidence was found for nonauditory activation in the A1 during visual processing [33] and during somatosensory processing [34]. Furthermore, Glick and Sharma [35] documented evidence of cross-modal plasticity in deaf humans and those with early-stage mild-moderate hearing loss, resulting in compensatory recruitment of frontal cortices for top-down modulation of sensory processing and cross-modal recruitment of auditory cortex by vision.

Using functional magnetic resonance imaging (fMRI), Bola et al. [36] instructed deaf and hearing adults to discriminate between sequences of rhythmic stimuli. Both deaf and hearing subjects performed the task visually, in the central visual field. In addition, hearing subjects performed the same task also in the auditory modality. The visual task robustly activated the auditory cortex in deaf subjects, peaking in the posterior–lateral part of high-level auditory areas. This activation pattern was strikingly similar to the pattern found in hearing subjects performing the auditory version of the task. Although performing the visual task in deaf subjects induced an increase in functional connectivity between the auditory cortex and the dorsal visual cortex, no such effect was found in hearing subjects. Bola et al. [36] concluded "that in deaf humans the high-level auditory cortex switches its input modality from sound to vision but preserves its task-specific activation pattern independent of input modality. Task-specific reorganization thus might be a general principle that guides cortical plasticity in the brain." This extends the findings of Meredith et al. [31] in cats to the human domain.

Noise Exposure-Induced Neural Plasticity

Here I limit myself largely to plastic changes in the adult auditory system following noise exposure, from traumatic to environmental, causing permanent hearing loss, temporary loss, or no audiometric hearing loss.

Types of Noise Exposure

From our previous review [37], I recall three types of noise exposures related to their effects on the auditory system:

1. 'Traumatic noise', defined as sound that causes a permanent threshold shift (PTS) with structural damage to the outer hair cells (OHC), reflected in reduced or absent otoacoustic emissions, and potentially also inner hair cells (IHC). Central consequences are hyperactivity in the cochlear nucleus, the inferior colliculus (IC), the medial geniculate body (MGB), and the auditory cortex [38] but also in nonclassical auditory-responsive cortical areas [39], such as the lateral amygdala and striatum. Whereas in the subthalamic areas only changes in SFR, neural synchrony, and neural gain have been observed, in MGB and A1 tonotopic map reorganization has been documented as well (for a recent review [40]).
2. 'Threatening noise' causes only temporary threshold shifts (TTS), but with potential damage to specific IHC ribbon synapses [41]. This results in subsequent degeneration of low spontaneous firing rate (SFR), high-threshold, and auditory nerve fibers (ANFs). This type of exposure results in auditory 'synaptopathy' [42], also called 'hidden hearing loss' [43].
3. 'Assumed safe' noise exposure is considered <80 dB(A) for 8 h exposure/day. A particular concern is what happens for more prolonged exposures as level-duration tradeoff curves have never been defined outside the 8 h/day exposure range [37]. Given that repeated TTS exposure

can result in a PTS [44], it is not clear what effect long exposure times, say of several weeks, at levels around 70 dB SPL will have. Animal experiments have shown that at these moderate sound levels, even for months of continuous exposure, there is no apparent effect on behavioral and auditory brainstem response (ABR) thresholds, otoacoustic emissions, or hair cell morphology [45, 46].

Traumatic Noise Exposure

Noreña et al. [47] presented the neural changes in cat A1 occurring within a few hours after a 1-h exposure to a 120-dB SPL pure tone (5 or 6 kHz). The exposure resulted in an ABR threshold increase that stabilized after a few hours to on average 40 dB in the frequency range of 6–32 kHz. The trauma induced a shift in characteristic frequency (CF) toward lower frequencies, an emergence of new, unmasked, responses, a broadening of the frequency-tuning curves, and an increase in the maximum of driven firing rate. In the same animals [48] it was found that immediately after the trauma, the SFR was not significantly changed. In contrast, neural synchrony—measured as pairwise spike-firing cross correlations—was increased immediately. The percentage of time that neurons were bursting, the mean burst duration, the number of spikes per burst, and the mean inter-spike interval in a burst were enhanced. A few hours post-trauma, the SFR was increased; however, burst-firing parameters returned to pre-exposure levels. The changes in excitation and inhibition that Scholl and Wehr [6] reported (section "Short-Term Plasticity") are therefore likely to play a role in the different mechanisms active of varying time courses. Sustained enhanced stimulus-driven and SFR across A1 were observed for weeks to months after the trauma [49, 50].

In addition to these changes, molecular studies [51–54] indicate that in the brainstem, after 2–5 days post-trauma, the glutamatergic activity is reduced, whereas glycinergic and GABAergic activity is largely unchanged. At 2 months post-trauma, excitatory activity remains decreased but the inhibitory activity is significantly increased. In contrast, protein assays related to inhibitory transmission are all decreased or unchanged in the brainstem, midbrain, and auditory cortex. Comparison of neurophysiological data [48–50] with the molecular findings during a timeline of changes following noise trauma suggests that increases in SFRs are related to decreases in inhibition and not to increases in excitation. Based on these studies, Eggermont [40] provided a detailed timeline of plastic molecular and electrophysiological changes in excitation, inhibition, SFR, and cross-correlation coefficient following noise trauma, which is slightly modified here—including data from Kalappa et al. [55] and Wu et al. [56] (Table 14.1).

Table 14.1 Changes in auditory structure activity with time after noise trauma

	0 h	2–5 days	16 days	32 days	59 days	145 days
VCN ipsi		⇩	⇑	↑	⇩	↑⇧
DCN ipsi	⇩↓≈	⇩↓⇑	⇑	⇧↑⇑	⇩⇑↑	⇩↑⇑
IC ipsi		↓	↓⇑			
IC contra	↓≈	↓	↓⇑	⇩	⇧⇑	⇧⇑↓
MGB					⇑↑	
A1 ipsi	⇩↓	↓⇑	↓⇑	↓⇑	⇑	
A1 contra	⇩≈↑	⇑↑	⇑↑	↓⇑↑	⇑↑	

⇩⇧ excitation (down, up); ↓↑ inhibition (down, up); ⇓ ⇑ ≈ SFR (down, up, no change); ↑ cross-corr (up)

It is known that tinnitus can occur immediately after acoustic trauma (e.g., [57]). Based on the observation that cross-correlation strengths for SFR were enhanced almost instantaneously following trauma ([48]; Table 14.1), and prior to the onset of SFR increase, correlated network spiking may be acting as a precursor to the ongoing plastic modulation of single cell and network response properties.

Noise Exposure Causing TTS

Peripheral Effects

Kujawa and Liberman [41] found that acoustic exposure—1-octave band of noise (8–16 kHz) at 100 dB SPL, for 2 h—caused moderate, but completely reversible, ABR-threshold elevation, left hair cells intact, but caused acute loss of afferent nerve terminals and delayed degeneration of ANFs. Specifically, there was a selective loss of ANFs with low- and medium-spontaneous rates, i.e., with high thresholds [58]. This suggested that noise-induced damage to the ear has progressive consequences that are considerably more widespread than are revealed by conventional threshold testing. Hickox and Liberman [59] showed that mice with such synaptopathy showed enhanced acoustic startle responses, while exposed mice without neuronal loss showed control-like responses.

Central, Subcortical Effects

Wu et al. [56] introduced a temporary-threshold shift in guinea pigs with exposure to a 7 kHz centered, half-octave noise at 97 dB SPL for 2 h. repeated after 1 week. Two months after exposure, they recorded SFRs from fusiform cells, the principle neurons of the DCN, in nonexposed and exposed (with or without tinnitus) animals with normal ABR thresholds. In tinnitus animals, increased synchrony and bursting were associated with increased SFR. Kalappa et al. [55] recorded from the MGB from unexposed and exposed rats an octave band of noise centered on 16 kHz, at of 116 dB, for 1 h. Two months after exposure, they found that animals with tinnitus exhibited increased SFRs and showed altered burst properties and increased rate-level function slope (sign of central gain), similar to the findings in DCN. Thus, changes in the DCN and MGB are very similar.

Findings in Primary Auditory Cortex

Exposing anesthetized adult cats to a 6 kHz tone at 115 dB SPL for 2 h produced variable ABR thresholds ranging from less than 20 to 60 dB at 10 kHz—the frequency expected to show the highest threshold elevation [60]. In accordance with findings by Rajan [61], we found a fairly sharp demarcation in the average amount of hearing loss (ABR thresholds 20–25 dB) that caused tonotopic map reorganization in A1 (Fig. 14.3 left). Thresholds at CF were correlated with the peripheral hearing loss at near CF frequencies as estimated from ABR measurements. Figure 14.3 right shows a scattergram of CF threshold vs. CF for cats showing reorganization (O) or absence of reorganization (+) of the tonotopic map. In the reorganized parts, thresholds at CF (33 ± 10 dB SPL) were significantly higher compared to parts that did not show reorganization (22 ± 18 dB SPL). In the same animals, Seki and Eggermont [50] found elevated SFRs and peak cross-correlations in frequency regions with reorganization of the tonotopic map compared to the neurons in the non-reorganized cortical frequency regions in the same animals. However, exposed animals showed higher SFRs compared to controls regardless of the presence of cortical reorganization. This may be a correlate of tinnitus in the presence of only minor (< 20 dB) hearing losses.

'Assumed Safe' Noise Exposure

I recently reviewed [45] the central effects of long-term exposure to multifrequency unstructured sounds, termed enhanced acoustic environment (EAE; 4–20 kHz; <80 dB SPL). There were no changes in ABR thresholds. In the A1 of cats exposed to this EAE, multiple sorted-units (MU) and LFP responses to frequencies of 4–20 kHz to sound were reduced to ~10% of normal values, i.e., showed the effect of reduced central gain (Fig. 14.4). In contrast, the 1-octave region above the 4–20 kHz region showed strongly increased MU and LFP responses to sound (increased gain). For frequencies <4 kHz, the increase in gain was most pronounced ~2 octaves below the 4 kHz border. In addition, we found that the cortical region original tuned to 4–20 kHz was now mostly responsive to frequencies above 20 kHz [62], i.e., the tonotopic map was reorganized. In a follow-up study using the same EAE but at lower exposure levels (~68 dB SPL), Pienkowski and Eggermont [63] reported basically the same pattern of findings as in the Noreña et al. [62] study—including normal ABRs and normal otoacoustic emissions—namely a strong reduction in the cortical response to 4–20 kHz sound, combined with a response enhancement for frequencies above and below this region. In addition, corresponding reductions and enhancements in the SFR were found in the 4–20 kHz range and outside this range, respectively. Recovery of these gain changes, reflected in the probability-distribution function of the CFs, took up to 12 weeks after cessation of the exposure. However, it was noticed that at the end of the 12-week recovery period, the tonotopic maps were still

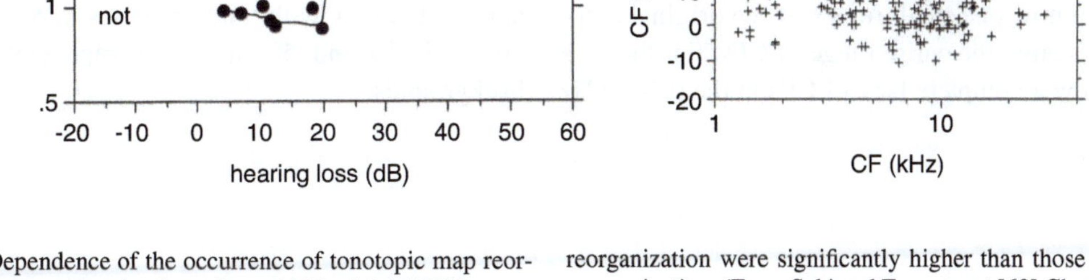

Fig. 14.3 Left. Dependence of the occurrence of tonotopic map reorganization of the average hearing loss above 6 kHz. A LOWESS curve is drawn in. Right. CF threshold as a function CF for cats showing cortical reorganization (a) and those that did not (+). Locally weighted average curves are drawn in. The thresholds for cats showing cortical reorganization were significantly higher than those that did not show reorganization. (From Seki and Eggermont [60] Changes in cat primary auditory cortex after minor-to-moderate pure-tone induced hearing loss Hear Res 173: 172–186, with permission from Elsevier)

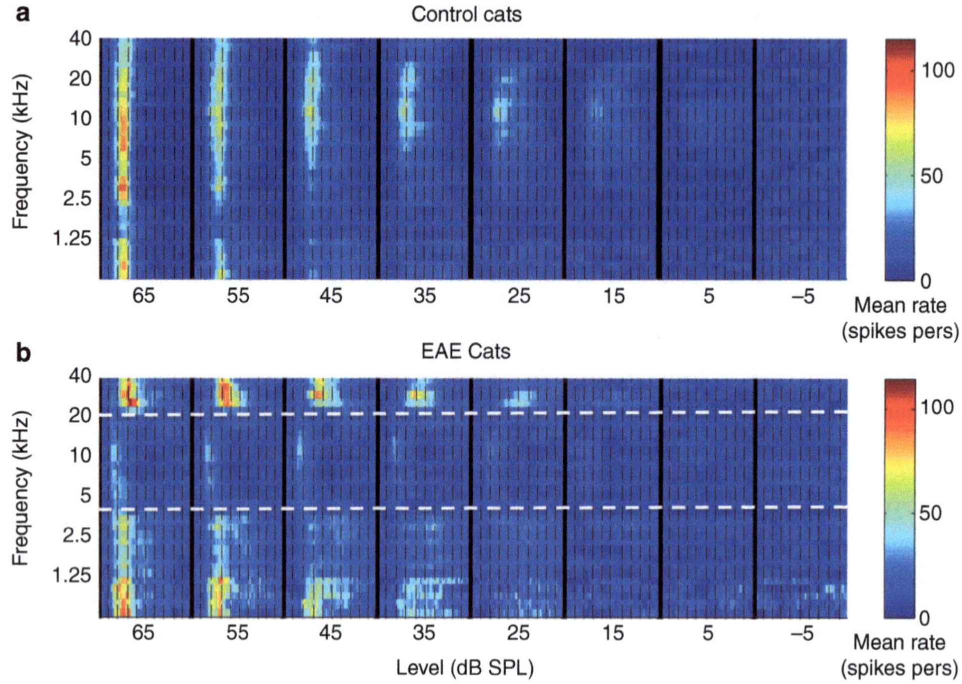

Fig. 14.4 Averaged post-stimulus-time histograms (2-ms time bins) as a function of frequency and SPL, each over a 100-ms time window, in the 15 controls and 4 exposed (EAE) cats. The exposure frequency range is indicated with dashed white lines. (**a**) In control cats, the mean response suggested that the highest sensitivity (lowest thresholds) was to frequencies around 10 kHz and that the largest responses were to frequencies between 2.5 kHz and 10 kHz. (**b**) In EAE cats, the most sensitive frequencies were those below 1.25 kHz and above 20 kHz. Note that neural responses in the EAE cats were much more spread out over time compared to those in control cats. Vertical dashed lines are at 10-ms intervals. Color bars indicate mean firing rate per 2 ms time bin. (From Noreña et al. [62]. Own copyright)

grossly reorganized, so that the center of gravity from all CFs between 4 and 9.9 kHz and the center of gravity for CFs in the octave above (10–20 kHz) were now overlapping in sharp contrast to the distribution in control animals [45, 64]. It appeared that these map changes occurred during the recovery period in a quiet room. This is elucidated in Fig. 14.5, which shows that immediately after the 6-week exposure, the tonotopic map in A1 based on LFPs was largely unchanged save for a downward expansion of the 20–40 kHz CF range, at the detriment of the 10–20 kHz range. This was not as clear for the single units. After 12 weeks recovery, quiet a dramatic change in the single unit data was observed; the location of the CFs was scrambled [45] so that now one small region of the original tonotopic axis represented the entire range of CFs. For the LFP data, there is now a complete lack of CFs in the 0.5–4 kHz range, with an overrepresentation of CFs in the 4–20 kHz range; the number of units that were tuned to frequencies >20 kHz was strongly reduced. Note again that none of these units had increased CF thresholds. One could conceive that the EAE caused a restoration of critical period plasticity (section "Reactivating Critical-Period Plasticity"), and that recovery in a low-noise environment deteriorated the previously existing tonototopic map.

Does this type of exposure cause tinnitus? Pienkowski [65] found that in rat after chronic exposure to 8–16 kHz noise at 70 dB SPL, there were no significant changes in acoustic startle reflex amplitudes evoked by sound at 85- and 105-dB SPL, and no changes in pre-pulse inhibition-amplitude ratios with tone prepulses at 50 and 70 dB SPL, nor with 20 and 50 ms silent gaps embedded in noise backgrounds.

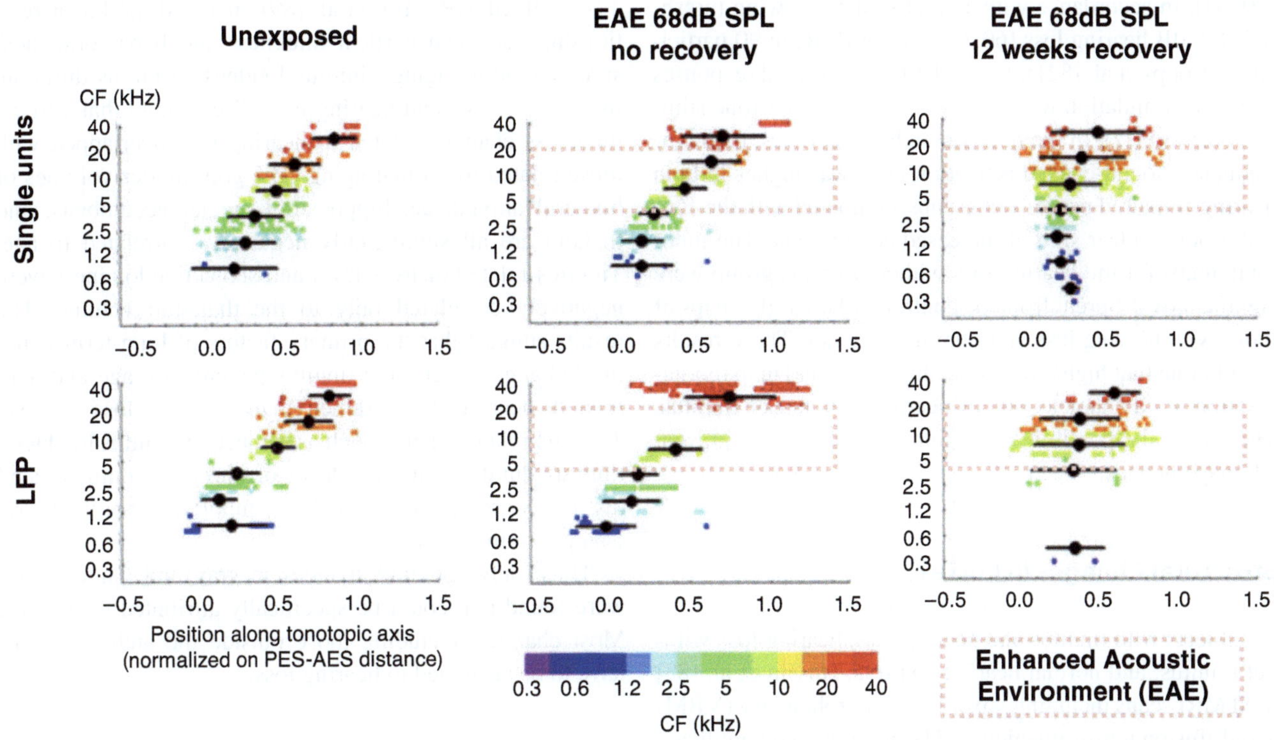

Fig. 14.5 Tonotopic maps, CF vs. location in A1, for a typical unexposed cat (left column), immediately after continuous exposure to a 4e20 kHz sound (middle column), and after 12 weeks recovery in quiet of the same cat (right column). Both single unit data and LFPs data are shown. The horizontal axis is arranged so that the tip of the PES is at coordinate 0.0 and the tip of the AES at 1.0. The positions of the centroids at each CF were estimated along the tonotopic axis. (From Eggermont [45] Effects of long-term non-traumatic noise exposure on the adult central auditory system. Hearing problems without hearing loss. Hear Res 352: 12–22, with permission from Elsevier)

Reactivating Critical-Period Plasticity

Chronic moderate intensity noise exposure in adult animals [66], likely also in our studies [62, 63], decreases cortical parvalbumin expression levels back to that observed in young animals and reinstates the tonotopic plasticity induced by pure tone rearing that is otherwise only observed during the first days after hearing onset. Other studies [67–69] also found a disorganization of tonotopic gradients and disruption of frequency processing in the adult rat A1. This phenomenon has been proposed to occur through a reopening of critical period (CP) plasticity since exposure to pure tones following noise exposure results in their exaggerated representation within the tonotopic map [70].

Critical periods are epochs of early postnatal development, when structural and functional neural circuits are shaped by passive experience with the external environment [71]. As an example, the tonotopic map is established during a CP for frequency tuning, when passive acoustic experiences influence map organization. The timing of CPs is itself plastic and can be influenced by the sensory environment [72]. As Persic et al. [73] wrote: "Unstructured, noisy environments postpone CP closure [74], whereas exposure to highly structured pulsed tones or pulsed white noise hastens CP closure [69, 75]. Enriched sensory environments also keep the CP open longer and have opposite effects to deprivation, stimulating dendritic growth and improving auditory response properties [76]. Effects of sound exposure on CP timing can be further restricted to specific functional regions within the auditory cortex. For example, band-limited noise delays tonotopic refinement only for portions of the tonotopic map within the noise band [77]. The presence of high-fidelity sensory inputs is, therefore, necessary for the normal progression of critical periods and the functional and structural maturation of the primary auditory cortex [78]."

Tinnitus and Maladaptive Plasticity

Tonotopic Map Changes

Early animal studies suggested a relation between hearing loss-induced tonotopic reorganization and tinnitus (e.g., [79]). In humans, fMRI studies have found no evidence of cortical tonotopic reorganization when examining subjects with tinnitus and normal or near-normal hearing thresholds

[80, 81], in accordance with animal studies showing threshold ≤20 dB hearing loss [60, 61]. Using fMRI in 90 participants, Koops et al. [82] measured bilateral cortical responses to sound stimulation with loudness-matched pure-tone stimuli (0.25–8 kHz). In the bilateral auditory cortices, the high-frequency sound-evoked activation level was higher in both hearing-impaired participant groups, compared with the control group, a clear sign of increased central gain. The tonotopic maps for the hearing loss without tinnitus group were significantly different from the controls, whereas the maps of those with hearing loss and tinnitus were not. These results corroborate that higher response amplitudes and map reorganization are a characteristic of hearing loss, not of tinnitus. This raises the possibility that tinnitus sufficient to prevent BF map changes.

Structural Changes in Cortex

In subjects with tinnitus and hearing loss, hearing loss without tinnitus, and normal hearing controls, Husain et al. [83] used MRI scans including voxel-based morphometry (VBM) and diffusion tensor imaging (DTI) and found no significant changes in the gray matter (GM; based on VBM) between the three groups. There were also no significant differences in white matter (WM, based on DTI) in subjects with tinnitus and hearing loss compared to those with hearing loss without tinnitus. Melcher et al. [84] and Boyen et al. [85] found no significant GM volume differences between controls and tinnitus groups either. Allan et al. [86] examined changes in VBM and surface-based morphometry associated with tinnitus and hearing loss, tinnitus with clinically (≤8 kHz) normal hearing, and non-tinnitus controls with clinically normal hearing. The main tinnitus-related significant findings were found outside sensory auditory structures. The results support the notion that structural changes in the brain are not specific to tinnitus, but rather result from auditory deafferentation [87].

Yoo et al. [88] used DTI to analyze how white matter is influenced by tinnitus-related factors. White matter integrity in chronic tinnitus patients was both directly affected by age and also mediated by the hearing loss. The most important changes in white matter regions were found bilaterally in the anterior corona radiata, anterior corpus callosum, and bilateral sagittal strata. In the tractography analysis, the white matter integrity values in tracts of right parahippocampus were correlated with the subjective tinnitus loudness. This DTI study shows that tinnitus is likely not related to any robust white matter changes, with the possible exception of right parahippocampal integrity decrease in a group of young patients without hearing loss. The white matter changes seen in tinnitus patients can be explained by the hearing loss, which is largely determined by age. Using T1-weighted MRI, Yoo et al. [89] analyzed the linear relationships between cortical thickness and behavioral measures including aging, tinnitus loudness, tinnitus duration, tinnitus distress, and hearing loss. They found that cortical thickness changes related to hearing loss overlapped with those related to normal aging. The gray matter volumes of bilateral amygdalae, hippocampi, nuclei accumbens, and thalami are all significantly negatively correlated to age. Tinnitus-related distress level and subjective loudness were negatively correlated only to the thalamic volume. The results suggest that the primary factors of long-term structural changes in chronic tinnitus patients are age and age-related hearing loss, rather than hearing loss per se. Tinnitus-related factors such as subjective tinnitus loudness, tinnitus duration, and the level of chronic tinnitus-related distress were not correlated to important morphometric changes in this study.

Thus, only sporadic changes in gray and white matter were found that could be specifically attributed to tinnitus. Most changes, including those outside the auditory areas, have to be attributed to hearing loss.

Network Connectivity Studies

Hearing Loss without Tinnitus

Luan et al. [90] studied 35 patients with long-term bilateral sensorineural hearing loss (SNHL) and 35 matched healthy controls using structural imaging, resting-state fMRI, diffusion tensor imaging, and neuropsychological assessments. They found "Higher functional coupling between the dorsolateral prefrontal cortex and auditory and visual areas, accompanied by decreased fractional anisotropy along the fronto-occipital fasciculus connecting the frontal cortex and the occipito-temporal area, might mediate cross-modal plasticity via top-down regulation and facilitate the involvement of the auditory cortex in higher-order cognitive processing following long-term SNHL."

Bonna et al. [91] compared the resting-state functional network organization of the brain in early deaf adults and hearing controls and examined global network segregation and integration. In the deaf, regions of the salience network were coupled with the fronto-parietal network, while in the hearing controls, they were coupled with other large-scale networks. Deaf adults showed weaker connections between auditory and somatomotor regions, stronger coupling between the fronto-parietal network and several other large-scale networks (visual, memory, cingulo-opercular, and somatomotor), and an enlargement of the default mode network. Thus, brain plasticity in deaf adults is not limited to changes in the auditory cortex, but additionally alters the coupling between other large-scale networks and the development of functional brain modules. This has consequences for interpreting such changes in tinnitus patients as shown in the next section where I will focus on the activity within, and connectivity between MGB and cortex.

Tinnitus without Hearing Loss

Animal studies show that sodium salicylate (SS) increases the evoked response in the rat auditory thalamus, and functional connectivity (FC) was increased (among others) between auditory cortex (ACx; seed) and MGB, IC, and amygdala. Between MGB (seed) and ACx and hippocampus, as well as for IC (seed) with MGB and hippocampus [92]. Vianney-Rodrigues et al. [93] recorded oscillations in the rat MGB and A1, before and after salicylate. In the MGB, SS reduced theta, alpha, and beta oscillations and decreased coherence (synchrony) between electrode pairs in theta, alpha, and beta bands, but increased coherence in the gamma band. Within A1, SS significantly increased gamma oscillations, decreased theta power, and decreased coherence between electrode pairs in theta and alpha bands, but increased coherence in the gamma band. When coherence was measured between one electrode in the MGB and another in A1, SS decreased coherence in beta, alpha, and theta bands but increased coherence in the gamma band.

In mice, after noise exposure (100-dB SPL white noise binaurally for 2 h.), Qu et al. [94] found increased fMRI responses with amplitude of low-frequency fluctuation (ALFF) in the auditory cortex and decreased ALFF in the amygdala and hippocampus at day 1, but decreased ALFF in the auditory cortex and increased ALFF in the amygdala at day 28 post-noise exposure in tinnitus mice. Decreased functional connectivity between ACx and MGB was demonstrated at day 28 in tinnitus mice.

In humans, connectivity studies between auditory areas have suggested reduced FC between the MGB and ACx based on the FC reduction between IC and ACx [85]. The same group [95] also found the same reduction in connectivity with ACx for IC, but could not substantiate this for the MGB. Using rs-fMRI, Zhang et al. [96] reported decreased FC between the thalamus and primary and associative auditory cortex. This was recently corroborated in an elegant 7 T fMRI study by Berlot et al. [80]. Zhang et al. [96] had found that the decrease in connectivity was significantly correlated with tinnitus duration and THQ score. Leaver et al. [97] identified one resting state network (RSN) not apparent in control data. This tinnitus RSN included auditory–sensory regions like inferior colliculus and medial Heschl's gyrus (no connectivity change), as well as classically nonauditory regions like the mediodorsal nucleus of the thalamus, striatum, lateral prefrontal, and orbitofrontal cortex. Table 14.2 shows a compilation of results from the above-cited tinnitus studies. It is clear that the animal data for salicylate [92, 93] and noise trauma [94] show opposite connectivity patterns for sub-gamma frequencies, but a similar one for gamma. It is also clear that the noise exposure data from animals and tinnitus data from humans are similar.

Table 14.2 Activity and connectivity within/between subcortical and cortical auditory structures

	IC animal	MGB animal	A1 animal	IC human	MGB human	A1 human
IC	$\uparrow^{a}$	$\uparrow^{a}$			$\approx^{b}$	$\Downarrow^{c}$ $\Downarrow^{d} \approx^{e}$
MGB	$\uparrow^{a}$	$\downarrow_{\alpha,\beta,\theta}{}^{f} \sim_{\gamma}{}^{f}$ $\uparrow^{a}$	$\downarrow_{\alpha,\beta,\theta}{}^{f}$ $\uparrow_{\gamma}{}^{f} \uparrow^{a} \downarrow^{g}$	$\approx^{b}$		$\Downarrow^{h}$ $\Downarrow^{b} \approx^{d}$
A1		$\downarrow_{\alpha,\beta,\theta}{}^{f} \uparrow_{\gamma}{}^{f}$ $\uparrow^{a} \downarrow^{g}$	$\downarrow_{\alpha,\beta,\theta}{}^{f} \uparrow_{\gamma}{}^{f}$ $\uparrow^{a} \downarrow^{g}$	$\Downarrow^{c}$ $\Downarrow^{d} \approx^{e}$	$\Downarrow^{h} \Downarrow^{b} \approx^{d}$	

$\uparrow \sim \downarrow$ (up, no change, down), $\Uparrow \approx \Downarrow$ (up, no change, down), $\alpha,\beta,\theta,\gamma$ brain rhythms
All human data based on fMRI
[a]Chen et al. [92] fMRI, salicylate
[b]Berlot et al. [80]
[c]Boyen et al. [85]
[d]Lanting et al. [95]
[e]Leaver et al. [97]
[f]Vianna-Rodriguez et al. [93] LFP, salicylate
[g]Qu et al. [94] fMRI, TTS
[h]Zhang et al. [96]

Maladaptive Plasticity

Common Hypothesis

A common hypothesis is that tinnitus results from a maladaptive imbalance between excitation and inhibition as a result of downregulation of inhibitory amino acid neurotransmission in the central auditory pathway. This loss of inhibition may be a compensatory response to loss of afferent input such as that caused by acoustic insult and/or age-related hearing loss, the most common causes of tinnitus in people. Compensatory plastic changes may result in pathologic neural activity that underpins tinnitus [98]. For example, Dehmel et al. [99] showed that increased efficacy of somatosensory inputs to DCN granule cells after hearing loss is potentially part of this upregulation of SFR. Knipper et al. [100] suggested that "two divergent kinds of hyperactivity at the level of the DCN may differently influence higher brain areas after auditory trauma. Hyperactivity in sound-driven pathways may be regarded in the context of a rather typical compensatory response of a healthy system that, after sensory deprivation, adapts the synaptic strength toward original levels through homeostatic scaling." Shore et al. [101] noted that "animal model studies have identified tinnitus-associated neural changes that commence at the cochlear nucleus and extend to the auditory cortex and other brain regions. Maladaptive neural plasticity seems to underlie these changes: it results in increased spontaneous firing rates and synchrony among neurons in central auditory structures, possibly generating the phantom percept." Wu et al. [14] once more emphasized that "a large body of evidence supports DCN as the site of tinnitus induction, where diminished auditory nerve input initiates hyperactivity, which then spreads to higher areas. … Somatosensory inputs provide a reservoir of excitatory drive that can be tapped during homeostatic changes. It is therefore not surprising that more than two thirds of tinnitus patients are able to modulate tinnitus perception by somatic maneuvers: an epitome of maladaptive auditory–somatosensory plasticity."

Does Analogy with Phantom Pain Refutes this?

I reiterate what I wrote previously [102]. The cause of phantom pain experience has also commonly been attributed to maladaptive plasticity: following loss of sensory input, e.g., the deprived hand area of the primary sensorimotor cortex becomes responsive to inputs from cortical neighbors (for example the face), thereby triggering pain representations relating to the hand. However, Makin et al. [103] showed that, while loss of sensory input is generally characterized by structural and functional degeneration in the deprived sensorimotor cortex, the experience of persistent pain is associated with preserved structure and functional organization in the former hand area. Furthermore, phantom pain is associated with reduced inter-regional functional connectivity in the primary sensorimotor cortex. Makin et al. [103] therefore proposed that contrary to the maladaptive model, cortical plasticity associated with phantom pain is driven by powerful and long-lasting subjective sensory experience, such as triggered by nociceptive or top-down inputs. They suggested that phantom pain be best understood in terms of experience-dependent plasticity, with chronic phantom pain providing the experience. In a maladaptive plasticity model, such reorganization has been associated with phantom limb pain. However, the previously assumed relationship between sensorimotor cortex remapping and pain requires further consideration and thus does not rule out the maladaptive model [104, 105].

Kikkert et al. [106] showed that representation of the missing hand's individual fingers persists in the primary somatosensory cortex even decades after arm amputation. By demonstrating stable topography despite amputation, our finding questions the extent to which continued sensory input is necessary to maintain organization in sensory cortex, thereby reopening the question what happens to a cortical territory once its main input is lost. Kikkert et al. [107] confirm that amputees suffering from worse chronic phantom limb pain have stronger activity in the primary sensorimotor missing hand cortex while performing phantom hand movements.

Makin et al. [103]'s suggestion and Kikkert et al.'s [107] findings, translated to tinnitus, imply that the chronic tinnitus experience, which may be triggered either by bottom-up increased SFRs and neural synchrony or by top-down inputs from auditory-related brain areas, including limbic areas, drives plasticity because it maintains local cortical representations and disrupts inter-regional connectivity. We have seen that tinnitus does occur in the absence of tonotopic map reorganization. Local cortical representation implies a somatic memory for pitch. In case of even severe hearing loss, the missing frequency region still generates the remembered pitch as reflected in the tinnitus spectrum. This would mean that it is the continuing input to the cortex from subcortical structures that activates the auditory frequency-representation memories prior to the hearing loss and so explains the pitch or tinnitus spectrum of tinnitus [81, 82, 108–110]. This does not violate the presence of a reorganized tonotopic map, defined as the representation of CFs on the cortex, which is basically a reflection of the sensitivity of how these neurons respond to sound, not how their spontaneous activity is perceived. The interpretation of disrupted inter-regional connectivity could then be that the connectivity between tonotopic areas and non-tonotopic areas becomes different for spontaneous activity compared to that for stimulus-induced activity [102].

Summarizing, homeostatic plasticity does not need to be maladaptive because the chronic tinnitus percept may either be caused by a malfunctioning gate downstream from auditory cortex or is the result of experience-dependent plasticity with a percept engrained in memory as a result of continuous attention to it [111].

Conclusions

Plasticity occurs at various time scales. In addition to neuronal spike-firing adaptation at a relatively short time scale, central neural responses can be decreased over much longer time periods, e.g., as in habituation. Other forms of synaptic plasticity on this time scale are long-term potentiation, long-term depression, and spike-timing-dependent plasticity and play important roles in determining neural responses. In particular, spectrotemporal receptive fields might have slower timescales of adaptation on the order of minutes to hours.

Critical periods (CPs) are epochs of early postnatal development, when structural and functional neural circuits are shaped by passive experience with the external environment. The timing of CPs is itself plastic and can be influenced by the sensory environment. Unstructured, noisy environments postpone CP closure, whereas exposure to highly structured pulsed tones or pulsed white noise hastens CP closure. Consistent with this, plastic changes in the adult auditory system do occur following noise exposure, from traumatic to environmental, causing permanent hearing loss, temporary loss, or no audiometric hearing loss. Tonotopic map changes are not required for tinnitus to occur; however, tonotopic maps in people with hearing loss without tinnitus group were significantly different from the normal hearing controls, whereas the maps of those with hearing loss and tinnitus were not. These results corroborate that map reorganization is a characteristic of hearing loss, not of tinnitus. This raises the possibility that tinnitus sufficient to prevent BF map changes.

A common hypothesis is that tinnitus results from a maladaptive imbalance between excitation and inhibition as a result of downregulation of inhibitory amino acid neurotransmission in the central auditory pathway. The cause of phantom pain experience has also commonly been attributed to maladaptive plasticity: following loss of sensory input, e.g., the deprived hand area of the primary sensorimotor cortex becomes responsive to inputs from cortical neighbors (for example the face), thereby triggering pain representations relating to the hand. Thus, the effects of neural plasticity underlying noise exposure do not need to be maladaptive because the chronic tinnitus percept may be the result of experience-dependent plasticity with a percept engrained in memory as a result of continuous attention to it.

References

1. Eggermont JJ. Peripheral auditory adaptation and fatigue: a model oriented review. Hear Res. 1985;18:57–71.
2. Eggermont JJ. Animal models of auditory temporal processing. Int J Psychophysiol. 2015;95:201–15.
3. Froemke RC, Schreiner CE. Synaptic plasticity as a cortical coding scheme. Curr Opin Neurobiol. 2015;35:185–99.
4. Gourévitch B, Eggermont JJ. Spectrotemporal sound density dependent long-term adaptation in cat primary auditory cortex. Eur J Neurosci. 2008;27:3310–21.
5. Calford MB, Rajan R, Irvine DRF. Rapid changes in the frequency tuning of neurons in cat auditory cortex resulting from pure-tone-induced temporary threshold shift. Neuroscience. 1993;55:953–64.
6. Scholl B, Wehr M. Disruption of balanced cortical excitation and inhibition by acoustic trauma. J Neurophysiol. 2008;100:646–56.
7. Turrigiano GG. Homeostatic plasticity in neuronal networks: the more things change, the more they stay the same. TINS. 1999;22(5):221–7.
8. Turrigiano GG. The self-tuning neuron: synaptic scaling of excitatory synapses. Cell. 2008;135:422–35.
9. Turrigiano G. Homeostatic synaptic plasticity: local and global mechanisms for stabilizing neuronal function. Cold Spring Harb Perspect Biol. 2012;4:a005736.
10. Wang J, Ding D, Salvi RJ. Functional reorganization in chinchilla inferior colliculus associated with chronic and acute cochlear damage. Hear Res. 2002;168:238–49.
11. Caspary DM, Ling L, Turner JG, Hughes LF. Inhibitory neurotransmission, plasticity and aging in the mammalian central auditory system. J Exp Biol. 2008;211:1781–91.
12. Sedley W. Tinnitus: does gain explain? Neuroscience. 2019;407:213–28.
13. Gütig R, Aharonov R, Rotter S, Sompolinsky H. Learning input correlations through nonlinear temporally asymmetric Hebbian plasticity. J Neurosci. 2003;23:3697–714.
14. Wu C, Stefanescu RA, Martel DT, Shore SE. Tinnitus: maladaptive auditory-somatosensory plasticity. Hear Res. 2016a;334:20–9.
15. Tzounopoulos T, Kim Y, Oertel D, Trussell LO. Cell-specific, spike timing-dependent plasticities in the dorsal cochlear nucleus. Nat Neurosci. 2004;7:719–25.
16. Tzounopoulos T, Rubio ME, Keen JE, Trussell LO. Coactivation of pre- and postsynaptic signaling mechanisms determines cell-specific spike-timing-dependent plasticity. Neuron. 2007;54:291–301.
17. Zhao Y, Tzounopoulos T. Physiological activation of cholinergic inputs controls associative synaptic plasticity via modulation of endocannabinoid signaling. J Neurosci. 2011;31:3158–68.
18. Shore SE, Wu C. Mechanisms of noise-induced tinnitus: insights from cellular studies. Neuron. 2019;103:8–20.
19. Huttenlocher PR, Dabholkar AS. Regional differences in synaptogenesis in human cerebral cortex. J Comp Neurol. 1997;387:167–78.
20. Paus T, Collins DL, Evans AC, Leonard G, Pike B, Zijdenbos A. Maturation of white matter in the human brain: a review of magnetic resonance studies. Brain Res Bull. 2001;54:255–66.
21. Fair DA, Cohen AL, Dosenbach NUF, Church JA, Miezin FM, Barch DM, et al. The maturing architecture of the brain's default network. Proc Natl Acad Sci U S A. 2008;105(10):4028–32.
22. Dubois J, Adibpour P, Poupon C, Hertz-Pannier L, Dehaene-Lambertz G. MRI and M/EEG studies of the white matter development in human fetuses and infants: review and opinion. Brain Plast. 2016a;2:49–69. https://doi.org/10.3233/BPL-160031.
23. Dubois J, Hertz-Pannier L, Dehaene-Lambertz G, Cointepas Y, Le Bihan D. Assessment of the early organization and maturation of infants' cerebral white matter fiber bundles: a feasibility study using quantitative diffusion tensor imaging and tractography. Neuroimage. 2006;30(4):1121–32.
24. Kulikova S, Hertz-Pannier L, Dehaene-Lambertz G, Buzmakov A, Poupon C, Dubois J. Multi-parametric evaluation of the white matter maturation. Brain Struct Funct. 2015;220(6):3657–72.
25. Geng X, Gouttard S, Sharma A, Gu H, Styner M, Lin W, et al. Quantitative tract-based white matter development from birth to age 2 years. NeuroImage. 2012;61(3):542–57.
26. Dubois J, Poupon C, Thirion B, Simonnet H, Kulikova S, Leroy F, et al. Exploring the early organization and maturation of linguistic pathways in the human infant brain. Cereb Cortex. 2016b;26:2283–98.
27. Fransson P, Åden U, Blennow M, Lagercrantz H. The functional architecture of the infant brain as revealed by resting-state fMRI. Cereb Cortex. 2011;21:145–54.
28. He L, Parikh NA. Brain functional network connectivity development in very preterm infants: the first six months. Early Hum Dev. 2016;98:29–35.
29. Striem-Amit E, Almeida J, Belledonne M, Chen Q, Fang Y, Han Z, et al. Topographical functional connectivity patterns exist in the congenitally, prelingually deaf. Sci Rep. 2016;6:29375. https://doi.org/10.1038/srep29375.
30. Meredith MA, Lomber SG. Somatosensory and visual crossmodal plasticity in the anterior auditory field of early-deaf cats. Hear Res. 2011;280(1–2):38–47.
31. Meredith MA, Kryklywy J, McMillan AJ, Malhotra S, Lum-Tai R, Lomber SG. Crossmodal reorganization in the early deaf switches sensory, but not behavioral roles of auditory cortex. Proc Natl Acad Sci U S A. 2011;108(21):8856–61.
32. Barone P, Lacassagne L, Kral A. Reorganization of the connectivity of cortical field DZ in congenitally deaf cat. PLoS One. 2013;8:e60093.

33. Finney EM, Fine I, Dobkins KR. Visual stimuli activate auditory cortex in the deaf. Nat Neurosci. 2001;4:1171–3.
34. Karns CM, Dow MW, Neville HJ. Altered cross-modal processing in the primary auditory cortex of congenitally deaf adults: a visual-somatosensory fMRI study with a double-flash illusion. J Neurosci. 2012;32:9626–38.
35. Glick G, Sharma A. Cross-modal plasticity in developmental and age-related hearing loss: clinical implications. Hear Res. 2017;343:191–201.
36. Bola Ł, Zimmermann M, Mostowski P, Jednoróg K, Marchewka A, Rutkowski P, Szwed M. Task-specific reorganization of the auditory cortex in deaf humans. Proc Natl Acad Sci U S A. 2017;114(4):E600–9.
37. Gourévitch B, Edeline JM, Occelli F, Eggermont JJ. Is the din really harmless? Long-term effects of non-traumatic noise on the adult auditory system. Nat Rev Neurosci. 2014;15:483–91.
38. Eggermont JJ. The neuroscience of tinnitus. Oxford: Oxford University Press; 2012.
39. Chen G-D, Sheppard A, Salvi R. Noise trauma induced plastic changes in brain regions outside the classical auditory pathway. Neuroscience. 2016;315:228–45.
40. Eggermont JJ. Acquired hearing loss and brain plasticity. Hear Res. 2017a;343:176–90.
41. Kujawa SG, Liberman MC. Adding insult to injury: cochlear nerve degeneration after 'temporary' noise-induced hearing loss. J Neurosci. 2009;29:14077–85.
42. Kujawa SG, Liberman MC. Synaptopathy in the noise-exposed and aging cochlea: primary neural degeneration in acquired sensorineural hearing loss. Hear Res. 2015;330:191–9.
43. Schaette R, McAlpine D. Tinnitus with a normal audiogram: physiological evidence for hidden hearing loss and computational model. J Neurosci. 2011;31:13452–7.
44. Wang Y, Ren C. Effects of repeated 'benign' noise exposures in young, CBA mice: shedding light on age-related hearing loss. J Assoc Res Otolaryngol. 2012;13:505–15.
45. Eggermont JJ. Effects of long-term non-traumatic noise exposure on the adult central auditory system. Hearing problems without hearing loss. Hear Res. 2017b;352:12–22.
46. Pienkowski M, Eggermont JJ. Reversible long-term changes in auditory processing in mature auditory cortex in the absence of hearing loss induced by passive, moderate-level sound exposure. Ear Hear. 2012;33:305–14.
47. Norena AJ, Tomita M, Eggermont JJ. Neural changes in cat auditory cortex after a transient pure-tone trauma. J Neurophysiol. 2003;90:2387–401.
48. Noreña AJ, Eggermont JJ. Changes in spontaneous neural activity immediately after an acoustic trauma: implications for neural correlates of tinnitus. Hear Res. 2003;183:137–53.
49. Noreña AJ, Eggermont JJ. Enriched acoustic environment after noise trauma abolishes neural signs of tinnitus. Neuroreport. 2006;17:559–63.
50. Seki S, Eggermont JJ. Changes in spontaneous firing rate and neural synchrony in cat primary auditory cortex after localized tone-induced hearing loss. Hear Res. 2003;180:28–38.
51. Muly SM, Gross JS, Potashner SJ. Noise trauma alters D-[^{3}H] aspartate release and AMPA binding in chinchilla cochlear nucleus. J Neurosci Res. 2004;75:585–96.
52. Potashner SJ, Suneja SK, Benson CG. Regulation of D-aspartate release and uptake in adult brain stem auditory nuclei after unilateral middle ear ossicle removal and cochlear ablation. Exp Neurol. 1997;148:222–35.
53. Suneja SK, Benson CG, Potashner SJ. Glycine receptors in adult guinea pig brain stem auditory nuclei: regulation after unilateral cochlear ablation. Exp Neurol. 1998a;154:473–88.
54. Suneja SK, Potashner SJ, Benson CG. Plastic changes in glycine and GABA release and uptake in adult brain stem auditory nuclei after unilateral middle ear ossicle removal and cochlear ablation. Exp Neurol. 1998b;151:273–88.
55. Kalappa BI, Brozoski TJ, Turner JG, Caspary DM. Single unit hyperactivity and bursting in the auditory thalamus of awake rats directly correlates with behavioural evidence of tinnitus. J Physiol. 2014;592(22):5065–78.
56. Wu C, Martel DT, Shore SE. Increased synchrony and bursting of dorsal cochlear nucleus fusiform cells correlate with tinnitus. J Neurosci. 2016b;36(6):2068–73.
57. Loeb M, Smith RP. Relation of induced tinnitus to physical characteristics of the inducing stimuli. J Acoust Soc Am. 1967;42:453–5.
58. Furman AC, Kujawa SG, Liberman MC. Noise-induced cochlear neuropathy is selective for fibers with low spontaneous rates. J Neurophysiol. 2013;110:577–86.
59. Hickox AE, Liberman MC. Is noise-induced cochlear neuropathy key to the generation of hyperacusis or tinnitus? J Neurophysiol. 2014;111:552–64.
60. Seki S, Eggermont JJ. Changes in cat primary auditory cortex after minor-to-moderate pure-tone induced hearing loss. Hear Res. 2002;173:172–86.
61. Rajan R. Receptor organ damage causes loss of cortical surround inhibition without topographic map plasticity. Nat Neurosci. 1998;1:138–43.
62. Noreña AJ, Gourévitch B, Aizawa N, Eggermont JJ. Spectrally enhanced acoustic environment disrupts frequency representation in cat auditory cortex. Nat Neurosci. 2006;9:932–9.
63. Pienkowski M, Eggermont JJ. Long-term, partially-reversible reorganization of frequency tuning in mature cat primary auditory cortex can be induced by passive exposure to moderate-level sounds. Hear Res. 2009;257:24–40.
64. Eggermont JJ. On the similarities and differences of non-traumatic sound exposure during the critical period and in adulthood. Front Syst Neurosci. 2013;7:12. https://doi.org/10.3389/fnsys.2013.00012.
65. Pienkowski M. Prolonged exposure of CBA/Ca mice to moderately loud noise can cause cochlear synaptopathy but not tinnitus or hyperacusis as assessed with the acoustic startle reflex. Trends Hear. 2018;22:2331216518758109. https://doi.org/10.1177/2331216518758109.
66. Zhou X, Panizzutti R, de Villers-Sidani E, Madeira C, Merzenich MM. Natural restoration of critical period plasticity in the juvenile and adult primary auditory cortex. J Neurosci. 2011;31:5625–34.
67. Thomas ME, Friedman NHM, Cisneros-Franco JM, Ouellet L, de Villers-Sidani E. The prolonged masking of temporal acoustic inputs with noise drives plasticity in the adult rat auditory cortex. Cereb Cortex. 2019;29:1032–46.
68. Zheng W. Auditory map reorganization and pitch discrimination in adult rats chronically exposed to low-level ambient noise. Front Syst Neurosci. 2012;6:65.
69. Zhou X, Merzenich MM. Environmental noise exposure degrades normal listening processes. Nat Commun. 2012;3:843.
70. Schreiner CE, Polley DB. Auditory map plasticity: diversity in causes and consequences. Curr Opin Neurobiol. 2014;24:143–56.
71. Hensch TK. Critical period plasticity in local cortical circuits. Nat Rev Neurosci. 2005;6(11):877–88.
72. Voss P, Thomas ME, Cisneros-Franco JM, de Villers-Sidani E. Dynamic brains and the changing rules of neuroplasticity: implications for learning and recovery. Front Psychol. 2017;8:1657.
73. Persic D, Thomas ME, Pelekanos V, Ryugo DK, Takesian AE, Krumbholz K, Pyott SJ. Regulation of auditory plasticity during critical periods and following hearing loss. Hear Res. 2020;397:107976.
74. Chang EF, Merzenich MM. Environmental noise retards auditory cortical development. Science. 2003;300:498–502.

75. Zhang LI, Bao S, Merzenich MM. Disruption of primary auditory cortex by synchronous auditory inputs during a critical period. Proc Natl Acad Sci U S A. 2002;99:2309–14.
76. Bures Z, Pysanenko K, Lindovsky J, Syka J. Acoustical enrichment during early development improves response reliability in the adult auditory cortex of the rat. Neural Plast. 2018;2018:5903720.
77. de Villers-Sidani E, Simpson KL, Lu YF, Lin RC, Merzenich MM. Manipulating critical period closure across different sectors of the primary auditory cortex. Nat Neurosci. 2008;11:957–65.
78. de Villers-Sidani E, Merzenich MM. Lifelong plasticity in the rat auditory cortex: basic mechanisms and role of sensory experience. Prog Brain Res. 2011;191:119–31.
79. Eggermont JJ, Roberts LE. The neuroscience of tinnitus. Trends Neurosci. 2004;27:676–82.
80. Berlot E, Arts R, Smitd J, George E, Gulban OF, Moerel M, Stokroos R, Formisano E, De Martino F. A 7 tesla fMRI investigation of human tinnitus percept in cortical and subcortical auditory areas. Neuroimage Clin. 2020;25:102166.
81. Langers DM, de Kleine E, van Dijk P. Tinnitus does not require macroscopic tonotopic map reorganization. Front Syst Neurosci. 2012;6:2.
82. Koops EA, Renken RJ, Lanting CP, van Dijk P. Cortical tonotopic map changes in humans are larger in hearing loss than in additional tinnitus. J Neurosci. 2020;40(16):3178–85.
83. Husain FT, Medina RE, Davis CW, Szymko-Bennett Y, Simonyan K, Pajor NM, et al. Neuroanatomical changes due to hearing loss and chronic tinnitus: a combined VBM and DTI study. Brain Res. 2011;1369:74–88.
84. Melcher JR, Knudson IM, Levine RA. Subcallosal brain structure: correlation with hearing threshold at supra-clinical frequencies (>8 kHz), but not with tinnitus. Hear Res. 2013;295:79–86.
85. Boyen K, de Kleine E, van Dijk P, Langers DRM. Tinnitus-related dissociation between cortical and subcortical neural activity in humans with mild to moderate sensorineural hearing loss. Hear Res. 2014;312:48–59.
86. Allan TW, Besle J, Langers DRM, Davies J, Hall DA, Palmer AR, Adjamian P. Neuroanatomical alterations in tinnitus assessed with magnetic resonance imaging. Front Aging Neurosci. 2016;8:221. https://doi.org/10.3389/fnagi.2016.00221.
87. Adjamian P, Hall DA, Palmer AR, Allan TW, Langers DR. Neuroanatomical abnormalities in chronic tinnitus in the human brain. Neurosci Biobehav Rev. 2014;45:119–33.
88. Yoo HB, De Ridder D, Vanneste S. White matter changes in tinnitus: is it all age and hearing loss? Brain Connect. 2016a;6(1):84–93. https://doi.org/10.1089/brain.2015.0380.
89. Yoo HB, De Ridder D, Vanneste S. The importance of aging in gray matter changes within tinnitus patients shown in cortical thickness, surface area and volume. Brain Topogr. 2016b;29(6):885–96.
90. Luan Y, Wang C, Jiao Y, Tang T, Zhang J, Teng G-J. Prefrontal-temporal pathway mediates the cross-modal and cognitive reorganization in sensorineural hearing loss with or without tinnitus: a multimodal MRI study. Front Neurosci. 2019;13:222. https://doi.org/10.3389/fnins.2019.00222.
91. Bonna K, Finc K, Zimmermann M, Bola L, Mostowski P, Szul M, et al. Early deafness leads to re-shaping of functional connectivity beyond the auditory cortex. Brain Imaging Behav. 2020;15(3):1469–82.
92. Chen Y-C, Li X, Liu L, Wang J, Lu C-Q, Yang M, et al. Tinnitus and hyperacusis involve hyperactivity and enhanced connectivity in auditory-limbic-arousal-cerebellar network. eLife. 2015;4:e06576. https://doi.org/10.7554/eLife.06576.
93. Vianney-Rodrigues P, Auerbach BD, Salvi R. Aberrant thalamocortical coherence in an animal model of tinnitus. J Neurophysiol. 2019;121:893–907.
94. Qu T, Qi Y, Yu S, Du Z, Wei W, Cai A, et al. Dynamic changes of functional neuronal activities between the auditory pathway and limbic systems contribute to noise-induced tinnitus with a normal audiogram. Neuroscience. 2019;408:31–45.
95. Lanting CP, de Kleine E, Langers DRM, van Dijk P. Unilateral tinnitus: changes in connectivity and response lateralization measured with fMRI. PLoS One. 2014;9(10):e110704. https://doi.org/10.1371/journal.pone.01107.
96. Zhang J, Chen Y-C, Feng X, Yang M, Liu B, Qian C, et al. Impairments of thalamic resting-state functional connectivity in patients with chronic tinnitus. Eur J Radiol. 2015;84:1277–84.
97. Leaver AM, Turesky TK, Seydell-Greenwald A, Morgan S, Kim HJ, Rauschecker JP. Intrinsic network activity in tinnitus investigated using functional MRI. Hum Brain Mapp. 2016;37:2717–35.
98. Wang H, Brozoski TJ, Caspary DM. Inhibitory neurotransmission in animal models of tinnitus: maladaptive plasticity. Hear Res. 2011;279:111–7.
99. Dehmel S, Eisinger D, Shore SE. Gap prepulse inhibition and auditory brainstem-evoked potentials as objective measures for tinnitus in guina pigs. Front Syst Neurosci. 2012;6:42.
100. Knipper M, Müller M, Zimmermann U. Molecular mechanisms of tinnitus. In: Eggermont JJ, Zeng F-G, Popper AN, Fay RR, editors. Springer handbook of auditory research 44. New York: Springer; 2012. p. 59–82.
101. Shore SE, Roberts LE, Langguth B. Maladaptive plasticity in tinnitus — triggers, mechanisms and treatment. Nat Rev Neurol. 2016;12(3):150–60.
102. Eggermont JJ. Tinnitus: maladaptive plasticity? In: Dau T, Santurette S, Dalgaard JC, Tranebjaerg L, Andersen T, Poulsen T, editors. Proceedings of ISAAR 2013, auditory plasticity-listening with the brain. 4th symposium on auditory and audiological research; 2014. p. 141–52.
103. Makin TR, Scholz J, Filippini N, Slater DH, Tracey I, Johansen-Berg H. Phantom pain is associated with preserved structure and function in the former hand area. Nat Commun. 2013;4:1570. https://doi.org/10.1038/ncomms2571.
104. Makin TR, Flor H. Brain (re)organisation following amputation: implications for phantom limb pain. NeuroImage. 2020;218:116943.
105. Raffin E, Richard N, Giraux P, Reilly KT. Primary motor cortex changes after amputation correlate with phantom limb pain and the ability to move the phantom limb. NeuroImage. 2016;130:134–44.
106. Kikkert S, Kolasinski J, Jbabdi S, Tracey I, Beckmann CF, Heidi Johansen-Berg H, Makin TR. Revealing the neural fingerprints of a missing hand. eLife. 2016;5:e15292. https://doi.org/10.7554/eLife.15292.
107. Kikkert S, Johansen-Berg H, Tracey I, Makin TR. Reaffirming the link between chronic phantomlimb pain and maintained missing hand representation. Cortex. 2018;106:174–84.
108. Mulders WH, Robertson D. Progressive centralization of midbrain hyperactivity after acoustic trauma. Neuroscience. 2011;192:753–60.
109. Noreña A, Micheyl C, Chery-Croze S, Collet L. Psychoacoustic characterization of the tinnitus spectrum: implications for the underlying mechanisms of tinnitus. Audiol Neurootol. 2002;7:358–69.
110. Roberts LE, Moffat G, Baumann M, Ward LM, Bosnyak DJ. Residual inhibition functions overlap tinnitus spectra and the region of auditory threshold shift. J Assoc Res Otolaryngol. 2008;9:417–35.
111. Hullfish J, Abenes I, Yoo HB, De Ridder D, Vanneste S. Frontostriatal network dysfunction as a domain-general mechanism underlying phantom perception. Hum Brain Mapp. 2019;40:2241–51.

Structural and Functional MRI-Based Neuroimaging in Tinnitus

15

Katherine Adcock, Dirk De Ridder, and Sven Vanneste

Abstract

Tinnitus, or the perception of phantom sound, affects millions of individuals worldwide. Tinnitus is characterized by a specific loudness, inducing emotional, autonomic, and cognitive responses. It can become chronic and be associated with suffering, resulting in tinnitus disorder. Tinnitus disorder is characterized by emotional, autonomic, and cognitive dysfunctioning. Structural and functional neuroimaging approaches have advanced the understanding of tinnitus pathology and its comorbidity. Here, we will discuss various neuroimaging studies that observe neuroanatomical and neurophysiological dysfunction in both auditory and non-auditory regions in patients with chronic tinnitus. We then extend this evidence to proposed models that aim to delineate dysfunctional interactions between whole brain networks that may ascribe complex tinnitus characteristics such as chronification and cognitive dysfunction. Network-based models can provide a testbed for evaluation and develop a foundation for future studies to capture the full portrayal of chronic tinnitus in the clinic.

K. Adcock (✉) · S. Vanneste
Global Brain Health Institute and Institute of Neuroscience, Trinity College Dublin, Dublin, Ireland

Lab for Clinical and Integrative Neuroscience, Trinity Institute for Neuroscience, School of Psychology, Trinity College Dublin, Dublin, Ireland
e-mail: Adcockk@tcd.ie; sven.vanneste@tcd.ie

D. De Ridder
Section of Neurosurgery, Department of Surgical Sciences, University of Otago, Dunedin, New Zealand
e-mail: dirk.deridder@otago.ac.nz

W. Schlee et al. (eds.), *Textbook of Tinnitus*, https://doi.org/10.1007/978-3-031-35647-6_15

Graphical Abstract

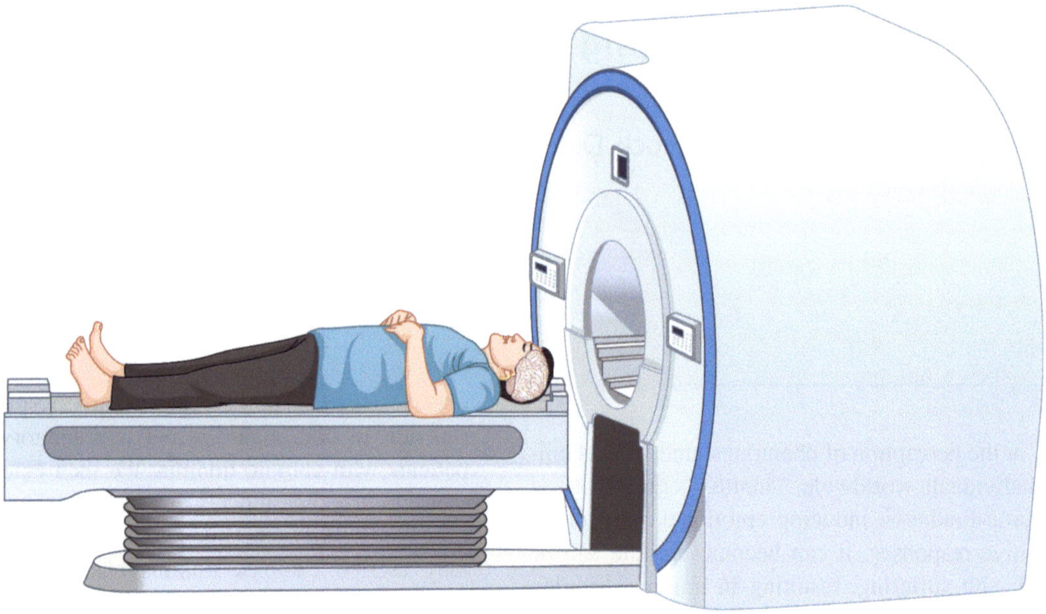

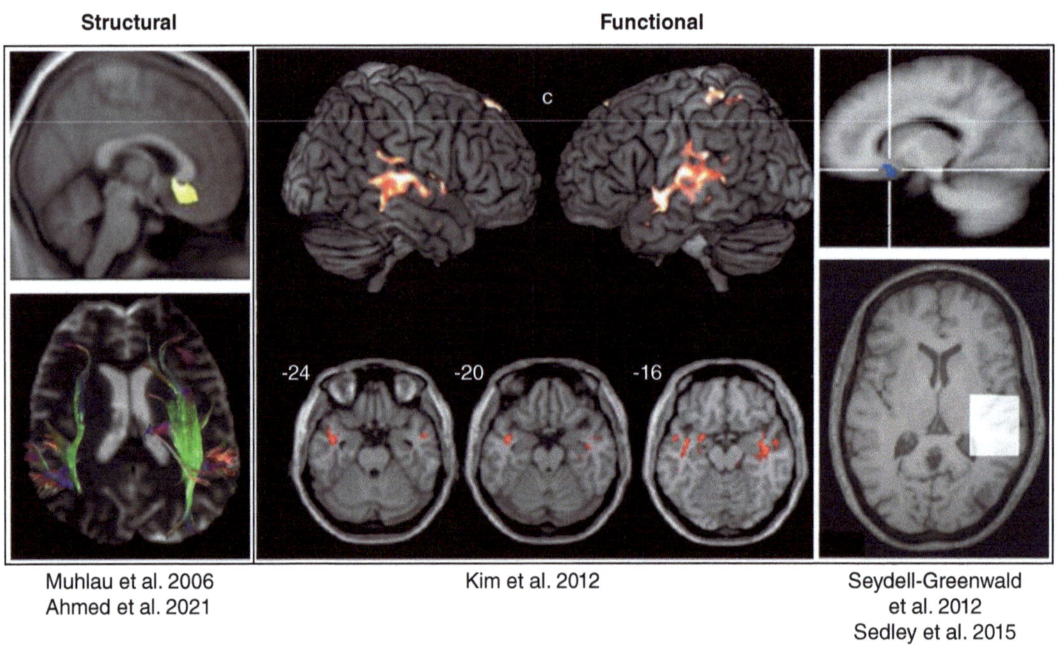

Highlights

- Tinnitus can consist of several characteristics such as tinnitus loudness, distress, hearing loss, duration (chronification), and cognitive disability.
- Structural and functional neuroimaging studies have identified anomalies in both auditory and non-auditory regions.
- VBM and DTI studies have identified age-related structural changes in tinnitus patients.
- Task-based and resting-state fMRI observed changes relating to distress, cognitive dysfunction, and chronification of tinnitus.
- Models may assist in discovering neural correlates to attribute complex tinnitus components.

Introduction

Chronic tinnitus has been defined as the conscious awareness of a tonal or composite noise for which there is no identifiable corresponding external acoustic source [1]. Tinnitus disorder, on the other hand, arises when the tinnitus sound component is associated with emotional distress, cognitive dysfunction, and/or autonomic arousal, leading to behavioural changes and functional disability [1]. In other words, "Tinnitus" describes the auditory or phantom sound component, whereas "Tinnitus Disorder" reflects the suffering associated with the phantom sound [1].

Tinnitus is characterized by a specific loudness, inducing emotional, autonomic, and cognitive responses [2]. Whereas acute tinnitus may be a symptom secondary trauma or disease, chronic tinnitus may be considered a primary disorder in its own right [1]. Tinnitus is often associated with hearing loss, and most pathophysiological treatments assume the hearing loss to be the trigger of the tinnitus [3, 4]. The technological advancement of structural and functional neuroimaging techniques has contributed greatly to our understanding of the tinnitus pathophysiology and its associated comorbidities. One of these techniques is functional resonance magnetic imaging (fMRI). fMRI uses blood oxygen level-dependent functional imaging (BOLD-fMRI), which identifies changes in blood oxygenation associated with neural activity that can be measured at rest (i.e., resting-state fMRI) or during a task (i.e., task-based fMRI). In tinnitus, task-based fMRI design commonly uses various sound stimuli to induce changes in blood oxygen to look at changes in specific brain areas. Resting-state fMRI is used to analyse functional brain network connectivity at rest. Magnetic resonance spectroscopy (MRS) can measure different metabolites. In addition to functional MRI methods, also structural MRI methods exist, such as diffusion weighted imaging (DWI), perfusion weighted imaging (PWI), susceptibility weighted imaging (SWI), voxel-based morphometry (VBM), and volume and thickness measures. Diffusion tensor imaging (DTI) is a form of DWI that can evaluate the anisotropy (having different properties in different directions) of white matter, thereby observing and tracking white matter fibre bundles. While these measures focus on white matter, common methods to look at grey matter changes are VBM and volume and thickness measures. In this chapter, we will highlight VBM, DTI, MRS, tasked-based fMRI, and resting-state fMRI methods in relationship to tinnitus and how they help to better understand the underlying neural mechanism related to tinnitus. We also extend these findings to previously proposed models of tinnitus.

Structural Imaging

Despite tinnitus being highly prevalent, with 15% of the population experiencing tinnitus, and 2–3% severely suffering from it [5, 6], the pathology of tinnitus remains poorly understood. Neuroimaging studies offer a way to identify tinnitus-related changes in the brain, and subsequently provide insight to potential mechanisms. Several studies have highlighted structural changes in both auditory and non-auditory regions affected by tinnitus. Notably, structural imaging studies have observed changes within gray and white matter that may elucidate the age-related hearing loss component in tinnitus.

Gray and White Matter Changes

Voxel-based morphometry (VBM) studies have revealed changes in gray matter concentration within the limbic system and auditory network. VBM in combination with high-resolution magnetic resonance imaging is one technique that can detect region-specific changes in concentration or volume of gray and white matter at a group level. However, the histological correlates of VBM are unknown and may include changes in the amount of cells (neurons and glial cells), changes in the size of cells (neurons or glial), but could also involve angiogenesis and endothelial cell proliferation, or shifts in dendritic spine size and density, and remodelling of axonal processes or alterations of the extracellular space (e.g. by changes in blood-perfusion and ultrafiltration, edema, glymphatic system) [7]. Within the limbic system, a significant decrease of gray-matter volume was observed in the subcallosal area, including the nucleus accumbens, of tinnitus patients [8]. This is corroborated in a separate study, in which tinnitus patients again displayed structural differences in the subcallosal region, specifically within the ventromedial prefrontal cortex (vmPFC) [9]. Tinnitus patients had significantly reduced signal intensity for gray matter area and led to a corresponding increase in signal intensity for white matter within the vmPFC compared to healthy controls. Within the auditory network of tinnitus patients, evidence revealed an increase in gray matter concentration in the right posterior thalamus, including the medial geniculate nucleus [8]. Another study found primary auditory cortex volume loss in the medial portion of Heschl's gyrus (HG) of tinnitus patients compared to healthy controls [10]. This is contradictory with other results demonstrating increased auditory cortex volume [11], in addition to several studies finding no changes in the auditory cortex of tinnitus patients [8, 9, 12–17].

Conflicting findings of tinnitus-related structural changes in the brain could be due to a number of confounding variables, including differences in methods, study design, or the control group used. Given this, studies have more recently begun controlling for variables such as hearing loss and age. Evidence supports that many structural differences observed within auditory, hippocampal, thalamic, and cerebellar areas were related to hearing loss, but not tinnitus, in tinnitus patients [18]. Furthermore, aging appears to play a significant role in gray matter changes. A study using surface-based image analyses to assess cortical thickness, surface-based areas, and gray matter volume found that aging, rather than hearing loss alone, appears to be the dominant factor in influencing structural changes in chronic tinnitus patients [19]. Both cortical thickness and gray matter volume were negatively correlated with age in widespread frontal regions and positively correlated with the bilateral entorhinal cortex and left rostral anterior cingulate cortex. In addition, gray matter volumes of limbic structures such as bilateral amygdalae, hippocampi, nuclei accumbens, and thalami were also all correlated to age. Tinnitus-related distress level and tinnitus loudness were negatively correlated to thalamic volume, suggesting that the thalamus may play a role in both the affective and sensory component of tinnitus [19]. Overall, findings have consistently shown that gray matter structural changes in chronic tinnitus patients are primarily explained by aging [19, 20].

Similarly, other studies using Diffusor Tensor Imaging (DTI) suggested that structural changes in white matter could be explained by age-related hearing loss, rather than tinnitus characteristics alone [21, 22]. DTI is a structural neuroimaging method used to assess white matter integrity through mapping the diffusion process of water molecules [23, 24]. Ahmed et al. assessed white matter integrity in two tracts: the arcuate fasciculus tract connecting auditory cortex with frontal and parietal cortices [25] and associated with cognitive expression of mood [26], and the acoustic radiation tract connecting the auditory thalamus to auditory cortex that conveys auditory information [27]. Tinnitus patients exhibited structural changes in white matter integrity, as seen by a reduction in tract density in both the arcuate fasciculus and acoustic radiation compared to healthy controls. Correlations controlled for hearing loss and loudness revealed that the left arcuate fasciculus changes are related with tinnitus distress. Additionally, correlations controlled for loudness and distress revealed that the left and right acoustic radiation changes are related to hearing loss [22]. These results provide initial evidence of the structural correlates within the white matter tracts in relation to tinnitus characteristics, after controlling for potential confounding variables. Furthermore, this study demonstrates that dysfunctional thalamic connections may contribute to hearing loss, and dysfunctional cortical connections may contribute to the cognitive or emotional component of tinnitus. In the same study, there was no relationship observed between the structural changes and tinnitus loudness. This is consistent with previous studies, showing structural changes may be due to hearing loss rather than the tinnitus loudness itself [19, 21, 28], suggesting that the sensory component of tinnitus may be due to functional changes rather than structural [22].

Functional Imaging

Functional imaging approaches aid in discovering complex neural mechanisms in tinnitus patients. Functional imaging techniques offer an avenue to delineate properties of neural activity such as location, strength, and functional connections that are temporally related within the central nervous system. One method of functional imaging is tracking blood oxygenation level-dependent (BOLD) signals with fMRI, which uses changes in blood oxygenation levels in the progress of neural activity. Fluctuations in BOLD signals can be measured during task-based fMRI, in which brain activity is examined when external stimuli such as sounds are presented, or resting-state fMRI, in which spontaneous brain activity is examined when no external stimuli are present. Compared to task-based fMRI, resting-state fMRI is considered advantageous in tinnitus patients since the tinnitus percept and distress is present constantly, even at rest.

fMRI can also be used to assess functional connectivity, which is utilized to demonstrate the operational interactions of brain areas that contribute to the neurophysiological mechanism of tinnitus. Functional connectivity is a method used to determine brain regions that have a consistent functional relationship, often highlighting distinct regions as networks. Brain regions are considered functionally connected when their corresponding neural activity is temporally correlated [29]. To assess functional connectivity, there are three common analyses for fMRI BOLD activity including seeding, graph connectivity, and independent component analysis [30]. In seeding, connectivity is correlated with a seed region selected by the researcher and the voxels in the whole brain or another specified region of interest. In graph connectivity, nodes are selected and correlated by the researcher to compare how the nodes are connected and the strength of the connection. Independent component analysis is data-driven and uses the time courses of voxels in the fMRI scans to spatially organize voxels into components to analyse whole brain networks.

Heterogeneity among studies exists partly due to differences in patient population or different analyses methods. Despite this, there have been two major themes in literature. Here, we outline evidence that depicts changes in two distinct non-auditory regions, the limbic system and attention system, which may contribute to tinnitus-related distress, cognitive dysfunction, and chronification of tinnitus.

Limbic System Changes

Similar to structural imaging studies, several fMRI studies have found a link between limbic areas with other brain areas. Specifically, studies have commonly observed dysregulation between the limbic and auditory system. A study evaluating both functional and structural abnormalities showed tones matched to the tinnitus frequency elicited hyperactivity in the left medial Heschl's gyrus (primary auditory cortex) and nucleus accumbens of tinnitus patients, which was positively correlated with tinnitus-related limbic abnormalities [9]. Consistent with this, both resting-state fMRI [31–33] and task-based fMRI [34] studies have demonstrated increased connectivity between the limbic and auditory regions of tinnitus patients. Tinnitus patients exhibited increased connectivity between primary auditory cortex and other limbic areas such as the dorsal anterior cingulate cortex, habenula, nucleus accumbens, posterior cingulate cortex, and subgenual anterior cingulate cortex when tinnitus matched tones were presented compared to non-tinnitus tones [34]. These studies illustrate increased connectivity with auditory cortex and areas pertaining to emotion and cognition. In a follow-up study, increased connectivity in tinnitus patients who had higher distress scores extended to more limbic areas, in which highly distressed patients displayed higher functional connectivity between auditory cortex and the amygdala, posterior cingulate cortex, parahippocampus and subgenual anterior cingulate cortex compared to patients with lower distress scores [35]. Studies consistently observe abnormal connectivity between auditory and limbic areas, but the exact consequence of the observed dysfunctional connectivity still needs to be elucidated.

While anatomical and physiological aberrations within the limbic system were originally linked to the emotional reaction of the tinnitus sound, there is speculation that the limbic system also plays a role in inhibiting the tinnitus signal [36]. Studies have proposed that the initial tinnitus signal may be generated by the auditory system, but general limbic system dysfunction and auditory-limbic connectivity dysfunction lead to chronic tinnitus [36, 37]. Furthermore, it is believed that the initial tinnitus signal can be blocked by the limbic system, so dysfunction within the limbic system would result in failure of inhibiting the tinnitus signal consequently mediating the chronification of tinnitus [9, 36].

Attention System Changes

Differences between the attention-processing regions with other brain areas are commonly observed in tinnitus patients [30]. A pilot study using resting-state fMRI showed increased connectivity between the dorsal medial prefrontal cortex, which plays a key role in attention processes, and auditory cortex [38]. Conversely, another study showed decreased correlations with attention-processing regions, suggesting that the attention network may mitigate the impact of the chronic internal sound [33]. Nevertheless, alterations in attention networks are seen in several studies, but results may vary due to the diverse analyses used.

It's also hypothesized that the tinnitus percept may be due to a lack in attentive cognitive control, resulting in cognitive dysfunction. In a separate study using task-based fMRI, tinnitus patients exhibited altered brain activity compared to healthy subjects while performing the Stroop test. Differences in brain activity were observed in the dorsolateral prefrontal cortex, ventromedial prefrontal cortex, and the cingulate cortex. Stroop test performance was correlated with brain activity level in the right dorsolateral prefrontal cortex and ventromedial prefrontal cortex in tinnitus patients, indicating that these areas may facilitate cognitive ability [39]. In addition to being involved in the emotional component, researchers posit that the dorsolateral prefrontal cortex and ventromedial prefrontal cortex may work together as part of a 'noise cancellation' pathway, as proposed by Rauschecker et al. 2010. Therefore, abnormal activity in the dorsolateral prefrontal cortex and ventromedial prefrontal cortex would result in a lack in tinnitus suppression.

Functional imaging approaches uncover neural correlates related to some components of tinnitus; however, it is likely that an interaction, or imbalance, between regions generates chronic tinnitus [9].

Ascending and Descending Pathways

Functional and structural research consistently implicates the involvement of limbic and auditory structures in chronic tinnitus. To augment this theory, studies have proposed a heuristic model in which chronic tinnitus can be structurally

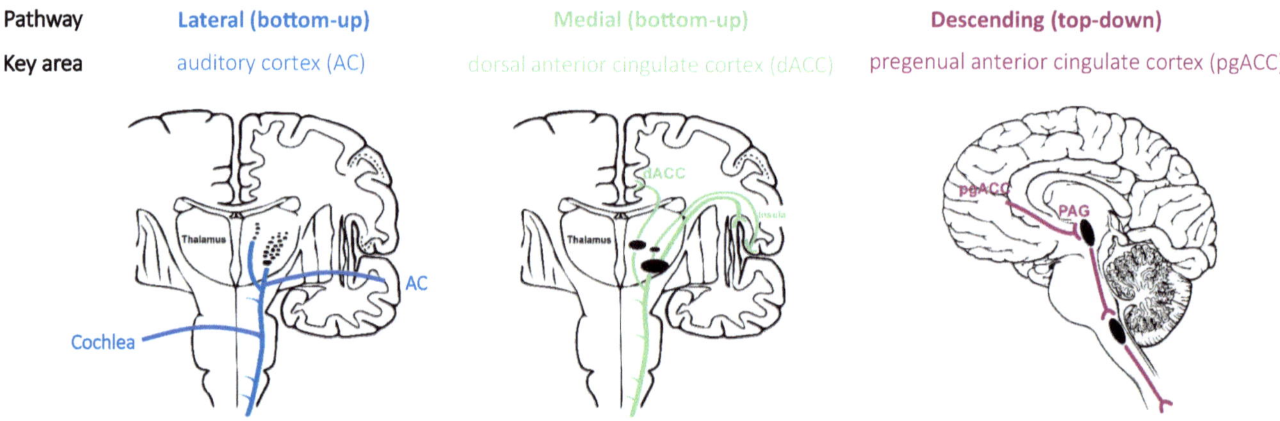

Fig. 15.1 Illustration of the anatomical pathway model separated into three interacting pathways: a lateral 'sound' pathway, a medial 'suffering' pathway, and a descending noise cancelling pathway

and functionally categorized into three pathways: two activating ascending pathways, and one deactivating descending pathway (Fig. 15.1) [2]. The pathways are functionally distinct in which each encodes a different tinnitus characteristic, and imbalance of these networks is believed to cause tinnitus. The two main tinnitus activating pathways include the lateral and medial pathway. The lateral pathway is proposed to primarily include the auditory cortex which generates the sound sensation and encodes loudness. Despite that tinnitus may be originally generated by alterations in the central auditory pathway, various regions of the brain are involved in persistent awareness and the associated distress. The medial pathway processes the affective component of tinnitus through the rostral to dorsal anterior cingulate (rdACC) and anterior insular cortex. Studies have shown a direct link between tinnitus distress and the medial pathway, in which distress was correlated with activity in the rdACC [40, 41]. The two activating pathways are balanced by the deactivating descending pathway, involving the ventromedial prefrontal cortex/pregenual anterior cingulate cortex (vmPFC/pgACC). The descending pathway is the brain's way of suppressing acute or chronic tinnitus, acting as a 'noise cancellation' system. When these pathways are imbalanced, often when the ascending pathways are overactive and the descending pathway is less active, the 'noise cancellation' is impaired and the brain is unable to block the tinnitus signal.

While initial studies attributed limbic activation for the emotional component of tinnitus, evidence supports that it has implications as a noise cancellation system in tinnitus at a thalamic level [36]. A previous fMRI study showed that changes in BOLD activity in vmPFC/pgACC were positively correlated with tinnitus characteristics such as loudness and percent of time during which tinnitus was perceived, but not the emotional component [42]. This evidence further illustrates how vmPFC/pgACC activity is related to strength of the tinnitus percept and not affective reaction to tinnitus. Both chronic pain and tinnitus studies suggest that the vmPFC/pgACC and NAc act as a 'gatekeeper', which assigns subjective or affective value to sensory signals, then act to minimize signals with negative values [37]. In short, this frontostriatal gating system is involved in evaluating the signal and modulating information flow through descending pathways. The compromised function of this system could affect sensory perception, mediated by a lack of suppression of irrelevant stimuli and dysfunctional evaluation of stimuli.

Neuromodulatory Changes

Frontostriatal gating is believed to be mediated by three main neuromodulators: dopamine, serotonin, and GABA [43–47]. Studies have hypothesized that the loss of inhibition in tinnitus may be due to lower GABA levels in the auditory pathway [46, 47]. Indirect evidence supports a GABAergic role in tinnitus, as seen by improvements in tinnitus characteristics in both animal and human studies after administration of GABA altering drugs [48–50]. Magnetic resonance spectroscopy (MRS) is a new emerging non-invasive neuroimaging method that can be used to assess GABA levels. In combination with MRI, it can be utilized to make brain neurochemical measurements by calculating the concentration of certain metabolite markers [51, 52].

This method was used in the bilateral auditory cortices of chronic tinnitus patients and age/hearing matched controls to quantify differences in GABA concentration linked to tinnitus only [51]. MRS measurements were made from a large voxel spanning almost all of auditory cortex, including primary and association areas, and including some non-auditory cortex. This study was the first to observe decreased GABA in auditory cortex of tinnitus patients. Researchers hypothesized that the GABA deficiency may affect the ability to inhibit and prevent spontaneous activity being perceived as tinnitus [51]. However, the exact role of GABA in tinnitus remains to be elucidated. Despite this, there is a clear importance of GABA in tinnitus pathology and lays a foundation for GABAergic treatments for tinnitus.

Networks

The ascending and descending pathways alone cannot attribute to the other complex components of tinnitus such as chronification or cognitive disability. Different models have been proposed to better delineate dysfunctional interactions among brain networks that may capture complex tinnitus characteristics. Network-based models, such as graph theory or the triple network model, can look at whole brain connectivity from a topological sense or the interaction between pre-defined set of networks, respectively. The models described lay a foundation for future studies to enable researchers to capture the full portrayal of chronic tinnitus in the clinic.

Graph Theory

Recently, graph theory has emerged as a method to assess dysfunctional network interactions in tinnitus, and how these dysfunctional networks contribute to tinnitus characteristics. Graph theory provides a mathematical framework to model and quantify pairwise relationships between objects and is often used to examine topological characteristics of brain networks, where brain regions correspond to nodes and functional connections to edges (Fig. 15.2) [53].

Findings show that tinnitus is associated with functional connectivity reorganization, with a correlation in connectivity patterns of the right executive control network and tinnitus distress. Since the central executive network is implicated in externally oriented attention and cognitive control abilities [54], these findings suggest that modification of these networks can alter how external information is perceived. Therefore, tinnitus distress is likely related to the paradoxical attention to the tinnitus sound.

A separate study utilized graph theory and resting-state fMRI to further analyse the relationship between tinnitus distress and network efficiency, by looking at network resilience and edge-between centrality [53]. Network resilience refers to the ability for a network to absorb change while preserving much of its original properties [55], whereas edge-betweenness centrality refers to the importance of a connection. The importance is measured as the number of shortest paths between pairs of rich-club nodes that are connected via a feeder edge [56, 57]. Rich-club organization is characterized by a high degree of above-average interconnected nodes, and feeder edges are the overlapping peripheral modules that connect to the rich-club regions [58]. Findings revealed that the relationship between tinnitus distress and network efficiency of tinnitus patients was mediated by the resilience and centrality of rich-club and feeder

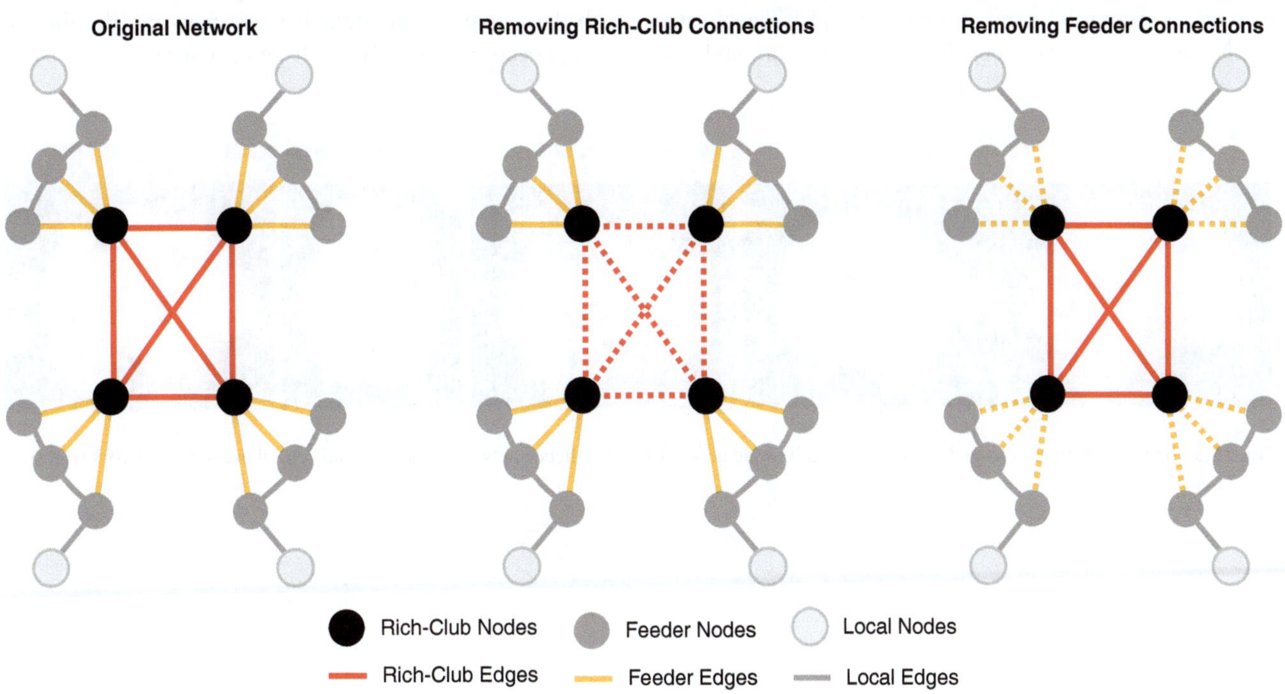

Fig. 15.2 A simplified representation of functional connectivity between rich-club and feeder regions [53]. The removal process of rich-club connections (middle) and feeder connections (right) is visualized, and the rate of change in efficiency was used to measure network resilience

connections. Higher network efficiency was associated with lower resilience of feeders and lower centrality of rich-club nodes, which manifests in higher distressed patients. Therefore, higher network efficiency equates to higher distress in patients, suggesting that network reorganization in tinnitus may support distress [53]. Conversely, a recent study demonstrated higher centrality with increased rich club connections and feeder connections in tinnitus patients [59]. These differences may arise due to discrepancies in distress levels. Further research is needed to delineate the impact of distress and cognitive disability.

Triple Network Model

The neural correlates behind the chronification and functional disability of tinnitus remains unknown. The triple network model, a model previously utilized to describe cognitive dysfunction, has been proposed to build the groundwork to investigate potential neural correlates at a network level. The triple network is a model that focuses on three major networks and how they interact, to find a common framework for understanding dysfunction across multiple cognitive and affective disorders [60]. This approach aims to identify aberrations within these network connections as a predictor of neuropsychiatric disorders.

The three major networks within the triple network model are the default mode network, the salience network, and the central executive network (Fig. 15.3). Anticorrelated with the salience and central executive networks, the default mode network is primarily active during rest and is deactivated during tasks [61]. Conversely, the salience network and central executive network are activated during tasks and deactivated at rest. The behavioural relevance encoding salient network acts as a 'switch' from the self-representational default mode network to the goal-oriented frontoparietal central executive network [61–68]. The salience network will detect an external behaviourally relevant stimulus, decrease activity of the default mode, and activate central executive network to address the stimulus.

The triple network model offers insight for the chronification of tinnitus and neural correlates of tinnitus. Studies have observed changes in the auditory, salience, default mode, and central executive network in patients with tinnitus. A study recently proposed that precuneus connectivity could serve as a marker for chronification or long duration tinnitus, as demonstrated by altered functional connectivity between the default mode network and the precuneus, in which the strength of the correlations between the precuneus and network could index tinnitus severity [69]. The reduced connectivity seen within the default mode network was accompanied with increased connectivity in the dorsal attention network and precuneus, indicating that patients are not in a true default resting-state but rather attending to the phantom sound. Furthermore, it was proposed that tinnitus treatment efficacy could be determined through connectivity between the default mode network and precuneus, in which reduced tinnitus severity would be correlated with increased connectivity between the default network and precuneus. Overall, these results suggest that the default mode network may become pathologically connected to tinnitus provoking networks. When the tinnitus percept becomes associated with the activity in the default mode network, the tinnitus percept becomes part of the self-percept at rest.

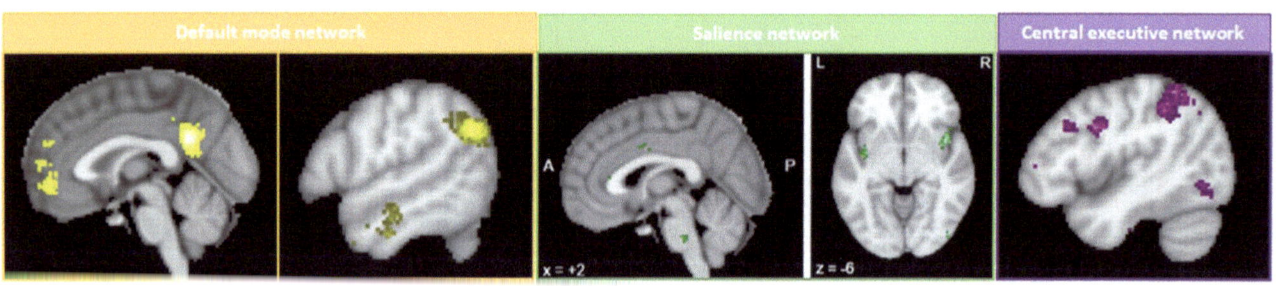

Fig. 15.3 Imaging of areas activated during the default mode network (left), salience network (middle), and central executive network (right)

Conclusion

Recent advances in neuroimaging have yielded more insight to the mechanism of tinnitus. Initial work suggested that chronic tinnitus is caused by damage to the auditory system. While the tinnitus signal may first develop because of auditory network dysfunction, evidence suggests that non-auditory regions play a large role in the emotional component, cognitive disability, and chronification of tinnitus.

Here, we highlighted some structural and functional imaging studies that have contributed to the field's understanding of anatomical and physiological aberrations in tinnitus patients and their potential roles in tinnitus characteristics. Structural imaging studies first elucidated the impact of age-related hearing loss in tinnitus-related structural changes. Moreover, functional imaging approaches aided in exploring brain changes and neural properties that may contribute to tinnitus-related distress, cognitive dysfunction, and chronification of tinnitus. Different tinnitus models have been proposed to illustrate complex characteristics of chronic tinnitus and create a framework for future studies to capture the full portrayal of chronic tinnitus in the clinic.

A number of limitations of neuroimaging studies merit consideration. Tinnitus studies have reported variable results, making it difficult to find consistent brain changes associated with tinnitus. First, scanner noise during neuroimaging could make tinnitus worse and techniques used to reduce scanner noise may vary. Second, the choice of control group is integral to avoid confounding variables that may exist. For example, initial research observed structural changes in tinnitus patients, but studies later confirmed that many structural changes are due to hearing loss, rather than tinnitus. This led researchers to control for multicollinear factors. Additionally, the patient population selected may have variable tinnitus characteristics since tinnitus is a heterogeneous disorder. Lastly, the use of many methods of analyses may lead to inconsistent results.

Altogether, further research with controlled methodology is needed to better delineate the complex tinnitus pathology. Neuroimaging approaches have the means to potentially predict treatment efficacy. Careful identification of anatomical and physiological tinnitus-related deficits will facilitate development of targeted therapeutic interventions to provide relief across all components of tinnitus.

References

1. De Ridder D, Schlee W, Vanneste S, Londero A, Weisz N, Kleinjung T, et al. Tinnitus and tinnitus disorder: theoretical and operational definitions (an international multidisciplinary proposal). Prog Brain Res. 2021;260:1–25.
2. De Ridder D, Vanneste S. The Bayesian brain in imbalance: medial, lateral and descending pathways in tinnitus and pain: a perspective. Prog Brain Res. 2021;262:309–34.
3. De Ridder D, Vanneste S, Weisz N, Londero A, Schlee W, Elgoyhen AB, et al. An integrative model of auditory phantom perception: tinnitus as a unified percept of interacting separable subnetworks. Neurosci Biobehav Rev. 2014;44:16–32.
4. De Ridder D, Vanneste S, Freeman W. The Bayesian brain: phantom percepts resolve sensory uncertainty. Neurosci Biobehav Rev. 2014;44:4–15.
5. Axelsson A, Ringdahl A. Tinnitus–a study of its prevalence and characteristics. Br J Audiol. 1989;23(1):53–62.
6. Shargorodsky J, Curhan GC, Farwell WR. Prevalence and characteristics of tinnitus among US adults. Am J Med. 2010;123(8):711–8.
7. Asan L, Falfan-Melgoza C, Beretta CA, Sack M, Zheng L, Weber-Fahr W, et al. Cellular correlates of gray matter volume changes in magnetic resonance morphometry identified by two-photon microscopy. Sci Rep. 2021;11(1):4234.
8. Mühlau M, et al. Structural brain changes in tinnitus. Cereb Cortex. 2006;16:1283–8.
9. Leaver AM, et al. Dysregulation of limbic and auditory networks in tinnitus. Neuron. 2011;69:33–43.
10. Schneider P, et al. Reduced volume of Heschl's gyrus in tinnitus. NeuroImage. 2009;45:927–39.
11. Boyen K, Langers DRM, de Kleine E, van Dijk P. Gray matter in the brain: differences associated with tinnitus and hearing loss. Hear Res. 2013;295:67–78.
12. Aldhafeeri FM, MacKenzie I, Kay T, Alghamdi J, Sluming V. Neuroanatomical correlates of tinnitus revealed by cortical thickness analysis and diffusion tensor imaging. Neuroradiology. 2012;54:883–92.
13. Lehner A, et al. Structural brain changes following left temporal low-frequency rTMS in patients with subjective tinnitus. Neural Plast. 2014;2014:132058.
14. Landgrebe M, et al. Structural brain changes in tinnitus: grey matter decrease in auditory and non-auditory brain areas. NeuroImage. 2009;46:213–8.
15. Mahoney CJ, et al. Structural neuroanatomy of tinnitus and hyperacusis in semantic dementia. J Neurol Neurosurg Psychiatry. 2011;82:1274–8.
16. Diesch E, Schummer V, Kramer M, Rupp A. Structural changes of the corpus callosum in tinnitus. Front Syst Neurosci. 2012;6:1–11.
17. Leaver AM, et al. Cortico-limbic morphology separates tinnitus from tinnitus distress. Front Syst Neurosci. 2012;6:1–14.
18. Vanneste S, Van DeHeyning P, DeRidder D. Tinnitus: a large VBM-EEG correlational study. PLoS One. 2015;10:1–26.
19. Yoo HB, De Ridder D, Vanneste S. The importance of aging in gray matter changes within tinnitus patients shown in cortical thickness, surface area and volume. Brain Topogr. 2016;29:885–96.
20. Cheng S, et al. A multimodal meta-analysis of structural and functional changes in the brain of tinnitus. Front Hum Neurosci. 2020;14:28.
21. Yoo HB, De Ridder D, Vanneste S. White matter changes in tinnitus: is it all age and hearing loss? Brain Connect. 2016;6:84–93.
22. Ahmed S, et al. Structural correlates of the audiological and emotional components of chronic tinnitus. In: Progress in brain research, vol. 262. Amsterdam: Elsevier; 2021.
23. Basser PJ, Mattiello J, Lebihan D. Estimation of the effective self-diffusion tensor from the NMR spin echo. J Magn Reson Ser B. 1994;103:247–54.
24. Neil J, Miller J, Mukherjee P, Hüppi PS. Diffusion tensor imaging of normal and injured developing human brain - a technical review. NMR Biomed. 2002;15:543–52.

25. Catani M, Mesulam M. The arcuate fasciculus and the disconnection theme in language and aphasia: history and current state. Cortex. 2008;44:953–61.
26. Pujol J, et al. Beck depression inventory factors related to demyelinating lesions of the left arcuate fasciculus region. Psychiatry Res Neuroimaging. 2000;99:151–9.
27. Maffei C, et al. Topography of the human acoustic radiation as revealed by ex vivo fibers micro-dissection and in vivo diffusion-based tractography. Brain Struct Funct. 2018;223:449–59.
28. Melcher JR, Knudson IM, Levine RA. Subcallosal brain structure: correlation with hearing threshold at supra-clinical frequencies (8 kHz), but not with tinnitus. Hear Res. 2013;295:79–86.
29. Adams ME, Huang TC, Nagarajan S, Cheung SW. Tinnitus neuroimaging. Otolaryngol Clin N Am. 2020;53:583–603.
30. Husain FT, Schmidt SA. Using resting state functional connectivity to unravel networks of tinnitus. Hear Res. 2014;307:153–62.
31. Maudoux A, et al. Auditory resting-state network connectivity in tinnitus: a functional MRI study. PLoS One. 2012;7:e36222.
32. Maudoux A, et al. Connectivity graph analysis of the auditory resting state network in tinnitus. Brain Res. 2012;1485:10–21.
33. Schmidt SA, Akrofi K, Carpenter-Thompson JR, Husain FT. Default mode, dorsal attention and auditory resting state networks exhibit differential functional connectivity in tinnitus and hearing loss. PLoS One. 2013;8:1–12.
34. Hullfish J, et al. Functional brain changes in auditory phantom perception evoked by different stimulus frequencies. Neurosci Lett. 2018;683:160–7.
35. Hullfish J, et al. Functional connectivity analysis of fMRI data collected from human subjects with chronic tinnitus and varying levels of tinnitus-related distress. Data Br. 2018;21:779–89.
36. Rauschecker JP, Leaver AM, Mühlau M. Tuning out the noise: limbic-auditory interactions in tinnitus. Neuron. 2010;66:819–26.
37. Rauschecker JP, May ES, Maudoux A, Ploner M. Frontostriatal gating of tinnitus and chronic pain. Trends Cogn Sci. 2015;19: 567–78.
38. Kim JY, et al. Alteration of functional connectivity in tinnitus brain revealed by resting-state fMRI? A pilot study. Int J Audiol. 2012;51:413–7.
39. Araneda R, et al. A key role of the prefrontal cortex in the maintenance of chronic tinnitus: an fMRI study using a Stroop task. NeuroImage Clin. 2018;17:325–34.
40. de Ridder D, Vanneste S, Congedo M. The distressed brain: a group blind source separation analysis on tinnitus. PLoS One. 2011;6:2–11.
41. Vanneste S, et al. The neural correlates of tinnitus-related distress. NeuroImage. 2010;52:470–80.
42. Seydell-Greenwald A, et al. Functional MRI evidence for a role of ventral prefrontal cortex in tinnitus. Brain Res. 2012;1485:22–39.
43. Lopez-Gonzalez MA, Santiago AM, Esteban-Ortega F. Sulpiride and melatonin decrease tinnitus perception modulating the auditolimbic dopaminergic pathway. J Otolaryngol. 2007;36:213–9.
44. Dobie RA. Depression and tinnitus. Otolaryngol Clin N Am. 2003;36:383–8.
45. Simpson JJ, Davies WE. A review of evidence in support of a role for 5-HT in the perception of tinnitus. Hear Res. 2000;145:1–7.
46. Sun W, et al. Salicylate increases the gain of the central auditory system. Neuroscience. 2009;159:325–34.
47. Richardson BD, Brozoski TJ, Ling LL, Caspary DM. Targeting inhibitory neurotransmission in tinnitus. Brain Res. 2012;1485: 77–87.
48. Brozoski TJ, Odintsov B, Bauer C. Gamma-aminobutyric acid and glutamic acid levels in the auditory pathway of rats with chronic tinnitus: a direct determination using high resolution point-resolved proton magnetic resonance spectroscopy (1H-MRS). Front Syst Neurosci. 2012;6:1–12.
49. Han SS, et al. Clonazepam quiets tinnitus: a randomised crossover study with Ginkgo biloba. J Neurol Neurosurg Psychiatry. 2012;83:821–7.
50. Zheng Y, Vagal S, McNamara E, Darlington CL, Smith PF. A dose-response analysis of the effects of L-baclofen on chronic tinnitus caused by acoustic trauma in rats. Neuropharmacology. 2012;62:940–6.
51. Sedley W, et al. Human auditory cortex neurochemistry reflects the presence and severity of tinnitus. J Neurosci. 2015;35:14822–8.
52. Hu J, et al. The neural mechanisms of tinnitus: a perspective from functional magnetic resonance imaging. Front Neurosci. 2021;15:1–8.
53. Bin YH, Mohan A, De Ridder D, Vanneste S. Paradoxical relationship between distress and functional network topology in phantom sound perception. Prog Brain Res. 2021;260:367–95.
54. Kandeepan S, et al. Tinnitus distress: a paradoxical attention to the sound? J Neurol. 2019;266:2197–207.
55. Holling CS. Resilience and stability of ecological systems. Annu Rev Ecol Syst. 1973;4:1–23.
56. Cuzzocrea A, Papadimitriou A, Katsaros D, Manolopoulos Y. Edge betweenness centrality: a novel algorithm for QoS-based topology control over wireless sensor networks. J Netw Comput Appl. 2012;35:1210–7.
57. Girvan M, Newman MEJ. Community structure in social and biological networks. Proc Natl Acad Sci U S A. 2002;99:7821–6.
58. van den Heuvel MP, Sporns O. Rich-club organization of the human connectome. J Neurosci. 2011;31:15775–86.
59. Lan L, et al. Topological features of limbic dysfunction in chronicity of tinnitus with intact hearing: New hypothesis for 'noise-cancellation' mechanism. Prog Neuro-Psychopharmacol Biol Psychiatry. 2022;113:110459.
60. Menon V. Large-scale brain networks and psychopathology: a unifying triple network model. Trends Cogn Sci. 2011;15:483–506.
61. Fox MD, et al. The human brain is intrinsically organized into dynamic, anticorrelated functional networks. Proc Natl Acad Sci U S A. 2005;102:9673–8.
62. Greicius MD, Krasnow B, Reiss AL, Menon V. Functional connectivity in the resting brain: a network analysis of the default mode hypothesis. Proc Natl Acad Sci U S A. 2003;100:253–8.
63. Buckner RL, Andrews-Hanna JR, Schacter DL. The brain's default network: anatomy, function, and relevance to disease. Ann N Y Acad Sci. 2008;1124:1–38.
64. Seeley WW, et al. Dissociable intrinsic connectivity networks for salience processing and executive control. J Neurosci. 2007;27:2349–56.
65. Vincent JL, Kahn I, Snyder AZ, Raichle ME, Buckner RL. Evidence for a frontoparietal control system revealed by intrinsic functional connectivity. J Neurophysiol. 2008;100:3328–42.
66. Goulden N, et al. The salience network is responsible for switching between the default mode network and the central executive network: replication from DCM. NeuroImage. 2014;99:180–90.
67. Menon V, Uddin LQ. Saliency, switching, attention and control: a network model of insula function. Brain Struct Funct. 2010;214:655–67.
68. Sridharan D, Levitin DJ, Menon V. A critical role for the right fronto-insular cortex in switching between central-executive and default-mode networks. Proc Natl Acad Sci U S A. 2008;105:12569–74.
69. Schmidt SA, Carpenter-Thompson J, Husain FT. Connectivity of precuneus to the default mode and dorsal attention networks: a possible invariant marker of long-term tinnitus. NeuroImage Clin. 2017;16:196–204.

The Electrophysiological Explorations in Tinnitus Over the Decades Using EEG and MEG

16

Anusha Yasoda-Mohan and Sven Vanneste

Abstract

Ever since animal studies confirmed a more central origin of tinnitus, there has been a constant search for an objective marker of tinnitus with a thirst to unravel its mechanism of action. Researchers have used sound-evoked and resting state electrophysiological measures such as auditory brainstem responses, auditory steady-state responses, middle and long latency responses and resting state brain activity recorded using both an electroencephalogram and magnetic encephalogram to understand the neural correlates of tinnitus. What started as an exploration of changes in brain activity between tinnitus and non-tinnitus participants has evolved into understanding how networks of brain regions encode different behavioural characteristics of tinnitus and segueing into mobilising big data to build models to predict the same characteristics based on neural data. In the current chapter, we take a deep dive into various electrophysiological studies that have tried to achieve this through the ages and summarise what we know about tinnitus and its neural correlates using EEG and MEG and where we think the field is headed.

A. Yasoda-Mohan (✉) · S. Vanneste
Global Brain Health Institute and Institute of Neuroscience, Trinity College Dublin, Dublin, Ireland

Lab for Clinical and Integrative Neuroscience, Trinity Institute for Neuroscience, School of Psychology, Trinity College Dublin, Dublin, Ireland
e-mail: Anusha.mohan@gbhi.org; sven.vanneste@tcd.ie

W. Schlee et al. (eds.), *Textbook of Tinnitus*, https://doi.org/10.1007/978-3-031-35647-6_16

Graphical Abstract

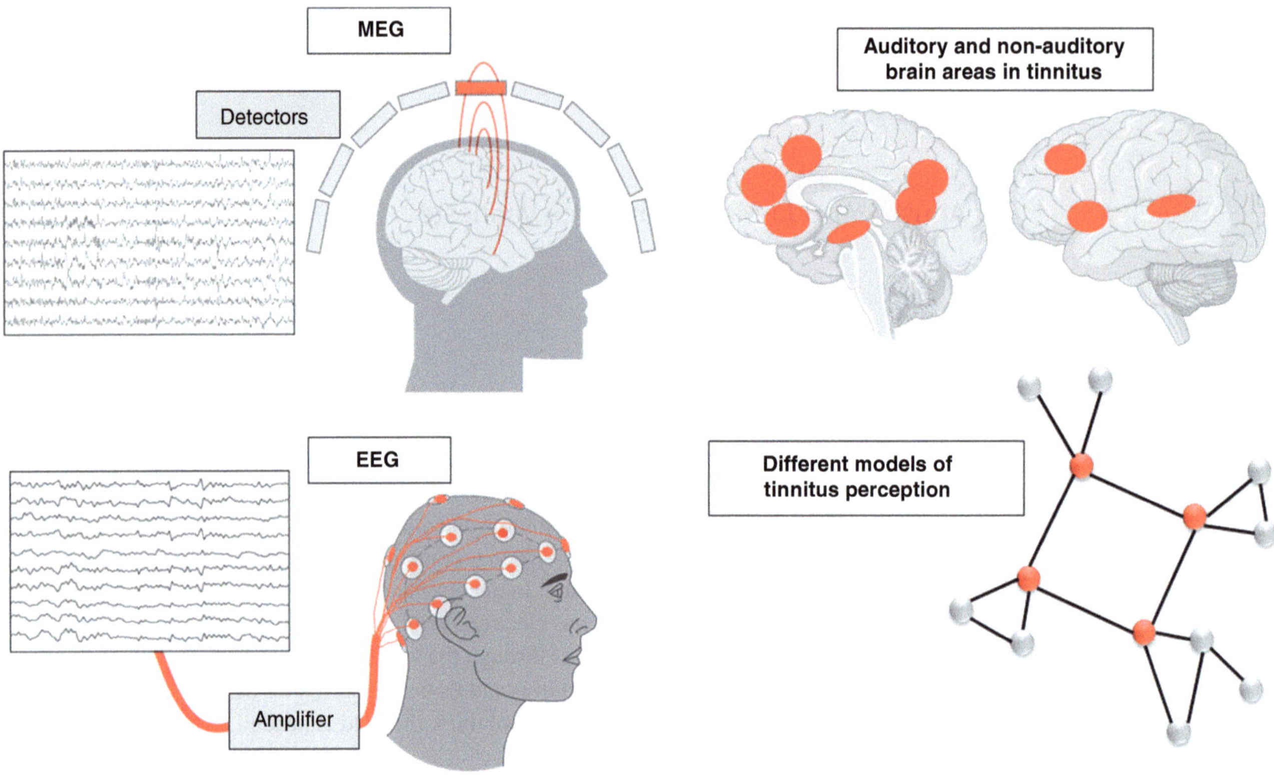

Highlights

- Tinnitus was initially studied as a symptom or side effect to other disorders
- Early neural correlates were investigated using ABRs, ASSRs, and other AEPs
- The breakthrough came with understanding spontaneous brain activity
- Resting-state electrophysiology helped empirically characterise behavioural measures
- Model-based and hypothesis-driven research then re-introduced AEP-related research
- The future lies in using neural correlates to predict behaviour and guide treatment

Introduction

For several decades, tinnitus (ringing in the ear) was associated with different disorders relating to the ear (e.g. labyrinthitis [1], otosclerosis [2], Meniere's disease [3], acoustic neuroma [4], medication-induced ototoxicity [5]), vestibular (balance) systems [6] (e.g. Neri-Barre syndrome [7], vestibular schwannoma [8]), and other disorders [9–15] etc.) as mostly a symptom or a side effect. However, following extensive work in the animal field [16], specifically with noise-induced hearing loss models [17–19], and analysis of several surgical techniques [20] including microvascular decompression [21], tinnitus is now classified as objective and subjective tinnitus. Subjective tinnitus, which is continuous and has no specific sound source, is shown in the animal literature, using single neuronal recordings, to have a more central origin [22]. Since then, scientists have been on the search for an objective marker for tinnitus using non-invasive electrophysiological techniques such as electroencephalography (EEG) and magnetoencephalography (MEG).

EEG is the summation of dendritic post-synaptic potentials that are picked up from the cortical surface through scalp electrodes [23]. MEG measures the magnetic field generated by these synchronised dendritic post-synaptic potentials and is recorded using very sensitive magnetometers [24]. According to the laws of physics, the electrical and magnetic fields generated by the neurons are perpendicular to each other essentially transmitting the same information but in different formats. From a more practical standpoint, EEG is cheaper and easier to measure than MEG, although MEG is more reliable in detecting the source of physiological activity than EEG. However, they have both been used quite extensively to study the neural correlates of tinnitus. In this chapter, we will review how EEG and MEG played a role in advancing the understanding of the mechanism of action of tinnitus and what their future use holds in store for us.

Types of Electrophysiological Recordings (Using Both EEG and MEG)

The auditory pathways start from the inner ear (cochlea) and reach the auditory cortex by passing through the medulla (cochlear nuclei), pons (superior olive), midbrain (lateral lemniscus, inferior colliculus), and medial geniculate body of the thalamus (Fig. 16.1) [25]. From the auditory cortex, auditory signals are processed by higher-order brain regions including the secondary auditory cortices and regions of cognitive functioning including those of the fronto-parietal network which bring the sound to conscious perception [26]. The neural activity from the auditory nerve in the cochlea to these higher brain regions is usually recorded in response to sounds by EEG and MEG and are called auditory-evoked potentials (AEP).

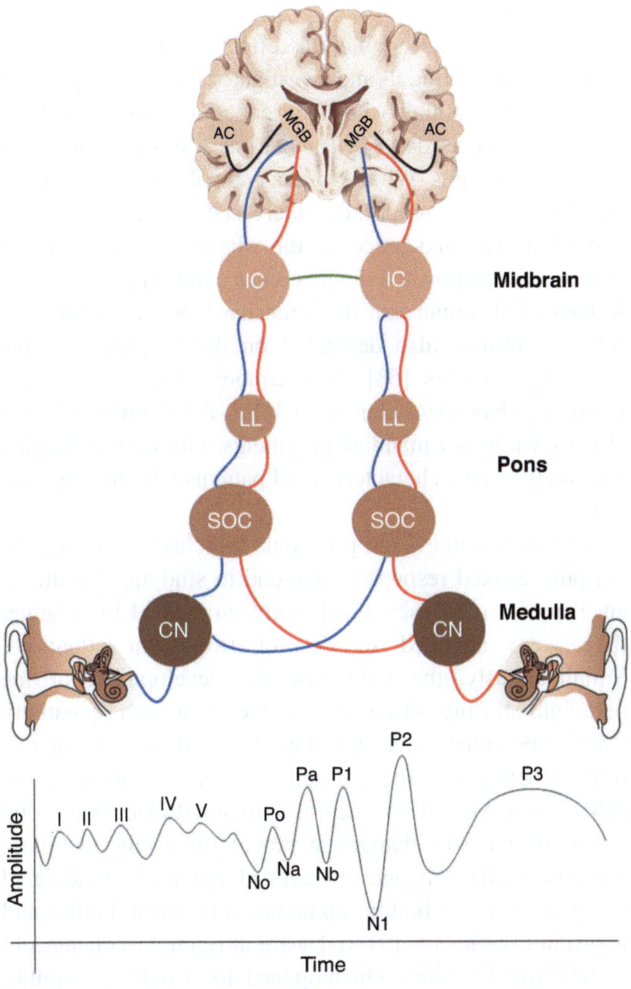

Fig. 16.1 The auditory pathways and auditory-evoked responses. (*Top*) Shows the simplified schematic of the bilateral auditory pathways leading up from the auditory nerve to the *CN* cochlear nucleus, *SOC* superior olivary complex, *LL* lateral lemniscus, *IC* inferior colliculus, *MGB* medial geniculate body up to the *AC* auditory cortex. The blue and red lines signify the input from the left and right ears, respectively. (*Below*) A schematic of the early, middle, and late latency responses evoked by different auditory stimuli

AEPs are divided into early, middle, and long latency potentials depending on the latency of the response to the sound. Early AEPs include auditory brainstem responses (ABRs) which reflect activity from the cochlear nerve up to the midbrain [27] and are divided into five distinct waves I–V which are all generated within the first 5–6 ms after signal presentation [28, 29]. The middle and long latency responses occur within 11–50 and 50–600 ms after stimulus presentation, respectively, and reflect both sensory and cognitive components. The middle latency potentials are still generated at a more subcortical level reflecting subcortical relays to the cortex [30], whereas the long latency potentials are generated by more cortical sources including the auditory cortex and higher brain regions [31, 32]. Another type of AEP is called the auditory steady-state response (ASSR). ASSR is the response to rapid stimuli whose timing follows the frequency of stimulation. The electrical activity is recorded by placing an electrode on the forehead or vertex (for ABRs and ASSRs) or the scalp (for other AEPs) in reference to another set of electrodes placed at a more neutral position (earlobes).

Brain activity can also be studied in the absence of sound stimulation, and this presents a more generalised view of spontaneous brain activity at any given moment in time. This is called resting state activity popularly measured using an electrode cap of 19, 32, 64, 128, or 256 channels placed around the scalp following the International 10–20 system electrode placement system. Analysing the resting brain activity in tinnitus exponentially advanced the field in terms of understanding the neural correlates of its different behavioural characteristics such as tinnitus pitch, loudness, laterality, associated distress, sex differences, and influence of hearing loss. It also gave rise to different models in understanding the mechanism of action of tinnitus and led to the transition from more exploratory to hypothesis-driven research.

Auditory Brainstem Response (ABR) and Auditory Steady-State Responses (ASSR)

ABRs and ASSRs are cost-effective methods that are primarily used for two purposes—estimating hearing thresholds [33] and diagnosing inconsistencies in the auditory pathways [34–36] (ABRs), specifically in populations that are unable to perform behavioural experiments. In tinnitus, ABRs were used to differentiate peripheral from central lesions [37], estimate treatment efficacy [38, 39], and identify noise-induced "hidden" hearing loss that does not manifest in traditional pure-tone audiometry [40]. ASSRs are also used to determine audiometric thresholds, not using peak detection, but more statistically advanced techniques that take into account the spectral information in the signal.

The reduction of wave I amplitude in the ABR (called cochlear synaptopathy) even in patients with normal audiometric thresholds of <20 dB HL, but a normal wave V, explains a central auditory compensation resulting in the normal auditory thresholds at a more systemic level [41, 42]. Some tinnitus patients show increase in wave V amplitude reflecting an increase in neural synchrony, which is one of the proposed mechanisms of tinnitus generation [43, 44]. This was postulated to be sufficient to produce a perception of a phantom sound by the higher cortical regions even in the absence of actual sound stimulation. In older tinnitus patients, reductions in wave III and wave V were noted even in the absence of wave I changes showing age-related changes in the neural pathways [45]. A meta-analysis of ABR studies in tinnitus patients to understand how changes in amplitude and latency of different waves impacted tinnitus generation in different populations of hearing loss showed that increase in wave I latency and decrease in wave I amplitude in normal hearing tinnitus patients compared to matched controls were consistent across several studies [46]. They also suggest the use of gap-in-noise ABR with different background noise frequencies in humans to further the understanding of tinnitus mechanisms using ABRs.

ASSRs have been used to understand not just the neural correlates of hearing loss, but also how the stimulus interacted with other input streams and internally generated signals like tinnitus [47]. ASSRs are usually studied alongside middle latency responses which occur in transition from early to late potentials and are induced typically by amplitude-modulated tones. The earliest research with ASSR used the tinnitus frequency as the carrier frequency and which lie above the frequency of their audiometric edge, i.e. the location on the frequency axis above which the hearing loss increases rapidly [48]. They observed that the ASSR amplitude increased in tinnitus patients and the field amplitude of the tinnitus frequency correlated with the tinnitus intensity and distress, even after controlling for hearing loss. The relationship between tinnitus distress and ASSR features was shown by other labs who also uncovered the network of areas which correlated with tinnitus distress [49, 50]. ASSRs were also used to compare the tonotopic frequency representation in the auditory cortex of tinnitus patients with controls and showed a degraded frequency representations replicating results of animal studies [51]. This was attributed to reflect the loss of intracortical inhibition in the deafferented regions.

Early Cortical Electrophysiology: Exploratory Research Using Long-Latency AEPs

The earliest electrophysiological studies in tinnitus were carried out using auditory-evoked MEG. Different groups examined amplitude and latency changes of the M100 and M200 (responses 100 and 200 ms post-stimulus presentation). Hoke et al. [52] only stimulated the non-tinnitus ear of unilateral tinnitus patients, whereas Jacobson et al. [53], stimulated both the tinnitus and non-tinnitus ears. Hoke and colleagues reported a significant reduction in amplitude of M100 and M200, a delay in the M200 latency, and reduction in the M200/M100 amplitude ratio in tinnitus patients [52]. These results were not replicated by Jacobson et al. [53] or Colding-Jorgensen [54] and colleagues, but were supported by Attias et al. using EEG [55] in both auditory and visual domains [56].

Other researchers studied the effect of stimulus intensity on the evoked potentials and investigated intensity-dependent N100-P200 amplitude (the electrical equivalent of the magnetic components described above) as a possible objective marker for tinnitus. While Norena and colleagues found that the N100-P200 amplitude increased in an intensity-dependent way and based on the whether patients showed improved or aggravated tinnitus when exposed to noise [57], Kander et al. found that the intensity-dependent change in N100 amplitude also depended on the frequency of the incoming stimulus [58]. Furthermore, this intensity and frequency-dependent change in N100-P200 amplitude was also shown to not manifest in patients with normal hearing and likely to be a characteristic of patients with hearing loss [59].

Research with evoked potentials switched from studying the pure evoked responses to sound to studying the difference in two responses which were modulated by whether they were attended to or not (top-down attention). Simultaneously, the field saw the development of the paradigm-shifting discovery of the mismatch negativity (MMN) potential by Naatanen et al. [60] defined as the difference between a frequent and infrequency stimulus. The MMN was known to record stimulus-driven bottom-up attention owing to changes in probability of the incoming auditory scene. Changes in evoked potentials modulated using top-down or bottom-up attention between tinnitus and non-tinnitus subjects [61–63] were attributed to changes in higher brain functions which opened doors to the possibility of other brain regions such as the limbic structures and the frontal cortex in addition to the primary and secondary auditory cortices to be involved in tinnitus. These studies were some of the first to start to explore other aspects of tinnitus such as tinnitus-related distress and its relationship with attention.

Breakthrough in Understanding Tinnitus: Exploratory Research Using Resting State Activity

The breakthrough to understanding tinnitus characteristics came with the study of spontaneous resting state EEG and MEG data together with that of brain oscillations. The brain transmits different kinds of information through different frequency bands, much like a radio. These range from slow waves, viz. delta (1–3.5 Hz), theta (4–8 Hz), alpha (8–12 Hz), to fast waves, viz. beta (13–30 Hz) and gamma (>30 Hz). Different studies looked at changes in local activity in different brain regions, synchronous activity between two regions called functional connectivity, directional flow of information from one region to the other called effective connectivity, and communication between two frequencies in the same region called cross-frequency coupling or nesting. These different neural signatures in the different frequency bands were used to estimate the neural correlates of various tinnitus characteristics.

The three main behavioural signatures of tinnitus patients are tinnitus loudness, tinnitus-related distress, and hearing loss. One of the seminal findings in the tinnitus literature is the decrease in alpha activity and simultaneous increase in delta/theta and gamma activity, specifically in the auditory cortex in patients with tinnitus compared to controls both in the acute [64] and chronic conditions [65–67]. Furthermore, researchers also found a decrease in functional connectivity between frontal, temporal, and parietal regions including the anterior and posterior cingulate cortex in the alpha frequency band and increase in functional connectivity in the gamma frequency band in tinnitus patients compared to controls [68]. Increased activity in the gamma frequency band was also attributed to the conscious auditory percept in tinnitus [69] which was brought to conscious awareness by the fronto-parietal global neuronal workspace [26]. Several studies were able to show that the loudness of this conscious percept was correlated with the strength of gamma activity in the auditory cortex [70, 71]. Progressively, research was able to show that the subjectively perceived loudness was correlated with the amount of cross-frequency coupling between the theta and gamma frequency bands in the auditory cortex [72, 73].

Tinnitus-related distress activated very different regions. In a seminal paper by Vanneste and colleagues, the team showed that tinnitus distress was correlated with an increase in alpha and beta activity in nonauditory brain regions such as the subgenual anterior cingulate cortex, insula, parahippocampus, and the amygdala and decreased alpha activity in the posterior cingulate cortex, precuneus, and dorsolateral prefrontal cortex [74] which was confirmed by other studies [75, 76]. These areas were found to overlap with the emotional component of the pain matrix raising the hypothesis that maybe tinnitus, similar to pain, had a lateral and medial pathway, where the lateral pathway delivered information about the conscious percept and medial pathway about the emotional component of the percept [77]. Furthermore, tinnitus-related distress and depression showed very different neural correlates as demonstrated by resting-state EEG [78], supporting the idea of a dedicated pathway to convey the emotional component of tinnitus.

Loudness and distress were shown to not have a direct relationship. While some researchers showed that they were two distinct independent components [79], others showed that there may be a nonlinear relationship based on the amount of distress [80]. Loudness and distress were linearly related at low distress levels, whereas they were not correlated at high distress levels [80]. In fact, based on the amount of distress the functional connectivity changed between the auditory cortex and other brain regions. In patients with high distress, there was increased functional connectivity between the auditory cortex and subgenual anterior cingulate cortex showing that patients with high distress probably start to associate the loudness of the sound to the amount of distress perceived making the tinnitus harder to modify in these patients [80, 81]. Furthermore, patients who were not able to cope with the tinnitus showed increased subjective loudness, distress, and depression scores. Maladaptive coping was also related to changes in alpha activity in the dorsolateral prefrontal cortex and increased alpha functional connectivity between the regions of the default mode network [82].

Hearing loss most commonly accompanies tinnitus with >80% of the patients showing some signs of degraded hearing. Schmidt and colleagues were one of the first to perform a comprehensive analysis of the neural correlates of tinnitus using fMRI with hearing loss as one of the variables [83]. Following this, several studies investigated changes in EEG and MEG activity in the presence and absence of hearing loss. In a seminal study by Vanneste and De Ridder, the authors showed that different regions were activated in tinnitus depending upon the amount of hearing loss [84]. In patients with little to no hearing loss, tinnitus patients showed increased gamma activity and functional connectivity between the left and right auditory cortices compared to controls, whereas in severe hearing loss, this was localised to increased theta activity in the parahippocampus and increased theta functional connectivity between the two parahippocampi and a directional connectivity from the left parahippocampus to the left auditory cortex. Furthermore, the mean and range of hearing loss was correlated to theta activity in the parahippocampus and increased theta functional connectivity between the auditory cortex and the parahippocampus. Compared to patients with hearing loss and no tinnitus, patients with hearing loss and tinnitus showed increased beta activity in the parahippocampus and gamma activity in the

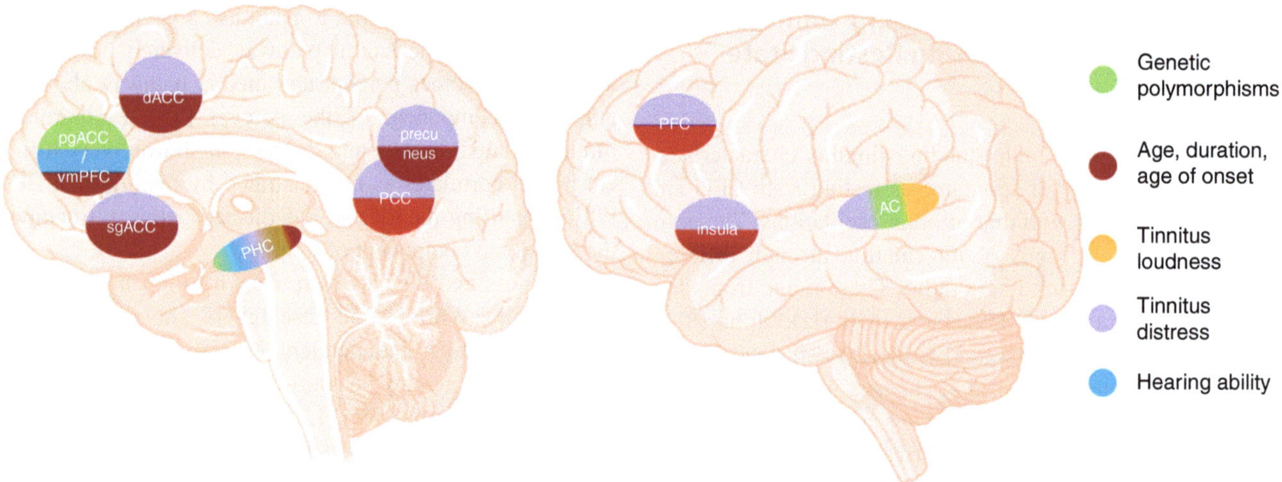

Fig. 16.2 Summary of brain regions involved in encoding different tinnitus characteristics. The different characteristics are shown in different colours. *dACC* dorsal anterior cingulate cortex; *pgACC/vmPFC* pregenual anterior cingulate cortex/ventromedial prefrontal cortex, *sgACC* subgenual anterior cingulate cortex, *PHC* parahippocampus, *PCC* posterior cingulate cortex, *PFC* prefrontal cortex, *AC* auditory cortex

inferior parietal lobule. Additionally, there was an increase in delta functional connectivity between the parahippocampus and inferior parietal lobule and in beta functional connectivity between the posterior cingulate cortex and inferior parietal lobule [85]. Here the authors theorised that the inferior parietal lobule may be acting as a "circuit breaker" to render tinnitus as a salient event in the presence of decreased sensory input and perceiving this salient event was the new normal, given the connection to the hub of the default mode network (i.e. posterior cingulate cortex). Hearing loss was also shown to interact with the polymorphism of COMT Val^{158}Met gene (whose main function is with the metabolise dopamine), where patients with hearing loss who were Met carriers demonstrated increased gamma activity in the parahippocampus and theta and gamma functional connectivity between the auditory cortex and parahippocampus [86]. Therefore, the parahippocampus becomes more involved in patients with hearing loss.

Resting state EEG and MEG studies also investigated the neural correlates to other tinnitus characteristics such as pitch of the tinnitus [87], low-frequency vs high-frequency tinnitus [88], narrow-band noise vs pure tinnitus [89], having unilateral vs bilateral phantom percept [90], laterality in unilateral tinnitus patients [91], sex differences in tinnitus perception [92], the role of sympathetic and parasympathetic activation on tinnitus using heart-rate variability markers [93, 94], changes in brain activity between acute and chronic tinnitus [95], and age of onset of tinnitus, i.e. early and late-onset of tinnitus [96, 97]. The auditory and nonauditory brain areas involved in tinnitus are summarised in Fig. 16.2.

Tinnitus as a Unified Phantom Percept of Individual Separable Subnetworks

From the above studies, researchers agreed that tinnitus was not a problem involving just the auditory regions, but was a whole-brain problem including auditory and nonauditory regions [98]. Tinnitus was thus proposed to be an integrated percept consisting of multiple subnetworks where each subnetwork encoded a different characteristic of tinnitus [99] (Fig. 16.3). The next set of studies in the field circled around this concept of tinnitus as a unified percept from multiple subnetworks.

With graph theory gaining traction in the neurosciences, understanding the neural correlates of a pathology received a different perspective. Here, the brain was considered a complex system whose network topology was balanced in a cost-effective way by short and long-distance connections [100, 101]. The regions were conceptualised as nodes, the connections between them were called edges, and the important regions through which many connections passed were called hubs [102]. Subnetworks were segregated through local connections and the hubs of the subnetworks were integrated through a "rich-club" network [103]. There was trade-off between cost and efficiency, segregation, and integration and any deviation from a "small-world" balanced topology towards a less efficient lattice topology or more efficient random topology was considered pathological [104]. Disorders with diametrically opposing behavioural characteristics were defined as deviation into one or the other topology.

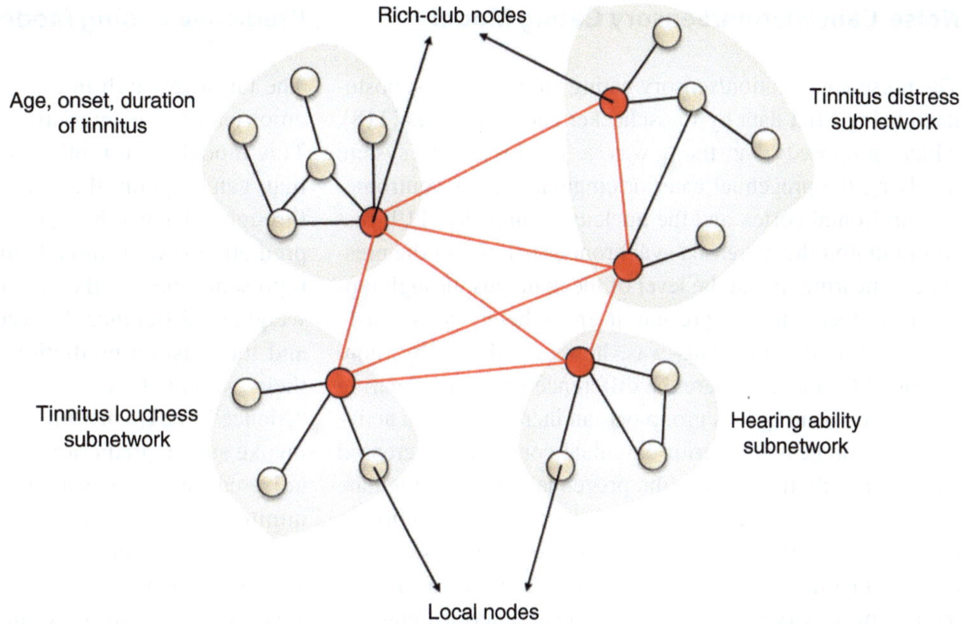

Fig. 16.3 A schematic of a whole brain network using graph theory modelling tinnitus as a unified percept of multiple separable subnetworks. The red circles denote hubs which are interconnected in a "rich-club network" which are in turn connected to local nodes. Each individual subnetwork characterises a different behavioural correlate of tinnitus

By applying graph theory to tinnitus, researchers were able to characterise tinnitus networks from a complex system perspective where there was a frequency-dependent deviation to a more lattice or random topology [105]. Furthermore, they were able to determine the hubs of the tinnitus network, how they were different from a control network [106, 107], and work out the resilience of the tinnitus network when different nodes of the network were attacked [108]. Graph theory was also instrumental in empirically determining the directional core tinnitus distress network [109]. Therefore, through these and other studies [110], researchers were able to empirically quantify the concept of behaviourally segregated tinnitus subnetworks that were integrated to produce the unified tinnitus percept. Further research with whole brain tinnitus networks also showed that these neural correlates, specifically the topology of the tinnitus network [111], were not static but dynamically changing even within a 5 to 7-minute resting state recording [112, 113]. In fact, the whole brain network correlate of tinnitus loudness and distress was dynamically modified by the parahippocampus, wherein high distress patients showed increased variability to connections with the parahippocampus with increasing loudness and decreased variability to connections with the parahippocampus with increasing distress [114]. This further confirmed that with networks of patients with higher distress was possibly more difficult to modify.

Other Models of Tinnitus Mechanisms from Electrophysiological Findings

More recent electrophysiological research in tinnitus has moved from exploratory to hypothesis-driven and model-based research. Below are some of the models inspired from or derived from the exploratory research.

Thalamocortical Dysrhythmia Model

One of the oldest models put forth in tinnitus by Rodolfo Llinas based on EEG and MEG findings was the thalamocortical dysrhythmia model [115]. This is a deafferentation-based model which shows that hearing loss is accompanied by decrease in alpha activity shifting to pathological theta activity and simultaneous increase in gamma activity in the auditory cortex [66]. The hearing loss induces decreased lateral inhibition, which is featured by the decrease in alpha activity, resulting in increased neural synchrony featured by the increase in theta-gamma activity [116]. Later, studies also showed that the gamma activity was tightly coupled to the phase of the theta activity which was related to the loudness of the tinnitus percept [72, 73]. This phenomenon was not only prevalent in tinnitus, but other pathologies that also presented with deafferentation such as chronic pain, Parkinson's Disease [117], etc.

Noise-Cancellation/Sensory Gating Model

The noise-cancellation/sensory gating model was first postulated using MRI data by Rauschecker and colleagues [118], which proposed that there was a fronto-striatal system involving the pregenual anterior cingulate cortex/ventromedial prefrontal cortex and the nucleus accumbens [119] that would inhibit the increased synchronous activity in the presence of hearing loss at the level of the thalamus through top-down connections, to prevent it from being consciously perceived as tinnitus. This was, however, shown by more recent EEG studies, where the difference between a hearing loss and no hearing loss group was an increased alpha activity in the pregenual anterior cingulate cortex and increased alpha connectivity between the pregenual anterior cingulate cortex and auditory cortex showing successful inhibition in the absence of tinnitus [120]. Furthermore, increased theta activity in the pregenual anterior cingulate and decreased theta connectivity between the pregenual anterior cingulate cortex and the auditory cortex correlate with the loudness of the tinnitus [86], and the decreased connectivity between the rostral anterior cingulate cortex and auditory cortex in the beta frequency band correlates with increased tinnitus awareness [121]. These studies show empirical evidence for a malfunctioning top-down inhibitory system in-line with the noise-cancelling model.

Top-Down and Bottom-Up Tinnitus: Moving Away from Categorical Subtypes to Dimensional Variation

Combining the deafferentation-based and noise-cancelling models, a new model was proposed by Vanneste and colleagues showing that depending on the amount of hearing loss there are possibly different neurological subtypes of tinnitus, viz. top-down and bottom-up-driven tinnitus [120]. This model postulates that in the absence of hearing loss, there is a more top-down type of tinnitus which is driven by maladaptive functioning of the noise cancellation system, and in the presence of hearing loss, the tinnitus is driven by more bottom-up mechanisms involving the parahippocampus. Additionally, as the hearing loss increases, there is accumulated maladaptive functioning across different top-down and bottom-up networks which then proposes the idea of tinnitus as a dimensional disorder rather than categorical subtypes [122], where there is an imbalance between bottom-up and top-down systems and this imbalance may be empirically characterised as a ratio of bottom-up to top-down activity. This raises a question for future studies to explore other possible dimensions of tinnitus such as loudness and distress to better understand the mechanism of action of tinnitus through electrophysiology.

Predictive Coding Model

The latest research in the tinnitus field is centered around empirically characterising the predictive coding model. This model is currently viewed as an overarching model that can explain the mechanism of action of tinnitus through all the other existing models. According to the predictive coding model, the brain maintains an internal representation of the external environment [123]. The weighted difference between the incoming information and the existing prediction is called prediction error and their weighted sum is the percept, whose default is "silence" [124]. In tinnitus, decreased sensory input can invoke such a prediction error. In the presence of a healthy noise cancellation system, this prediction error is usually minimised and the percept is retained as "silence", also known as no phantom percept. However, when there is an aberration in the predictive coding system, even in the absence of hearing loss, an auditory prediction error can over-ride the existing percept of "silence" to perceive a phantom percept.

According to the predictive coding model, prediction error is encoded in gamma oscillations [125]. Based on the explained electrophysiological findings in this chapter, De Ridder and colleagues postulated that in the presence of no hearing loss, the prediction error is compensated by increased activity in the auditory cortex, whereas in the presence of moderate to severe hearing loss, the missing information is replayed from the auditory memory also known as the parahippocampus [126]. Furthermore, Sedley and colleagues postulated that over time, the brain learns through experience-dependent plasticity that perceiving tinnitus is the "new normal" and updates its prediction to perceive tinnitus, and not silence [124].

Future of Electrophysiology in Tinnitus

Currently, research is being undertaken to show empirical evidence for the predictive coding model [127–130], thereby moving the research in the field back to more evoked response-based research questions [131, 132], but this time more hypothesis and model-driven rather than being exploratory. Over the last 40 years, the evoked response field has also grown exponentially to investigate time-frequency responses, phase locking, phase synchrony, and connectivity measures in other pathologies, specifically in the cognitive domain that can be applied to tinnitus. Additionally, the tinnitus field can also take inspiration from the application of big data and machine learning to data-mine static and dynamic electrophysiological correlates to build predictive models of objectively determining the loudness and distress of patients.

The more intriguing questions that electrophysiology can answer surround its clinical application. Electrophysiological correlates are already currently in use to guide transcranial electrical and magnetic stimulation and neurofeedback-based treatments. However, also understanding whether we can use electrophysiological correlates of auditory perception in healthy adults [133–135] to identify populations that may be vulnerable to developing tinnitus will be next step in advancing medicine towards preventative care to reduce burden on the healthcare system.

References

1. Barkwill D, Arora R. Labyrinthitis. Tampa: StatPearls; 2021.
2. Skarżyński PH, et al. Prevalence and severity of tinnitus in otosclerosis: preliminary findings from validated questionnaires. J Int Adv Otol. 2019;15:277.
3. Sajjadi H, Paparella MM. Meniere's disease. Lancet. 2008;372:406–14. https://doi.org/10.1016/S0140-6736(08)61161-7.
4. Bell JR, Anderson-Kim SJ, Low C, Leonetti JP. The persistence of tinnitus after acoustic neuroma surgery. Otolaryngology. 2016;155:317–23.
5. Seligmann H, Podoshin L, Ben-David J, Fradis M, Goldsher M. Drug-induced tinnitus and other hearing disorders. Drug Saf. 1996;14:198–212.
6. Agrup C, Gleeson M, Rudge P. The inner ear and the neurologist. J Neurol Neurosurg Psychiatry. 2007;78:114–22.
7. Pearce J. Barré-Liéou "syndrome". J Neurol Neurosurg Psychiatry. 2004;75:319.
8. Wang J-J, et al. Changes in tinnitus after vestibular schwannoma surgery. Sci Rep. 2019;9:1–12.
9. Pegge SA, Steens SC, Kunst HP, Meijer FJ. Pulsatile tinnitus: differential diagnosis and radiological work-up. Curr Radiol Rep. 2017;5:5.
10. Oliveira CA, Negreiros J, Cavalcante IC, Bahmad F, Venosa AR. Palatal and middle-ear myoclonus: a cause for objective tinnitus. Int Tinnitus J. 2003;9:37–41.
11. Folmer RL, Griest SE. Chronic tinnitus resulting from head or neck injuries. Laryngoscope. 2003;113:821–7.
12. Farmer JC. Diving injuries to the inner ear. Ann Otol Rhinol Laryngol. 1977;86:1–20.
13. Migliori G, Battisti E, Pari M, Vitelli N, Cingolani C. A shifty diagnosis: Cogan's syndrome. A case report and review of the literature. Acta Otorhinolaryngol Ital. 2009;29:108–13.
14. Monsell EM. The mechanism of hearing loss in Paget's disease of bone. Laryngoscope. 2004;114:598–606.
15. Huang Y-S, Koo M, Chen J-C, Hwang J-H. The association between tinnitus and the risk of ischemic cerebrovascular disease in young and middle-aged patients: a secondary case-control analysis of a nationwide, population-based health claims database. PLoS One. 2017;12:e0187474.
16. Noreña AJ. Revisiting the cochlear and central mechanisms of tinnitus and therapeutic approaches. Audiol Neurotol. 2015;20:53–9.
17. Eggermont JJ. Animal models of spontaneous activity in the healthy and impaired auditory system. Front Neural Circuits. 2015;9:19.
18. Noreña AJ, Eggermont JJ. Enriched acoustic environment after noise trauma reduces hearing loss and prevents cortical map reorganization. J Neurosci. 2005;25:699–705.
19. Norena A, Eggermont J. Changes in spontaneous neural activity immediately after an acoustic trauma: implications for neural correlates of tinnitus. Hear Res. 2003;183:137–53.
20. Silverstein H, Haberkamp T, Smouha E. The state of tinnitus after inner ear surgery. Otolaryngology. 1986;95:438–41.
21. De Ridder D, et al. Microvascular decompression for tinnitus: significant improvement for tinnitus intensity without improvement for distress. A 4-year limit. Neurosurgery. 2010;66:656–60.
22. Noreña AJ, Farley BJ. Tinnitus-related neural activity: theories of generation, propagation, and centralization. Hear Res. 2013;295:161–71.
23. Wadman W, Da Silva F. Biophysical aspects of EEG and MEG generation. In: Niedermeyer's electroencephalography: basic principles, clinical applications, and related fields. Oxford: Oxford Univ Press; 2017. p. 89–103.
24. Hämäläinen M, Hari R, Ilmoniemi RJ, Knuutila J, Lounasmaa OV. Magnetoencephalography—theory, instrumentation, and applications to noninvasive studies of the working human brain. Rev Mod Phys. 1993;65:413.
25. Purves D, et al. Neuroscience. Sunderland: Sinauer Accociates Inc; 2012.
26. Sadaghiani S, Hesselmann G, Kleinschmidt A. Distributed and antagonistic contributions of ongoing activity fluctuations to auditory stimulus detection. J Neurosci. 2009;29:13410–7.
27. Parkkonen L, Fujiki N, Mäkelä JP. Sources of auditory brainstem responses revisited: contribution by magnetoencephalography. Hum Brain Mapp. 2009;30:1772–82. https://doi.org/10.1002/hbm.20788.
28. Jewett DL, Williston JS. Auditory-evoked far fields averaged from the scalp of humans. Brain. 1971;94:681–96.
29. Møller AR, Jannetta PJ, Jho HD. Click-evoked responses from the cochlear nucleus: a study in human. Electroencephalogr Clin Neurophysiol. 1994;92:215–24.
30. Deiber M, Ibanez V, Fischer C, Perrin F, Mauguiere F. Sequential mapping favours the hypothesis of distinct generators for Na and Pa middle latency auditory evoked potentials. Electroencephalogr Clin Neurophysiol. 1988;71:187–97.
31. Woods DL, Clayworth C, Knight RT, Simpson G, Naeser M. Generators of middle-and long-latency auditory evoked potentials: implications from studies of patients with bitemporal lesions. Electroencephalogr Clin Neurophysiol. 1987;68:132–48.
32. Polich J. Updating P300: an integrative theory of P3a and P3b. Clin Neurophysiol. 2007;118:2128–48.
33. Sininger YS. Auditory brain stem response for objective measures of hearing. Ear Hear. 1993;14:23–30.
34. Starr A, Picton TW, Sininger Y, Hood LJ, Berlin CI. Auditory neuropathy. Brain. 1996;119:741–53.
35. Hall JW. Handbook of auditory evoked responses. Boston: Allyn & Bacon; 1992.
36. Hood LJ. Clinical applications of the auditory brainstem response. San Diego: Singular; 1998.
37. Kehrle HM, et al. Comparison of auditory brainstem response results in normal-hearing patients with and without tinnitus. Arch Otolaryngol. 2008;134:647–51.
38. Bayar N, Böke B, Turan E, Belgin E. Efficacy of amitriptyline in the treatment of subjective tinnitus. J Otolaryngol. 2001;30:300–3.
39. Gopal KV, Thomas BP, Mao D, Lu H. Efficacy of carnitine in treatment of tinnitus: evidence from audiological and MRI measures—a case study. J Am Acad Audiol. 2015;26:311–24.
40. Liberman MC, Kujawa SG. Cochlear synaptopathy in acquired sensorineural hearing loss: manifestations and mechanisms. Hear Res. 2017;349:138–47.
41. Schaette R, McAlpine D. Tinnitus with a normal audiogram: physiological evidence for hidden hearing loss and computational model. J Neurosci. 2011;31:13452–7.

42. Gu JW, Herrmann BS, Levine RA, Melcher JR. Brainstem auditory evoked potentials suggest a role for the ventral cochlear nucleus in tinnitus. J Assoc Res Otolaryngol. 2012;13:819–33.
43. Eggermont J. Tinnitus: some thoughts about its origin. J Laryngol Otol. 1984;98:31–7.
44. Møsller AR. Pathophysiology of tinnitus. Ann Otol Rhinol Laryngol. 1984;93:39–44.
45. Konrad-Martin D, et al. Age-related changes in the auditory brainstem response. J Am Acad Audiol. 2012;23:018–35.
46. Milloy V, Fournier P, Benoit D, Noreña A, Koravand A. Auditory brainstem responses in tinnitus: a review of who, how, and what? Front Aging Neurosci. 2017;9:237.
47. Diesch E, Andermann M, Flor H, Rupp A. Interaction among the components of multiple auditory steady-state responses: enhancement in tinnitus patients, inhibition in controls. Neuroscience. 2010;167:540–53. https://doi.org/10.1016/j.neuroscience.2010.02.003.
48. Diesch E, et al. Enhancement of steady-state auditory evoked magnetic fields in tinnitus. Eur J Neurosci. 2004;19:1093–104.
49. Schlee W, Weisz N, Dohrmann K, Hartmann T, Elbert T. Unravelling the tinnitus distress network using single trial auditory steady-state responses. Int Congr Ser. 2007;1300:73–6. https://doi.org/10.1016/j.ics.2006.12.059.
50. Schlee W, Weisz N, Bertrand O, Hartmann T, Elbert T. Using auditory steady state responses to outline the functional connectivity in the tinnitus brain. PLoS ONE. 2008;3:e3720. https://doi.org/10.1371/journal.pone.0003720.
51. Wienbruch C, Paul I, Weisz N, Elbert T, Roberts LE. Frequency organization of the 40-Hz auditory steady-state response in normal hearing and in tinnitus. NeuroImage. 2006;33:180–94. https://doi.org/10.1016/j.neuroimage.2006.06.023.
52. Hoke M, Feldmann H, Pantev C, Lütkenhöner B, Lehnertz K. Objective evidence of tinnitus in auditory evoked magnetic fields. Hear Res. 1989;37:281–6.
53. Jacobson GP, et al. Auditory evoked cortical magnetic field (M100—M200) measurements in tinnitus and normal groups. Hear Res. 1991;56:44–52.
54. Colding-Jørgensen E, Lauritzen M, Johnsen N, Mikkelsen K, Saermark K. On the evidence of auditory evoked magnetic fields as an objective measure of tinnitus. Electroencephalogr Clin Neurophysiol. 1992;83:322–7.
55. Attias J, Urbach D, Gold S, Shemesh Z. Auditory event related potentials in chronic tinnitus patients with noise induced hearing loss. Hear Res. 1993;71:106–13. https://doi.org/10.1016/0378-5955(93)90026-W.
56. Attias J, Furman V, Shemesh Z, Bresloff I. Impaired brain processing in noise-induced tinnitus patients as measured by auditory and visual event-related potentials. Ear Hear. 1996;17:327–33.
57. Norena A, Cransac H, Chéry-Croze S. Towards an objectification by classification of tinnitus. Clin Neurophysiol. 1999;110:666–75. https://doi.org/10.1016/S1388-2457(98)00034-0.
58. Kadner A, et al. Lateral inhibition in the auditory cortex: an EEG index of tinnitus? Neuroreport. 2002;13:443–6.
59. Lee C-Y, Jaw F-S, Pan S-L, Lin M-Y, Young Y-H. Auditory cortical evoked potentials in tinnitus patients with normal audiological presentation. J Formos Med Assoc. 2007;106:979–85.
60. Näätänen R, Paavilainen P, Titinen H, Jiang D, Alho K. Attention and mismatch negativity. Psychophysiology. 1993;30:436–50.
61. Jacobson GP, et al. Electrophysiological indices of selective auditory attention in subjects with and without tinnitus. Hear Res. 1996;97:66–74. https://doi.org/10.1016/S0378-5955(96)80008-6.
62. Weisz N, Voss S, Berg P, Elbert T. Abnormal auditory mismatch response in tinnitus sufferers with high-frequency hearing loss is associated with subjective distress level. BMC Neurosci. 2004;5:8. https://doi.org/10.1186/1471-2202-5-8.
63. Delb W, et al. Alterations in event related potentials (ERP) associated with tinnitus distress and attention. Appl Psychophysiol Biofeedback. 2008;33:211–21. https://doi.org/10.1007/s10484-008-9065-y.
64. Ortmann M, Müller N, Schlee W, Weisz N. Rapid increases of gamma power in the auditory cortex following noise trauma in humans. Eur J Neurosci. 2011;33:568–75.
65. Weisz N, Moratti S, Meinzer M, Dohrmann K, Elbert T. Tinnitus perception and distress is related to abnormal spontaneous brain activity as measured by magnetoencephalography. PLoS Med. 2005;2:e153.
66. Weisz N, et al. The neural code of auditory phantom perception. J Neurosci. 2007;27:1479–84.
67. Ashton H, et al. High frequency localised "hot spots" in temporal lobes of patients with intractable tinnitus: a quantitative electroencephalographic (QEEG) study. Neurosci Lett. 2007;426:23–8.
68. Schlee W, Hartmann T, Langguth B, Weisz N. Abnormal resting-state cortical coupling in chronic tinnitus. BMC Neurosci. 2009;10:1–11.
69. Sedley W, Cunningham MO. Do cortical gamma oscillations promote or suppress perception? An under-asked question with an over-assumed answer. Front Hum Neurosci. 2013;7:595. https://doi.org/10.3389/fnhum.2013.00595.
70. Van Der Loo E, et al. Tinnitus intensity dependent gamma oscillations of the contralateral auditory cortex. PLoS One. 2009;4:e7396.
71. Balkenhol T, Wallhäusser-Franke E, Delb W. Psychoacoustic tinnitus loudness and tinnitus-related distress show different associations with oscillatory brain activity. PLoS One. 2013;8:e53180.
72. De Ridder D, et al. Theta-gamma dysrhythmia and auditory phantom perception: case report. J Neurosurg. 2011;114:912–21.
73. De Ridder D, Congedo M, Vanneste S. The neural correlates of subjectively perceived and passively matched loudness perception in auditory phantom perception. Brain Behav. 2015;5:e00331.
74. Vanneste S, et al. The neural correlates of tinnitus-related distress. NeuroImage. 2010;52:470–80. https://doi.org/10.1016/j.neuroimage.2010.04.029.
75. Mohsen S, Mahmoudian S, Talbian S, Pourbakht A. Correlation analysis of the tinnitus handicap inventory and distress network in chronic tinnitus: an EEG study. Basic Clin Neurosci. 2019;10:499–514. https://doi.org/10.32598/bcn.9.10.215.
76. De Ridder D, Vanneste S, Congedo M. The distressed brain: a group blind source separation analysis on tinnitus. PLoS ONE. 2011;6:e24273. https://doi.org/10.1371/journal.pone.0024273.
77. De Ridder D, Vanneste S. Progress in brain research, vol. 262. Amsterdam: Elsevier; 2021. p. 309–34.
78. Meyer M, et al. EEG oscillatory power dissociates between distress- and depression-related psychopathology in subjective tinnitus. Brain Res. 2017;1663:194–204. https://doi.org/10.1016/j.brainres.2017.03.007.
79. Meyer M, Luethi MS, Neff P, Langer N, Büchi S. Disentangling tinnitus distress and tinnitus presence by means of EEG power analysis. Neural Plast. 2014;2014:468546. https://doi.org/10.1155/2014/468546.
80. Vanneste S, De Ridder D. Stress-related functional connectivity changes between auditory cortex and cingulate in tinnitus. Brain Connect. 2015;5:371–83. https://doi.org/10.1089/brain.2014.0255.
81. Vanneste S, Congedo M, De Ridder D. Pinpointing a Highly Specific Pathological Functional Connection That Turns Phantom Sound into Distress. Cereb Cortex. 2014;24:2268–82. https://doi.org/10.1093/cercor/bht068.
82. Vanneste S, Joos K, Langguth B, To WT, De Ridder D. Neuronal correlates of maladaptive coping: an EEG-study in tinnitus patients. PLoS One. 2014;9:e88253.
83. Schmidt SA, Akrofi K, Carpenter-Thompson JR, Husain FT. Default mode, dorsal attention and auditory resting state net-

works exhibit differential functional connectivity in tinnitus and hearing loss. PLoS ONE. 2013;8:e76488. https://doi.org/10.1371/journal.pone.0076488.
84. Vanneste S, De Ridder D. Deafferentation-based pathophysiological differences in phantom sound: tinnitus with and without hearing loss. NeuroImage. 2016;129:80–94. https://doi.org/10.1016/j.neuroimage.2015.12.002.
85. Lee S-Y, et al. Is the posterior cingulate cortex an on-off switch for tinnitus? A comparison between hearing loss subjects with and without tinnitus. Hear Res. 2021;411:108356. https://doi.org/10.1016/j.heares.2021.108356.
86. Vanneste S, Alsalman O, De Ridder D. COMT and the neurogenetic architecture of hearing loss induced tinnitus. Hear Res. 2018;365:1–15. https://doi.org/10.1016/j.heares.2018.05.020.
87. Adamchic I, Hauptmann C, Tass PA. Changes of oscillatory activity in pitch processing network and related tinnitus relief induced by acoustic CR neuromodulation. Front Syst Neurosci. 2012;6:18. https://doi.org/10.3389/fnsys.2012.00018.
88. Zhang J, et al. Differences in clinical characteristics and brain activity between patients with low- and high-frequency tinnitus. Neural Plast. 2020;2020:5285362. https://doi.org/10.1155/2020/5285362.
89. Vanneste S, Plazier M, van der Loo E, Van de Heyning P, De Ridder D. The differences in brain activity between narrow band noise and pure tone tinnitus. PLoS ONE. 2010;5:e13618. https://doi.org/10.1371/journal.pone.0013618.
90. Vanneste S, Plazier M, van der Loo E, Van de Heyning P, De Ridder D. The difference between uni- and bilateral auditory phantom percept. Clin Neurophysiol. 2011;122:578–87. https://doi.org/10.1016/j.clinph.2010.07.022.
91. Vanneste S, Van de Heyning P, De Ridder D. Contralateral parahippocampal gamma-band activity determines noise-like tinnitus laterality: a region of interest analysis. Neuroscience. 2011;199:481–90. https://doi.org/10.1016/j.neuroscience.2011.07.067.
92. Vanneste S, Joos K, De Ridder D. Prefrontal cortex based sex differences in tinnitus perception: same tinnitus intensity, same tinnitus distress, different mood. PLoS ONE. 2012;7:e31182. https://doi.org/10.1371/journal.pone.0031182.
93. van der Loo E, Congedo M, Vanneste S, De Heyning PV, De Ridder D. Insular lateralization in tinnitus distress. Auton Neurosci Basic Clin. 2011;165:191–4. https://doi.org/10.1016/j.autneu.2011.06.007.
94. Vanneste S, De Ridder D. Brain areas controlling heart rate variability in tinnitus and tinnitus-related distress. PLoS ONE. 2013;8:e59728. https://doi.org/10.1371/journal.pone.0059728.
95. Vanneste S, van de Heyning P, De Ridder D. The neural network of phantom sound changes over time: a comparison between recent-onset and chronic tinnitus patients. Eur J Neurosci. 2011;34:718–31. https://doi.org/10.1111/j.1460-9568.2011.07793.x.
96. Song J-J, Vanneste S, Schlee W, Van de Heyning P, De Ridder D. Onset-related differences in neural substrates of tinnitus-related distress: the anterior cingulate cortex in late-onset tinnitus, and the frontal cortex in early-onset tinnitus. Brain Struct Funct. 2015;220:571–84. https://doi.org/10.1007/s00429-013-0648-x.
97. Song J-J, De Ridder D, Schlee W, Van de Heyning P, Vanneste S. "Distressed aging": the differences in brain activity between early- and late-onset tinnitus. Neurobiol Aging. 2013;34:1853–63. https://doi.org/10.1016/j.neurobiolaging.2013.01.014.
98. Vanneste S, De Ridder D. The auditory and non-auditory brain areas involved in tinnitus. An emergent property of multiple parallel overlapping subnetworks. Front Syst Neurosci. 2012;6:31. https://doi.org/10.3389/fnsys.2012.00031.
99. De Ridder D, et al. An integrative model of auditory phantom perception: tinnitus as a unified percept of interacting separable subnetworks. Neurosci Biobehav Rev. 2014;44:16–32. https://doi.org/10.1016/j.neubiorev.2013.03.021.
100. Bullmore E, Sporns O. Complex brain networks: graph theoretical analysis of structural and functional systems. Nat Rev Neurosci. 2009;10:186–98. https://doi.org/10.1038/nrn2575.
101. Achard S, Bullmore E. Efficiency and cost of economical brain functional networks. PLoS Comput Biol. 2007;3:e17. https://doi.org/10.1371/journal.pcbi.0030017.
102. Rubinov M, Sporns O. Complex network measures of brain connectivity: uses and interpretations. NeuroImage. 2010;52:1059–69. https://doi.org/10.1016/j.neuroimage.2009.10.003.
103. van den Heuvel MP, Sporns O. Rich-club organization of the human connectome. J Neurosci. 2011;31:15775. https://doi.org/10.1523/JNEUROSCI.3539-11.2011.
104. Stam CJ. Modern network science of neurological disorders. Nat Rev Neurosci. 2014;15:683–95. https://doi.org/10.1038/nrn3801.
105. Mohan A, De Ridder D, Vanneste S. Graph theoretical analysis of brain connectivity in phantom sound perception. Sci Rep. 2016;6:19683. https://doi.org/10.1038/srep19683.
106. Mohan A, De Ridder D, Vanneste S. Emerging hubs in phantom perception connectomics. NeuroImage Clin. 2016;11:181–94. https://doi.org/10.1016/j.nicl.2016.01.022.
107. Schlee W, et al. Mapping cortical hubs in tinnitus. BMC Biol. 2009;7:80. https://doi.org/10.1186/1741-7007-7-80.
108. Mohan A, De Ridder D, Vanneste S. Robustness and dynamicity of functional networks in phantom sound. NeuroImage. 2017;146:171–87. https://doi.org/10.1016/j.neuroimage.2016.04.033.
109. Mohan A, Davidson C, De Ridder D, Vanneste S. Effective connectivity analysis of inter- and intramodular hubs in phantom sound perception – identifying the core distress network. Brain Imaging Behav. 2020;14:289–307. https://doi.org/10.1007/s11682-018-9989-7.
110. Mohan A, Moreno N, Song J-J, De Ridder D, Vanneste S. Evidence for behaviorally segregated, spatiotemporally overlapping subnetworks in phantom sound perception. Brain Connect. 2017;7:197–210. https://doi.org/10.1089/brain.2016.0459.
111. Mohan A, Alexandra SJ, Johnson CV, De Ridder D, Vanneste S. Effect of distress on transient network dynamics and topological equilibrium in phantom sound perception. Prog Neuro-Psychopharmacol Biol Psychiatry. 2018;84:79–92. https://doi.org/10.1016/j.pnpbp.2018.01.025.
112. Cai Y, et al. Deviant dynamics of resting state electroencephalogram microstate in patients with subjective tinnitus. Front Behav Neurosci. 2018;12:122. https://doi.org/10.3389/fnbeh.2018.00122.
113. Cao W, et al. Microstate in resting state: an EEG indicator of tinnitus? Acta Otolaryngol. 2020;140:564–9. https://doi.org/10.1080/00016489.2020.1743878.
114. Mohan A, De Ridder D, Idiculla R, Dsouza C, Vanneste S. Distress-dependent temporal variability of regions encoding domain-specific and domain-general behavioral manifestations of phantom percepts. Eur J Neurosci. 2018;48:1743–64. https://doi.org/10.1111/ejn.13988.
115. Llinás RR, Ribary U, Jeanmonod D, Kronberg E, Mitra PP. Thalamocortical dysrhythmia: a neurological and neuropsychiatric syndrome characterized by magnetoencephalography. Proc Natl Acad Sci. 1999;96:15222. https://doi.org/10.1073/pnas.96.26.15222.
116. De Ridder D, Vanneste S, Langguth B, Llinas R. Thalamocortical dysrhythmia: a theoretical update in tinnitus. Front Neurol. 2015;6:124. https://doi.org/10.3389/fneur.2015.00124.
117. Vanneste S, Song J-J, De Ridder D. Thalamocortical dysrhythmia detected by machine learning. Nat Commun. 2018;9:1103. https://doi.org/10.1038/s41467-018-02820-0.

118. Rauschecker JP, Leaver AM, Mühlau M. Tuning out the noise: limbic-auditory interactions in tinnitus. Neuron. 2010;66:819–26. https://doi.org/10.1016/j.neuron.2010.04.032.
119. Rauschecker JP, May ES, Maudoux A, Ploner M. Frontostriatal gating of tinnitus and chronic pain. Trends Cogn Sci. 2015;19:567–78. https://doi.org/10.1016/j.tics.2015.08.002.
120. Vanneste S, Alsalman O, De Ridder D. Top-down and bottom-up regulated auditory phantom perception. J Neurosci. 2019;39:364–78. https://doi.org/10.1523/JNEUROSCI.0966-18.2018.
121. Song JJ, Vanneste S, De Ridder D. Dysfunctional noise cancelling of the rostral anterior cingulate cortex in tinnitus patients. PLoS One. 2015;10:e0123538. https://doi.org/10.1371/journal.pone.0123538.
122. Mohan A, Leong SL, De Ridder D, Vanneste S. Symptom dimensions to address heterogeneity in tinnitus. Neurosci Biobehav Rev. 2021;134:104542.
123. Hullfish J, Sedley W, Vanneste S. Prediction and perception: insights for (and from) tinnitus. Neurosci Biobehav Rev. 2019;102:1–12. https://doi.org/10.1016/j.neubiorev.2019.04.008.
124. Sedley W, Friston KJ, Gander PE, Kumar S, Griffiths TD. An integrative tinnitus model based on sensory precision. Trends Neurosci. 2016;39:799–812. https://doi.org/10.1016/j.tins.2016.10.004.
125. Arnal LH, Giraud A-L. Cortical oscillations and sensory predictions. Trends Cogn Sci. 2012;16:390–8.
126. De Ridder D, Vanneste S, Freeman W. The Bayesian brain: phantom percepts resolve sensory uncertainty. Neurosci Biobehav Rev. 2014;44:4–15. https://doi.org/10.1016/j.neubiorev.2012.04.001.
127. Sedley W, Alter K, Gander PE, Berger J, Griffiths TD. Exposing pathological sensory predictions in tinnitus using auditory intensity deviant evoked responses. J Neurosci. 2019;39:10096. https://doi.org/10.1523/JNEUROSCI.1308-19.2019.
128. Mohan A, Luckey A, Weisz N, Vanneste S. Predisposition to domain-wide maladaptive changes in predictive coding in auditory phantom perception. NeuroImage. 2021;248:118813.
129. Mohebbi M, et al. The potential role of auditory prediction error in decompensated tinnitus: an auditory mismatch negativity study. Brain Behav. 2019;9:e01242. https://doi.org/10.1002/brb3.1242.
130. Partyka M et al. Phantom auditory perception (tinnitus) is characterised by stronger anticipatory auditory predictions. bioRxiv. 2019. 869842. https://doi.org/10.1101/869842.
131. Hong SK, Park S, Ahn M-H, Min B-K. Top-down and bottom-up neurodynamic evidence in patients with tinnitus. Hear Res. 2016;342:86–100. https://doi.org/10.1016/j.heares.2016.10.002.
132. Mahmoudian S, et al. Central auditory processing during chronic tinnitus as indexed by topographical maps of the mismatch negativity obtained with the multi-feature paradigm. Brain Res. 2013;1527:161–73. https://doi.org/10.1016/j.brainres.2013.06.019.
133. Mohan A, et al. Investigating functional changes in the brain to intermittently induced auditory illusions and its relevance to chronic tinnitus. Hum Brain Mapp. 2020;41:1819–32. https://doi.org/10.1002/hbm.24914.
134. Norena A, Micheyl C, Chery-Croze S. An auditory negative after-image as a human model of tinnitus. Hear Res. 2000;149:24–32. https://doi.org/10.1016/S0378-5955(00)00158-1.
135. Leske S, et al. The strength of alpha and beta oscillations parametrically scale with the strength of an illusory auditory percept. NeuroImage. 2014;88:69–78. https://doi.org/10.1016/j.neuroimage.2013.11.014.

Part III

Pathophysiological Models

The Bayesian Brain and Tinnitus

17

Dirk De Ridder, Sven Vanneste, William Sedley, and Karl Friston

Abstract

There is strong and growing evidence for 'Bayesian' accounts of brain function, such as predictive coding, in which perception depends upon internally generated models of the sensorium, which are updated and refined based on sensory input.

Bayesian perception involves both automatic stimulus-based perceptual inference and active time-based inference that underwrites the active sampling of predicted sensory stimuli.

Predictions in perceptual inference are associated with beta band activity, the precision of predictions with alpha activity and prediction errors with gamma oscillatory activity in sensory cortex, where prediction errors are propagated to other brain areas. Predictions in active inference are associated with theta activity, precision with delta and prediction errors with gamma activity in hippocampus and other cortical areas.

Activity in these frequency bands, in auditory and other cortical areas, has been linked to tinnitus, but not yet specifically to Bayesian processes in this context.

Different pathophysiological models have been proposed to explain the emergence of tinnitus, two of which are based on Bayesian processes. One account postulates that tinnitus is the result of memory-based prior beliefs about sounds, which are mobilised in compensation for the absence of evidence from sensory input. This model is based on active inference. Alternatively, spontaneous activity in the ascending auditory pathway (a 'tinnitus precursor') is usually ignored as noise, which conflicts with the default prediction of 'no sound', and chronic tinnitus occurs when this activity gains sufficient 'precision' to influence perceptual inference.

Stress may influence perceptual inference in various ways, favouring the initial emergence of tinnitus and/or its perpetuation.

In both accounts, incorporation of the tinnitus percept into default predictions leads to chronification of the condition.

Anatomical and electrophysiological data in tinnitus research are compatible with a Bayesian brain model, but are largely circumstantial and also compatible with alternative formulations.

D. De Ridder (✉)
Section of Neurosurgery, Department of Surgical Sciences, University of Otago, Dunedin, New Zealand
e-mail: Dirk.deridder@otago.ac.nz; http://www.brai3n.com

S. Vanneste
Global Brain Health Institute, Institute of Neuroscience, Trinity College Dublin, Dublin, Ireland
e-mail: Sven.vanneste@tcd.ie

W. Sedley
Translational and Clinical Research Institute, Newcastle University, Newcastle upon Tyne, UK
e-mail: william.sedley@newcastle.ac.uk

K. Friston
Wellcome Trust Centre for Neuroimaging, University College London, London, UK
e-mail: k.friston@ucl.ac.uk

W. Schlee et al. (eds.), *Textbook of Tinnitus*, https://doi.org/10.1007/978-3-031-35647-6_17

Graphical Abstract

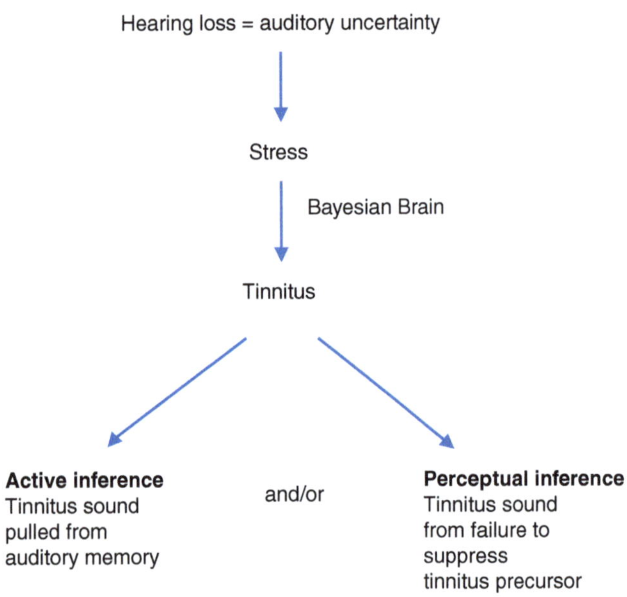

Highlights

- There is compelling evidence that perception operates in a Bayesian manner, combining prior expectations with sensory input to minimise uncertainty about the environment.
- Bayesian perception involves both perceptual and active inference:
  - Perceptual inference involves stimulus-based prediction error computations between sensory input and prior predictions.
  - Active inference involves time-based prediction error computations that underwrite sampling the environment for predicted stimuli.
  - The temporal (oscillatory) and spatial (anatomically specialised) processes likely differ between perceptual and active inference.
- It is highly likely that tinnitus emerges as an aspect of Bayesian perception.
- Two contemporary theories explain the emergence of tinnitus as an emergent property of aberrant Bayesian inference under conditions of increased sensory uncertainty due to hearing loss:
  - In one account, auditory information that fails to be delivered through input to the ear(s) due to hearing loss is instead retrieved from top-down predictions derived from auditory memory.
  - In the other account, compensation for hearing loss increases spontaneous neuronal activity in the auditory pathway, and tinnitus occurs when Bayesian inference fails to infer these signals are noise.
- Stress, caused by auditory sensory uncertainty itself and/or other unrelated causes, undergirds the initial emergence of tinnitus, and drives the transition from acute to chronic tinnitus, i.e. chronification.
- In chronification, the tinnitus becomes incorporated into the (generative) model of the sensed world.
- The neural correlates of Bayesian inference are putatively known, which may shed light on the computational mechanisms of tinnitus.
- Computational models of Bayesian inference in the brain may help to develop, test and refine theories of tinnitus, and predict the effects of treatments.

Introduction

Chronic tinnitus has been defined as the conscious awareness of a tonal or composite noise for which there is no identifiable corresponding external acoustic source [1]. In about 20% of people with tinnitus, the tinnitus sound is associated with emotional distress, cognitive dysfunction and/or autonomic arousal, leading to behavioural changes and functional disability, with the term 'tinnitus disorder' recently proposed to refer to these patients [1]. In other words, 'Tinnitus' describes the auditory or phantom sound component, and 'Tinnitus Disorder' reflects the suffering associated with the phantom sound [1]. Tinnitus can have various causes, though these causes tend to involve some degree of hearing loss, which is the principal risk factor, and is present in 80% of elderly tinnitus patients [2]. However, tinnitus may occur remotely from the onset of hearing loss, yet once present for 4 weeks is usually persistent long-term [3]. Taken together, these observations suggest that additional factors—beyond hearing loss—are responsible for the onset of tinnitus, and that these factors tend to become self-perpetuating.

Phantom perceptions are common in people who sustain sensory deafferentation, in various sensory domains (such as tinnitus in hearing loss, phantom limb pain in amputation or Charles Bonnet syndrome in visual loss), suggesting there exist generic, amodal pathophysiological mechanisms that generate phantom percepts. The explanation proposed here advocates that the brain works in a Bayesian fashion, and that its main function is to infer causes of sensations and implicitly reduce uncertainty about (hidden) states of the environment—an uncertainty that is confounded by sensory deprivation [4]. Importantly, in the face of deafferentation, the very imperative to reduce uncertainty can be achieved by creating phantom percepts, even though these percepts can themselves create other problems [4].

We summarise two alternative—and perhaps complementary—accounts of how phantom percepts can resolve uncertainty: in one account, sensory cortex is unable to find the requisite information in sensory afferents, and therefore retrieves compatible information from auditory memory [4]; in the other account, deafferentation leads to increased spontaneous activity in the ascending sensory pathway, and phantom perception occurs when higher predictive processes fail to override this evidence for a percept, in favour of the default 'no percept' prediction [5]. Both models further posit that if the sensory deprivation persists for a certain time, the phantom percept will become the new default, leading to chronic persistence of the phantom perception, even if some of the initial conditions triggering its onset are reversed.

Active Perception

Perception differs from sensation. Whereas sensation can be defined as the detection and processing of sensory information, perception is the act of interpreting and organising this sensory information to produce a meaningful experience of the world and of oneself [6, 7]. In other words, perception is the assimilation of sensory data from the environment into our model of the world, which depends on the meaning [8] and context [9, 10] of the sensory information, and on prior experience and expectations.

Perception involves both automatic stimulus-based perceptual inference, and active inference, related to targeted sampling of predicted or anticipated sensory stimuli. In perceptual inference, the brain compares sensory stimuli with predicted stimuli, based on a model it has of the environment or world. This model is referred to as a world model or generative model, in the sense it can generate predictions of (observable) sensory input from (unobservable) causes (e.g. sound objects). In active inference, the brain actively explores the world and samples the environment for stimuli it expects to find in the environment. In the context of auditory perception, this kind of active sensing may be covert; in the sense it can be understood as selectively attending to various aspects of auditory afferents. Together perceptual and active inference constitute a sensorimotor perceptual loop (c.f., perception action cycle), in the service of trying to minimise prediction errors and implicit uncertainty about the causes of sensations.

Bayesian Inference, Perception and the Free Energy Principle

The ultimate function of the brain is to reduce the inherent uncertainty present in a changing environment. In order to survive—and function effectively in an uncertain world—any self-organising system must maintain a boundary that individuates it from the embedding environment. This existential separation is required to differentiate a biological entity from the environment. To be alive as 'me' means I have a structure, a pattern, a form, separate from the environment: in short, I possess characteristics states that are distinct from those of my eco-niche. Everything within the membrane or skin, i.e. everything within the boundary, is 'me'. Mathematically this is represented as a Markov blanket [11]. 'I' survive only if 'I' am capable to resist the tendency to disorder/entropy, famously celebrated as the second law of thermodynamics [11]. Survival then just is the maintenance of my Markov blanket that, crucially, mediates an exchange with my environment. In other words, I am an open system exchanging energy and information with the environment where, to survive, means to maintain one's inner states (and blanket states) within the domain of the states that characterise me [11].

Consequently, this requires the external environment to be internally represented, by creating an inner model of the environment that needs to be constantly updated via processes such as inference and learning. This model enables me to maintain physiological states within characteristic bounds (i.e. homeostasis) and, more generally, ensures living entities occupy a small number of characteristic states [11]. This is sometimes cast in terms of minimising prediction errors, based on predictions that enable me to predict what will happen next (good or bad), and increase my chances of survival and procreation. In short, the goal of the brain is to minimise prediction errors or minimise uncertainty about the lived world.

Minimising 'prediction error' is effectively minimising 'free energy'. In the context of the free energy principle, variational free energy scores the surprise inherent in sensory exchanges with the environment and is exactly the same quantity used in statistics and machine learning to do Bayesian inference. Minimising variational free energy is the same as maximising the evidence for one's generative model of the world (a.k.a., marginal likelihood). This means that minimising prediction error or free energy can be neatly summarised as self-evidencing [12]; namely, seeking evidence for one's model of the world and changing one's model of the world to fit the sensory evidence that is garnered.

Free energy or prediction errors can be reduced by changing predictions through perception, i.e. perceptual inference. Or, by selectively sampling sensory inputs that are predicted, through overt or covert action, i.e. active inference [13].

Perceptual inference thus entails inferring the causes of sensory input, i.e. what object or event caused this input [13]? As such, perceptual inference relates to the past. These inferred causes update prior beliefs about the environment, to form of posterior beliefs that best predict time-varying sensory input. Active inference, on the other hand, relates to the future: how can I change my sensory input to confirm the prediction, i.e. to reduce prediction error [13]? As such, the sensory input is adapted to accommodate posterior expectations, by actively sampling the environment in a way that best corresponds to what is expected or predicted. If these posterior expectations are sufficiently constrained by prior beliefs, I will sample the kind of inputs I expect to encounter and thereby securing sensory evidence that my generative model is apt for my world and, coincidentally, ensuring my sensory inputs (and their inferred causes) are characteristic of the sort of creature 'I am'.

The pursuit of reducing uncertainty, in a changing environment, has been argued to constitute the singular act of minimising 'free energy' [14, 15]. Free energy is a mathematically defined measure of disorder, related to entropy, which scores the inaccuracy and complexity of predictions under a generative model (c.f., sensory and prior prediction errors, respectively). As noted above, the negative free energy corresponds to model evidence, which is simply accuracy minus complexity. Here, we foreground the principal role of free energy, namely to quantify 'surprise' [14].

Mathematically, surprise is the improbability of a particular sensory input or event based on posterior predictions [14]. Minimising surprise entails accurately anticipating current and upcoming sensory inputs, based on predictions that are generated from internal models of the environment. Surprise is often equated with 'prediction error', as it indicates the inaccuracy of predictions, and acts to optimise internal models—and ensuing predictions—in light of new sensory information. Minimising surprise, therefore, involves optimising the accuracy of predictions (while minimising prior prediction errors—higher in hierarchical generative models—optimises complexity).

In 'predictive coding' implementations of hierarchical inference [16], predictions within a particular perceptual dimension (e.g. pitch) are encoded as Gaussian probability distributions, characterised by their mean and variance. 'Precision' (i.e. inverse variance) describes the confidence or reliability placed in a particular representation (e.g. prior or sensory prediction errors). The 'posterior' is the inferred expectation (or percept) and corresponds to the prior updated by new sensory information, each weighted by their precision. Precision is dynamically and adaptively modulated, so as to provide the optimal balance between prior predictions and sensory input, depending on factors such as the reliability of sensory input (e.g. clear hearing conditions vs. hearing in noisy environments, or even a lack of input altogether), past experience (e.g. a stimulus that has just been repeating is likely to repeat again) and attentional state (attention increasing the precision or reliability of sensory input). In other words, depending on the context, e.g. arousal or stress, the precision of the priors or precision of the sensory input may itself be updated [17].

Bayes' rule is a mathematical formulation of inference under uncertainty, where prior beliefs are reconciled with new evidence, and is the basis for reaching optimal conclusions in all settings from criminal culpability to medical diagnoses.

Mathematically, Bayes rule is expressed as

$$P(A|B) = \frac{P(B|A)P(A)}{P(B)}$$

With $P(A|B)$ = the posterior probability, i.e. the probability P that the prediction or hypothesis A is correct, given the evidence B. $P(A)$ = the prior probability of the prediction or hypothesis, $P(B)$ = the probability of the evidence B, and $P(B|A)$ = likelihood = the probability that the evidence B is correct given the prediction or hypothesis. $P(B|A)/P(B)$ reflects the support for the prediction or hypothesis A. In sum, the posterior probability, which equals the percept, thought, action, feeling, etc., is the result of the prior hypothesis or prediction A, adjusted by the support coming from evidence B.

The Bayesian brain casts perception as a constructive process, based on internal generative models of the world [14]. A generative model comprises a prior belief and the likelihood [17]. Generative models in the brain can therefore predict sensory data, based upon posterior expectations [17]. The ensuing prediction is compared to the observed sensation, and the difference between the two constitutes the prediction error, which is used to update the prior belief into a posterior belief, i.e. percept [17]. This is known as perceptual inference. In short, the brain has a model of the world that it constantly updates using sensory information [14], as to reduce uncertainty, inherently present in a changing environment [4]. The animal or human will then actively sample the sensory environment that it expects based on the prediction [4, 18], as to update its model of the world, so that it can make better predictions in the future. This is known as active inference.

So how the model of the world is updated? This depends on the precision of various expectations or prediction errors [19], where precise prediction errors have a greater influence on Bayesian belief updating with less precision. The Bayesian brain is constantly performing Bayesian computa-

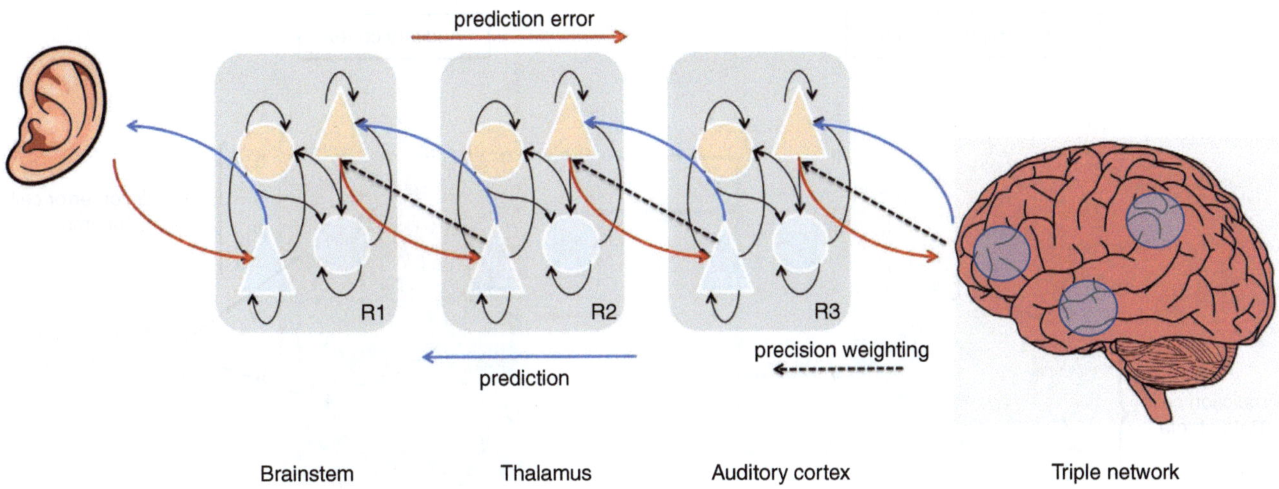

Fig. 17.1 R(epresentation) units in hierarchical levels. Figure modified from [20]

tions, in a hierarchical manner. At each level of the hierarchy, top-down predictions are generated from representations in the level above, and compared with input at the level below (which, at the lowest level, is the sensory organ itself). The resulting prediction error is then passed back in the form of an ascending prediction error. In a hierarchical setting, higher hierarchical levels represent the sensorium at increasingly abstract levels (Fig. 17.1).

The efficiency of this kind of predictive coding scheme is due to the bottom-up passing of information that is needed to update higher-level representations—i.e. prediction error—and the top-down transmission of requisite predictions. Unpredicted changes in the sensory environment result in prediction errors and Bayesian belief updating (which are reflected in stimulus-evoked brain responses).

The Neurobiology of Bayesian Belief Updating

Bayesian inference is argued to underwrite perceptual synthesis, and therefore to occur at every level in the cortical hierarchies. The local neocortical circuitry within brain areas has been interpreted in terms of predictive coding schemes [21] (Fig. 17.2). In these accounts, ascending prediction error arrives in the granular layer (layer 4). Prediction-generating neurons are located in infragranular (deep) layers, fire with low-frequency rhythmicity and send predictions to lower hierarchical levels. Prediction error neurons are thought to be located in supragranular (superficial) layers, fire with high-frequency rhythmicity and send prediction errors to hierarchically higher levels. The laminar segregation of these processes has been demonstrated by direct recordings from multiple layers simultaneously [22].

Specific oscillatory frequencies of the local field potential in sensory cortex have also been linked to pre-attentive predictive processes, with the gamma band (>35 Hz) linked to surprise (i.e. elaboration of prediction errors) [23–29], beta band (around 15 Hz) linked to changing predictions [30, 31] and alpha band linked to the precision of predictions (Fig. 17.3).

Yet, these frequencies may be specific to stimulus-based perceptual inference in sensory cortex. For inference in deep generative models (i.e. hierarchical models with temporal depth), active inference may entail processing over extended periods of time, and different frequencies may be implicated. For example, deep (active) inference may involve hippocampal predictions encoded in the theta frequency band [32] and precision in delta [33], where prediction errors may still be conveyed in the gamma frequency band, as in lower levels of perceptual inference (Fig. 17.3).

The mismatch negativity (MMN) is a ubiquitous neurophysiological response generated by unexpected or changing stimuli in various sensory modalities [34, 35], so-called because of its negative polarity at the vertex. The MMN reflects the unpredicted nature of stimuli [36], based on priors, and is therefore often considered to be a response to prediction violation, encompassing prediction error and updating of priors. The principal neuronal generators of the MMN are the sources in a recurrent network, encompassing primary and secondary sensory cortex and inferior frontal gyrus [36]; the latter believed to generate and/or oversee the generation and updating of predictions [37]. The MMN is often used to detect abnormalities of predictive processing in psychiatric and neuropsychiatric disorders [schizophrenia research, etc.]. Crucially, the MMN does not require attention, but can be modulated by attention [34]. Conversely, a later positive polarity potential evoked by unexpected stim-

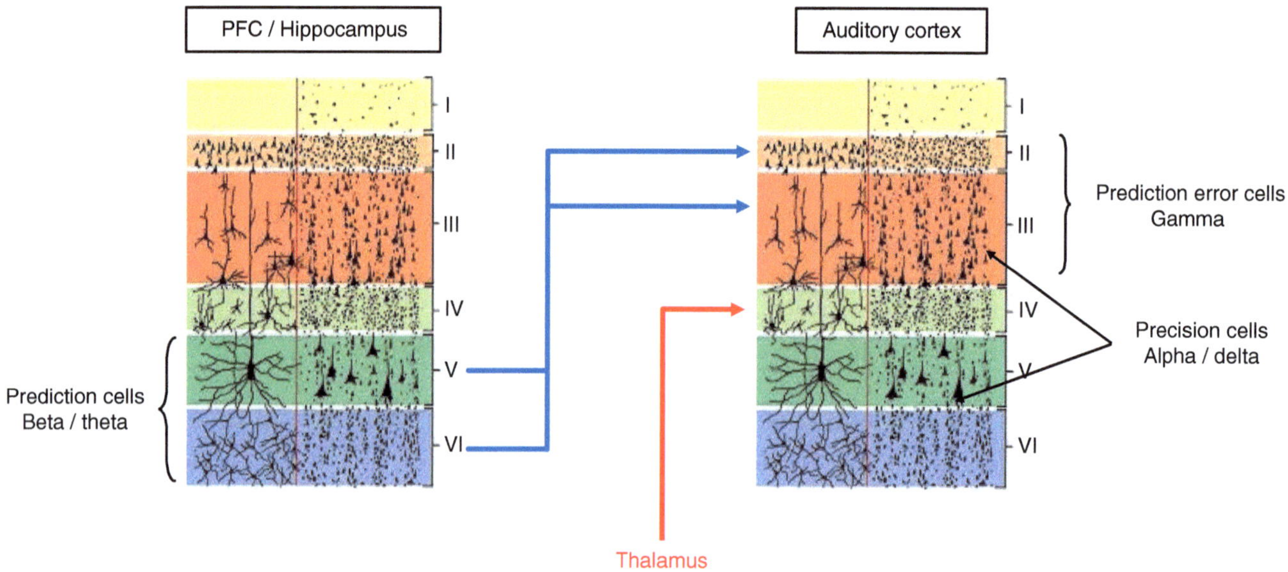

Fig. 17.2 Layer-specific prediction and prediction error

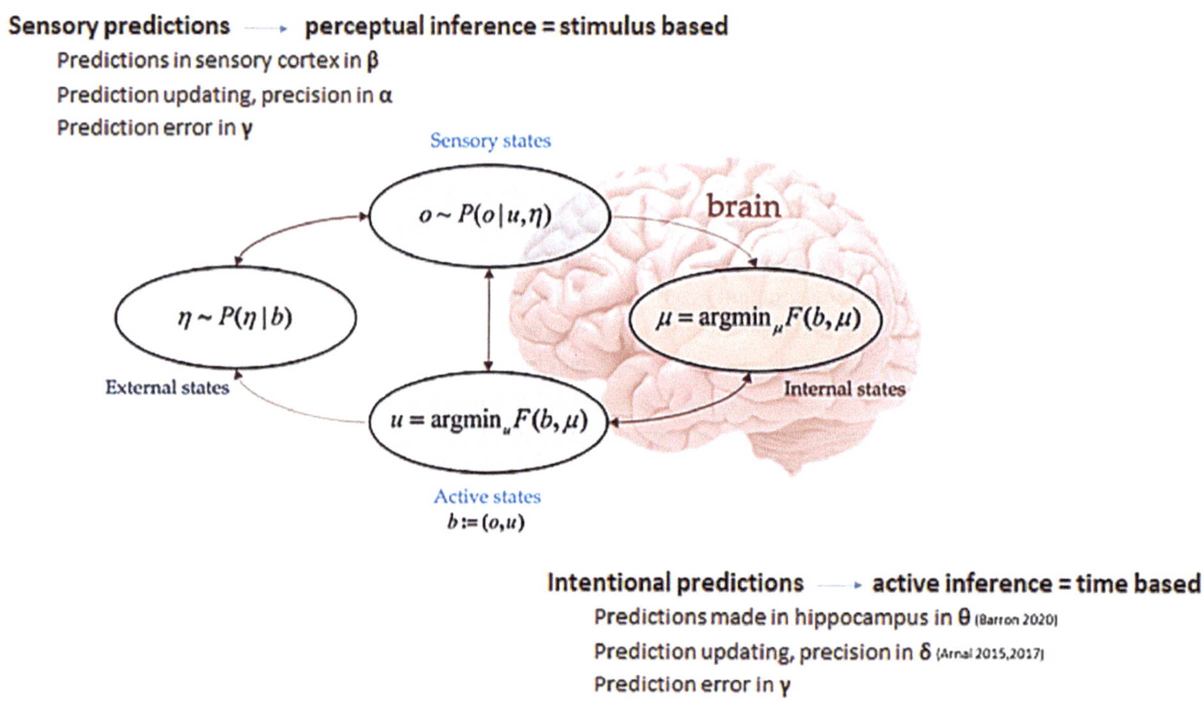

Fig. 17.3 Two kinds of predictions. Stimulus-based perceptual inference and intentional or active inference with temporal depth may involve different oscillatory frequencies for predictions and precision, but similar frequencies for prediction errors

uli, the P300, specifically requires attention or an active task. The distinction between the MMN and P300 reflects the difference in temporal scales implicit in perceptual inference at lower levels of the auditory hierarchy, relative to deep (active) inference that implicates recurrent exchange of predictions and prediction errors at higher levels [38]. Much of the phenomenology of the MMN is thought to reflect changes in the precision of prediction errors at different levels of the auditory hierarchy, based upon predictions of precision. These predictions of precision can be regarded as mediating attentional gain, in the face of an unpredicted change in the auditory stream.

Precision is, neurobiologically, thought to be encoded by the postsynaptic gain of populations broadcasting prediction errors (e.g. superficial pyramidal cells in the upper layers of cortex). Whilst other factors—such as neural synchrony may be important— a major dynamic mechanism of precision control in neocortex is the local action of acetylcholine, which is released by projections from the basal forebrain cholinergic system [39–41]. Attention can therefore be considered a form of gain control via this system, with increased attention amounting to increasing the gain on prediction errors within the attended regime of sensory space.

The Bayesian Brain and Tinnitus

If Bayesian processes are the basis of normal perception, then tinnitus must, from first principles, be explained within such a framework. Furthermore, the prevalence of tinnitus is so high that it should be explicable as an emergent phenomenon, under certain conditions, of a normally functioning Bayesian system. As mentioned above, tinnitus is commonly associated with hearing loss (80%). Furthermore, a normal audiogram does not exclude auditory deafferentation [42], suggesting that deprivation of auditory input, whether measurable or not, may be a general underlying cause for tinnitus.

One main reason why auditory deafferentation may be relevant is that it subverts the dynamics of the sensory states that constitute the Markov blanket; namely, the boundary between the self and the auditory environment, resulting in an altered model of the self-auditory world interaction. Yet, only when the brain considers the ensuing lack of auditory information behaviourally relevant will that lead to a filling in mechanism, i.e. tinnitus [43]. If the brain does not consider the auditory deafferentation behaviourally relevant, it will not change its self-auditory environment interactions [43]. Tinnitus is commonly associated with stress and distress, which may make any change in sensations more salient.

We now consider two alternative accounts of how otherwise normal Bayesian mechanisms might lead to tinnitus as an unintended consequence of otherwise adaptive compensation for hearing loss [4, 6, 43] (Fig. 17.4). These differ fundamentally as to whether tinnitus arises from an erroneous top-down prediction—which 'fills in' missing sensory information due to hearing loss—or whether hearing loss leads to increased spontaneous firing in the ascending auditory pathway and higher predictive mechanisms reject the default hypothesis of 'no sound'. Both accounts share the common feature that when tinnitus is present for an extended time, the tinnitus may become the new norm, the new prior [4, 5, 44], and the tinnitus becomes part of the self-percept, i.e. part of who you are. This could be the phenomenological consequence of the electrophysiological putative 'tinnitus network' becoming functionally connected to the self-perceptual network, analogous to what has been proposed for pain [45, 46]. Additionally, the brain may have stored sounds in memory and must be able to actively explore the sensory environ-

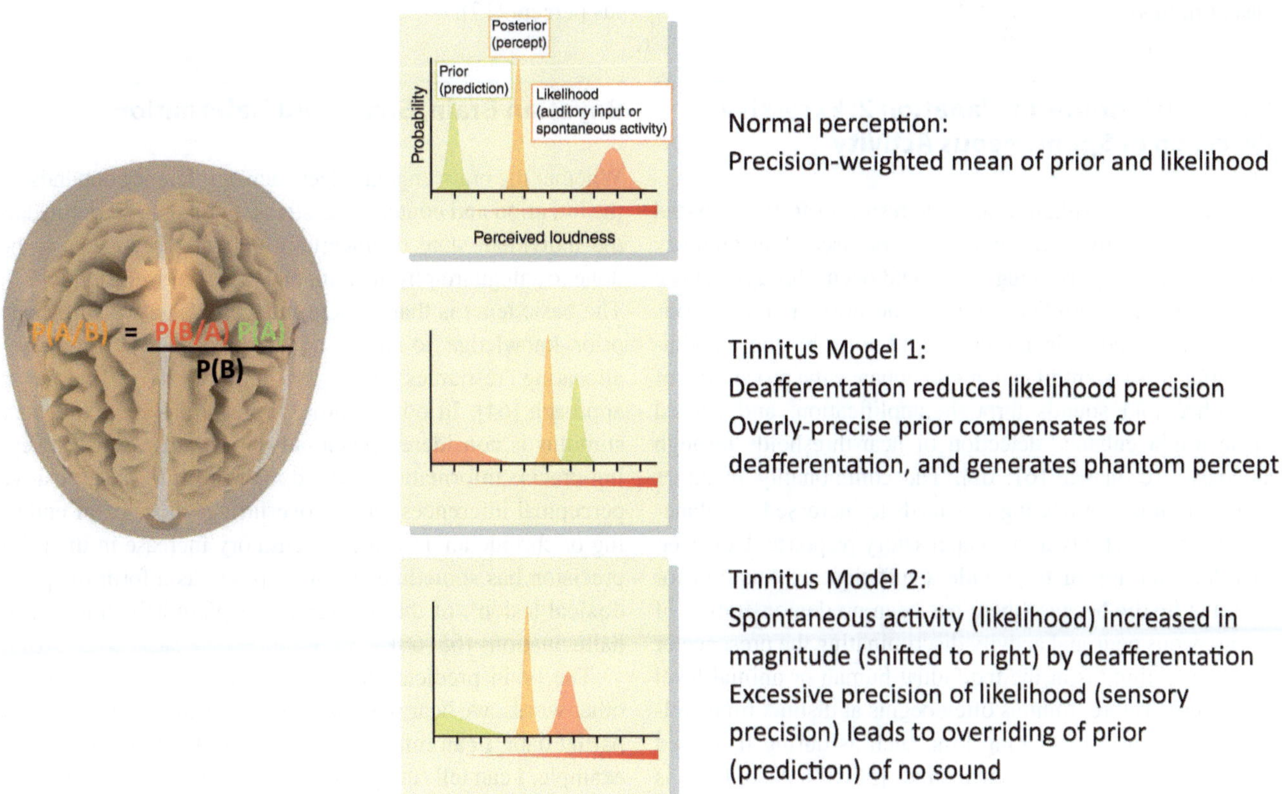

Fig. 17.4 Precision or reliability of the sound signal is different in the two tinnitus models

ment for auditory input. Indeed, children with congenital hearing loss do not develop tinnitus, as they have not built up a deep model of the auditory world that can be used to generate apt auditory predictions [47].

Bayesian Tinnitus Explanation 1: Tinnitus by Filling in Missing Auditory Information

Auditory deafferentation leads to tonotopically restricted prediction errors based on temporal or spatial incongruity [4, 48, 49]. This creates an increase in tonotopically restricted uncertainty, which could be adaptively addressed by plastic repair mechanisms in the auditory cortex or via (para)hippocampal involvement, if the missing auditory information cannot be retrieved from the auditory cortex adjacent to the deafferented thalamocortical column [4, 43, 46–54].

Tinnitus often develops during a period of stress, or is worsened by stress [55–57]. It can be envisioned that during stress, the brain adjusts its predictions of precision, reducing the relative precision of sensory prediction errors in a noisy, volatile and unpredictable context: i.e. analogous to what has been postulated for the emergence of auditory hallucinations [58]. This kind of covert active inference may lead to false beliefs that can lead to maladaptive inferences by relying too much on the precision or reliability of predictions. Consequently, people may perceive sound in the environment that is predicted but not necessarily present (in this case, tinnitus).

Bayesian Tinnitus Explanation 2: Excessive Precision of Spontaneous Activity

Various models explain tinnitus as resulting from increased spontaneous activity of neurons in the ascending auditory pathway. Broadly speaking, this could occur through central gain having a multiplicative effect on normal spontaneous activity [59] and/or increased central noise having an additive effect [60]. Central gain might enhance the processing of suprathreshold sounds through amplification, and central noise might enhance detection of near-thresholds through stochastic resonance [61, 62]. The commonality in either explanation is that hearing loss leads to increased spontaneous neuronal activity as a compensatory response. However, this does not appear to provide a sufficient explanation for tinnitus; firstly, because there has been no demonstration of spontaneous neuronal activity discriminating the presence or absence of tinnitus at the individual human or animal level [63]. Furthermore, tinnitus often begins at distinct times following the onset of hearing loss, such as during increased physiological or psychological stress [55–57]. Also, there is only a limited correlation between degree of hearing loss and presence or intensity of tinnitus, including individuals with minimal hearing loss who yet have tinnitus, and those with marked hearing loss but no tinnitus.

This second Bayesian account of tinnitus regards increased spontaneous activity in the auditory pathway as a tinnitus 'precursor', but not the tinnitus itself [5]. In Bayesian inference, this precursor affects the likelihood of various posterior beliefs, which leads to a prediction error insofar as it does not accord with auditory priors. However, tinnitus—as a percept—relates to the posterior, which results from an interplay between this precursor and auditory priors, each weighted by its precision. If the precision of the precursor is increased sufficiently to bring the posterior over the threshold for perception, then tinnitus occurs. Furthermore, if tinnitus persists as the posterior explanation, for a sufficient period of time, then the prior adapts to conform to it and thereby further reduce prediction errors. This is adaptive from a Bayesian or free energy perspective, in that it minimises prediction error at lower hierarchical levels of processing, but maladaptive in that it involves accepting an erroneous and information-poor auditory object at a higher hierarchical level.

This account also ties in with stress as a precipitant of tinnitus. Stress involves heightened awareness of external inputs, including unexpected ones, as part of a state of hypervigilance and being ready to detect threats. In Bayesian terms, this relates to increased precision of prediction errors that initially generate, and subsequently maintain, the tinnitus percept [17].

Bayesian Brain, Stress and Habituation

Whether the brain engages deep, active inference depends on the intention and context, e.g. stress. Stress can be defined as the individual state of uncertainty about what needs to be done to safeguard physical, mental or social well-being [17]. The basic tenet is that anxiety induces a putative shift from prior knowledge to incoming sensory data [17, 64], re-allocating resources from a top-down to a bottom-up approach [64]. In other words, in uncertain contexts every stimulus is considered potentially informative (i.e. conveying precise information), which may result in false positive perceptual inferences, due to overfitting. In states of enduring or chronic anxiety, a compensatory increase in the prior precision has sometimes been proposed as a form of 'paradoxical lesion', of the sort used to explain hallucinosis and hallucinations [65–68].

The brain predicts the sensory input it expects [69]. In other words, we hear what we expect to hear. Even with only partial data, I can infer the person I predict to be there. For example, I can tell 'my partner' is arriving home, based only on the sound she makes when entering the house.

In rapidly changing, unpredictable environments, we should not rely too much on our prior model of the world, and we should thus prioritise incoming signals [17]. Uncertainty of this sort induces a state of active exploration of the environment and risky decision making [70, 71], as a Bayes optimal response to an unpredictable world [64]. Exploring the sensorium more intensively is possible by increasing sensory precision, i.e. the gain or signal to noise ratio of postsynaptic responses, as mediated by neuromodulators, such as acetylcholine and noradrenaline [17, 19]. These theoretical interpretations are, however, not confirmed by clinical studies. Stress-inducing procedures, even when successfully eliciting subjective stress ratings as well as stress-relevant physiological parameters, do not necessarily change reliance on sensory information [64]. A possible explanation is that stress creates an inverted-U curve response in the brain [72] in relation to noradrenaline [73], dopamine [74] and glucocorticoid levels [75], changing information processing [12] and behaviour [76].

Exaggerated prior precision may lead one to falsely infer the presence of expected events. For example, prior beliefs that are very strong may lead to hearing voices that are not present, i.e. auditory hallucinations [58]. In short, people can perceive stimuli in the environment that are predicted but not necessarily present [77]. Mechanistically, this could be explained via stress-mediated reversible atrophy of the vmPFC [78]. The associated dysfunction of the vmPFC may result in decreased suppression of sensory input [46, 49, 79]. When accompanied by an increased noradrenaline-mediated sensory gain [17], this could trigger perceptions unaccounted for by sensory evidence. This may explain the development and persistence of tinnitus under stressful circumstances [55, 57, 80–82].

The only option left if the stress is maintained is to update prior beliefs and habituate to the stressful stimuli [17], i.e. reduce the stress by changing prior expectations. This approach is commonly used by health care providers in the setting of tinnitus, when they tell the patient that nothing can be done about the tinnitus, and the patient should learn to live with it.

Belief-Free and Belief-Based Behaviour

Model-based and model-free learning and decision-making systems have been described [83–85]. Under normal circumstances, a model-based, goal-oriented system is used, whereas under stress, a model-free approach is employed, because it is more reliable [86, 87]. This is in keeping with the above description: under normal conditions or low stress circumstances, the model of the world can be adjusted based on deep inference, yet, under uncertainty, when energy expenditure and speed of response are more critical, a model-free approach can be engaged by suspending the precision of deep priors.

A model-based approach employs a deep model of the world to make its decisions by using sequential predictions (e.g. tree searches), chaining together short-term predictions about immediate consequences of each action in a sequence. The model-based approach effectively deliberates about the potential outcomes of all options, is therefore computationally expensive, carries a heavy memory load, is time consuming and slow, error prone, but flexible and adaptive, ideal for goal-directed control [88]. In this setting, active inference is key, evaluating the consequences of action over extended periods of time. Under stress, a model-free approach may be more apt. Model-free behaviour and learning involves reflexive repetition of previously successful choices, is computationally simple and inexpensive, based on simple memory, is quick, without errors, but inflexible, and ideal for habitual control [78, 88, 89].

The distinction between model-based and model-free schemes is found in computational neuroscience and reinforcement learning in psychology. From an active inference point of view, this distinction may be better cast as belief-based versus belief-free [90], as the model of the world results in a belief of what sensory input will be detected in the environment [90], which drives the next action (based on preferences and implicit intentions). Belief-free schemes are useful when there is no ambiguity [90], or ambiguity cannot be tolerated, i.e. in very stressful situations [91–94]. In summary, under moderate uncertainty, the brain resorts to active inference, exploring the environment in an attempt to resolve uncertainty. This is accompanied by increasing sensory precision to pick up relevant information. However, if uncertainty cannot be resolved, this irreducibility may itself be learned, leading to chronic uncertainty and stress—and a persistent imbalance between prior and sensory precision. Having said this, this formulation may need refinement to account for the inverted-U curve of stress [72, 76]. Thus, without ambiguity belief-free (habitual) approaches may suffice, but with ambiguity and moderate stress creative belief-based (goal-oriented) approaches may be more optimal. Yet, under high stress, the automatic fast and efficient belief-free approach may predominate again, especially after negative outcome of a belief-based approach [93]. The argument here is that these changes in the deployment of precision may precipitate or maintain the tinnitus percept.

Irrespective of the nature of changes in predicted precision—at various levels of hierarchical inference—we would expect to see the neuronal correlates of changes in postsynaptic gain. Because these changes are effectively differences in synaptic rate constants, one would expect to see characteristic changes in the frequency content of electrophysiological correlates of neuronal message passing; e.g. recurrent exchange of prediction errors and predictions among levels of the auditory hierarchy. We now turn to the empirical evidence for these kinds of correlates.

Bayesian Interpretations of Functional Brain Changes in Tinnitus

Resting-state studies of brain activity in people with tinnitus associated with hearing loss have shown a pattern of changes in oscillatory power in auditory cortex, comprising increased delta/theta, reduced alpha and increased gamma band activity [50, 95–99]. Most of these studies do not feature control groups matched for hearing loss, and one such study found only delta band activity to associate with tinnitus, once hearing loss was controlled for [95]. However, successful tinnitus treatment has shown changes in all of these frequency bands in the reverse direction [100], and transient suppression of tinnitus (residual inhibition) is associated with reversal of delta and gamma changes [95, 101, 102].

Neurofeedback to increase alpha activity has had some success in at least temporarily suppressing tinnitus [103]. Furthermore, the amplitude of gamma power has been positively correlated to perceived tinnitus intensity [104, 105]. Interestingly, transient increases in tinnitus loudness following acoustic stimulation have been associated with decreases in gamma power (a.k.a., residual excitation) [102]. The delta/theta increase has been interpreted as a dysfunctional thalamocortical rhythm resulting from deafferentation and resultant hyperpolarisation, termed 'thalamocortical dysrhythmia' [97]. Gamma oscillations were originally posited to result at the interface between dysfunctional theta/delta and normal alpha activity in auditory cortex, and to generate the tinnitus percept. Alpha reduction was posited to indicate reduced inhibition, and loss of normal 'idling' rhythm [106].

In a predictive coding framework, these oscillations inherit a complementary explanation. Although the role of delta/theta oscillations is still not entirely clear, these oscillations may resemble activity seen during sensory input [107, 108], and also in deafferentation [50, 96–98] and in sleep [109]. They can thus be considered indicative of increased thalamocortical input (driving tinnitus), or of cortical deafferentation (leaving a 'void' for tinnitus to fill). Another explanation is that theta reflects a memory-based prediction from the (para)hippocampus [32, 50], and delta reflects the precision of these predictions [33].

Alpha oscillations have been linked to the precision of prior sensory predictions in the auditory cortex [110], during perceptual inference, and therefore a reduction could indicate reduced precision of auditory priors, which are associated with increased precision of ascending prediction errors. Beta oscillations are linked to the updating of predictions [5, 110]. There is relatively little evidence of altered beta activity in tinnitus, compared to other frequency bands, and the beta activity is related to distress [111–115], rather than the tinnitus sound. This might reflect that rapidly changing predictions are not thought to be part tinnitus pathophysiology.

Gamma oscillations are linked to tinnitus by a large number of studies [50, 99, 102, 116–128]. In a predictive coding framework, increased gamma oscillations indicate elevated prediction errors in association with hearing loss and tinnitus. It is not clear whether tinnitus is associated with increased spontaneous gamma activity, once hearing loss is considered, but this does not necessarily matter for its role in a Bayesian framework. If gamma oscillations indicate prediction errors, then they can be seen as reflecting a discrepancy between auditory priors and sensory input or spontaneous ascending activity. They could indicate that an auditory prior of a sound (tinnitus) is present but there is no corresponding sensory input, or, alternatively, that there is spontaneous ascending auditory activity that does not (fully) accord with priors. Both Bayesian explanations of tinnitus would accord with this notion in broad terms. However, in Explanation 1 (tinnitus is primarily driven by a precise prior), hearing loss without tinnitus should not necessarily be associated with increased gamma oscillations, and the presence of tinnitus should increase gamma oscillations. Conversely, if chronic tinnitus occurs following to increased spontaneous ascending activity (Explanation 2), then hearing loss itself should correlate with gamma oscillations, and, if anything, occurrence of tinnitus should be associated with at least a partial reduction in gamma, indication reconciliation of these prediction errors. Available data lack the granularity to distinguish between these possibilities.

Activity beyond the auditory cortex has also been linked to tinnitus. Altered theta activity has been observed in the medial temporal cortex, i.e. the hippocampal and parahippocampal area, extending to the inferior and middle temporal area, i.e. the parabelt of the auditory cortex, contralateral to the tinnitus percept [50, 104, 122, 123, 126, 129]. This suggests that the auditory cortex gamma activity may subsequently become cross-frequency coupled—not only to thalamic slowed alpha—but also to theta from the hippocampus [50]. Consequently, tinnitus may derive from (para)hippocampal auditory memory, encoded in theta frequency, as previously suggested [50, 104], which is compatible with memory-based predictions in tinnitus [4].

Tinnitus has been considered a unified percept related to interaction of dynamically changing, partially overlapping subnetworks, each representing a different aspect of the tinnitus, e.g. loudness, location, distress, etc. [130]. A small tinnitus core network [130] has been proposed recently, comprising the posterior cingulate cortex, parahippocampus and auditory cortex, extending to the temporoparietal area, and communicating in the predictive beta range [43, 51]. The functional connectivity of the tinnitus network will thus change, depending on the tinnitus specifics, but it should involve gamma band changes, as a reflection of a prediction error that is propagated throughout the extended tinnitus network, involving both the salience network, and other intrinsic brain networks [126, 131–133]. Furthermore, in resting-state, the larger the gamma-related prediction error, the louder the tinnitus is perceived [105].

Tinnitus Without Deafferentation

Whilst hearing loss seems the major risk factor and initiating factor, for most cases of tinnitus, up to 10% of cases have clinically normal hearing thresholds. A number of studies suggest there is simply more subtle (or higher frequency) hearing loss in these cases [42]. However, tinnitus also occurs as part of the visual snow syndrome (VSS) [134], in which people experience visual noise resembling the 'static' of a badly tuned analogue television. The majority of these patients also experience persistent tinnitus, which does not require clinically detectable hearing loss. Also, notably, the visual experience, equivalent to tinnitus, does not require visual deafferentation either. VSS has been explained as a visual analogue of thalamocortical dysrhythmia [135], but could also, alternatively, be considered as resulting from altered Bayesian inference akin to that in tinnitus [136]. The major difference between this Bayesian explanation and the two we have described above is that in VSS there is no compensation for—or belief updating after—deafferentation, and the percept is generalised across the sensory domains, rather than localised to specific topographic regions (e.g. specific high frequencies or retinotopic locations). Therefore, while tinnitus might result from compensation for deafferentation (likely in combination with other factors such as stress), it may also be possible for these other non-deafferentation factors, like hypersensitivity, based on altered perceptual inference, to cause tinnitus.

VSS also might offer some insight into the way in which Bayesian processes are altered in tinnitus. While the auditory experience in tinnitus could plausibly result from either a low-level prediction error not being 'ignored', or from maladaptive priors 'making up' a tinnitus percept, in VSS, the origin of the phantom visual percepts is related to the retina itself. This is because one cardinal feature, termed the 'blue field entoptic phenomenon', is the perception of small white dots in vision that move quickly along a curving path, especially against a blue background (e.g. sky). These are known to correspond to white blood cells passing through retinal capillaries. A heightened perceptual awareness of these indicates a failure of higher perceptual mechanisms to 'ignore' these sensory fluctuations as one ordinarily would.

Evidence for Altered Predictive Processes in Tinnitus

So far, we have considered post-hoc explanations of how altered activity in association with tinnitus and/or hearing loss can be interpreted in light of current Bayesian models of perceptual function. However, if Bayesian explanations of tinnitus are to be evaluated scientifically for their correctness or incorrectness, then testable hypotheses need to be generated and tested.

Some components of Bayesian or predictive coding systems are not uniquely explained within these frameworks. For instance, the precision of prediction errors could also be simply considered in terms of gain or synchrony, which is already a phenomenon of interest in tinnitus [137]. Stimulus-evoked responses such as MMN are not solely influenced by prediction violations, but also in part respond to straightforward changes in stimulus properties [36, 138]. Similarly, neuronal activity in the entire auditory pathway shows a hierarchical organisation of prediction errors [139] and stimulus-specific adaptation [140], which is context dependent [141]. Nonetheless, with careful, hypothesis-driven, experimental design, it should be possible to use empirical responses to probe the auditory hierarchy in people with and without tinnitus, and evidence of altered precision and/or priors.

With this aim, auditory deviant stimuli have been compared, either increasing or decreasing in intensity, to become more or less similar to the perceived tinnitus (and therefore the tinnitus prediction) [137]. Compared to hearing-matched controls, people with tinnitus showed larger MMN responses to upward (away from tinnitus) intensity deviants, and smaller responses to downward (towards tinnitus) deviants, in-line with hypotheses of chronically altered auditory predictions. However, further work is required to reproduce this effect, and rule out alternative explanations such as difference in dynamic range adaptation.

A key question—with respect to Bayesian accounts of tinnitus—is what individual traits or states determine whether an individual, as a result of hearing loss, develops tinnitus or not. An attempt to address this has examined the formation of automatic auditory predictions, based on the transition probabilities in sequences of pure tones varying in frequency but keeping well away from frequencies affected by tinnitus or hearing loss. As the predictability of sequences increased, subjects with tinnitus showed stronger patterns of brain activity that (correctly) represented the upcoming stimulus [142]. Using an auditory oddball paradigm with omission of global deviants increased a pre-stimulus response (=predictions) associated with increased alpha connectivity between the parahippocampus, dorsal anterior cingulate cortex and parahippocampus, pregenual anterior cingulate cortex and posterior cingulate [143]. Increased prediction errors were identified by gamma activity and increased theta connectivity between auditory cortices, parahippocampus and dorsal anterior cingulate cortex in the tinnitus group [143]. This was associated with increased effective connectivity in theta from the auditory cortex and parahippocampus to the dorsal anterior cingulate cortex [143]. Further analyses showed correlations of pre-stimulus theta activity to tinnitus loudness and alpha activity to tinnitus distress [143]. These results strongly suggest that tinnitus patients with minimal to no hearing loss are predisposed to domain-wide maladaptive changes in predictive coding [143]. Whilst work to target predictive processes in tinnitus specifically is at an early stage, this emerging field could help to confirm or refute the existence of a Bayesian basis to tinnitus, and thereby elucidate its mechanisms and networks involved.

Computational Modelling of Bayesian Processes in Tinnitus

Rather than relying on direct examination of spontaneous or sound-driven brain activity, and linking it to proposed Bayesian processes, an alternative or complementary approach is to generate and compare computational models of underlying perceptual processes, and determine which model best explains observed behavioural and/or neural responses recorded from people with tinnitus. There are limitations to these approaches: for example, they rely on a clear set of hypotheses about the possible models and how they operate. Nonetheless, such models may offer much deeper insights into underlying mechanisms, and might in future be useful for modelling and predicting the results of interventions [144].

Whilst several non-Bayesian computational models of tinnitus have been tested, we are aware of one Bayesian computational model [145]. This was based on Explanation 2 [5], and used a hierarchical Gaussian filter, incorporating an interplay between spontaneous auditory activity (a 'tinnitus precursor'), auditory priors, external auditory input and their precision. Based on optimisation of model parameters to individual tinnitus subjects' phenomenology, this model was able to demonstrate internal consistency and computational plausibility of this particular Bayesian account of tinnitus—and use individual parameters to successfully predict individual subjects' residual inhibition functions. Further work in this area might include building in long-term plasticity to model the chronification of tinnitus, comparing different Bayesian models of tinnitus, comparing model performance to non-Bayesian models, and fitting to (or explaining) spontaneous and/or sound-driven brain activity as well as psychophysical data.

Conclusions

Bayesian models of perceptual function, such as predictive coding, are increasingly popular. From first principles, tinnitus should occur within such a framework. Furthermore, Bayesian models of tinnitus offer solutions to numerous paradoxical observations about tinnitus symptomatology and its neural correlates, which are otherwise hard to reconcile. Existing brain data are compatible with such models, though have other possible interpretations. Studies directly examining predictive processes in tinnitus are starting to emerge, with tentative findings of enhanced formation of auditory predictions in people prone to tinnitus, and altered auditory intensity predictions in association with chronic tinnitus. Computational models are also starting to emerge, which might—in the future—link directly to observed brain activity. Ultimately, Bayesian models of tinnitus need to be specified to a degree where they can be confirmed, refuted or refined, based on testing of specific process theories. However, if these aims are met, then these models might provide a useful way forward in gaining a deeper understanding of the underlying basis of tinnitus, and may also help to inspire, improve and predict response to tinnitus treatments.

References

1. De Ridder D, et al. Tinnitus and tinnitus disorder: theoretical and operational definitions (an international multidisciplinary proposal). Prog Brain Res. 2021;260:1–25.
2. Gibrin PC, Melo JJ, Marchiori LL. Prevalence of tinnitus complaints and probable association with hearing loss, diabetes mellitus and hypertension in elderly. Codas. 2013;25(2):176–80.
3. Wallhausser-Franke E, et al. Transition from acute to chronic tinnitus: predictors for the development of chronic distressing tinnitus. Front Neurol. 2017;8:605.
4. De Ridder D, Vanneste S, Freeman W. The Bayesian brain: phantom percepts resolve sensory uncertainty. Neurosci Biobehav Rev. 2014;44C:4–15.
5. Sedley W, et al. An integrative tinnitus model based on sensory precision. Trends Neurosci. 2016;39(12):799–812.
6. De Ridder D, et al. Phantom percepts: tinnitus and pain as persisting aversive memory networks. Proc Natl Acad Sci U S A. 2011;108(20):8075–80.
7. Freeman WJ. How brains make up their minds. London: Phoenix; 1999.
8. Nanay B. Perception is not all-purpose. Synthese. 2021;198(Suppl 17):4069–80.
9. Freeman WJ. The wave packet: an action potential for the 21st century. J Integr Neurosci. 2003;2(1):3–30.
10. Merleau-Ponty M. Phénomènologie de la Perception. Paris: Gallimard; 1945.
11. Friston K. Life as we know it. J R Soc Interface. 2013;10(86):20130475.
12. Hohwy J. The self-evidencing brain. Noûs. 2016;50(2):259–85.
13. Parr T, Friston KJ. Generalised free energy and active inference. Biol Cybern. 2019;113(5–6):495–513.
14. Friston K. The free-energy principle: a unified brain theory? Nat Rev Neurosci. 2010;11(2):127–38.
15. Friston K. The free-energy principle: a rough guide to the brain? Trends Cogn Sci. 2009;13(7):293–301.
16. Rao RP, Ballard DH. Predictive coding in the visual cortex: a functional interpretation of some extra-classical receptive-field effects. Nat Neurosci. 1999;2(1):79–87.
17. Peters A, McEwen BS, Friston K. Uncertainty and stress: why it causes diseases and how it is mastered by the brain. Prog Neurobiol. 2017;156:164–88.
18. Freeman WJ. Neurodynamic models of brain in psychiatry. Neuropsychopharmacology. 2003;28(Suppl 1):S54–63.
19. Yon D, Frith CD. Precision and the Bayesian brain. Curr Biol. 2021;31(17):R1026–32.

20. Seth AK. Interoceptive inference, emotion, and the embodied self. Trends Cogn Sci. 2013;17(11):565–73.
21. Bastos AM, et al. Canonical microcircuits for predictive coding. Neuron. 2012;76(4):695–711.
22. Spaak E, et al. Layer-specific entrainment of gamma-band neural activity by the alpha rhythm in monkey visual cortex. Curr Biol. 2012;22(24):2313–8.
23. Strube A, et al. Alpha-to-beta- and gamma-band activity reflect predictive coding in affective visual processing. Sci Rep. 2021;11(1):23492.
24. Strube A, et al. The temporal and spectral characteristics of expectations and prediction errors in pain and thermoception. elife. 2021;10:62809.
25. Nickel MM, et al. Temporal-spectral signaling of sensory information and expectations in the cerebral processing of pain. Proc Natl Acad Sci U S A. 2022;119(1):e2116616119.
26. Gueguen MCM, et al. Anatomical dissociation of intracerebral signals for reward and punishment prediction errors in humans. Nat Commun. 2021;12(1):3344.
27. Hein TP, Herrojo Ruiz M. State anxiety alters the neural oscillatory correlates of predictions and prediction errors during reward-based learning. NeuroImage. 2022;249:118895.
28. Lewis AG, Bastiaansen M. A predictive coding framework for rapid neural dynamics during sentence-level language comprehension. Cortex. 2015;68:155–68.
29. Roehe MA, et al. Early alpha/beta oscillations reflect the formation of face-related expectations in the brain. PLoS One. 2021;16(7):e0255116.
30. Chao ZC, et al. Large-scale cortical networks for hierarchical prediction and prediction error in the primate brain. Neuron. 2018;100(5):1252–1266 e3.
31. Auksztulewicz R, Friston KJ, Nobre AC. Task relevance modulates the behavioural and neural effects of sensory predictions. PLoS Biol. 2017;15(12):e2003143.
32. Barron HC, Auksztulewicz R, Friston K. Prediction and memory: a predictive coding account. Prog Neurobiol. 2020;192:101821.
33. Arnal LH, Doelling KB, Poeppel D. Delta-beta coupled oscillations underlie temporal prediction accuracy. Cereb Cortex. 2014;25(9):3077–85.
34. Naatanen R, et al. Attention and mismatch negativity. Psychophysiology. 1993;30(5):436–50.
35. Naatanen R, et al. Development of a memory trace for a complex sound in the human brain. Neuroreport. 1993;4(5):503–6.
36. Garrido MI, et al. The mismatch negativity: a review of underlying mechanisms. Clin Neurophysiol. 2009;120(3):453–63.
37. Donoso M, Collins AG, Koechlin E. Human cognition. Foundations of human reasoning in the prefrontal cortex. Science. 2014;344(6191):1481–6.
38. Garrido MI, et al. Evoked brain responses are generated by feedback loops. Proc Natl Acad Sci U S A. 2007;104(52):20961–6.
39. Moran RJ, et al. Free energy, precision and learning: the role of cholinergic neuromodulation. J Neurosci. 2013;33(19):8227–36.
40. Thiel CM, Friston KJ, Dolan RJ. Cholinergic modulation of experience-dependent plasticity in human auditory cortex. Neuron. 2002;35(3):567–74.
41. Vossel S, et al. Cholinergic stimulation enhances Bayesian belief updating in the deployment of spatial attention. J Neurosci. 2014;34(47):15735–42.
42. Weisz N, Hartmann T, Dohrmann K, Schlee W, Norena A. High-frequency tinnitus without hearing loss does not mean absence of deafferentation. Hear Res. 2006;222(1–2):108–14.
43. Lee SY, et al. Is the posterior cingulate cortex an on-off switch for tinnitus? A comparison between hearing loss subjects with and without tinnitus. Hear Res. 2021;411:108356.
44. Hullfish J, Sedley W, Vanneste S. Prediction and perception: insights for (and from) tinnitus. Neurosci Biobehav Rev. 2019;102:1–12.
45. De Ridder D, et al. Pain and the triple network model. Front Neurol. 2022;13:757241.
46. De Ridder D, Adhia D, Vanneste S. The anatomy of pain and suffering in the brain and its clinical implications. Neurosci Biobehav Rev. 2021;130:125–46.
47. Lee SY, et al. No auditory experience, no tinnitus: lessons from subjects with congenital- and acquired single-sided deafness. Hear Res. 2017;354:9–15.
48. De Ridder D, Joos K, Vanneste S. The enigma of the tinnitus-free dream state in a Bayesian world. Neural Plast. 2014;2014:612147.
49. De Ridder D, Vanneste S. The Bayesian brain in imbalance: medial, lateral and descending pathways in tinnitus and pain: a perspective. Prog Brain Res. 2021;262:309–34.
50. De Ridder D, et al. Thalamocortical dysrhythmia: a theoretical update in tinnitus. Front Neurol. 2015;6:124.
51. Lee SY, et al. Cortical oscillatory signatures reveal the prerequisites for tinnitus perception: a comparison of subjects with sudden sensorineural hearing loss with and without tinnitus. Front Neurosci. 2020;14:596647.
52. Mohan A, et al. Distress-dependent temporal variability of regions encoding domain-specific and domain-general behavioral manifestations of phantom percepts. Eur J Neurosci. 2018;48(2):1743–64.
53. Song JJ, et al. The balance between Bayesian inference and default mode determines the generation of tinnitus from decreased auditory input: a volume entropy-based study. Hum Brain Mapp. 2021;42(12):4059–73.
54. Vanneste S, De Ridder D. Deafferentation-based pathophysiological differences in phantom sound: Tinnitus with and without hearing loss. NeuroImage. 2016;129:80–94.
55. Ciminelli P, et al. Tinnitus: the sound of stress? Clin Pract Epidemiol Ment Health. 2018;14:264–9.
56. Hebert S. Psychological comorbidities of tinnitus. Curr Top Behav Neurosci. 2021;51:349–59.
57. Hebert S, Lupien SJ. The sound of stress: blunted cortisol reactivity to psychosocial stress in tinnitus sufferers. Neurosci Lett. 2007;411(2):138–42.
58. Corlett PR, et al. Hallucinations and strong priors. Trends Cogn Sci. 2019;23(2):114–27.
59. Schaette R, McAlpine D. Tinnitus with a normal audiogram: physiological evidence for hidden hearing loss and computational model. J Neurosci. 2011;31(38):13452–7.
60. Zeng FG, Fu QJ, Morse R. Human hearing enhanced by noise. Brain Res. 2000;869(1-2):251–5.
61. Krauss P, et al. Adaptive stochastic resonance for unknown and variable input signals. Sci Rep. 2017;7(1):2450.
62. Krauss P, et al. Stochastic resonance controlled upregulation of internal noise after hearing loss as a putative cause of tinnitus-related neuronal hyperactivity. Front Neurosci. 2016;10:597.
63. Galazyuk A, Brozoski TJ. Animal models of tinnitus: a review. Otolaryngol Clin N Am. 2020;53(4):469–80.
64. Trapp S, Vilares I. Bayesian decision-making under stress-preserved weighting of prior and likelihood information. Sci Rep. 2020;10(1):21456.
65. Powers AR, Mathys C, Corlett PR. Pavlovian conditioning–induced hallucinations result from overweighting of perceptual priors. Science. 2017;357(6351):596–600.
66. Sterzer P, et al. The predictive coding account of psychosis. Biol Psychiatry. 2018;84(9):634–43.
67. Benrimoh D, et al. Hallucinations both in and out of context: an active inference account. PLoS One. 2019;14(8):e0212379.

68. Lyndon S, Corlett PR. Hallucinations in posttraumatic stress disorder: insights from predictive coding. J Abnorm Psychol. 2020;129(6):534–43.
69. Hohwy J. The predictive mind. 1st ed. New York: Oxford University Press; 2013. p. 282.
70. Starcke K, et al. Anticipatory stress influences decision making under explicit risk conditions. Behav Neurosci. 2008;122(6):1352–60.
71. Pabst S, Brand M, Wolf OT. Stress and decision making: a few minutes make all the difference. Behav Brain Res. 2013;250:39–45.
72. Sapolsky RM. Stress and the brain: individual variability and the inverted-U. Nat Neurosci. 2015;18(10):1344–6.
73. Aston-Jones G, Cohen JD. An integrative theory of locus coeruleus-norepinephrine function: adaptive gain and optimal performance. Annu Rev Neurosci. 2005;28:403–50.
74. Cools R, D'Esposito M. Inverted-U-shaped dopamine actions on human working memory and cognitive control. Biol Psychiatry. 2011;69(12):113–25.
75. Gray JD, et al. Genomic and epigenomic mechanisms of glucocorticoids in the brain. Nat Rev Endocrinol. 2017;13(11):661–73.
76. Yerkes R, Dodson J. The relation of strength of stimulus to rapidity of habit-formation. J Comp Neurol Psychol. 1908;18:459–82.
77. Benrimoh D, et al. Active inference and auditory hallucinations. Comput Psychiatr. 2018;2:183–204.
78. Soares JM, et al. Stress-induced changes in human decision-making are reversible. Transl Psychiatry. 2012;2:e131.
79. De Ridder D, et al. Psychosurgery reduces uncertainty and increases free will? A review. Neuromodulation. 2016;19(3):239–48.
80. Hasson D, et al. Stress and prevalence of hearing problems in the Swedish working population. BMC Public Health. 2011;11:130.
81. Kim HJ, et al. Analysis of the prevalence and associated risk factors of tinnitus in adults. PLoS One. 2015;10(5):e0127578.
82. Elarbed A, et al. Tinnitus and stress in adults: a scoping review. Int J Audiol. 2021;60(3):171–82.
83. Dayan P, Berridge KC. Model-based and model-free Pavlovian reward learning: revaluation, revision, and revelation. Cogn Affect Behav Neurosci. 2014;14(2):473–92.
84. Glascher J, et al. States versus rewards: dissociable neural prediction error signals underlying model-based and model-free reinforcement learning. Neuron. 2010;66(4):585–95.
85. Lee SW, Shimojo S, O'Doherty JP. Neural computations underlying arbitration between model-based and model-free learning. Neuron. 2014;81(3):687–99.
86. Schwabe L, et al. Preventing the stress-induced shift from goal-directed to habit action with a beta-adrenergic antagonist. J Neurosci. 2011;31(47):17317–25.
87. Schwabe L, Wolf OT. Stress prompts habit behavior in humans. J Neurosci. 2009;29(22):7191–8.
88. Daw ND, Niv Y, Dayan P. Uncertainty-based competition between prefrontal and dorsolateral striatal systems for behavioral control. Nat Neurosci. 2005;8(12):1704–11.
89. Doll BB, Simon DA, Daw ND. The ubiquity of model-based reinforcement learning. Curr Opin Neurobiol. 2012;22(6):1075–81.
90. Friston K, et al. Active inference and learning. Neurosci Biobehav Rev. 2016;68:862–79.
91. Friedel E, Sebold M, Kuitunen-Paul S, et al. How accumulated real life stress experience and cognitive speed interact on decision-making processes. Front Hum Neurosci. 2017;11:302.
92. Otto AR, Raio CM, Chiang A, Phelps EA, Daw ND. Working-memory capacity protects model-based learning from stress. Proc Natl Acad Sci U S A. 2013;110(52):20941–6.
93. Park H, Lee D, Chey J. Stress enhances model-free reinforcement learning only after negative outcome. PLoS One. 2017;12(7):e0180588.
94. Radenbach C, Reiter AM, Engert V, et al. The interaction of acute and chronic stress impairs model-based behavioral control. Psychoneuroendocrinology. 2015;53:268–80.
95. Adjamian P, et al. Neuromagnetic indicators of tinnitus and tinnitus masking in patients with and without hearing loss. J Assoc Res Otolaryngol. 2012;13(5):715–31.
96. De Ridder D, et al. Theta-gamma dysrhythmia and auditory phantom perception. J Neurosurg. 2011;114(4):912–21.
97. Llinas RR, et al. Thalamocortical dysrhythmia: a neurological and neuropsychiatric syndrome characterized by magnetoencephalography. Proc Natl Acad Sci U S A. 1999;96(26):15222–7.
98. Vanneste S, Song JJ, De Ridder D. Thalamocortical dysrhythmia detected by machine learning. Nat Commun. 2018;9(1):1103.
99. Weisz N, et al. The neural code of auditory phantom perception. J Neurosci. 2007;27(6):1479–84.
100. Tass PA, et al. Counteracting tinnitus by acoustic coordinated reset neuromodulation. Restor Neurol Neurosci. 2012;30(2):137–59.
101. Kahlbrock N, Weisz N. Transient reduction of tinnitus intensity is marked by concomitant reductions of delta band power. BMC Biol. 2008;6:4.
102. Sedley W, et al. Single-subject oscillatory gamma responses in tinnitus. Brain. 2012;135(10):3089–100.
103. Dohrmann K, et al. Neurofeedback for treating tinnitus. Prog Brain Res. 2007;166:473–85.
104. De Ridder D, Congedo M, Vanneste S. The neural correlates of subjectively perceived and passively matched loudness perception in auditory phantom perception. Brain Behav. 2015;5:e00331.
105. van der Loo E, et al. Tinnitus intensity dependent gamma oscillations of the contralateral auditory cortex. PLoS ONE. 2009;4(10):e7396.
106. Llinas R, et al. Rhythmic and dysrhythmic thalamocortical dynamics: GABA systems and the edge effect. Trends Neurosci. 2005;28(6):325–33.
107. Doelling KB, et al. Acoustic landmarks drive delta-theta oscillations to enable speech comprehension by facilitating perceptual parsing. NeuroImage. 2014;85(Pt 2):761–8.
108. Kubetschek C, Kayser C. Delta/Theta band EEG activity shapes the rhythmic perceptual sampling of auditory scenes. Sci Rep. 2021;11(1):2370.
109. Steriade M. Sleep oscillations in corticothalamic neuronal networks and their development into self-sustained paroxysmal activity. Rom J Neurol Psychiatry. 1993;31(3-4):151–61.
110. Sedley W, et al. Neural signatures of perceptual inference. elife. 2016;5:e11476.
111. De Ridder D, Joos K, Vanneste S. Anterior cingulate implants for tinnitus: report of 2 cases. J Neurosurg. 2016;124(4):893–901.
112. De Ridder D, Vanneste S, Congedo M. The distressed brain: a group blind source separation analysis on tinnitus. PLoS One. 2011;6(10):e24273.
113. Meyer M, et al. Disentangling tinnitus distress and tinnitus presence by means of EEG power analysis. Neural Plast. 2014;2014:468546.
114. Vanneste S, De Ridder D. Stress-related functional connectivity changes between auditory cortex and cingulate in tinnitus. Brain Connect. 2015;5(6):371–83.
115. Vanneste S, et al. The neural correlates of tinnitus-related distress. NeuroImage. 2010;52(2):470–80.
116. Adamchic I, Hauptmann C, Tass PA. Changes of oscillatory activity in pitch processing network and related tinnitus relief induced by acoustic CR neuromodulation. Front Syst Neurosci. 2012;6:18.
117. Adamchic I, et al. Reversing pathologically increased EEG power by acoustic coordinated reset neuromodulation. Hum Brain Mapp. 2014;35(5):2099–118.
118. Lan L, et al. Alterations of brain activity and functional connectivity in transition from acute to chronic tinnitus. Hum Brain Mapp. 2021;42(2):485–94.

119. Vanneste S, de Heyning PV, Ridder DD. Contralateral parahippocampal gamma-band activity determines noise-like tinnitus laterality: a region of interest analysis. Neuroscience. 2011;199:481–90.
120. Vanneste S, De Ridder D. The use of alcohol as a moderator for tinnitus-related distress. Brain Topogr. 2012;25(1):97–105.
121. Vanneste S, et al. Pairing sound with vagus nerve stimulation modulates cortical synchrony and phase coherence in tinnitus: an exploratory retrospective study. Sci Rep. 2017;7(1):17345.
122. Vanneste S, et al. The differences in brain activity between narrow band noise and pure tone tinnitus. PLoS One. 2010;5(10):e13618.
123. Vanneste S, et al. The difference between uni- and bilateral auditory phantom percept. Clin Neurophysiol. 2011;122(3):578–87.
124. Vanneste S, Song JJ, De Ridder D. Tinnitus and musical hallucinosis: the same but more. NeuroImage. 2013;82C:373–83.
125. Vanneste S, To WT, De Ridder D. Tinnitus and neuropathic pain share a common neural substrate in the form of specific brain connectivity and microstate profiles. Prog Neuro-Psychopharmacol Biol Psychiatry. 2019;88:388–400.
126. Vanneste S, van de Heyning P, De Ridder D. The neural network of phantom sound changes over time: a comparison between recent-onset and chronic tinnitus patients. Eur J Neurosci. 2011;34(5):718–31.
127. Zhang J, et al. Switching tinnitus-on: maps and source localization of spontaneous EEG. Clin Neurophysiol. 2021;132(2):345–57.
128. Schlee W, et al. Abnormal resting-state cortical coupling in chronic tinnitus. BMC Neurosci. 2009;10:11.
129. De Ridder D, Vanneste S. Targeting the parahippocampal area by auditory cortex stimulation in tinnitus. Brain Stimul. 2014;7(5):709–17.
130. De Ridder D, et al. An integrative model of auditory phantom perception: tinnitus as a unified percept of interacting separable subnetworks. Neurosci Biobehav Rev. 2014;44:16–32.
131. Mohan A, De Ridder D, Vanneste S. Graph theoretical analysis of brain connectivity in phantom sound perception. Sci Rep. 2016;6:19683.
132. Mohan A, De Ridder D, Vanneste S. Emerging hubs in phantom perception connectomics. Neuroimage Clin. 2016;11:181–94.
133. Zobay O, et al. Source space estimation of oscillatory power and brain connectivity in tinnitus. PLoS One. 2015;10(3):e0120123.
134. Renze M. Visual snow syndrome and its relationship to tinnitus. Int Tinnitus J. 2017;21(1):74–5.
135. Lauschke JL, Plant GT, Fraser CL. Visual snow: a thalamocortical dysrhythmia of the visual pathway? J Clin Neurosci. 2016;28:123–7.
136. Fraser CL. Visual snow: updates on pathology. Curr Neurol Neurosci Rep. 2022;22(3):209–17.
137. Sedley W, et al. Exposing pathological sensory predictions in tinnitus using auditory intensity deviant evoked responses. J Neurosci. 2019;39(50):10096–103.
138. Garrido MI, et al. The functional anatomy of the MMN: a DCM study of the roving paradigm. NeuroImage. 2008;42(2):936–44.
139. Parras GG, et al. Neurons along the auditory pathway exhibit a hierarchical organization of prediction error. Nat Commun. 2017;8(1):2148.
140. Ayala YA, Malmierca MS. The effect of inhibition on stimulus-specific adaptation in the inferior colliculus. Brain Struct Funct. 2018;223(3):1391–407.
141. Ayala MN, Henriques DYP. Context-dependent concurrent adaptation to static and moving targets. PLoS One. 2018;13(2):e0192476.
142. Partyka M, et al. Phantom auditory perception (tinnitus) is characterised by stronger anticipatory auditory predictions. BioRxiv, 2022.
143. Mohan A, et al. Predisposition to domain-wide maladaptive changes in predictive coding in auditory phantom perception. NeuroImage. 2022;248:118813.
144. Schwartenbeck P, Friston K. Computational phenotyping in psychiatry: a worked example. eNeuro. 2016;3(4):16.
145. Hu S, et al. Bayesian brain in tinnitus: computational modeling of three perceptual phenomena using a modified hierarchical Gaussian filter. Hear Res. 2021;410:108338.

18 Central Gain Model for Tinnitus: A Review on Noise-Induced Plasticity or When Less at the Periphery Is More in the Center

Vinay Parameshwarappa and Arnaud J. Norena

Abstract

Hearing loss represents a major sensory deficit as it is largely prevalent in the general population and can dramatically impair quality of life. One of the most prevalent causes of sensorineural hearing loss is noise exposure. Noise-induced hearing loss (NIHL) is the second most common form of the sensorineural hearing deficit, after age-related hearing loss. Importantly, it induces neuropathophysiological alterations in the auditory system, which can result in the generation of "aberrant auditory perceptions" such as tinnitus or hyperacusis. Here, we review the central plasticity that is triggered by noise-induced hearing loss. In brief, there is overwhelming evidence that noise-induced hearing loss is associated to compensatory mechanisms in the auditory centers: while the sensory inputs are reduced at the periphery (i.e., in the cochlear nerve), they are enhanced at virtually all levels of the auditory centers. A vast repertoire of molecular mechanisms are involved in these functional changes. It is plausible that these peripherally triggered central changes can result in tinnitus and/or hyperacusis.

V. Parameshwarappa · A. J. Norena (✉)
UMR CNRS 7291, Aix-Marseille University, Marseille, France
e-mail: arnaud.norena@univ-amu.fr

W. Schlee et al. (eds.), *Textbook of Tinnitus*, https://doi.org/10.1007/978-3-031-35647-6_18

Graphical Abstract

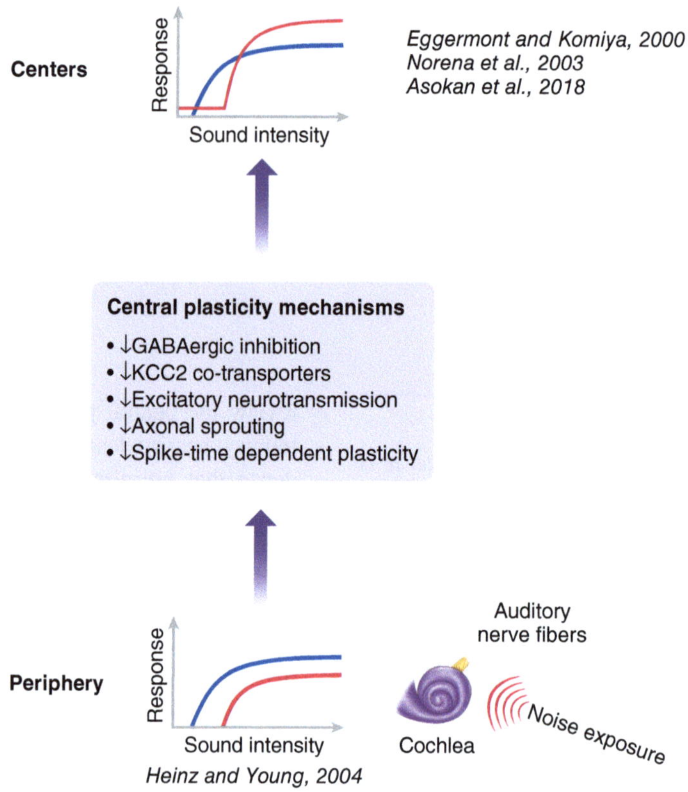

Highlights

- Noise-induced hearing loss is associated to compensatory central changes due to loss of sensory inputs from the cochlea.
- Neural hyperactivity in the auditory centers result from an increase in central gain which might serve to maintain mean neural activity at a set value.
- Increase in central gain may trigger tinnitus and/or hyperacusis.

Introduction

Hearing loss represents a major sensory deficit as it is largely prevalent in the general population, and can dramatically impair quality of life; its social and economic impacts in developed countries is also considerable [1]. One of the most prevalent causes of sensorineural hearing loss is noise exposure. Noise-induced hearing loss (NIHL) is the second most common form of the sensorineural hearing deficit, after age-related hearing loss [2]. NIHL represents a significant form of sensory impairment in the general population, mainly caused by occupational and recreational acoustic overstimulation. In fact, a significant amount of younger adults are affected by noise exposure through activities such as attending concerts or overuse of personal music players [3]. It severely affects their communication, sustainably reducing their quality of life and presents a social burden [4]. More importantly, it induces neuropathophysiological alterations in the auditory system, which can result in the generation of "aberrant auditory perceptions" such as tinnitus or hyperacusis [5].

At the cochlear level, intense noise exposure induces loss of hearing sensitivity (raising the auditory threshold) which can be reversible [6, 7] or permanent with death of hair cells, loss of hair cell stereocilia, damage to the basilar membrane, and neural degeneration of auditory nerve fibers [8]. Electrophysiological studies in animal models have shown that cochlear damage induced by noise exposure is usually followed by a dramatic reduction of spontaneous firing-rate and stimulus-induced activity in the cochlear nerve [9, 11]. That is to say, noise-induced hearing loss results in cochlear nerve providing reduced activity to the central auditory system. Interestingly, despite the decrease in peripheral drive associated with cochlear damage, recordings made from higher levels of the ascending auditory pathway reveal an increase in stimulus-induced and spontaneous activity.

One proposal is that neural hyperactivity could result from an increase in central gain which might serve to maintain mean neural activity at a set value [11, 12]. However, these compensatory central changes due to loss of sensory inputs from the cochlea may come at a price: increase in central neural gain is proposed to cause or act as a trigger in generation of tinnitus and/or hyperacusis.

Enhanced neural response in auditory centers after auditory deafferentation is not at all a new phenomenon. One of the earliest indication of compensatory central changes after sensory deprivation comes from the study examining the acute and chronic metabolic changes of the auditory pathway using 2-deoxyglucose after deafferentation of the mammalian auditory pathway [13]. After acute left cochlear removal, increased uptake of glucose was observed in the cochlear nucleus connected to the intact cochlea while reduction was observed in other structures contralateral to the cochlear ablation. Interestingly, after chronic cochlear ablation, the levels of glucose uptake commensurate with those seen in the structures connected to the intact side. This increase glucose uptake is suggested to be related to increased neuronal activity after chronic cochlear ablation. Roughly at the same time, Gerken studied the behavioral detection thresholds for pulsatile electrical stimuli delivered at different levels of the central auditory system, i.e., the cochlear nucleus, the superior olivary complex, the inferior colliculus, and the medial geniculate body, before and after cochlear destruction [14]. He reported an increased sensitivity to electrical stimulation in most regions of the subcortical auditory system in deafened animals.

Reviewing these early studies carried out in animals after cochlear hearing loss [13–15], Jastreboff and Hazell were among the first to use the expression "increased gain" to describe the kind of compensatory mechanisms just described [16]:

> Plasticity in the auditory system has been clearly demonstrated (...) Importantly, even a temporal decrease in auditory input results in an increase of sensitivity of neurons within the subcortical centres (...). These observations provide an explanation to the well-recognized phenomenon that if a person with normal hearing is deprived of auditory input in an anechoic chamber, the person will experience increased hearing sensitivity, start to hear extremely weak sounds, and frequently experience tinnitus. The implication of these findings and the postulate of the involvement of subcortical processing in tinnitus is that in certain cases tinnitus might be due to such an increased gain within the subcortical centres of the auditory system. As such it can be treated by a method aimed at decreasing this gain; that is, hearing aids or white noise generators incorporated into a protocol which employs a very gradual increase of such auditory input over prolonged periods of time. (...) Another ramification of this hypothesis is that hyperacusis can be regarded as a pretinnitus state. Hyperacusis is a manifestation of increased central gain (...).

The acute (*see* Table 18.1) and chronic (*see* Table 18.2) effects of sensory deprivation caused by noise exposure on stimulus-induced and spontaneous activity have been extensively documented at different levels of the auditory system. We look at some of these interesting studies across the auditory pathway.

Table 18.1 Summary of acute studies

Structure	Exposure stimulus	Species	Results	Reference
DCN	Broadband white noise (5–20 kHz), 115 dB SPL, 3 h (bilateral)	Mice	**Increase** in SFR	Gröschel et al. [17]
	Tone matched to BF or center of the high-frequency inhibitory sideband of recorded neuron, 85- or 109-dB SPL, 2 min (unilateral)	Hamsters	**Increase** in SFR and **decrease** rate-intensity function (RIF) at the BF tone/**decrease** in SFR and **increase** in RIF at non-BF tone	Gao et al. [19]
VCN	One-half octave above the neuron's CF, 80–105 dB SPL, 3–5 min	Chinchillas	**Increase** in evoked activity	Boettcher and Salvi [19]
	Broadband white noise (5–20 kHz), 115 dB SPL, 3 h (bilateral)	Mice	**Increase** in SFR	Gröschel et al. [17]
IC	2 kHz pure tone, 105 dB SPL (bilateral)	Chinchillas	**Increase** in evoked LFP	Salvi et al. [15]
	Pure tone frequency above neuron's CF, 95–115 dB SPL, 15–25 min (ipsilateral ear exposed)	Chinchillas	**Increase** in evoked activity, **alteration** in tuning curve	Wang et al. [20]
	0.5 octave band of noise with a CF of 16 kHz, 103 dB SPL, 1 h (unilateral and bilateral)	Mice	**Increase** in SFR in CNIC/no changes in bursting activity in bilateral exposure Changes in temporal pattern of firing in unilateral exposure	Ma et al. [21]
	Narrow band noise centered at 12 kHz, 120 dB SPL, 1 h (bilateral)	Rats	**Decrease** of sound evoked potential	Sun et al. [22]
	10 kHz tone, 124 dB SPL, 2 h (unilateral)	Guinea pig	No changes in SFR after 4 h/**increased** SFR after 12 h	Mulders and Robertson [23]
	Broadband white noise (5–20 kHz), 115 dB SPL, 3 h (bilateral)	Mice	**No significant change** in SFR immediately after exposure	Gröschel et al. [17]
AC	Pure tone 0.5 octaves above the highest CF, 93–123 dB SPL, 30 min (contralateral ear exposed)	Cats	SFR **increased** in A1, **decreased** in AII, and did not change in AAF Mean CF threshold **increased** for LFP and **decreased** for units/**decrease** in CF in A1	Kimura and Eggermont [24]
	5–6 kHz pure tone, 120 dB SPL, 1 h (contralateral ear exposed)	Cats	**Increase** in SFR after 2 h **Increase** in spike-synchrony and bursting properties	Noreña and Eggermont [25]
	5-6 kHz pure tone, 120 dB SPL, 1 h (contralateral ear exposed)	Cats	**Alteration** in tuning curves and temporal pattern, **increase** in evoked activity and monotonicity index	Noreña et al. [26]
	Narrow-band noise, 120 dB SPL, 1 h (unilateral)	Rats	**Increase** in evoked activity	Sun et al. [27]
	White noise, 125 dB SPL, 5 min	Mice	**Alteration** in PV+ and SST+ inhibitory interneurons. **Increase** in spontaneous and sound-evoked activity of SST+ in layer 4, and in layer 2/3 for PV+	Novák et al. [28]

Table 18.2 Summary of chronic studies

Structure	Exposure stimulus	Species	Results	Reference
DCN	10 kHz continuous tone at 127 dB SPL for 4 h (unilateral)	Hamsters	**Increase** in evoked potential amplitudes/**Increase** in SFR	Kaltenbach and Afman [29]
	4 kHz tone for 30–60 min at 80 dB SPL (unilateral)	Chinchillas	**Increase** in SFR/**increase** in rate-intensity function at 1 kHz and CF	Brozoski et al. [30]
	250 Hz band of noise centered at 10 Hz, 105–120 dB SPL, 4 h (bilateral)	Mice	**Changes** in tuning curve/**Increase** in SFR	Ma and Young [31]
	10 kHz tone, 115 dB for 4 h (bilateral)	Hamsters	**Increase** in SFR and bursting activity	Finlayson and Kaltenbach [32]
	7 kHz centered, half-octave noise, 97 dB SPL, 2 h (unilateral)	Guinea pig	**Increase** in SFR, synchrony, and bursting for frequencies above exposure frequency	Wu et al. [33]
VCN	10 kHz tone, 124 dB SPL, 2 h (unilateral)	Guinea pig	**Increase** in SFR (primary and onset neurons)	Vogler et al. [34]
	Broadband white noise (5–20 kHz), 115 dB SPL, 3 h (bilateral)	Mice	No significant change in SFR 7 and 14 days after noise exposure	Gröschel et al. [17]
	7 kHz centered, half-octave noise, 97 dB SPL, 2 h (unilateral)	Guinea pig	**Increase** in rate-intensity functions at high sound levels/**Increase** in sound-evoked cross-unit synchrony of bushy cell	Martel and Shore [35]
IC	4kHz tone, 85 dB SPL, 1 h (unilateral)	Chinchillas	**Increase** in SFR and synchrony	Bauer et al. [36]
	5 or 8 kHz pure tone, 110–121 dB SPL, 3.3–16 h (bilateral)	Rats	**Increase** in response threshold/**Residual responses** in the damaged region	Izquierdo et al. [37]
	10 kHz tone, 124 dB SPL, 1h	Guinea Pig	**Increase** in SFR	Mulders and Robertson [38]
	10 kHz tone, 124 dB SPL, 1 h (unilateral)	Guinea pig	**Increase** in CAP threshold and SFR	Dong et al. [39]
	1/3 octave narrow band noise at 4 kHz, 120 dB 4 h (bilateral)	Guinea pig	**Alteration** in different types of frequency response areas/**Increase** in SFR	Wang et al. [40]
	10 kHz tone, 124 dB, 2 h (unilateral)	Guinea pig	**Increase** in SFR above the exposure frequency, **Increase** in monotonicity	Vogler et al. [41]
	16 kHz tone, 116 dB SPL, 2 h (unilateral)	Rats	**Increase** in SFR	Ropp et al. [42]
MGB	Cochlear lesion	Cats	**Reorganization** of the tonotopic map	Kamke et al. [43]
	Octave noise band centered around 16 kHz, 116 dB SPL, 1 h (unilateral)	Rats	**Increase** in SFR and bursting properties in both the Lemniscal and non-lemniscal/**Increase** in evoked activity	Kalappa et al. [44]
AC	Unilateral cochlear lesion	Cats	**Reorganization** of the tonotopic map	Rajan et al. [45]
	6 kHz pure tone, 126 dB SPL, 1 h (bilateral)	Cats	**Reorganization** of the tonotopic map/**Increase** in SFR and synchrony	Eggermont and Komiya [46]
	6 kHz pure tone, 115 dB SPL, 2 h (bilateral)	Cats	**Increase** in threshold/**Reorganization** of the tonotopic map correlated with hearing loss	Seki and Eggermont [47]
	One-third octave band noise centered at 5 kHz, 120 dB SPL, 2 h (bilateral)	Cats	**Reorganization** of the tonotopic map in exposed animals without additional exposure to enriched acoustic environment	Noreña and Eggermont [48]
	One-third octave band of noise centered at 8 kHz, 115 dB SPL, 2 h (bilateral)	Guinea pigs	**Increase** in evoked local field potential and alterations in frequency-intensity response area/**Decrease** in spectral power	Noreña et al. [49]
	Narrow-band noise centered at 12 kHz, 120 dB SPL, 1 h (bilateral)	Rats	**Increase** in evoked potential amplitude for frequencies above exposure frequency	Sun et al. [22]
	Octave band noise (OBN, 10–20 kHz) or narrow-band noise (16–20 kHz) at 104 dB SPL for several days (bilateral)	Rats	**Increase** in SFR and evoked activity	Chen et al. [50]
	Octave band of noise (8–16 kHz), 100 dB SPL, 2 h (bilateral)	Mice	**Increase** in evoked corticocollicular response	Asokan et al. [48]

Central Plasticity Changes After Noise Trauma

Dorsal Cochlear Nucleus (DCN)

Acute Noise Exposure

Single and multiunit recordings in DCN fusiform cells of anesthetized hamsters showed an increase in spontaneous firing rate (SFR) twenty minutes after moderately intense tone noise exposure (85- or 109-dB SPL for 2 min) [18]. When the exposure frequency matched the best frequency (BF) of unit clusters, SFR significantly enhanced with a mean ratio of post- to pre-exposure (Po/Pr) of 2.74 at 20 min. However, SFR decreased (mean Po/Pr at 16 kHz = 0.25 at 20 min) in the lower frequency regions (4–7 kHz) when the exposure frequency fell inside the inhibitory sideband (10 kHz tone at 109 dB SPL for 2 min). The above finding suggests that the SFR increases when the exposure frequency and BF of the unit clusters match; on the other hand, it decreases when there is a significant gap between the exposure frequency and the cluster's BF. Furthermore, in the same study, the peak activity in the rate-intensity function decreased in response to a subsequent BF tone, whereas it was enhanced when exposed to a non-BF tone (tone frequency that activated the inhibitory sideband). Similarly, Gröschel et al. [17] showed an increase (12.6 ± 1.8 imp/s for 13 recorded neurons) in SFR in the DCN of anesthetized mice immediately after noise exposure (broadband white noise (5–20 kHz) at 115 dB SPL for 3 h) compared to controls (8.8 ± 1.4 imp/s for 95 recorded neurons).

Chronic Noise Exposure

Kaltenbach and Afman [29], measured spontaneous multiunit activity and response thresholds at 2 and 30 days after noise exposure (10 kHz continuous tone at 127 dB SPL for 4 h). Two days after noise exposure, response thresholds were elevated but the SFR decreased throughout the DCN. At 30 days after noise exposure, the response threshold did not differ from those observed at 2 days. However, SFR was significantly elevated at 30 days in cells with best frequencies close to the noise exposure spectrum. Overall, the study suggests that spontaneous hyperactivity in the DCN is a slowly developing phenomenon that is delayed relative to the appearance of neural threshold shift. Similarly, Brozoski et al. [30], showed an increase in SFR in the DCN fusiform cells of noise-exposed chinchillas (mean 24–28 spikes/s) with behavioral evidence of tinnitus compared with unexposed animals (mean 15–17 spikes/s). Further, the dynamic range and slope of the rate-intensity function significantly enhanced at the frequency for which there was maximum effect of noise trauma. Finlayson and Kaltenbach [32], also showed an increase in SFR in single units from the DCN fusiform cell layer of hamsters (15.9 spikes/s) exposed to 10 kHz tone at a level of 115 dB for 4 h compared to hearing controls (8.7 spikes/s). Approximately half of the increase in spontaneous activity in exposed animals was accounted for by an increase in bursting activity.

In addition to increase in SFR in the frequency region above exposure frequency, Wu et al. [33] showed an increase in spontaneous properties such as spike synchrony and bursting in guinea pigs several weeks following unilateral noise exposure (7 kHz centered, half-octave noise, 97 dB SPL, 2 h). Increase in SFR was higher in the tonotopic regions one octave above the exposure frequency. Furthermore, changes in synchrony and SFR were strongly correlated with tinnitus behavior. Using noise parameters similar to that in the above studies, Zacharek et al. [52] showed that removal of the ipsilateral cochlear input to DCN by partial or complete cochlear ablation had no significant effect on the SFR in noise-exposed (10 kHz pure tone at a sound level of 122–127 dB SPL for 4 h) hamsters. This result suggests that hyperactivity in the DCN is not dependent on inputs coming from the ipsilateral cochlea but may originate centrally.

Ma and Young [31], recorded single neurons in the DCN of unanesthetised cats one month after exposure to a 250 Hz band of noise centered at 10 Hz presented at 105–120 dB SPL for 4 h. The threshold shift, determined from compound action potentials audiograms, showed an elevated threshold of about 60 dB for neurons at BFs above an edge frequency of 5–10 kHz. Additionally, the study showed that the SFR was not higher in fusiform cells with elevated thresholds relative to controls. This finding contrasts with those observed in the previous studies using similar noise exposure parameters, suggesting that changes in SFR are species-specific or are sensitive to anesthesia.

Ventral Cochlear Nucleus (VCN)

Acute Noise Exposure

Gröschel et al. [17] showed a significant increase in SFR from 10.6 ± 2.1 imp/s (53 recorded neurons) in the control group to 14.2 ± 1.8 imp/s (24 recorded neurons) immediately after noise exposure (broadband white noise (5–20 kHz), 115 dB SPL, 3 h) in the VCN of mice. The study did not report location-specific increase in SFR. On the other hand, Boettcher and Salvi [19], showed a 25% increase in maximum discharge rate at characteristic frequency (CF) compared to the maximum pre-exposure firing rate in the VCN of chinchillas exposed (3- to 5-min, 90–105 dB SPL) to a tone above the neuron's CF.

Chronic Noise Exposure

Contrary to the study from Gröschel et al. [17], single neuron recordings in the VCN of pigmented guinea pigs showed a reduction in SFR immediately after noise exposure (10 kHz tone at 124 dB SPL for 2 h) [34]. However, the mean SFR significantly elevated about a factor of two compared to sham control two weeks after noise exposure. This hyperactivity in the VCN was more evident in primary-like and onset types of neurons. Also, an increase in SFR was more widely distributed across CF regions, i.e., independent of the frequencies corresponding to threshold elevation. These results were also in contrast with the study of Gröschel et al. [17]. Using the same above animal model, Martel and Shore [35] showed an enhanced stimulus-driven response at suprathreshold sound levels after noise exposure (7 kHz centered, half-octave noise, 97 dB SPL). Additionally, sound-evoked cross-unit synchrony as a function of intensity increased across a wide range of frequencies. On the other hand, mean SFR increased in bushy cells across all BFs in exposed animals with behavioral evidence of tinnitus compared to those that did not show tinnitus-like behavior and controls. Further, cross-unit spontaneous synchrony increased, but this increase did not correlate with an animal's tinnitus index (TI). Overall, the findings suggested that VCN bushy cells in noise-overexposed guinea pigs show hyperacusis-like neural firing patterns. Unlike the fusiform cells in the DCN, bushy cells did not show an association between SFR, synchrony, and behavioral measures of tinnitus.

Inferior Colliculus (IC)

Acute Noise Exposure

Ma et al. [21] investigated the changes in spontaneous activity in the central nucleus of the inferior colliculus (CNIC) of CBA/J mice subjected to either bilateral or unilateral noise exposure. The exposure stimulus was a 0.5-octave band of noise with a center frequency of 16 kHz presented for one hour at a maximum sound level of 103 dB SPL. Unilaterally exposed neurons showed less hearing loss near the exposure frequency than bilaterally exposed neurons. However, bilaterally exposed mice showed a significant increase in median SFR (6.0 sp/s ± 10.4 sp/s) shortly after the exposure compared to controls (4.1 sp/s ± 8.9 sp/s). This increase in SFR was limited to frequencies (with elevated thresholds) near the trauma frequency. Additionally, bursting activity did not change in the CNIC for bilaterally exposed mice. But in the unilaterally exposed mice, changes in temporal aspects of firing were found in the protected ear. Similar to the findings in the SFR in the above study, Gröschel et al. [17] showed average SFRs of 4.9 ± 0.4 (56 recorded neurons) in controls and 5.9 ± 0.5 (40 recorded neurons) immediately after exposure to 3 h of broadband white noise (5–20 kHz) at 115 dB SPL. This increase in SFR was not significant and the study did not differentiate between low and high frequency neurons.

Mulders and Robertson [23] studied the time of onset of spontaneous hyperactivity by single neuron recordings in the CNIC of guinea pigs subjected to unilateral noise exposure (10 kHz tone at 124 dB SPL for 1 h). No changes in SFR were found 4 h after the cessation of noise exposure but significantly increased after 12 h compared to sham controls. SFR was elevated across all CF and there was no significant difference between neurons with normal and elevated thresholds. This finding suggested that plastic changes in the IC are rapid, beginning some hours after noise exposure.

Wang et al. [20], investigated acute changes in sound-induced activity in the IC of Chinchillas. Exposure to continuous trauma tone frequency (at 95–115 dB SPL, 15–25 min) above the neurons CF resulted in a significant increase in driven discharge rate in 70% of all neurons studied in comparison to before the exposure. Additionally, traumatizing exposure drastically altered the tuning curves of most of the IC neurons (40% of units), with an expansion of the low-frequency tail of the excitatory response area of the turning curve. In another study on the same animal model, local field potential (LFP) amplitude for frequencies below the trauma frequency increased by a factor of 4 [15]. Furthermore, the amplitudes at frequencies above the trauma frequency increased slightly at a moderate intensity level. In contrast to the above study, Sun et al. [22] found no obvious changes in sound-evoked potentials in the IC of rats 1 h after noise exposure (narrow band noise, 12 kHz, 120 dB SPL, 1 h).

Chronic Noise Exposure

Vogler et al. [41] performed single-neuron spontaneous recordings in the CNIC of guinea pigs exposed to 10 kHz tone at 124 dB SPL for 2 h. After a recovery period of 2 weeks, mean SFR in the trauma group significantly increased (4.32 ± 0.36) relative to the sham group (1.44 ± 0.36). This increase was higher for neurons with CF above the trauma frequency and was not confined to a particular cell type. Similarly, Ropp et al. [42] showed spontaneous hyperactivity in the contralateral and ipsilateral CNIC of rats 1–4 months after noise exposure (continuous 16 kHz tone at 116 dB SPL for 2 h). The increase in spontaneous activity was found below and above the region of maximum threshold shift.

Mulders and Robertson [38], showed increased SFR 2 weeks after noise exposure (10 kHz tone at 124 dB SPL for 1 h) in the CNIC neurons corresponding to cochlear threshold loss compared to control animals. On the other hand, blocking spontaneous firing of primary afferents and cochlear ablation resulted in reduced SFR in the CNIC at all recovery times. This result suggests that hyperactivity induced in the IC after noise exposure is dependent on the activity in the contralateral cochlea. Using the same noise exposure and animal model, Dong et al. [39], showed elevated thresholds of compound action potential around and above 8 kHz. SFR did not change immediately after noise exposure (0.92 ± 0.23 spk/s) compared to controls (1.15 ± 0.16 spk/s). But increased two (6.05 ± 0.55 spk/s) to four (5.41 ± 0.47 spk/s) weeks after noise exposure compared to controls. This increase in SFR was particularly higher in the frequency range of peripheral hearing loss. In addition to increase in SFR, Bauer et al. [36], also showed an increase in cross-fiber synchrony in the contralateral IC of chinchillas after noise exposure (4 kHz tone, 85 dB SPL, 1 h) with behavioral evidence of tinnitus.

Wang et al. [40], recorded single-units from the IC of guinea pigs to demonstrate acute and chronic effects of noise exposure (narrow band noise at 4 kHz, 120 dB, 4 h) on both the spontaneous and sound-induced activity. Immediately after noise exposure, the percentage of V-shaped tuning curves decreased significantly but recovered after chronic changes. The W-shaped tuning curves (double-peaked) significantly increased immediately and after recovery period. Plotting CF as a function of depth showed a gap at 4 kHz immediately after noise exposure correlating with the noise exposure frequency. This gap was reduced in the chronic group. SFR increased in acute (31.6 ± 3.6) and chronic (40.5 ± 13.8) group compared to normal group (15.3 ± 3.0).

Medial Geniculate Body (MGB)

Kalappa et al. [44], studied the spontaneous discharge properties of MGB neurons from awake unexposed hearing controls and noise-exposed (unilateral exposure for 1 h at 116 dB SPL centered on 16 kHz octave band) rats with behavioral evidence of tinnitus. Two months after exposure, single-unit recordings from MGB neurons revealed an increased SFR in both the lemniscal (mean 5.6 ± 0.3) and non-lemniscal (3.5 ± 0.7) subdivisions of the MGB compared to the control (mean 4.68 ± 0.48 spikes/s). Also, spontaneous bursting properties including bursts per minute (9.2 in control and 37.1 in exposed), mean spikes in burst (5.1 in control and 6.13 exposed), mean bust duration (60 ms in control and 90 ms after noise exposure) significantly enhanced in tinnitus animals compared to unexposed control animals. Rate-level functions were steeper in tinnitus animals compared to units recorded from unexposed control groups. Driven firing rates were significantly elevated at suprathreshold sound levels and correlated with tinnitus score.

Auditory Cortex (AC)

Acute Noise Exposure

Kimura and Eggermont [24] investigated changes in spontaneous activity and frequency tuning in primary auditory cortex (A1), anterior auditory field (AAF), and secondary auditory cortex (AII) of cats before and immediately after noise exposure (pure tone, 93–123 dB SPL, 30 min). SFR in the A1 increased (from 0.54 to 1.08 spk/s) 20 min after exposure to a tone frequency 0.5 octaves above the highest CF. SFR did not change in the AAF (from 0.98 to 0.84 spks/s) and decreased in the AII (from 1.22 to 0.76 spks/s). Furthermore, LFP and single-unit (SU) mean threshold significantly increased in A1 when the trauma tone frequency was close to the CF. However, the mean threshold increased only for LFP in AAF, while it did not change in AII. In addition, the mean CF for all units in A1 decreased significantly, whereas there was no significant effect in AAF and AII.

Noreña and Eggermont [25], performed multiunit recordings in the A1 of cats before and after noise exposure (5–6 kHz pure tone, 120 dB SPL, 1 h). Immediately after exposure (3.74 spk/s), SFR did not differ compared to pre-exposure (3.5 spk/s) but significantly elevated 2 h after noise exposure (5.12 spk/s). Furthermore, peak cross-correlation coefficients increased immediately (0.021) and few hours (0.024) after exposure to a 5 kHz pure tone compared to pre-exposure (0.02). The changes in cross-correlation coefficients did not correlate with changes in SFR.

Calford et al. [53] studied changes in receptive fields of single neurons in the A1 of anesthetized cats before and after short exposure to an intense pure tone frequency 0.5 octaves below the CF of the studied neurons. In their study, tuning curves of 41% neurons expanded; that is, new frequency inputs which were previously insensitive, due to strong inhibition, were unmasked. On the other hand, the tuning curve of 18% of neurons contracted, and in some cases, the neurons were unresponsive after the intense tone exposure. Noreña et al. [26], reported similar changes in receptive fields of multiunit activity in anesthetized cats after noise exposure (5 or 6 kHz tone, at 115–120 dB SPL, 1 h). Immediately after noise exposure, the CF was shifted toward lower frequencies, MU receptive fields expanded, and, in some cases, they contracted after noise exposure. The results from the two above studies suggest that noise exposure induces both an increase and decrease in inhibition. In addition, the later study also showed that noise exposure significantly increased the monotonicity index and the maximum driven firing rate (by a factor of 2) in neurons with a CF below the trauma-tone frequency. Enhancement of evoked potential amplitude a few hours after noise exposure (narrowband noise, 120 dB SPL, 1 h) was shown in the AC of rats [27].

In a more recent study, Novák et al. [28], showed layer-specific changes in auditory cortical inhibitory interneurons (parvalbumin-positive (PV+) and somatostatin-positive (SST+)) within minutes after noise exposure (125 dB SPL, white noise, 5 min). Spontaneous and pure-tone-evoked firing rates of SST+ interneurons increased in layer 4 and remained unchanged in layer 2/3. In contrast, PV+ interneurons with high best frequencies increased in layer 2/3 while it did not change in layer 4.

Chronic Noise Exposure

Eggermont and Komiya [46], exposed 5-week-old kittens to a loud 6 kHz pure tone at 126 dB SPL for 1 h. Two to five months after noise exposure, the mean threshold shift for frequencies above 8 kHz was between 25 dB and 35 dB. This moderate hearing loss induced reorganization of the frequency map in the auditory cortex. In the cortical reorganized region, neurons having their best frequency above the traumatizing frequency no longer responded. Instead, these neurons now respond to a narrow frequency range corresponding to the low-frequency boundary of hearing loss. Therefore, the edge frequency of hearing loss is overrepresented in the reorganized region of the cortex. Surprisingly, the sharpness of the frequency tuning curves in the reorganized area was normal or with near-normal thresholds. The SFR significantly increased in the reorganized region of the cortex (mean 2.33 ± 2.43 spk/s) compared to the non-reorganized region (1.36 ± 1.50 spikes/s). Similar to the above study, tonotopic map was reorganized 2–11 months after unilateral cochlear lesions in adult cats [45]. The new CF threshold in the reorganized cortical region in most cases did not differ significantly from those in the normal cortical region.

To evaluate potential age effects on the reorganization of the cortical tonotopic map, Seki and Eggermont [47], exposed cats of different age groups (36 days, 56 days, and 118 days after birth) to a 6 kHz pure tone presented at a level of 115 dB SPL for 2 h. Cortical changes in these exposed cats were compared to age-matched controls. Peripheral hearing threshold measured using auditory brainstem responses (ABR) increased by 20–60 dB, but there was no significant dependence of induced hearing loss on the age of exposure. However, the presence of cortical reorganization correlated with the average amount of hearing loss. That is, the cortical map reorganized in exposed cats having a hearing threshold above 20–25 dB. Immediate and long-term changes in local field potential (LFP) amplitude after noise exposure (one-third octave band of noise with a center frequency of 8 kHz, 115 dB SPL, 2 h) was addressed by Noreña et al. [49]. Immediately after noise exposure, LFP amplitudes rapidly increased for frequencies below 8 kHz and recovered few days after the trauma. Furthermore, the frequency intensity response area (FIRA) displayed significant reduction in cortical responses in the high-frequency band. In addition, spontaneous power spectra decreased immediately after noise exposure. In a more recent study, Asokan et al. [51], showed that corticocollicular response gain of cortical layer 5 neurons strongly depresses hours after noise exposure (8–16 kHz, 100 dB SPL for 2 h) but rebounded above baseline levels by the following day and remained elevated for several weeks.

Mechanisms of Central Changes After Sensory Deprivation

Several neural mechanisms have been proposed to account for the observed changes in the auditory centers after noise-induced hearing loss. Understanding these mechanisms is important for developing therapies aiming to suppress abnormal neural activity that may be associated to tinnitus.

GABAergic Inhibition

In the primary sensory cortex, GABAergic neurons play a critical role in cortical circuit refinement and stabilization to adapt to any changes in the environment. They are a variety of GABAergic interneurons with distinct physiological characteristics, anatomical locations, and capacities for plasticity. GABAergic interneurons are highly interconnected, with connections to local excitatory neurons and local inhibitory neurons. The interaction between inhibitory and excitatory neurons is fundamental in maintaining neural networks in a balanced state, favoring neural computations necessary for accurate processing of acoustic information. Under normal conditions, the ratio of excitatory–inhibitory inputs in the cortical circuits is stable; that is, excitatory–inhibitory networks receive balanced responses from all subsets of presynaptic inputs. Such balanced excitatory–inhibitory circuits, for instance in the AC, are involved in shaping the temporal and spectral selectivity and intensity tuning. However, it is proposed that disruption of the tight balance of excitation and inhibition underlies rapid neuronal changes in the cortical circuits, such as changes in the receptive field and enhanced spontaneous and evoked activity. To better understand the neurobiological mechanisms underpinning cortical changes after noise-induced hearing loss, several studies over the past few years have focused on investigating the role of GABAergic inhibition.

In the cochlear nucleus (CN) of several animal species, noise exposure is shown to result in elevation of spontaneous and stimulus-induced activity. These neuronal changes are attributed, at least in part, from reduced levels of inhibitory neurotransmitters, such as glycine and GABA. In the fusiform cells of the DCN, the protein levels of α_1 and α_3 glycine receptor subunits (GlyRs) were reduced in the middle and high frequency regions of rats with behavioral evidence of tinnitus several months after noise exposure [54]. Similarly, reduction in GABAergic inhibition was shown by electrical stimulation of glutamatergic axons in DCN slices from mice with behavioral evidence of tinnitus compared to controls [55]. In the IC, cytosolic levels of glutamic acid decarboxylase (GAD) decreased immediately following noise exposure, with complete recovery after 30 days post-exposure [56]. Furthermore, increased spontaneous firing rate in the frequency region affected by noise exposure is shown to be accompanied by downregulation of mRNA levels of the α_1 subunits of the GlyR and $GABA_AR$'s [39]. GABA1 was significantly reduced in both the contralateral and ipsilateral IC compared to controls immediately (59% reduction) and 4 weeks (40% reduction) after noise exposure.

In contrast to the CN and IC, noise exposure is shown to increase tonic extrasynaptic $GABA_A$ R by elevating $GABA_AR$ δ-subunit mRNA levels in the thalamocortical MGB neurons [57]. In the AC, Yang et al. [58], have shown reduction in tonic and phasic $GABA_A$ R current amplitudes and frequency along with decreases in presynaptic GAD levels in the frequency region above exposure frequency. Similarly, $GABA_A\alpha 1$ expression levels in the ipsilateral and contralateral AC are reduced after noise exposure [59].

In summary, peripheral deafferentation induced by noise exposure results in plastic changes in the inhibitory mechanism through downregulation or altering of ligand-gated inhibitory receptors and their associated proteins. Changes in GABAergic neurotransmission could disrupt the balance between the inhibitory–excitatory ratio. Consequently, this could potentially mediate hyperexcitability, such as an increase in evoked and spontaneous activity and changes in temporal firing patterns in the central auditory system. "*Lateral inhibition*" or "*surround inhibition*" is a well-known inhibitory model proposed to explain neuronal hyperexcitability or the complex changes in receptive field properties [60, 61]. Lateral inhibition is inhibition between neighboring neurons in a neuronal structure and has been suggested as an important mechanism for balancing neural networks [62]. This mechanism exists at many levels of the auditory system. In the AC, lateral inhibition is supposed to be involved in the sharpening of the receptive field (RF) (but see [63]). Here, pyramidal neurons of the AC receive inhibitory inputs covering much of the audible spectrum and hence exhibiting border tuning rather than excitation. This difference in tuning broadness of excitation and inhibition could generate a stronger inhibition in frequency regions at the flanks of the excitation peak and thus narrowing the tuning curve. However, in the event of cochlear damage restricted to the high-frequency base of the cochlea, inhibition is reduced at nearby and distant frequencies resulting in the loss of surround inhibition. This loss of surround/side-band inhibition would later unmask previously inhibited excitatory inputs, therefore, resulting in broader excitatory tuning curves and potentially inducing hyperexcitability in the low-frequency region.

KCC2 Co-transporters

GABAA receptors which mediate fast synaptic inhibition in the brain are ligand-gated receptors associated with an anion-permeable conductance [64]. GABAA receptor currents are carried by chloride ions. The net ion flux through the GABAA receptor channels depend on the transmembrane chloride gradients and the neuronal resting membrane potential, which determine the driving force of GABAA receptor currents. The transmembrane chloride gradient is regulated by the opposing actions of two cation-chloride co-transporters: KCC2 and NKCC1. While NKCC1 is responsible for inward movement of chloride ions, KCC2 is responsible for chloride ion extrusion and for the generation of chloride-dependent hyperpolarizing postsynaptic currents mediated by GABAA receptors. The inhibitory effect of GABA is dependent on the intracellular chloride concentration [65]. In mature neurons, KCC2 is the primary determinant in maintaining intracellular chloride concentration below electrochemical equilibrium [66]. However, when KCC2 co-transporters are downregulated, chloride extrusion is reduced leading to higher intracellular chloride ion concentration. As a result, the transmembrane chloride gradient is reduced or even reversed [67].

Downregulation of KCC2 has been found in several neurological disorders, such as epilepsy [68] and neuropathic pain [67]. In the auditory system, Tighilet et al. [69], showed downregulation of KCC2 (by 50%) in the ipsilateral cochlear nucleus (CN) after unilateral cochlear nerve section. Their results suggest that changes in KCC2 density on the neuronal membrane after auditory deafferentation would eventually switch the role of GABA from inhibitory to excitatory or reduce the inhibitory effect of GABA.

In summary, KCC2 activity regulates the polarity of GABA action of membrane potential. Any downregulation in KCC2 expression would result in decrease of GABA inhibition and/or switch to an excitatory action of GABA. Either way, this can lead to an imbalance of excitation and inhibition than can potentially induce abnormal neuronal activity.

Excitatory Neurotransmission

In contrast to the downregulation of GABAergic neurotransmission following sensory deafferentation, several studies reported upregulation of excitatory neurotransmission at many levels of the auditory system. In the CN, Barker et al. [70] investigated the changes in vesicular glutamate transporters VGLUT-1 and VGLUT-2 in DCN of rats exposed to 15 kHz pure tone at 110 dB SPL for 6 h. Five days after noise exposure, VGLUT-2 expression increased in the DCN and VCN. In contrast, VGLUT-1 expression decreased in the VCN and within the molecular layer of the DCN. Upregulation of VGLUT-2 expression in the CN may result in an increased release of glutamate, resulting in hyperactivity in the CN.

Similar findings on changes in vesicular glutamate transporter expression in the CN of guinea pigs after noise exposure (narrowband noise centered at 7 kHz, 0.4-octave bandwidth, 97 dB SPL, 2 h) was reported by Heeringa et al. [71]. Animals with behavioral evidence of tinnitus showed a significant increase in VGLUT-2 density in the ipsilateral AVCN compared to non-tinnitus animals and controls. However, in the DCN, VGLUT-2 density increased on the contralateral side. This study demonstrated that increased glutamatergic excitatory neurotransmission is restricted to animals with behavioral evidence of tinnitus.

Increased excitatory neurotransmission in the AC following cochlear damage has also been reported by several studies. In the study of Yang et al. [58], the amplitude and frequency of the miniature excitatory postsynaptic currents (mEPSCs) increased in the low-CF area and did not alter in the high-CF area. Kotak et al. [72] reported increased mEPSCs amplitude and duration in gerbil after sensorineural hearing loss (SNHL) induced by cochlear ablation. This increase in synaptic excitation suggests being due to the upregulation of both AMPA and NMDA receptors. In addition, both these studies reported decreased amplitude of mIPSCs, indicating that enhanced synaptic excitation is accompanied by diminished inhibition.

Axonal Sprouting

Axonal sprouting plays a crucial role in cortical remapping after sensory deafferentation in almost all sensory cortices [73–75]. In the visual cortex, monocular laser lesions produce a lesion projection zone (LPZ) [76] where neurons are initially unresponsive to visual stimuli but would regain their activity over time. Immediately after the lesion induction, the receptive fields of the neurons in the LPZ shift to parts of the retina surrounding the lesion. However, when the visually driven activity gets restored over months, the visuotopic remapping progresses toward the center of the LPZ. Now the responsive neurons within the LPZ receive inputs from regions of the retina adjacent to the lesion via long-range horizontal connections. These horizontal connections cover the entire cortical reorganized area and undergo axonal sprouting after sensory deprivation. Axonal sprouting occurs rapidly in a matter of hours after retinal lesion [79] and possibly after cochlear lesion. Under normal conditions, the density of long-range horizontal axonal arbors is stable with dynamic boutons. However, sensory deafferentation triggers dynamic changes in axonal arbors overtime, involving concurrent sprouting and pruning. Over weeks, horizontal axonal density increases and rises to about twofold after six months to 1 year compared to the normal cortex.

To the best of our knowledge, there is no study investigating axonal sprouting in the auditory cortex after cochlear hearing loss. However, some functional findings are consistent with an increase of axonal sprouting in auditory cortex. The increase in axonal density after cochlear damage could account for the shift in CF and expansion of the receptive field of neurons within the damaged region in the AC. Moreover, axonal sprouting may account for the cortical sink in the supragranular layers that has been shown to emerge after acute and chronic noise trauma [77].

Spike-Time-Dependent Plasticity (STDP)

STDP is a common form of synaptic plasticity in many neuronal cell types in different regions of the brain and drives several forms of developmental plasticity and adult learning. STDP changes synaptic strength as a function of the timing between the presynaptic and postsynaptic action potentials [78]. Importantly, it is sensitive to the time interval between the pre-and postsynaptic action potentials. The occurrence of a presynaptic action potential a few milliseconds before the postsynaptic action potential leads to long-term potentiation (LTP) of the synapses. LTP involves the sustained strengthening of synaptic connections between neurons [79] and this mechanism gives rise to a long-lasting increase in neuronal excitability. In contrast to LTP, occurrence of a postsynaptic action potential a few milliseconds before a presynaptic action potential leads to long-term depression (LTD) of the synapses. LTD weakens the synaptic strength between two neurons. LTP is shown to be involved in central changes in the visual cortex [80] and may contribute to some of the plasticity changes in the auditory cortex after noise-induced hearing loss. In the DCN fusiform cells, LTP is suggested to play an important role in increased synchronization [81]. On the other hand, LTD is found to be involved in central changes in the somatosensory cortex after whisker deprivation [82].

Discussion

There is overwhelming evidence that noise-induced hearing loss is associated to compensatory mechanisms in the auditory centers: while the sensory inputs are reduced at the periphery (i.e., in the cochlear nerve), neural activity is enhanced at virtually all levels of the auditory centers. This increase in neural responses can result from a vast repertoire of mechanisms. The plastic mechanisms that are triggered by noise-induced hearing loss can be divided into two broad categories: those that can be interpreted in terms of central gain and those that can be thought as resulting from "new" inputs or connections. The mechanisms that are involved in the central gain can be seen as neural changes amplifying given sensory inputs. These mechanisms are those involved in central inhibition and excitation. An analogy for the central gain is represented by an amplifier: the neural signal is enhanced or reduced in such a way that there is an optimal use of the full range of the neural firing rate [83]. On the other hand, other central changes are better described by "new" inputs rather than an amplification. These mechanisms are axonal sprouting, the unmasking of excitatory inputs, or spike-time dependent plasticity. An analogy for these mechanisms is represented by "rerouting" of sensory information: a new "route" is created that can propagate the neural activity. This is, for instance, the case for the unmasking of excitatory responses coming from remote frequencies, and when non-auditory activity can activate and propagate through the auditory system. It is unclear whether tinnitus and/or hyperacusis result from central gain and/or rerouting of inputs.

It has been suggested that an increase in central gain may result in tinnitus and/or hyperacusis. However, the latter hypothesis must be tempered. First, not all tinnitus sufferers have hearing loss (and reduced sensory inputs) and many other mechanisms can account for the tinnitus generation [84]. Second, while the approaches that are aimed at compensating for the reduced sensory inputs can improve the tinnitus condition (acoustic stimulation, hearing aid amplification, cochlear implants) [85–85], they are rarely efficient enough to suppress the tinnitus percept completely. The "resistance" of tinnitus to the acoustic approaches (like to the pharmacological approaches) is not consistent with a simple explanation based on central gain. In this context, it is possible that "rerouting" mechanisms can play a role in tinnitus and/or hyperacusis. These mechanisms (axonal sprouting, for instance) may be hardly reversible and may account for the fact that tinnitus is resistant to most treatments.

An important point to consider when discussing the mechanisms of tinnitus and hyperacusis is that neural activity is critical but does not represent the entire story accounting for these clinical conditions. Indeed, beside the "amount" of neural activity (in terms of firing rate), neural activity must be transmitted to the next stages of the central auditory system [11]. In a recent study carried out in anesthetized animals exposed to noise trauma, we addressed this question specifically using cortical recordings over an entire cortical column [77]. The current sinks and sources were derived from the current source density analysis method. We found a new cortical sink in supragranular layers (possibly resulting from axonal sprouting and/or quick unmasking of excitatory inputs coming from parallel fibers). Moreover, in the animals exposed to noise trauma, our results are consistent with the interpretation that neural activity is propagating through the cortical column and auditory cortex during resting state activity. On control animals, on the other hand, the spontaneous activity reaches the granular layer but seems to stop there since no synaptic activity can be detected thereafter. These results suggest that neural changes intrinsic to cortex (new current sink in supragranular layer), that are partially independent from central gain increase, may alter the propagation of neural activity.

Finally, it is well known that a given percept is associated to the activation of a distributed cortical network [89]. An enhanced propagation of cortical activity, as the one reported above [77], is likely to facilitate the recruitment of a distributed network. In this context, the emotional valence of tinnitus and/or hyperacusis and the resulting attentional focus on tinnitus/hyperacusis are also likely to make tinnitus/hyperacusis network more salient.

References

1. Mackenzie I, Smith A. Deafness—the neglected and hidden disability. Ann Trop Med Parasitol. 2009;103(7):565–71. https://doi.org/10.1179/000349809X12459740922372.
2. Van Eyken E, Van Camp G, Van Laer L. The complexity of age-related hearing impairment: contributing environmental and genetic factors. Audiol Neuro-Otol. 2007;12(6):345–58. https://doi.org/10.1159/000106478.
3. Keppler H, Dhooge I, Vinck B. Hearing in young adults. Part II: the effects of recreational noise exposure. Noise Health. 2015;17(78):245–52. https://doi.org/10.4103/1463-1741.165026.
4. Seidman MD, Standring R. Noise and quality of life. Int J Environ Res Public Health. 2010;7(10):3730–8. https://doi.org/10.3390/ijerph7103730.
5. Shore SE, Wu C. Mechanisms of noise-induced tinnitus: insights from cellular studies. Neuron. 2019;103(1):8–20. https://doi.org/10.1016/j.neuron.2019.05.008.
6. Kujawa SG, Liberman MC. Acceleration of age-related hearing loss by early noise exposure: evidence of a misspent youth. J Neurosci. 2006;26(7):2115–23. https://doi.org/10.1523/JNEUROSCI.4985-05.2006.
7. Kujawa SG, Liberman MC. Adding insult to injury: cochlear nerve degeneration after "temporary" noise-induced hearing loss. J Neurosci. 2009;29(45):14077. https://doi.org/10.1523/JNEUROSCI.2845-09.2009.
8. Wang Y, Hirose K, Liberman MC. Dynamics of noise-induced cellular injury and repair in the mouse cochlea. JARO. 2002;3(3):248–68. https://doi.org/10.1007/s101620020028.
9. Heinz MG, Young ED. Response growth with sound level in auditory-nerve fibers after noise-induced hearing loss. J Neurophysiol. 2004;91(2):784–95. https://doi.org/10.1152/jn.00776.2003.
10. Liberman MC, Dodds LW. Single-neuron labeling and chronic cochlear pathology. II. Stereocilia damage and alterations of spontaneous discharge rates. Hear Res. 1984;16(1):43–53.
11. Noreña AJ, Farley BJ. Tinnitus-related neural activity: theories of generation, propagation, and centralization. Hear Res. 2013;295:161–71. https://doi.org/10.1016/j.heares.2012.09.010.
12. Schaette R, Kempter R. Development of tinnitus-related neuronal hyperactivity through homeostatic plasticity after hearing loss: a computational model. Eur J Neurosci. 2006;23(11):3124–38. https://doi.org/10.1111/j.1460-9568.2006.04774.x.
13. Sasaki CT, Kauer JS, Babitz L. Differential [14C]2-deoxyglucose uptake after deafferentation of the mammalian auditory pathway—

a model for examining tinnitus. Brain Res. 1980;194(2):511–6. https://doi.org/10.1016/0006-8993(80)91233-0.
14. Gerken GM. Central denervation hypersensitivity in the auditory system of the cat. J Acoust Soc Am. 1979;66(3):721–7. https://doi.org/10.1121/1.383222.
15. Salvi RJ, Saunders SS, Gratton MA, Arehole S, Powers N. Enhanced evoked response amplitudes in the inferior colliculus of the chinchilla following acoustic trauma. Hear Res. 1990;50(1–2):245–57. https://doi.org/10.1016/0378-5955(90)90049-U.
16. Jastreboff PJ, Hazell JW. A neurophysiological approach to tinnitus: clinical implications. Br J Audiol. 1993;27(1):7–17. https://doi.org/10.3109/03005369309077884.
17. Gröschel M, Ryll J, Götze R, Ernst A, Basta D. Acute and long-term effects of noise exposure on the neuronal spontaneous activity in cochlear nucleus and inferior colliculus brain slices. Biomed Res Int. 2014;2014:909260. https://doi.org/10.1155/2014/909260.
18. Gao Y, Manzoor N, Kaltenbach JA. Evidence of activity-dependent plasticity in the dorsal cochlear nucleus, in vivo, induced by brief sound exposure. Hear Res. 2016;341:31–42. https://doi.org/10.1016/j.heares.2016.07.011.
19. Boettcher FA, Salvi RJ. Functional changes in the ventral cochlear nucleus following acute acoustic overstimulation. J Acoust Soc Am. 1993;94(4):2123–34. https://doi.org/10.1121/1.407484.
20. Wang J, Salvi RJ, Powers N. Plasticity of response properties of inferior colliculus neurons following acute cochlear damage. J Neurophysiol. 1996;75(1):171–83. https://doi.org/10.1152/jn.1996.75.1.171.
21. Ma W-LD, Hidaka H, May BJ. Spontaneous activity in the inferior colliculus of CBA/J mice after manipulations that induce tinnitus. Hear Res. 2006;212(1–2):9–21. https://doi.org/10.1016/j.heares.2005.10.003.
22. Sun W, Deng A, Jayaram A, Gibson B. Noise exposure enhances auditory cortex responses related to hyperacusis behavior. Brain Res. 2012;1485:108–16. https://doi.org/10.1016/j.brainres.2012.02.008.
23. Mulders WHAM, Robertson D. Development of hyperactivity after acoustic trauma in the guinea pig inferior colliculus. Hear Res. 2013;298:104–8. https://doi.org/10.1016/j.heares.2012.12.008.
24. Kimura M, Eggermont JJ. Effects of acute pure tone induced hearing loss on response properties in three auditory cortical fields in cat. Hear Res. 1999;135(1-2):146–62. https://doi.org/10.1016/s0378-5955(99)00104-5.
25. Noreña AJ, Eggermont JJ. Changes in spontaneous neural activity immediately after an acoustic trauma: Implications for neural correlates of tinnitus. Hear Res. 2003;183(1–2):137–53. https://doi.org/10.1016/S0378-5955(03)00225-9.
26. Noreña AJ, Tomita M, Eggermont JJ. Neural changes in cat auditory cortex after a transient pure-tone trauma. J Neurophysiol. 2003;90(4):2387–401. https://doi.org/10.1152/jn.00139.2003.
27. Sun W, Zhang L, Lu J, Yang G, Laundrie E, Salvi R. Noise exposure–induced enhancement of auditory cortex response and changes in gene expression. Neuroscience. 2008;156(2):374–80. https://doi.org/10.1016/j.neuroscience.2008.07.040.
28. Novák O, Zelenka O, Hromádka T, Syka J. Immediate manifestation of acoustic trauma in the auditory cortex is layer specific and cell type dependent. J Neurophysiol. 2016;115(4):1860–74. https://doi.org/10.1152/jn.00810.2015.
29. Kaltenbach JA, Afman CE. Hyperactivity in the dorsal cochlear nucleus after intense sound exposure and its resemblance to tone-evoked activity: a physiological model for tinnitus. Hear Res. 2000;140(1-2):165–72. https://doi.org/10.1016/S0378-5955(99)00197-5.
30. Brozoski TJ, Bauer CA, Caspary DM. Elevated fusiform cell activity in the dorsal cochlear nucleus of chinchillas with psychophysical evidence of tinnitus. J Neurosci. 2002;22(6):2383–90. https://doi.org/10.1523/JNEUROSCI.22-06-02383.2002.
31. Ma W-LD, Young ED. Dorsal cochlear nucleus response properties following acoustic trauma: Response maps and spontaneous activity. Hear Res. 2006;216–217:176–88. https://doi.org/10.1016/j.heares.2006.03.011.
32. Finlayson PG, Kaltenbach JA. Alterations in the spontaneous discharge patterns of single units in the dorsal cochlear nucleus following intense sound exposure. Hear Res. 2009;256(1–2):104–17. https://doi.org/10.1016/j.heares.2009.07.006.
33. Wu C, Martel DT, Shore SE. Increased synchrony and bursting of dorsal cochlear nucleus fusiform cells correlate with tinnitus. J Neurosci. 2016;36(6):2068–73. https://doi.org/10.1523/JNEUROSCI.3960-15.2016.
34. Vogler DP, Robertson D, Mulders WHAM. Hyperactivity in the ventral cochlear nucleus after cochlear trauma. J Neurosci. 2011;31(18):6639–45. https://doi.org/10.1523/JNEUROSCI.6538-10.2011.
35. Martel DT, Shore SE. Ventral cochlear nucleus bushy cells encode hyperacusis in guinea pigs. Sci Rep. 2020;10(1):20594. https://doi.org/10.1038/s41598-020-77754-z.
36. Bauer CA, Turner JG, Caspary DM, Myers KS, Brozoski TJ. Tinnitus and inferior colliculus activity in chinchillas related to three distinct patterns of cochlear trauma. J Neurosci Res. 2008;86(11):2564–78. https://doi.org/10.1002/jnr.21699.
37. Izquierdo MA, Gutiérrez-Conde PM, Merchán MA, Malmierca MS. Non-plastic reorganization of frequency coding in the inferior colliculus of the rat following noise-induced hearing loss. Neuroscience. 2008;154(1):355–69. https://doi.org/10.1016/j.neuroscience.2008.01.057.
38. Mulders WHAM, Robertson D. Hyperactivity in the auditory midbrain after acoustic trauma: dependence on cochlear activity. Neuroscience. 2009;164(2):733–46. https://doi.org/10.1016/j.neuroscience.2009.08.036.
39. Dong S, Mulders WHAM, Rodger J, Woo S, Robertson D. Acoustic trauma evokes hyperactivity and changes in gene expression in guinea-pig auditory brainstem: brainstem plasticity after acoustic trauma. Eur J Neurosci. 2010;31(9):1616–28. https://doi.org/10.1111/j.1460-9568.2010.07183.x.
40. Wang F, Zuo L, Hong B, Han D, Range EM, Zhao L, Sui Y, Guo W, Liu L. Tonotopic reorganization and spontaneous firing in inferior colliculus during both short and long recovery periods after noise overexposure. J Biomed Sci. 2013;20(1):91. https://doi.org/10.1186/1423-0127-20-91.
41. Vogler DP, Robertson D, Mulders, W. H. a. M. Hyperactivity following unilateral hearing loss in characterized cells in the inferior colliculus. Neuroscience. 2014;265:28–36. https://doi.org/10.1016/j.neuroscience.2014.01.017.
42. Ropp T-JF, Tiedemann KL, Young ED, May BJ. Effects of unilateral acoustic trauma on tinnitus-related spontaneous activity in the inferior colliculus. JARO. 2014;15(6):1007–22. https://doi.org/10.1007/s10162-014-0488-2.
43. Kamke MR, Brown M, Irvine DRF. Plasticity in the tonotopic organization of the medial geniculate body in adult cats following restricted unilateral cochlear lesions. J Comp Neurol. 2003;459(4):355–67. https://doi.org/10.1002/cne.10586.
44. Kalappa BI, Brozoski TJ, Turner JG, Caspary DM. Single unit hyperactivity and bursting in the auditory thalamus of awake rats directly correlates with behavioural evidence of tinnitus. J Physiol. 2014;592(Pt 22):5065–78. https://doi.org/10.1113/jphysiol.2014.278572.
45. Rajan R, Irvine DRF, Wise LZ, Heil P. Effect of unilateral partial cochlear lesions in adult cats on the representation of lesioned and

unlesioned cochleas in primary auditory cortex. J Comp Neurol. 1993;338(1):17–49. https://doi.org/10.1002/cne.903380104.
46. Eggermont JJ, Komiya H. Moderate noise trauma in juvenile cats results in profound cortical topographic map changes in adulthood. Hear Res. 2000;142(1–2):89–101. https://doi.org/10.1016/S0378-5955(00)00024-1.
47. Seki S, Eggermont JJ. Changes in cat primary auditory cortex after minor-to-moderate pure-tone induced hearing loss. Hear Res. 2002;173(1-2):172–86. https://doi.org/10.1016/S0378-5955(02)00518-X.
48. Noreña AJ, Eggermont JJ. Enriched acoustic environment after noise trauma reduces hearing loss and prevents cortical map reorganization. J Neurosci. 2005;25(3):699–705. https://doi.org/10.1523/JNEUROSCI.2226-04.2005.
49. Noreña AJ, Moffat G, Blanc JL, Pezard L, Cazals Y. Neural changes in the auditory cortex of awake guinea pigs after two tinnitus inducers: salicylate and acoustic trauma. Neuroscience. 2010;166(4):1194–209. https://doi.org/10.1016/j.neuroscience.2009.12.063.
50. Chen G-D, Sheppard A, Salvi R. Noise trauma induced plastic changes in brain regions outside the classical auditory pathway. Neuroscience. 2016;315:228–45. https://doi.org/10.1016/j.neuroscience.2015.12.005.
51. Asokan MM, Williamson RS, Hancock KE, Polley DB. Sensory overamplification in layer 5 auditory corticofugal projection neurons following cochlear nerve synaptic damage. Nat Commun. 2018;9(1):2468. https://doi.org/10.1038/s41467-018-04852-y.
52. Zacharek MA, Kaltenbach JA, Mathog TA, Zhang J. Effects of cochlear ablation on noise induced hyperactivity in the hamster dorsal cochlear nucleus: implications for the origin of noise induced tinnitus. Hear Res. 2002;172(1–2):137–43. https://doi.org/10.1016/s0378-5955(02)00575-0.
53. Calford MB, Rajan R, Irvine DRF. Rapid changes in the frequency tuning of neurons in cat auditory cortex resulting from pure-tone-induced temporary threshold shift. Neuroscience. 1993;55(4):953–64. https://doi.org/10.1016/0306-4522(93)90310-C.
54. Wang H, Brozoski TJ, Turner JG, Ling L, Parrish JL, Hughes LF, Caspary DM. Plasticity at glycinergic synapses in dorsal cochlear nucleus (DCN) of rats with behavioral evidence of tinnitus. Neuroscience. 2009;164(2):747–59. https://doi.org/10.1016/j.neuroscience.2009.08.026.
55. Middleton JW, Kiritani T, Pedersen C, Turner JG, Shepherd GMG, Tzounopoulos T. Mice with behavioral evidence of tinnitus exhibit dorsal cochlear nucleus hyperactivity because of decreased GABAergic inhibition. Proc Natl Acad Sci. 2011;108(18):7601–6. https://doi.org/10.1073/pnas.1100223108.
56. Milbrandt JC, Holder TM, Wilson MC, Salvi RJ, Caspary DM. GAD levels and muscimol binding in rat inferior colliculus following acoustic trauma. Hear Res. 2000;147(1–2):251–60. https://doi.org/10.1016/s0378-5955(00)00135-0.
57. Sametsky EA, Turner JG, Larsen D, Ling L, Caspary DM. Enhanced GABAA mediated tonic inhibition in auditory thalamus of rats with behavioral evidence of tinnitus. J Neurosci. 2015;35(25):9369–80. https://doi.org/10.1523/JNEUROSCI.5054-14.2015.
58. Yang S, Weiner BD, Zhang LS, Cho S-J, Bao S. Homeostatic plasticity drives tinnitus perception in an animal model. Proc Natl Acad Sci. 2011;108(36):14974–9. https://doi.org/10.1073/pnas.1107998108.
59. Browne CJ, Morley JW, Parsons CH. Tracking the expression of excitatory and inhibitory neurotransmission-related proteins and neuroplasticity markers after noise induced hearing loss. PLoS ONE. 2012;7(3):e33272. https://doi.org/10.1371/journal.pone.0033272.
60. Irvine DR, Rajan R. Injury-induced reorganization of frequency maps in adult auditory cortex: the role of unmasking of normally-inhibited inputs. Acta Otolaryngol. 1997;532:39–45. https://doi.org/10.3109/00016489709126143.
61. Schaette R, Kempter R. Computational models of neurophysiological correlates of tinnitus. Front Syst Neurosci. 2012;6:34. https://doi.org/10.3389/fnsys.2012.00034.
62. Isaacson JS, Scanziani M. How inhibition shapes cortical activity. Neuron. 2011;72(2):231–43. https://doi.org/10.1016/j.neuron.2011.09.027.
63. Wehr M, Zador AM. Balanced inhibition underlies tuning and sharpens spike timing in auditory cortex. Nature. 2003;426(6965):442–6. https://doi.org/10.1038/nature02116.
64. Goutierre M, Al Awabdh S, Donneger F, François E, Gomez-Dominguez D, Irinopoulou T, Menendez de la Prida L, Poncer JC. KCC2 regulates neuronal excitability and hippocampal activity via interaction with task-3 channels. Cell Rep. 2019;28(1):91–103. https://doi.org/10.1016/j.celrep.2019.06.001.
65. Jacob TC, Moss SJ, Jurd R. GABA A receptor trafficking and its role in the dynamic modulation of neuronal inhibition. Nat Rev Neurosci. 2008;9(5):331–43. https://doi.org/10.1038/nrn2370.
66. Rivera C, Voipio J, Payne JA, Ruusuvuori E, Lahtinen H, Lamsa K, Pirvola U, Saarma M, Kaila K. The K+/Cl− co-transporter KCC2 renders GABA hyperpolarizing during neuronal maturation. Nature. 1999;397(6716):251–5. https://doi.org/10.1038/16697.
67. Coull JAM, Boudreau D, Bachand K, Prescott SA, Nault F, Sík A, De Koninck P, De Koninck Y. Trans-synaptic shift in anion gradient in spinal lamina I neurons as a mechanism of neuropathic pain. Nature. 2003;424(6951):938–42. https://doi.org/10.1038/nature01868.
68. Chen L, Wan L, Wu Z, Ren W, Huang Y, Qian B, Wang Y. KCC2 downregulation facilitates epileptic seizures. Sci Rep. 2017;7(1):156. https://doi.org/10.1038/s41598-017-00196-7.
69. Tighilet B, Dutheil S, Siponen MI, Noreña AJ. Reactive neurogenesis and down-regulation of the potassium-chloride cotransporter KCC2 in the cochlear nuclei after cochlear deafferentation. Front Pharmacol. 2016;7:281. https://doi.org/10.3389/fphar.2016.00281.
70. Barker M, Solinski HJ, Hashimoto H, Tagoe T, Pilati N, Hamann M. Acoustic overexposure increases the expression of VGLUT-2 mediated projections from the lateral vestibular nucleus to the dorsal cochlear nucleus. PLoS ONE. 2012;7(5):e35955. https://doi.org/10.1371/journal.pone.0035955.
71. Heeringa AN, Wu C, Chung C, West M, Martel D, Liberman L, Liberman MC, Shore SE. Glutamatergic projections to the cochlear nucleus are redistributed in tinnitus. Neuroscience. 2018;391:91–103. https://doi.org/10.1016/j.neuroscience.2018.09.008.
72. Kotak VC, Fujisawa S, Lee FA, Karthikeyan O, Aoki C, Sanes DH. Hearing loss raises excitability in the auditory cortex. J Neurosci. 2005;25(15):3908–18. https://doi.org/10.1523/JNEUROSCI.5169-04.2005.
73. Calford MB, Wright LL, Metha AB, Taglianetti V. Topographic plasticity in primary visual cortex is mediated by local corticocortical connections. J Neurosci. 2003;23(16):6434–42. https://doi.org/10.1523/JNEUROSCI.23-16-06434.2003.
74. Ramirez JJ. The role of axonal sprouting in functional reorganization after CNS injury: lessons from the hippocampal formation. Restor Neurol Neurosci. 2001;19(3–4):237–62.
75. Yamahachi H, Marik SA, McManus JNJ, Denk W, Gilbert CD. Rapid axonal sprouting and pruning accompany functional reorganization in primary visual cortex. Neuron. 2009;64(5):719. https://doi.org/10.1016/j.neuron.2009.11.026.
76. Calford MB, Wang C, Taglianetti V, Waleszczyk WJ, Burke W, Dreher B. Plasticity in adult cat visual cortex (area 17) following circumscribed monocular lesions of all retinal layers. J Physiol. 2000;524(Pt 2):587–602. https://doi.org/10.1111/j.1469-7793.2000.t01-1-00587.x.

77. Parameshwarappa V, Pezard L, Noreña AJ. Changes in the spatiotemporal pattern of spontaneous activity across a cortical column after noise trauma. J Neurophysiol. 2022;127(1):239–54. https://doi.org/10.1152/jn.00262.2021.
78. Fröhlich F. Chapter 4—synaptic plasticity. In: Fröhlich F, editor. Network neuroscience. New York: Academic; 2016. p. 47–58. https://doi.org/10.1016/B978-0-12-801560-5.00004-5.
79. Citri A, Malenka RC. Synaptic plasticity: multiple forms, functions, and mechanisms. Neuropsychopharmacology. 2008;33(1):18–41. https://doi.org/10.1038/sj.npp.1301559.
80. Cooke SF, Bear MF. How the mechanisms of long-term synaptic potentiation and depression serve experience-dependent plasticity in primary visual cortex. Philos Trans R Soc B Biol Sci. 2014;369(1633):20130284. https://doi.org/10.1098/rstb.2013.0284.
81. Marks KL, Martel DT, Wu C, Basura GJ, Roberts LE, Schvartz-Leyzac KC, Shore SE. Auditory-somatosensory bimodal stimulation desynchronizes brain circuitry to reduce tinnitus in guinea pigs and humans. Sci Transl Med. 2018;10(422):3175. https://doi.org/10.1126/scitranslmed.aal3175.
82. Drew PJ, Feldman DE. Intrinsic signal imaging of deprivation-induced contraction of whisker representations in rat somatosensory cortex. Cereb Cortex. 2009;19(2):331–48. https://doi.org/10.1093/cercor/bhn085.
83. Noreña AJ. An integrative model of tinnitus based on a central gain controlling neural sensitivity. Neurosci Biobehav Rev. 2011;35(5):1089–109.
84. Noreña AJ. Revisiting the cochlear and central mechanisms of tinnitus and therapeutic approaches. Audiol Neuro-Otol. 2015;20(suppl 1):53–9. https://doi.org/10.1159/000380749.
85. Baguley DM, Atlas MD. Cochlear implants and tinnitus. Prog Brain Res. 2007;166:347–55. https://doi.org/10.1016/S0079-6123(07)66033-6.
86. Parazzini M, Del Bo L, Jastreboff M, Tognola G, Ravazzani P. Open ear hearing aids in tinnitus therapy: an efficacy comparison with sound generators. Int J Audiol. 2011;50(8):548–53. https://doi.org/10.3109/14992027.2011.572263.
87. Quaranta N, Wagstaff S, Baguley DM. Tinnitus and cochlear implantation. Int J Audiol. 2004;43(5):245–51.
88. Tyler RS, Noble W, Coelho CB, Ji H. Tinnitus retraining therapy: mixing point and total masking are equally effective. Ear Hear. 2012;33(5):588–94. https://doi.org/10.1097/AUD.0b013e31824f2a6e.
89. Dehaene S, Changeux J-P. Experimental and theoretical approaches to conscious processing. Neuron. 2011;70(2):200–27. https://doi.org/10.1016/j.neuron.2011.03.018.

The Frontostriatal Gating Model of Tinnitus

19

Josef P. Rauschecker

Abstract

Research on tinnitus over the past decade has made it abundantly clear that this highly prevalent disorder is not just due to changes in the peripheral and central auditory system, but also involves affective centers of the limbic system. Current research now focuses on the question of which of these brain regions are the drivers of the bothersome experience that is tinnitus. In other words, does chronic tinnitus originate from a learned association between auditory and affective signals, or is tinnitus the result of a failing frontostriatal gating system? In healthy individuals, the gating system has the ability to cancel the tinnitus signal via brain mechanisms involving medial prefrontal cortex (PFC) and ventral striatum (VS). Studies of tinnitus patients using different neuroimaging modalities, as well as theoretical considerations, make the existence of such a brain-based "noise cancellation" system likely. Neurostimulation approaches, some of which show promise for the treatment of mood disorders, may prove successful for the treatment of tinnitus as well.

J. P. Rauschecker (✉)
Georgetown University Medical Center, Washington, DC, USA
e-mail: rauschej@georgetown.edu

W. Schlee et al. (eds.), *Textbook of Tinnitus*, https://doi.org/10.1007/978-3-031-35647-6_19

Graphical Abstract

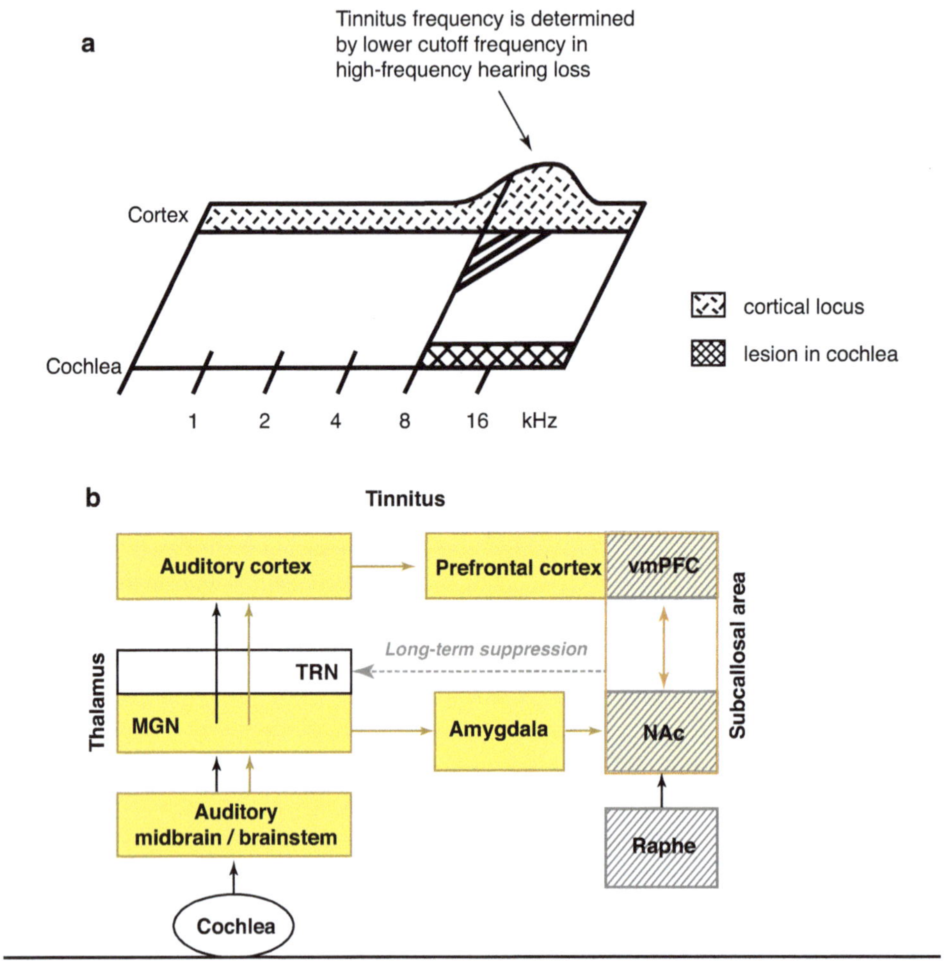

1. (a) Loud-noise exposure kills hair cells in the inner ear.
   (b) This triggers a reorganization (remapping) of the tonotopic map in auditory cortex and an expansion in the representation of lesion-edge frequencies, which underlies the tinnitus sensation.
2. At the same time, another brain system that would be in a position to cancel out the tinnitus signal in healthy individuals is also compromised and is unable to habituate to the phantom sound.
3. Tinnitus is exacerbated by stress and insomnia and is sometimes comorbid with mild to moderate depression.

Highlights
- Tinnitus is an auditory phantom sensation without external sound source.
- The tinnitus perception originates from lesion-induced plasticity in the auditory cortex after damage to the hair cells of the inner ear, which can result from loud-noise exposure or aging.
- In addition, there is involvement of limbic regions: (a) volume loss in the subgenual (SG) area of the anterior cingulate cortex (which is part of the ventromedial prefrontal cortex, vmPFC) can be shown with voxel-based morphometry, and (b) hyperactivity in the nucleus accumbens (NAc) of the ventral striatum (VS) is apparent from functional imaging studies in tinnitus patients.
- Our main hypothesis is that tinnitus consists of auditory-limbic dysregulation, where a circuit normally cancels the noise originating from hyperactivity in the auditory cortex. When this noise cancellation system becomes dysfunctional (for other reasons), chronic tinnitus is the result.

The Nature of Phantom Perception

The term "phantom sensation" refers to the perception of sensory events in the absence of a physical stimulus [1]. Phantom sensations are not the same as hallucinations. The latter come with an assumption of reality (or a firm denial of nonexistence), whereas phantom sensations come with the insight of their lack of reality and are rarely or never confused with actual, non-phantom perceptions. An exception are rare cases of musical hallucinosis [2], where people experience a phantom sensation so realistically that they initially assume an objective experience, but immediately have the insight that they are dealing with a phantom when shown the evidence. Phantom sensations, like tinnitus or certain forms of chronic pain [3, 4], carry the experience of a real sensation that can be assigned a stimulus intensity and quality in terms of pitch or degree of pain. The suffering that comes with this experience may or may not be directly proportional to the intensity of the perceived sensation. Brain imaging studies have shown that the two parameters are largely independent and are even mediated by discrete brain regions [5]. Recent overviews make this distinction even clearer [6].

Tinnitus sensations are generally rather simple sounds [7], from tones (27%) through hissing noise (31%), to amplitude-modulated chirping or "cricket sounds" (34%). This is one reason why their origin has commonly been assigned to brain regions in early parts of auditory cortex, where neuronal responses of this kind prevail, whereas more complex sounds reside in nonprimary regions of the auditory cortex [8, 9].

Cortical Reorganization After Peripheral Lesions: Lesion-Induced Plasticity of the Auditory Cortex

Another hypothesis is that phantom sensations are a result of lesion-induced plasticity [10], as has been observed in the visual and somatosensory cortex of adult animals. In the somatosensory cortex of nonhuman primates, for instance, such results have been obtained after peripheral deafferentation of the arms or fingers [11–13], which leads to massive reorganization in the corresponding brain regions and hyperactivity resulting from disinhibition. Expansion from neighboring body-part representations into the vacated territory is found, such that neurons in the area formerly representing the hand or arm are now activated by touching areas of the face. This can explain the phantom sensations experienced by upper-limb amputees, who often report feeling their phantom limb when touched in the face [14, 15].

Similarly, small lesions of the cochlea, in a restricted region of the frequency axis of the basilar membrane in the inner ear, lead to a missing frequency representation in the auditory cortex of adult cats [16]. The same region is now occupied by input from neighboring frequencies, which expands into the vacated space. Two testable predictions can be made: (1) by analogy with the "blind spot" in vision, subjects might not be aware of the missing frequency range, unless specifically tested; (2) by analogy with touch, they might be expected to perceive phantom sensations that come from the deafferented frequency region. In the somatosensory system, stimulation of specific finger regions has been shown to lead to an expansion of the corresponding areas of representation in the somatosensory cortex [17]. Similarly, training of monkeys at a particular tone frequency (the equivalent of place in the sensory periphery) leads to an expansion of the corresponding frequency representation in the auditory cortex [18]. In these animal models, loss of a finger, for instance, results in the loss of peripheral input to the corresponding region of somatosensory cortex without the loss of neuronal activity from the deafferented region. In the case of tinnitus, loss of hair cells in the inner ear (through aging or loud-noise exposure) leads to reorganization of auditory cortex in the sense that the deafferentation leads to shrinkage of the deprived frequency region and expansion of neighboring regions. This expansion results in an overrepresentation of the corresponding frequency—the tinnitus frequency. Functional imaging studies have generally verified this hypothesis [19] (but see [20]). In fact, the expanded frequency region extends beyond primary auditory cortex into nonprimary belt regions, as one would predict from the most common response characteristics (hissing and other complex sounds) of nonprimary auditory cortex, and not pure tones characteristic of the primary region (Fig. 19.1) [21].

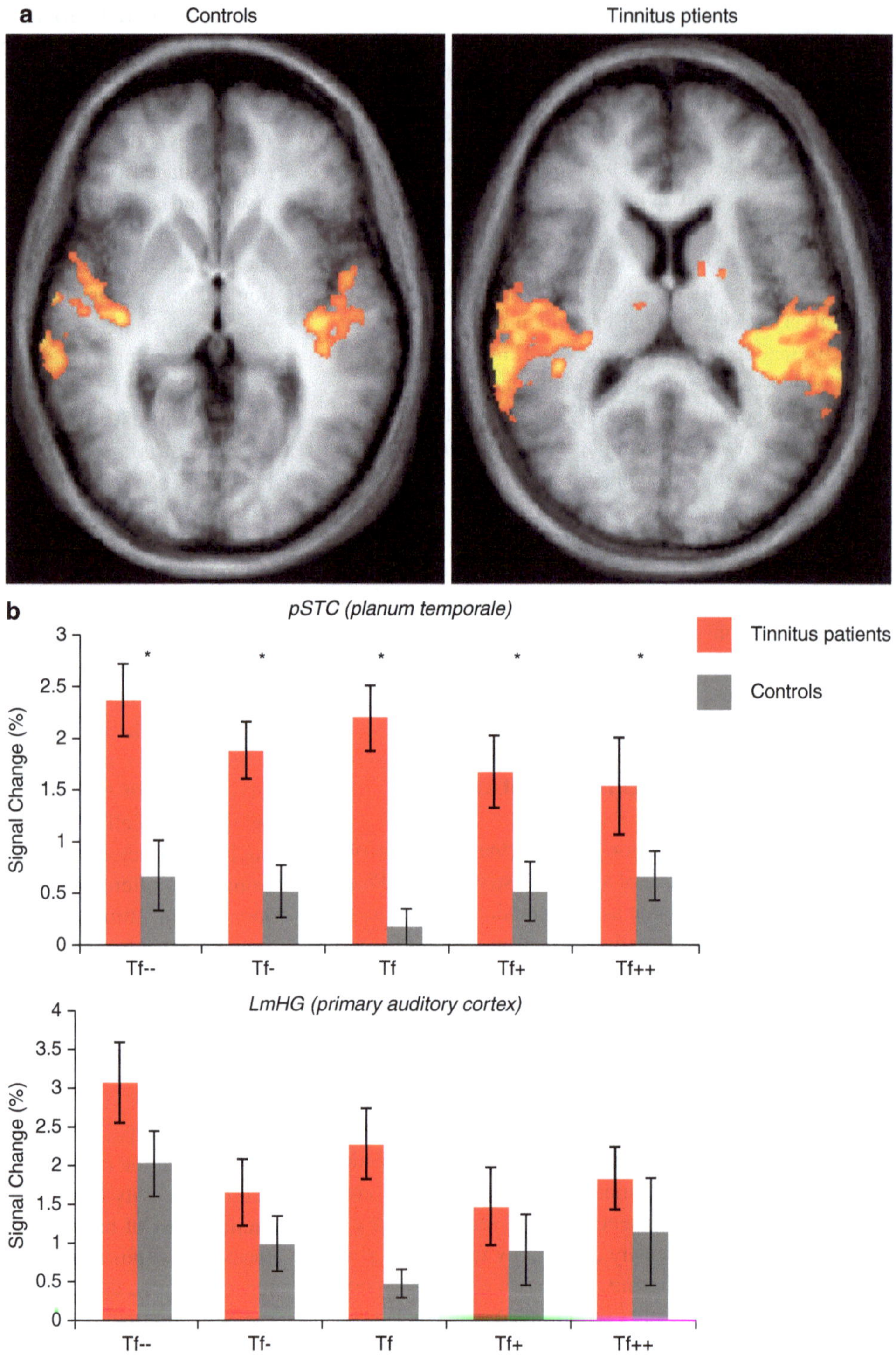

Fig. 19.1 Functional changes in the auditory cortex of tinnitus patients. (**a**) Functional MRI studies demonstrate the expansion/distortion of the auditory cortical map as a form of lesion-induced plasticity, similar to studies in the somatosensory cortex of monkeys [11]. (**b**) Signal change in primary auditory cortex is largely confined to the tinnitus frequency, whereas activation extending into nonprimary areas is more broadly tuned, indicating involvement of nonprimary auditory cortex in tinnitus as well [21] [and unpublished]

Structural Changes in the Medial Prefrontal Cortex (mPFC) and Anterior Cingulate Indicate Involvement of the Limbic System

When searching for correlates of tinnitus in structural MRI scans, fewer studies than not have found changes in the auditory system. An exception was a study by Schneider et al. [22] which found reduced volume of Heschl's gyrus in tinnitus patients using high-field MRI. Such results could be an indication of the reorganization found with functional MRI, possibly relating to degenerative changes from auditory deprivation. More commonly, structural MRI studies using voxel-based morphometry (VBM) [23] have found brain changes indicative of structural plasticity in regions outside the auditory system, including limbic structures and medial prefrontal cortex (mPFC). In particular, a significant volume loss was found in the subgenual (SG) area of the anterior cingulate, which is considered a part of ventromedial prefrontal cortex (vmPFC) (Fig. 19.2) [24]. This finding was later replicated with more refined techniques by other studies [21, 28].

While it is currently unknown what a statistical volume loss (or shrinkage) of brain tissue relates to in microanatomical terms, one may assume that it corresponds to a reduction in the number or density of cells. What cell types (neurons, glia, or neuropil) are primarily affected and whether the volume loss actually corresponds to atrophy or cell death is equally unknown. Only postmortem studies (or studies in animals with experimentally induced tinnitus) can provide a definitive answer.

The result of a volume loss in the subgenual (SG) region (also: Brodmann area 25) is intriguing, because it is associated with the perception of unpleasant sounds [29] and is implicated in mood disorders, including clinical depression [30, 31]. Clinical trials applying deep-brain stimulation (DBS) and closed-loop neuromodulation to this region have established it as a node in the depression network [32, 33]. Although not all tinnitus patients have clinical depression or anxiety, a strong association between these disorders and tinnitus has been demonstrated [34]. DBS of the caudate has also been shown to modulate tinnitus [35].

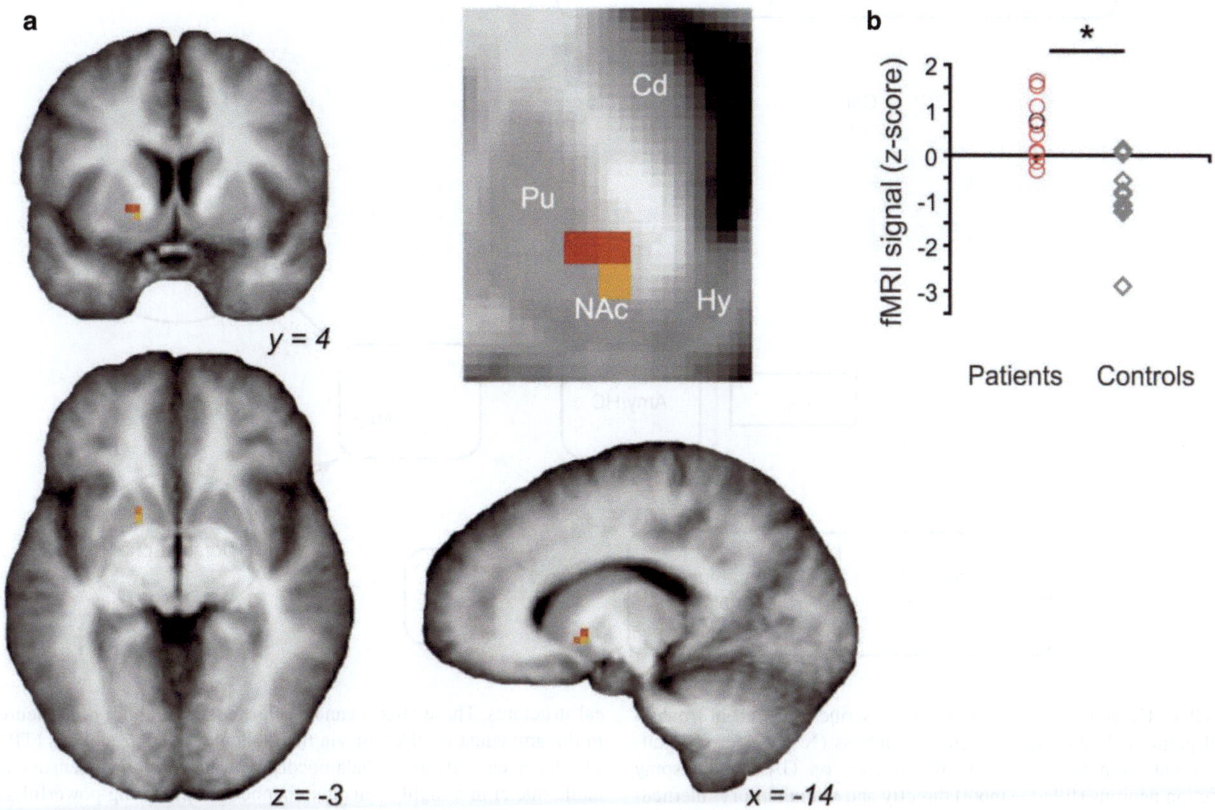

Fig. 19.2 Structural changes in the ventral part of medial prefrontal cortex (vmPFC) of tinnitus patients have been found using voxel-based morphometry [24, 25]. The subgenual (SG) area (in yellow) has a significant volume loss ($z = 4.9$; $p < 0.05$ corrected) in the study by Mühlau et al. [24], shown in (**a**). The same location (in blue) was reported by Leaver et al. [21] using more refined techniques, independent of age and hearing loss ($t > 4.65$ $p < 0.0001$) (**b**). On the right of panel (**b**) is a close-up of the sagittal image, showing the position of anatomical differences located in vmPFC inferior to the corpus callosum (CC). The position of basal ganglia structures is also indicated (*Cd* caudate, *NAc* nucleus accumbens). Patients with chronic pain also show volume loss in regions of the mPFC [26]; see also [27]. Panel (**a**) reproduced from Rauschecker et al. [25], with permission. Panel (**b**) from Leaver et al. [21], with permission

Other structural correlates of tinnitus in the brain have been found with diffusion tensor imaging (DTI) [36, 37] and cortical thickness measurements [38], all indicating rewiring of central auditory-limbic circuitry [39, 40].

Functional Changes in the Nucleus Accumbens (NAc) of the Ventral Striatum (VS): Dysregulation of Auditory-Limbic Networks

The structural changes in nonauditory regions of the brain bring to mind that tinnitus is not a purely auditory disorder to begin with. A prominent functional change is also found in the nucleus accumbens (NAc) of the ventral (or limbic) striatum (VS), which shows significant hyperactivity in tinnitus patients on the basis of functional MRI [21] (Fig. 19.3). In fact, the NAc exhibited an even greater degree of hyperactivity than auditory cortex, specifically to sounds frequency-matched to patients' tinnitus. The vmPFC/SG region with volume loss (see above) is heavily connected to the NAc. Furthermore, tinnitus-related anomalies were intercorrelated in the two limbic regions and between limbic and primary auditory areas, indicating the importance of auditory-limbic interactions in tinnitus. Neuroimaging studies utilizing connectivity methods like resting-state fMRI and diffusion MRI have uncovered (and continue to uncover) tinnitus-related anomalies throughout auditory, limbic, and other brain systems [41, 42].

Besides the hallmark auditory phantom sound, severe forms of tinnitus are commonly accompanied by emotional side effects, which reach from a simple annoyance to severe depression [43, 44]. What is equally striking is that tinnitus is by no means an automatic consequence of hearing loss: only

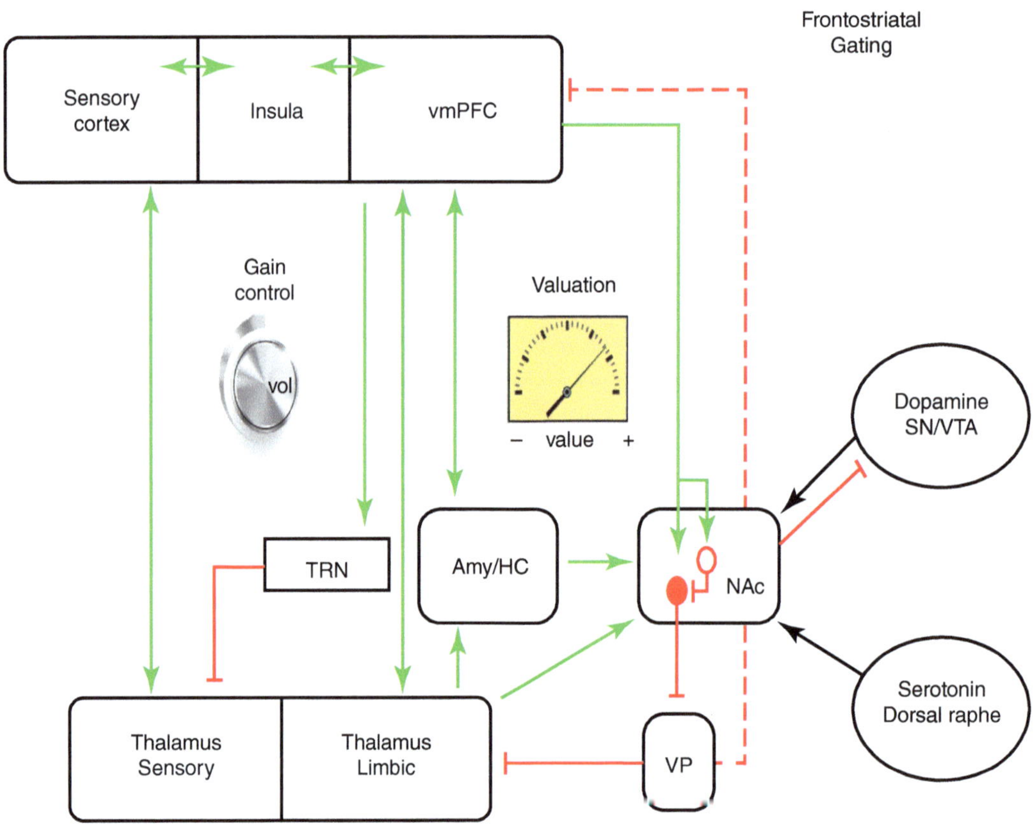

Fig. 19.3 The noise cancellation model describes a deficit in frontostriatal gating [25, 26]. The nucleus accumbens (NAc) receives excitatory input from the neocortex, which ends on GABAergic spiny projection neurons (filled symbol) directly and via inhibitory interneurons [55]. In addition, the NAc receives modulatory input from (among others) dopaminergic [56] and serotonergic [57] structures, and forms a processing loop for the valuation of sensory stimuli with the subgenual region (SG) of ventromedial prefrontal cortex (vmPFC) and, via the ventral pallidum (VP), with thalamic nuclei in the limbic system, such as the mediodorsal nucleus [21]. The amygdala (shown here without subdivisions and intrinsic circuitry) can bias this valuation system by providing emotional information [58]. The result of this valuation is used by the vmPFC to send a descending inhibitory signal to subcortical structures. These effects can be achieved via inhibitory interneurons in the amygdala or NAc, or via the thalamic reticular nucleus (TRN). The latter can attenuate thalamocortical transmission in sensory thalamic nuclei in a highly selective manner, thus exerting powerful gain control [25, 59–61]. See [62] for more details on corticostriatal connectivity. Abbreviations as in Fig. 19.1; in addition: *GABA* g-aminobutyric acid, *Vol* volume, *VTA* ventral tegmental area. Lines in green (with pointed endings) represent excitatory connections (glutamate); lines in red (with flat endings) refer to inhibitory connections (GABA). A direct GABAergic projection from the basal ganglia back to frontal cortex is currently hotly debated [63] and is shown as a broken red line. From Rauschecker et al. [26], with permission

about one-third of patients with sensorineural hearing loss end up with chronic tinnitus. The remaining two-thirds are somehow protected against ever getting tinnitus. Thus, it seems that central hearing loss is a frequent and perhaps even necessary precondition for developing tinnitus, but it is by no means sufficient. Other risk factors in tinnitus involve a (potentially genetic) vulnerability, whereas others are protected by a strong resilience against the disorder (see [26] for a discussion).

A more likely interpretation is, therefore, that morphological changes in vmPFC, including atrophy or cell death, are caused by factors independent of the process leading to hyperactivity in early sensory areas. One such factor could be stress, which is known to modulate both tinnitus and chronic pain [45], and which can even lead to their onset. Indeed, extensive studies in animal models have demonstrated that specifically vmPFC undergoes dramatic structural modification when animals are exposed to long-lasting stress [46]. Interestingly, dopamine release upon stress is increased in the PFC and inhibited in the NAc [47]. Prolonged sleep-deprivation and insomnia are also inversely correlated with grey matter volume of the brain in humans, specifically orbitofrontal cortex and hippocampus [48]. These effects may relate to dysregulation in cortisol levels [46, 49] which could, in tinnitus subjects, reflect a disturbance of the neuroendocrine reaction to stress [50]. There is indeed a high prevalence of organic sleep disorders in tinnitus patients [51, 52] and restoration of normal sleep patterns may be helpful for the treatment of tinnitus and chronic pain.

Dysregulation of Auditory-Limbic Networks: Reaction or Cause?

In discussions with my colleagues in the field, I often beg them: please do not call the affective correlates of tinnitus a "reaction" to the tinnitus sound, as if there was a causal relationship only in one direction (from the tinnitus sound to its affective coloration). In reality, the relationship between the tinnitus sound and its affective component is at the very least a two-way street, if not principally a causal relationship in the other direction: an affective disorder that prevents the cancellation of the phantom sound.

The traditional interpretation of affective or emotional sequelae of tinnitus is that they are a consequence or "reaction" to the perception of tinnitus sound [53]. Who would not become angry, anxious, or depressed if he or she is exposed to the constant tinnitus noise one cannot escape from? Who would not have problems falling asleep if they had to deal with constant exposure to hissing or ringing noise? Even the latest Tinnitus Functional Index (TFI) questionnaire [54] still asks: "*Does the tinnitus sound keep you up at night?*", and does not consider the alternative that a sleep disorder might actually cause the tinnitus and its persistence.

If one follows the neuroimaging findings presented in this chapter, one might come up with a very different reading. According to the counter-hypothesis reiterated here, there is evidence for top-down modulation of tinnitus by frontal and limbic brain structures (Fig. 19.4). Stress, for instance, or sleep deprivation can clearly exacerbate tinnitus, almost as if the tinnitus sound can serve as an indicator for the degree of stress. Accordingly, relaxation techniques not only make tinnitus more tolerable, they can measurably reduce tinnitus loudness. The observation alone that tinnitus can vary day-by-day, or that tinnitus affects only some people with hearing loss but not others, should be reason enough to consider the importance of top-down influences. What proponents of conventional tinnitus theories may counter is that these top-down influences are mediated by attention [64]. If this were the case, the tinnitus sound would become louder or more bothersome if the patient pays more attention to it, and the sound should disappear if it is ignored and attention is directed to a different target. Effects of that kind are quite small and certainly cannot explain cases of intermittent tinnitus, where the tinnitus sound can disappear for days as if it was switched off, only to come back with a vengeance after a stressful day or a sleepless night. Thus, the top-down model advocated here is more in line with the type of mood disorder that causes anhedonia or dysthymia, fundamentally different from an attention-related mechanism.

Other models of tinnitus have emphasized the effects of learning [1], where the tinnitus sound generated in the afferent branch is amplified and made chronic by salience networks [65] including the hippocampus. While learning effects cannot be excluded, these models ignore the crucial role of vmPFC and the striatum, or interpret them differently. Salience keeps the maladaptive learning going, whereas a broken gating system lacks the habituation (perhaps via the thalamic reticular nucleus (TRN) (Fig. 19.4)) to the tinnitus sound.

Bottom-up and top-down models may not have to be mutually exclusive [66]. The auditory-limbic circuit may form a closed-loop system, where sensory amplification in the afferent branch, which is generated by lesion-induced plasticity (see part 1), produces a limbic response ("reaction"). In a person with an uncompromised system, this reaction will be attenuated and controlled by habituation-like mechanisms [25, 26]. In tinnitus patients, where the "noise cancellation system" is less effective, however, the tinnitus signal remains in force. In order to develop treatments and come closer to a cure from this devastating disorder, empirically tested approaches from cognitive behavioral or mindfulness therapy [67–70] should be measured in relation to neurobiological knowledge about their effects on brain anatomy. This convergence would ultimately permit a more systematic way of drug therapy or treatment through stimulation

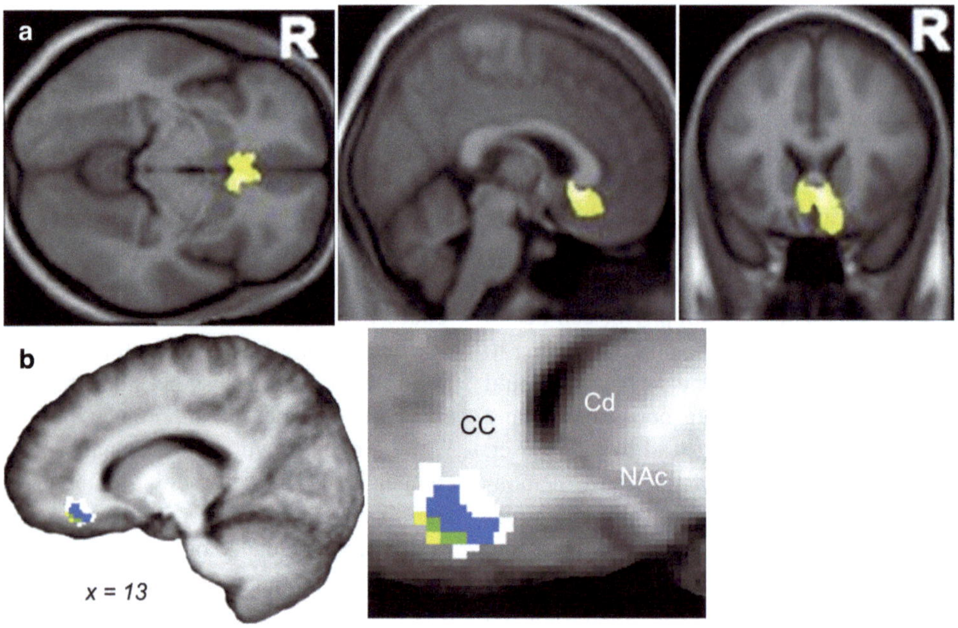

Fig. 19.4 Functional changes in the limbic system. Hyperactivity in tinnitus patients was found in the ventral striatum (VS) near the nucleus accumbens (NAc) [21]. (**a**) Voxels exhibiting significant (p(corr) < 0.05) between-group differences in fMRI signal are shown on group averaged anatomical images. Inset in (**a**) shows a close-up of the coronal image, emphasizing the position of the cluster in the VS. Mean fMRI signal for each subject is plotted for tinnitus patients (red circles) and stimulus-matched control participants (gray diamonds) in (**b**). Asterisk denotes statistical significance at the single-voxel level demonstrated in (**a**). This functional difference in NAc was not related to participant age or mean hearing loss. *Cd* caudate, *Pu* putamen, *Hy* hypothalamus. Reproduced from Leaver et al. [21], with permission

or neuromodulation. Finally, building on that, animal models of cognitive aspects of tinnitus are sorely missing and deserve greater attention [71].

Acknowledgments I would like to dedicate this review chapter to my colleagues and coauthors on the original papers that this chapter is based upon, especially Amber Leaver, Anna Seydell-Greenwald, and Mark Mühlau, and many others without whose help the present results would not have been possible. I also thank the funders, including NIDCD, ATA, TRC, TRI, and the Skirball Foundation.

References

1. Jastreboff PJ. Phantom auditory perception (tinnitus): mechanisms of generation and perception. Neurosci Res. 1990;8:221–54.
2. Griffiths TD. Musical hallucinosis in acquired deafness phenomenology and brain substrate. Brain. 2000;123:2065–76.
3. Tonndorf J. The analogy between tin & us and pain: a suggestion for a physiological basis of chronic tinnitus. Hear Res. 1987;28:271–5.
4. Møller A. Similarities between chronic pain and tinnitus. Am J Otolaryngol. 1997;18:577–85.
5. Leaver AM, Seydell-Greenwald A, Turesky TK, Morgan S, Kim HJ, Rauschecker JP. Cortico-limbic morphology separates tinnitus from tinnitus distress. Front Syst Neurosci. 2012;6:1–14.
6. Elgoyhen AB, Langguth B, De Ridder D, Vanneste S. Tinnitus: perspectives from human neuroimaging. Nat Rev Neurosci. 2015;16:632–42.
7. Kojima T, Kanzaki S, Oishi N, Ogawa K. Clinical characteristics of patients with tinnitus evaluated with the tinnitus sample case history questionnaire in Japan: a case series. PLoS One. 2017;12:1–11.
8. Rauschecker JP, Scott SK. Maps and streams in the auditory cortex: nonhuman primates illuminate human speech processing. Nat Neurosci. 2009;12:718–24.
9. DeWitt I, Rauschecker JP. Phoneme and word recognition in the auditory ventral stream. Proc Natl Acad Sci U S A. 2012;109:E505–14.
10. Rauschecker JP. Auditory cortical plasticity: a comparison with other sensory systems. Trends Neurosci. 1999;22:74–80.
11. Merzenich MM, Kaas JH. Reorganization of mammalian somatosensory cortex following peripheral nerve injury. Trends Neurosci. 1982;5:434–6.
12. Pons TP, Garraghty PE, Ommaya AK, Kaas JH, Taub ET, Mishkin M. Massive cortical reorganization after sensory deafferentation in adult macaques. Science. 1991;252:1857–60.
13. Calford M, Tweedale R. Acute changes in cutaneous receptive fields in primary somatosensory cortex after digit denervation in adult flying fox. J Neurophysiol. 1991;65:178–87.
14. Ramachandran VS, Rogers-Ramachandran D, Stewart M. Perceptual correlates of massive cortical reorganization. Science. 1992;258:1159–60.
15. Ramachandran VS, Rogers-Ramachandran D, Cobb S. Touching the phantom limb. Nature. 1995;377:489–90.
16. Rajan R, Irvine D. Neuronal responses across cortical field A1 in plasticity induced by peripheral auditory organ damage. Audiol Neurotol. 1998;3:123–44.
17. Recanzone GH, Merzenich MM, Schreiner CE. Changes in the distributed temporal response properties of SI cortical neurons reflect improvements in performance on a temporally based tactile discrimination task. J Neurophysiol. 1992;67:1071–91.
18. Recanzone GH, Merzenich MM, Schreiner CE. Plasticity in the frequency representation of primary auditory cortex follow-

ing discrimination training in adult owl monkeys. J Neurosci. 1993;13:87–103.
19. Arnold W, Bartenstein P, Oestreicher E, Römer W, Schwaiger M. Focal metabolic activation in the predominant left auditory cortex in patients suffering from tinnitus: a PET study with [18F]Deoxyglucose. ORL J Otorhinolaryngol Relat Spec. 1996;58:195–9.
20. Langers DRM, de Kleine E, van Dijk P. Tinnitus does not require macroscopic tonotopic map reorganization. Front Syst Neurosci. 2012;6:1–15.
21. Leaver AM, Renier L, Chevillet MA, Morgan S, Kim HJ, Rauschecker JP. Dysregulation of limbic and auditory networks in tinnitus. Neuron. 2011;69:33–43.
22. Schneider P, Andermann M, Wengenroth M, Goebel R, Flor H, Rupp A, et al. Reduced volume of Heschl's gyrus in tinnitus. NeuroImage. 2009;45:927–39.
23. Ashburner J, Friston KJ. Voxel-based morphometry - the methods. NeuroImage. 2000;11:805–21.
24. Mühlau M, Rauschecker JP, Oestreicher E, Gaser C, Röttinger M, Wohlschläger A, et al. Structural brain changes in tinnitus. Cereb Cortex. 2006;16:1283–8.
25. Rauschecker JP, Leaver A, Mühlau M. Tuning out the noise: limbic-auditory interactions in tinnitus. Neuron. 2010;66:819–26.
26. Rauschecker JP, May ES, Maudoux A, Ploner M. Frontostriatal gating of tinnitus and chronic pain. Trends Cogn Sci. 2015;19:567–78.
27. Landgrebe M, Langguth B, Rosengarth K, Braun S, Koch A, Kleinjung T, et al. Structural brain changes in tinnitus: grey matter decrease in auditory and non-auditory brain areas. NeuroImage. 2009;46:213–8.
28. Meyer M, Neff P, Liem F, Kleinjung T, Weidt S, Langguth B, et al. Differential tinnitus-related neuroplastic alterations of cortical thickness and surface area. Hear Res. 2016;342:1–12.
29. Blood AJ, Zatorre RJ, Bermudez P, Evans AC. Emotional responses to pleasant and unpleasant music correlate with activity in paralimbic brain regions. Nat Neurosci. 1999;2:382–7.
30. Drevets WC, Price JL, Simpson JR Jr, Todd RD, Reich T, Vannier M, et al. Subgenual prefrontal cortex abnormalities in mood disorders. Nature. 1997;386:824–7.
31. Price JL, Drevets WC. Neurocircuitry of mood disorders. Neuropsychopharmacology. 2010;35:192–216.
32. Mayberg HS, Lozano AM, Voon V, McNeely HE, Seminowicz D, Hamani C, et al. Deep brain stimulation for treatment-resistant depression. Neuron. 2005;45:651–60.
33. Scangos KW, Khambhati AN, Daly PM, Makhoul GS, Sugrue LP, Zamanian H, et al. Closed-loop neuromodulation in an individual with treatment-resistant depression. Nat Med. 2021;27:1696–700.
34. Bhatt J, Bhattacharyya N, Lin H. Relationships between tinnitus and the prevalence of anxiety and depression. Laryngoscope. 2017;127:466–9.
35. Cheung SW, Larson PS. Tinnitus modulation by deep brain stimulation in locus of caudate neurons (area LC). Neuroscience. 2010;169:1768–78.
36. Crippa A, Lanting CP, van Dijk P, Roerdink JBT. A diffusion tensor imaging study on the auditory system and tinnitus. Open Neuroimaging J. 2010;4:16–25.
37. Seydell-Greenwald A, Raven EP, Leaver AM, Turesky TK, Rauschecker JP. Diffusion imaging of auditory and auditory-limbic connectivity in tinnitus: preliminary evidence and methodological challenges. Neural Plast. 2014;2014:145943.
38. Hullfish J, Abenes I, Bin YH, De Ridder D, Vanneste S. Frontostriatal network dysfunction as a domain-general mechanism underlying phantom perception. Hum Brain Mapp. 2019;40:2241–51.
39. Adjamian P, Hall D, Palmer A, Allan T, Langers D. Neuroanatomical abnormalities in chronic tinnitus in the human brain. Neurosci BioRev. 2014;45:119–33.
40. Aldhafeeri FM, MacKenzie I, Kay T, Alghamdi J, Sluming V. Neuroanatomical correlates of tinnitus revealed by cortical thickness analysis and diffusion tensor imaging. Neuroradiology. 2012;54:883–92.
41. Leaver AM, Seydell-Greenwald A, Rauschecker JP. Auditory-limbic interactions in chronic tinnitus: challenges for neuroimaging research. Hear Res. 2016;334:49–57.
42. Leaver AM, Turesky TK, Seydell-Greenwald A, Morgan S, Kim HJ, Rauschecker JP. Intrinsic network activity in tinnitus investigated using functional MRI. Hum Brain Mapp. 2016;37:2717–35.
43. Dobie RA. Depression and tinnitus. Otolaryngol Clin N Am. 2003;36:383–8.
44. Simpson JJ, Davies WE. A review of evidence in support of a role for 5-HT in the perception of tinnitus. Hear Res. 2000;145:1–7.
45. Folmer R, Griest S, Martin W. Chronic tinnitus as phantom auditory pain. Otolaryngol Neck Surg. 2001;124:394–400.
46. Sousa N, Almeida OFX. Disconnection and reconnection: the morphological basis of (mal)adaptation to stress. Trends Neurosci. 2012;35:742–51.
47. Charney DS. Psychobiological mechanisms of resilience and vulnerability: implications for successful adaptation to extreme stress. Am J Psychiatry. 2004;161:195–216.
48. Wallhäusser-Franke E, Schredl M, Delb W. Tinnitus and insomnia: is hyperarousal the common denominator? Sleep Med Rev. 2013;17:65–74.
49. Hébert S, Fullum S, Carrier J. Polysomnographic and quantitative electroencephalographic correlates of subjective sleep complaints in chronic tinnitus. J Sleep Res. 2011;20:38–44.
50. Simoens VL, Hébert S. Cortisol suppression and hearing thresholds in tinnitus after low-dose dexamethasone challenge. BMC Ear Nose Throat Disord. 2012;12:4.
51. Crönlein T, Langguth B, Geisler P, Hajak G. Tinnitus and insomnia. Prog Brain Res. 2007;166:227–33.
52. Asplund R. Sleepiness and sleep in elderly persons with tinnitus. Arch Gerontol Geriatr. 2003;37:139–45.
53. Tyler R, Coelho C, Tao P, Ji H, Noble W, Gehringer A, et al. Identifying tinnitus subgroups with cluster analysis. Am J Audiol. 2008;17:176–84.
54. Meikle M, Henry J, Griest S, Stewart B, Abrams H, McArdle R, et al. The tinnitus functional index: development of a new clinical measure for chronic, intrusive tinnitus. Ear Hear. 2012; 33:153–76.
55. Tepper JM, Koós T, Wilson CJ. GABAergic microcircuits in the neostriatum. Trends Neurosci. 2004;27:662–9.
56. Yim C, Mogenson G. Response of ventral pallidal neurons to amygdala stimulation and its modulation by dopamine projections to nucleus accumbens. J Neurophysiol. 1983;50:148–61.
57. Azmitia EC, Segal M. An autoradiographic analysis of the differential ascending projections of the dorsal and median raphe nuclei in the rat. J Comp Neurol. 1978;179:641–67.
58. Quirk GJ, Beer JS. Prefrontal involvement in the regulation of emotion: convergence of rat and human studies. Curr Opin Neurobiol. 2006;16:723–7.
59. Crick F. Function of the thalamic reticular complex: the searchlight hypothesis. Proc Natl Acad Sci U S A. 1984;81:4586–90.
60. Halassa MM, Chen Z, Wimmer RD, Brunetti PM, Zhao S, Zikopoulos B, et al. State-dependent architecture of thalamic reticular subnetworks. Cell. 2014;158:808–21.
61. Yu XJ, Xu XX, He S, He J. Change detection by thalamic reticular neurons. Nat Neurosci. 2009;12:1165–70.Shepherd GMG. Corticostriatal connectivity and its role in disease. Nat Rev Neurosci. 2013;14:278–91.
62. Saunders A, Oldenburg IA, Berezovskii VK, Johnson CA, Kingery ND, Elliott HL, et al. A direct GABAergic output from the basal ganglia to frontal cortex. Nature. 2015;521:85–9.

63. Eggermont JJ, Roberts LE. The neuroscience of tinnitus. Trends Neurosci. 2004;27:676–82.
64. De Ridder D, Elgoyhen AB, Romo R, Langguth B. Phantom percepts: tinnitus and pain as persisting aversive memory networks. Proc Natl Acad Sci U S A. 2011;108:8075–80.
65. De Ridder D, Vanneste S. The Bayesian brain in imbalance: medial, lateral and descending pathways in tinnitus and pain: a perspective. Prog Brain Res. 2021;262:309–34.
66. Gans JJ, O'Sullivan P, Bircheff V. Mindfulness based tinnitus stress reduction pilot study: a symptom perception-shift program. Mindfulness. 2014;5:322–33.
67. Martinez-Devesa P, Perera R, Theodoulou M, Waddell A. Cognitive behavioural therapy for tinnitus. Cochrane Database Syst Rev. 2010;9:CD005233.
68. Baguley DM. Mechanisms of tinnitus. Br Med Bull. 2002;63:195–212.
69. McKenna L, Marks EM, Vogt F. Mindfulness-based cognitive therapy for chronic tinnitus: evaluation of benefits in a large sample of patients attending a tinnitus clinic. Ear Hear. 2018;39:359–66.
70. Shore SE, Wu C. Mechanisms of noise-induced tinnitus: insights from cellular studies. Neuron. 2019;103:8–20.

The Neurophysiological Model of Tinnitus and Decreased Sound Tolerance

20

Pawel J. Jastreboff

Abstract

This chapter presents an outline of the neurophysiological model of tinnitus and decreased sound tolerance (hyperacusis and misophonia). The main postulates of the model are as follows: (1) Tinnitus is a phantom auditory perception, i.e., perception of tinnitus is not linked to any vibratory activity within the cochlea; (2) the model distinguishes tinnitus as an experience from bothersome (clinically significant) tinnitus because separate mechanisms are involved in the perception of tinnitus and in evoked by it negative reactions; (3) the auditory system is secondary for clinically significant tinnitus and for misophonia; (4) the spreading of tinnitus signal to other systems in the brain (particularly to the limbic and autonomic nervous systems) is responsible for negative reactions evoked by tinnitus; and (5) the subconscious connections, governed by the principles of conditioned reflexes, play a dominant role. It is postulated that hyperacusis results from an increased gain within the subconscious part of the auditory pathways and is determined solely by physical characteristics of sound. Misophonia results from enhanced subconscious functional connections between the auditory and limbic and autonomic nervous systems, with reactions occurring to a particular, for a given patient, patterns of sound—the sound energy being secondary or irrelevant. The neurophysiological model of tinnitus is a basis for habituation-based treatment (tinnitus retraining therapy).

P. J. Jastreboff (✉)
Department Otolaryngology, School of Medicine, Emory University, Atlanta, GA, USA

JHDF, Inc., Ellicott City, MD, USA

W. Schlee et al. (eds.), *Textbook of Tinnitus*, https://doi.org/10.1007/978-3-031-35647-6_20

Graphical Abstract

The Neurophysiological Model of Tinnitus & Misophonia

Conscious path of activation of the Limbic and Autonomic nervous systems

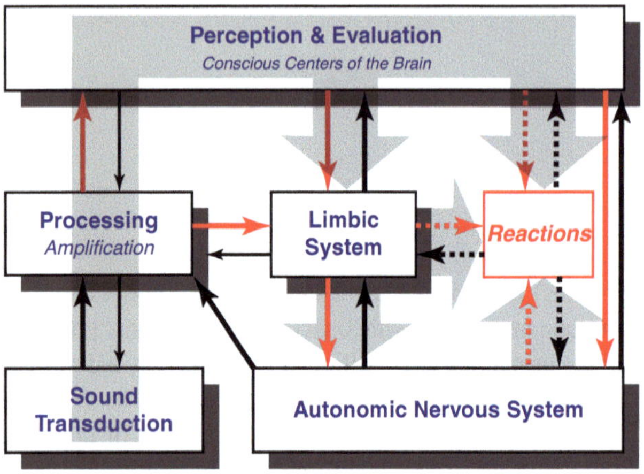

Conscious path is significant at the initial stage of tinnitus and misophonia

Subconscious path of activation of the Limbic and Autonomic nervous systems

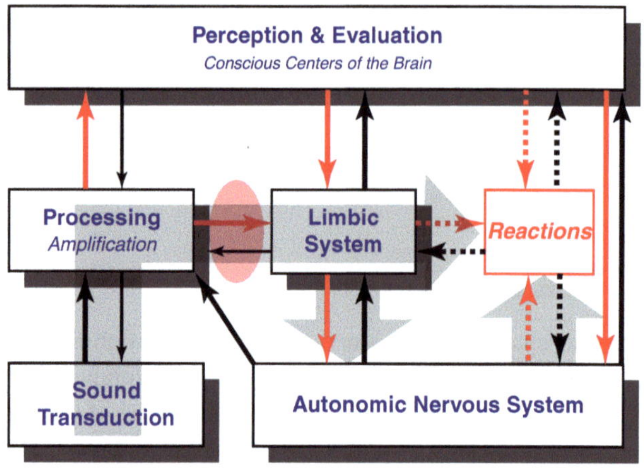

Subconscious connections (in red oval), between the auditory and limbic and autonomic nervous systems, governed by conditioned reflexes, play a dominant role in presence of negative reactions in chronic tinnitus and misophonia

Abbreviations

DST Decreased Sound Tolerance
LDL Loudness Discomfort Level
TRT Tinnitus Retraining Therapy

Highlights

- Tinnitus is a phantom auditory perception; i.e., perception of tinnitus is not linked to any vibratory activity within the cochlea.
- It is crucial to differentiate and separate tinnitus as experience versus tinnitus evoking negative physiological and behavioral reactions (clinically significant tinnitus, i.e., tinnitus that bothers people, affects their life, to the extent that they frequently seek professional help and become patients).
- The auditory system, while needed for perception of tinnitus, is secondary for clinically relevant tinnitus.
- The functional strength of connections between the auditory system and various centers in the brain plays a crucial role in clinically relevant tinnitus with the dominant role of subconscious connections.
- Connections within the neural networks, which are involved in the adverse effects of tinnitus, are governed by the principles of conditioned reflexes.
- The limbic and autonomic nervous systems are the main systems responsible for negative tinnitus-evoked reactions.
- Tinnitus is frequently accompanied by a decreased sound tolerance, consisting of hyperacusis and misophonia.
  - Hyperacusis results from an increased gain within the auditory pathways and is determined solely by physical characteristics of sound (i.e., its intensity and spectrum).
  - Misophonia results from enhanced functional connections between the auditory and the limbic and autonomic nervous systems, and reactions occur to specific patterns of sound, with the total spectral energy being secondary or irrelevant.
  - In misophonia, the meaning of sound and an individual's past history of encountering is crucial, with the auditory characteristics of the sound playing a secondary role.

- There are two loops in network processing tinnitus signal and activity evoked by bothersome sounds:
  - The high loop, which involves cognitive processing of the signal, and which is dominant at the initial stages of tinnitus or misophonia.
  - The low, subconscious loop, governed by principles of conditioned reflexes, and appears to be dominant in chronic tinnitus or misophonia.
- The neurophysiological model of tinnitus is a basis for habituation-based treatment, aimed at modification of neuronal connections involved in clinically significant tinnitus reversing a patient into a person experiencing tinnitus.
- Tinnitus retraining therapy is a specific implementation of habituation-oriented treatment with the use of counseling (to reclassify tinnitus to a category of neutral stimuli) and sound therapy (to decrease the strength of tinnitus signal within the brain).

History and the Outline of the Neurophysiological Model of Tinnitus

Knowing the history of how and when the neurophysiological model of tinnitus was developed is helpful for a better understanding of the principles of the model. The model was created in about 1984, when the consensus was that tinnitus results exclusively from dysfunction of the inner ear, and perhaps the auditory nerve, without other parts of the brain involved. There was no distinction made between people who experienced tinnitus without having a problem because of this and people who suffered from it while discussing potential mechanisms of tinnitus. No attempts were made to study mechanisms involved in creating negative reactions evoked by tinnitus.

During this time, an animal model of tinnitus was not yet proposed, and only clinical results were available. These results were conflicting, and the dominant treatments used were medications and masking. The focus was entirely on tinnitus perception, with the belief that psychoacoustic characterization of tinnitus is crucial, and tinnitus loudness has to decrease to achieve successful treatment outcome, with consensus that total removal of tinnitus perception should be the goal of treatment. The role of the sound used was to suppress tinnitus perception.

Clinical data contradicted the common belief of psychoacoustical parameters of tinnitus as crucial factor in determining tinnitus severity and a treatment outcome. There was no difference in psychoacoustic description of tinnitus (its loudness, pitch match, and tinnitus maskability) in population of subjects who experienced tinnitus vs. patients who suffered because of it [1, 2].

Perception and Detection of a Signal: Terminological Note

In psychology, the term "perception" covers a situation when a stimulus is detected but a subject is not necessarily aware of its presence. This concept has been proposed for tinnitus as well [3, 4].

In tinnitus field, the dominant understanding of the term "perception" is when the subject detects and is aware of the presence of tinnitus or external sound. The term "detection" denotes a subconscious process with the nervous system separating a signal from spontaneous neural activity, and activity evoked by other sensory stimuli, and may occur without corresponding perception. Perception necessitates detection of a signal. The definition of detection and perception, as described above, will be used in this chapter.

Definition of Tinnitus

During the 1980s, the most common tinnitus definitions used were "ringing in the ears" [5] or "conscious experience of sound that originates in the head of its owner" [6]. In this, and many other subsequent definitions of tinnitus, it was assumed to be the same as a physical, external sound and it was automatically assumed that interaction of tinnitus with external sounds follows the rules of interaction of two external sounds.

The neurophysiological model of tinnitus introduced a different view on tinnitus, starting from the definition of tinnitus as a phantom auditory perception, i.e., perception of sound without corresponding vibratory and mechanical activity in the cochlea [7, 8]. The perception is absolutely real and can be viewed similarly as phantom pain and the phantom limb phenomena. It was postulated that there is a tinnitus signal in the form of neural activity in the brain that is perceived as a sound, and it is labeled tinnitus. Consequent to this approach, the term "objective tinnitus" is considered to be somatosound and excluded from tinnitus, while auditory imagery (auditory hallucinations) is classified as a tinnitus, which originates in the high level of the auditory system.

Realizing the phantom aspect of tinnitus is fundamental for understanding the interaction of tinnitus with external sounds, and as such, it is essential for predicting usefulness of different forms of sound therapies. As mentioned above, during the 1980s, the suppression of tinnitus perception by external sound was used predominantly and it was known as "tinnitus masking." Unfortunately, the basis for this approach arose from misunderstanding of the mechanisms of interaction of an external sound and tinnitus, while considering tinnitus as physical sound and not phantom perception [9].

> Tinnitus is a phantom auditory perception, i.e., perception of sound without corresponding vibratory, mechanical activity in the cochlea

Experimental Support for Postulate that Tinnitus Is a Phantom Auditory Perception

Masking represents interaction of two traveling waves at the basilar membrane of the cochlea. Therefore, it exhibits a "V-shaped" masking curve and follows the phenomenon of the critical band (i.e., it is impossible to mask one sound by a second if there is larger than critical band frequency difference between the two sounds). None of these phenomena exists in connection with tinnitus, which can be equally easily suppressed by sounds from wide range of frequencies, and there is no critical band observed in case of suppressing tinnitus perception [10] (see Fig. 20.1). Furthermore, it is sometimes easier to suppress tinnitus by contralateral stimulation which further supports the postulate that "masking" of tinnitus is in reality neuronal suppression occurring in the auditory pathways at the level above the auditory nerve.

The Neurophysiological Model of Tinnitus and Generator of Tinnitus Signal

Specific mechanisms responsible for the emergence of tinnitus-related neuronal activity are irrelevant to the model. It is crucial, however, to distinguish between mechanisms involved in the generation of tinnitus perception and mechanisms involved in tinnitus-evoked negative reactions [11, 12]. As long as tinnitus-related neuronal activity is constrained within the auditory system, people experience a sound sensation, but they are not bothered by it, and the presence of tinnitus will not induce negative behavioral and physiological responses. Tinnitus evokes negative reactions and is bothersome in only about 20% of people with tinnitus [3]. The psychoacoustic characteristics of tinnitus in these two subpopulations are indistinguishable and are not related to the severity of the tinnitus. Moreover, treatment outcome does not depend on the psychoacoustic of tinnitus [13].

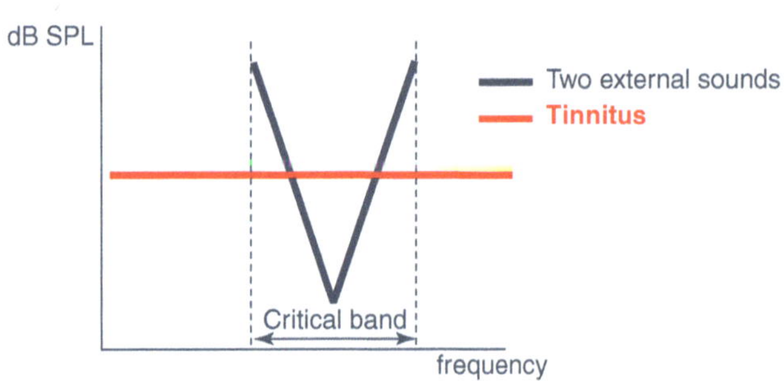

Fig. 20.1 Experiment showing that tinnitus is a phantom auditory perception and not physical sound. Vertical axis: external sound level needed to suppress perception of another external sound (black, V-curve) or tinnitus (pink, flat line). Lack of V-shaped curve and of critical band in the case of tinnitus proves that there is no vibratory activity in the cochlea corresponding to tinnitus perception. Therefore, tinnitus is a phantom auditory perception

> - Specific mechanisms responsible for the emergence of tinnitus-related neuronal activity is irrelevant to the model.

The Role of Auditory System in Tinnitus

These observations prove that the auditory system plays only a secondary role in the case of bothersome, clinically significant tinnitus, that there are different mechanisms involved in the generation of the neural signal that causes tinnitus perception, and that there are other mechanisms responsible for evoking negative reactions to this signal. Recognition of this difference is important. It offers the possibility of rectifying tinnitus-induced negative reactions without modifying or removing tinnitus perception, by using treatments aimed at the mechanism of tinnitus-induced negative reactions.

In the past, dominant treatments aimed at removing, or at least decreasing, tinnitus perception, especially its loudness. These approaches were not particularly successful. Notably, a decrease in tinnitus perception does not automatically translate into a decrease in tinnitus severity, and actually, there is no relation between tinnitus loudness match and the perceived severity of the tinnitus [14, 15].

> - It is crucial to distinguish between mechanisms involved in the generation of tinnitus perception and mechanisms involved in tinnitus-evoked negative reactions.

The Main Postulate of the Neurophysiological Model of Bothersome Tinnitus

All these observations lead to the conclusion, which underlies the neurophysiological model of tinnitus, that **in clinically significant tinnitus (i.e., tinnitus that bothers people, affects their life, to the extent that they frequently seek professional**

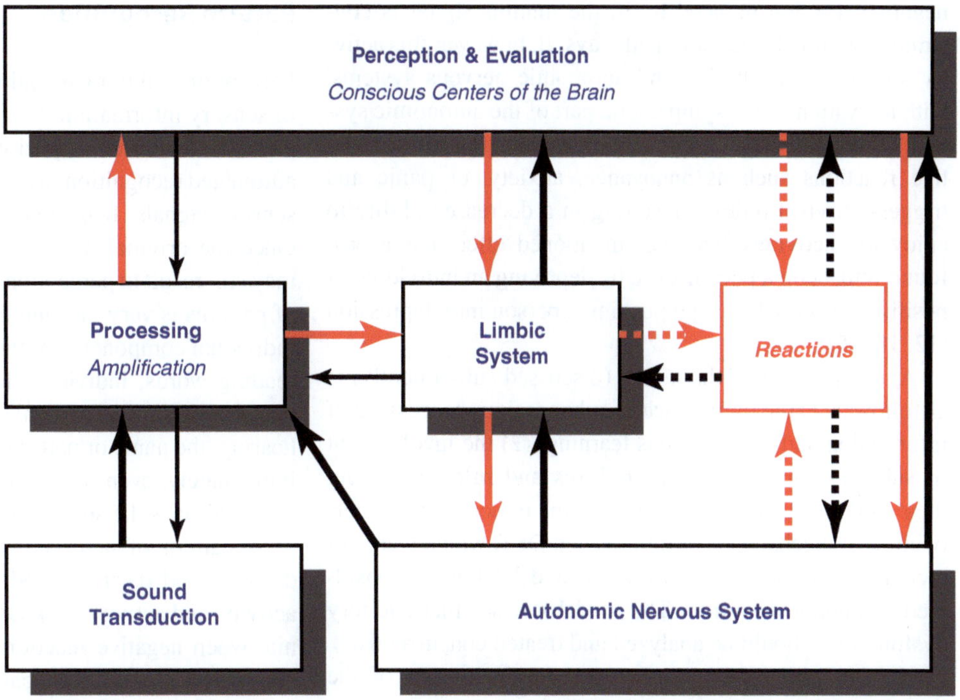

Fig. 20.2 Block diagram outlining the neurophysiological model of tinnitus

help and become patients), the auditory system plays a secondary role and other systems in the brain are dominant.

The neurophysiological model of tinnitus postulates that many systems in the brain are involved in tinnitus and other auditory disorders which evoke negative reactions and are bothersome. Since tinnitus-related neuronal activity (i.e., tinnitus signal) is perceived as sound, obviously the auditory system has to be involved in tinnitus perception, but it plays a secondary role in clinically significant problems.

> In clinically-significant tinnitus (i.e., tinnitus that bothers people, affects their life, to the extent that they frequently seek professional help and become patients), the auditory system plays a secondary role and other systems in the brain are dominant.

System that Needs to be Included in Mechanisms of Clinically Significant Tinnitus

The analysis of the negative reactions evoked by tinnitus provides information about which other systems in the brain are involved and are crucial in bothersome tinnitus and in decreased sound tolerance (DST) (defined as a condition when sounds tolerated by the average person are bothersome to a subject). These reactions (e.g., annoyance, anxiety, panic, disturbance of concentration, sleep, and decreased ability to enjoy life activities) clearly indicate that the limbic and autonomic nervous systems have to be included and they are playing a significant role. It is postulated that the negative reactions evoked by tinnitus are a consequence of sustained activation of the limbic and autonomic nervous systems (particularly of the sympathetic part of the autonomic nervous system). The auditory system, while needed for perception of tinnitus, plays a secondary role in clinically relevant tinnitus. In the past, most studies and treatments of tinnitus were predominantly cochleocentric and focused on the periphery of the auditory system. The neurophysiological model of tinnitus shifts the attention away not only from the cochlea, but also from the auditory nervous system toward other systems in the brain. The main focus of the model is presented in the form of a diagram, which was first published in the end of the 1990s [16] (see Fig. 20.2).

> The negative reactions evoked by tinnitus are a consequence of sustained activation of the limbic and autonomic nervous systems (particularly of the sympathetic part of the autonomic nervous system).

According to the model, the tinnitus signal—the generation of which is typically linked to the periphery of the auditory system (see explanation of the discordant dysfunction theory in accompanying Chapter on TRT [17])—is detected and processed by subconscious centers of the auditory pathways and finally perceived at the highest level of the auditory system. If a person just perceives tinnitus without having a negative reaction induced by it, the tinnitus signal is constrained within the auditory pathways. If, however, this activity spreads to the limbic and autonomic nervous systems, with activation of the sympathetic part of the autonomic system being particularly important, it evokes a number of negative reactions such as annoyance, anxiety, or panic and triggers survival reflexes resulting in a decreased ability to enjoy life activities. This last mentioned effect has a profound impact on a person's life by depriving an individual of positive aspects of life and pushing a person into depression [12, 18–25].

Another aspect of the model (discussed subsequently) is as follows: (1) the importance of subconscious processing of information and subconscious learning, (2) the involvement of subconscious conditioned reflexes and rules governing their creation and extinction, and (3) the importance of intertwining of mechanisms of tinnitus and DST, which were not recognized in the past, and tinnitus and DST were considered as unrelated entities. The model stresses that auditory dysfunctions should be analyzed and treated concurrently.

Notably, the model stresses the dominant role of the strength of functional connections between the brain structures involved and consequently aiming a treatment at modification of these connections. The individual structures may work perfectly within the norms, but emergence of abnormal functional connections between different brain structures results in tinnitus or external sounds becoming bothersome.

Important aspect of the model

1. Importance of subconscious processing of information and subconscious learning.
2. Involvement of subconscious conditioned reflexes and rules governing their creation and extinction.
3. Importance of intertwining of mechanisms of tinnitus and DST.
4. Strength of functional connections between the brain structures involved plays the dominant role; consequently, treatment aims at modification of these connections.
5. Normality of functional properties of the involved brain center is secondary.

In-Depth Presentation of the Neurophysiological Model of Tinnitus

The presentation of the neurophysiological model of tinnitus will be facilitated by a brief review of the relevant neurophysiological principles used in the model.

Pattern Recognition

Perception is the organization, identification, and awareness of sensory information. It is governed by pattern recognition principle. Pattern recognition in physiology is defined as the automated recognition of patterns and regularities in received sensory signals. It involves previous learning and memory. Once the original pattern is learned, an incomplete signal may still result in perception of the learned pattern. Detection of patterns is very fast and does not require identification of individual components of the whole pattern. For example, in reading words, individual letters are not separately identified, but a word is recognized and detected as a pattern. In hearing, the name or pattern of native language is recognized immediately, even in the presence of noise or hearing loss, which distorts the spectrum of the sound [12].

A pattern of neuronal activity perceived as tinnitus is detected and discriminated from background, spontaneous activity, and activity evoked by external sounds. In misophonia, when negative reactions are evoked by sounds, which are specific for a given patient (labeled "misophonic triggers"), these are immediately recognized without need for thinking or analyzing sound. The pattern may include, for example, a category of sounds made during eating, and the sound of eating of a new person will evoke an automatic reaction.

Pattern recognition in physiology is defined as the automated recognition of patterns and regularities in received sensory signals. It involves previous learning and memory.

The Role of Subconscious Brain Vs. Conscious Parts of the Brain

Functioning of the brain can be divided into two: conscious and subconscious. For the purpose of this chapter, it is not important to assign specific anatomical structures involved in conscious and subconscious functions. It is crucial, however, to recognize functional differences between these two systems and that these two systems are, to a large extent, independent from each other. The conscious brain is involved in perception (as defined in this chapter), cognition, attention, verbalization, thinking, and planning. It has a limitation of not being able to handle more than one task requiring full attention (e.g., it is impossible to read a book and write a letter at the same time, listening with understanding two people talking simultaneously).

Subconscious brain does not have this limitation and simultaneously performs many tasks. It provides homeostasis for functioning of the brain and all of the body (via autonomic nervous system). It is involved in emotions, learning, memory recall, detection, and further processing of sensory signals. It has its own judgment and ranking system to determine the relative importance of incoming information, which is independent of the judgment of conscious brain. It is a "gatekeeper," deciding which sensory stimuli we are aware about, to which we are responding, and which are blocked at subconscious level. As such, it controls habituation of reactions and of perception [20].

Reaction to a stimulus can be evoked by conscious, cognitive thinking or can be carried on by subconscious, conditioned reflexes. In the second scenario, the reaction occurs much faster and without necessity of awareness and analyzing the stimulus.

There are crucial differences between conscious and subconscious part of the brain which are, to a large extent, independent from each other.

1. Conscious brain has a limitation of not being able to handle more than one task requiring full attention.
2. Subconscious brain can simultaneously perform many tasks.
3. Subconscious brain is a "gatekeeper," deciding which sensory stimuli we are aware about, to which we are responding, and which are blocked at subconscious level. Consequently, it controls habituation of reactions and of perception.

Habituation

Habituation of reactions and habituation of perception are a necessity to survive due to the fact that we can perform only one task requiring our full attention at the time. Considering that we are immersed in many sensory signals, and we need to consciously think and make decisions, this limitation necessitates that the majority of signals that do not require reactions have to be blocked from being perceived. This process cannot be achieved by conscious effort (it would contradict the goal of this action) and has to be done independently from the conscious brain, at a subconscious level which necessitates that the subconscious brain must have a system of judging the importance of incoming stimuli.

Habituation of reactions and habituation of perception is a necessity to survive due to the fact that we can perform only one task requiring our full attention at the time while we are immersed in many sensory signals which need to be handled.

Assigning the Level of Importance to a Stimulus

The subconscious brain continuously makes decisions ranking all stimuli present at the moment and the tasks requiring action and creates a hierarchy of importance on a continuous scale. Then, the few most important stimuli [5–7] are attended by the conscious brain with fast switching from one stimulus to the other, creating an impression of doing a number of tasks simultaneously. The remaining stimuli are habituated, i.e., there is no awareness of their presence and there are no reactions to them. If stimulus is judged by the subconscious brain as important and requiring action, there is no habituation of reaction, and we may be aware of its presence. Note that the stimuli may evoke reactions without their perception. Depending on the situation, the same signal may be at the top of importance or may be considered not important depending on the presence of other stimuli (e.g., perception of tinnitus when there is no important task to be done vs. a situation when a person is significantly engaged in challenging work). Learning and past experiences play a crucial role in developing and modifying the ranking.

The main role of the subconscious brain is keeping the functionality of the brain and body and keeping us safe. It preserves the homeostasis of biochemical and physiological pathways in our body. Therefore, all signals that are indicating potential danger or negativity, which may happen, are getting high priority and are not habituated. The judgments performed at conscious and subconscious levels can be dramatically different. The same stimulus can be recognized and consciously judged as benign, e.g., perception of tinnitus similar to the perception of innocent external sounds and perception of misophonic triggers where the majority of misophonic patients realize that the sound of triggers is benign. Nevertheless, these benign sounds can evoke strong negative reactions if they are judged by the subconscious brain to be linked with something negative. While behavioral reactions to these sounds can be controlled, the emotional and autonomic reactions are outside the control of the conscious brain.

The subconscious brain continuously makes decisions ranking all stimuli present at the moment and the tasks requiring action, and creates a hierarchy of importance on a continuous scale and decides which are habituated.

Brain Systems Involved in Tinnitus

Since tinnitus-related neuronal activity is perceived as a sound, obviously the auditory system has to be involved in tinnitus perception. Analysis of the negative effects of tinnitus on individuals provides information about systems in the brain involved in this process that cannot be ignored. It is possible to distinguish between two main categories of negative effects: (1) physiological responses to tinnitus (e.g., anxiety, depression, sleep problems, and increased stress level) and (2) behavioral responses and consequences (e.g., attention and concentration problems, decreased ability to enjoy life activities, and affected life activities resulting in poor social interactions, work impairment, or family problems). These observations indicate that two major systems in the brain are involved in generating the negative effects of tinnitus, namely the limbic and autonomic nervous systems. There are other systems involved as well, such as the prefrontal cortex, thalamus, reticular formation, and cerebellum [20, 26–29]. While these other brain systems may be involved, by utilizing the Ockham Razor principle ("Plurality should not be posited without necessity," i.e., this principle gives precedence to simplicity—of two competing theories, the simpler explanation of an entity is to be preferred). Therefore, for presentation of the basis of the model of tinnitus, it is sufficient to consider the involvement of these two main systems. It has been proposed that it is actually necessary to include these systems in the analysis of the generation of tinnitus and in peoples' reaction to the tinnitus and its treatment [12].

> Analysis of the complaints of tinnitus patients reveals that two major systems in the brain are involved in generating the negative effects of tinnitus, namely the limbic and autonomic nervous systems.

The Limbic System

There is discussion regarding the definition of the limbic system and which structures should be included in it, but there is general agreement that the limbic system deals with emotions, emotional behavior, motivations, learning, and memory. It regulates autonomic or endocrine function in response to emotional stimuli and also is involved in reinforcing behavior [30, 31]. The main structures considered to be part of the limbic system are as follows: amygdala (which is related to a number of emotional processes); hypothalamus (which is considered to be a center for the limbic system and is connected with the frontal lobes, septal nuclei, the brain stem, reticular formation, the hippocampus, and with the thalamus. It regulates many autonomic processes); hippocampus (consolidation of new memories); septal nuclei (considered a pleasure zone); and anterior nuclei of thalamus (involved in memory processing).

Of particular importance is the observation that the limbic system handles behaviors needed for survival: feeding, reproduction, and "fight-or-flight" responses. Operation of the limbic system includes influencing the endocrine system and the autonomic nervous system. It interacts strongly with the prefrontal cortex.

Autonomic Nervous System

The autonomic nervous system is a part of the peripheral nervous system, which controls and regulates bodily functions, such as the heart rate, digestion, respiratory rate, pupillary response, urination, and sexual arousal. It acts at the unconscious level and is regulated by reflexes through the brainstem to the spinal cord and organs. The hypothalamus acts as an integrator for autonomic functions, receiving autonomic regulatory input from the limbic system.

The autonomic nervous system consists of three parts: the sympathetic nervous system, the parasympathetic nervous system, and the enteric nervous system (which is involved in gastrointestinal functions). The sympathetic nervous system is often labeled as responsible for the fight-or-flight, and it reacts fast and is considered as having excitatory action. The parasympathetic nervous system is often considered the "rest and digest" or "feed and breed" system, and it is slower and has a dampening effect. As such, the sympathetic and parasympathetic systems generally have opposite actions (except for sexual arousal and orgasm). Their synchronized action provides homeostasis of body functions.

Symptoms of an overactive sympathetic nervous system are anxiety, panic attacks, nervousness, insomnia, breathlessness, palpitations, inability to relax, poor digestion, fear, and high blood pressure. If the sympathetic nervous system is overstimulated for longer period of time, then a number of problems are observed, e.g., anxiety, shallow breathing, increased heart rate, poor sleep quality, restlessness, night sweats, decreased libido, fatigue, nervousness, increased agitation/irritability, increased muscle tension, increased inflammation, increased susceptibility to infections (i.e., frequent illness), indigestion, and constipation [12]. It is postulated that the overactivation of the sympathetic part of the autonomic nervous system, by tinnitus signal or neural activity evoked by misophonic triggers, is a factor responsible for problems linked to tinnitus or to misophonia [12, 32, 33].

Both limbic and autonomic nervous systems are involved in stress and are activated in a stressful situation. Typically, tinnitus is getting louder and more bothersome when the level of stress increases. One of the consequences of "strain-to-hear" observed in people with hearing loss is the increase in the stress level and consequently tinnitus. Furthermore, reactions evoked by bothersome sounds are enhanced by stress. Note that stress works as a modulator, enhancing the negative reaction caused by tinnitus or DST, and is not responsible for their occurrence.

Incorporating Presented Above Principles of the Neuroscience Into the Neurophysiological Model of Tinnitus

As pointed out previously, the basic concept of the neurophysiological model of tinnitus is that for clinically significant tinnitus it is necessary to include a variety of systems in the brain and their functional interactions in addition to the auditory system, in study of, and in treatment of tinnitus [7, 12]. There are, however, other important specific postulates of the model, which are presented as follows.

Two Loops

It is important to analyze pathways involved in tinnitus-related activation of these systems. Firstly, continuous activation of connections illustrated in Fig. 20.2 results in their strengthening and consequently causes stronger activation of the limbic and autonomic nervous systems by the same tinnitus signal, according to the general rules of neural plasticity.

The term neural plasticity was first proposed by Konorski in 1948 [34, 35]. It is crucial for learning memory, and it is a basic brain function. One of the potential mechanisms of neural plasticity was proposed by Hebb in 1949 and is known as Hebbian theory, which postulates that an increase in synaptic efficacy between neurons (weight of synaptic connection) is caused when a presynaptic cell repeatedly stimulates a postsynaptic cell [36]. Currently, this theory is generalized to postulate that if a connection is frequently activated, it becomes stronger; if it is not activated, it gradually becomes weaker, which explains associative learning and creation and extinction of conditioned reflexes [37].

> Neural plasticity, first proposed by Konorski in 1948 is crucial for learning, memory and it is a basic brain function.

Secondly, the limbic and autonomic nervous systems are interconnected, and connections with other systems in the brain involve reciprocal connections (feedback). Consequently, the increase in activity causes an increase in activity of the system from which the initial signal was coming. For example, autonomic nervous system activation via a backward feedback can increase the activity in the limbic system, in cognitive brain areas, and in the auditory system. Therefore, the term "loop" is used to emphasize the feedback aspects of the interaction between the different systems.

The tinnitus signal activates the limbic and autonomic nervous systems via two loops (see Fig. 20.3). The upper one ("high loop" labeled the "high route" by LeDoux [38]) involves conscious areas of the cerebral cortex, perception, evaluation, verbalization, and conscious associations. It induces negative emotions and autonomic reactions as well. This loop is crucial at the initial stage of developing clinically significant tinnitus. The second, lower one ("low loop," labeled the "low route" by LeDoux [38]), involves subcon-

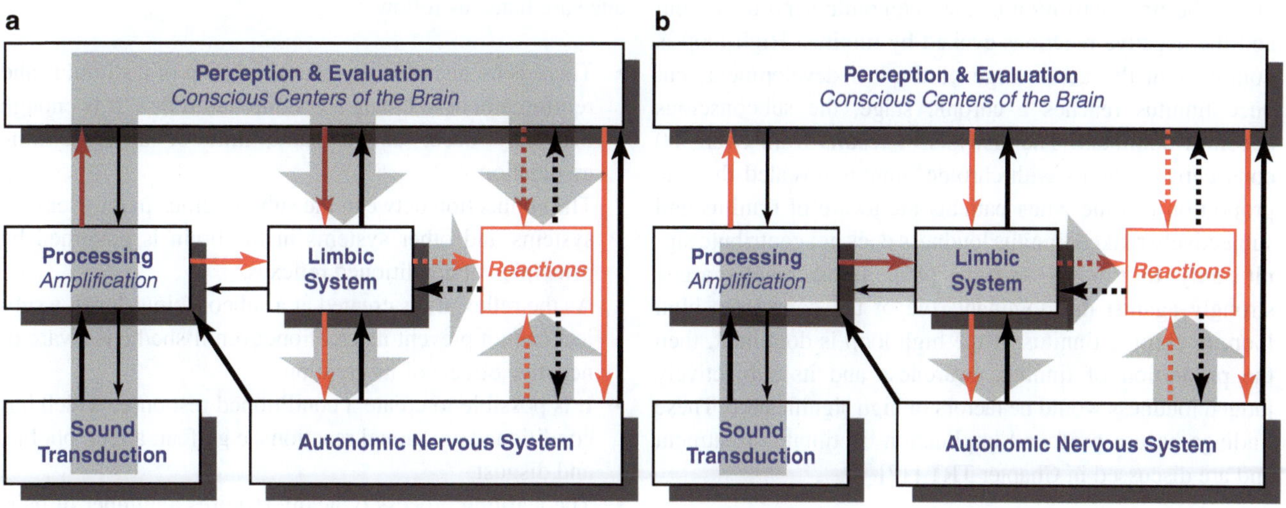

Fig. 20.3 Two loops involved in evoking negative reactions by tinnitus or by DST. (**a**) High loop, involving cognition, evaluation, and awareness; (**b**) low, subconscious loop. Red arrows show flow of the neuronal activity from the auditory system, and black arrows represent feedback connections between systems. High loop is important at the initial stage of tinnitus or DST, while low loop is dominant in chronic stage. Note that these loops are identical for tinnitus and for misophonia with the difference in tinnitus signal being generated internally within the auditory pathways in tinnitus, while in the case of misophonia, the neuronal activity is evoked by external sounds (misophonic triggers)

scious centers in the brain. It branches from the auditory system at the level of extralemniscal subnuclei of the medial geniculate body, reaches the lateral nucleus of amygdala, and, via other parts of the limbic system, reaches centers of the autonomic nervous system [12, 39–41]. Documented anatomical connections link the amygdala with the inferior colliculus, and therefore, both connections (from auditory system to limbic system and back) are included in the diagram [42–44]. The connection transferring tinnitus signal, or activity evoked by bothersome sound, from the medial geniculate body to the amygdala would be responsible for modifying the emotional state of a subject by tinnitus (or external sound, e.g., misophonic trigger), even when a person is not aware of its presence. On the other hand, the connection from the amygdala to the inferior colliculi [12, 44] modifies the processing of tinnitus signal (or activity evoked by misophonic trigger), depending on the emotional state of a person.

> The tinnitus signal activates the limbic and autonomic nervous systems via two loops. The upper "high loop" involves conscious areas of the cerebral cortex, perception, evaluation, verbalization, and conscious associations and it is crucial at the initial stage of developing clinically-significant tinnitus. The second, "low loop" involves subconscious centers in the brain and is crucial in chronic tinnitus and in misophonia.

It has been postulated that tinnitus as a problem results mainly from overactivation of the sympathetic part of the autonomic system [12, 24]. Both high and low loops contribute to the final activation of the autonomic nervous system and the negative reactions evoked by tinnitus. High loop is dominant in the acute stage of tinnitus development, but once tinnitus reaches a chronic stage, the subconscious becomes dominant. The analysis of results from over 300 consecutive patients with chronic tinnitus revealed that the proportion of time when patients are aware of tinnitus and subjectively ranked tinnitus loudness does not contribute significantly to tinnitus severity [45]. These results argue strongly against the dominant role of the conscious, high loop, in chronic tinnitus. If the high loop is dominant, then the proportion of tinnitus awareness and its subjectively judged loudness would be factors of high significance. These findings have a profound implication on tinnitus treatment and are discussed in Chapter TRT [17].

The Role of Conditioned Reflexes

The connections between the brain systems involved in the processing of the tinnitus signal are governed by principles of conditioned reflexes. The tinnitus signal in the auditory pathways (or neuronal activity evoked by misophonic trigger) acts as a conditioning stimulus, which, via one or more subconscious reflex arcs, activates the limbic and autonomic nervous systems and thereby evokes a variety of negative reactions.

> The connections between the brain systems involved in the processing of the tinnitus signal are governed by principles of conditioned reflexes which have a specific set of rules.

Principles of Conditioned Reflexes

The term classical conditioning describes a learning procedure during which a neutral sensory stimulus (conditioned stimulus, e.g., a sound) is paired with biologically significant positive or negative stimulus (unconditioned stimulus, e.g., food and electrical shock). Unconditioned stimulus alone evokes an unconditioned response, which is an unlearned, reflex response. Due to neuronal plasticity, a "reflex arc" is created, causing that conditioned stimulus, without unconditioned stimulus, evokes unconditioned response.

Classical conditioning was first studied and described by Ivan Pavlov, and "Pavlov's dog" becomes proverbial—ringing a bell, associated several times with giving of food, resulted in a situation wherein the sound of the bell alone was sufficient to evoke salivation. Classical conditioning has been intensively studied and described, and only selected, crucial features of rules governing conditioned reflexes relevant to mechanisms of tinnitus and decreased sound tolerance are listed as follows:

- There is no need for any causal relation of a stimulus and reinforcement to create a conditioned reflex. It is enough that they occur at the same time or in close time association.
- The connection between the subconscious part of sensory systems and other systems in the brain is governed by principles of conditioned reflexes.
- As the reflex arc is created at a subconscious level, a subject cannot prevent its creation, even if she/he is aware of negative effects of its creation.
- It is possible to create a conditioned response, which has conditioned emotional reactions, e.g., fear, anger, phobia, and disgust.
- The learning process typically requires a number of pairings of sensory stimulus with reinforcement, but a reflex can be established even as a result of one pairing of a stimulus and reinforcement.
- It is not necessary that every presentation of a conditioned stimulus is paired with an unconditioned stimulus; it is

sufficient that only some presentations are paired, but it is required that if an unconditioned stimulus is present, it occurs in close time association with a conditioned stimulus.

- Typically, the length of training has an inverse relation to the strength of reinforcement; i.e., reflex with stronger (particularly negative) reinforcement requires less time to be established.
- Usually, the conditioned response is similar to the unconditioned response, but sometimes different.
- All reflexes resulting from classical conditioning can be extinguished (abolished) when the conditioned stimulus is presented repeatedly without the unconditioned stimulus (labeled as "passive extinction" or habituation of reaction).
- It is possible to extinguish a previously created reflex by a pairing conditioned stimulus with an unconditioned stimulus of the opposite type of reinforcement; e.g., if the original unconditioned stimulus used for training was negative (e.g., electrical shock), then for extinguishing trained response, the conditioned stimulus is now paired with positive reinforcement (e.g., food) (the procedure labeled as "active extinction").
- Once the reflex is established, the anticipation of occurrence of the conditioned stimulus is sufficient to evoke unconditioned response.
- Once the reflex is established to a given conditioned stimulus, the unconditioned response will occur to other stimuli, similar to a conditioned stimulus (Principle of Stimulus Generalization).
- Fear generalization is a specific type of generalization, which occurs when a person associates fears learned in the past through classical conditioning to similar situations, events, people, and objects in the present. Fear generalization is important for survival, as humans and animals need to be able to assess potentially dangerous situations and respond appropriately and fast based on generalizations made from past experiences.
- Fear generalization may become maladaptive (described then as overgeneralization of fear), and it is connected to many anxiety disorders. It can also lead to the development of posttraumatic stress disorder.
- Brain regions involved in fear generalization include the amygdala and the hippocampus.
- The amygdala is fundamental in developing a classically conditioned fear response to either a stimulus or the context in which it is found.
- Reflexes based on negative reinforcement are more difficult to extinguish.
- It is easier and faster to create a conditioned reflex to a novel conditioned stimulus (latent inhibition).
- Reactions occurring as a result of subconscious conditioned reflexes are faster than if the conscious brain is involved.
- The strength of reaction evoked by a conditioned stimulus depends mainly on the strength of reinforcement (unconditioned stimulus); the physical characteristics and the strength of conditioned stimulus are secondary.
- The conscious brain cannot control emotional and autonomic reactions resulting from actions of subconscious conditioned reflexes.
- Strength of functional connections between the centers in the brain controlled by conditioned reflexes is the dominant factor; the functional properties of centers are secondary, and these centers may work within the norm.

All these features of conditioned reflexes are incorporated and used in the neurophysiological model of tinnitus. They are playing a crucial role in the model and in the explanation of specifics of tinnitus and misophonia.

Several different scenarios may create conditioned reflexes linking neuronal activity within the auditory system with enhancement activity in the limbic and autonomic nervous systems. One common situation is "negative counseling"; i.e., a person is told something which links tinnitus with a threatening, unpleasant, or dangerous situation such as "nothing can be done, you will have tinnitus up to the end of your life, you need to learn to cope with it, and we need to do a brain scan to eliminate the possibility of a brain tumor." The negative counseling provides a negative reinforcement, which creates a conditioned reflex arc, causing the tinnitus signal to subsequently evoke strong reactions of the limbic and sympathetic autonomic nervous systems. This causes physiological and behavioral reactions such as anxiety, tension, annoyance, fear, and decreased ability of enjoying life activities. The last effect has a tendency of pushing people to depression, and indeed, depression and anxiety are observed routinely in patients with tinnitus and/or decreased sound tolerance. Notably, many patients state that they have not experienced depression or anxiety before getting significant tinnitus or decreased sound tolerance. Other patients distinguish a new part of depression or anxiety evoked by their hearing problem.

Another common scenario occurs when a person with tinnitus is under strong emotionally negative stress, such as during retirement, divorce, or from non-related to tinnitus or decreased sound tolerance health problems. Indeed, a study ranking ordered factors present when a person's tinnitus became a clinical problem revealed that in the top 20 most frequent situations linked to emergence of clinically significant tinnitus, the auditory-related factors were ranked number 4 and 9 (8% and 6%, respectively) out of 100 studied cases [46]. On the top were retirement/work problems (18%), domestic problems (10%), and negative counseling (9%). While noise exposure is regarded as a frequent cause of the appearance of tinnitus perception, it is not the case for the emergence of tinnitus as a problem. Non-bothersome tinnitus may be present for years, and only when it becomes associated with something negative, it becomes a problem.

It should be stressed that no causal link is necessary for the creation of a conditioned reflex of any kind, and a close temporal association of a conditioning signal and reinforcement is sufficient to create the reflex. For example, retirement, which is listed as a number one triggering situation, may be explained by a combination of existence of stress related to cessation of regular work, decreased number of other tasks that need to be taken care of, potential increase in tinnitus level due to decreased environmental sound levels related to spending more time at home, more time to explore potential health problems, and a high probability of receiving negative counseling from a contacted professional.

The neurophysiological model described above predicts that a sudden appearance of tinnitus perception combined with a high level of the emotional stress is particularly effective in evoking clinically significant tinnitus. Indeed, bothersome tinnitus is typically observed in cases of sudden hearing loss since tinnitus starts rapidly at a very specific time and a person is in the state of highly negative emotions due to concerns and fears evoked by sudden hearing loss. Similarly, clinically significant tinnitus can be expected to be more prevalent in professions where there is a combination of a high level of noise, particularly impulsive noise (e.g., gunfire), with a high level of negative emotional stress. Policeman, firefighters, and soldiers are typical examples of members of such professions.

This prediction has been confirmed by the fact that tinnitus occurs in a high rate (49%) of soldiers returning from Iraq and Afghanistan who were exposed to blast noise, the occurrence of which is even higher than the reported proportion of soldiers with blast-induced hearing loss (25%). As of September 2020, over 2 million veterans are receiving disability because of tinnitus, nearly twice as many as receiving disability because of hearing loss [47, 48].

Once the reflex is established, a negative reaction can be evoked without the presence of negative reinforcement, which means that while general health may improve and work problems may be resolved, a person's tinnitus will keep evoking negative reactions—a situation commonly observed in clinical practice. A potential explanation for this observation is that as tinnitus-evoked negative reaction acts as the reinforcement to created reflex arc, these reactions continue to enhance the strength of this conditioned reflex. This self-enhancing aspect of tinnitus explains the very low rate of spontaneous recovery, since the perception of clinically significant tinnitus is constantly present, it evokes constant negative reactions; therefore, the passive extinction of this reflex will not occur, and the reflex may actually become even stronger.

- Importantly, no causal link is necessary for the creation of a conditioned reflex, and a close temporal association of a conditioning signal and reinforcement is sufficient to create the reflex. Consequently, appearance of tinnitus perception combined with a high-level of the emotional stress is sufficient in evoking clinically-significant tinnitus.
- As tinnitus-evoked negative reaction acts as the reinforcement to created reflex arc, this results in self-enhancing aspect of tinnitus which explains the very low rate of spontaneous recovery - the clinically-significant tinnitus is constantly present, it evokes constant negative reactions; therefore, the passive extinction of classical conditioning of this reflex does not occur.

Proposed Mechanisms of Clinically Significant Tinnitus and Decreased Sound Tolerance Based on the Neurophysiological Model of Tinnitus

Tinnitus, hyperacusis, misophonia, and tensor tympani syndrome involve auditory and other systems in the brain. These disorders have intertwined mechanisms with all the main systems in common. Clinical practice showed their frequent comorbidity and necessity to treat them concurrently to achieve positive results. For example, if misophonia coexists with tinnitus and if it is not treated, then the probability of a successful outcome of tinnitus treatment is significantly decreased. The neurophysiological model of tinnitus provides a frame of reference to analyze all these disorders and to propose mechanism-based treatments.

Discussed auditory disorders have intertwined mechanisms with all the main systems in common.

Tinnitus

Tinnitus is defined as a phantom auditory perception, namely perception of sound without corresponding vibratory and mechanical activity in the cochlea [7, 8, 12]. Tinnitus signal (i.e., the neuronal activity perceived as tinnitus) originates in the auditory system, and in subjects who only experience tinnitus, it is restricted to the auditory system. Typically, it seems to originate in the auditory periphery, but it may result from central processes triggered by a decreased neural signal from the auditory periphery, as what happens in case of the cochlea or auditory nerve being destroyed or damaged. Decreased auditory input can create or enhance tinnitus as well. The observation that the majority of people who are, for even few minutes, in low-level sound environment start to experience tinnitus [49, 50] can be explained by postulating that a decreased auditory input triggers enhancement of the gain within the auditory pathways, resulting in the perception of the spontaneous neuronal activity constantly present in the auditory system. This postulate has been supported by results from electrophysiological finding from animal experiments [51, 52]. Notably, this central "automatic gain control" mechanism yields enhancement of preexisting tinnitus when the environmental sound level is low, or when a sound transmission to the inner ear is impaired by, e.g., otosclerosis or subject using ear protection.

Another central mechanism involves reverberation, the internal replaying patterns of sound stored in memory. It has been proposed that it is the basis for auditory imagery (auditory hallucinations) and can exist without any psychiatric problems [53–64] and has been linked to hearing loss [65].

Therefore, auditory imagery/musical hallucination should be considered a central type of tinnitus. There is a need to separate this phenomenon from auditory verbal hallucinations in schizophrenia, where people clearly perceive and understand a voice commanding them to do something.

A variety of mechanisms may contribute to perceived tinnitus, and there is no restriction on its complexity. For example, discordant dysfunction theory [7, 12, 17] postulates that local discordance dysfunction of outer and inner hair cells at a given portion of the basilar membrane of the cochlea provides micro-sources of tinnitus signal and allows for creating perception of sound of unlimited complexity.

It has been postulated that the increase in spontaneous activity within the auditory pathways is the tinnitus signal [66, 67]. Measurements of neuronal activity of single neurons in animals with sound-induced tinnitus and hearing loss strongly suggested that epileptic-like, bursting activity is correlated with the extent of behavioral manifestation of tinnitus, while increase in spontaneous activity was related to hearing loss [68, 69].

- Observation that majority of people who are in low level sound environment start to experience tinnitus, can be explained by postulating that a decreased auditory input triggers enhancement of the gain within the auditory pathways, resulting in the perception of the spontaneous neuronal activity. Neurophysiological model proposes that neuronal activity measurements are constantly present in the auditory system. This central "automatic gain control" mechanism yields enhancement of pre-existing tinnitus when the environmental sound level is low, or when a sound transmission to the inner ear is impaired by e.g., otosclerosis or subject using ear protection.
- One of central mechanisms of brain function involves reverberation and replaying patterns of sound stored in memory. It has been proposed that it is the basis for auditory imagery (auditory hallucinations) is considered a central type of tinnitus. There is a need to separate this phenomenon from auditory verbal hallucinations in schizophrenia, where people clearly perceive a voice commanding them to do something. The study of people with auditory imagery showed that they did not have any psychological or psychiatric disorders.
- Measurements of neuronal activity of single neurons in animals with sound-induced tinnitus and hearing loss strongly suggested that epileptic-like, bursting activity is correlated with the extent of behavioral manifestation. Neurophysiological model proposes that bursting neuronal activity relates to tinnitus, while increase of spontaneous activity was related to hearing loss.

Hyperacusis

It has been proposed that the neural mechanisms of hyperacusis involve abnormally high amplification within the auditory system, with only secondary activation of other centers of the brain responsible for negative reactions (i.e., the limbic and autonomic nervous systems) [12, 33] (see Fig. 20.4a). In other words, the activity that is evoked in the auditory pathways by stimulation with, e.g., 80 dB HL sound in a person with hyperacusis would be similar to that occurring in an individual who does not have hyperacusis, and is exposed to a much louder sound, e.g., 120 dB HL. Studies in animals support a proposed mechanism [51, 52]; however, lack of an animal model of hyperacusis hinders researchers from performing more specific studies.

Abnormally high amplification within the auditory system, is proposed as the neural mechanisms of hyperacusis, with only secondary activation of other centers of the brain responsible for negative reactions

Misophonia

The mechanism of misophonia involves creation of a conditioned reflex linking specific for a given patient patterns of sound with a negative reinforcement [12, 33] (see Fig. 20.4b). The auditory system is perfectly normal in persons with pure misophonia; however, selective connections from the auditory

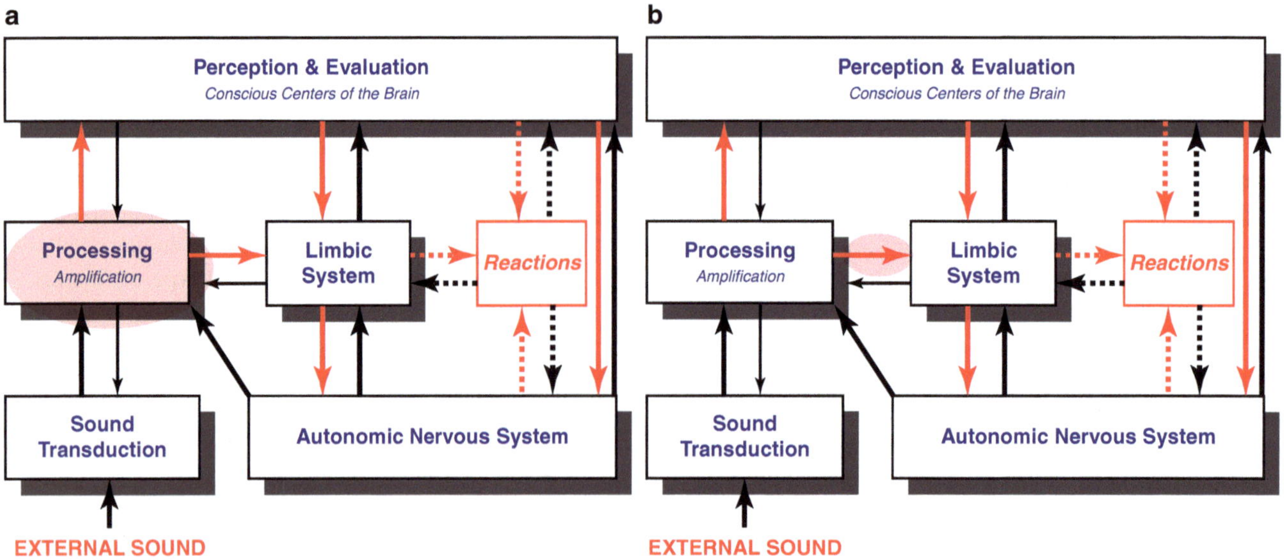

Fig. 20.4 Postulated mechanisms of hyperacusis (**a**) and misophonia (**b**). Red areas and connections point out crucial mechanisms acting in hyperacusis and in misophonia

system to the limbic and autonomic nervous systems for specific for a given patient patterns of sound are abnormally created or enhanced. Functional properties of these connections are governed by principles of conditioned reflexes. Consequently, the strength of the reactions they cause depends on the strength of the reinforcement, and the sound level plays a secondary role. These sounds are associated with an increased emotional negative status, which will be sufficient to create a conditioned reflex arc evoking misophonic reaction to these sounds. If tinnitus is present together with hyperacusis, bothersome sounds, by enhancing negative activation of the limbic and autonomic nervous systems, will enhance tinnitus, typically yielding increase in tinnitus loudness. Analogically, the presence of tinnitus will enhance reactions evoked by bothersome sounds.

Significant hyperacusis, even present for a short period of time, will automatically create misophonia, because exposure to the sound will create discomfort/pain and it will consequently provide the negative reinforcement associated with the sound. Once this reflex is created, it will persist, even when hyperacusis ceases to exist.

Notably, the reactions caused by presence of hyperacusis and of misophonia are the same, or very similar, in spite of their postulated different mechanisms, as the reactions reflect overactivation of the limbic and autonomic nervous systems evoked by external sounds. A common feature for hyperacusis and misophonia is that sound restricted in time is a trigger. In the case of tinnitus, physiological and behavioral reactions are the same but occur to a constantly present perception of sound. The neuronal networks involved in tinnitus and misophonia are identical—the difference is that in case of tinnitus, the neuronal signal perceived as tinnitus is generated within the auditory pathways, while in the case of misophonia, specific for a given patient sounds, which have been associated with negative status, evokes neuronal activity, which spreads from the auditory system to other systems in the brain. Note, that there is nothing particular or specific about the misophonic triggers themselves, and any sound can become a bothersome misophonic trigger. "Specific/particular" is directed to the relation of "a sound" to "a patient," i.e., that bothersome sounds are particular to a given patient.

This observation has ramifications on the approach to treatment of misophonia and its duration. Note, on the base of reactions only, it is impossible to differentiate tinnitus, hyperacusis and misophonia.

Importantly, because of fundamental differences in mechanisms of hyperacusis and misophonia, there is a dramatic difference in treatment approach and different treatments are needed for hyperacusis and for misophonia. These treatments and their justification are presented in Chapter on TRT [17].

- The mechanism of misophonia involves creation of a conditioned reflex linking specific, for a given patient, patterns of sound with a negative reinforcement
- Notably, the reactions caused by presence of hyperacusis and of misophonia are the same, or very similar, in spite of their postulated different mechanisms, as the reactions reflect overactivation of the limbic and autonomic nervous systems evoked by external sounds. Note, on the base of reactions only, it is impossible to differentiate tinnitus, hyperacusis and misophonia.
- The neuronal networks involved in tinnitus and misophonia are identical—the difference is that in case of tinnitus, the neuronal signal perceived as tinnitus is generated within the auditory pathways, while in the case of misophonia, misophonic triggers evoke neuronal activity which spreads from the auditory system to other systems in the brain.
- Importantly, because of fundamental differences in mechanisms of hyperacusis and misophonia, there is a dramatic difference in treatment approach and different treatments are needed for hyperacusis and for misophonia.

Tensor Tympani Syndrome

Tensor tympani syndrome describes an involuntary condition where the tensor tympani muscle in the middle ear spontaneously contracts, yielding a number of behavioral symptoms, e.g., fullness in the ear, pulsation, perception of abnormal hearing, feeling of vibration, dysacusis (various abnormal acoustic sensations, e.g., murmurs, clicks, tickling sensation, or may involve perception of distortions), tension headache, vertigo, dizziness, disequilibrium, and pain [70–74]. It frequently accompanies misophonia but may occur alone.

There are two muscles in the tympanic cavity: stapedius and tensor tympani. They are innervated by different cranial nerves and have different functions. The tensor tympani muscle is not a part of the acoustic reflex in humans. It is controlled by a neuronal network, which controls the Eustachian tube, and it is innervated by the trigeminal nerve. Contrary to the stapedius muscle (innervated by facial nerve), tensor tympani muscle is influenced by the higher level centers of the brain and by the autonomic nervous system and as such is affected by stress, anxiety, and panic. It is activated by sound as part of startle response, but it can contract spontaneously as well. Sounds perceived as unpleasant or dangerous are particularly strong activators, and consequently, tensor tympani syndrome is triggered by hyperacusis and misophonic reactions to sounds. Presence of tinnitus, by general increase in stress and anxiety, further enhances tensor tympani syndrome. Misophonia tends to facilitate the presence of the tensor tympani syndrome [33], which may become a significant, or even a dominant problem, particularly when pain is one of its syndromes.

Acoustic reflex in humans is based on the contraction of the stapedius muscle without contribution from the tensor tympani. The tensor tympani is part of a system cleaning the middle ear and contracts when the Eustachian tube opens and pulls the malleus medially, tensing the tympanic membrane and helping in pushing mucosa from the middle ear.

Sometimes, this syndrome is labeled as tonic tensor tympani syndrome (TTTS). It is misleading, as "tonic" describes constant contraction, which is maintained from several minutes up to hours at a time, while the contraction of tensor tympani can be fast and can change rapidly in time.

- The tensor tympani muscle is part of a system cleaning the middle ear, and contracts when the Eustachian tube opens. Tensor Tympani Syndrome describes an involuntary condition where the tensor tympani muscle contracts, yielding a number of behavioral symptoms, e.g., fullness in the ear, pulsation, perception of abnormal hearing, feeling of vibration, dysacusis, tension headache, vertigo, dizziness, disequilibrium, and pain. It frequently accompanies misophonia but may occur alone.
- Tensor tympani muscle is influenced by the higher level centers of the brain and by the autonomic nervous system, and as such is affected by stress, anxiety, panic. It is activated by sound as part of startle response, but it can contract spontaneously as well. Misophonia tends to facilitate the presence of the Tensor Tympani Syndrome, which may become a significant, or even a dominant problem, particularly when pain is one of its syndromes.

General Properties of Potential Treatments Based on the Neurophysiological Model of Tinnitus

The neurophysiological model of tinnitus proposes a general approach to tinnitus, which is not oriented toward elimination or even attenuation of tinnitus signal, but works outside of the source of this signal, aiming at disrupting the spread of neuronal activity to the part of the brain responsible for negative reactions evoked by tinnitus—habituation of tinnitus-evoked negative reactions [12, 24]. The model furthermore stresses the dominant role of the subconscious connections in chronic tinnitus, which are governed by the principles of

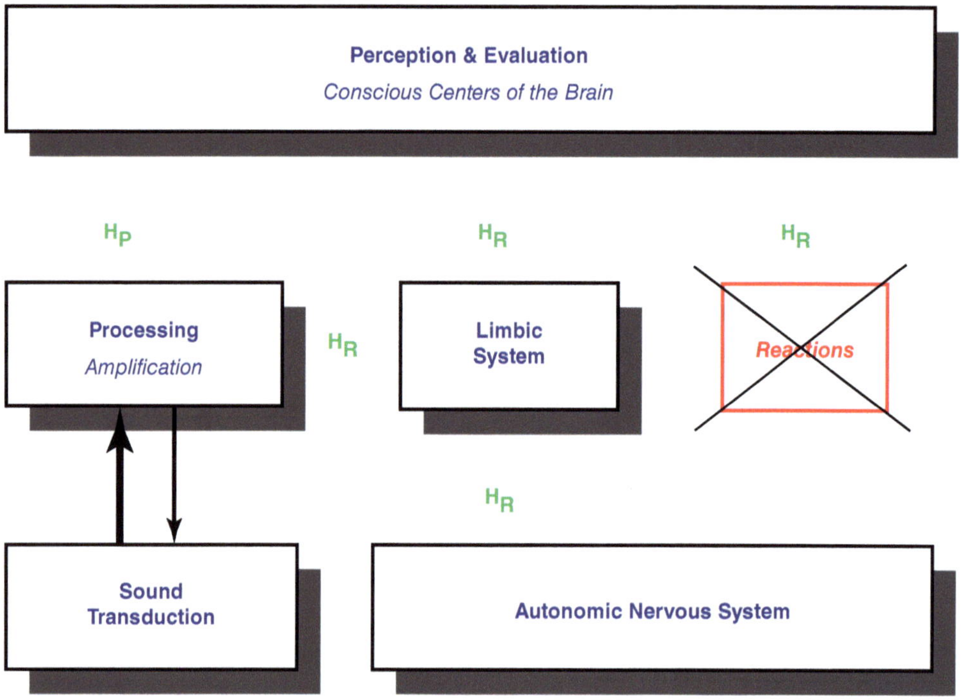

Fig. 20.5 The goals of habituation-based treatment. H_R habituation of reactions, H_P habituation of perception

conditioned reflexes, and generally the crucial role that the subconscious plays in tinnitus severity. The consciousness plays a significant role in acute tinnitus, but later on, while still contributing, ceases to be the dominant factor. Consequently, it is postulated that an effective treatment should involve retraining of subconscious conditioned reflexes linking the auditory system (the source of tinnitus signal) with other systems of the brain. The goal of habituation-based treatment is the habituation of reactions evoked by tinnitus or external sound (in case of DST) without attempting to change the tinnitus signal. Once habituation of reactions is even partially achieved, the habituation of perception occurs automatically without need for any additional procedures.

The neurophysiological model of tinnitus proposes a general approach to tinnitus, which is not oriented toward elimination or even attenuation of tinnitus signal, but works outside of the source of this signal, aiming at disrupting the spread of neuronal activity to the part of the brain responsible for negative reactions evoked by tinnitus—habituation of tinnitus-evoked negative reactions (see Fig. 20.5).

- The model stresses the dominant role of the subconscious connection in chronic tinnitus, governed by the principles of conditioned reflexes. The consciousness pathway plays a significant role in acute tinnitus, but later on, while still contributing, ceases to be the dominant factor.
- Consequently, an effective treatment should involve retraining of subconscious conditioned reflexes linking the auditory system (the source of tinnitus signal) with other systems of the brain.
- The goal of habituation-based treatment is the habituation of reactions evoked by tinnitus or external sound without attempting to change the tinnitus signal.
- Once habituation of reactions is even partially achieved, the habituation of perception occurs automatically without need for any additional procedures.
- Etiology of tinnitus is irrelevant and habituation-based methods are effective for any type of tinnitus, and even for somatosound.

One logical consequence of Habituation-based approaches is that the etiology of tinnitus is irrelevant, and these methods are effective for any type of tinnitus and even for somatosound. Habituation of reactions can be achieved by implementing a variety of approaches. One specific approach became known as tinnitus retraining therapy (TRT) and is described in chapter on TRT [17].

The main difference is that in the case of tinnitus, the neuronal activity is generated within the auditory system, while in the case of misophonia, the activity is evoked by external sounds. However, as it is possible to control external sounds, treatment of misophonia can be expanded to involve complex conditioning stimuli and active extinction of conditioned reflexes. In addition to modifying counseling to cover these differences, specific protocols of sound use are implemented.

According to the model, the treatment of hyperacusis needs to be substantially different. In the case of hyperacusis, an abnormal increase in the gain within the subconscious auditory pathways is responsible for this problem, and it is necessary to reverse this elevated gain to achieve successful treatment. Therefore, counseling is abbreviated accordingly, and sound therapy is focused on desensitization of subconscious auditory pathways of a sound by constant 24/7 exposure to sound.

Hyperacusis and misophonia frequently coexist, and then, it is necessary to treat both phenomena concurrently. According to a prediction from the model, and confirmed by practice, the treatment that is effective for hyperacusis is not providing help for misophonia, as it is not addressing the issue of modification of conditioned reflexes linking the auditory system with other systems in the brain, which is crucial in misophonia. On the other hand, treatment for misophonia has a limited efficiency for hyperacusis, where it is necessary to provide continuous, stimulation with neutral sound.

> The treatment which is effective for hyperacusis is not providing help for misophonia. On the other hand, treatment for misophonia has a limited efficiency for hyperacusis.

Summary and Conclusions

The neurophysiological model of tinnitus provides a frame of reference to understanding and treating a variety of disorders, which involve the subconscious part of the brain. Stress is placed at the significance of connections, particularly the subconscious, rather than the functioning of individual centers in the brain. The model points out that even if all centers are working within the norm, but the connections are improper, this may result in a disorder, e.g., tinnitus, misophonia, tensor tympani syndrome. The model can be applied to other health problems outside of the auditory modality.

The crucial part of the model is postulating the importance of the involvement of subconscious conditioned reflexes. Including the conditioned reflexes in mechanisms of tinnitus and misophonia explains why there are problems with tinnitus or misophonic triggers. It also explains why a person is unable to avoid creating tinnitus or misophonia if it is placed in a specific situation. Namely, when sensory stimulus is occurring concurrently with negative reinforcement (e.g., high emotional negative emotional stress, general health problem, and highly stressful situation), the reflex would be created automatically. Even when patients are fully aware of this process, they still cannot prevent it.

The process of habituation is controlled by the subconscious part of the brain, and therefore it is impossible, by definition, to block the development of these conditioned reflexes. Perception of tinnitus and of misophonic triggers cannot be blocked by conscious processes. Attempting to do so will yield the opposite result—even more attention is put on the signal and the signal becomes even more difficult to ignore.

The model points out the importance of the observation that the conscious and subconscious parts of the brain are working, to a large extent, independent from each other. The judgments done at cognitive level have no bearing on the decision made by the subconscious part of the brain.

Utilizing the principles outlined above allowed to propose an effective treatment, which follows the rules of creating and modifying the conditioned reflexes, which is described in separate chapter [17].

Specifically, treatment focuses on the modification of connections (without trying to change the functioning of the centers and systems involved), to achieve habituation of reactions evoked by a tinnitus or misophonic triggers. For example, in the case of tinnitus, there is no attempt to modify tinnitus signal. An exception is hyperacusis when the stress is on modifying abnormal gain in the subconscious auditory pathways while still recognizing contributions of connections between the auditory and other centers in the brain. Habituation of perception is a secondary goal, which is achieved automatically once habituation of reactions reaches a sufficient level.

References

1. Andersson G, Lyttkens L, Larsen HC. Distinguishing levels of tinnitus distress. Clin Otolaryngol Allied Sci. 1999;24(5):404–10.
2. Ward LM, Baumann M. Measuring tinnitus loudness using constrained psychophysical scaling. Am J Audiol. 2009;18(2):119–28.
3. De Ridder D, Schlee W, Vanneste S, Londero A, Weisz N, Kleinjung T, et al. Tinnitus and tinnitus disorder: theoretical and operational

definitions (an international multidisciplinary proposal). Prog Brain Res. 2021;260:1–25.
4. Dehaene S, Naccache L, Le Clec HG, Koechlin E, Mueller M, Dehaene-Lambertz G, et al. Imaging unconscious semantic priming. Nature. 1998;395(6702):597–600.
5. Hazell JWP. Tinnitus. Edinburgh: Churchill Livingstone; 1987.
6. McFadden D. Tinnitus: facts, theories, and treatments. Washington: National Academy Press; 1982.
7. Jastreboff PJ. Phantom auditory perception (tinnitus): mechanisms of generation and perception. Neurosci Res. 1990;8:221–54.
8. Jastreboff PJ. Tinnitus as a phantom perception: theories and clinical implications. In: Vernon J, Moller AR, editors. Mechanisms of tinnitus. Boston: Allyn & Bacon; 1995. p. 73–94.
9. Vernon J. Attemps to relieve tinnitus. J Am Audiol Soc. 1977;2:124–31.
10. Feldmann H. Homolateral and contralateral masking of tinnitus by noise-bands and by pure tones. Audiology. 1971;10:138–44.
11. Jastreboff PJ, Gray WC, Gold SL. Neurophysiological approach to tinnitus patients. Am J Otol. 1996;17:236–40.
12. Jastreboff PJ, Hazell JWP. Tinnitus retraining therapy: implementing the neurophysiological model. Cambridge: Cambridge University Press; 2004. p. 276.
13. Jastreboff PJ, Hazell JW, Graham RL. Neurophysiological model of tinnitus: dependence of the minimal masking level on treatment outcome. Hear Res. 1994;80(2):216–32.
14. Monzani D, Genovese E, Marrara A, Gherpelli C, Pingani L, Forghieri M, et al. Validity of the Italian adaptation of the tinnitus handicap inventory; focus on quality of life and psychological distress in tinnitus-sufferers. Acta Otorhinolaryngol Ital. 2008;28(3):126–34.
15. Andersson G. Tinnitus loudness matchings in relation to annoyance and grading of severity. Auris Nasus Larynx. 2003;30(2):129–33.
16. Jastreboff PJ. The neurophysiological model of tinnitus and hyperacusis. In: Hazell JWP, editor. Proceedings of the sixth international tinnitus seminar. Cambridge: THC; 1999. p. 32–8.
17. Jastreboff PJ, Jastreboff MM. Tinnitus retraining therapy. In: Moller A, editor. Textbook of tinnitus. 2nd ed. Cham: Springer; 2022.
18. Jastreboff PJ. Tinnitus retraining therapy. Prog Brain Res. 2007;166:415–23.
19. Jastreboff PJ, Jastreboff MM. Tinnitus retraining therapy: a different view on tinnitus. ORL J Otorhinolaryngol Relat Spec. 2006;68(1):23–9.
20. Jastreboff PJ. The neurophysiological model of tinnitus. In: Snow JB, editor. Tinnitus: theory and management. Hamilton: BC Decker; 2004. p. 96–106.
21. Jastreboff PJ. Tinnitus retraining therapy. In: Snow JB, editor. Tinnitus: theory and management. Hamilton: BC Decker; 2004. p. 295–309.
22. Jastreboff PJ, Jastreboff MM. Tinnitus retraining therapy for patients with tinnitus and decreased sound tolerance. Otolaryngol Clin N Am. 2003;36(2):321–36.
23. Jastreboff PJ, Jastreboff MM. The neurophysiological model of tinnitus and its practical implementation: current status. In: Myers EN, Bluestone CD, Brackman DE, Krause CJ, Tutchko MJ, editors. Advances in otolaryngology-head and neck surgery, vol. 15. St. Louis: Mosby; 2001. p. 135–47.
24. Jastreboff PJ. Tinnitus habituation therapy (THT) and tinnitus retraining therapy (TRT). In: Tyler R, editor. Tinnitus handbook. Singular, Thomson Learning: San Diego; 2000. p. 357–76.
25. Jastreboff PJ, Jastreboff MM. Tinnitus retraining therapy (TRT) as a method for treatment of tinnitus and hyperacusis patients. J Am Acad Audiol. 2000;11(3):156–61.
26. Bauer CA, Kurt W, Sybert LT, Brozoski TJ. The cerebellum as a novel tinnitus generator. Hear Res. 2013;295:130–9.
27. Mennink LM, van Dijk JMC, van Dijk P. The cerebellar (para)flocculus: a review on its auditory function and a possible role in tinnitus. Hear Res. 2020;398:108081.
28. Lanting CP. Neural activity underlying tinnitus generation: results from PET and fMRI. Hear Res. 2009;255(1-2):1–13.
29. Leaver AM, Seydell-Greenwald A, Turesky TK, Morgan S, Kim HJ, Rauschecker JP. Cortico-limbic morphology separates tinnitus from tinnitus distress. Front Syst Neurosci. 2012;6:21.
30. Torrico TJ, Abdijadid S. Neuroanatomy, limbic system. Treasure Island: StatPearls; 2021.
31. LeDoux JE. Emotion circuits in the brain. Annu Rev Neurosci. 2000;23:155–84.
32. Gibbons CH. Basics of autonomic nervous system function. Handb Clin Neurol. 2019;160:407–18.
33. Jastreboff P, Jastreboff M. Treatment for decreased sound tolerance (hyperacusis and misophonia). Semin Hear. 2014;35:105–20.
34. Konorski J. Conditioned reflexes and neuron organization. Cambridge: Cambridge University Press; 1948. p. 267.
35. Livingston RB. Brain mechanisms in conditioning and learning. Neurosci Res Program Bull. 1966;4(3):349–54.
36. Hebb DO. The organization of behavior; a neuropsychological theory. New York: Wiley; 1949. p. 335.
37. Konorski J. Integrative activity of the brain. Chicago: University of Chicago Press; 1967.
38. LeDoux JE. Brain mechanisms of emotion and emotional learning. Curr Opin Neurobiol. 1992;2(2):191–7.
39. Shinonaga Y, Takada M, Mizuno N. Direct projections from the non-laminated divisions of the medial geniculate nucleus to the temporal polar cortex and amygdala in the cat. J Comp Neurol. 1994;340:405–26.
40. LeDoux JE, Sakaguchi A, Iwata J, Reis DJ. Interruption of projections from the medial geniculate body to an archi-neostriatal field disrupts the classical conditioning of emotional responses to acoustic stimuli. Neuroscience. 1986;17(3):615–27.
41. Chen YC, Li X, Liu L, Wang J, Lu CQ, Yang M, et al. Tinnitus and hyperacusis involve hyperactivity and enhanced connectivity in auditory-limbic-arousal-cerebellar network. elife. 2015;4:e06576.
42. Woodson W, Farb CR, LeDoux JE. Afferents from the auditory thalamus synapse on inhibitory interneurons in the lateral nucleus of the amygdala. Synapse. 2000;38(2):124–37.
43. Farb CR, LeDoux JE. NMDA and AMPA receptors in the lateral nucleus of the amygdala are postsynaptic to auditory thalamic afferents. Synapse. 1997;27(2):106–21.
44. Marsh RA, Fuzessery ZM, Grose CD, Wenstrup JJ. Projection to the inferior colliculus from the basal nucleus of the amygdala. J Neurosci. 2002;22(23):10449–60.
45. Jastreboff PJ. The role of subconscious pathways in tinnitus and decreased sound tolerance. 9th International Tinnitus Seminar, Goeteborg, Sweden. 2008.
46. Hazell JWP, McKinney CJ. Support for a neurophysiological model of tinnitus. In: Vernon JA, Reich G, editors. Proceedings of the Fifth International Tinnitus Seminar. Portland: American Tinnitus Association; 1996. p. 51–7.
47. Carlson KF, Gilbert TA, O'Neil ME, Zaugg TL, Manning CA, Kaelin C, et al. Health care utilization and mental health diagnoses among veterans with Tinnitus. Am J Audiol. 2019;28(1):181–90.
48. Affairs USDoV. Annual benefits report. Fiscal year 2020. VA Administration 2020.
49. Heller MF, Bergman M. Tinnitus in normally hearing persons. Ann Otolaryngol. 1953;62:73–93.

50. Tucker DA, Phillips SL, Ruth RA, Clayton WA, Royster E, Todd AD. The effect of silence on tinnitus perception. Otolaryngol Head Neck Surg. 2005;132(1):20–4.
51. Boettcher FA, Salvi RJ. Functional changes in the ventral cochlear nucleus following acute acoustic overstimulation. J Acoust Soc Am. 1993;94:2123–34.
52. Gerken GM. Alteration of central auditory processing of brief stimuli: a review and a neural model. J Acoust Soc Am. 1993;93:2038–49.
53. Goodwin PE. Tinnitus and auditory imagery. Am J Otol. 1980;2:5–9.
54. Kraemer DJ, Macrae CN, Green AE, Kelley WM. Musical imagery: sound of silence activates auditory cortex. Nature. 2005;434(7030):158.
55. Crompton L, Lahav Y, Solomon Z. Auditory hallucinations and PTSD in ex-POWS. J Trauma Dissociation. 2017;18(5):663–78.
56. Bohlken MM, Hugdahl K, Sommer IE. Auditory verbal hallucinations: neuroimaging and treatment. Psychol Med. 2017;47(2):199–208.
57. Miller EE, Grosberg BM, Crystal SC, Robbins MS. Auditory hallucinations associated with migraine: case series and literature review. Cephalalgia. 2015;35(10):923–30.
58. Marschall TM, Brederoo SG, Ćurčić-Blake B, Sommer IEC. Deafferentation as a cause of hallucinations. Curr Opin Psychiatry. 2020;33(3):206–11.
59. Maijer K, Begemann MJH, Palmen S, Leucht S, Sommer IE. Auditory hallucinations across the lifespan: a systematic review and meta-analysis. Psychol Med. 2018;48(6):879–88.
60. Wheeler ME, Petersen SE, Buckner RL. Memory's echo: vivid remembering reactivates sensory-specific cortex. Proc Natl Acad Sci U S A. 2000;97(20):11125–9.
61. Linszen MMJ, van Zanten GA, Teunisse RJ, Brouwer RM, Scheltens P, Sommer IE. Auditory hallucinations in adults with hearing impairment: a large prevalence study. Psychol Med. 2019;49(1):132–9.
62. Blom JD. Auditory hallucinations. Handb Clin Neurol. 2015;129:433–55.
63. Zatorre RJ, Halpern AR. Mental concerts: musical imagery and auditory cortex. Neuron. 2005;47(1):9–12.
64. Berrios GE. Musical hallucinations. A historical and clinical study. Br J Psychiatry. 1990;156:188–94.
65. Marschall TM, Ćurčić-Blake B, Brederoo SG, Renken RJ, Linszen MMJ, Koops S, et al. Spontaneous brain activity underlying auditory hallucinations in the hearing-impaired. Cortex. 2021;136:1–13.
66. Kaltenbach JA. Tinnitus: models and mechanisms. Hear Res. 2011;276(1-2):52–60.
67. Theodoroff SM, Kaltenbach JA. The role of the brainstem in generating and modulating tinnitus. Am J Audiol. 2019;28(1):225–38.
68. Kwon O, Jastreboff MM, Hu S, Shi J, Jastreboff PJ. Modification of single-unit activity related to noise-induced tinnitus in rats. In: Hazell JWP, editor. Proceedings of the sixth international tinnitus seminar. Cambridge: THC; 1999. p. 459–62.
69. Chen G-D, Jastreboff PJ. Salicylate-induced abnormal activity in the inferior colliculus of rats. Hear Res. 1995;82:158–78.
70. Klochoff I. Impedance fluctuation and a "Tensor tympani syndrome" 1979 9/25/1979. Lisbon: Universidad Nova de Lisboa Ed Penha & Pizarro; 1979.
71. Keidar E, De Jong R, Kwartowitz G. Tensor tympani syndrome. In: StatPearls. Treasure Island: StatPearls Publishing; 2023.
72. Klockhoff I. Diagnosis of Menière's disease. Arch Otorhinolaryngol. 1976;212(4):309–14.
73. Westcott M, Sanchez TG, Diges I, Saba C, Dineen R, McNeill C, et al. Tonic tensor tympani syndrome in tinnitus and hyperacusis patients: a multi-clinic prevalence study. Noise Health. 2013;15(63):117–28.
74. Noreña AJ, Fournier P, Londero A, Ponsot D, Charpentier N. An integrative model accounting for the symptom cluster triggered after an acoustic shock. Trends Hear. 2018;22:2331216518801725.

Psychological Models of Tinnitus

21

Nicolas Dauman, Lise Hobeika, Soly Erlandsson, Rilana Cima, Laurence McKenna, Severine Samson, and Alain Londero

Abstract

This chapter presents three psychological models with the purpose to comprehend patients' struggle with tinnitus and how their tolerance to tinnitus can be improved. The intention is to give clinicians landmarks to rely on when meeting patients in need for guidance and hope. First, the neural networks involved in the salience of tinnitus are discussed in the light of current neuropsychological research. Second, the cognitive and behavioural reactions to the tinnitus signal are addressed in a model of tinnitus-related distress. Third, the fluctuation of tinnitus intrusiveness is enlightened in relation to patients' frustration, goal fulfilment and search for meaning throughout their journey towards tolerance. With distinct emphases, these models share the following assumptions: (1) The alleviation of intrusiveness requires patients' commitment to change their attitude towards their suffering, (2) the worsening of tinnitus-induced suffering results from self-perpetuating mechanisms that can be softened through the therapeutic alliance and (3) long-term tolerance of tinnitus is mediated by the strengthening of non-auditory factors such as attention, working memory and the fulfilment of valuable goals. Understanding the interaction between the perception of tinnitus and the patients' attitude towards it can help them to resume with a sense of responsibility in the alleviation of distress, although tinnitus, initially, was perceived as being out of control. Psychological research suggests that situations that fuel self-focused thinking would increase the level of frustration in suffering patients and, at the same time, the salience of tinnitus. A goal-directed focus on valued aims and improved control of attention may promote new pathways to nurture patients' ability to reduce their attention to tinnitus.

N. Dauman (✉)
Département de Psychologie, Université de Poitiers, Univ Rennes, Univ Angers, Univ Brest, RPPSY, Poitiers, France
e-mail: nicolas.dauman@univ-poitiers.fr

L. Hobeika
Univ. Lille, ULR 4072 - PSITEC - Psychologie: Interactions Temps Émotions Cognition, Lille, France

Institut du Cerveau et de la Moelle épinière–ICM, INSERM U 1127, CNRS UMR 7225, Sorbonne Université, Paris, France

S. Erlandsson
Department of Social and Behavioural Science, University West, Trollhättan, Sweden
e-mail: soly.erlandsson@hv.se

R. Cima
Department of Clinical Psychological Science, Maastricht University, Maastricht, Netherlands

Adelante, Centre for Expertise in Rehabilitation and Audiology, Hoensbroek, Limburg, Netherlands
e-mail: r.cima@maastrichtuniversity.nl

L. McKenna
Royal National ENT and Eastman Dental Throat Nose and Ear Hospitals, University College Hospitals, London, UK

Ear Institute, UCL, London, UK
e-mail: laurence.mckenna@nhs.net

S. Samson
Univ. Lille, ULR 4072 - PSITEC - Psychologie: Interactions Temps Émotions Cognition, Lille, France

Institut du Cerveau et de la Moelle épinière–ICM, INSERM U 1127, CNRS UMR 7225, Sorbonne Université, Paris, France

AP-HP, GH Pitié-Salpêtrière-Charles Foix, Unité d'Epileptologie, Paris, France
e-mail: severine.samson@univ-lille.fr

A. Londero
Hôpital Européen Georges Pompidou, Assistance Publique - Hôpitaux de Paris, Paris, France

Faculté de Médecine Paris Descartes - Université de Paris, Paris, France

W. Schlee et al. (eds.), *Textbook of Tinnitus*, https://doi.org/10.1007/978-3-031-35647-6_21

Graphical Abstract

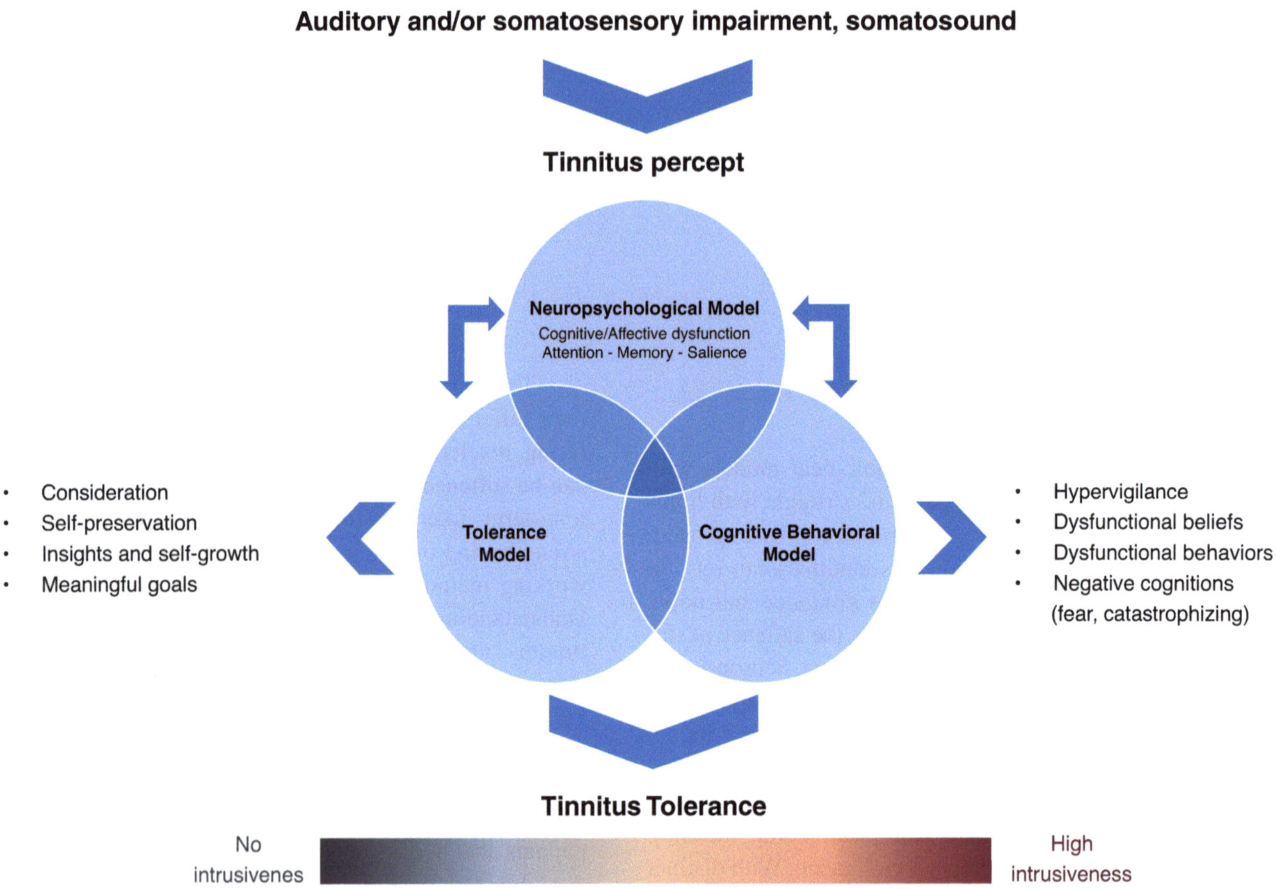

Highlights

- Chronic tinnitus may severely disrupt quality of life in a subset of individuals.
- A variety of pre-existing or induced psychological factors have been put forward to explain such intolerance.
- A variety of comprehensive psychological models of chronic tinnitus have been proposed.
- Neuropsychological models highlight the dysfunction of salience, attention, memory and emotion networks, which can be targeted by neuropsychological rehabilitations.
- Cognitive behavioural models highlight the role of dysfunctional cognitions and behaviours, which can be adapted by means of cognitive behavioural therapy.
- The tolerance model supports a dynamic approach to patients' suffering by promoting self-growth and the integration of tinnitus into the individual's sense of identity within a therapeutic alliance.
- These psychological models are partially overlapping and are not mutually exclusive.

Introduction

While most individuals experience tinnitus from time to time in their life, for some people the sensation is chronic; this is usually defined as a perception for more than 3 months [1]. Chronic tinnitus can have a tremendous impact on individuals' quality of life. For some, the sensation is painful and distressing and is associated with deterioration of the individuals' health, well-being and social life [2]. In most of the cases, tinnitus cannot be perceived by others, which makes this auditory experience elusive [3]. In addition, any perception is hard to communicate and patients who suffer from tinnitus, whether in subjective and objective forms (i.e. somatosounds), usually consider that other people who do not have it cannot understand what it is to live with chronic tinnitus. Patients may have to strive to make their suffering acknowledged in the workplace, with their relatives or even in health encounters [4] and feel relieved to share their experience in self-help groups and patient associations [5, 6]. Meanwhile, many people who acknowledge having tinnitus do not even seek any help from physicians. Among those who do seek help, clear information about tinnitus delivered in primary and secondary care is often enough to reassure most patients. The huge discrepancy between individuals' *reaction* to tinnitus was central to the first psychological model of tinnitus-related distress proposed by Hallam et al. [7]. This model suggested that *habituation* was the natural history of individuals' perception of tinnitus and that clinicians could help patients remove putative barriers to habituation (stress arousal and emotional significance) in order to pay less attention to the tinnitus signal. Habituation was also promoted in the neurophysiological model proposed by Jastreboff et al. [8]. This popularized a medical discourse according to which patients could *learn* to habituate to their tinnitus. Unfortunately, physicians rarely elaborated within this discourse about *how* patients should gain tolerance [9]. The present chapter aims to address this issue. In the first part, the authors will present three psychological models that analyse the complexity of patients' struggle with their tinnitus and potential factors that help alleviate distress that is related to its unwanted presence. The neural networks involved in the salience of tinnitus will be discussed in light of current neuropsychological research. The cognitive and behavioural reactions to the tinnitus signal will be addressed in a model of tinnitus-related distress. The fluctuation of tinnitus intrusiveness will be enlightened in relation to patients' frustration, goal fulfilment and search for meaning throughout their journey towards tolerance. In the final part, the authors will consider shared perspectives between these models and some distinctive features in their approach to tinnitus-induced suffering.

Part I: Understanding the Experience of Tinnitus—A Diversity of Focuses in Psychology

Neuropsychological Approaches to Tinnitus

Tinnitus and Cognitive Functioning

A large literature has described the psychological distress linked to the experience of tinnitus. Although less documented than the emotional disturbances, impaired cognitive functioning seems to be frequently associated with the presence of a chronic tinnitus. Although these cognitive difficulties can be self-reported, they are generally objectively measured by task performances assessing response time and accuracy providing objective behavioural data.

People suffering from chronic tinnitus often report difficulties in concentration. As a distractor, tinnitus captures their attention throughout the day [10]. Moreover, sleep deprivation that is often associated with chronic tinnitus can also have negative effects on basic cognitive processes such as memory and concentration. Thus, concentration issues are at the root of most daily life difficulties, being particularly disabling in professional and social life. Their presence constitutes a significant part of the rating of tinnitus severity [11]. Scientific studies have been conducted to better understand these concentration difficulties and identify the underlying cognitive mechanisms, by targeting first the evaluation of attention processes [12]. One interpretation of the concentration difficulties associated with this auditory sensation is to consider that tinnitus is a salient event capturing people's attentional resources. Thus, fewer cognitive resources are available to perform other attention-demanding tasks, explaining the poorer performances compared to people without tinnitus. By using divided attention tasks that require switching of attention from one task to another, several studies reported that persons with chronic tinnitus obtained slower and less accurate responses than persons without tinnitus in the most demanding dual-task contexts [13–15]. To further investigate these attentional deficits, Heeren et al. assessed the functioning of the three subcomponents of the attentional system: alerting, orienting and executive control with the Attentional Network Test [16]. The results suggest that tinnitus sufferers do not have a global impairment of the attentional system, but rather a specific deficit in executive control of attention. The observations indicate that tinnitus sufferers have difficulty focusing attentional resources on task-relevant information and in inhibiting the processing of distracting or task-irrelevant stimuli. It is interesting to note that some studies found that the importance of the attentional deficits was correlated with the severity of the tinnitus distress [15, 16]. This suggests that the defective cognitive processes targeted in these experiments might be at the root of the concentration difficulties reported by tinnitus sufferers. The cognitive dysfunctions linked to tinnitus may go beyond the attentional system and might involve memory and executive functions as well. Several memory deficits have been reported. Working memory in verbal domain that requires temporarily storing and managing the information to carry out complex tasks (i.e. reasoning, understanding) can be impaired [14, 17–19]. Long-term memory and in particular autobiographical memory can also be degraded; people with chronic tinnitus recall fewer specific memories and showed longer retrieval latencies than people without tinnitus [20]. Moreover, deficits in executive function have been demonstrated in these people using the classical colour word or the spatial Stroop tests [15, 21, 22] and the Trail Making Test [23] suggesting impaired inhibition and switching processes. All these findings indicate that bothersome tinnitus can be associated with subtle changes in attention, memory and executive functions, which might be explained by an inadequate utilization of attention resources rather than a global alteration of the cognitive system. Even if these tasks seem to capture the deficits reported by tinnitus patients, it remains difficult to identify which specific cognitive function is impaired. Indeed, neuropsychological tasks are multifaceted and generally involve several cognitive functions. For example, the Stroop test, known to rely on executive functions, also requires attentional resources and cognitive control. To overcome the limitations of task impurity, Clarke et al. performed a meta-analysis with the aim to identify the cognitive function deficits associated with tinnitus [24]. These authors screened over 3000 references to include 38 studies involving a large panel of cognitive tasks. They subsequently classified the cognitive tasks according to seven broad cognitive domains including fluid intelligence, crystalized intelligence, visual processing, long-term storage and retrieval, general short-term memory, speed processing and executive functions. In this latter case, the authors distinguished three core executive functions (i.e. inhibition, shifting and updating) as defined by Miyake and Friedman [25]. In agreement with previously reported data, the meta-analysis was performed on those classified functions. Globally, the results showed an association between chronic tinnitus and poorer executive function (and particularly inhibition and shifting), processing speed, short-term and working memory and learning and retrieval in long-term memory. Those results clearly indicated that even if tinnitus is an auditory percept, it interferes with a variety of brain functions involving non-auditory brain networks.

The Attention-Switching Model

The emergence of chronic and bothersome tinnitus is usually divided into two components: first the generation of a conscious tinnitus signal and second the persistence of this conscious percept in time [26]. While the generation of tinnitus is attributed to a deregulation in the auditory pathway (i.e. damage in the periphery or central auditory system), the maintenance of the sensation appears to involve non-auditory brain networks. At the cerebral level, chronic tinnitus is characterized by functional differences in the auditory cortex, but also in the emotional, attention and memory-related networks [27, 28]. The attention-switching model developed by Trevis et al. [19] proposes an explanation of persistent awareness of tinnitus in terms of disruptive brain connectivity. The model focused on four cerebral networks previously described in the literature: salience network (SN), cognitive control network (CCN), autobiographical memory network (AMN) and affective network (AN). The SN, using key nodes in the dorsal anterior cingulate cortex and the insula [29], allows relevant sensory inputs in the environment to be identified for further processing. The CCN orientates the cognitive, attention and memory resources towards a goal, with key nodes in the prefrontal cortex and the intraparietal sulcus [30]. The AMN, also called the default mode network, is activated during a resting state [31]. Its activation is linked to introspection and rumination and is antithetical to the CCN. Its key nodes are in the ventral prefrontal cortex, the hippocampus and the posterior cingulate cortex. Finally, the AN regulates emotional experiences, with key nodes in the amygdala, the cingulate cortex, the prefrontal cortex and the nucleus accumbens [32]. According to the attention-switching model, the psychological difficulties linked to chronic tinnitus are explained by dysfunctional interactions between those large-scale cognitive brain networks (Fig. 21.1). To switch attention from one event to another, the SN needs to recruit the CCN to direct attentional resources towards salient information. A tinnitus sufferer encounters difficulties switching attention from the tinnitus sound. This phenomenon could be the result of a failure of the SN to identify the relevant input, leading to a hypoactive CCN. As the CCN is antithetical from the AMN, a hypoactivation of the CCN may provoke a hyperactivation of the AMN. As already described, the AMN is linked to internal focus and rumination. Its hyperactivation could lead to excessive attention to the internal sound that is tinnitus, which increases the salience of the negative thoughts related to its presence.

This model proposes that two separated processes mediate the maintenance and the affective dimension of the tinnitus. While the persistence of a tinnitus perception is related to defective activation of the CCN mediated by the SN and the AMN, the affective component linked to tinnitus is underpinned by altered coupling of the AMN, the AN and the SN. This distinction between awareness and valence of the perception is similar in models proposed for chronic pain, where attentional factors mediate the perception of the pain, whereas affective factors as mood modulate the perceived unpleasantness of the pain [33]. Such a distinction might also provide an explanation to the disparity in tinnitus-related distresses. As previously mentioned, two persons can describe similarly their tinnitus in terms of pitch and loudness, but they will not necessarily experience similar distress. The possible dissociation between awareness and emotions might be explained by the involvement of these two different brain networks.

Causal Link Between Psychological Profiles and Chronic Tinnitus

The psychological distress and cognitive dysfunction are usually understood as a reaction to chronic tinnitus. The presence of tinnitus negatively impacts affective state and distracts attention. The deterioration of this psychological profile in turn aggravates the tinnitus severity and creates a vicious cycle of events. Conversely, other psychological models [19] interpret differently the relations between the tinnitus severity and the altered emotional and cognitive functioning. As mentioned above, chronic tinnitus is not necessarily distressing. Indeed, most people get used to this auditory sensation. The persistence of the intrusive tinnitus and its associated distress might depend on pre-existing individual psychological profiles. Individuals with high anxiety or attentional deficits might fail to habituate to the tinnitus percept. The emotional and cognitive functioning gets worse

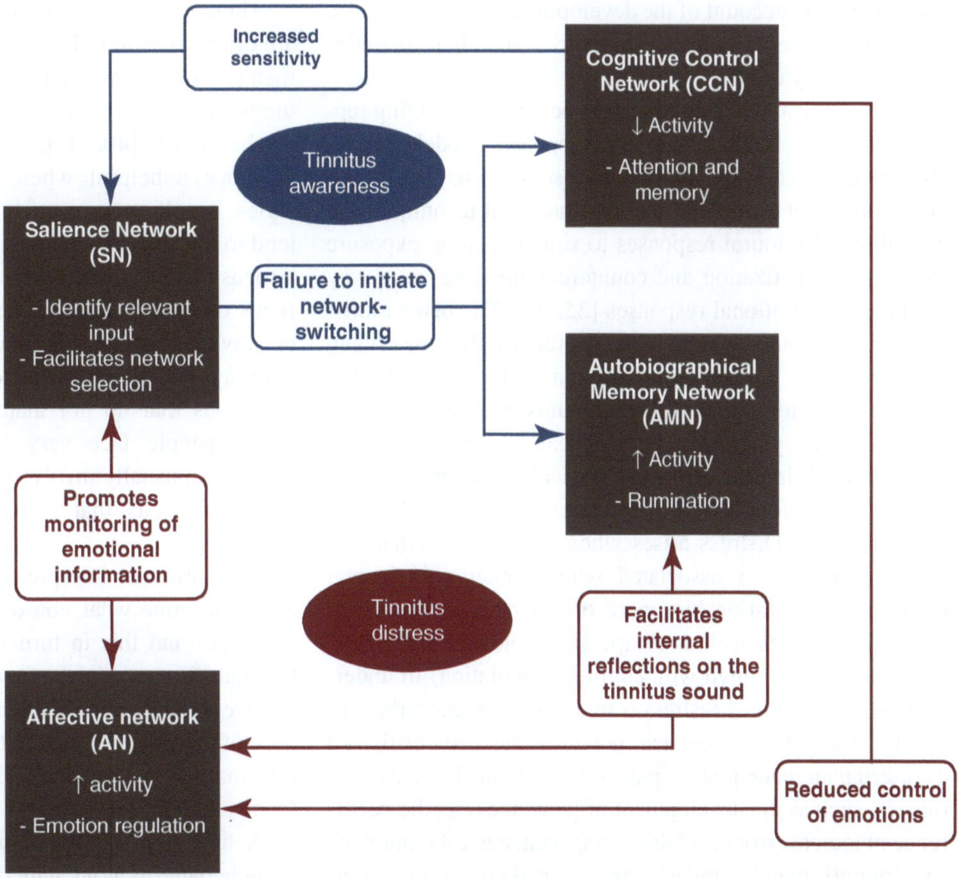

Fig. 21.1 Attention-switching model adapted from Trevis et al. [19]. The model explains the tinnitus awareness and tinnitus distress by the functioning of separated brain networks and cognitive processes

with the tinnitus severity, and the situation may worsen until reaching a catastrophic impact. All these findings underline the importance of evaluating the affective and cognitive psychological profiles linked with chronic tinnitus, to unravel causal relationships between psychological functioning, tinnitus awareness and tolerance using appropriate self-reported questionnaires and neuropsychological tests.

Cognitive Behavioural Models for Tinnitus

History of Cognitive Behavioural Approaches

Cognitive behaviour therapy has its roots in the interplay between psychology and philosophy in the early twentieth century. This period saw an attempt to bring a scientific approach to psychology; introspection and concepts such as consciousness were rejected in favour of observable, measurable, events, i.e. behaviour. Historic mind–body problems were side-stepped by removing the concept of mind as a proper object of study [34]. In this, there was an attempt to apply the same approaches used in physics and chemistry at the time. John Watson (1878–1958) of Chicago University and later Johns Hopkins University is described as the father of behaviourism. This school of thought owes much to the learning theories of Pavlov (classical conditioning) [35] and later Skinner (operant conditioning) [36]. Classical conditioning stems from Pavlov's observations that pairing a neutral stimulus such as the sound of a bell with the presentation of food led a dog to respond to the bell in the same way it naturally responded to food, viz. by salivating. In this process, the food is referred to as an unconditioned stimulus and the natural response to it as an unconditioned response. The bell acquires the status of a conditioned stimulus and the response it produces is known as a conditioned response. Repeated exposure to the conditioned stimulus in the absence of the unconditioned one leads to the conditioned response being extinguished [37]. Operant conditioning emphasizes the role of rewards or punishments in determining how likely a behaviour is to happen again. If a laboratory rat receives positive reinforcement (e.g. food and water) or negative reinforcement (e.g. it escapes an electric shock) when it presses a lever, the probability that it will press the lever again increases. If the animal receives a punishment (e.g. an electric shock) when it pushes the lever, then the chances of the behaviour recurring are reduced. Again, if the reinforcement or punishment is no longer contingent on the behaviour then the conditioning is lost [37]. In the early and mid-twentieth century, both classical learning and operant learning were seen to offer an account of the development and maintenance of a wide range of human experiences including anxieties about everyday events.

Both classical conditioning and operant conditioning represented "black box" or "stimulus-response" models of psychological functioning. In a clinical setting, they led to the development of behaviour therapy that used techniques for changing behavioural responses to situations (e.g. exposure therapy, desensitization and counterconditioning) as a way of changing emotional responses [35, 36]. The behaviourist concepts continue to offer very useful insights into many problems such as addiction, trauma and education (e.g. rewards are more powerful than punishments in shaping behaviour). They have also been appealed to in our attempts to understand tinnitus distress. Classical conditioning forms the theoretical foundation of the neurophysiological model of tinnitus [8]: Distress arises when tinnitus (an otherwise neutral stimulus) is associated with another coincidental stress such as relationship, work or other health problems. Operant processes such as escape and avoidance are important concepts (although with cognitive mediation) in understanding how tinnitus distress is maintained or exacerbated.

The "black box" approach, however, has been criticized as offering an inadequate explanation for many human experiences, such as the development of language (e.g. the occurrence of logical errors in children's speech; e.g. cat [singular], cats [plural]; man [singular] mans [logical but incorrect plural]) or the resistance of some psychological problems to behaviour therapy techniques such as exposure therapy. In the later part of the twentieth century, such inadequacies provoked people to explore the content of the "black box."

Two particularly influential figures in this endeavour were Albert Ellis [38] and Aaron Beck [39]. Both had been psychoanalytic psychotherapists and expanded on the behaviourist understanding of psychology to recognize the role of cognition. Their fundamental premise was that individuals are affected not only by external events but also, and more importantly, by the way they perceive and interpret such events. Thus, an individual's response to any situation depends more upon how they think about that situation than on the situation itself. This can be illustrated using an "everyday" event; you wave to someone you know on the other side of the street, but the other person keeps walking without making a response. If you tell yourself that the other person is deliberately ignoring you, then you are likely to feel an upsetting emotion such as sadness or anger; if, however, you interpret the lack of response as reflecting the other person's preoccupation with worries, you may experience a more compassionate emotion. Clearly, different people can think differently about the same event at the same time. It is also the case that the same person can think differently about the same event at different times.

Thoughts arise in our mind automatically and quickly and are often taken to reflect a "truth" of a situation to which we then react. Such automatic thinking can allow us to navigate the world intuitively using little effort and judgments based on heuristics [40, 41]. This "quick thinking" approach becomes unhelpful when it involves particular thinking styles. People are prone to information processing biases that tend to intensify in a context of threat and loss. For example, a focus on threat will lead to more anxiety-filled thoughts; a focus on loss or negative self-evaluation will lead to more negative and depressive thoughts. Thus, the biases in information processing intrinsic to our brains often result in interpretations that do not match the available evidence [40]. While people face very "real" challenges, anxiety and depression usually involve *overly* negative interpretations of these situations that result from information processing biases.

The particular interpretation you place on the event will also determine what you do about it (i.e. your behavioural response) and this in turn will strengthen or weaken your thoughts. For example, a focus on threat can lead someone to believe a situation is very dangerous; this can motivate avoidance of the situation that, in turn, can keep the threat-focused information processing alive by preventing accurate feedback.

A first step in intervention is the identification of the thought patterns along with the associated information biases (or cognitive distortions). The veracity of these thoughts is then evaluated through discussion and information gathering, the latter often involving experimenting with changes in behaviour. The resulting insights reduce the strength and influence of the overly negative thinking.

CBT was originally developed to treat psychiatric disorders [42, 43]. It is also effective at alleviating distress and improving quality of life across a range of other distressing long-term physical health conditions such as chronic pain [44], somatic complaints [45], insomnia [46] and tinnitus [47]. Thinking styles affect how we perceive physical sensations. While most people would prefer not to have tinnitus, profound distress emerges only in about 10% of tinnitus sufferers. A CBT approach postulates that suffering is worsened through information processing biases that lead to overly negative interpretations of tinnitus and in turn to unhelpful behavioural responses to it.

Cognitive Behavioural Models in Tinnitus Care

The role of cognition in tinnitus distress was proposed by Hallam et al. [7] as part of the habituation model. These authors suggested that the natural history of tinnitus is characterized by habituation and that distress arises because of a failure of that process. They suggested that when tinnitus acquires emotional significance (i.e. there is a negative evaluation of it) and there are elevated levels of stress arousal then habituation is impeded. These ideas inspired the use of CBT in managing tinnitus [48–52], before the development of a more coherent CBT model of tinnitus distress.

Kröner-Herwig et al. [52] advanced the development of a model by including operant conditioning in the habituation model; this was in order to account for learning and the emergence of avoidant behaviour. For example, if someone with tinnitus becomes anxious when exposed to loud noise, and experiences a reduction in that anxiety when they avoid or escape from the noise, then that behaviour will be reinforced and is likely to become part of their pattern of responding to tinnitus and noise. This, however, may limit their activity in life and maintain their anxiety. This model suggests reciprocal interactions between thinking, behaviour, emotion and tinnitus sensation. There is, however, no clear primacy attributed to any one of these factors, and the model seems difficult to test.

In 2014, McKenna et al. [53] proposed a cognitive behavioural model of tinnitus (Fig. 21.2) This suggested that an overly negative interpretation of tinnitus leads to increased sympathetic autonomic arousal and to selective attention and monitoring of tinnitus. The resulting increased detection of tinnitus leads to an iterative process. When overly negative thinking and stress arousal are sustained, they may cause

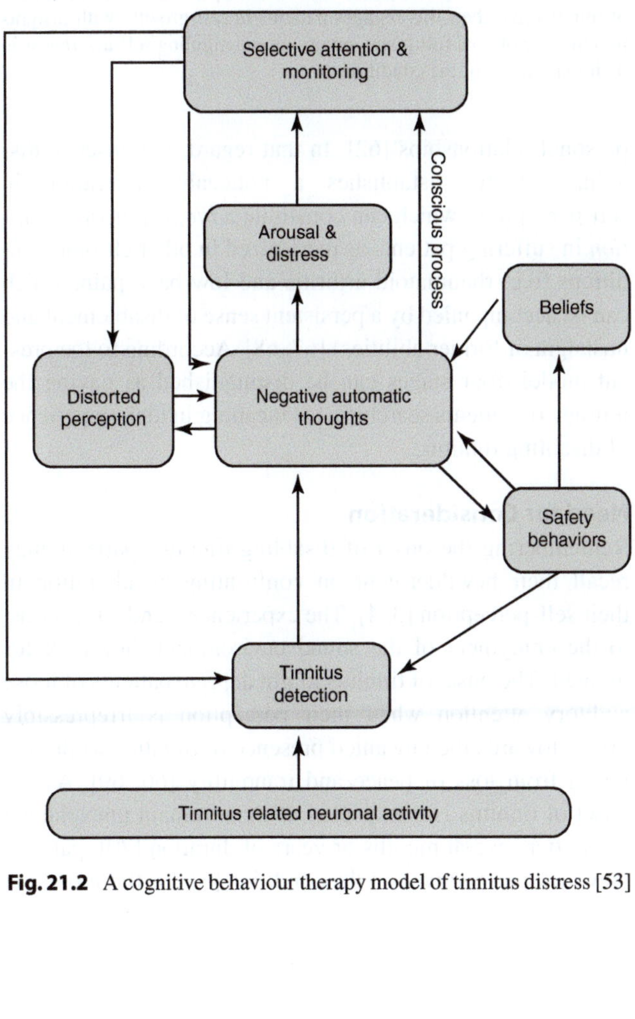

Fig. 21.2 A cognitive behaviour therapy model of tinnitus distress [53]

increasing levels of anxiety or low mood. These processes, in turn, worsen the overly negative cognition. The individual engages in behaviours that attempt to keep her safe and usually involve avoidance, suppression and escape. These "safety-seeking behaviours" reduce anxiety immediately but are unhelpful in the long term as they prevent the person from discovering that their thoughts are the product of an information processing bias and are overly negative. Selective attention is known to distort perception in other areas of life [54], and the model suggests that it can distort the perception of tinnitus; this would account for the catastrophic descriptions of tinnitus commonly heard in clinic.

The model gives a clear primacy to the role of cognition. Behavioural processes are seen as important in that they maintain or negate the cognitive processes. The model involves both psychosomatic and somatopsychic processes. It differs from Hallam et al.'s [7] focus in that a greater emphasis is placed on vigilance and orientation to tinnitus rather than simply a failure of habituation. There is good evidence pointing to the existence of the component parts of this model although the studies themselves were not designed to test the model itself and certainly stronger evidence is needed for the idea that perception is distorted.

A similar model has been proposed by Cima et al. [2, 55]. This fear-avoidance model, however, attributes a more central role to *avoidance behaviour* motivated by catastrophic fear beliefs. It is based on the fear-avoidance model of pain. The role of negative cognitive appraisals of tinnitus is again seen as critical in the process of producing distress. This appraisal is again seen as leading to aversive emotional reactions (e.g. fear) and to behavioural safety responses. The model also appeals to the behavioural processes of classical and operant conditioning recognizing that conditioned responses can generalize to other situations.

The clinical implication of both these models is that unhelpful, overly negative, beliefs about tinnitus and its implications need to be weakened and corrected [56]. This can be achieved through a variety of means [55]. The "talking therapy" component of the therapy usually helps to weaken the strength with which unhelpful beliefs are held. This often lays the foundation for a change in behaviour that, in turn, consolidates the cognitive shift. This is sometimes expressed in terms of the cognitive component leading to a new "intellectual understanding" and the behavioural change bringing about a new "emotional understanding". In the model proposed by Cima et al. [2, 55], anxious beliefs and avoidance behaviour are seen as the key processes involved in creating and maintaining distress. This model therefore suggests that exposure therapy is a key strategy in resolving that distress. Exposure to tinnitus in a controlled context allows a patient to test their catastrophic (mis)interpretations and learn that there is less to fear than anticipated. While anxious thoughts and avoidance behaviour are undoubtedly central to a great deal of tinnitus distress, they may not be the only processes and a clear understanding of the function of behaviour in terms of the cognitive context is crucial. These models therefore predict that "a one-size-fits-all" approach to tinnitus therapy may be counter-productive. For example, sound therapy may be unhelpful for a person who believes that tinnitus will overwhelm her and therefore uses her sound generators to avoid it as much as possible; the use of sound therapy may prevent her from testing this overly negative belief.

Cognitive behaviour therapy is one of the most extensively studied approaches to tinnitus management, and meta-analyses have indicated the beneficial effects of CBT on tinnitus-related distress [47, 57]. A Cochrane review of CBT for tinnitus [58] concluded that this therapy approach had a greater impact in reducing the negative impact of tinnitus on quality of life than audiological care, tinnitus retraining therapy and other types of treatment. It is also noteworthy that the available clinical guidelines in tinnitus management all recommend CBT as part of that management [59, 60]. Although the benefits of CBT in tinnitus management cannot be regarded as a test of the cognitive models, those benefits might nonetheless be regarded as offering indirect support for these models.

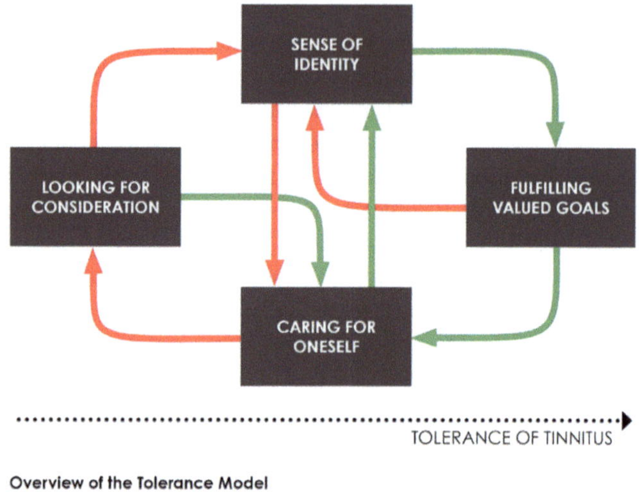

Fig. 21.3 Tolerance model is grounded on qualitative interviews with patients, in which individuals accounted for the intrusiveness of tinnitus according to situations they were involved in. The model describes patients' journey searching for meaning as a process of restoration of their *sense of identity* that may have been disrupted by the onset of tinnitus. Variability of intrusiveness is explained by the fluctuation of levels of frustration in patients whether they were able, with the help of others, to fulfil three basic needs: (a) looking for consideration, (b) caring for oneself and (c) fulfilling valued goals. Green arrows and red arrows account, respectively, for *progress towards tolerance* (i.e. softened frustration for having tinnitus through goal fulfilment) and *worsened intrusiveness of tinnitus* (i.e. increased frustration and sense of disablement in trying to resume a desirable way of life). The integration of tinnitus into their life engages patients in self-growth, with insights into the role of goal fulfilment, emotions and niggling self-awareness in their experience of the condition

Patients' Journey Searching for Meaning: A Model of Tinnitus Tolerance

The tolerance model explained in this chapter broadens the findings of Dauman et al. [3, 61] by the implementation of a humanistic perspective that includes a narrative psychological approach [62] and psychotherapy research involving both group and individual therapy [63, 64]. Figure 21.3 presents an overview of the model that is characterized by three main features. First, the model follows a salutogenic approach [65] to the suffering induced by tinnitus, in that it emphasizes the role of helpful attitudes and resources that *promote health* in living with tinnitus, rather than focusing on maladaptive behaviours and cognitions to be challenged according to a more traditional pathogenic approach. Finding meaning and coherence in life is essential to health promotion, for it maintains perspectives for the individual who must allocate her/his resources effectively when dealing with stressful events [65]. Second, the model is based on the daily experience of suffering patients over time (i.e. intra-individual variability) [66], which suggests that *fluctuations* of intrusiveness are an important aspect of chronic tinnitus. The model further relates fluctuations to the level of *frustration* individuals may encounter in interactions with their social surroundings [3]. Third, the model suggests pathways towards the integration of tinnitus into patients' *sense of identity*, which is closely related to self-narration and interpersonal relationships [62]. In that regard, the onset of disabling tinnitus establishes a noticeable alteration in self-perception, which can constitute a *biographical disruption* in suffering patients as recognized in other chronic conditions (e.g. rheumatoid arthritis and low back pain, which can be accompanied by a persistent sense of disablement and nostalgia of former abilities) [67, 68]. According to the present model, four stages can be distinguished as paving the journey of patients searching for meaning in their experience of disabling tinnitus.

Need for Consideration

Remembering the onset of disabling tinnitus, patients may recall their bewilderment on confronting an alteration in their self-perception [3, 4]. The experience stands in contrast to the enjoyment of the sound environment they took for granted. The onset of tinnitus might deprive patients of loose auditory attention when their perception is irrepressibly driven towards the unwanted presence of tinnitus, while suffering from loss of peace and tranquility [66, 69]. As the onset of tinnitus is unexpected and can remain unexplained even after several months or years of duration [70], patients may lack perspectives on the condition [3]. Furthermore, the unwanted presence of tinnitus thwarts basic psychological needs and well-being, such as relatedness to others, autonomy and competence [71]. Chronic tinnitus may isolate suffering patients from people who are unable to understand their distress [72], a situation that can diminish the patients' sense of initiative [4] and willpower to fulfil personal goals [3]. It is recognized that individuals who are confused seek multiple medical consultations. Thereby, Brüggemann et al. [73] reported that the number of physicians consulted by patients with tinnitus was found to be the second-best predictor of their level of distress. The higher the patients' distress, the more they searched for interlocutors to help them to come to grips with tinnitus.

Many patients find it difficult to explain what tinnitus is and what it means to them, and they also find it hard to convince others of the seriousness of their burden [69, 74]. Patients may feel that health professionals do not validate their struggle by suggesting they adapt to the condition as early as possible [5]. In accordance with Marks et al. [4], the present tolerance model supports the idea that lack of consideration for tinnitus-induced confusion may leave patients in a state of roaming, worsening their feelings of helplessness and frustration in the belief that "nothing is being done" [61]. However, clinicians who engage in an authentic dialogue about patients' experience of distress nurture a *hope for improvement* [63, 64]. Patients who overcome their anguish after the onset of tinnitus associate this improvement with the clinician's thorough validation of their first reactions [75]. Self-help groups may also support the importance of validation regarding the seriousness of the participants' confusion and worries [5]. As most tinnitus sufferers must come to terms with a long-standing condition, meeting their individual needs requires time, patience and self-confidence from clinicians [62, 66]. Professionals' attentive listening can contribute to the recovery of self-worth in those who feel isolated and abandoned in their attempts to normalize life. Listening to patients when they feel discouraged trying to adapt to tinnitus can promote a sense of responsibility in caring for themselves and offer hope for improvement [66].

Need for Self-Preservation

Even if habituation may occur in many individuals as a natural process of adaptation that can be retarded or fail due to the emotional load of the tinnitus percept [7], struggling against the presence of tinnitus can also be considered as a natural and spontaneous reaction to tinnitus. Especially for someone who perceives tinnitus as threatening or who is deeply concerned and worried about its presence relatedly to the emotional significance of tinnitus and the tinnitus signal changing. Indeed, the continuation of an intrusive bodily stimulus may naturally induce a defensive reflex leading to a flight reaction over time [6]. When patients cannot fulfil their wish for an *immediate detachment* from the intrusiveness of tinnitus, the reaction becomes thwarted and nourishes frustration [3]. Persistent frustration may be accompanied by hopelessness, anger and fear of endless torment, due to perceived lack of professional help, especially if the consultation implies a narrow and cure-focused discourse on tinnitus [4]. Instead, clinicians can consider patients' own experiences by focusing more on unsatisfactory parts of their life. Although very few narrative case studies are being published in international journals, it is likely that some clinicians are familiar with the occurrence of stressful situations in the life of their patients, prior to the onset of tinnitus [62]. By allowing those patients to talk about significant life situations, clinicians are encouraging them to use self-reflection in their work situation, family life and relationships in general.

Prolonged suffering in their patients should require clinicians to make a deeper exploration, searching for a possible inner turmoil, for which a narrative approach might provide some light. Erlandsson et al. [62] illustrated, using a narrative study approach, how ongoing struggles and unresolved prejudices intervened with the personal histories of chronic tinnitus sufferers. The study results showed that intrusiveness of tinnitus was associated with personal issues and behaviours that the patients were unable to bring to closure. With time and in the context of tinnitus, these issues became a threat towards their self-worth and social status. The narratives gave voice to ruminations, loss of agency, feelings of guilt and blame towards others and the thwarting of goal fulfilments by life circumstances. By understanding that tinnitus is part of the patient's personal history, an existential meaning and sense of agency can be rebuilt. This aspect of self-narration is relevant, especially in patients who fear not being able to manage tinnitus and worry that it might become worse no matter their attitude towards the disorder [2]. Self-narration can help patients to view tinnitus from a different angle and realize that caring for themselves might have been neglected prior to tinnitus onset [66]. The loss of tranquility can contribute to patients' reflection on the negative consequences of a stressful lifestyle that collides with the presence of tinnitus and demands moderation of their situation [3]. Exploring the limitations and adjustments that tinnitus imposes on the patients' life governs them in their search for self-preservation. Self-awareness and life adjustments can lead to an increased level of control over tinnitus suffering in a long-term perspective.

The detrimental influence that *exhaustion* can have on the intrusiveness of tinnitus should be considered when caring for the patients. The observation that tiredness makes tinnitus harder to endure [76] was elaborated in research associating energy depletion to increased inefficiency in filtering out tinnitus [70]. Lack of energy was also associated with ceaseless efforts of patients to endure the taxing presence of tinnitus on their social participation [4]. Those findings are consistent with the positive influence of a moderated lifestyle that allows patients to further regulate their resources [61]. Temporary withdrawal from participation in social life may contribute to the conservation of autonomy, known to preserve individuals from the accumulation of stress [77]. In addition to those strategies, the common use of sound enrichment [76, 78, 79] can soften the patients' tension towards tinnitus. Moreover, sound enrichment can allow them to act more spontaneously and break a vicious circle of involuntary isolation.

Relief Through Meaningful Goals

Most important for both sufferers and clinicians is to understand the following paradox: *to wish for* tinnitus to be silenced only reinforces its intrusiveness; relief is the result from being absorbed by the fulfilment of some *other* valued goal. Basically, patients can experience a temporary relief when they are fully engrossed in doing something else than dwelling on the unwanted presence of tinnitus. Dauman et al. [61] suggested that the most efficient way to alleviate the patient's frustration would be to help them carry on searching for gratifying goals. Moreover, patients can free themselves from observing tinnitus when they are engaged in something meaningful enough to outweigh *niggling self-awareness*. Observations from several research studies support a similar approach to tinnitus intrusiveness [3, 70, 78, 79]. Slater et al. [76] were first to emphasize the *mediating* role that pleasant and meaningful activities play for patients' motivation to reach a state of tinnitus tolerance (e.g. going to the theatre, walking outdoors and crafting at home). Consistent with this is the opposite observation that *boredom* tends to induce self-monitoring [80], coupled with increased rumination and tension towards the invasive symptom [81]. Hence, tolerance can be reached by the fulfilment of valued goals allowing patients to withdraw their attention from tinnitus.

In their study on chronic pain, Eccleston and Crombez [82] emphasized the importance of recovering from interruption in the pursuit of a meaningful life despite patients' diminished agency. The fluctuating self-experience of both patients with pain and patients with tinnitus illustrates the dynamic of attention that was studied by psychologist Csikszentmihalyi and collaborators [83, 84] who defined the state of a conscious *flow* as an optimal experience of attention. According to these authors, meaningful situations requiring sustained motivation might allow for patients to attenuate self-awareness when full absorption of attention in goal fulfilment occurs [83]. To reconnect the patients with meaningful goals can be one gratifying outcome of psychotherapy. Moreover, it may allow them to renew their sense of spontaneity similar to what they experienced prior to the onset of tinnitus [85].

Searching for a New Self

An integration of tinnitus-induced changes in self-perception can contribute to progress in tinnitus tolerance and self-growth. Patients who took part in psychotherapy studies and in self-help groups support the view of a growing tolerance, which enlightens the *interpersonal* dimension in their search for a new self. Sharing the experience of victimization with other participants in a group psychotherapy regime can facilitate new insights into the association between emotional reactions in various social contexts and tinnitus annoyance [63]. Patients may also gain insight about the role of self-confidence, as they understand how interpersonal conflicts can influence tinnitus intrusiveness [66]. Instead of blaming others for a passive attitude, they begin to challenge their own attitude in different social contexts. Consistent with this finding, Andersson and Edvinsson [74] reported that patients may recognize that tinnitus led them to become more independent-minded, which contributed to a positive outcome of the condition. In psychotherapy, behind the initial complaint of tinnitus, stories of unrecognized prejudices that patients suffer in silence can be disclosed [66]. Further studies should focus on the significant analogy between the absence of an external stimulus corresponding to tinnitus and the lack of social recognition of traumatic events that some sufferers have endured without external assistance. Although the prevalence of prejudices is inherently difficult to estimate in a population of patients with tinnitus, the association between traumatic events and disabling tinnitus requires special attention from clinicians [86]. These prejudices may include threats of violence, rape and incest that have attacked patients' self-worth and weakened their resources to cope with life during months or years before the onset of tinnitus [62]. In a psychodynamic case study, Dauman and Erlandsson [64] explored the relationship between a patient's disclosure of a succession of threats and how she was able to end her preoccupation on tinnitus.

Patients may improve their control over the intrusiveness of tinnitus, when they begin to realize the negative consequences of resentment and irritation over other's lack of understanding for the precarious condition. They can also lower their conflictual attitude towards tinnitus by becoming more tolerant towards themselves. Stories of successful adaptation to tinnitus narrated in self-help groups may likewise provide hope for improvement in suffering patients [5]. Dauman et al. [3] found that a greater congruence between the interviewees' personal choices and social interactions could alleviate emotional conflicts and frustration. To better understand the reasons behind tinnitus fluctuations can help patients to restore a sense of responsibility and self-confidence, as Zöger et al. [63] showed in their study investigating the efficacy of group psychotherapy. Some patients expressed at the follow-up interview how tinnitus varied with emotional distress, as recognized in the two citations as follows:

> It varies how disturbed I am by the sound, but the periods when I feel hopeless are shorter. I understand that I must work with the emotional crisis that tinnitus has triggered…have more hope that this will go in the right direction.

> I have understood that I must learn how to take care of myself, have too high expectations. I have also realized that tinnitus, in my case, is triggered by emotional factors.

Working with self-images, worries, beliefs and desires in a group psychotherapy format can allow patients to be more self-reflective encouraging them to continue their search for answers within themselves. To summarize, suffering that the individual is able to express through emotional pain is more accessible and, therefore, easier to communicate and find words for [72]. A narrow approach to tinnitus cannot help us to move the patients towards insight into their state of mind and health, neither insight about the interplay between emotions and tinnitus suffering [72].

Part II: Psychological Models of Tinnitus Contrasted and Related One to Another

From a clinical perspective, the development of psychological models of tinnitus raises two conceptual questions not fully resolved by the scientific debate, so far. The first issue is the lack of a consensual theoretical or operational definition of tinnitus [1]. Indeed, the umbrella term tinnitus encompasses a wide variety of clinical situations even when leaving out associated symptoms such as hearing loss, hyperacusis, vertigo or pain [87, 88]. Basically, the simplest definition of tinnitus is "the conscious perception of an auditory sensation in the absence of a corresponding external stimulus", but this does not account for the obvious difference between (a) subjective tinnitus (i.e. abnormal neuronal activity in the auditory system) [89, 90], (b) somatosounds (e.g. blood turbulence or muscle contraction) [91, 92], (c) sounds produced by a device (e.g. vascular valve) [93] and (d) musical or psychiatric hallucinations [94]. For the first three subtypes, it seems disputable to claim that the perception is exclusively caused by cognitive or psychological impairments, which are generally disregarded by clinicians when tinnitus can be silenced. On the other hand, defining the tinnitus condition exclusively as a sound perception (whatever its spectral, loudness or rhythmic characteristics) is a misleading simplification. Patients do not seek medical advice just because they are hearing a sound but rather because they eventually suffer from it. Indeed, not all persons experiencing tinnitus become tinnitus patients seeking healthcare professionals' help [95]. When tinnitus becomes an intrusive disorder affecting patients' quality of life, the interaction with pre-existing or induced cognitive and psychological factors is evident as this is true for every other auditory object [96]. Indeed, people suffering from chronic tinnitus tend to present more mood disorders than people without tinnitus, being more anxious [97, 98] and depressed [81].

Indeed, anxiety and depression levels are predictors of tinnitus severity [99]. As for chronic pain [100], these mood disorders are mediators worsening intrusiveness of the bothersome sensation. Chronic tinnitus is also associated with the presence of other psychological distresses, such as sleep disturbances [101], confusion, rumination, lack of motivation and irritability [102]. All these symptoms lead to social withdrawal and work hindrance [103]. Elevated levels of some personality traits have been observed in tinnitus populations. For example, it has been reported that chronic tinnitus can be associated with higher rates of persistent pessimism, hypochondriasis and hysteria [104], increased psychasthenia [105] and introversion and neuroticism [106]. Moreover, the prevalence of psychiatric problems such as phobias and of obsessive–compulsive disorder is higher in the presence of chronic tinnitus [107]. In addition to these mood and personality differences, individuals with chronic tinnitus may also present cognitive dysfunction as discussed below. These neuropsychological disturbances lead people with chronic tinnitus to seek help in primary and secondary care settings [48]. Nevertheless, it is important to emphasize that all people with chronic tinnitus do not present such emotional suffering. Some individuals experience chronic tinnitus with no particular distress and therefore are less inclined to look for clinical help. It remains, however, difficult to understand why some individuals suffer from chronic tinnitus, whereas others do not present such difficulties with everyday life. This justifies the efforts to develop explanatory psychological models of tinnitus-induced intolerance, but this highlights the second issue, which is about the actuality of the causal link between the persistence of tinnitus as an intrusive percept and the associated psychopathological traits or states [56]. Indeed, the consistent correlation between tinnitus and cognitive or psychological disorders [95, 108] does not say much about the causality link and its direction. Do patients feel stressed, hypervigilant, anxious and depressed because they have tinnitus, or do they experience an intrusive tinnitus because of these neuropsychological conditions? Animal [109, 110] and human data [99] support both these non-exclusive explanations. There could even be a third party explaining both the susceptibility to develop a tinnitus and a neuropsychological disorder (e.g. abnormal GABA neurotransmission) [111, 112]. Deciphering this complex and multidirectional interplay may be of crucial importance to develop efficient therapies.

The psychological models that are presented in this chapter share perspectives that are worth considering. First, these models require *patients' commitment* to changing their attitude towards tinnitus in order to alleviate their suffering. Such a perspective contrasts with patients' wish for the suppression of tinnitus and, therefore, clinicians must be confident enough with an alternative approach to the problem. The presented models explain the benefits of changing their attitude to tinnitus with clear perspectives on their experience. Understanding the interaction between their attitude and the perception of tinnitus can help them to resume with a sense of responsibility in the alleviation of distress, whereas tinnitus may have been initially perceived as being out of control. By applying psychological models, clinicians help patients to broaden their experience of tinnitus. They give them landmarks to rely on that meet their need for improvement in the tolerance of tinnitus. The presented models also agree that increased intrusiveness of tinnitus results from *self-perpetuating* mechanisms. A similar perspective was proposed by Wagenaar et al. [113] who suggested that exhaustion, resulting from the accumulation of stress, mediates the patients' overburdening. This perspective was originally proposed in the habituation model [7] in which tinnitus-related distress results from the maintained orientation towards the presence of tinnitus. This was further elaborated by McKenna et al. [53] that suggested an iterative process between negative thoughts about tinnitus and increased levels of arousal and selective attention, which, in turn, worsen the salience of tinnitus. Cima et al. [2] also suggested that behavioural avoidance of tinnitus, through sound enrichment and distraction, maintained awareness to tinnitus in the long term. Similarly, Trevis et al. [19] described the salience of tinnitus as a result of an iterative process between antithetical neural networks. They suggested that lack of proficiency in switching attention away from tinnitus (i.e. hypoactivity of the cognitive control network) contributes to self-focused thinking and rumination that is associated with hyperactivity of the autobiographical memory network (AMN). The tolerance model considers the worsening of the intrusiveness of tinnitus in the context of patients' expectancies towards health professionals. The model describes a vicious circle between lack of consideration for disabling tinnitus and increased frustration in suffering patients who lack perspectives in the context of ceaseless efforts to cope with the condition. The attenuation of self-perpetuating mechanisms is a common pathway to the presented models in promoting tolerance of tinnitus. A third agreement is that the intrusiveness of tinnitus is *mediated by non-auditory factors* such as attention, working memory or executive functions. As indicated earlier, the cognitive behavioural models consider that events and perceptions are mediated by the individuals' *interpretation* that attributes them emotional valence and meaning. Furthermore, the model emphasizes the interplay between individuals' behaviours and beliefs about events, which reinforce each other according to short-term benefits (e.g. avoidance of anxiety). The attention-switching model enlightens the interplay between *goal-directed* behaviour and *self-focused* thinking in the interference of tinnitus with daily activities. The mediation of goal fulfilment in tinnitus-induced annoyance enriches findings about negative thoughts and behavioural avoidance of tinnitus in accounting for high levels of anxiety and depression in suffering patients [12]. In that regard, these emotional consequences can be related to the persistent *interruption* of the patients' ongoing behaviour with their surroundings. Such a goal-directed perspective on intrusiveness was previously proposed by Eccleston and Crombez [82] for understanding anxiety and depression in patients with chronic pain. The tolerance model shares this perspective, suggesting that the *meaning* of the situations in which patients are involved underlies their willingness to maintain attention away from tinnitus. Thereby, this model emphasizes the importance of valued goals, pleasure and spontaneity in alleviating the struggle with tinnitus. These topics of psychological research could contribute to further understanding factors that influence negative emotional consequences associated with disabling tinnitus.

Conversely, two main differences can be noticed in the assumptions of the presented models. The first concerns the definition of the tinnitus *percept*. In accordance with the habituation model [7], cognitive behavioural models [2, 53] consider that tinnitus per se is a meaningless and non-threatening signal that is not *intrinsically* a source of suffering. Epidemiological studies and psychoacoustic tinnitus matching support this perspective. It is well documented that the majority of people with tinnitus do not suffer from it [53] and that in most cases tinnitus matching does not exceed 10 dB above hearing thresholds [48, 114]. These observations, however, do not exclude that more severe forms may exist in suffering patients, including noise-reactive tinnitus [115] and disabling tinnitus that cannot be masked with sounds up to 90 dB above hearing thresholds [116]. The tolerance model was based on patients' experience of such disabling forms of tinnitus, for which the fluctuation of intrusiveness was essential to their suffering. In that regard, the notion of *salience* of tinnitus percept in the attention-switching model [19] may offer an interesting alternative to the usual analogy between tinnitus and a constant sound [17] for which it should be eventually possible to achieve an "habituation", meaning the loss of the "orienting response" towards it. The use of these psychophysiological concepts drawn from experimental research with highly controlled stimulus and response parameters is attractive, but it seems hazardous to overuse them in our attempts to understand the complex clinical symptomatology displayed by tinnitus patients. Indeed, the salience of tinnitus *may vary* according to the goal-directed attention that individuals are able to dedicate to their daily activities. Schlee et al. [117] reported similar findings about moment-to-moment changes in tinnitus-induced annoyance according to the time of the day. This fluctuation may substantially contribute to the threatening experience that tinnitus is inescapable and interferes with activities *whatever* the patients try in order to flee from its unwanted presence. Therefore, Trevis et al. [12, 19] suggested that the alleviation of tinnitus interference with goal-directed behaviour, through attention training and emotion regulation, may strengthen the effectiveness of cognitive strategies that target patients' attitude and beliefs towards tinnitus. The notion of salience of tinnitus percept is also consistent with the importance of valued goal fulfilment in the tolerance model. Indeed, tinnitus salience and individual frustration can be seen as both sides of the same coin, since both vary from moment-to-moment according to the ongoing activities that patients are involved in and changes in their physical surroundings. In that regard, situations that *fuel self-focused thinking* (e.g. loneliness in a quiet room or difficulties to participate in noisy group meetings) would increase tinnitus salience and frustration in suffering patients, at the same time. Further research on the fluctuations of intrusiveness is needed in order to contribute to the implementation of clinical strategies according to subtypes of tinnitus.

The second difference between the presented models reflects a diversity of approaches to suffering in *psychology*. Covering this issue is beyond the scope of the present chapter; however, some clinical implications can be briefly outlined. It is well acknowledged that cognitive behavioural therapies are the most influential psychological approaches in tinnitus and the most evidence-based treatment options for tinnitus-related distress [58, 118]. However, this successful contribution to the help provided to patients with tinnitus contrasts with the almost *absence* of other approaches to tinnitus-induced suffering, among the most established ones in clinical psychology. Indeed, cognitive behavioural therapies do recognize the importance of historical and existential processes in influencing how a patent thinks about tinnitus. The current thinking is seen as a reflection of the history. Issues are primarily addressed in the current context, and there is usually an implicit assumption that the current changes will modify the historical influences. While "schema"-based work is undertaken in a CBT context, it is perhaps less common. Existential therapies [119], patient-centred therapies [120] and psychodynamic psychotherapies [121] address these historical influences more directly. It is noted that some evidence of their effectiveness has been provided. A common feature of these humanistic approaches is the *validation* of the patients' experience as the foundation of therapeutic progresses. These approaches also emphasize the links between the alleviation of individuals' suffering, self-growth and the *search for meaning and dignity* as distinctive drives of human behaviour (compared to animal behaviour). Rooted in the mechanisms of conditioning, cognitive and behavioural approaches to tinnitus have traditionally challenged the patients' experience in order to correct putative misinterpretations of suffering individuals about tinnitus threat. In this chapter, different approaches to sound enrichment are illustrative of such distinct views on the patients' experience (i.e. validation or challenge). On the one hand, it can be advocated within the CBT models that the use of sounds (e.g. music) as distractors from tinnitus allows for short-term benefits only and rather maintains the patients' avoidance of tinnitus in the long term [2, 13]. On the other hand, taking into account the patients' exhaustion induced by disabling tinnitus, sound enrichment allows for moments of relief, softens the frustration associated with lack of control and prevents the accumulation of stress. Thereby, sound enrichment may also be considered a suitable strategy to deal with tinnitus in the long term [61].

The tolerance model presented in this chapter provides a theoretical foundation for testable hypotheses of a humanistic perspective in tinnitus-induced suffering. Interestingly, the frustration fulfilment (of valued goals) hypothesis is consistent with the goal-directed perspective of neuropsychological research, since both identify niggling self-awareness as being persistent hindrance to patients' commitment to helpful activities. Such approach to tinnitus is also in agreement with basic assumptions of acceptance and commitment therapy (ACT) [122], which were applied to tinnitus-induced annoyance [123]. The hypothesis of self-perpetuating frustration (lack of involvement in meaningful activities) also fits with a mindfulness-based approach to tinnitus, which enlightens the role of attentional flexibility and patients' insights into rumination in reconnecting with others and pleasant activities [124]. In that regard, depletion of physical resources was suggested to increase the impact of tinnitus on sufferers [62, 64] and may be explored further through narratives of life events prior to tinnitus onset [70, 125]. As indicated by Fagelson et al. [86], the investigation of potential post-traumatic stress disorder (PTSD) associated with tinnitus is essential in order to adjust therapeutic means to the diversity of patients' histories. As suggested by Biehl et al. [126] research on biographical disruptions should explain further the cumulative effects of emotional distress, individual vulnerability and the salience of tinnitus, which are common focuses in the psychological models presented in this chapter.

Conclusion

In the absence of a cure for each patient with annoying tinnitus, psychological approaches to the struggle of sufferers remain at the core of therapeutic strategies. It can even be advocated that every clinical approach to tinnitus incorporates some psychology in the very act of interacting with suffering patients. In that regard, the use of psychological frameworks not only contribute to the clinical dialogue about the subjective experience of tinnitus, but also prove rewarding for both patients and practitioners who can share perspectives of improvement in the tolerance of tinnitus. In this chapter, the diversity of psychological models that provide an account of patients' experience of tinnitus is in line with the authors' conviction that there is not "a one-size-fits-all" approach to the psychological needs of patients with tinnitus. Many of them will benefit from a structured, step-by-step, approach to their distress, enabling them to challenge their fear and worries about tinnitus through practical exercises and behavioural exposure. Others will rather benefit from neuropsychological rehabilitation that does not confront their cognitions about tinnitus, but help them strengthen their attentional resources and reinforce their ability to pursue goal-directed behaviours. Still, others will express, in psychotherapy, the need of a deeper exploration of personal and traumatic issues that have been aggravated by the onset of their tinnitus. In fact, the diversity of patients' needs supports the need of a diversity of psychological practices in the tinnitus field. Most of the time, suffering patients will consult practitioners that are not psychologists themselves, but ENT or audiologists who have professional interest in counselling individuals confronted with the confusion induced by tinnitus. This chapter would have achieved its goal if it had provided some light about the usefulness of understanding the individuals' struggle with tinnitus in gaining their trust in the therapeutic alliance. The current psychological models in the literature thus contribute to the resources that each clinician can use in supporting patients who seek their help.

References

1. De Ridder D, Schlee W, Vanneste S, Londero A, Weisz N, Kleinjung T, et al. Tinnitus and tinnitus disorder: theoretical and operational definitions (an international multidisciplinary proposal). In: Progress in brain research. Amsterdam: Elsevier; 2021. p. 1–25. Available from https://linkinghub.elsevier.com/retrieve/pii/S0079612320302326.
2. Cima RFF, Crombez G, Vlaeyen JWS. Catastrophizing and fear of tinnitus predict quality of life in patients with chronic tinnitus. Ear Hear. 2011;32(5):634–41.
3. Dauman N, Erlandsson SI, Albarracin D, Dauman R. Exploring Tinnitus-induced disablement by persistent frustration in aging individuals: a grounded theory study. Front Aging Neurosci. 2017;9:272.
4. Marks E, Smith P, McKenna L. Living with tinnitus and the health care journey: an interpretative phenomenological analysis. Br J Health Psychol. 2019;24(2):250–64.
5. Pryce H, Moutela T, Bunker C, Shaw R. Tinnitus groups: a model of social support and social connectedness from peer interaction. Br J Health Psychol. 2019;24(4):913–30.
6. Dauman N, Erlandsson S, Carlsson S. Habituation theories in current models of chronic tinnitus: evidence and criticism. In: Buskirk A, editor. Habituation: theories, characteristics and biological mechanisms. New York: Nova Biomedical; 2013. p. 55–90.
7. Hallam RS, Rachman S, Hinchcliffe R. Psychological aspects of tinnitus. Contrib Med Psychol. 1984;3:31–53.
8. Jastreboff PJ, Hazell JW. A neurophysiological approach to tinnitus: clinical implications. Br J Audiol. 1993;27(1):7–17.
9. Erlandsson S, Dauman N. Categorization of tinnitus in view of history and medical discourse. Int J Qual Stud Health Well-being. 2013;8:23530. Available from http://www.ncbi.nlm.nih.gov/pmc/articles/PMC3873117/.
10. Hall DA, Fackrell K, Li AB, Thavayogan R, Smith S, Kennedy V, et al. A narrative synthesis of research evidence for tinnitus-related complaints as reported by patients and their significant others. Health Qual Life Outcomes. 2018;16(1):61.
11. Fackrell K, Hall DA, Barry JG, Hoare DJ. Psychometric properties of the tinnitus functional index (TFI): assessment in a UK research volunteer population. Hear Res. 2016;335:220–35.
12. Trevis KJ, Mclachlan NM, Wilson SJ. A systematic review and meta-analysis of psychological functioning in chronic tinnitus. Clin Psychol Rev. 2018;60(January):62–86.
13. Hallam RS, McKenna L, Shurlock L. Tinnitus impairs cognitive efficiency. Int J Audiol. 2004;43(4):218–26.
14. Rossiter S, Stevens C, Walker G. Tinnitus and its effect on working memory and attention. J Speech Lang Hear Res. 2006;49(1):150–60.
15. Stevens C, Walker G, Boyer M, Gallagher M. Severe tinnitus and its effect on selective and divided attention. Int J Audiol. 2007;46(5):208–16.
16. Heeren A, Maurage P, Perrot H, De Volder A, Renier L, Araneda R, et al. Tinnitus specifically alters the top-down executive control sub-component of attention: evidence from the Attention Network Task. Behav Brain Res. 2014;269:147–54.
17. Andersson G, Khakpoor A, Lyttkens L. Masking of tinnitus and mental activity. Clin Otolaryngol. 2002;27(4):270–4.
18. Pierce KJ, Kallogjeri D, Piccirillo JF, Garcia KS, Nicklaus JE, Burton H. Effects of severe bothersome tinnitus on cognitive function measured with standardized tests. J Clin Exp Neuropsychol. 2012;34(2):126–34.
19. Trevis KJ, McLachlan NM, Wilson SJ. Cognitive mechanisms in chronic tinnitus: psychological markers of a failure to switch attention. Front Psychol. 2016;7:1262.
20. Andersson G, Ingerholt C, Jansson M. Autobiographical memory in patients with tinnitus. Psychol Health. 2003;18(5):667–75.
21. Andersson G, Eriksson J, Lundh LG, Lyttkens L. Tinnitus and cognitive interference: a Stroop paradigm study. J Speech Lang Hear Res. 2000;43(5):1168–73.
22. Araneda R, De Volder AG, Deggouj N, Philippot P, Heeren A, Lacroix E, et al. Altered top-down cognitive control and auditory processing in tinnitus: Evidences from auditory and visual spatial Stroop. Restor Neurol Neurosci. 2015;33(1):67–80.
23. Pajor AM, Ormezowska EA, Jozefowicz-Korczynska M. The impact of co-morbid factors on the psychological outcome of tinnitus patients. Eur Arch Otorhinolaryngol. 2013;270(3):881–8.
24. Clarke NA, Henshaw H, Akeroyd MA, Adams B, Hoare DJ. Associations between subjective tinnitus and cognitive performance: systematic review and meta-analyses. Trends Hear. 2020;24:2331216520918416.
25. Miyake A, Friedman NP. The nature and organization of individual differences in executive functions: four general conclusions. Curr Dir Psychol Sci. 2012;21(8):8–14.
26. Georgiewa P, Klapp BF, Fischer F, Reisshauer A, Juckel G, Frommer J, et al. An integrative model of developing tinnitus based on recent neurobiological findings. Med Hypotheses. 2006;66(3):592–600.
27. Husain FT. Neural networks of tinnitus in humans: elucidating severity and habituation. Hear Res. 2016;334:37–48.

28. Ridder DD, Elgoyhen AB, Romo R, Langguth B. Phantom percepts: Tinnitus and pain as persisting aversive memory networks. PNAS. 2011;108(20):8075–80.
29. Seeley WW, Menon V, Schatzberg AF, Keller J, Glover GH, Kenna H, et al. Dissociable intrinsic connectivity networks for salience processing and executive control. J Neurosci. 2007;27(9):2349–56.
30. Corbetta M, Shulman GL. Control of goal-directed and stimulus-driven attention in the brain. Nat Rev Neurosci. 2002;3:201–15.
31. Gusnard DA, Akbudak E, Shulman GL, Raichle ME. Medial prefrontal cortex and self-referential mental activity: relation to a default mode of brain function. Proc Natl Acad Sci. 2001;98(7):4259–64.
32. Ochsner K, Gross J. The cognitive control of emotion. Trends Cogn Sci. 2005;9(5):242–9.
33. Rauschecker JP, May ES, Maudoux A, Ploner M. Frontostriatal gating of tinnitus and chronic pain. Trends Cogn Sci. 2015;19(10):567–78.
34. Grayling AC. The history of philosophy. London: Penguin; 2019.
35. Pavlov IP. Lectures on conditioned reflexes: twenty-five years of objective study of the higher nervous activity (behaviour) of animals. New York: Liverwright Publishing Corporation; 1928. Available from http://content.apa.org/books/11081-000.
36. Skinner BF. Operant behavior. Am Psychol. 1963;18(8):503–15.
37. Rachlin H. Behaviour and learning. San Francisco: Freeman; 1976.
38. Ellis A. Rational psychotherapy and individual psychology. J Individ Psychol. 1957;13(1):38.
39. Beck AT. Depression: causes and treatment. Philadelphia: University of Pennsylvania Press; 1967.
40. Kahneman D. Thinking, fast and slow. New York: Farrar, Straus and Giroux; 2011.
41. Tversky A, Kahneman D. Judgment under uncertainty: heuristics and biases. Science. 1974;185(4157):1124–31.
42. Persons JB, Davidson J, Tompkins MA. Essential components of cognitive-behavior therapy for depression. Washington: American Psychological Association; 2001.
43. Butler A, Chapman J, Forman E, Beck A. The empirical status of cognitive-behavioral therapy: a review of meta-analyses. Clin Psychol Rev. 2006;26(1):17–31.
44. Morley S, Eccleston C, Williams A. Systematic review and meta-analysis of randomized controlled trials of cognitive behaviour therapy and behaviour therapy for chronic pain in adults, excluding headache. Pain. 1999;80(1):1–13.
45. Kroenke K. Efficacy of treatment for somatoform disorders: a review of randomized controlled trials. Psychosom Med. 2007;69(9):881–8.
46. Morin C, Culbert J, Schwartz S. Nonpharmacological interventions for insomnia: a meta-analysis of treatment efficacy. AJP. 1994;151(8):1172–80.
47. Hesser H, Weise C, Westin VZ, Andersson G. A systematic review and meta-analysis of randomized controlled trials of cognitive–behavioral therapy for tinnitus distress. Clin Psychol Rev. 2011;31(4):545–53.
48. Scott B, Lindberg P. Psychological profile and somatic complaints between help-seeking and non-help-seeking tinnitus subjects. Psychosomatics. 2000;41(4):347–52.
49. Sweetow RW. Cognitive aspects of tinnitus patient management. Ear Hear. 1986;7(6):390–6.
50. Henry JL, Wilson PH. Tinnitus: a self-management guide for the ringing in your ears. 1st ed. Boston: Allyn & Bacon; 2001.
51. Andersson G. Psychological aspects of tinnitus and the application of cognitive–behavioral therapy. Clin Psychol Rev. 2002;22(7):977–90.
52. Kröner-Herwig B, Frenzel A, Fritsche G, Schilkowsky G, Esser G. The management of chronic tinnitus. J Psychosom Res. 2003;54(4):381–9.
53. McKenna L, Handscomb L, Hoare DJ, Hall DA. A scientific cognitive-behavioral model of tinnitus: novel conceptualizations of tinnitus distress. Front Neurol. 2014;5:196. Available from http://www.ncbi.nlm.nih.gov/pmc/articles/PMC4186305/.
54. Tuschen-Caffier B, Bender C, Caffier D, Klenner K, Braks K, Svaldi J. Selective visual attention during mirror exposure in anorexia and bulimia nervosa. PLoS ONE. 2015;10(12):e0145886.
55. Cima RFF, Andersson G, Schmidt CJ, Henry JA. Cognitive-behavioral treatments for tinnitus: a review of the literature. J Am Acad Audiol. 2014;25(1):29–61.
56. Langguth B, Kleinjung T, Landgrebe M. Severe tinnitus and depressive symptoms: a complex interaction. Otolaryngol Head Neck Surg. 2011;145(3):519; author reply 520.
57. Andersson G, Lyttkens L. A meta-analytic review of psychological treatments for tinnitus. Br J Audiol. 1999;33(4):201–10.
58. Fuller T, Cima R, Langguth B, Mazurek B, Vlaeyen JW, Hoare DJ. Cognitive behavioural therapy for tinnitus. Cochrane Database Syst Rev. 2020;1:CD012614.
59. Fuller TE, Haider HF, Kikidis D, Lapira A, Mazurek B, Norena A, et al. Different teams, same conclusions? a systematic review of existing clinical guidelines for the assessment and treatment of tinnitus in adults. Front Psychol. 2017;8:206. Available from https://www.ncbi.nlm.nih.gov/pmc/articles/PMC5319986/.
60. National Institute for health and Care Excellence (NICE). Tinnitus: assessment and management guideline [NG155]. Available from https://www.nice.org.uk/guidance/ng155.
61. Dauman N, Dauman R. An empowerment model for individuals with chronic tinnitus. Ear Hear. 2021;42(2):425–42.
62. Erlandsson SI-M, Lundin L, Dauman N. The experience of tinnitus and its interaction with unique life histories—life events, trauma and inner resources narrated by patients with tinnitus. Front Psych. 2020;11:136. https://doi.org/10.3389/fpsyt.2020.00136/full.
63. Zöger S, Erlandsson S, Svedlund J, Holgers K-M. Benefits from group psychotherapy in the treatment of severe refractory tinnitus. Audiol Med. 2008;6(1):62–72.
64. Dauman N, Erlandsson SI. Learning from tinnitus patients' narratives—a case study in the psychodynamic approach. Int J Q Stud Health Well-being. 2012;7(1):19540.
65. Antonovsky A. The salutogenic model as a theory to guide health promotion. Health Promot Int. 1996;11(1):11–8.
66. Dauman N, Erlandsson S, Lundlin L, Dauman R. Intra-individual variability in tinnitus patients: current thoughts and perspectives. HNO. 2015;63(4):302–6.
67. Bury M. Chronic illness as biographical disruption. Sociol Health Illn. 1982;4(2):167–82.
68. Smith JA, Osborn M. Interpretative phenomenological analysis. In: Doing social psychology research. Hoboken: Wiley; 2008. p. 229–54. https://doi.org/10.1002/9780470776278.ch10.
69. Pryce H, Chilvers K. Losing silence, gaining acceptance: a qualitative exploration of the role of thoughts in adult patients with subjective tinnitus. Int J Audiol. 2018;57(11):801–8.
70. Colagrosso EMG, Fournier P, Fitzpatrick EM, Hébert S. A qualitative study on factors modulating tinnitus experience. Ear Hear. 2018;40(3):636–44.
71. Ryan RM, Deci EL. Self-determination theory and the facilitation of intrinsic motivation, social development, and well-being. Am Psychol. 2000;55(1):68–78.
72. Erlandsson S. Psychological profiles of tinnitus patients. In: Tyler RS, editor. Tinnitus handbook. Clifton Park: Thomson Delmar Learning; 2000.
73. Brüggemann P, Szczepek AJ, Rose M, McKenna L, Olze H, Mazurek B. Impact of multiple factors on the degree of tinnitus distress. Front Hum Neurosci. 2016;10:341. Available from https://www.ncbi.nlm.nih.gov/pmc/articles/PMC4925660/.
74. Andersson G, Edvinsson E. Mixed feelings about living with tinnitus: a qualitative study. Audiol Med. 2008;6(1):48–54.

75. Erlandsson SI. Psychological counselling in the medical setting – some clinical examples given by patients with tinnitus and Ménière's disease. Int J Adv Couns. 1998;20(4):265–76.
76. Slater R, Terry M, Davis B. Tinnitus: a guide for sufferers and professionals. Beckenham: Croon Helm; 1987.
77. Hobfoll SE. Conservation of resources: a new attempt at conceptualizing stress. Am Psychol. 1989;44(3):513–24.
78. Adams J, Verrier E, Walsh M, Lind C. Adults' perceptions of their tinnitus and a tinnitus information service. Aust N Z J Audiol. 2010;32(2):83–94.
79. Beukes EW, Manchaiah V, Andersson G, Allen PM, Terlizzi PM, Baguley DM. Situationally influenced tinnitus coping strategies: a mixed methods approach. Disabil Rehabil. 2018;40(24):2884–94.
80. Eastwood JD, Frischen A, Fenske MJ, Smilek D. The unengaged mind: defining boredom in terms of attention. Perspect Psychol Sci. 2012;7(5):482–95.
81. Trevis KJ, McLachlan NM, Wilson SJ. Psychological mediators of chronic tinnitus: the critical role of depression. J Affect Disord. 2016;204:234–40.
82. Eccleston C, Crombez G. Pain demands attention: a cognitive–affective model of the interruptive function of pain. Psychol Bull. 1999;125(3):356–66.
83. Csikszentmihalyi M. Flow: the psychology of optimal experience. New York: Harper [and] Row; 2009. p. 303.
84. Delle Fave A, Massimini F. The investigation of optimal experience and apathy: developmental and psychosocial implications. Eur Psychol. 2005;10(4):264–74.
85. Erlandsson S, Dauman N. Reaction to tinnitus. In: Tyler RS, editor. The consumer handbook on tinnitus. Sedona: Auricle Ink Publishers; 2015. p. 53–70.
86. Fagelson MA. The association between tinnitus and posttraumatic stress disorder. Am J Audiol. 2007;16(2):107–17.
87. Genitsaridi E, Hoare DJ, Kypraios T, Hall DA. A review and a framework of variables for defining and characterizing tinnitus subphenotypes. Brain Sci. 2020;10(12):938. Available from https://www.ncbi.nlm.nih.gov/pmc/articles/PMC7762072/.
88. Baguley D, McFerran D, Hall D. Tinnitus. Lancet. 2013;382(9904):1600–7.
89. Eggermont JJ, Roberts LE. The neuroscience of tinnitus: understanding abnormal and normal auditory perception. Front Syst Neurosci. 2012;6:53.
90. Noreña AJ. Revisiting the cochlear and central mechanisms of tinnitus and therapeutic approaches. Audiol Neurootol. 2015;20(1):53–9.
91. Mattox DE, Hudgins P. Algorithm for evaluation of pulsatile tinnitus. Acta Otolaryngol. 2008;128(4):427–31.
92. Sinclair CF, Gurey LE, Blitzer A. Palatal myoclonus: algorithm for management with botulinum toxin based on clinical disease characteristics. Laryngoscope. 2014;124(5):1164–9.
93. Hong Z-N, Huang J-S, Huang L-Q, Cao H, Chen Q. The effect of valve noise on the quality of life of patients after mechanical mitral valve replacement in a Chinese population. J Cardiothorac Surg. 2019;14:137. Available from https://www.ncbi.nlm.nih.gov/pmc/articles/PMC6642469/.
94. Moseley P, Alderson-Day B, Kumar S, Fernyhough C. Musical hallucinations, musical imagery, and earworms: a new phenomenological survey. Conscious Cogn. 2018;65:83–94.
95. Bhatt JM, Lin HW, Bhattacharyya N. Prevalence, severity, exposures, and treatment patterns of tinnitus in the United States. JAMA Otolaryngol Head Neck Surg. 2016;142(10):959–65.
96. Brefczynski-Lewis JA, Lewis JW. Auditory object perception: a neurobiological model and prospective review. Neuropsychologia. 2017;105:223–42.
97. Andersson G, Vretblad P. Anxiety sensitivity in patients with chronic tinnitus. Scand J Behav Ther. 2000;29(2):57–64.
98. Ooms E, Vanheule S, Meganck R, Vinck B, Watelet J-B, Dhooge I. Tinnitus severity and its association with cognitive and somatic anxiety: a critical study. Eur Arch Otorhinolaryngol. 2012;269(11):2327–33.
99. Boecking B, von Sass J, Sieveking A, Schaefer C, Brueggemann P, Rose M, et al. Tinnitus-related distress and pain perceptions in patients with chronic tinnitus – do psychological factors constitute a link? PLoS One. 2020;15(6):e0234807. Available from https://www.ncbi.nlm.nih.gov/pmc/articles/PMC7316290/.
100. Bushnell MC, Ceko M, Low LA. Cognitive and emotional control of pain and its disruption in chronic pain. Nat Rev Neurosci. 2013;14(7):502–11.
101. Hébert S, Carrier J. Sleep complaints in elderly tinnitus patients: a controlled study. Ear Hear. 2007;28:649–55.
102. Tyler RS, Baker LJ. Difficulties experienced by tinnitus sufferers. J Speech Hear Disord. 1983;48(2):150–4.
103. Zeman F, Koller M, Langguth B, Landgrebe M, Figueiredo R, Aazevedo A, et al. Which tinnitus-related aspects are relevant for quality of life and depression: results from a large international multicentre sample. Health Qual Life Outcomes. 2014;12(1):1–10.
104. Marciano E, Carrabba L, Giannini P, Sementina C, Verde P, Bruno C, et al. Psychiatric comorbidity in a population of outpatients affected by tinnitus. Int J Audiol. 2003;42:4–9.
105. Bayar N, Oguztürk Ö, Koç C. Minnesota multiphasic personality inventory profile of patients with subjective tinnitus. J Otolaryngol. 2002;31(5):317–22.
106. Rutter DR, Stein MJ. Psychological aspects of tinnitus: a comparison with hearing loss and ear, nose and throat disorders. Psychol Health. 1999;14(4):711–8.
107. Andersson G, Carlbring P, Kaldo V, Ström L. Screening of psychiatric disorders via the Internet. A pilot study with tinnitus patients. Nord J Psychiatry. 2004;58(4):287–91.
108. Durai M, Searchfield G. Anxiety and depression, personality traits relevant to tinnitus: a scoping review. Int J Audiol. 2016;55(11):605–15.
109. Guitton MJ, Pujol R, Puel J-L. m-Chlorophenylpiperazine exacerbates perception of salicylate-induced tinnitus in rats. Eur J Neurosci. 2005;22(10):2675–8.
110. Guitton MJ. Tinnitus-provoking salicylate treatment triggers social impairments in mice. J Psychosom Res. 2009;67(3):273–6.
111. Sedley W, Parikh J, Edden RA, Tait V, Blamire A, Griffiths TD. Human auditory cortex neurochemistry reflects the presence and severity of tinnitus. J Neurosci. 2015;35(44):14822–8.
112. Nuss P. Anxiety disorders and GABA neurotransmission: a disturbance of modulation. Neuropsychiatr Dis Treat. 2015;11:165–75.
113. Wagenaar O, Wieringa M, Verschuure H. A cognitive model of tinnitus and hyperacusis; a clinical tool for patient information, appeasement and assessment. Int Tinnitus J. 2010;16(1):66–72.
114. Zenner HP, Pfister M, Birbaumer N. Tinnitus sensitization: sensory and psychophysiological aspects of a new pathway of acquired centralization of chronic tinnitus. Otol Neurotol. 2006;27(8):1054–63.
115. Greenberg BS, Carlos MC. The sound-sensitive tinnitus index: psychometric properties of a scale to assess the impact of tinnitus exacerbated by sound. Noise Health. 2019;21(100):98–107.
116. Penner MJ, Brauth S, Hood L. The temporal course of the masking of tinnitus as a basis for inferring its origin. J Speech Lang Hear Res. 1981;24(2):257–61.
117. Schlee W, Pryss RC, Probst T, Schobel J, Bachmeier A, Reichert M, et al. Measuring the moment-to-moment variability of tinnitus: the TrackYourTinnitus Smart Phone App. Front Aging Neurosci. 2016;8:294.
118. Cima RFF, Maes IH, Joore MA, Scheyen DJWM, El Refaie A, Baguley DM, et al. Specialised treatment based on cognitive behaviour therapy versus usual care for tinnitus: a randomised controlled trial. Lancet. 2012;379(9830):1951–9.

119. Vos J, Craig M, Cooper M. Existential therapies: a meta-analysis of their effects on psychological outcomes. J Consult Clin Psychol. 2015;83(1):115–28.
120. Kim SK, Park M. Effectiveness of person-centered care on people with dementia: a systematic review and meta-analysis. CIA. 2017;12:381–97.
121. Shedler J. The efficacy of psychodynamic psychotherapy. Am Psychol. 2010;65(2):98–109.
122. Hayes SC, Luoma JB, Bond FW, Masuda A, Lillis J. Acceptance and commitment therapy: model, processes and outcomes. Behav Res Ther. 2006;44(1):1–25.
123. Westin VZ, Schulin M, Hesser H, Karlsson M, Noe RZ, Olofsson U, et al. Acceptance and commitment therapy versus tinnitus retraining therapy in the treatment of tinnitus: a randomised controlled trial. Behav Res Ther. 2011;49(11):737–47.
124. Marks E, Smith P, McKenna L. I wasn't at war with the noise: how mindfulness based cognitive therapy changes patients' experiences of tinnitus. Front Psychol. 2020;11:483.
125. Alpini D, Cesarani A. Tinnitus as an alarm bell: stress reaction tinnitus model. ORL. 2006;68(1):31–7.
126. Biehl R, Boecking B, Brueggemann P, Grosse R, Mazurek B. Personality traits, perceived stress, and tinnitus-related distress in patients with chronic tinnitus: support for a vulnerability-stress model. Front Psychol. 2020;10:3093.

Neuroinflammation Model of Tinnitus

22

Weihua Wang and Shaowen Bao

Abstract

Tinnitus is a widespread and potentially debilitating hearing disorder with a diverse clinical etiology. Here, we review evidence that neuroinflammation may be a mechanism leading to tinnitus-related cellular and synaptic pathologies. In clinical studies, elevated pro-inflammatory cytokine levels and reduced anti-inflammatory cytokine levels are observed in tinnitus patients. Genetic polymorphisms of inflammatory cytokines are associated with the risk of noise-related tinnitus. Many neuroinflammation-related nonauditory pathologies and health conditions are associated with an increased risk for tinnitus. Animal studies indicate that noise-induced hearing loss, a risk factor for tinnitus, induces neuroinflammation in the central auditory pathway. Neuroinflammation promotes noise-induced parvalbumin-positive inhibitory neuron loss in the auditory cortex and causes an excitation–inhibition imbalance in the central auditory pathway. Blocking neuroinflammation prevents noise-induced tinnitus in animal models. Based on these findings, we propose a neuroinflammation model of tinnitus, in which neuroinflammation in the central auditory pathway is triggered by noise trauma, hearing loss, and other neuroinflammation-related brain disorders and health conditions. Neuroinflammation in turn leads to an excitation–inhibition imbalance, which is an underlying mechanism for tinnitus.

W. Wang · S. Bao (✉)
Department of Physiology, University of Arizona, Tucson, AZ, USA
e-mail: sbao@email.arizona.edu

W. Schlee et al. (eds.), *Textbook of Tinnitus*, https://doi.org/10.1007/978-3-031-35647-6_22

Graphical Abstract

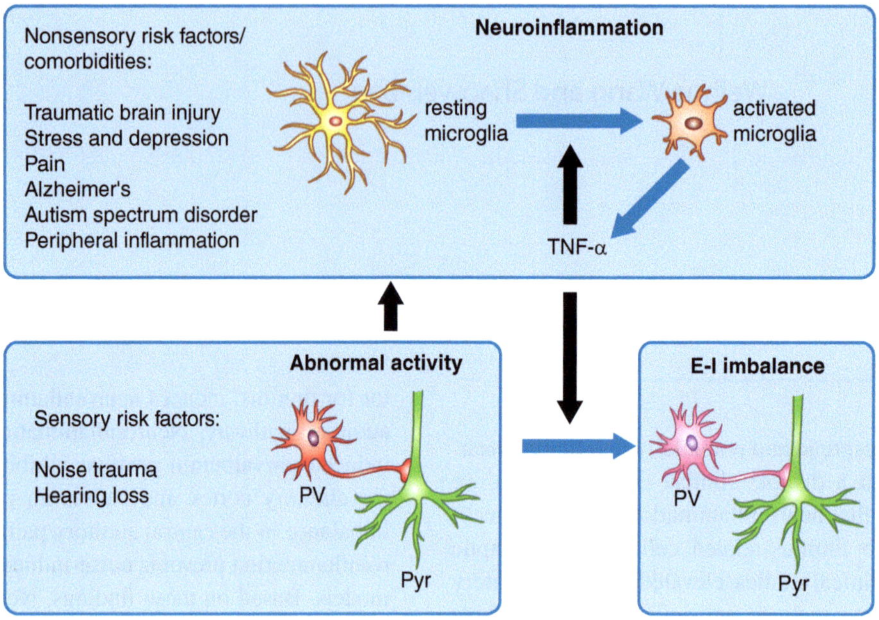

Highlights

- Tinnitus in humans is correlated with pro- and anti-inflammatory cytokine levels and polymorphisms of pro-inflammatory cytokine genes.
- Noise trauma induces neuroinflammation in the central auditory pathway.
- Blocking neuroinflammation prevents noise-induced tinnitus in animal models.
- Diffusible pro-inflammatory cytokines in the brain increase the risk of tinnitus.
- Strain differences in noise-induced tinnitus correlate with neuroinflammation.
- Tinnitus is correlated with reduced inhibitory neuron function.
- Noise trauma results in parvalbumin-positive (PV) neuron loss, which is correlated with neuroinflammation and tinnitus.

Introduction

Tinnitus is the perception of phantom sounds in the absence of corresponding external sound. Although its clinical etiology is diverse, the biggest risk factor is hearing loss due to aging or acoustic trauma [1–7]. Hearing loss can cause a range of cellular and physiological changes in the auditory pathway, including neuronal cell loss, altered synaptic transmission and ion channel function, distorted sensory maps, and abnormal neuronal firing patterns [8–20]. All these changes have been proposed as potential mechanisms for tinnitus [7, 21]. Attempts have been made to treat hearing loss-related tinnitus by targeting specific cellular and physiological changes, but success has been limited [22]. The failure to alleviate tinnitus by targeting individual molecular and cellular mechanisms suggests that tinnitus could be mediated by multiple, parallel mechanisms [7–10, 21]. Blocking only one of the mechanisms might be ineffective as the other mechanisms can still lead to tinnitus perception. Upstream events that link hearing loss to the subsequent cellular and physiological pathologies need to be examined in order to develop effective tinnitus treatments. Here, we discuss evidence that neuroinflammation in the central auditory pathway may play a pivotal role in triggering many of the pathological mechanisms underlying tinnitus.

Neuroinflammation as a Risk Factor for Human Tinnitus

Tinnitus in humans has long been associated with increased serum pro-inflammatory cytokine levels and inflammation biomarkers [23–25]. The level of interleukin 10, an anti-inflammatory cytokine also known as human cytokine synthesis inhibitory factor, was reduced in people with tinnitus, but not in people who had hearing loss without tinnitus [25]. These changes in pro-inflammatory and anti-inflammatory cytokines in tinnitus patients were often interpreted as consequences of tinnitus-related stress and depression, but not risk factors for tinnitus [23]. Peripheral inflammatory cytokines can enter the brain either through circumventricular organs [26] or via transporters across the blood–brain barrier [27, 28]. Through pro-inflammatory cytokines, peripheral immune responses could act as a risk factor for tinnitus by activating neuroinflammation in the brain [29]. Alternatively, peripheral cytokine levels may also be a measure of tinnitus-related neuroinflammation in the brain. Inflammation as a risk factor for tinnitus was implicated in studies showing that, in humans, genetic polymorphisms of inflammatory cytokines TNF-α, interleukin 1α, and interleukin 6 are associated with the risk of noise-related tinnitus [30–32]. A recent genome-wide association study found that a single nucleotide polymorphism in the intron of the *TNFRSF1A* gene, which encodes TNF receptor 1, is significantly associated with the risk of noise-induced tinnitus, supporting a role of TNF-α signaling in tinnitus [33].

Neuroinflammation as a risk factor for tinnitus is consistent with finding that several neuroinflammation-related nonauditory pathologies and health conditions are associated with increased risk for tinnitus, including autoimmune/inflammatory diseases [34], traumatic brain injury [35, 36], stress [37–39], depression and pain [40–48], schizophrenia [49–51], and autism spectrum disorder [52, 53]. These diverse nonauditory risk factors could signify genetic propensity to developing neuroinflammatory responses or may directly increase diffusible pro-inflammatory cytokine levels in the brain to promote neuroinflammatory responses in the central auditory pathway [54–58].

In the following sections, we will review research that uses animal models to elucidate potential mechanisms by which neuroinflammation contributes to tinnitus.

Noise Trauma Induces Neuroinflammation in the Central Auditory Pathway

Increasing evidence indicates that noise-induced hearing loss and conductive hearing loss can lead to inflammatory responses in the central auditory pathway, which is often manifested as the activation of microglia and the release of pro-inflammatory cytokines [59–61]. For example, in a recent study, monaural exposure to a continuous 8-kHz tone at 112–114 dB SPL for 2 h was found to rapidly increase the expression of pro-inflammatory cytokines such as TNF-α (Fig. 22.1), IL-1β, and IL-18 [62]. Microglia were also activated as exemplified by their morphological transition from ramified to deramified, amoeboid shapes [62–66]. In addition to noise trauma-induced tinnitus, salicylate-induced tinnitus is also associated with increased expression of pro-inflammatory cytokines and activation of microglia in the central auditory pathway [67–70]. Neuroinflammatory responses profoundly influence neuronal functions. For example, microglia play an important role in neural development, maturation, plasticity, and aging [71–73]. Pro-inflammatory cytokines also modulate neuronal functions such as synaptic transmission, plasticity, and membrane excitability [18, 74–77]. Many of these processes are implicated in tinnitus [7, 21], raising the possibility that neuroinflammation contributes to pathologies underlying tinnitus.

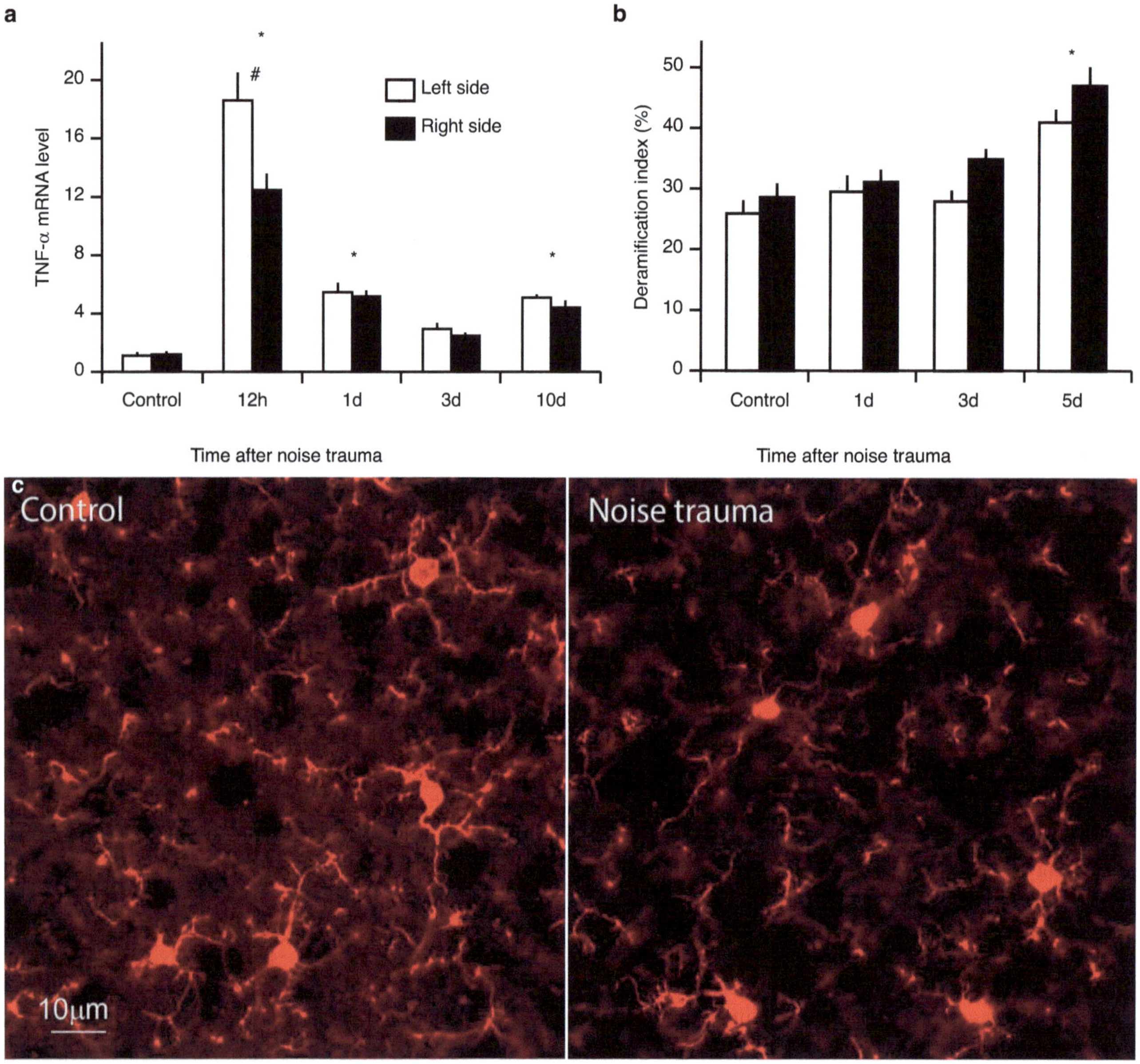

Fig. 22.1 Noise exposure results in elevated TNF-α expression and microglial deramification in the primary auditory cortex. (**a**) TNF-α mRNA level increased rapidly within 12 hours of noise exposure, with a stronger ipsilateral than contralateral increase. The increase was also significant at 1 day and 10 days post-noise exposure. (**b**) The soma-to-whole cell size ratio of microglia was used to measure microglial deramification as an index of microglial activation. There was a significant increase in the microglial deramification 5 days after noise exposure, and the deramification was stronger for the right than the left side. (**c**) Representative images of IBA1 antibody-stained microglia in AI of control and noise-exposed mice. Error bars represent SEM. * depicts $p < 0.01$ compared to control; # indicates $p < 0.01$ comparing left and right hemispheres

Blocking Neuroinflammation Prevents Noise-Induced Tinnitus in Animal Models

The notion that neuroinflammation is involved in tinnitus etiologies is supported by evidence that blocking neuroinflammation prevents behavioral evidence of noise-induced tinnitus in rodent models [62]. In one experiment, mice were given PLX3397 to block the CSF1 receptor, which is expressed in microglia and required for microglial survival. Administration of PLX3397 for 21 days, which had been shown to deplete most of the microglia [78–81], suppressed basal TNF-α expression and prevented the noise-induced increase in TNF-α expression (Fig. 22.2). The treatment with PLX3397 also prevented noise-induced tinnitus as assessed with a gap detection test (Fig. 22.2). Furthermore, blocking TNF-α expression with 3,6′-dithiothalidomide alleviated

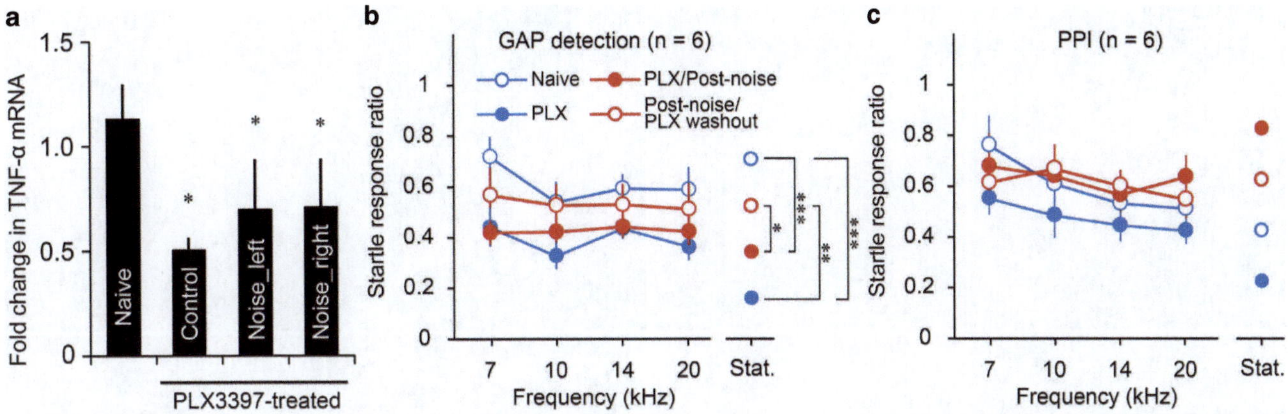

Fig. 22.2 Depleting microglia prevents noise trauma-induced TNF-α expression and behavioral evidence of tinnitus. (**a**) Treatment with PLX3397 suppressed the TNF-α mRNA level in AI and prevented noise-induced increases in TNF-α expression 12 hours after noise exposure. Control mice that had undergone PLX3397 treatment and sham exposure had a lower TNF-α mRNA level compared to naïve mice. In PLX 3397-treated mice, noise exposure did not significantly increase TNF-α expression in AI of either hemisphere. * indicates $p < 0.05$ compared to Naïve. (**b**) Behavioral evidence of tinnitus was evaluated with gap detection. Behavioral tests were conducted at four-time points: (1) before PLX 3397 treatment (Naïve); (2) after 21 days of PLX3397 treatment (PLX); (3) after noise exposure and still with PLX 3397 treatment (PLX/Post-noise); and (4) after 7 days of washout of PLX3397 (Post-noise/PLX washout). Microglial depletion improved basal level gap detection and prevented noise exposure-induced impairment in gap detection as observed in wild-type mice in Fig. 22.4b. *, ** and *** indicate $p < 0.05$, $p < 0.01$ and $p < 0.001$, respectively. (**c**) Animals' ability to hear tones, which was measured with prepulse inhibition (PPI), was not altered by PLX treatment or noise exposure (treatment effect, $p = 0.15$)

noise-induced tinnitus in mouse models assessed by a gap detection test and in a rat model assessed by a conditioned lick suppression test [62, 82]. Administration of TNF-α blockers also alleviated salicylate-induced tinnitus in mouse models [82, 83].

Diffusible Pro-Inflammatory Cytokines Increase the Risk of Tinnitus

In addition to hearing loss, several nonauditory pathologies and health conditions that are known to be associated with neuroinflammation can also increase the risk of tinnitus. For example, traumatic brain injury (TBI), which causes neuroinflammatory responses [35], increases the risk of tinnitus. The incidence of tinnitus is higher in military personnel with TBI compared to those without TBI [36]. Stress, which causes neuroinflammation in many brain regions [37, 38], is also a risk factor and modulator for tinnitus [39]. Depression and pain, which are not only mere comorbidities, but also risk factors of tinnitus [40–45], are also associated with neuroinflammation [46–48]. All these diverse nonauditory risk factors could potentially increase pro-inflammatory cytokine concentration in the cerebrospinal fluid [54–57], providing a diffusible signal to influence the function of the central auditory system. A recent study examined whether the infusion of recombinant TNF-α into the right lateral cerebral ventricle would increase the risk of tinnitus [58]. The report showed microglial activation in the auditory cortex and evidence of tinnitus in mice that had received both TNF-α infusion and exposure to an 86-dB noise, but not in mice that had received either TNF-α infusion or noise exposure alone. These results suggest that disease-related increases in brain pro-inflammatory cytokine release could be a risk factor for tinnitus (Fig. 22.3).

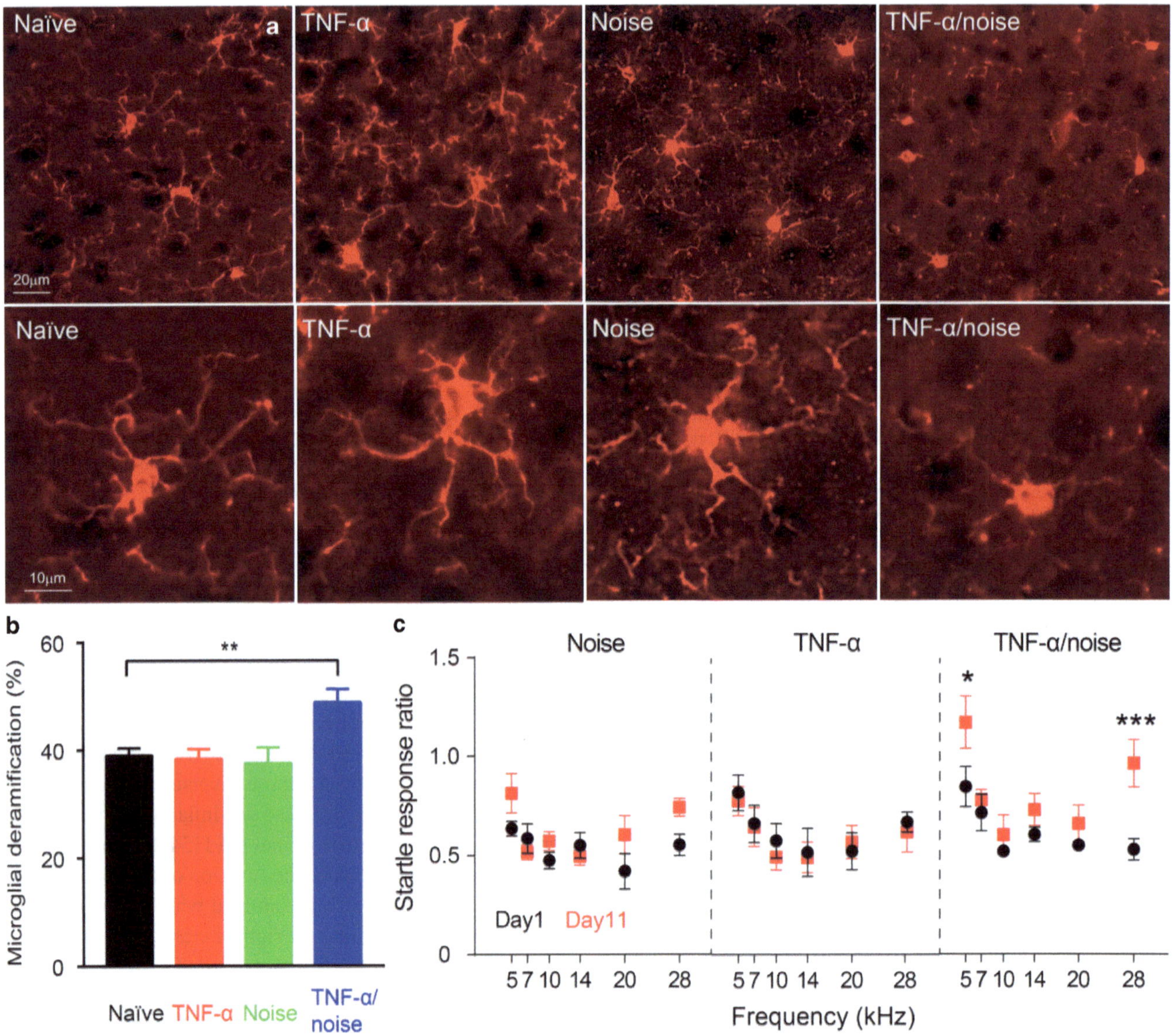

Fig. 22.3 TNF-α infusion and noise exposure synergistically induce microglial deramification and tinnitus. (**a**) Representative images of microglia stained with an IBA1 antibody. The bottom roll shows enlarged images of individual microglial cells. (**b**) Microglial deramification index was enhanced only in mice that had received both TNF-α infusion and exposure to a moderately loud noise at 86 dB SPL. (**c**) Animals' performances in gap detection before (Day 1) and after (Day 11) noise exposure (Noise), TNF-α infusion (TNF-α) and combined TNF-α infusion and noise exposure (TNF-α + Noise). Data are presented as mean ± SEM. * indicates $p < 0.05$, ** $p < 0.01$ and *** $p < 0.005$. Gap detection was impaired in mice that had received combined TNF-α infusion and noise exposure

Strain Differences in Noise-Induced Tinnitus Correlate with Neuroinflammation

Strain differences in immune and neuroinflammatory responses have been widely reported in common mouse strains [84–86]. For example, the C57BL/6 and the FVB strains exhibit different immune response profiles, with C57BL/6 mice being type 1 T helper cell-dominant (Th1-dominant) and FVB mice being Th2-dominant [87]. Th1 cells promote the secretion of pro-inflammatory cytokines, and Th2 cells promote the secretion of anti-inflammatory cytokines [88]. When challenged with experimentally induced stroke and reperfusion, the two strains showed different profiles of immune cell activation [89]. In addition, C57BL/6 mice displayed greater neurological and motor deficits from the stroke than FVB mice did [89]. Interestingly, strain differences were also reported between C57BL/6 and FVB mice in noise-induced neuroinflammation and tinnitus [90, 91]. Exposure to loud noises resulted in microglial deramification in the auditory cortex and behavioral evidence of tinnitus in C57BL/6 but not FVB mice (Fig. 22.4). These results suggest that genetic variability in immune response profiles contributes to differences in tinnitus susceptibility.

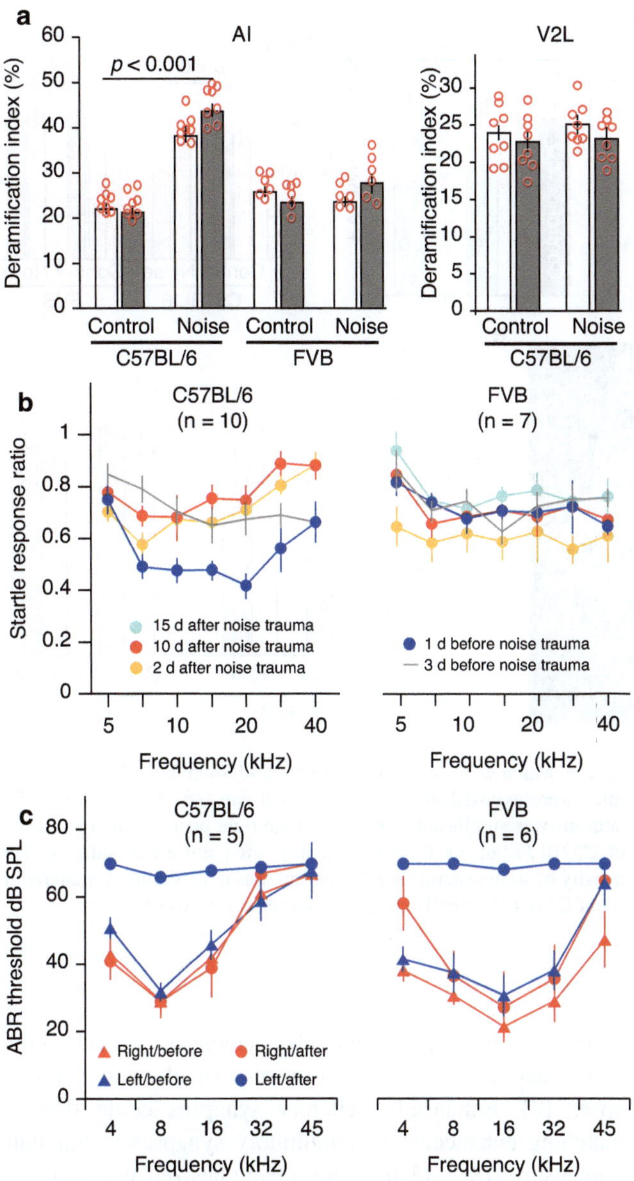

Fig. 22.4 Strain differences in noise trauma-induced microglial activation and tinnitus. (**a**) Microglial deramification was observed 5 days after noise trauma in C57BL/6 but not FVB mice. Noise trauma-induced microglial deramification was not observed in the lateral area of the secondary visual cortex (V2L), which is located dorsal to AI. (**b**) C57BL/6 mice exhibited gap detection deficit over a broad frequency range 2 and 10 days after noise trauma. The same noise trauma did not significantly alter gap detection performances in FVB mice 2, 10, and 15 days after the trauma. (**c**) Noise exposure produced similar levels of ABR threshold increases in C57BL/6 and FVB mice

Neuroinflammation in Noise-Induced Excitation-Inhibition Imbalance

Following noise trauma, excitatory synapses in the auditory cortex are strengthened and inhibitory synapses are weakened [8, 62]. This disruption of excitation–inhibition balance has been hypothesized as a mechanism underlying tinnitus. The pro-inflammatory cytokine TNF-α, which is upregulated after noise trauma, can strengthen excitatory synapses and weaken inhibitory synapses [18, 74–77]. A recent study investigated whether increased TNF-α expression is required for noise trauma-induced excitatory–inhibitory imbalance [62]. The report showed that blocking TNF-α expression by 3,6′-dithiothalidomide (dTT) prevented noise trauma-induced enhancement of excitatory synapse and weakening of inhibitory synapses, i.e., prevented noise trauma-induced excitation–inhibition imbalance (Fig. 22.5a, b). The homeostatic recovery of sensory-evoked auditory cortical responses following conductive hearing loss, which presumably involves an increase in synaptic excitation–inhibition ratio, also requires TNF-α [92].

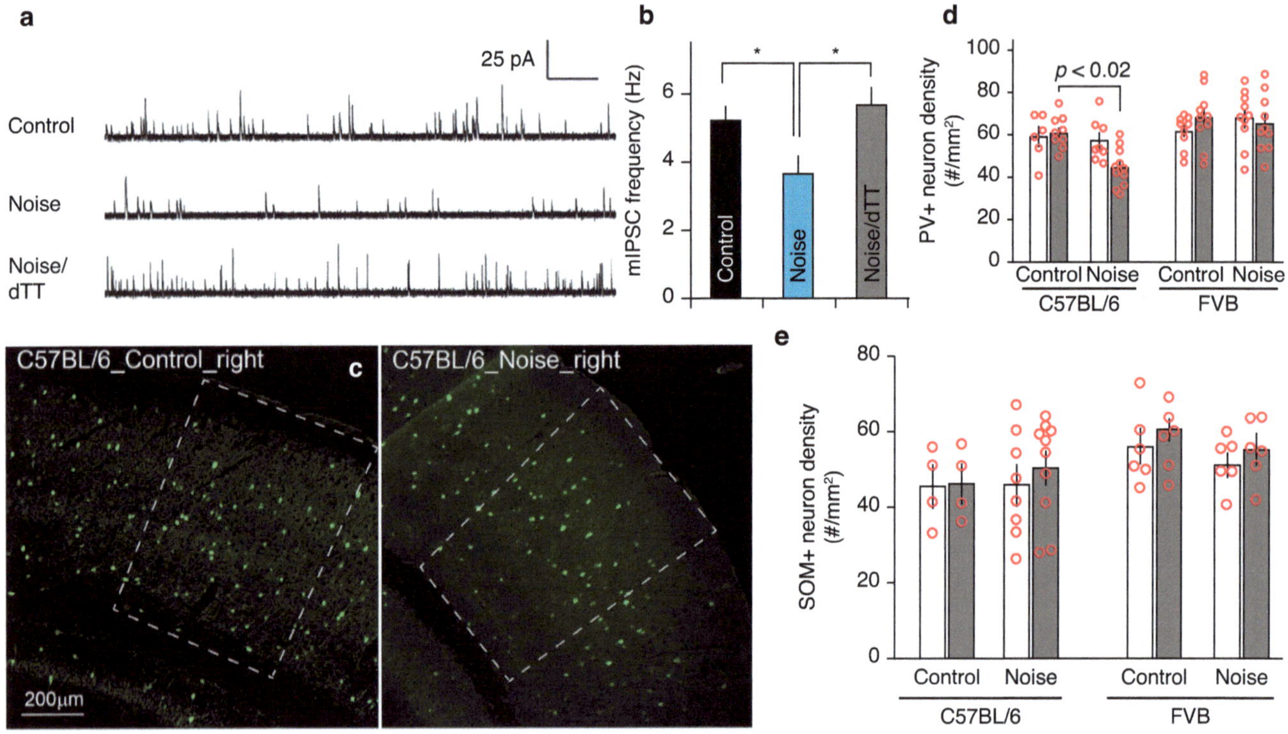

Fig. 22.5 Noise trauma results in neuroinflammation-dependent PV neuron loss in the auditory cortex. (**a**, **b**) Noise trauma weakened inhibitory synapses in the auditory cortex. Panel A shows example traces of miniature inhibitory postsynaptic current (mIPSC), and panel B shows that noise trauma resulted in reduced mIPSC frequency, which was prevented by dTT, a TNF-α blocker. * indicates $p < 0.05$. (**c**) Example images of PV neurons in the primary auditory cortex of the right hemisphere, which were delineated with white-dashed lines. Noise-exposed mice were exposed to noise in their left ears. (**d**) The density of PV neurons was significantly reduced in the right primary auditory cortex of C57BL/6 but not FVB mice 5 days after noise exposure. (**e**) The density of somatostatin (SOM) neurons was not significantly altered in AI of C57BL/6 or FVB mice 5 days after noise exposure

Neuroinflammation-Dependent PV Neuron Loss in Tinnitus

Although noise trauma both enhances excitatory synapses and weakens inhibitory synapses, evidence implicates the reduction of inhibitory tone as a major correlate of tinnitus [8, 15, 90, 93]. Enhancement of the excitatory synapses, which often transmit sensory input, may lead to an increase in sensory-driven responses. This could result in sensory map reorganization if the neurons with reduced sensory input enhance their latent responses to previously non-optimal stimuli. By contrast, a reduction of inhibition could lead to elevated excitability/spontaneous activity, possibly in addition to enhanced sensory-driven responses. It is conceivable that reduced inhibition may lead to tinnitus, which is the perception of sounds in the absence of external input, whereas enhanced excitation could result in hyperacusis, which is an increased sensitivity to external sound input. This notion was supported by evidence that tinnitus is correlated with reduced inhibitory synaptic function, but not sensory map reorganization [90]. Also, tinnitus in a rodent model was alleviated by an enhancement of cortical inhibitory synapses but not inhibition of cortical excitatory synapses [8]. Enhanced excitatory synapses could drive a matching enhancement of inhibitory synapses to maintain homeostasis [8], which has been hypothesized as a treatment of hearing loss-related tinnitus [94].

Noise trauma-induced tinnitus in rodent models has been correlated with reduced inhibitory tone in the auditory cortex [8, 90]. Different subtypes of inhibitory neurons are differentially impacted by noise trauma. For example, the density of PV neurons was reduced in the auditory cortex following noise trauma, whereas the density of somatostatin (SOM)-expressing inhibitory neurons was not altered (Fig. 22.5c–e) [91]. PV neurons account for 8–12% of neurons in the cortex [95, 96]. PV is a slow calcium buffer protein that regulates dynamic intracellular calcium concentration, which in turn influences membrane excitability and synaptic transmission [97]. PV neurons also have the unique expression of the KV3.1 potassium channel [98], whose fast channel kinetics contribute to the characteristic, fast-spiking phenotype of the PV neurons [99]. In addition, these neurons form inhibitory synapses onto the somas and axonal initial segments of cortical principal neurons to powerfully modulate the excitation–inhibition balance of the cortical network [100–104]. Dysfunction of PV neurons likely contributes to noise trauma-induced cortical excitation–inhibition imbalance.

Although the mechanisms underlying noise trauma-induced PV neuron loss are still unknown, some evidence implicates neuroinflammation as a potential player. Noise trauma-induced PV neuron loss was observed in the pro-inflammatory, Th1-dominant strain C57BL/6, but not the anti-inflammatory Th1-dominant strain FVB (Fig. 22.5d) [91]. In addition, intracerebroventricular infusion of the pro-inflammatory cytokine TNF-α lowered the threshold of noise-induced PV neuron loss to 87 dB SPL, which by itself does not cause PV neuron loss [58]. It should be noted that both the strain difference in noise trauma-induced PV neuron loss and the TNF-α-dependent PV neuron loss were correlated with behavioral evidence of tinnitus in rodent models (Figs. 22.3 and 22.4) [58, 90, 91]. Furthermore, chemogenetic activation of cortical PV neurons alleviated noise trauma-induced behavioral evidence of tinnitus [105].

A Neuroinflammation Model of Tinnitus

Based on recent development in animal and human research, we propose a neuroinflammation model of tinnitus. In this model, neuroinflammation in the central auditory pathway is triggered by noise trauma, hearing loss, and other neuroinflammation-related brain disorders and health conditions. Neuroinflammation in the central auditory system results in an excitation–inhibition imbalance by enhancing excitatory synapses, weakening inhibitory synapses, and increasing membrane excitability. The disrupted excitation–inhibition balance is an underlying mechanism for tinnitus. Different neuroinflammation-related circuit changes are being investigated for their contributions to tinnitus. Initial evidence implicates PV neuron dysfunction in tinnitus. The role of neuroinflammation in tinnitus is only beginning to be understood. The model proposed here will undoubtedly be revised as we gain new insights into how neuroinflammation in the central auditory pathway is initiated, sustained, and modulated, how neuroinflammation alters neural circuits, and what circuit deficits give rise to the phantom sound perception.

References

1. Henry JA, Dennis KC, Schechter MA. General review of tinnitus: prevalence, mechanisms, effects, and management. J Speech Lang Hear Res. 2005;48(5):1204–35.
2. Langguth B, et al. Tinnitus: causes and clinical management. Lancet Neurol. 2013;12(9):920–30.
3. Salvi RJ, Wang J, Ding D. Auditory plasticity and hyperactivity following cochlear damage. Hear Res. 2000;147(1–2):261–74.
4. Eggermont JJ, Roberts LE. The neuroscience of tinnitus. Trends Neurosci. 2004;27(11):676–82.
5. Heffner HE, Koay G. Tinnitus and hearing loss in hamsters (Mesocricetus auratus) exposed to loud sound. Behav Neurosci. 2005;119(3):734–42.
6. Elgoyhen AB, Langguth B. Pharmacological approaches to the treatment of tinnitus. Drug Discov Today. 2010;15(7–8):300–5.
7. Shore SE, Roberts LE, Langguth B. Maladaptive plasticity in tinnitus—triggers, mechanisms and treatment. Nat Rev Neurol. 2016;12(3):150–60.
8. Yang S, et al. Homeostatic plasticity drives tinnitus perception in an animal model. Proc Natl Acad Sci U S A. 2011;108(36):14974–9.
9. Li S, Choi V, Tzounopoulos T. Pathogenic plasticity of Kv7.2/3 channel activity is essential for the induction of tinnitus. Proc Natl Acad Sci U S A. 2013;110(24):9980–5.
10. Li S, Kalappa BI, Tzounopoulos T. Noise-induced plasticity of KCNQ2/3 and HCN channels underlies vulnerability and resilience to tinnitus. elife. 2015;4:4.
11. Kotak VC, et al. Hearing loss raises excitability in the auditory cortex. J Neurosci. 2005;25(15):3908–18.
12. Abbott SD, et al. Detection of glutamate decarboxylase isoforms in rat inferior colliculus following acoustic exposure. Neuroscience. 1999;93(4):1375–81.
13. Milbrandt JC, et al. GAD levels and muscimol binding in rat inferior colliculus following acoustic trauma. Hear Res. 2000;147(1–2):251–60.
14. Browne CJ, Morley JW, Parsons CH. Tracking the expression of excitatory and inhibitory neurotransmission-related proteins and neuroplasticity markers after noise induced hearing loss. PLoS One. 2012;7(3):e33272.
15. Llano DA, Turner J, Caspary DM. Diminished cortical inhibition in an aging mouse model of chronic tinnitus. J Neurosci. 2012;32(46):16141–8.
16. Engineer ND, et al. Reversing pathological neural activity using targeted plasticity. Nature. 2011;470(7332):101–4.
17. Yang S, Su W, Bao S. Long-term, but not transient, threshold shifts alter the morphology and increase the excitability of cortical pyramidal neurons. J Neurophysiol. 2012;108(6):1567–74.
18. Stellwagen D, et al. Differential regulation of AMPA receptor and GABA receptor trafficking by tumor necrosis factor-alpha. J Neurosci. 2005;25(12):3219–28.
19. Sturm JJ, et al. Noise trauma-induced behavioral gap detection deficits correlate with reorganization of excitatory and inhibitory local circuits in the inferior colliculus and are prevented by acoustic enrichment. J Neurosci. 2017;37(26):6314–30.
20. Krauss P, et al. Stochastic resonance controlled upregulation of internal noise after hearing loss as a putative cause of tinnitus-related neuronal hyperactivity. Front Neurosci. 2016;10:597.
21. Roberts LE, et al. Ringing ears: the neuroscience of tinnitus. J Neurosci. 2010;30(45):14972–9.
22. Langguth B, Salvi R, Elgoyhen AB. Emerging pharmacotherapy of tinnitus. Expert Opin Emerg Drugs. 2009;14(4):687–702.
23. Weber C, et al. Impact of a relaxation training on psychometric and immunologic parameters in tinnitus sufferers. J Psychosom Res. 2002;52(1):29–33.
24. Demir M. Does inflammation play a role in the pathophysiology of tinnitus? Niger J Clin Pract. 2021;24(2):199–204.
25. Haider HF, et al. Tinnitus, hearing loss and inflammatory processes in an older Portuguese population. Int J Audiol. 2020;59(5):323–32.
26. Roth J, et al. Signaling the brain in systemic inflammation: role of sensory circumventricular organs. Front Biosci. 2004;9:290–300.
27. Banks WA. Blood-brain barrier transport of cytokines: a mechanism for neuropathology. Curr Pharm Des. 2005;11(8):973–84.

28. Gutierrez EG, Banks WA, Kastin AJ. Murine tumor necrosis factor alpha is transported from blood to brain in the mouse. J Neuroimmunol. 1993;47(2):169–76.
29. Yang G, et al. Peripheral elevation of TNF-alpha leads to early synaptic abnormalities in the mouse somatosensory cortex in experimental autoimmune encephalomyelitis. Proc Natl Acad Sci U S A. 2013;110(25):10306–11.
30. Marchiori LLM, et al. Association between polymorphism of tumor necrosis factor alpha (TNF-alpha) in the region −308 g/a with tinnitus in the elderly with a history of occupational noise exposure. Noise Health. 2018;20(93):37–41.
31. Doi MY, et al. Association between polymorphism of interleukin-6 in the region -174G/C and tinnitus in the elderly with a history of occupational noise exposure. Noise Health. 2015;17(79):406–10.
32. Marchiori LLM, et al. Interleukin-1 alpha gene polymorphism (IL-1alpha) and susceptibility to tinnitus in the elderly. Noise Health. 2019;21(99):77–82.
33. Xie C, et al. Genome-wide association study identifies new loci associated with noise-induced tinnitus in Chinese populations. BMC Genom Data. 2021;22(1):31.
34. Schubert NMA, et al. A retrospective cross-sectional study on tinnitus prevalence and disease associations in the Dutch population-based cohort lifelines. Hear Res. 2021;411:108355.
35. Simon DW, et al. The far-reaching scope of neuroinflammation after traumatic brain injury. Nat Rev Neurol. 2017;13(3):171–91.
36. Lew HL, et al. Auditory dysfunction in traumatic brain injury. J Rehabil Res Dev. 2007;44(7):921–8.
37. Calcia MA, et al. Stress and neuroinflammation: a systematic review of the effects of stress on microglia and the implications for mental illness. Psychopharmacology. 2016;233(9):1637–50.
38. Grippo AJ, Scotti MA. Stress and neuroinflammation. Mod Trends Pharmacopsychiatry. 2013;28:20–32.
39. Mazurek B, Szczepek AJ, Hebert S. Stress and tinnitus. HNO. 2015;63(4):258–65.
40. Isaacson JE, et al. Clinical associations between tinnitus and chronic pain. Otolaryngol Head Neck Surg. 2003;128(5):706–10.
41. Walker AK, et al. Neuroinflammation and comorbidity of pain and depression. Pharmacol Rev. 2014;66(1):80–101.
42. Wright EF, Gullickson DC. Dental pulpalgia contributing to bilateral preauricular pain and tinnitus. J Orofac Pain. 1996;10(2):166–8.
43. Durai M, Searchfield G. Anxiety and depression, personality traits relevant to tinnitus: a scoping review. Int J Audiol. 2016;55(11):605–15.
44. Langguth B, et al. Tinnitus and depression. World J Biol Psychiatry. 2011;12(7):489–500.
45. Popeo DM, Tobias KG, Kellner CH. Tinnitus as a symptom of psychotic depression successfully treated with electroconvulsive therapy. J ECT. 2011;27(1):e7–8.
46. DeLeo JA, Yezierski RP. The role of neuroinflammation and neuroimmune activation in persistent pain. Pain. 2001;90(1–2):1–6.
47. Ellis A, Bennett DL. Neuroinflammation and the generation of neuropathic pain. Br J Anaesth. 2013;111(1):26–37.
48. Kiguchi N, Kobayashi Y, Kishioka S. Chemokines and cytokines in neuroinflammation leading to neuropathic pain. Curr Opin Pharmacol. 2012;12(1):55–61.
49. Dolberg D, Schaaf H, Hesse G. Tinnitus in primarily schizophrenic patients. HNO. 2008;56(7):719–26.
50. Nam EC. Is it necessary to differentiate tinnitus from auditory hallucination in schizophrenic patients? J Laryngol Otol. 2005;119(5):352–5.
51. Muller N, et al. The role of inflammation in schizophrenia. Front Neurosci. 2015;9:372.
52. Danesh AA, et al. Tinnitus and hyperacusis in autism spectrum disorders with emphasis on high functioning individuals diagnosed with Asperger's syndrome. Int J Pediatr Otorhinolaryngol. 2015;79(10):1683–8.
53. El-Ansary A, Al-Ayadhi L. Neuroinflammation in autism spectrum disorders. J Neuroinflammation. 2012;9:265.
54. Bianchi M, et al. Increased tumor necrosis factor-alpha and prostaglandin E2 concentrations in the cerebrospinal fluid of rats with inflammatory hyperalgesia: the effects of analgesic drugs. Anesth Analg. 2007;104(4):949–54.
55. Levine J, et al. Cerebrospinal cytokine levels in patients with acute depression. Neuropsychobiology. 1999;40(4):171–6.
56. Lerman I, et al. Posttraumatic stress disorder influences the nociceptive and intrathecal cytokine response to a painful stimulus in combat veterans. Psychoneuroendocrinology. 2016;73:99–108.
57. Juengst SB, et al. Exploratory associations with tumor necrosis factor-alpha, disinhibition and suicidal endorsement after traumatic brain injury. Brain Behav Immun. 2014;41:134–43.
58. Deng D, Wang W, Bao S. Diffusible tumor necrosis factor-alpha (TNF-α) promotes noise-induced parvalbumin-positive (PV+) neuron loss and auditory processing impairments. Front Neurosci. 2020;14:573047.
59. Fuentes-Santamaria V, et al. Glia-related mechanisms in the anteroventral cochlear nucleus of the adult rat in response to unilateral conductive hearing loss. Front Neurosci. 2014;8:319.
60. Baizer JS, et al. Effects of acoustic trauma on the auditory system of the rat: the role of microglia. Neuroscience. 2015;303:299–311.
61. Fuentes-Santamaria V, et al. The role of glia in the peripheral and central auditory system following noise overexposure: contribution of TNF-alpha and IL-1beta to the pathogenesis of hearing loss. Front Neuroanat. 2017;11:9.
62. Wang W, et al. Neuroinflammation mediates noise-induced synaptic imbalance and tinnitus in rodent models. PLoS Biol. 2019;17(6):e3000307.
63. Ziebell JM, Morganti-Kossmann MC. Involvement of pro- and anti-inflammatory cytokines and chemokines in the pathophysiology of traumatic brain injury. Neurotherapeutics. 2010;7(1):22–30.
64. Donat CK, et al. Microglial activation in traumatic brain injury. Front Aging Neurosci. 2017;9:208.
65. Dang DK, et al. Apocynin prevents mitochondrial burdens, microglial activation, and pro-apoptosis induced by a toxic dose of methamphetamine in the striatum of mice via inhibition of p47phox activation by ERK. J Neuroinflammation. 2016;13:12.
66. Hovens IB, et al. Postoperative cognitive dysfunction and microglial activation in associated brain regions in old rats. Neurobiol Learn Mem. 2015;118:74–9.
67. Xia C, et al. Neuroglial activation in the auditory cortex and medial geniculate body of salicylate-induced tinnitus rats. Am J Transl Res. 2020;12(10):6043–59.
68. Chen XH, Zheng LL. Expression of pro-inflammatory cytokines in the auditory cortex of rats with salicylate-induced tinnitus. Mol Med Rep. 2017;16(4):5643–8.
69. Hwang JH, et al. Expression of tumor necrosis factor-alpha and interleukin-1beta genes in the cochlea and inferior colliculus in salicylate-induced tinnitus. J Neuroinflammation. 2011;8:30.
70. Hu SS, et al. Effects of salicylate on the inflammatory genes expression and synaptic ultrastructure in the cochlear nucleus of rats. Inflammation. 2014;37(2):365–73.
71. Wolf SA, Boddeke HW, Kettenmann H. Microglia in physiology and disease. Annu Rev Physiol. 2017;79:619–43.
72. Salter MW, Beggs S. Sublime microglia: expanding roles for the guardians of the CNS. Cell. 2014;158(1):15–24.

73. Allen NJ, Barres BA. Signaling between glia and neurons: focus on synaptic plasticity. Curr Opin Neurobiol. 2005;15(5):542–8.
74. Di Filippo M, et al. Neuroinflammation and synaptic plasticity: theoretical basis for a novel, immune-centred, therapeutic approach to neurological disorders. Trends Pharmacol Sci. 2008;29(8):402–12.
75. Stellwagen D, Malenka RC. Synaptic scaling mediated by glial TNF-alpha. Nature. 2006;440(7087):1054–9.
76. Steinmetz CC, Turrigiano GG. Tumor necrosis factor-alpha signaling maintains the ability of cortical synapses to express synaptic scaling. J Neurosci. 2010;30(44):14685–90.
77. Bellinger FP, Madamba S, Siggins GR. Interleukin 1 beta inhibits synaptic strength and long-term potentiation in the rat CA1 hippocampus. Brain Res. 1993;628(1–2):227–34.
78. Qu W, et al. Inhibition of colony-stimulating factor 1 receptor early in disease ameliorates motor deficits in SCA1 mice. J Neuroinflammation. 2017;14(1):107.
79. Cuccarese MF, et al. Heterogeneity of macrophage infiltration and therapeutic response in lung carcinoma revealed by 3D organ imaging. Nat Commun. 2017;8:14293.
80. Spiller KJ, et al. Microglia-mediated recovery from ALS-relevant motor neuron degeneration in a mouse model of TDP-43 proteinopathy. Nat Neurosci. 2018;21(3):329–40.
81. Butowski N, et al. Orally administered colony stimulating factor 1 receptor inhibitor PLX3397 in recurrent glioblastoma: an ivy Foundation early phase clinical trials consortium phase II study. Neuro Oncol. 2016;18(4):557–64.
82. Gonzalez-Gonzalez S, Cazevieille C. 3,6'-Dithiothalidomide reduces tinnitus phenotype in two different mouse preclinical models of tinnitus. J Community Prev Med. 2020;3(1):1–8.
83. Hwang JH, et al. Effects of tumor necrosis factor blocker on salicylate-induced tinnitus in mice. Int Tinnitus J. 2017;21(1):24–9.
84. Browne CA, et al. Differential lipopolysaccharide-induced immune alterations in the hippocampus of two mouse strains: effects of stress. Neuroscience. 2012;225:237–48.
85. Perez CJ, et al. Several classical mouse inbred strains, including DBA/2, NOD/Lt, FVB/N, and SJL/J, carry a putative loss-of-function allele of Gpr84. J Hered. 2013;104(4):565–71.
86. Tacchini-Cottier F, et al. An immunomodulatory function for neutrophils during the induction of a CD4+ Th2 response in BALB/c mice infected with Leishmania major. J Immunol. 2000;165(5):2628–36.
87. Whitehead GS, et al. Allergen-induced airway disease is mouse strain dependent. Am J Physiol Lung Cell Mol Physiol. 2003;285(1):L32–42.
88. Arumugam TV, Granger DN, Mattson MP. Stroke and T-cells. NeuroMolecular Med. 2005;7(3):229–42.
89. Kim HA, et al. Brain immune cell composition and functional outcome after cerebral ischemia: comparison of two mouse strains. Front Cell Neurosci. 2014;8:365.
90. Miyakawa A, et al. Tinnitus correlates with downregulation of cortical glutamate decarboxylase 65 expression but not auditory cortical map reorganization. J Neurosci. 2019;39(50):9989–10001.
91. Zinsmaier AK, et al. Resistance to noise-induced GAP detection impairment in FVB mice is correlated with reduced Neuroinflammatory response and Parvalbumin neuron loss. Sci Rep. 2020;10:20445.
92. Teichert M, et al. Homeostatic plasticity and synaptic scaling in the adult mouse auditory cortex. Sci Rep. 2017;7(1):17423.
93. Deng D, et al. Increasing endogenous activity of NMDARs on GABAergic neurons increases inhibition, alters sensory processing and prevents noise-induced tinnitus. Sci Rep. 2020;10(1):11969.
94. Yang S, Bao S. Homeostatic mechanisms and treatment of tinnitus. Restor Neurol Neurosci. 2013;31(2):99–108.
95. Hu H, Gan J, Jonas P. Interneurons. Fast-spiking, parvalbumin(+) GABAergic interneurons: from cellular design to microcircuit function. Science. 2014;345(6196):1255263.
96. Fogaca MV, Duman RS. Cortical GABAergic dysfunction in stress and depression: new insights for therapeutic interventions. Front Cell Neurosci. 2019;13:87.
97. Orduz D, et al. Parvalbumin tunes spike-timing and efferent short-term plasticity in striatal fast spiking interneurons. J Physiol. 2013;591(13):3215–32.
98. Chow A, et al. K(+) channel expression distinguishes subpopulations of parvalbumin- and somatostatin-containing neocortical interneurons. J Neurosci. 1999;19(21):9332–45.
99. Erisir A, et al. Function of specific K(+) channels in sustained high-frequency firing of fast-spiking neocortical interneurons. J Neurophysiol. 1999;82(5):2476–89.
100. Moore AK, Wehr M. Parvalbumin-expressing inhibitory interneurons in auditory cortex are well-tuned for frequency. J Neurosci. 2013;33(34):13713–23.
101. Cruikshank SJ, et al. Pathway-specific feedforward circuits between thalamus and neocortex revealed by selective optical stimulation of axons. Neuron. 2010;65(2):230–45.
102. Kubota Y, et al. The diversity of cortical inhibitory synapses. Front Neural Circuits. 2016;10:27.
103. Moore AK, et al. Rapid rebalancing of excitation and inhibition by cortical circuitry. Neuron. 2018;97(6):1341–1355 e6.
104. Ferguson BR, Gao WJ. PV Interneurons: critical regulators of E/I balance for prefrontal cortex-dependent behavior and psychiatric disorders. Front Neural Circuits. 2018;12:37.
105. Masri S, et al. Chemogenetic activation of cortical parvalbumin-positive Interneurons reverses noise-induced impairments in gap detection. J Neurosci. 2021;41:8848.

Part IV

Animal Research for Tinnitus

Animal Models of Hyperacusis: Neural Hyperactivity in Auditory, Emotional, Arousal, Memory, and Motor Networks

23

Richard Salvi, Guang-Di Chen, Xiaopeng Liu, Ben Auerbach, Dalian Ding, Yu-Chen Chen, and Senthilvelan Manohar

Abstract

High doses of salicylate, the active ingredient in aspirin, are ototoxic resulting in behavioral evidence of tinnitus and hyperacusis and electrophysiological increases in auditory thresholds of 20–25 dB at the auditory nerve (AN), cochlear nucleus (CN), inferior colliculus (IC), medial geniculate body (MGB), and auditory cortex (AC). High doses of salicylate reduce suprathreshold neural response by more than 60% at the AN (hypoactivity). However, suprathreshold responses are progressively amplified as neural responses are relayed from CN, to IC, MGB, and AC so that suprathreshold neural responses are enhanced nearly 100% at the AC (hyperactivity). Remarkably, high-dose salicylate also enhances suprathreshold sound-evoked responses in brain regions outside the classical auditory pathway in brain regions involved with emotion (amygdala), memory and spatial navigation (hippocampus), arousal (reticular formation), and motor coordination and tinnitus gating (parafloccular lobe of cerebellum). Functional magnetic resonance imaging and connectome network analysis revealed increased functional connectivity of AC, MGB, and IC with the amygdala, hippocampus, reticular formation and parafloccular lobe of the cerebellum, structures that link and embellish auditory perceptual activity to other brain regions involved with memory, spatial navigation, emotion, arousal, motor coordination, and tinnitus. Tinnitus and hyperacusis likely have their origins in a complex neural network involving both auditory and non-auditory brain regions.

R. Salvi (✉) · G.-D. Chen · X. Liu · B. Auerbach · D. Ding · S. Manohar
Center for Hearing and Deafness, 137 Cary Hall, University at Buffalo, Buffalo, NY, USA
e-mail: salvi@buffalo.edu; xpliu369@illinois.edu; bda5@illinois.edu; dding@buffalo.edu

Y.-C. Chen
Department of Radiology, Nanjing First Hospital, Nanjing Medical University, Nanjing, China

W. Schlee et al. (eds.), *Textbook of Tinnitus*, https://doi.org/10.1007/978-3-031-35647-6_23

Graphical Abstract

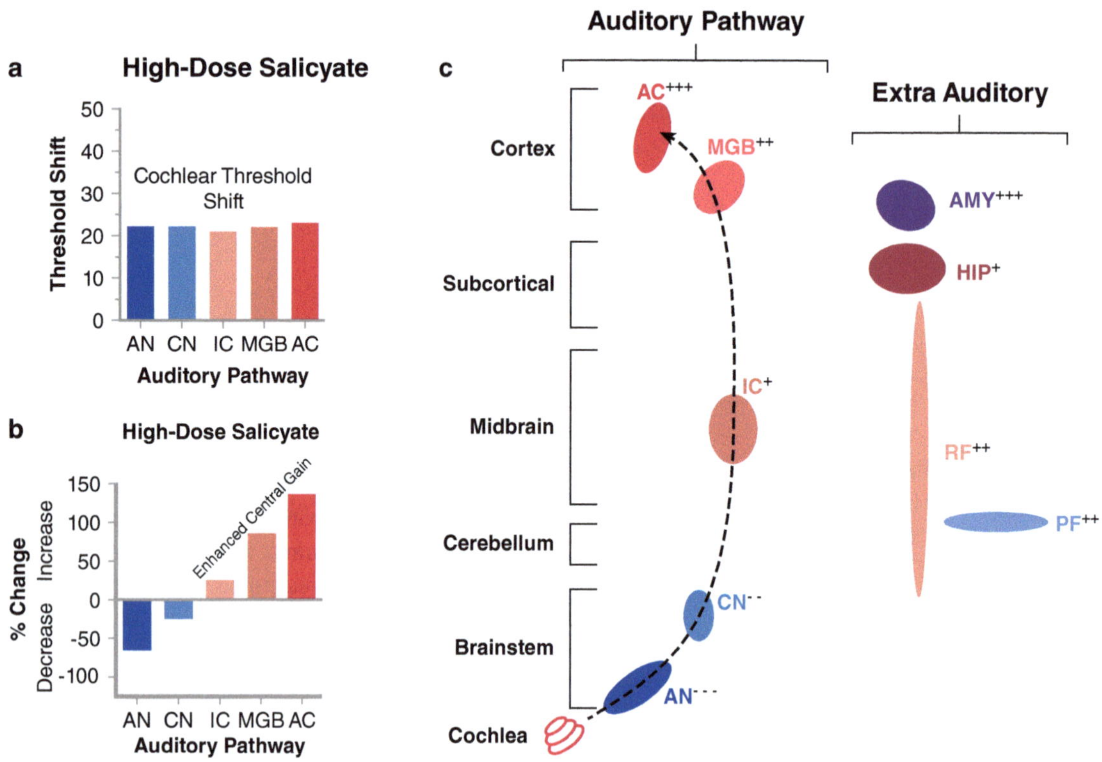

(a) High-dose salicylate elevates auditory thresholds approximately 20–25 dB at all levels of the peripheral (AN) and central auditory pathway (CN, IC, MGB, and AC). (b) Salicylate reduces suprathreshold, sound-evoked responses more than 60% in the auditory periphery (AN), but enhances responses in higher auditory centers. (c) Schematic shows connectome model of salicylate-induced hyperacusis and sound-evoked neural hyperactivity. Up arrows next to text identifies brain regions where suprathreshold sound-evoked activity increased (up arrows = hyperactivity) or decreased (down arrows = hypoactivity). In the classical auditory pathway (blue-red color gradient), suprathreshold sound-evoked activity greatly depressed in cochlea and slightly depressed in the cochlear nucleus (down blue arrows) and slightly enhanced in inferior colliculus and greatly enhanced in medial geniculate body and auditory cortex (up red arrows). Brain regions outside the classical auditory pathway where suprathreshold sound-evoked activity was enhanced (as indicated by up arrows) by salicylate included the amygdala (emotional valence), hippocampus (memory, spatial localization), reticular formation (arousal area) and paraflocular lobe of cerebellum (motor coordination, tinnitus gating).

Abbreviations

AC	Auditory cortex
AN	Auditory nerve
ASD	Autism spectrum disorder
CAP	Compound action potential
CN	Cochlear nucleus
IC	Inferior colliculus
HPA	Hypothalamic–pituitary–adrenal
KO	Knockout
MGB	Medial geniculate body (MGB)
ULL	Uncomfortable loudness level
WT	Wild type

Highlights

- Noise, salicylate, and genetic models of loudness and avoidance hyperacusis.
- Reaction time–intensity function assessment of loudness hyperacusis and recruitment.
- Sound aversion assessment with active sound avoidance paradigm.
- Salicylate-induced hyperacusis linked to hyperactivity in auditory and emotional centers.
- Hyperacusis associated with increased corticosterone stress hormone.
- Hyperacusis-hyperactive auditory, emotional, arousal, memory, and motor planning network.

Introduction

At its core, hyperacusis is a loudness intolerance disorder that can manifest in different ways [1]. The most common and widely recognized form is loudness hyperacusis characterized by uncomfortable loudness levels (ULL) that are far below the typical 100 dB SPL ULL of normal listeners [2]. A less common, but more debilitating type is pain hyperacusis, a condition in which sounds are not only perceived as excessively loud, but which evoke painful sensations around the ear and face. The sound levels needed to evoke these painful sensations are far below the typical aural threshold of pain which occurs around 120–130 dB SPL [3]. Annoyance hyperacusis is another type which has been defined as a persistent negative emotional reaction to sounds that induce anxiety or tension. Finally, fear hyperacusis is manifested by behaviors aimed at avoiding situation where loud sounds might occur.

Prevalence

The prevalence of hyperacusis obtained from various surveys ranges from 8–15% (please see also Chap.4). Hyperacusis is more common in females than males and its prevalence increases with age [4–7]. Hyperacusis is often associated with tinnitus and hearing loss. Among patients whose primary complaint is hyperacusis, the prevalence of tinnitus is as high as 86% [7, 8]. Among those whose primary complaint was tinnitus, approximately 40% also reported hyperacusis [9]. However, the percentage of tinnitus patients with hyperacusis may be much higher because many tinnitus patients are unaware that they are intolerant of loud sounds [10].

Comorbidities

Although hyperacusis is primarily considered an audiological disorder, it is associated with a broad spectrum of neurological and genetic disorders (please see also the Chaps. 5 and 42). Hyperacusis is associated with several pain-related disorders such as fibromyalgia, migraine, pain associated with temporomandibular disorders, and complex regional pain syndrome [7, 11, 12]. Mechanical and nociceptive circuits in multisensory regions of the nervous system can become sensitized resulting in hyperactive responses to weak inputs from touch, temperature, and auditory and mechanical stimulation. Imaging studies of subjects with pain-related temporomandibular disorders show unexpected activation of auditory cortex, the amygdala, an emotional area, and cingulate cortex in response to innocuous touch stimulation [11]. Hyperacusis is associated with several neurological disorders such as multiple sclerosis [13], herpes zoster [14], neuropathies [15], and dementia [16]. Individuals with genetic disorders such as autism [17, 18] and Williams syndrome frequently suffer from hyperacusis [19, 20]. When viewed in this large context, hyperacusis is not simply an auditory problem, but rather a complex neurological disorder that likely results from aberrant neural activity in many different parts of the central nervous system.

Animal Behavioral Models of Hyperacusis

A detailed understanding of the biological mechanisms that give rise to hyperacusis would benefit from the development of animal behavioral models which recapitulate many of the core features associated with hyperacusis such as the avoidance, fear, anxiety, arousal, loudness intolerance, and sound-evoked pain. Over that past decade, a number animal models have been developed that recapitulate some of the features of loudness growth and hyperacusis as described in recent review [21]. In order to accurately assess hyperacusis in an animal model, objective behavioral readouts of the testing paradigm must correlate with an animal's subjective experience of loudness intolerance or sound-evoked pain, fear, annoyance, or avoidance (please see also Chap.24 for a general overview of animal models).Loudness is the subjective experience that is most closely related to the acoustic measure of sound pressure level, i.e., loudness increases with sound pressure level (please see also the Chaps. 3 and 41 on hyperacusis in humans). However, the subjective experience of loudness is affected by many other acoustic variables such as frequency, stimulus bandwidth, stimulus duration, stimulus rise time, binaural versus monaural presentation, and background noise (i.e., masker) [22–26] Sounds can also evoke pain, fear, and anxiety. Acoustic stimuli can acquire emotional significance, for example, when a sound is paired with positive (i.e., food) or negative (e.g., foot shock) reinforcement administered in a particular environment (e.g., dentist office). In such cases, neutral environments or situations can acquire a positive or negative valence [27, 28]. The negative emotions and stress associated with auditory stimulation can act on emotional and memory centers in the brain such as the amygdala and hippocampus which in turn can lead to the release of stress hormones that can disrupt the hypothalamic–pituitary–adrenal (HPA) axis [29, 30] and influence neural activity in the auditory pathway [31, 32].

Enhanced Acoustic Startle Reflex Amplitude and Hyperacusis

The acoustic startle reflex is a short-latency, robust motoric response that is elicited by the onset of an acoustic stimulus with a short rise time [33, 34]. The muscle stiffening, which occurs during the startle reflex, represents a rapid protective response mediated primarily by a brainstem network comprised of the auditory nerve, cochlear nerve root neurons, giant neurons in the caudal pontine reticular nucleus, and the reticulospinal motor neurons [35] although some have suggested a contribution from neurons in the cochlear nucleus [36, 37]. Because the startle reflex is mainly driven by neural circuits in the auditory, arousal, and motor circuits in the brainstem, with some top-down influence, conditions that enhance or depress startle responses amplitudes largely reflect functional changes in the periphery and may not accurately represent all the neural elements that give rise to all forms of hyperacusis. The amplitude of the startle reflex is much larger for binaural stimulation than monaural stimulation, evidence of binaural summation [35]. Similarly, neurons in the caudal pontine reticular nucleus response more robustly to binaural than monaural stimulation.The amplitude of the acoustic startle reflex evoked by the startle stimulus has been used to infer the presence of hyperacusis in cases where the amplitude of the response has increased significantly above the normal amplitude [38]. For example, high doses of salicylate, the active ingredient in aspirin, which induces cochlear hearing loss and tinnitus, cause a temporary increase in startle amplitudes at intensities above 90 dB SPL. Startle reflex amplitudes return to normal several days after drug washout [39–41]. Increased startle reflex amplitudes have also been observed after some noise exposures [38, 42] and with age-related hearing loss [43]. The main advantage of using startle reflex amplitudes to screen for hyperacusis is that the startle reflex is an innate response that does not require any training. However, the method has some disadvantages and limitations. Relatively high sound levels (≥90 dB SPL) are needed to test for the presence of enhanced startle response. Therefore, it is not possible to test for hyperacusis at lower intensities. The amplitude of the startle reflex is reduced in animals with significant unilateral hearing loss limiting the ability to test for hyperacusis in the opposite intact ear [44, 45]. However, startle amplitudes appear to be enhanced in animals with moderate thresholds (50–70 dB SPL), but not in those with thresholds above 70 dB SPL [38]. In addition, the amplitude of the acoustic startle response depends on acoustic and environmental factors [27, 38].

Loudness Recruitment and Hyperacusis Measured by Reaction Time–Intensity Function

Reaction time has been used to assess the brightness and loudness of visual and auditory stimuli in humans and animals for many years [46–49]. In humans, reaction time has been shown to decrease in a systematic manner as intensity increases [50]. Reaction time estimates of loudness are also in good agreement with loudness values estimated by magnitude estimation [47]. Auditory reaction time has also been used to develop equal loudness contours and estimate the loudness of acoustic stimuli in several different species including rats [49, 51–53]. Reaction time measures of loudness perception recapitulate the main features of loudness perception in humans. For example, the loudness of a sound increases with stimulus duration (i.e., temporal integration of loudness) and loudness grows with increasing bandwidth of the stimulus (i.e., spectral integration of loudness) [22, 54, 55]. Based on these results, it is clear that reaction time–intensity functions provide a powerful tool for detecting changes in loudness growth associated with background masking noise, loudness recruitment, and hyperacusis [54, 56, 57]. In subjects with cochlear hearing loss and loudness recruitment, reaction times are longer than normal at low intensities, but as intensity increases, reaction times recovers to normal at high intensities. However, in subjects with hyperacusis, reaction times are shorter than normal at moderate to high intensities. Hyperacusis-like reaction time–intensity functions have been observed in canaries with a hereditary, high-frequency permanent hearing loss [52].

High doses of salicylate have long been known to cause a temporary cochlear hearing loss and to reliably induce tinnitus in human and animals [58–61]. The drug also increases acoustic startle reflex amplitudes at intensities greater than 90 dB SPL [41] suggesting that it might also disrupt reaction time–intensity function of loudness growth. Radziwon carefully addressed these issues by measuring reaction time–intensity functions with tone bursts and noise bursts before and after treating rats with wide range of salicylate doses (50 to 300 mg/kg) [62, 63]. Baseline reaction time–

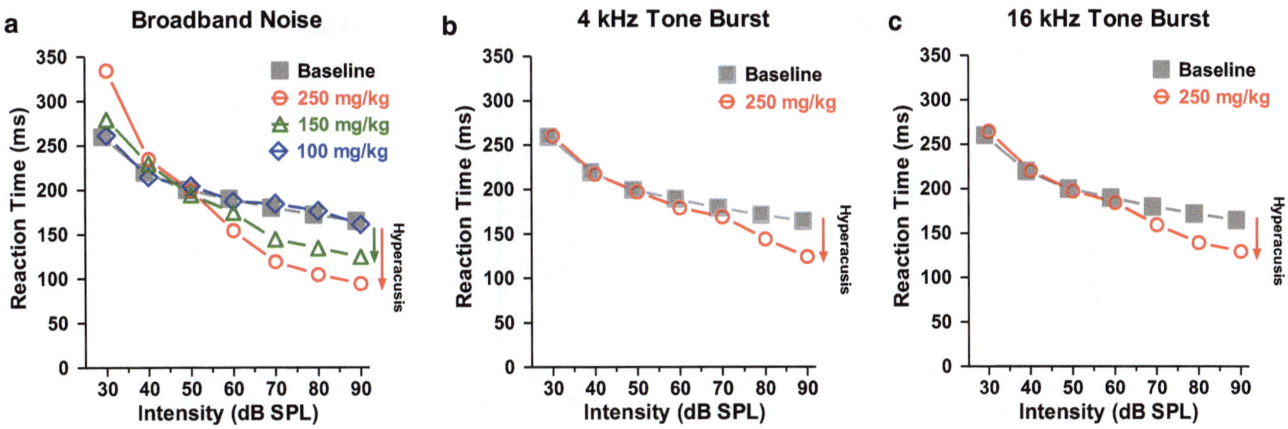

Fig. 23.1 Schematic of reaction time–intensity function pre- and post-salicylate. (**a**) Reaction time–intensity functions measured with broadband noise at baseline and after 250, 150, or 100 mg/kg treatment with sodium salicylate. Reaction times from 70–90 dB SPL are much shorter than baseline after treatment with 250 and 150 mg/kg sodium salicylate, behavior indicative of hyperacusis. Reaction times at 30 dB SPL following the 250 mg/kg dose were longer than baseline due to a hearing loss of ~20 dB. Reaction times after treatment with 100 mg/kg were similar to baseline. Reaction time–intensity functions for (**b**) 4 kHz tone burst and (**c**) 16 kHz tone bursts during baseline and after treatment with 250 mg/kg of sodium salicylate. After salicylate treatment, reaction times were shorter than baseline at 80 and 90 dB SPL, behavior consistent with hyperacusis

intensity functions were used to estimate loudness growth for broadband noise bursts from 30 to 90 dB SPL. Reaction time decreased in an orderly manner as the intensity of the broadband noise increased (Fig. 23.1a). The reaction time–intensity function was unchanged when rats were treated with 50 or 100 mg/kg of salicylate. However, when the dose was increased to 150 mg/kg, the reaction times evoked by 70 to 90 dB SPL noise bursts were shorter than normal indicating that these intensities were perceived as louder than normal. Reaction times were largely unchanged at lower intensities. When the dose of salicylate was increased to 250 mg/kg or higher, the reaction time at 30 dB SPL became longer than normal indicating that it was perceived as quieter than normal. This increase in reaction time at 30 dB SPL was attributed to the ~20 dB drug-induced hearing loss which "pushed" the 30 dB SPL stimulus close to the threshold of hearing. As intensity increased, reaction time decreased rapidly and became shorter than normal from 60–90 dB SPL, behaviors indicative of loudness hyperacusis. Reaction time–intensity functions were also measured with tone bursts to identify potential frequency-dependent effects of salicylate on hyperacusis behavior (Fig. 23.1b–c). Following treatment with 250 mg/kg of salicylate, reaction times became shorter than normal at intensities from 80 to 90 dB SPL, whereas reaction times were similar to baseline at lower intensities. Salicylate doses equal to or greater than 150 mg/kg consistently induced hyperacusis; these are the same doses that cause hearing loss and tinnitus [59, 62, 64]. Hyperacusis was induced over a broad range of frequencies consistent with the fact that salicylate induces hearing loss across the full audiometric range.

Intense noise exposures have long been known to induce loudness recruitment at frequencies located in the region of hearing loss [53, 65, 66], but there have been few reports of noise-induced hyperacusis. A recent study reported that intense, long-duration noise exposure (102 dB SPL, 16–20 kHz) induced both loudness recruitment and hyperacusis. Loudness recruitment was exclusively present during the long-duration noise exposure. Two months after the noise exposure, loudness recruitment was still present in the region of maximum hearing loss around 20 kHz (Fig. 23.2a); however, hyperacusis emerged at frequencies below the region of maximum hearing loss [67]. Hyperacusis was present at 16 kHz, a frequency near the low-frequency edge of the hearing loss (Fig. 23.2b); reaction times were shorter than normal at intensities from 70 to 90 dB SPL. Thresholds remained normal at 4 kHz after the high-frequency noise exposure. Interestingly, reaction times were shorter than normal at intensities between 30 and 90 dB SPL (Fig. 23.2c). Thus, hyperacusis emerged several months after the exposure, but only at low frequencies below the region of hearing loss. In this study, hyperacusis had a spectral profile which differs from the broad spectrum hyperacusis reported in other studies [52, 68]. A major advantage of using the reaction time–intensity technique is that it can detect loudness hyperacusis over a range of intensities (Fig. 23.2c), at intensities far below that are possible using the startle reflex. In addition, many of the acoustic variables can be manipulated to assess the effect of stimulus frequency, duration, and bandwidth on loudness perception and hyperacusis [54]. A disadvantage of the reaction time method is that it takes considerable time to train and test animals.

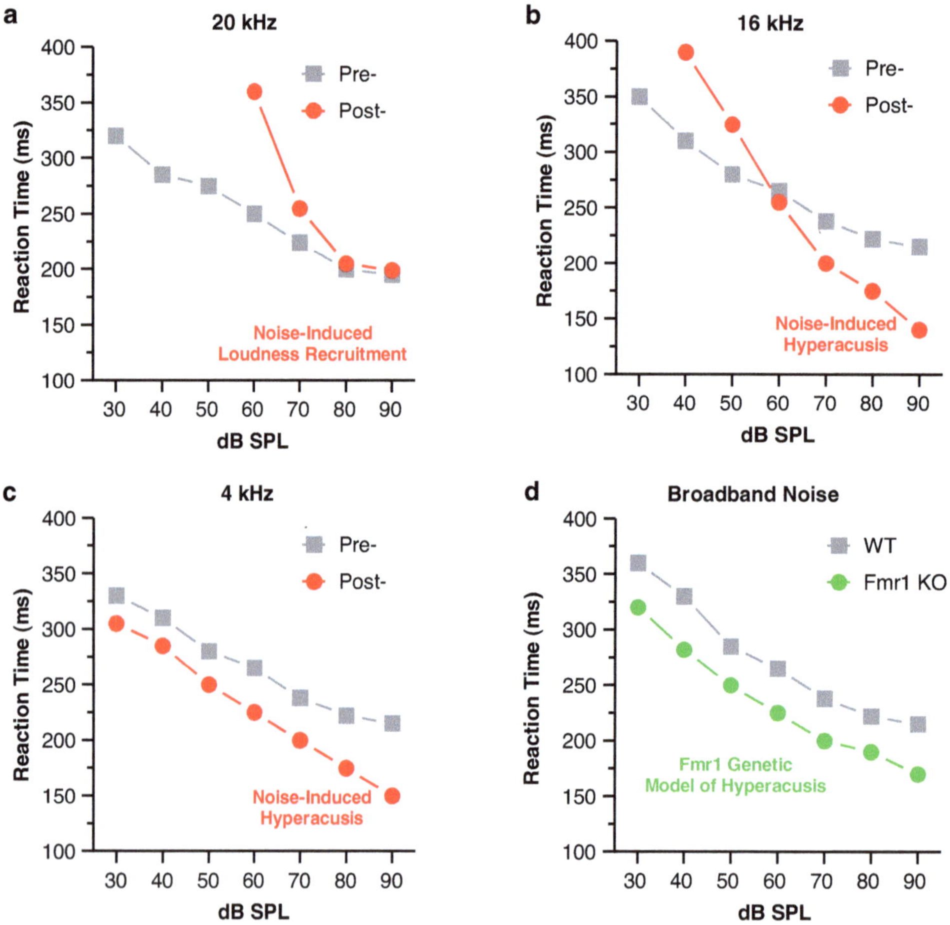

Fig. 23.2 Schematics of reaction time–intensity functions measured in rats with noise-induced high-frequency hearing loss pre- and post-exposure (**a–c**). (**a**) Post-exposure reaction time–intensity function in region of significant hearing loss (20 kHz). Post-exposure reaction time–intensity function exhibits loudness recruitment features. Note post-exposure reaction times at 80–90 dB SPL equal pre-exposure reaction times. (**b**) The post-exposure reaction time–intensity function at 16 kHz, near the low-frequency edge of the high-frequency hearing loss. Reaction times were longer than normal at low intensities due to the hearing loss. However, reaction times were much shorter than normal at high intensities indicating that the sounds were perceived as louder than normal indicative of hyperacusis. (**c**) Post-exposure reaction time–intensity function at 4 kHz, a frequency where hearing thresholds were normal. Reaction times were shorter than normal over a broad range of intensities, behaviors indicative of loudness hyperacusis at intensities from ~50 to 90 dB SPL. (**d**) Schematic of reaction time–intensity functions measured with broadband noise in normal wild-type (WT) rat and in an Fmr1 knockout (KO) rat model of autism spectrum disorder. Reaction times were shorter in Fmr1 KO rats than normal WT at all intensities

Loudness Intolerance in a Fragile X Animal Model of Autism

Auditory hypersensitivity is one of the most common and debilitating features of autism spectrum disorder (ASD) [69]. In an ASD case study, ULLs and reaction time–intensity functions were measured at 1 and 4 kHz in a single subject with ASD [52]. ULLs in the ASD subject were approximately 20 lower than those in a normal hearing control subject. Reaction times at 1 and 4 kHz were much shorter in the ASD subject than the normal control subject over a broad range of intensities; these reaction time differences were greater at 4 kHz than 1 kHz. These results suggest that reaction time–intensity measures of loudness growth might be useful to test for loudness intolerance disorders in an animal model of ASD.

Fragile X syndrome (FX) is the leading inherited causes of ASD and several animal models of FX have been developed. These animal models could provide new insights on the biological bases of auditory hypersensitivity disorders provided that one can demonstrate that an FX animal model shows behavioral evidence of loudness hyperacusis. To address this issue, preliminary reaction time–intensity functions were measured in normal wild-type (WT) rats and *Fmr1* knockout (KO) rats, an animal model that exhibits many of the core pathophysiological features of ASD [70, 71]. *Fmr1* KO rats exhibited shorter reaction times than WT rats across a wide range of sound intensities (Fig. 23.2d). The shorter reaction times in *Fmr1* KO rats could not be accounted for by differences in learning, task performance, generalized hyperactivity, or abnormal motor activity. These results suggest that Fmr1 KO rats exhibit loudness hyperacusis over a wide range of intensities consistent with the sensory hypersensitivity disorders seen ASD. This compelling auditory phenotypic behavior could be used to screen for drugs that reverse sensory hypersensitivity disorders, determine the neural correlates of loudness hyperacusis, and identify genetic and biological variables that contribute to hyperacusis.

Active Sound Avoidance Paradigm and Avoidance Hyperacusis

Hyperacusis has considerable phenotypic diversity [1, 72]. One form of hyperacusis is characterized by behaviors that involve avoiding or escaping from sounds perceived as aversive, dangerous, anxiety-provoking, or annoying. To evaluate this more complex form of hyperacusis, an active sound avoidance paradigm (ASAP) was developed in which rats were acoustically "driven out" of a comfortable enclosure to one that they naturally disliked [73]. The ASAP apparatus consists of a brightly illuminated arena connected to dark, sound-attenuating enclosure equipped with a loudspeaker through which sounds of various intensities can be presented. Rats have a natural aversion of bright open spaces and prefer to stay in a dark enclosure [74]. Therefore, when normal hearing rats are tested on the dark/light apparatus, they spent more than 90% of the time in the dark chamber during the no-stimulus (NS) condition (Fig. 23.3a). However, when a 2–8 kHz low-frequency noise is presented through the loudspeaker to the dark chamber, the normal hearing rats spend progressively less time in the dark chamber as the noise level is increased from 60 to 90 dB SPL presumably because the noise is perceived as annoying, aversive, or fear-evoking.

To determine if noise-induced hearing loss would affect sound avoidance behavior, the rats were exposed to a 16–20 kHz noise presented at 102 dB SPL for 4 weeks in order to induce a permanent high-frequency hearing loss of approximately 50 dB SPL at 16 and 32 kHz while retaining normal low-frequency hearing (Fig. 23.3b) [73]. The rats with high-frequency hearing loss were then retested on the ASAP paradigm. During the no-stimulus condition, the rats with high-frequency hearing loss continued to spend more than 90% of the time in the dark chamber (Fig. 23.3a). However, when the 2–8 kHz noise was presented at 60 and 90 dB SPL, the high-frequency hearing loss rats spent considerably less time in the dark box than when their hearing was normal (Fig. 23.3a). These results suggest that after the rats developed a high-frequency hearing loss, they now perceived the 2–8 kHz low-frequency noise as more annoying, aversive, or fearful than when their hearing was normal.

Humans with ASD and Williams syndrome exhibit a range of sensory processing disorders and often perceive auditory stimuli as aversive, annoying, or anxiety-provoking [75, 76]. To determine if Fmr1 KO rats would perceive broadband noise as aversive, preliminary studies were carried with WT and Fmr1 KO rats to assess sound aversion with ASAP. During the no-stimulus condition, both normal

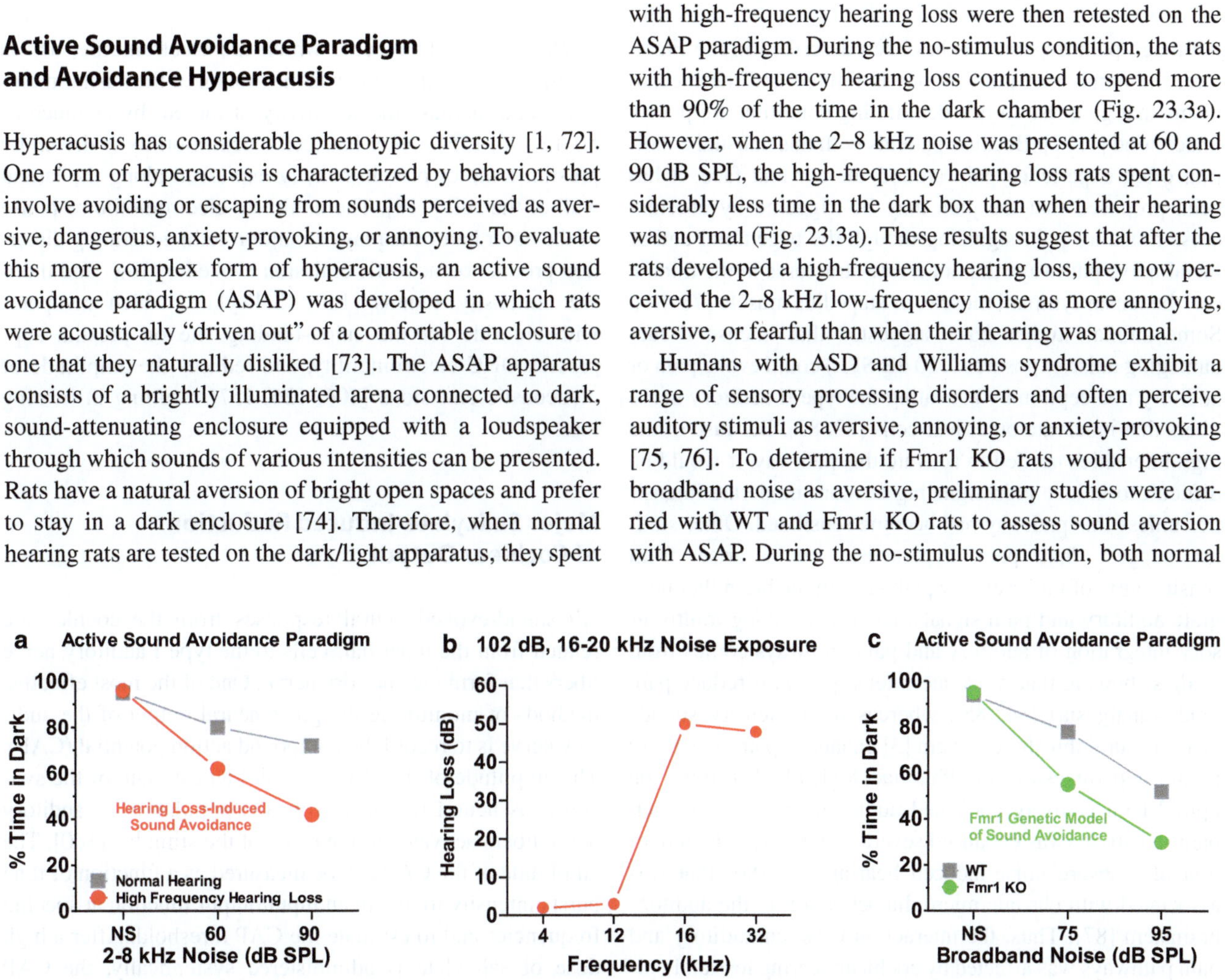

Fig. 23.3 (**a**) Schematic illustrating results of the active sound avoidance paradigm (ASAP) before and after rats develop a high-frequency noise-induced hearing loss. In the no-stimulus (NS) condition, normal hearing rats spend more than 90% of the time in the dark box. As the intensity of the low frequency 2–8 kHz noise stimulus presented through the loudspeaker is increased from 60 to 90 dB SPL, normal hearing loss spend progressively less time in the dark box. (**b**) Rats exposed to noise develop a high-frequency hearing loss at 16–20 kHz. The rats with noise-induced high-frequency hearing loss spend less time in the dark box as the low-frequency noise stimulus is increased from 60 to 90 dB SPL. The high-frequency hearing loss did not affect the percent time spent in the dark box for the NS condition. (**c**) Schematic comparing active sound avoidance in Fmr1 KO rats compared to normal WT rats. Both Fmr1 KO and WT rats spent equal amount of time in the dark on NS trials indicating that both genotypes found the brightly open arena equally aversive. However, when broadband noise was presented at 60 and 90 dB, the Fmr1 KO rats spent less time in the dark than WT rats indicating that the KO rats found the sounds more aversive than WT rats

WT and Fmr1 KO rats spent approximately 93% of the time in the dark chamber indicating that both genotypes found the brightly illuminated arena equally aversive. However, when broadband noise was introduced into the dark chamber, the Fmr1 KO rats spent significantly less time in the dark than WT rats at 60 and 90 dB SPL (Fig. 23.3c). These preliminary studies suggest that the Fmr1 KO rats perceive the noise as more annoying, aversive, or anxiety-provoking than normal WT rats.

Pain Hyperacusis Interaction of Auditory and Pain Pathways

Although pain hyperacusis has been described in the literature, the number of publications is limited and the mechanisms that give rise to this debilitating condition are poorly understood [1, 77]. Because patients with this unusual condition often experience pain around the ear and face, it has been proposed that the pain may be triggered by aberrant cross-modality pain signaling though the trigeminal and/or facial nerve pathways that innervate structures in the middle ear, the tensor tympani muscle, or stapedius muscle [78–81]. Some animal studies have suggested that intense tissue-damaging noise exposures (120 dB SPL) could evoke pain or auditory nociception by activating the type II auditory nerve fibers that innervate outer hair cells [82, 83]. Because of the high intensities needed to activate this pathway, it would be difficult to induce pain signaling at more moderate intensities unless this pathway had become sensitized. Other studies suggest that pain hyperacusis could arise from sensitization of multisensory pathways in the brain that integrate auditory and pain signals. Evidence linking multisensory integration of auditory and pain pathways comes from studies showing that moderate-intensity sounds reduce pain (audio-analgesia) [84, 85], whereas high-intensity sounds near the aural threshold of pain [3] enhanced pain sensitivity (audio-hyperalgesia) [86]. Pharmacologically disrupting the opioid pain pathway abolished audio-analgesia. Moreover, pain sensitivity was enhanced several weeks after the induction of a severe noise-induced hearing loss [86] that was associated with chronic microglia activation in the auditory brainstem [87]. Thus, the interaction between auditory and pain pathways was affected by cochlear hearing loss and opioid pain signaling.

Neural Correlates of Hyperacusis

The development of animal behavioral models of hyperacusis has made it possible to investigate the neural correlates of hyperacusis at multiple sites along the central auditory pathway. Sound-evoked neural responses increase with intensity in much the same way as loudness perception does. Therefore, it is reasonable to assume that loudness hyperacusis is caused by excessive sound-evoked neural activity to moderate and intense sounds. Because high-dose salicylate is one of the most reliable methods of inducing hyperacusis, it has been used extensively to study the biological mechanism that gives rise to hyperacusis. Salicylate readily crosses the blood–brain barrier [88, 89]; therefore, it is capable of disrupting sound-evoked neural activity in the cochlea as well as the central nervous system as described below.

Otoacoustic Emissions Suppressed by Salicylate

Cochlear outer hair cells, which are electromotile, act as tuned amplifiers that enhance the motion of the basilar membrane and increase the sensitivity of the ear by as much as 50 dB [90, 155]. Outer hair cell electromotility is driven by prestin, a motor protein heavily expressed along the lateral wall of the cell [118]. The nonlinear electromotile response of the outer hair cells plays a major role in generating distortion product otoacoustic emission evoked by low- and moderate-intensity sounds [130]. Salicylate, which competes with chloride for the anion-binding site on prestin, suppresses OHC electromotility, and reduces the amplitude of otoacoustic emissions [106, 126, 157] resulting in hearing loss.

Major Salicylate-Induced Reduction of Cochlear Output

All sound-evoked neural responses from the cochlea are related from the inner hair cells to the type I auditory nerve fibers that form the auditory nerve. One of the most effective methods of monitoring the gross neural output of the auditory nerve is to record the compound action potential (CAP). The amplitude of the CAP provides an estimate of the synchronous neural response from the population of auditory nerve fibers activated to the onset of the stimulus [100]. The amplitude of the CAP can be measured as a function of tone bursts intensity to obtain an input/output function at specific frequencies and to estimate the CAP threshold. After a high dose of salicylate is administered systemically, the CAP threshold increases approximately 20 dB, reflected in a rightward shift of the input/output function at low intensities (Fig. 23.4a, horizontal arrow). The slope of the post-salicylate input/output function is much shallower than baseline and the maximum amplitude of the post-salicylate response is reduced by more than 60% relative to baseline (down arrow, Fig. 23.4a). Changes similar to this occur across a broad range of frequencies. The large reduction in the output of the cochlea cannot account for salicylate-induced hyperacusis.

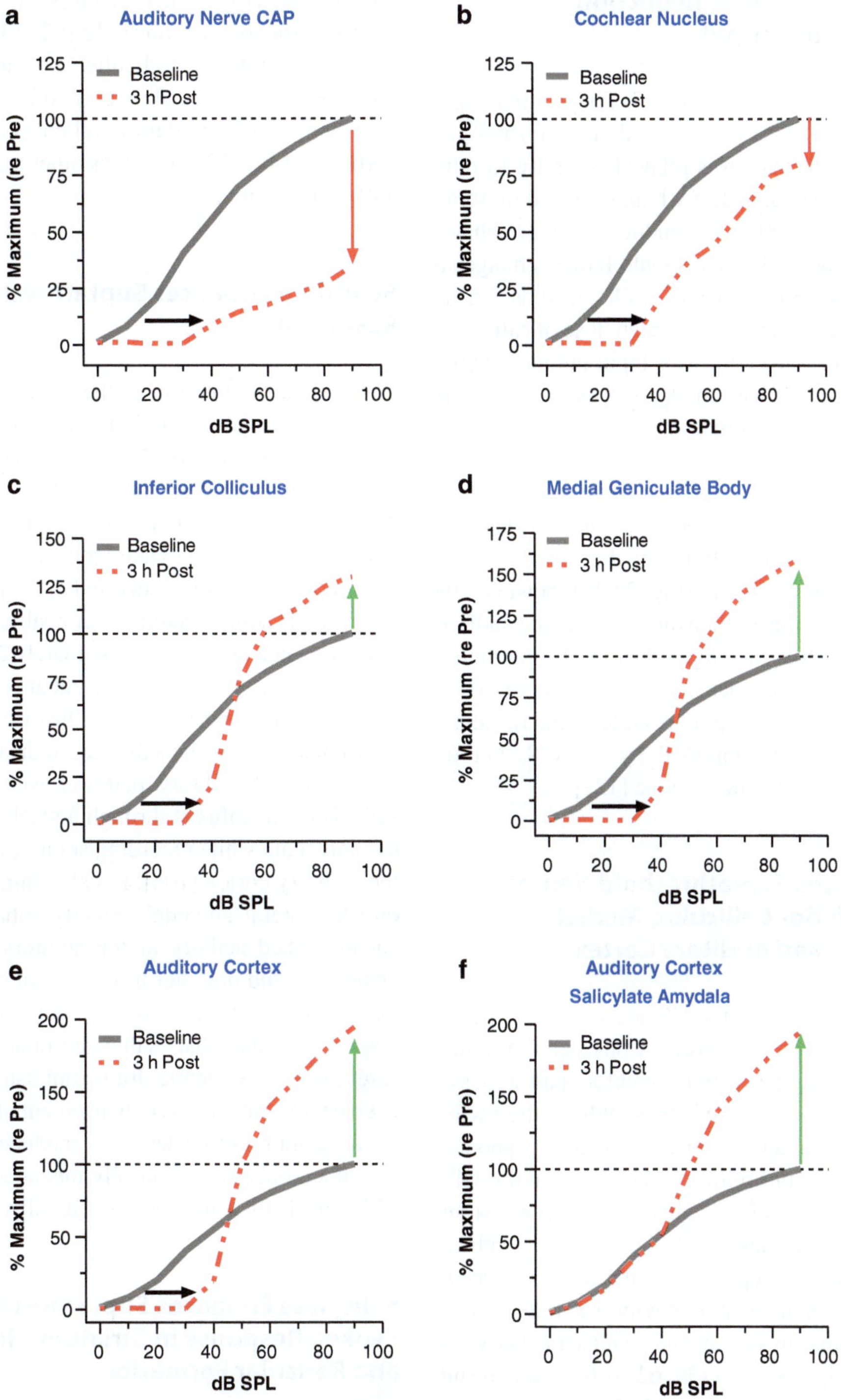

Fig. 23.4 Schematics of neural input/output functions from different levels of the auditory pathway at baseline and approximately 3-h following treatment with a high dose of salicylate administered systemically (**a–e**) or after salicylate was infused locally into the amygdala (**f**). Ordinate scaled at % of maximum baseline amplitude at 90 dB SPL (dashed horizon line at 100%). (**a**) Schematic of auditory nerve compound action potential (CAP) input/output functions. Post-exposure input/output function at low intensities shifted to the right about 20 dB (20 threshold shift, black horizontal arrow). Note large decrease in suprathreshold amplitude (down red arrow). (**b**) Schematic of cochlear nucleus input/output function at baseline and 3-h post-salicylate. Note 20 dB salicylate-induced threshold shift (horizontal black line) similar to auditory nerve. Post-salicylate response amplitudes in cochlear nucleus were significantly less than baseline (down red arrow), but the reductions were much less in the cochlear nucleus than in the auditory nerve. Schematics of (**c**) inferior colliculus, (**d**) medial geniculate body, and (**e**) auditory cortex input/output functions at baseline and 3-h post-salicylate. Note 20 dB salicylate-induced threshold shift (horizontal black line) similar to auditory nerve. Post-salicylate response amplitudes in the inferior colliculus, medial geniculate body, and auditory cortex were larger than baseline (up, blue arrow). (**f**) Schematics of auditory cortex input/output functions at baseline and 3-h after salicylate was infused into the amygdala. Local infusion of salicylate into amygdala significantly increased suprathreshold response in the auditory cortex, but unlike systemic administration, it did not cause a threshold shift

Modest Salicylate-Induced Reduction in Cochlear Nucleus Output

The neural output of the auditory nerve is relayed to the ipsilateral cochlear nuclei (CN) where it undergoes further processing before the information is relayed centrally to other ipsilateral and contralateral auditory brainstem and midbrain nuclei [103, 160, 168, 178]. If the auditory system behaved as a linear system, then salicylate should induce changes in CN input/output functions that are similar to those in the auditory nerve. After administering a high dose of salicylate, the low-intensity portion of the CN input/output function was shifted to the right of baseline by approximately 20 dB (Fig. 23.4b). Thus, the magnitude of the salicylate-induced threshold shift in the CN was nearly identical to the CAP threshold shift suggesting that the hearing loss (i.e., threshold shift) in the CN was inherited from the cochlea. The suprathreshold response amplitudes in the CN were also reduced after salicylate treatment (Fig. 23.4b); however, the reductions were much smaller than those seen in the auditory nerve due to the fact that the slope of the CN input/output function was much steeper than the auditory nerve. These results indicate that the weak suprathreshold neural responses leaving the cochlea were amplified by the CN, but the responses were still well below baseline [121].

Salicylate Enhances Suprathreshold Neural Responses in Inferior Colliculus, Medial Geniculate Body, and Auditory Cortex

The neural responses leaving the CN are relayed to higher levels of the central auditory pathway. Consistent with measurements made at lower levels of the auditory pathway, systemic salicylate treatment caused thresholds in the medial geniculate body and auditory cortex to increase approximately 20 dB. These results reinforce the view that the salicylate-induced threshold shifts originate in the cochlea and are inherited by higher levels of the auditory pathway (Fig. 23.4c–e). However, suprathreshold responses became progressively larger as the neural activity was relayed from the inferior colliculus, to the medial geniculate body and then the auditory (Fig. 23.4c–e) [39, 62, 166]. These results are generally in good agreement with functional imaging studies which show enhanced sound-evoked activity in the inferior colliculus and auditory cortex [174]. Taken together, these results indicate that each successive stage of the auditory pathway from the cochlear nucleus to the auditory cortex appears to provide a small amount of amplification so that by the time the signal reaches the auditory cortex the neural output is much larger than normal. This serial amplification process can be thought of as the "central auditory amplifier" which boosts suprathreshold neural activity as opposed to the so-called outer hair cell "cochlear amplifier" which enhances the neural output of the cochlea to low-intensity sound near threshold [92, 139]. The hyperactivity observed in inferior colliculus and medial geniculate body could be due to descending corticofugal circuits which modulate activity in the inferior colliculus and medial geniculate body [93, 144, 173] as well as other areas such as the amygdala and striatum.

Salicylate Enhances Suprathreshold Amygdala Response

The amygdala, a region of the brain that assigns emotional valence to sensory stimuli, has neuroanatomical connections with several region within the auditory pathway such as the medial geniculate body and auditory cortex [99, 102, 128]. Neurons in the lateral amygdala respond to sound [98, 113] and high dose of salicylate increase the expression of c-fos immunolabeling in the amygdala [171]. After a high dose of salicylate is administered systemically, thresholds in the lateral amygdala increase approximately 20 dB, whereas suprathreshold response are greatly enhanced similar to that seen in the medial geniculate and auditory cortex [105].

To determine if the salicylate-induced changes occurring in the central auditory pathway were mediated centrally, salicylate was infused through a small cannula directly into the amygdala while recording sound-evoked responses from the auditory cortex [104]. Local administration of salicylate into the lateral amygdala greatly enhanced suprathreshold sound-evoked activity in the auditory cortex (Fig. 23.4f); however, it did not alter thresholds or the low-intensity portion of the auditory cortex input/output function. These results indicate that salicylate-induced threshold shifts resulting from systemic drug administration originate in the cochlea. In contrast, the enhancement of sound-evoked activity at suprathreshold levels is mediated centrally, possibly due to a reduction in centrally mediated inhibition [41, 154, 172, 176, 180] or increased excitability [125, 177].

Salicylate Enhances Suprathreshold Sound-Evoked Response in Striatum, Hippocampus, and Reticular Formation

The auditory pathway conveys acoustic information to many other parts of the brain where information from other sensory, motor, cognitive, and emotional information is integrated in order to interpret and respond to events in the external environment as well as internal conditions. The striatum receives acoustic information from the auditory cortex and thalamus and integrates this information with expected reward outcomes to drive motor behaviors [97, 115, 148]. Neuroanatomical studies have revealed that high-dose salicylate increases the expression of c-fos expression in many brain regions such as the striatum, a motor control region that regulates vocal output [162, 170, 171]. When high-dose salicylate was administered systemically, sound-evoked thresholds in the striatum increased approximately 20 dB due to the cochlear hearing loss. However, suprathreshold sound-evoked responses became larger than normal [105]. It is unclear if the hyperactivity results from a direct effect of salicylate on the striatum and/or an indirect effect mediated by hyperactivity in the auditory cortex relayed back to the striatum by descending corticofugal circuits [144].

The hippocampus, an integrative center involved in memory and spatial navigation [140, 165] has been implicated in clinical studies of hyperacusis [120, 149]. Sensory inputs from the auditory system contribute to short- and long-term memory and aid in spatial navigation [110, 127, 142, 143, 152]. Because cochlear hearing loss disrupts memory and spatial navigation [111, 131, 136], salicylate was expected to induce hyperactivity in the hippocampus. Salicylate elevated sound-evoked thresholds in the hippocampus approximately 20 dB, consistent with results from the cochlea, whereas suprathreshold sound-evoked responses in the hippocampus were greatly enhanced similar to that seen in higher auditory center [105].

Salicylate-Induced Hyperactivity in Reticular Formation and Cerebellum

There is growing recognition that hyperacusis arises from neural hyperactivity in a network that extends to brain regions linked to arousal and anxiety, such as the reticular formation [124, 135]. Neurons in the caudal pontine reticular nucleus form part of the neural circuit responsible for the acoustic startle reflex. Neurons in the caudal pontine nucleus have relatively high thresholds similar to intensities needed to elicit the startle reflex. High doses of salicylate enhance the amplitude of the acoustic startle reflex, one of the behavioral measures used to infer hyperacusis [38, 41, 105]. Consistent with these behavioral results, salicylate also enhanced the suprathreshold firing rates of caudal pontine reticular neurons 10 ms or more after stimulus onset [107]. The salicylate-induced hyperactivity in these reticular neuron was minimal at short interstimulus intervals (<1 s), but hyperactivity increased significantly as the interstimulus interval increased. The effect of interstimulus interval on these reticular neurons is similar to that seen for the startle reflex [129, 151].

The cerebellum, which integrates sensory information from many parts of the body, plays a major roles fine-tuning head and arm motor activity and coordinating head and eye movement [150, 153]. Selective regions of the paraflocculus lobe of the cerebellum, however, also respond to acoustic stimulation [94, 132] and recent studies suggest it may be involved in the generation or gating of tinnitus and hyperacusis [95, 107]. Systemic treatment with high-dose salicylate significantly enhanced the local field potential and spike discharge rate of multiunit clusters recorded from the parafloccular lobe of the cerebellum [107]. The increased firing in the parafloccular lobe of the cerebellum could be due to locally mediated effects or reflect the salicylate-induced hyperactivity in higher auditory centers that are relayed back through descending pathways [94, 101].

Role of Stress in Salicylate-Induced Hyperacusis

Hyperacusis is often associated with hearing loss, but not everyone with hearing loss develops hyperacusis suggesting that other comorbidities such as stress and anxiety may be required for this condition to emerge [96, 116, 145]. It has been suggested stress combined with hearing loss interact to increase the likelihood of developing tinnitus, hyperacusis, and sound-evoked hyperactivity [91, 123, 138, 170]. High-dose salicylate increases c-fos expression in the regions of the brain associated with stress, anxiety, and pain [134, 170]. Imaging studies indicate that high doses of salicylate activate the anterior hypothalamus, which releases the corticotrophin-releasing hormone [114] which stimulates the release of adrenocorticotropic hormone. This is consistent with the fact that a high dose of salicylate causes a rapid increase of plasma adrenocorticotropic hormone, which is released from the pituitary gland into the bloodstream [109]. Circulating adrenocorticotropic hormone binds to receptors in the adrenal gland causing the adrenal glands to secrete corticosterone, a stress hormone, into the bloodstream. This sequence of events likely accounts for the rapid rise in plasma corticosterone stress hormone levels that occur for salicylate doses ≥150 mg/kg [107]. These same doses of salicylate not only cause a cochlear hearing loss, but also consistently induce hyperacusis and tinnitus [59, 63]. Taken together, these results suggest that high doses of salicylate disrupt the HPA axis consistent with previous studies showing that the HPA axis is dysregulated in tinnitus subjects with abnormally low ULLs indicative of loudness hyperacusis [164]. Tinnitus subjects with hyperacusis exhibit normal basal cortisol stress hormones, but when tested under stressful conditions, they exhibit a blunted cortisol stress response indicative of a dysregulated HPA axis [119].

The corticosterone stress hormone (cortisol in humans) binds with high and low affinity respectively to mineralocorticoid and glucocorticoid receptors. The hippocampus, which contains one of the highest concentrations of glucocorticoid receptors in the brain, is an important structure which provides negative feedback to the HPA axis which aids in terminating the adrenocortical stress response [158, 159]. Intense noise exposure, which causes significant hearing loss in rats, significantly upregulates the expression of glucocorticoid receptors, but not the mineralocorticoid receptors, in the hippocampus and tends to reduce reactive corticosterone stress hormones levels (i.e., a slightly blunted stress response), but not basal corticosterone levels [117]. The noise-induced upregulation of hippocampal glucocorticoid receptors presumably contributes to this blunted reactive stress response similar to the blunting seen in humans with tinnitus and loudness intolerance disorders [119, 164]. Please see also Chap. 6 for the influence of work-related stress on tinnitus.

Tinnitus–Hyperacusis Connectome

Sensory perceptions evoked by a real sound or the phantom sound of tinnitus result in dynamic coordinated activity in a distributed brain network or connectome that binds together neural responses in the auditory pathway with activity in other brain regions that encode other features or responses to the acoustic input such as its spatial location, emotional reactions, memories, behavioral arousal and motor responses, and neural activity that allows an organism to interact with the external environment or its internal biological states [108, 141, 163, 167].

Behavioral, electrophysiological, and functional imaging and connectivity data from rats treated with high doses of salicylate have been used to the identify some of the major changes that occur in key neural structures associated with the onset of hyperacusis, tinnitus, and hearing loss [39] as schematized in Fig. 23.5. The hearing loss associated with high doses of salicylate and ototraumatic agents such as noise exposure or aging invariably damage or disrupts the function of cochlear outer and inner hair cells and auditory nerve fibers that relay acoustic information to the central auditory system. High doses of salicylate reduce the electromotile response of outer hair cells and disrupt the transmission of sound-evoked activity from the inner hair cells to the auditory nerve; these two pathophysiological changes result in a salicylate-induced hearing loss of 20–25 dB and a large reduction of suprathreshold, sound-evoked activity that

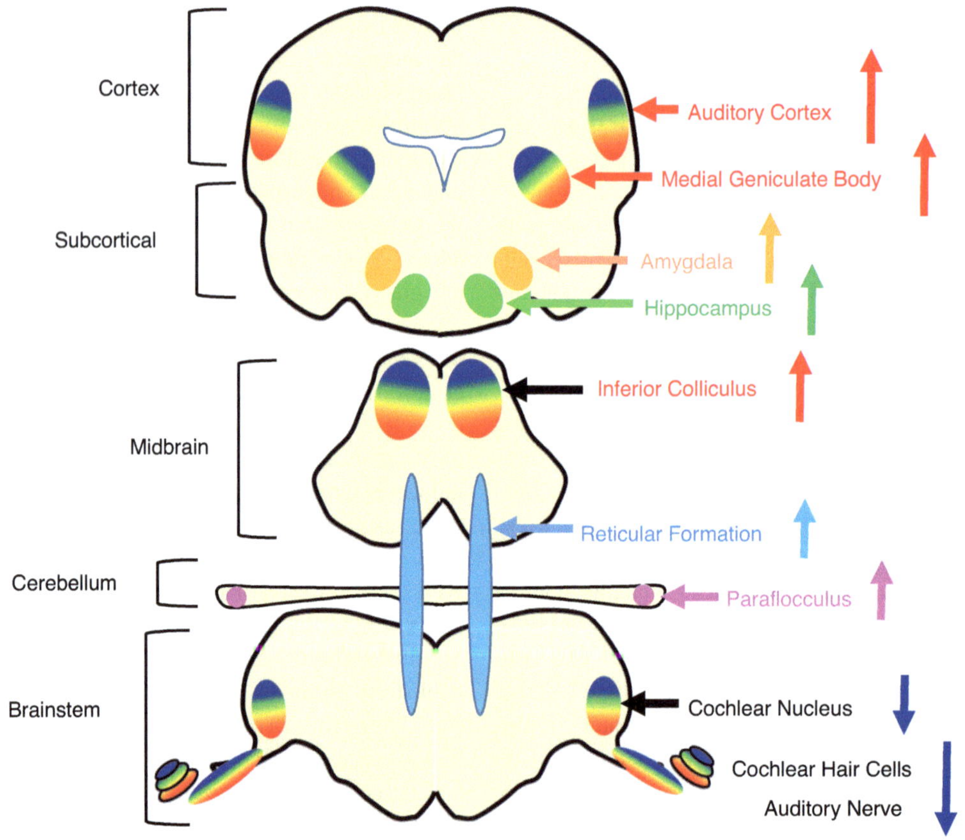

Fig. 23.5 Connectome model of salicylate-induced hyperacusis and sound-evoked neural hyperactivity. Up arrows next to text identifies brain regions where suprathreshold sound-evoked activity increased (up arrows = hyperactivity) or decreased (down arrows = hypoactivity). In the classical auditory pathway (blue-red color gradient), suprathreshold sound-evoked activity greatly depressed in cochlea and slightly depressed in the cochlear nucleus (down blue arrows), slightly enhanced in inferior colliculus and greatly enhanced in medial geniculate body and auditory cortex (up red arrows). Brain regions outside the classical auditory pathway where suprathreshold sound-evoked activity was enhanced (indicated by up arrows) by salicylate in the amygdala (emotional valence), hippocampus (memory, spatial localization), reticular formation (arousal area) and parafloccular lobe of cerebellum (motor coordination, tinnitus gating)

depresses neural output by more than 60%. Neural thresholds in the cochlear nucleus are elevated 20–25 dB, consistent with the cochlear hearing loss. While suprathreshold responses are below normal, the maximum output of the cochlear nucleus is only reduced by approximately 25%, substantially less than the 60% reduction seen in the auditory nerve. Neural response from the cochlear nucleus is relayed to the inferior colliculus in the midbrain where threshold shifts are again 20–25 dB, but now suprathreshold responses are slightly enhanced rather than depressed. Suprathreshold responses become progressively larger in the medial geniculate and auditory cortex. Suprathreshold responses are also enhanced in regions which receive information from various parts of the classically defined auditory pathway [179]. Responses are enhanced in the reticular formation, which regulates arousal and the amplitude of the acoustic reflex [34]; the parafloccular lobe of the cerebellum, hypothesized to be a tinnitus generator [95] and involved in head and eye movements [169]. Hyperactivity also occurs in the amygdala, which assigns emotional valence and cognitive attributes to auditory stimuli [146, 161] and the hippocampus, which in involved in spatial navigation, encoding auditory cues, and memory [111, 142, 156].

Summary

Hearing loss from high-dose salicylate and other ototraumatic insults typically damages the sensory hair cells and neurons in the cochlea. Cochlear damage to the hair cells and auditory nerve raises the threshold for hearing and reduces the neural output of the cochlea. Left unchecked, the weak neural output from the cochlea would make suprathreshold sounds seem muffled and impair auditory perception. While the central auditory system is unable to compensate for the cochlear hearing loss, once the neural responses rise above threshold, the central nervous system compensates for these weak neural signals by increasing the gain at multiple sites along the auditory pathway. In most cases, this serial amplification process boosts the signals reaching the cochlea back into the normal, homeostatic range resulting in loudness recruitment. However, when the serial amplification process in the central auditory pathway is excessive, as in cases of salicylate-ototoxicity, suprathreshold sound-evoked response becomes hyperactive at higher levels of the auditory pathway resulting in loudness hyperacusis. High-dose salicylate is one of the most reliable methods of inducing tinnitus and hyperacusis. One reason for this is that salicylate not only causes a cochlear hearing loss, but also disrupts neural activity at many sites within the central nervous system presumably because it causes a large upsurge in corticosterone stress hormones and alters the balance between excitation and inhibition in the central nervous system [112, 122, 133, 147, 172, 175]. Acoustic stress increases the amplitude of the auditory brainstem response, plasma corticosterone levels, and glucocorticoid receptor gene expression in the inferior colliculus [137], while chronic treatment with corticosteroid stress hormone disrupts auditory fear conditioning and dendritic arbors in the inferior colliculus [32]. Taken together, these results suggest that hyperacusis is most likely to develop in cases that involve hearing loss in combination with stress that disrupts the HPA axis [119, 164].

References

1. Tyler RS, Pienkowski M, Roncancio ER, Jun HJ, Brozoski T, Dauman N, Dauman N, Andersson G, Keiner AJ, Cacace AT, Martin N, Moore BC. A review of hyperacusis and future directions: part I. Definitions and manifestations Am J Audiol. 2014;23(4):402–19. https://doi.org/10.1044/2014_AJA-14-0010.
2. Sherlock LP, Formby C. Estimates of loudness, loudness discomfort, and the auditory dynamic range: normative estimates, comparison of procedures, and test-retest reliability. J Am Acad Audiol. 2005;16(2):85–100. https://doi.org/10.3766/jaaa.16.2.4.
3. Gierke HEV, Davis H, Eldredge DH, Hardy JD. Aural pain produced by sound. In: Benox report, an exploratory study of the biological effects of noise. Project NR 144079. Chicago: Office of Naval Research. University of Chicago Press; 1953.
4. Andersson G, Lindvall N, Hursti T, Carlbring P. Hypersensitivity to sound (hyperacusis): a prevalence study conducted via the internet and post. Int J Audiol. 2002;41(8):545–54. https://doi.org/10.3109/14992020209056075.
5. Baguley DM. Hyperacusis. J R Soc Med. 2003;96(12):582–5. https://doi.org/10.1258/jrsm.96.12.582.
6. Dauman R, Bouscau-Faure F. Assessment and amelioration of hyperacusis in tinnitus patients. Acta Otolaryngol. 2005;125(5):503–9. https://doi.org/10.1080/00016480510027565.
7. Paulin J, Andersson L, Nordin S. Characteristics of hyperacusis in the general population. Noise Health. 2016;18(83):178–84. https://doi.org/10.4103/1463-1741.189244.
8. Anari M, Axelsson A, Eliasson A, Magnusson L. Hypersensitivity to sound—questionnaire data, audiometry and classification. Scand Audiol. 1999;28(4):219–30. https://doi.org/10.1080/010503999424653.
9. Jastreboff PJ, Jastreboff MM. Tinnitus retraining therapy (TRT) as a method for treatment of tinnitus and hyperacusis patients. J Am Acad Audiol. 2000;11(3):162–77.
10. Gu JW, Halpin CF, Nam EC, Levine RA, Melcher JR. Tinnitus, diminished sound-level tolerance, and elevated auditory activity in humans with clinically normal hearing sensitivity. J Neurophysiol. 2010;104(6):3361–70. https://doi.org/10.1152/jn.00226.2010.
11. Nebel MB, Folger S, Tommerdahl M, Hollins M, McGlone F, Essick G. Temporomandibular disorder modifies cortical response to tactile stimulation. J Pain. 2010;11(11):1083–94. https://doi.org/10.1016/j.jpain.2010.02.021.
12. Suhnan AP, Finch PM, Drummond PD. Hyperacusis in chronic pain: neural interactions between the auditory and nociceptive systems. Int J Audiol. 2017;56(11):801–9. https://doi.org/10.1080/14992027.2017.1346303.
13. Weber H, Pfadenhauer K, Stohr M, Rosler A. Central hyperacusis with phonophobia in multiple sclerosis. Mult Scler. 2002;8(6):505–9. https://doi.org/10.1191/1352458502ms814oa.

14. Adour KK. Otological complications of herpes zoster. Ann Neurol. 1994;35(Suppl):S62–4. https://doi.org/10.1002/ana.410350718.
15. Gilchrist JM. Seventh cranial neuropathy. Semin Neurol. 2009;29(1):5–13. https://doi.org/10.1055/s-0028-1124018.
16. Mahoney CJ, Rohrer JD, Goll JC, Fox NC, Rossor MN, Warren JD. Structural neuroanatomy of tinnitus and hyperacusis in semantic dementia. J Neurol Neurosurg Psychiatry. 2011;82(11):1274–8. https://doi.org/10.1136/jnnp.2010.235473.
17. Khalfa S, Bruneau N, Roge B, Georgieff N, Veuillet E, Adrien JL, Barthelemy C, Collet L. Increased perception of loudness in autism. Hear Res. 2004;198(1–2):87–92. https://doi.org/10.1016/j.heares.2004.07.006.
18. Rosenhall U, Nordin V, Sandstrom M, Ahlsen G, Gillberg C. Autism and hearing loss. J Autism Dev Disord. 1999;29(5):349–57. https://doi.org/10.1023/a:1023022709710.
19. Levitin DJ, Cole K, Lincoln A, Bellugi U. Aversion, awareness, and attraction: investigating claims of hyperacusis in the Williams syndrome phenotype. J Child Psychol Psychiatry. 2005;46(5):514–23. https://doi.org/10.1111/j.1469-7610.2004.00376.x.
20. Zarchi O, Attias J, Gothelf D. Auditory and visual processing in Williams syndrome. Isr J Psychiatry Relat Sci. 2010;47(2):125–31.
21. Hayes SH, Radziwon KE, Stolzberg DJ, Salvi RJ. Behavioral models of tinnitus and hyperacusis in animals. Front Neurol. 2014;5:179. https://doi.org/10.3389/fneur.2014.00179.
22. Florentine M, Buus S, Robinson M. Temporal integration of loudness under partial masking. J Acoust Soc Am. 1998;104(2 Pt 1):999–1007.
23. Gjaevenes K, Rimstad ER. The influence of rise time on loudness. J Acoust Soc Am. 1972;51(4):1233–9. https://doi.org/10.1121/1.1912966.
24. Henning GB, Zwicker E. Loudness perception for short-duration tones in masking noise. Hear Res. 1990;47(1–2):17–23.
25. Scharf B. Loudness of complex sounds as a function of the number of components. J Acoust Soc Am. 1985;11(4):783–5.
26. Zwicker E, Zwicker UT. Dependence of binaural loudness summation on interaural level differences, spectral distribution, and temporal distribution. J Acoust Soc Am. 1991;89(2):756–64.
27. Davis M, Falls WA, Campeau S, Kim M. Fear-potentiated startle: a neural and pharmacological analysis. Behav Brain Res. 1993;58(1–2):175–98. https://doi.org/10.1016/0166-4328(93)90102-v.
28. Gilboa A, Sekeres M, Moscovitch M, Winocur G. Higher-order conditioning is impaired by hippocampal lesions. Current biology : CB. 2014;24(18):2202–7. https://doi.org/10.1016/j.cub.2014.07.078.
29. Horner KC. The emotional ear in stress. Neurosci Biobehav Rev. 2003;27(5):437–46. https://doi.org/10.1016/s0149-7634(03)00071-x.
30. Kraus KS, Canlon B. Neuronal connectivity and interactions between the auditory and limbic systems. Effects of noise and tinnitus. Hear Res. 2012;288(1–2):34–46. https://doi.org/10.1016/j.heares.2012.02.009.
31. Chavez CM, McGaugh JL, Weinberger NM. The basolateral amygdala modulates specific sensory memory representations in the cerebral cortex. Neurobiol Learn Mem. 2009;91(4):382–92. https://doi.org/10.1016/j.nlm.2008.10.010.
32. Dagnino-Subiabre A, Perez MA, Terreros G, Cheng MY, House P, Sapolsky R. Corticosterone treatment impairs auditory fear learning and the dendritic morphology of the rat inferior colliculus. Hear Res. 2012;294(1–2):104–13. https://doi.org/10.1016/j.heares.2012.09.008.
33. Lee Y, Lopez DE, Meloni EG, Davis M. A primary acoustic startle pathway: obligatory role of cochlear root neurons and the nucleus reticularis pontis caudalis. J Neurosci. 1996;16(11):3775–89.
34. Yeomans JS, Frankland PW. The acoustic startle reflex: neurons and connections. Brain Res Brain Res Rev. 1995;21(3):301–14.
35. Gomez-Nieto R, Horta-Junior Jde A, Castellano O, Millian-Morell L, Rubio ME, Lopez DE. Origin and function of short-latency inputs to the neural substrates underlying the acoustic startle reflex. Front Neurosci. 2014;8:216. https://doi.org/10.3389/fnins.2014.00216.
36. Davis M, Gendelman DS, Tischler MD, Gendelman PM. A primary acoustic startle circuit: lesion and stimulation studies. J Neurosci. 1982;2(6):791–805.
37. Meloni EG, Davis M. The dorsal cochlear nucleus contributes to a high intensity component of the acoustic startle reflex in rats. Hear Res. 1998;119(1–2):69–80.
38. Salloum RH, Yurosko C, Santiago L, Sandridge SA, Kaltenbach JA. Induction of enhanced acoustic startle response by noise exposure: dependence on exposure conditions and testing parameters and possible relevance to hyperacusis. PLoS One. 2014;9(10):e111747. https://doi.org/10.1371/journal.pone.0111747.
39. Chen YC, Li X, Liu L, Wang J, Lu CQ, Yang M, Jiao Y, Zang FC, Radziwon K, Chen GD, Sun W, Krishnan Muthaiah VP, Salvi R, Teng GJ. Tinnitus and hyperacusis involve hyperactivity and enhanced connectivity in auditory-limbic-arousal-cerebellar network. elife. 2015;4:e06576. https://doi.org/10.7554/eLife.06576.
40. Lu J, Lobarinas E, Deng A, Goodey R, Stolzberg D, Salvi RJ, Sun W. GABAergic neural activity involved in salicylate-induced auditory cortex gain enhancement. Neuroscience. 2011;189:187–98. https://doi.org/10.1016/j.neuroscience.2011.04.073.
41. Sun W, Lu J, Stolzberg D, Gray L, Deng A, Lobarinas E, Salvi RJ. Salicylate increases the gain of the central auditory system. Neuroscience. 2009;159(1):325–34. https://doi.org/10.1016/j.neuroscience.2008.12.024.
42. Chen G, Lee C, Sandridge SA, Butler HM, Manzoor NF, Kaltenbach JA. Behavioral evidence for possible simultaneous induction of hyperacusis and tinnitus following intense sound exposure. J Assoc Res Otolaryngol. 2013a;14(3):413–24. https://doi.org/10.1007/s10162-013-0375-2.
43. Xiong B, Alkharabsheh A, Manohar S, Chen GD, Yu N, Zhao X, Salvi R, Sun W. Hyperexcitability of inferior colliculus and acoustic startle reflex with age-related hearing loss. Hear Res. 2017;350:32–42. https://doi.org/10.1016/j.heares.2017.03.011.
44. Lobarinas E, Hayes SH, Allman BL. The gap-startle paradigm for tinnitus screening in animal models: limitations and optimization. Hear Res. 2013;295:150–60. https://doi.org/10.1016/j.heares.2012.06.001.
45. Longenecker RJ, Galazyuk AV. Methodological optimization of tinnitus assessment using prepulse inhibition of the acoustic startle reflex. Brain Res. 2012;1485:54–62. https://doi.org/10.1016/j.brainres.2012.02.067.
46. Cardello AV. Reaction time and visual brightness: within-subject correlations. Percept Mot Skills. 1979;48(1):107–15. https://doi.org/10.2466/pms.1979.48.1.107.
47. Marshall L, Brandt JF. The relationship between loudness and reaction time in normal hearing listeners. Acta Otolaryngol. 1980;90(3–4):244–9. https://doi.org/10.3109/00016488009131721.
48. Pins D, Bonnet C. On the relation between stimulus intensity and processing time: Pieron's law and choice reaction time. Percept Psychophys. 1996;58(3):390–400.
49. Stebbins WC. Auditory reaction time and the derivation of equal loudness contours for the monkey. J Exp Anal Behav. 1966;9(2):135–42. https://doi.org/10.1901/jeab.1966.9-135.
50. Kohfeld DL. Simple reaction time as a function of stimulus intensity in decibels of light and sound. J Exp Psychol. 1971;88(2):251–7. https://doi.org/10.1037/h0030891.
51. Dooling RJ, Zoloth SR, Baylis JR. Auditory sensitivity, equal loudness, temporal resolving power, and vocalizations in the house finch (Carpodacus mexicanus). J Comp Physiol Psychol. 1978;92(5):867–76.

52. Lauer AM, Dooling RJ. Evidence of hyperacusis in canaries with permanent hereditary high-frequency hearing loss. Semin Hear. 2007;28(4):319–26.
53. May BJ, Little N, Saylor S. Loudness perception in the domestic cat: reaction time estimates of equal loudness contours and recruitment effects. J Assoc Res Otolaryngol. 2009;10(2):295–308. https://doi.org/10.1007/s10162-009-0157-z.
54. Radziwon K, Salvi R. Using auditory reaction time to measure loudness growth in rats. Hear Res. 2020;395:108026. https://doi.org/10.1016/j.heares.2020.108026.
55. Scharf B. Comparison of normal and impaired hearing. I. Loudness, localization. Scand Audiol Suppl. 1978;6:49–79.
56. Feitosa AG, Moody DB, Stebbins WC. Loudness recruitment in the dihydrostreptomycin-treated patas monkey. J Acoust Soc Am. 1981;70:s27.
57. Hellman RP. Relation between the growth of loudness and high-frequency excitation. J Acoust Soc Am. 1994;96(5 Pt 1):2655–63. https://doi.org/10.1121/1.411445.
58. Jastreboff PJ, Brennan JF, Sasaki CT. An animal model for tinnitus. Laryngoscope. 1988;98(3):280–6. https://doi.org/10.1288/00005537-198803000-00008.
59. Lobarinas E, Sun W, Cushing R, Salvi R. A novel behavioral paradigm for assessing tinnitus using schedule-induced polydipsia avoidance conditioning (SIP-AC). Hear Res. 2004;190(1–2):109–14. https://doi.org/10.1016/S0378-5955(04)00019-X.
60. McCabe PA, Dey FL. The effect of aspirin upon auditory sensitivity. Ann Otol Rhinol Laryngol. 1965;74:312–25. https://doi.org/10.1177/000348946507400203.
61. Myers EN, Bernstein JM. Salicylate ototoxicity; a clinical and experimental study. Arch Otolaryngol. 1965;82(5):483–93. https://doi.org/10.1001/archotol.1965.00760010485006.
62. Auerbach BD, Radziwon K, Salvi R. Testing the central gain model: loudness growth correlates with central auditory gain enhancement in a rodent model of hyperacusis. Neuroscience. 2019;407:93–107. https://doi.org/10.1016/j.neuroscience.2018.09.036.
63. Radziwon K, Holfoth D, Lindner J, Kaier-Green Z, Bowler R, Urban M, Salvi R. Salicylate-induced hyperacusis in rats: dose- and frequency-dependent effects. Hear Res. 2017;350:133–8. https://doi.org/10.1016/j.heares.2017.04.004.
64. Radziwon KE, Stolzberg DJ, Urban ME, Bowler RA, Salvi RJ. Salicylate-induced hearing loss and gap detection deficits in rats. Front Neurol. 2015;6:31. https://doi.org/10.3389/fneur.2015.00031.
65. Moody DB. Behavioral studies of noise-induced hearing loss in primates: loudness recruitment. Adv Otorhinolaryngol. 1973;20:82–101.
66. Pugh JE Jr, Moody DB, Anderson DJ. Electrocochleography and experimentally induced loudness recruitment. Arch Otorhinolaryngol. 1979;224(3–4):241–55.
67. Radziwon K, Auerbach BD, Ding D, Liu X, Chen GD, Salvi R. Noise-induced loudness recruitment and hyperacusis: insufficient central gain in auditory cortex and amygdala. Neuroscience. 2019;422:212–27. https://doi.org/10.1016/j.neuroscience.2019.09.010.
68. Sheldrake J, Diehl PU, Schaette R. Audiometric characteristics of hyperacusis patients. Front Neurol. 2015;6:105. https://doi.org/10.3389/fneur.2015.00105.
69. Sinclair D, Oranje B, Razak KA, Siegel SJ, Schmid S. Sensory processing in autism spectrum disorders and fragile X syndrome-from the clinic to animal models. Neurosci Biobehav Rev. 2017;76(Pt B):235–53. https://doi.org/10.1016/j.neubiorev.2016.05.029.
70. Hamilton SM, Green JR, Veeraragavan S, Yuva L, McCoy A, Wu Y, Warren J, Little L, Ji D, Cui X, Weinstein E, Paylor R. Fmr1 and Nlgn3 knockout rats: novel tools for investigating autism spectrum disorders. Behav Neurosci. 2014;128(2):103–9. https://doi.org/10.1037/a0035988.
71. Till SM, Asiminas A, Jackson AD, Katsanevaki D, Barnes SA, Osterweil EK, Bear MF, Chattarji S, Wood ER, Wyllie DJ, Kind PC. Conserved hippocampal cellular pathophysiology but distinct behavioural deficits in a new rat model of FXS. Hum Mol Genet. 2015;24(21):5977–84. https://doi.org/10.1093/hmg/ddv299.
72. Pienkowski M, Tyler RS, Roncancio ER, Jun HJ, Brozoski T, Dauman N, Coelho CB, Andersson G, Keiner AJ, Cacace AT, Martin N, Moore BC. A review of hyperacusis and future directions: part II. Measurement, mechanisms, and treatment. Am J Audiol. 2014;23(4):420–36. https://doi.org/10.1044/2014_AJA-13-0037.
73. Manohar S, Spoth J, Radziwon K, Auerbach BD, Salvi R. Noise-induced hearing loss induces loudness intolerance in a rat active sound avoidance paradigm (ASAP). Hear Res. 2017;353:197–203. https://doi.org/10.1016/j.heares.2017.07.001.
74. Bourin M, Hascoet M. The mouse light/dark box test. Eur J Pharmacol. 2003;463(1–3):55–65. https://doi.org/10.1016/s0014-2999(03)01274-3.
75. Charbonneau G, Bertone A, Lepore F, Nassim M, Lassonde M, Mottron L, Collignon O. Multilevel alterations in the processing of audio-visual emotion expressions in autism spectrum disorders. Neuropsychologia. 2013;51(5):1002–10. https://doi.org/10.1016/j.neuropsychologia.2013.02.009.
76. Reiss AL, Freund L. Behavioral phenotype of fragile X syndrome: DSM-III-R autistic behavior in male children. Am J Med Genet. 1992;43(1–2):35–46. https://doi.org/10.1002/ajmg.1320430106.
77. Pollard B. Unravelling the mystery of hyperacusis with pain. ENT Audiol News. 2018;6:61–2.
78. Collard ME, Parker W. Exaggerated acoustic reflex response in a patient with transient facial palsy and hyperacusis. Am J Otol. 1984;5(5):355–9.
79. McCandless GA, Schumacher MH. Auditory dysfunction with facial paralysis. Arch Otolaryngol. 1979;105(5):271–4.
80. Norena AJ, Fournier P, Londero A, Ponsot D, Charpentier N. An integrative model accounting for the symptom cluster triggered after an acoustic shock. Trends Hear. 2018;22:2331216518801725. https://doi.org/10.1177/2331216518801725.
81. Westcott M, Sanchez TG, Diges I, Saba C, Dineen R, McNeill C, Chiam A, O'Keefe M, Sharples T. Tonic tensor tympani syndrome in tinnitus and hyperacusis patients: a multi-clinic prevalence study. Noise Health. 2013;15(63):117–28. https://doi.org/10.4103/1463-1741.110295.
82. Flores EN, Duggan A, Madathany T, Hogan AK, Marquez FG, Kumar G, Seal RP, Edwards RH, Liberman MC, Garcia-Anoveros J. A non-canonical pathway from cochlea to brain signals tissue-damaging noise. Curr Biol. 2015;25(5):606–12. https://doi.org/10.1016/j.cub.2015.01.009.
83. Liu C, Glowatzki E, Fuchs PA. Unmyelinated type II afferent neurons report cochlear damage. Proc Natl Acad Sci U S A. 2015;112(47):14723–7. https://doi.org/10.1073/pnas.1515228112.
84. Gardner WJ, Licklider JC, Weisz AZ. Suppression of pain by sound. Science. 1960;132(3418):32–3.
85. Helmstetter FJ, Bellgowan PS. Hypoalgesia in response to sensitization during acute noise stress. Behav Neurosci. 1994;108(1):177–85.
86. Manohar S, Adler HJ, Radziwon K, Salvi R. Interaction of auditory and pain pathways: effects of stimulus intensity, hearing loss and opioid signaling. Hear Res. 2020b;393:108012. https://doi.org/10.1016/j.heares.2020.108012.
87. Baizer JS, Wong KM, Manohar S, Hayes SH, Ding D, Dingman R, Salvi RJ. Effects of acoustic trauma on the auditory system of the rat: the role of microglia. Neuroscience. 2015;303:299–311. https://doi.org/10.1016/j.neuroscience.2015.07.004.
88. Boettcher FA, Bancroft BR, Salvi RJ. Concentration of salicylate in serum and perilymph of the chinchilla. Arch Otolaryngol Head Neck Surg. 1990;116(6):681–4. https://doi.org/10.1001/archotol.1990.01870060039005.

89. Jastreboff PJ, Hansen R, Sasaki PG, Sasaki CT. Differential uptake of salicylate in serum, cerebrospinal fluid, and perilymph. Arch Otolaryngol Head Neck Surg. 1986;112(10):1050–3. https://doi.org/10.1001/archotol.1986.03780100038004.
90. Dallos P, Harris D. Properties of auditory nerve responses in absence of outer hair cells. J Neurophysiol. 1978;41(2):365.
91. Alpini D, Cesarani A. Tinnitus as an alarm bell: stress reaction tinnitus model. ORL J Otorhinolaryngol Relat Spec. 2006;68 (1):31-36:discussion 36-37. https://doi.org/10.1159/000090488.
92. Ashmore JF. A fast motile response in Guinea-pig outer hair cells: the cellular basis of the cochlear amplifier. J Physiol (London). 1987;388:323–47.
93. Asokan MM, Williamson RS, Hancock KE, Polley DB. Sensory overamplification in layer 5 auditory corticofugal projection neurons following cochlear nerve synaptic damage. Nat Commun. 2018;9(1):2468. https://doi.org/10.1038/s41467-018-04852-y.
94. Azizi SA, Burne RA, Woodward DJ. The auditory corticopontocerebellar projection in the rat: inputs to the paraflocculus and midvermis. An anatomical and physiological study. Exp Brain Res. 1985;59(1):36–49. https://doi.org/10.1007/BF00237663.
95. Bauer CA, Kurt W, Sybert LT, Brozoski TJ. The cerebellum as a novel tinnitus generator. Hear Res. 2013;295:130–9. https://doi.org/10.1016/j.heares.2012.03.009.
96. Blaesing L, Kroener-Herwig B. Self-reported and behavioral sound avoidance in tinnitus and hyperacusis subjects, and association with anxiety ratings. Int J Audiol. 2012;51(8):611–7. https://doi.org/10.3109/14992027.2012.664290.
97. Bordi F, LeDoux J. Sensory tuning beyond the sensory system: an initial analysis of auditory response properties of neurons in the lateral amygdaloid nucleus and overlying areas of the striatum. J Neurosci. 1992;12(7):2493–503.
98. Bordi F, LeDoux J, Clugnet MC, Pavlides C. Single-unit activity in the lateral nucleus of the amygdala and overlying areas of the striatum in freely behaving rats: rates, discharge patterns, and responses to acoustic stimuli. Behav Neurosci. 1993;107(5):757–69.
99. Bordi F, LeDoux JE. Response properties of single units in areas of rat auditory thalamus that project to the amygdala. II. Cells receiving convergent auditory and somatosensory inputs and cells antidromically activated by amygdala stimulation. Exp Brain Res. 1994;98(2):275–86. https://doi.org/10.1007/BF00228415.
100. Bourien J, Tang Y, Batrel C, Huet A, Lenoir M, Ladrech S, Desmadryl G, Nouvian R, Puel JL, Wang J. Contribution of auditory nerve fibers to compound action potential of the auditory nerve. J Neurophysiol. 2014;112(5):1025–39. https://doi.org/10.1152/jn.00738.2013.
101. Broch-Smith T, Brodal P. Organization of the cortico-ponto-cerebellar pathway to the dorsal paraflocculus. An experimental study with anterograde and retrograde transport of WGA-HRP in the cat. Arch Ital Biol. 1990;128(2-4):249–71.
102. Budinger E, Heil P, Scheich H. Functional organization of auditory cortex in the Mongolian gerbil (Meriones unguiculatus). IV. Connections with anatomically characterized subcortical structures. Eur J Neurosci. 2000;12(7):2452–74. https://doi.org/10.1046/j.1460-9568.2000.00143.x.
103. Cant NB, Benson CG. Parallel auditory pathways: projection patterns of the different neuronal populations in the dorsal and ventral cochlear nuclei. Brain Res Bull. 2003;60(5–6):457–74. https://doi.org/10.1016/s0361-9230(03)00050-9.
104. Chen GD, Manohar S, Salvi R. Amygdala hyperactivity and tonotopic shift after salicylate exposure. Brain Res. 2012;1485:63–76. https://doi.org/10.1016/j.brainres.2012.03.016.
105. Chen GD, Radziwon KE, Kashanian N, Manohar S, Salvi R. Salicylate-induced auditory perceptual disorders and plastic changes in nonclassical auditory centers in rats. Neural Plast. 2014;2014:658741. https://doi.org/10.1155/2014/658741.
106. Chen GD, Stolzberg D, Lobarinas E, Sun W, Ding D, Salvi R. Salicylate-induced cochlear impairments, cortical hyperactivity and re-tuning, and tinnitus. Hear Res. 2013b;295(1–2):100–13. https://doi.org/10.1016/j.heares.2012.11.016.
107. Chen YC, Chen GD, Auerbach BD, Manohar S, Radziwon K, Salvi R. Tinnitus and hyperacusis: contributions of paraflocculus, reticular formation and stress. Hear Res. 2017;349:208–22. https://doi.org/10.1016/j.heares.2017.03.005.
108. Dolan RJ, Morris JS, de Gelder B. Crossmodal binding of fear in voice and face. Proc Natl Acad Sci U S A. 2001;98(17):10006–10. https://doi.org/10.1073/pnas.171288598.
109. Eades CH Jr, King JS Jr. Detectable amounts of ACTH in blood following salicylate administration. Endocrinology. 1953;52(5):594–6.
110. Gener T, Perez-Mendez L, Sanchez-Vives MV. Tactile modulation of hippocampal place fields. Hippocampus. 2013;23(12):1453–62. https://doi.org/10.1002/hipo.22198.
111. Goble TJ, Moller AR, Thompson LT. Acute high-intensity sound exposure alters responses of place cells in hippocampus. Hear Res. 2009;253(1–2):52–9. https://doi.org/10.1016/j.heares.2009.03.002.
112. Gong N, Zhang M, Zhang XB, Chen L, Sun GC, Xu TL. The aspirin metabolite salicylate enhances neuronal excitation in rat hippocampal CA1 area through reducing GABAergic inhibition. Neuropharmacology. 2008;54(2):454–63. https://doi.org/10.1016/j.neuropharm.2007.10.017.
113. Grimsley JM, Hazlett EG, Wenstrup JJ. Coding the meaning of sounds: contextual modulation of auditory responses in the basolateral amygdala. J Neurosci. 2013;33(44):17538–48. https://doi.org/10.1523/JNEUROSCI.2205-13.2013.
114. Groschel M, Gotze R, Muller S, Ernst A, Basta D. Central Nervous Activity upon Systemic Salicylate Application in Animals with Kanamycin-Induced Hearing Loss—a Manganese-Enhanced MRI (MEMRI) Study. PLoS One. 2016;11(4):e0153386. https://doi.org/10.1371/journal.pone.0153386.
115. Guo L, Weems JT, Walker WI, Levichev A, Jaramillo S. Choice-selective neurons in the auditory cortex and in its striatal target encode reward expectation. J Neurosci. 2019;39(19):3687–97. https://doi.org/10.1523/JNEUROSCI.2585-18.2019.
116. Hasson D, Theorell T, Bergquist J, Canlon B. Acute stress induces hyperacusis in women with high levels of emotional exhaustion. PLoS One. 2013;8(1):e52945. https://doi.org/10.1371/journal.pone.0052945.
117. Hayes SH, Manohar S, Majumdar A, Allman BL, Salvi R. Noise-induced hearing loss alters hippocampal glucocorticoid receptor expression in rats. Hear Res. 2019;379:43–51. https://doi.org/10.1016/j.heares.2019.04.013.
118. He DZ, Beisel KW, Chen L, Ding DL, Jia S, Fritzsch B, Salvi R. Chick hair cells do not exhibit voltage-dependent somatic motility. J Physiol. 2003;546(Pt 2):511–20. https://doi.org/10.1113/jphysiol.2002.026070.
119. Hebert S, Lupien SJ. The sound of stress: blunted cortisol reactivity to psychosocial stress in tinnitus sufferers. Neurosci Lett. 2007;411(2):138–42. https://doi.org/10.1016/j.neulet.2006.10.028.
120. Hwang JH, Chou PH, Wu CW, Chen JH, Liu TC. Brain activation in patients with idiopathic hyperacusis. Am J Otolaryngol. 2009;30(6):432–4. https://doi.org/10.1016/j.amjoto.2008.08.005.
121. Jiang C, Luo B, Manohar S, Chen GD, Salvi R. Plastic changes along auditory pathway during salicylate-induced ototoxicity: hyperactivity and CF shifts. Hear Res. 2017;347:28–40. https://doi.org/10.1016/j.heares.2016.10.021.
122. Jin Y, Luo B, Su YY, Wang XX, Chen L, Wang M, Wang WW, Chen L. Sodium salicylate suppresses GABAergic inhibitory activity in neurons of rodent dorsal raphe nucleus. PLoS One. 2015;10(5):e0126956. https://doi.org/10.1371/journal.pone.0126956.

123. Kim YH, Jung HJ, Kang SI, Park KT, Choi JS, Oh SH, Chang SO. Tinnitus in children: association with stress and trait anxiety. Laryngoscope. 2012;122(10):2279–84. https://doi.org/10.1002/lary.23482.
124. Kornetsky C, Eliasson M. Reticular stimulation and chlorpromazine: an animal model for schizophrenic overarousal. Science. 1969;165(3899):1273–4. https://doi.org/10.1126/science.165.3899.1273.
125. Kotak VC, Fujisawa S, Lee FA, Karthikeyan O, Aoki C, Sanes DH. Hearing loss raises excitability in the auditory cortex. J Neurosci. 2005;25(15):3908–18. https://doi.org/10.1523/JNEUROSCI.5169-04.2005.
126. Kujawa SG, Fallon M, Bobbin RP. Intracochlear salicylate reduces low-intensity acoustic and cochlear microphonic distortion products. Hear Res. 1992;64(1):73–80. https://doi.org/10.1016/0378-5955(92)90169-n.
127. Kumar S, Joseph S, Gander PE, Barascud N, Halpern AR, Griffiths TD. A brain system for auditory working memory. J Neurosci. 2016;36(16):4492–505. https://doi.org/10.1523/JNEUROSCI.4341-14.2016.
128. LeDoux JE. Emotion circuits in the brain. Annu Rev Neurosci. 2000;23:155–84. https://doi.org/10.1146/annurev.neuro.23.1.155.
129. Leitner DS, Hammond GR, Springer CP, Ingham KM, Mekilo AM, Bodison PR, Aranda MT, Shawaryn MA. Parameters affecting gap detection in the rat. Percept Psychophys. 1993; 54(3):395–405.
130. Liberman MC, Zuo J, Guinan JJ Jr. Otoacoustic emissions without somatic motility: can stereocilia mechanics drive the mammalian cochlea? J Acoust Soc Am. 2004;116(3):1649–55. https://doi.org/10.1121/1.1775275.
131. Liu L, Shen P, He T, Chang Y, Shi L, Tao S, Li X, Xun Q, Guo X, Yu Z, Wang J. Noise induced hearing loss impairs spatial learning/memory and hippocampal neurogenesis in mice. Sci Rep. 2016;6:20374. https://doi.org/10.1038/srep20374.
132. Lockwood AH, Salvi RJ, Coad ML, Arnold SA, Wack DS, Murphy BW, Burkard RF. The functional anatomy of the normal human auditory system: responses to 0.5 and 4.0 kHz tones at varied intensities. Cereb Cortex. 1999;9(1):65–76. https://doi.org/10.1093/cercor/9.1.65.
133. Lu YG, Tang ZQ, Ye ZY, Wang HT, Huang YN, Zhou KQ, Zhang M, Xu TL, Chen L. Salicylate, an aspirin metabolite, specifically inhibits the current mediated by glycine receptors containing alpha1-subunits. Br J Pharmacol. 2009;157(8):1514–22. https://doi.org/10.1111/j.1476-5381.2009.00321.x.
134. Mahlke C, Wallhausser-Franke E. Evidence for tinnitus-related plasticity in the auditory and limbic system, demonstrated by arg3.1 and c-fos immunocytochemistry. Hear Res. 2004;195(1–2):17–34. https://doi.org/10.1016/j.heares.2004.03.005.
135. Mandell AJ, Bach LM. Production of anxiety behavior and avoidance conditioning by stimulation of bulbar reticular formation. Proc Soc Exp Biol Med. 1958;97(4):880–1. https://doi.org/10.3181/00379727-97-23908.
136. Manohar S, Adler HJ, Chen GD, Salvi R. Blast-induced hearing loss suppresses hippocampal neurogenesis and disrupts long term spatial memory. Hear Res. 2020a;395:108022. https://doi.org/10.1016/j.heares.2020.108022.
137. Mazurek B, Haupt H, Joachim R, Klapp BF, Stover T, Szczepek AJ. Stress induces transient auditory hypersensitivity in rats. Hear Res. 2010;259(1–2):55–63. https://doi.org/10.1016/j.heares.2009.10.006.
138. Mazurek B, Haupt H, Olze H, Szczepek AJ. Stress and tinnitus-from bedside to bench and back. Front Syst Neurosci. 2012;6:47. https://doi.org/10.3389/fnsys.2012.00047.
139. Mills DM, Rubel EW. Development of the cochlear amplifier. J Acoust Soc Am. 1996;100:428–41.
140. Mishkin M. A memory system in the monkey. Philos Trans R Soc Lond Ser B Biol Sci. 1982;298(1089):83–95.
141. Mohan A, De Ridder D, Vanneste S. Robustness and dynamicity of functional networks in phantom sound. NeuroImage. 2017;146:171–87. https://doi.org/10.1016/j.neuroimage.2016.04.033.
142. Moita MA, Rosis S, Zhou Y, LeDoux JE, Blair HT. Hippocampal place cells acquire location-specific responses to the conditioned stimulus during auditory fear conditioning. Neuron. 2003;37(3): 485–97. https://doi.org/10.1016/s0896-6273(03)00033-3.
143. Moita MA, Rosis S, Zhou Y, LeDoux JE, Blair HT. Putting fear in its place: remapping of hippocampal place cells during fear conditioning. J Neurosci. 2004;24(31):7015–23. https://doi.org/10.1523/JNEUROSCI.5492-03.2004.
144. Moriizumi T, Hattori T. Pyramidal cells in rat temporoauditory cortex project to both striatum and inferior colliculus. Brain Res Bull. 1991;27(1):141–4. https://doi.org/10.1016/0361-9230(91)90297-w.
145. Nelson JJ, Chen K. The relationship of tinnitus, hyperacusis, and hearing loss. Ear Nose Throat J. 2004;83(7):472–6.
146. Nishijo H, Hori E, Tazumi T, Ono T. Neural correlates to both emotion and cognitive functions in the monkey amygdala. Behav Brain Res. 2008;188(1):14–23. https://doi.org/10.1016/j.bbr.2007.10.013.
147. Patel CR, Zhang H. Local application of sodium salicylate enhances auditory responses in the Rat's dorsal cortex of the inferior colliculus. Front Neurol. 2014;5:235. https://doi.org/10.3389/fneur.2014.00235.
148. Ponvert ND, Jaramillo S. Auditory Thalamostriatal and Corticostriatal pathways convey complementary information about sound features. J Neurosci. 2019;39(2):271–80. https://doi.org/10.1523/JNEUROSCI.1188-18.2018.
149. Ponzetto E, Vinetti M, Grandin C, Duprez T, van Pesch V, Deggouj N, Lhommel R, Hantson P. Partly reversible central auditory dysfunction induced by cerebral vasospasm after subarachnoid hemorrhage. J Neurosurg. 2013;119(5):1125–8. https://doi.org/10.3171/2013.7.JNS13674.
150. Prevosto V, Graf W, Ugolini G. Cerebellar inputs to intraparietal cortex areas LIP and MIP: functional frameworks for adaptive control of eye movements, reaching, and arm/eye/head movement coordination. Cereb Cortex. 2010;20(1):214–28. https://doi.org/10.1093/cercor/bhp091.
151. Putnam LE, Roth WT. Effects of stimulus repetition, duration, and rise time on startle blink and automatically elicited P300. Psychophysiology. 1990;27(3):275–97. https://doi.org/10.1111/j.1469-8986.1990.tb00383.x.
152. Quirk GJ, Muller RU, Kubie JL. The firing of hippocampal place cells in the dark depends on the rat's recent experience. J Neurosci. 1990;10(6):2008–17.
153. Rambold H, Churchland A, Selig Y, Jasmin L, Lisberger SG. Partial ablations of the flocculus and ventral paraflocculus in monkeys cause linked deficits in smooth pursuit eye movements and adaptive modification of the VOR. J Neurophysiol. 2002;87(2):912–24. https://doi.org/10.1152/jn.00768.2000.
154. Resnik J, Polley DB. Fast-spiking GABA circuit dynamics in the auditory cortex predict recovery of sensory processing following peripheral nerve damage. Elife. 2017;6:e21452. https://doi.org/10.7554/eLife.21452.
155. Ryan A, Dallos P. Effect of absence of cochlear outer hair cells on behavioural auditory threshold. Nature. 1975;253(5486):44–6. https://doi.org/10.1038/253044a0.
156. Sakurai Y. Coding of auditory temporal and pitch information by hippocampal individual cells and cell assemblies in the rat. Neuroscience. 2002;115(4):1153–63. https://doi.org/10.1016/s0306-4522(02)00509-2.

157. Santos-Sacchi J, Song L, Zheng J, Nuttall AL. Control of mammalian cochlear amplification by chloride anions. J Neurosci. 2006;26(15):3992–8. https://doi.org/10.1523/JNEUROSCI.4548-05.2006.
158. Sapolsky RM, Krey LC, McEwen BS. Glucocorticoid-sensitive hippocampal neurons are involved in terminating the adrenocortical stress response. Proc Natl Acad Sci U S A. 1984a;81(19):6174–7.
159. Sapolsky RM, Krey LC, McEwen BS. Stress down-regulates corticosterone receptors in a site-specific manner in the brain. Endocrinology. 1984b;114(1):287–92. https://doi.org/10.1210/endo-114-1-287.
160. Schofield BR, Cant NB. Projections from the ventral cochlear nucleus to the inferior colliculus and the contralateral cochlear nucleus in Guinea pigs. Hear Res. 1996;102(1–2):1–14.
161. Schultz W. Predictive reward signal of dopamine neurons. J Neurophysiol. 1998;80(1):1–27.
162. Schulz GM, Greer M, Friedman W. Changes in vocal intensity in Parkinson's disease following pallidotomy surgery. J Voice. 2000;14(4):589–606. https://doi.org/10.1016/s0892-1997(00)80015-6.
163. Sepulcre J. Functional streams and cortical integration in the human brain. Neuroscientist. 2014;20(5):499–508. https://doi.org/10.1177/1073858414531657.
164. Simoens VL, Hebert S. Cortisol suppression and hearing thresholds in tinnitus after low-dose dexamethasone challenge. BMC ear, nose, and throat disorders. 2012;12:4. https://doi.org/10.1186/1472-6815-12-4.
165. Sinnamon HM, Freniere S, Kootz J. Rat hippocampus and memory for places of changing significance. J Comp Physiol Psychol. 1978;92(1):142–55.
166. Stolzberg D, Chen GD, Allman BL, Salvi RJ. Salicylate-induced peripheral auditory changes and tonotopic reorganization of auditory cortex. Neuroscience. 2011;180:157–64. https://doi.org/10.1016/j.neuroscience.2011.02.005.
167. Tobyne SM, Somers DC, Brissenden JA, Michalka SW, Noyce AL, Osher DE. Prediction of individualized task activation in sensory modality-selective frontal cortex with 'connectome fingerprinting'. NeuroImage. 2018;183:173–85. https://doi.org/10.1016/j.neuroimage.2018.08.007.
168. Voigt HF, Young ED. Neural correlations in the dorsal cochlear nucleus: pairs of units with similar response properties. J Neurophysiol. 1988;59(3):1014–32.
169. Voogd J, Barmack NH. Oculomotor cerebellum. Prog Brain Res. 2006;151:231–68. https://doi.org/10.1016/S0079-6123(05)51008-2.
170. Wallhausser-Franke E. Salicylate evokes c-fos expression in the brain stem: implications for tinnitus. Neuroreport. 1997;8(3):725–8.
171. Wallhausser-Franke E, Mahlke C, Oliva R, Braun S, Wenz G, Langner G. Expression of c-fos in auditory and non-auditory brain regions of the gerbil after manipulations that induce tinnitus. Exp Brain Res. 2003;153(4):649–54. https://doi.org/10.1007/s00221-003-1614-2.
172. Wang HT, Luo B, Huang YN, Zhou KQ, Chen L. Sodium salicylate suppresses serotonin-induced enhancement of GABAergic spontaneous inhibitory postsynaptic currents in rat inferior colliculus *in vitro*. Hear Res. 2008;236(1–2):42–51. https://doi.org/10.1016/j.heares.2007.11.015.
173. Winer JA. Decoding the auditory corticofugal systems. Hear Res. 2006;212(1–2):1–8. https://doi.org/10.1016/j.heares.2005.06.014.
174. Wong E, Radziwon K, Chen GD, Liu X, Manno FA, Manno SH, Auerbach B, Wu EX, Salvi R, Lau C. Functional magnetic resonance imaging of enhanced central auditory gain and electrophysiological correlates in a behavioral model of hyperacusis. Hear Res. 2020;389:107908. https://doi.org/10.1016/j.heares.2020.107908.
175. Wu C, Bao W, Yi B, Wang Q, Wu X, Qian M, Zuo C, Huang Z. Increased metabolic activity and hysteretic enhanced GABAA receptor binding in a rat model of salicylate-induced tinnitus. Behav Brain Res. 2019;364:348–55. https://doi.org/10.1016/j.bbr.2019.02.037.
176. Xu H, Gong N, Chen L, Xu TL. Sodium salicylate reduces gamma aminobutyric acid-induced current in rat spinal dorsal horn neurons. Neuroreport. 2005;16(8):813–6. https://doi.org/10.1097/00001756-200505310-00007.
177. Yang S, Su W, Bao S. Long-term, but not transient, threshold shifts alter the morphology and increase the excitability of cortical pyramidal neurons. J Neurophysiol. 2012;108(6):1567–74. https://doi.org/10.1152/jn.00371.2012.
178. Young E. Response characteristics of neurons of the cochlear nucleus. In: Berlin C, editor. Hearing science. San Diego: College-Hill; 1984. p. 423–60.
179. Zhao Z, Ma L, Wang Y, Qin L. A comparison of neural responses in the primary auditory cortex, amygdala, and medial prefrontal cortex of cats during auditory discrimination tasks. J Neurophysiol. 2019;121(3):785–98. https://doi.org/10.1152/jn.00425.2018.
180. Zugaib J, Ceballos CC, Leao RM. High doses of salicylate reduces glycinergic inhibition in the dorsal cochlear nucleus of the rat. Hear Res. 2016;332:188–98. https://doi.org/10.1016/j.heares.2015.10.008.

Translating Animal Findings to Humans in Tinnitus Research

24

Yiwen Zheng and Paul F. Smith

Abstract

Animal models of tinnitus have made significant contributions to the current understanding of its neurobiological mechanisms and to the evaluation of potential tinnitus treatments. They have also played an important role in identifying biomarkers for tinnitus diagnosis and treatment. Nonetheless, translating findings from animal studies to humans remains a challenge due to the different and complex pathophysiologies of tinnitus, heterogeneity of the testing population, different methodologies and outcome measures, and differences in drug pharmacokinetics between animals and humans. Future translational studies that employ stricter subject selection criteria, appropriate calculations for human equivalent doses (HEDs) based on body mass, more precise control of electrode locations and stimulation parameters, and a set of comprehensive outcome measures could be expected to achieve more consistent results that may translate more readily to humans suffering from tinnitus. Considering the heterogeneity of tinnitus, developing personalised treatments based on sensitive and reliable biomarkers is urgently needed for both animal and human studies.

Y. Zheng (✉) · P. F. Smith
Department of Pharmacology and Toxicology, School of Biomedical Sciences, University of Otago, Dunedin, New Zealand

Brain Health Research Centre, University of Otago, Dunedin, New Zealand

Brain Research New Zealand, Christchurch, New Zealand

Eisdell Moore Centre for Hearing and Balance Research, University of Auckland, Auckland, New Zealand
e-mail: yiwen.zheng@otago.ac.nz

W. Schlee et al. (eds.), *Textbook of Tinnitus*, https://doi.org/10.1007/978-3-031-35647-6_24

Graphical Abstract

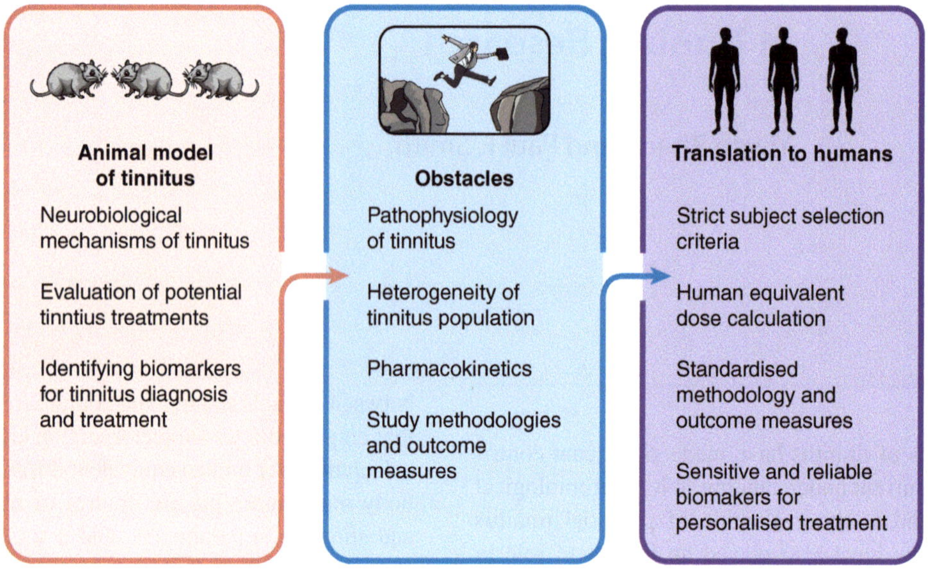

Highlights

- Animal models of tinnitus have made significant contributions to the current understanding of the neurobiological mechanisms of tinnitus and to the evaluation of potential tinnitus treatments. Animal models have also played an important role in identifying biomarkers for tinnitus diagnosis and treatment.
- Translating findings from animal studies to humans remains a challenge due to the different pathophysiologies of tinnitus, heterogeneity of the testing population, different methodologies and outcome measures, and differences in drug pharmacokinetics between animals and humans.
- Future translational studies that employ more strict subject selection criteria, appropriate calculations for human equivalent doses, precise control of the electrode locations and stimulation parameters and a set of comprehensive outcome measures are expected to achieve more consistent results.
- Considering the heterogeneity of tinnitus, developing personalised treatment based on sensitive and reliable biomarkers is urgently needed for both animal and human studies.

Abbreviations

FDA	US Food and Drug Administration
GABA	γ-aminobutyric acid
NMDA	N-methyl-D-aspartate

Introduction

Despite the increase in the global effort to understand the underlying mechanisms and to search for effective treatments, tinnitus is still an incurable condition. Apart from cognitive behavioural therapy, none of the currently available approaches, such as hearing aids, sound masking, drug treatments, acupuncture, and neuromodulation, showed beneficial effects following meta-analysis [1–4]. Cognitive behavioural therapy was effective only in improving the quality of life of tinnitus patients, but not in reducing the actual tinnitus loudness [3] (please also see Chap. 44). This is because we still do not fully understand the pathophysiology of tinnitus. Over the last 30 years, animal models of tinnitus have played an important role in characterising the pathophysiology of tinnitus, identifying therapeutic targets and biomarkers and evaluating potential therapies for tinnitus treatment. Two types of animal models of tinnitus have been used, namely the salicylate model [5–7] and the acoustic trauma model [8–16]. Using animal models, neuronal hyperactivity, increased neuronal synchrony and tonotopic map reorganisation have been reported in multiple brain areas associated with tinnitus, including the dorsal cochlear nucleus, the inferior colliculus, the medial geniculate body and the auditory cortex [17–22] (please also see Chaps. 15 and 23). Animal models have also shown neuronal activity and metabolic profile changes in both auditory and non-auditory brain areas [23–25]. These results are in general agreement with the findings from clinical imaging studies that tinnitus is associated with changes in neuronal activity and connectivity involving multiple interactive, dynamically changing neural networks [26–36]. Animal models have been used to evaluate various treatment options for tinnitus, including pharmaceuticals [37] and various stimulation techniques [38–40]. One of the problems is that almost all of the treatments tested that have been effective in animal models have failed to be replicated in clinical trials [41]. Potential reasons for that include the different pathophysiologies of tinnitus, heterogeneity of the testing population, different methodologies and outcome measures, and different drug pharmacokinetics between animals and humans, as well as intolerable side effects observed in humans that did not occur in animals.

Translating Pharmacological Treatments from Animals to Humans

Although no FDA (US Food and Drug Administration)-approved drug is currently available for tinnitus, medications are still rated as the most preferred form of treatment over external devices, cochlear implants, brain surface implants or intra-brain implants by patients [42]. There are not many drugs that have been tested both in animal models and in human clinical trials for the treatment of tinnitus. Evidence from animal studies using molecular, neurochemical or electrophysiological approaches suggests that an imbalance between inhibitory and excitatory neurotransmission may play an important role in tinnitus development [20, 33, 43, 44]. Therefore, testing drugs that modulate either excitatory or inhibitory neurotransmission has been the main focus of tinnitus research.

Based on the evidence that the NMDA (N-methyl-D-aspartate) receptor was upregulated in the cochlea and the auditory brain regions of animals following salicylate-induced tinnitus [45–48] and in limited animal studies following acoustic trauma [49, 50], many NMDA receptor antagonists have been tested in tinnitus animal models. For example, MK-801 (also known as dizocilpine, a channel blocker), 7-chlorokynurenate (a glycine-site antagonist), gacyclidine (a phencyclidine-site antagonist) and memantine (an uncompetitive NMDA receptor antagonist) have been tested in the salicylate-induced tinnitus model and showed promising effects in reducing tinnitus-like behaviour in three of the studies [45, 48, 51], but one, which used a much lower dose of memantine compared to the other studies [52]. Memantine has also been shown to reduce the number of rats exhibiting tinnitus-like behaviour in the acoustic trauma-induced tinnitus model [53]. Of those NMDA receptor antagonists tested in animals, memantine is the only one that has been tested in humans for the treatment of tinnitus [54], since memantine has been approved to be used in humans for the treatment of Alzheimer's disease [55]. However, in this prospective, randomised, placebo-controlled, double-blind crossover trial, memantine did not show significant improvement in tinnitus [54]. A number of factors could contribute to the discrepancy between the animal and human studies. In animal studies, memantine was only effective in reducing tinnitus at a dose of 5 mg/kg [48, 51, 53], but not at 3 mg/kg [52]. Using the body surface area normalisation method, the human equivalent dose for a 70 kg human for 3 mg/kg and 5 mg/kg of memantine should be approximately 34 mg/kg and 56 mg/kg, respectively. However, the dose of memantine used in the clinical trial was 20 mg/day [54], which was even lower than the ineffective dose in animals. Differences also exist in the drug administration route, i.e. subcutaneous or intraperitoneal injection in animals versus oral administration in humans. It is generally accepted that subcutaneous or intraperitoneal injection offers better bioavailability than oral administration due to variable absorption and first-pass metabolism by the liver associated with oral administration. Although there is no study directly comparing subcutaneous injection with oral administration for memantine, differences in the bioavailability of memantine between oral and patch (transdermal) administration were examined in a pharmacokinetic study in rats [56]. This study showed that memantine bioavailability was 41% and 63% for oral and patch administration, respectively [56]. Therefore, a much lower plasma concentration of memantine would be expected in the subjects in the abovementioned clinical trial than in animals.

In addition to the upregulation of glutamatergic neurotransmission, animal studies also support the association between tinnitus and a downregulation of GABAergic (γ-aminobutyric acid) neurotransmission at multiple levels along the auditory pathways. For example, $GABA_A$ receptor expression and the expression of the enzyme responsible for the synthesis of GABA, glutamic acid decarboxylase-67, were significantly reduced in the auditory brain regions following acoustic trauma or salicylate treatment [57–61]. Therefore, drugs with GABAergic-enhancing properties may be effective in the treatment of tinnitus. Since there are many GABAergic medications on the market that have already been used clinically for the treatment of epilepsy [62] and neuropathic pain [63], repurposing them for the treatment of tinnitus will maximise the therapeutic utility of these drugs and reduce the costs for new drug development.

One example is gabapentin, which is an anticonvulsant and an antinociceptive drug and has been suggested to act as a $GABA_B$ receptor agonist in the brain [64, 65]. However, more recent studies suggested that gabapentin also binds to voltage-gated calcium channels [66] and inhibits glutamatergic neurotransmission in the CA1 area of the hippocampus through presynaptic NMDA autoreceptors [67]. Nevertheless, the effect of gabapentin on tinnitus was first reported on a patient experiencing tinnitus for 10 months and gabapentin (500 mg/day) managed to keep the patient tinnitus-free during the 2-year follow-up [68]. This prompted the study that investigated gabapentin's effect on chronic tinnitus induced by unilateral acoustic trauma in rats [69]. In this study, tinnitus was induced by exposing the rats to unilateral acoustic trauma (a narrowband noise centred at 16 kHz, at 105 dB for 1 or 2 h) and confirming the perception of tinnitus in rats using a lever-pressing procedure [69]. Gabapentin was delivered in the drinking water for 10 days for each of the doses used (equivalent to 115 mg/kg and 351 mg/kg, respectively), and gabapentin significantly reduced the behavioural evidence of tinnitus at both doses [69]. However, results from the subsequent clinical trials were disappointing. In a prospective, placebo-controlled, single-blind clinical trial [70], different doses of gabapentin (800 mg–2400 mg/day) were tested in tinnitus patients with and without the association with acoustic trauma. Gabapentin was given in an ascending–descending dose series with the duration of the treatment for each dose being 4 weeks. The results showed that gabapentin improved only tinnitus annoyance in the acoustic trauma group but showed no significant effects on objective psychoacoustic tinnitus loudness in either group [70]. Four more clinical trials were conducted thereafter, and none of them supported the use of gabapentin for tinnitus [71–74]. Comparing the differences among these clinical trials, one factor that stood out is the heterogeneity of the sample populations. In Bauer (2006), tinnitus subjects were subdivided into those whose tinnitus was associated with acoustic trauma and those whose tinnitus was not associated with acoustic trauma and they reported an improvement in tinnitus annoyance that was specifically related to the acoustic trauma group. This is similar to the animal study where tinnitus was induced by acoustic trauma [69]. However, in other clinical trials, the subjects were all classified as having idiopathic tinnitus without further subdivision [71–74]. Nevertheless, gabapentin did not reduce tinnitus loudness according to objective measures in any of these studies.

Another GABAergic drug that has been tested in both animals and humans is baclofen, which is a $GABA_B$ receptor agonist and has been used as an antispastic drug for more than 40 years [75]. In the only published double-blind, placebo-controlled clinical trial with baclofen [76], patients in the baclofen group received 3 weeks of treatment with an ascending dose regimen (10 mg twice daily for week 1, 20 mg twice daily for week 2 and 30 mg twice daily for week 3). At the conclusion of the study, there was no significant difference in either the subjective or objective ratings of tinnitus between the baclofen and placebo groups [76]. However, it was argued that this study might be underpowered due to the difference in the severity of tinnitus between the baclofen and placebo groups and the inclusion of highly heterogeneous tinnitus subjects [77]. It is also noteworthy that the baclofen used in the clinical trial would be in a racemic form, which contains equal amounts of R- and L-baclofen. It has been shown that R-baclofen can reduce the effects of L-baclofen in the trigeminal nucleus [78, 79] and antagonise the effects of L-baclofen in the spinal cord [80]. Furthermore, L-baclofen was five times more effective in relieving the symptoms of trigeminal neuralgia than racemic baclofen in a double-blind crossover trial [81]. In order to investigate the potential of L-baclofen in the treatment of tinnitus, it was tested in animals with acoustic trauma-induced tinnitus [82]. In this study, animals all received vehicle, or 1, 3 or 5 mg/kg (s.c) of L-baclofen 30 min before tinnitus behavioural testing using a conditioned lick suppression paradigm with a 2-week washout period in between each dose. The results showed that both 3 and 5 mg/kg L-baclofen significantly reduced tinnitus-like behaviour in animals [82]. Comparing the doses used in animals (equivalent to 56 mg/day in humans for the highest dose) with those used in the clinical trial (60 mg/day for the highest dose), they are comparable. However, if L-baclofen is five times more effective than racemic baclofen [81], it would suggest that baclofen could have potentially been effective in the previous clinical trial if the dose was increased by five times. This is not practical as high doses of baclofen are associated with severe side effects, even causing tinnitus [83]. Therefore, future studies should see L-baclofen being tested again in clinical trials.

Another drug that has caused considerable controversy over its effectiveness for tinnitus treatment is the *Ginkgo biloba* extract, one of the most commonly used herbal supplements in the world. Although there is no FDA-approved indication, *Ginkgo biloba* has been used as an over-the-counter medication for dementia, cognitive impairment, cardiovascular diseases, psychiatric disorders, sexual dysfunction, vertigo, tinnitus, glaucoma, macular degeneration and altitude sickness [84], and recently, it has been suggested for influenza and COVID-19 infections [85]. The standardised extract, EGb-761, contains 24% flavonoids, 7% proanthocyanidins and 6% terpenoids and has been shown to have anti-oxidant, anti-inflammatory, anti-platelet aggregation and vasodilatory properties [86, 87]. The anti-oxidant, anti-inflammatory and vasodilatory effects of the *Ginkgo biloba* extract are probably the main reasons motivating the investigations for its effectiveness in reducing tinnitus. The first animal test was conducted by Jastreboff (1997) in the salicylate-induced tinnitus model, where EGb-671 was administered to the animals in a series of doses from 10 mg/kg/day to 100 mg/kg/day 2 weeks before tinnitus was induced by salicylate [88]. It was found that EGb-671 significantly reduced tinnitus-like behaviour at doses of 25, 50 and 100 mg/kg/ day [88]. This study has inspired many clinical trials to test the effectiveness of EGb-671 in tinnitus patients; however, the results have been controversial and inconclusive (see [89–94] for examples). In 2011, von Boetticher published a review analysing the randomised, placebo-controlled clinical trials published at the time and concluded that the inconsistent results could be due to the quality of the design and reporting of those trials and there was still insufficient evidence supporting the use of *Ginkgo biloba* for the treatment of tinnitus [95]. Subsequently, two animal studies were conducted investigating the effects of EGb-671 in tinnitus prevention [96] and treatment [97], respectively, in the acoustic trauma-induced tinnitus model. In the study to prevent acoustic trauma-induced tinnitus, EGb-761 (100 mg/kg/day in drinking water) was delivered to Mongolian gerbils 2 weeks before acoustic trauma and behavioural evidence of tinnitus was measured using a gap detection paradigm before and after acoustic trauma [96]. EGb-761 significantly reduced the number of tinnitus animals following acoustic trauma compared to vehicle treatment [96]. Based on this finding, they conducted the second study to investigate the effects of EGb-761 on chronic tinnitus induced by acoustic trauma, where they showed that EGb-761(100 mg/kg/day in drinking water) administered from 1 week after acoustic trauma for 3 weeks, significantly reduced the number of tinnitus animals, compared to vehicle, at 2 weeks and 3 weeks following the treatment [97]. However, tinnitus reappeared in the fourth week after EGb-761 treatment was stopped for a week [97]. While these two animal studies provided additional evidence to support the use of *Ginkgo biloba* extract for tinnitus prevention and treatment, results from recent clinical trials with tinnitus as the primary complaint are still controversial. In an open-label, randomised, crossover study, the effects of clonazepam and EGb-761 on tinnitus were compared in 39 tinnitus patients [98]. The patients received either clonazepam or EGb-761 for 3 weeks and then crossed over after 2 weeks of washout. The severity of tinnitus was measured using visual analogue scales (VAS) for subjectively perceived tinnitus loudness, annoyance and awareness, objective psychoacoustic measurements for tinnitus pitch and loudness matching and the Tinnitus Handicap Inventory (THI) for the impact of tinnitus on everyday life. It was found that clonazepam significantly improved tinnitus in terms of tinnitus loudness, tinnitus awareness, tinnitus annoyance and THI scores, whereas EGb-761 did not show any beneficial effects [98]. By contrast, another randomised, double-blind clinical trial showed the opposite. In this study, the effects of EGb-761 on tinnitus were compared with that of pentoxifylline, which is a competitive nonselective phosphodiesterase inhibitor for muscle pain [99]. Patients in this study received either EGb-761 or pentoxifylline for 12 weeks and the therapeutic effects were evaluated by a numeric analogue scale (11-Point Box Scales) for tinnitus loudness and annoyance, a self-rating scale (Mini-TQ) for the psychological burden of tinnitus and the Hospital Anxiety and Depression scale (HADS) for anxiety and depression. Both treatments resulted in significant improvements in all tinnitus-related scores and scores for anxiety and disability [99]. It is notable that different outcome measures were used in the two studies, especially the inclusion of psychoacoustic measurement for tinnitus loudness in Han et al. (2018) [98], but not in Procházková et al. (2018) [99]. It needs to be mentioned that the two studies employed different experimental designs. While the first one used a crossover design [98], the second one used a parallel group design [99]. One of the disadvantages of a crossover study is that the treatment effects of the first drug may be carried over to the phase of the second drug. In Han et al. (2018) [98], they did notice the carryover effects of clonazepam on EGb-761 treatment in the clonazepam first group. However, despite the residual improvement in tinnitus associated with clonazepam, EGb-761 treatment actually increased tinnitus loudness during the assessment period [98], which suggests that the lack of effect of EGb-761 on tinnitus could be a replicable phenomenon. The discrepancy between the two studies could also be due to the lower dose and shorter treatment duration of EGb-761 used in Han et al. (2018) [98]. Therefore, more clinical trials using comparable designs and dosage are needed in order to assess the effectiveness of the *Ginkgo biloba* extract in tinnitus treatment (please also see Chap. 48 on pharmacotherapy in tinnitus).

Translating Brain Stimulation Therapies from Animals to Humans

Another area that has stimulated a considerable amount of animal and human research is the use of various stimulation techniques to achieve neuromodulation for tinnitus treatment. Although the neuropathology of tinnitus is still not fully understood, research from both animals and humans suggests that tinnitus is a result of changes in multiple neural networks. For example, peripheral auditory damage has been shown to cause long-term plasticity in the brain auditory pathways evidenced by neuronal hyperactivity, hypersynchrony and tonotopic map reorganisation, i.e. the “bottom-up” theory [18–22, 100]. Although it is true that the majority of tinnitus patients have some degree of sensorineural hearing loss [101], the fact that not everyone with sensorineural hearing loss develops tinnitus [101] suggests changes in the auditory system alone are not sufficient for the perception of tinnitus. Increasing evidence from both human and animal studies points to the involvement of non-auditory brain structures in tinnitus generation and perception [23, 26–28, 30–32, 102, 103]. In particular, the frontal–limbic–striatal structures have been proposed to act as a "noise cancellation" system to block the repetitive unwanted noises within the auditory pathways from reaching conscious perception. Therefore, tinnitus has been suggested to be a result of a breakdown of this "noise cancellation" system, i.e. the "top-down" theory [104]. Therefore, it seems conceivable that restoring normal brain network activity through neuromodulation may provide an effective therapeutic avenue in tinnitus treatment. Although there are many clinical trials in humans testing various stimulation protocols (intracochlear stimulation, direct electrical brain stimulation, transcranial direct current stimulation, transcranial magnetic stimulation, somatosensory stimulation and bimodal stimulation) [105–111], animal studies are very limited [38]. Earlier animal studies on stimulation-induced neuromodulation and tinnitus were focused on the stimulation of the auditory system, mainly the cochlear nucleus [112] and the auditory cortex [113, 114]. Electrical stimulation of either the cochlear nucleus or the auditory cortex suppressed tinnitus-like behaviour in animals [112, 113], which in general supported the clinical studies showing promising effects from stimulation of the same structures on tinnitus [115–119]. However, no animal study has investigated the underlying neurobiological mechanisms in order to optimise the stimulation parameters for auditory cortex stimulation, which could be further explored in future studies.

By comparison, the recent development of bimodal stimulation, i.e. pairing vagus nerve or somatosensory stimulation with sound stimulation for the treatment of tinnitus, offers a great example of translating animal studies to humans. Although vagus nerve stimulation has been approved by the FDA for the treatment of epilepsy and depression, its potential application in tinnitus treatment was only suggested by Engineer et al. (2011) [39] in an animal study. The study showed that vagus nerve stimulation paired with tones of multiple non-tinnitus frequencies significantly reversed acoustic trauma-induced tinnitus in animals and reversed the tonotopic map reorganisation, reduced neuronal hyperactivity and decreased neuronal synchrony in the auditory cortex [39]. This has stimulated a series of studies to assess the effectiveness and safety of this type of stimulation, optimising the stimulation parameters and exploring the mechanisms of action, over the last 20 years. However, based on the two most recent reviews, the clinical studies all suffered from critical limitations, such as a considerable risk of bias in participant selection, small sample sizes and lack of detail on methodology; therefore, there is no strong evidence to support the effectiveness of vagus nerve stimulation in reducing tinnitus [107, 120]. In addition to the general poor quality of the available clinical studies, different studies employed different vagus nerve stimulation locations, different stimulation parameters and different outcome measures, which made it even more difficult to draw any conclusions confidently [120]. Therefore, more clinical studies are needed to refine and optimise the technique. For example, the effects of different rates and duration of vagus nerve stimulation when paired with tones on cortical plasticity have been investigated in animals and a specific set of paired stimulation parameters that could drive effective cortical remapping have been identified [121]; however, this information has not been incorporated into clinical studies, which could result in better clinical outcomes.

In addition to the vagus nerve stimulation, somatosensory stimulation paired with auditory stimulation as a potential treatment for tinnitus has also made significant progress in translation from animals to humans. Based on animal studies showing that stimulation-timing-dependent plasticity could be achieved by precisely pairing somatosensory stimulation with auditory stimulation [122–124] and that the timing rules were altered in tinnitus animals compared to either sham or tinnitus-free animals [125], paired stimulation of the somatosensory and auditory systems was tested in an a guinea pig model of acoustic trauma-induced tinnitus and in a small sample of participants with somatic tinnitus [40]. It was found that paired stimulation was known to induce long-term depression, reduced neuronal hypersynchrony in the cochlear nucleus and reversed behavioural evidence of tinnitus in animals [40]. It also reduced tinnitus loudness and tinnitus-related distress in tinnitus patients [40]. Although this type of paired stimulation was only tested in a very small number of patients with somatic tinnitus, it provided promising results in supporting further investigations, especially in large randomised, controlled clinical trials.

Another form of bimodal stimulation that has not been tested in animals, but showed promising clinical efficacy in reducing tinnitus, is paired somatosensory auditory stimulation through the stimulation of the trigeminal nerve via the tongue. It was first tested in an open-label feasibility and safety study in participants with constant subjective tinnitus for more than 6 months. In this study, the auditory stimulation and the tongue stimulation were delivered simultaneously, and following 10 weeks of 30–60 min daily stimulation, there were significant improvements on the THI scores and minimal masking level but no significant reduction in the tinnitus loudness matching [126]. The stimulation was well tolerated, and there were no adverse effects reported. Based on these results, a randomised, double-blind clinical trial was conducted [110]. This study included 326 participants that were further divided into three treatment arms and subjects in each arm received a different stimulation parameter

60 min daily for 12 weeks. They reported a very impressive outcome with overall tinnitus improvement in 81% of the participants at the end of the 12-week treatment period and 77% at 12 months after the treatment [110]. They also showed that two of the three stimulation parameters demonstrated sustained effects in reducing tinnitus [110], which is supported by the neurophysiological evidence from animal studies [122–124]. One of the limitations of this study was the lack of control groups, e.g. placebo control, sound stimulation only and tongue stimulation only groups, although they are difficult to conduct blind under these conditions. In addition, the primary endpoints were THI and TFI scores and changes in tinnitus loudness were not measured objectively. Nevertheless, both animal and human studies suggest that bimodal stimulation is a promising therapy for tinnitus treatment (Please also see Chap. 54). It is interesting to note that transcutaneous vagus nerve stimulation for tinnitus treatment has been performed by placing the stimulating electrode(s) on the auricular branch of the vagus nerve, i.e. at tragus, cymba concha and/or cavum of the external ear [120]. However, innervation at those places is complicated by somatogenic fibres, such as the trigeminal nerve, the facial nerve and the superficial branches of the cervical plexus originating from the C2 and C3 spinal nerves [127], which are also the targets for the paired somatosensory auditory stimulation. Therefore, it seems impossible to separate the effects of transcutaneous vagus nerve stimulation from that of somatosensory stimulation from the current clinical studies. It has been shown that transcutaneous vagus nerve stimulation-induced multiple neural network changes, including not only the activation of the vagus-related brainstem nuclei, but also the deactivation of the auditory and limbic systems [128] and the modulation of tinnitus-related beta- and gamma-band activity [129]. Further animal and clinical studies should investigate the neural network changes induced by paired somatosensory stimulation and compare them with those of paired transcutaneous vagus nerve stimulation, in order to understand the similarities/differences between these two techniques and to improve the outcomes of tinnitus treatment (please also see Chaps. 52 and 53 for non-invasive and invasive brain stimulation in humans).

Challenges and Future Directions

Animal models of tinnitus are indispensable in tinnitus research to understand the underlying pathophysiology of tinnitus, to screen, evaluate and optimise potential therapies and to explore the mechanism of action of those therapies. However, as for many other animal models of human disease, animal models of tinnitus are often criticised for their validity in reproducing the clinical symptoms of tinnitus and the reliability of the methods to detect and quantify the perception of the phantom tinnitus sound in animals [130]. The currently available tinnitus animal models all have their advantages and drawbacks, and there is no consensus on which animal model of tinnitus, as well as which tinnitus assessment method, is the best to use. However, it is very important for tinnitus research using animals to objectively confirm the perception of tinnitus in those animals, as not every animal would develop tinnitus following the intervention [131]. It is also important for animal studies to include proper control groups to be tested in parallel with other experimental groups. For example, a group of control animals receiving the tested treatment to control for any nonspecific effects of the treatment on the animal's behaviour [132], which is often omitted in animal studies. In general, the main advantage of using animal models is the ability to control the homogeneity of the aetiology and experimental conditions, to have a comprehensive experimental design and statistical analysis and to use a range of technologies, non-invasive and invasive, to investigate the underlying mechanisms. However, these advantages of animal studies also become limitations when translating the treatment to humans, as tinnitus is a highly heterogeneous condition with many different causes and comorbidities [133]. The participant inclusion criteria for most of the clinical trials have not distinguished different subtypes of tinnitus, which may explain the overall low translatability of tinnitus treatment from animals to humans. In addition, the inappropriate drug dose translation from animals to humans and the less precise control of the electrode locations and stimulation parameters in human studies compared to that in animals may also account for discrepancies between animal and human studies.

Another challenge for the translation from animal to human studies is the different outcome measures. In animal studies, tinnitus severity and any therapeutic effect on tinnitus are exclusively measured by the "objective" perception of tinnitus, i.e. the changes in animal's behaviour in response to certain frequencies and intensities of sound. However, tinnitus evaluation in clinical trials is often made by a combination of objective pitch/loudness matching, subjective tinnitus ratings or self-assessment questionnaires. While there is no consensus on the correlation between these measurements [134–138], the subjective tinnitus ratings and self-assessment questionnaires are the most frequently used outcome measures due to their simplicity and ease of administration. Since tinnitus is a subjective condition with multidimensional changes covering auditory, emotional and attentional aspects, it is recommended to use both objective and subjective measurements that take different aspects of tinnitus into account [139]. In addition, much effort has been made to identify objective markers, such as biochemical [140, 141], electrophysiological [142] and neuroanatomical [143] measurements, for tinnitus diagnosis and treatment assessment. The advancement in the development of sensitive and accurate objective outcome measures of tinnitus in humans will greatly improve the quality of future clinical trials.

Since tinnitus can be caused and influenced by many factors, developing personalised treatment should be the future focus in both animal and human tinnitus research. A recent study showed that an individual's demographic, tinnitus and treatment characteristics collected through a survey from an Internet Web platform could be used to make a modest prediction of the treatment outcomes, which suggests that the heterogeneity of tinnitus could be used to develop personalised treatment [144]. Another technique that could be used to subtype tinnitus patients and develop personalised treatment is metabolomics, which is the large-scale study of small molecule metabolites within cells, biofluids, tissues or organisms and has been used to identify biomarkers for many diseases [145–151]. Metabolic profiling has also been proposed to subtype diseases, such as breast cancer [152], stroke [153] and Alzheimer's disease [154], for better diagnosis and treatment. Animal studies have shown that acoustic trauma altered multiple metabolic pathways not only in the auditory brain regions [24, 25], but also in the hippocampus and serum [24]. Based on these findings, a pilot study using serum samples from 30 tinnitus patients and 30 control subjects revealed a significant metabolic profile shift in tinnitus patients (unpublished observations by the authors). Although these are very preliminary results, they suggest that metabolomics may be a useful technology in identifying tinnitus biomarkers, tinnitus subtyping and developing personalised tinnitus treatment.

References

1. Liu F, Han X, Li Y, Yu S. Acupuncture in the treatment of tinnitus: a systematic review and meta-analysis. Eur Arch Otorhinolaryngol. 2016;273(2):285–94.
2. Hoare DJ, Kowalkowski VL, Kang S, Hall DA. Systematic review and meta-analyses of randomized controlled trials examining tinnitus management. Laryngoscope. 2011;121(7):1555–64.
3. Hesser H, Weise C, Westin VZ, Andersson G. A systematic review and meta-analysis of randomized controlled trials of cognitive-behavioral therapy for tinnitus distress. Clin Psychol Rev. 2011;31(4):545–53.
4. Song JJ, Vanneste S, Van de Heyning P, De Ridder D. Transcranial direct current stimulation in tinnitus patients: a systemic review and meta-analysis. ScientificWorldJournal. 2012;2012:427941.
5. Stolzberg D, Hayes SH, Kashanian N, Radziwon K, Salvi RJ, Allman BL. A novel behavioral assay for the assessment of acute tinnitus in rats optimized for simultaneous recording of oscillatory neural activity. J Neurosci Methods. 2013;219(2):224–32.
6. Jastreboff PJ, Brennan JF, Sasaki CT. An animal model for tinnitus. Laryngoscope. 1988;98(3):280–6.
7. Lobarinas E, Sun W, Cushing R, Salvi R. A novel behavioral paradigm for assessing tinnitus using schedule-induced polydipsia avoidance conditioning (SIP-AC). Hear Res. 2004;190(1–2):109–14.
8. Brozoski TJ, Spires TJD, Bauer CA. Vigabatrin, a GABA transaminase inhibitor, reversibly eliminates tinnitus in an animal model. J Assoc Res Otolarnygol. 2007;8(1):105–18.
9. Turner J, Larsen D, Hughes L, Moechars D, Shore S. Time course of tinnitus development following noise exposure in mice. J Neurosci Res. 2012;90(7):1480–8.
10. Zheng Y, Hamilton E, Stiles L, McNamara E, de Waele C, Smith PF, et al. Acoustic trauma that can cause tinnitus impairs impulsive control but not performance accuracy in the 5-choice serial reaction time task in rats. Neuroscience. 2011;180:75–84.
11. Heffner HE. A two-choice sound localization procedure for detecting lateralized tinnitus in animals. Behav Res Methods. 2011;43(2):577–89.
12. Zuo H, Lei D, Sivaramakrishnan S, Howie B, Mulvany J, Bao J. An operant-based detection method for inferring tinnitus in mice. J Neurosci Methods. 2017;291:227–37.
13. Dehmel S, Eisinger D, Shore SE. Gap prepulse inhibition and auditory brainstem-evoked potentials as objective measures for tinnitus in Guinea pigs. Front Syst Neurosci. 2012;6:42.
14. Brozoski TJ, Bauer CA, Caspary DM. Elevated fusiform cell activity in the dorsal cochlear nucleus of chinchillas with psychophysical evidence of tinnitus. J Neurosci. 2002;22:2383–90.
15. Nowotny M, Remus M, Kossl M, Gaese BH. Characterization of the perceived sound of trauma-induced tinnitus in gerbils. J Acoust Soc Am. 2011;130(5):2827–34.
16. Heffner HE, Koay G. Tinnitus and hearing loss in hamsters (Mesocricetus auratus) exposed to loud sound. Behav Neurosci. 2005;119(3):734–42.
17. Kaltenbach JA, Zhang J, Afman CE. Plasticity of spontaneous neural activity in the dorsal cochlear nucleus after intense sound exposure. Hear Res. 2000;147:282–92.
18. Chang H, Chen K, Kaltenbach JA, Zhang J, Godfrey DA. Effects of acoustic trauma on dorsal cochlear nucleus neuron activity in slices. Hear Res. 2002;164:59–68.
19. Kaltenbach JA, Zacharek MA, Zhang J, Frederick S. Activity in the dorsal cochlear nucleus of hamsters previously tested for tinnitus following intense tone exposure. Neurosci Lett. 2004;355:121–5.
20. Eggermont JJ, Roberts LE. The neuroscience of tinnitus. Trends Neurosci. 2004;27(11):676–82.
21. Brozoski TJ, Ciobanu L, Bauer CA. Central neural activity in rats with tinnitus evaluated with manganese-enhanced magnetic resonance imaging (MEMRI). Hear Res. 2007;228(1–2):168–79.
22. Kalappa BI, Brozoski TJ, Turner JG, Caspary DM. Single unit hyperactivity and bursting in the auditory thalamus of awake rats directly correlates with behavioural evidence of tinnitus. J Physiol. 2014;592(Pt 22):5065–78.
23. Chen YC, Li X, Liu L, Wang J, Lu CQ, Yang M, et al. Tinnitus and hyperacusis involve hyperactivity and enhanced connectivity in auditory-limbic-arousal-cerebellar network. elife. 2015;4:e06576.
24. He J, Aa JY, Sun JG, Smith PF, De Ridder D, Wang GJ, et al. Metabolic changes in the brain and blood of rats following acoustic trauma, tinnitus and hyperacusis. Prog Brain Res. 2021;262;399–430.
25. He J, Zhu YJ, Aa JY, Smith PF, De Ridder D, Wang GJ, et al. Brain metabolic changes in rats following acoustic trauma. Front Neurosci. 2017;11:260.
26. Boyen K, de Kleine E, van Dijk P, Langers DRM. Tinnitus-related dissociation between cortical and subcortical neural activity in humans with mild to moderate sensorineural hearing loss. Hear Res. 2014;312:48–59.
27. Husain FT, Schmidt SA. Using resting state functional connectivity to unravel networks of tinnitus. Hear Res. 2014;307:153–62.
28. Leaver AM, Renier L, Chevillet MA, Morgan S, Kim HJ, Rauschecker JP. Dysregulation of limbic and auditory networks in tinnitus. Neuron. 2011;69(1):33–43.

29. Maudoux A, Lefebvre P, Cabay JE, Demertzi A, Vanhaudenhuyse A, Laureys S, et al. Auditory resting-state network connectivity in tinnitus: a functional MRI study. PLoS One. 2012;7(5):e36222.
30. Song JJ, De Ridder D, Van de Heyning P, Vanneste S. Mapping tinnitus-related brain activation: an activation-likelihood estimation metaanalysis of PET studies. J Nucl Med. 2012;53(10):1550–7.
31. Vanneste S, de Heyning PV, De Ridder D. The neural network of phantom sound changes over time: a comparison between recent-onset and chronic tinnitus patients. Eur J Neurosci. 2011;34(5):718–31.
32. Vanneste S, De Ridder D. The auditory and non-auditory brain areas involved in tinnitus. An emergent property of multiple parallel overlapping subnetworks. Front Syst Neurosci. 2012;6:31.
33. Roberts LE, Eggermont JJ, Caspary DM, Shore SE, Melcher JR, Kaltenbach JA. Ringing ears: the neuroscience of tinnitus. J Neurosci. 2010;30(45):14972–9.
34. Henry JA, Roberts LE, Caspary DM, Theodoroff SM, Salvi RJ. Underlying mechanisms of tinnitus: review and clinical implications. J Am Acad Audiol. 2014;25(1):5–22.
35. Leaver AM, Turesky TK, Seydell-Greenwald A, Morgan S, Kim HJ, Rauschecker JP. Intrinsic network activity in tinnitus investigated using functional MRI. Hum Brain Mapp. 2016;37(8):2717–35.
36. Simonetti P, Oiticica J. Tinnitus neural mechanisms and structural changes in the brain: the contribution of neuroimaging research. Int Arc Otorhinolaryngol. 2015;19(3):259–65.
37. Zheng Y, McTavish J, Smith PF. Pharmacological evaluation of drugs in animal models of tinnitus. Curr Top Behav Neurosci. 2021;51:51–82.
38. Zhang J, Firestone E, Elattma A. Animal models of tinnitus treatment: cochlear and brain stimulation. Curr Top Behav Neurosci. 2021;51:83–129.
39. Engineer ND, Riley JR, Seale JD, Vrana WA, Shetake JA, Sudanagunta SP, et al. Reversing pathological neural activity using targeted plasticity. Nature. 2011;470(7332):101–U14.
40. Marks KL, Martel DT, Wu C, Basura GJ, Roberts LE, Schvartz-Leyzac KC, et al. Auditory-somatosensory bimodal stimulation desynchronizes brain circuitry to reduce tinnitus in Guinea pigs and humans. Sci Transl Med. 2018;10(422):eaal3175.
41. McFerran DJ, Stockdale D, Holme R, Large CH, Baguley DM. Why is there no cure for tinnitus? Front Neurosci. 2019;13:802.
42. Tyler RS. Patient preferences and willingness to pay for tinnitus treatments. J Am Acad Audiol. 2012;23(2):115–25.
43. Eggermont JJ. Tinnitus: neurobiological substrates. Drug Discov Today. 2005;10(19):1283–90.
44. Wang H, Brozoski TJ, Caspary DM. Inhibitory neurotransmission in animal models of tinnitus: maladaptive plasticity. Hear Res. 2011;279(1–2):111–7.
45. Guitton MJ, Caston J, Ruel J, Johnson RM, Pujol R, Puel J-L. Salicylate induces tinnitus through activation of cochlear NMDA receptors. J Neurosci. 2003;23(9):3944–52.
46. Hu SS, Mei L, Chen JY, Huang ZW, Wu H. Expression of immediate-early genes in the dorsal cochlear nucleus in salicylate-induced tinnitus. Eur Arch Otorhinolaryngol. 2015;273:325.
47. Hwang JH, Chen JC, Chan YC. Effects of c-phycocyanin and spirulina on salicylate-induced tinnitus, expression of NMDA receptor and inflammatory genes. PLoS One. 2013;8(3):e58215.
48. Jang CH, Lee S, Park IY, Song A, Moon C, Cho GW. Memantine attenuates salicylate-induced tinnitus possibly by reducing NR2B expression in auditory cortex of rat. Exp Neurobiol. 2019;28(4):495–503.
49. Godfrey DA, Kaltenbach JA, Chen K, Ilyas O, Liu X, Licari F, et al. Amino acid concentrations in the hamster central auditory system and long-term effects of intense tone exposure. J Neurosci Res. 2012;90(11):2214–24.
50. Dong S, Mulders WH, Rodger J, Woo S, Robertson D. Acoustic trauma evokes hyperactivity and changes in gene expression in Guinea-pig auditory brainstem. Eur J Neurosci. 2010;31(9):1616–28.
51. Ralli M, Troiani D, Podda MV, Paciello F, Eramo SL, de Corso E, et al. The effect of the NMDA channel blocker memantine on salicylate-induced tinnitus in rats. Acta Otorhinolaryngol Ital. 2014;34(3):198–204.
52. Lobarinas E, Yang G, Sun W, Ding D, Mirza N, Dalby-Brown W, et al. Salicylate- and quinine-induced tinnitus and effects of memantine. Acta Otolaryngol Suppl. 2006;126(sup556):13–9.
53. Zheng Y, McNamara Y, Stiles L, Darlington CL, Smith PF. Evidence that memantine reduces chronic tinnitus caused by acoustic trauma in rats. Front Neurol. 2012;3:127.
54. Figueiredo RR, Langguth B, Mello de Oliveira P, Aparecida de Azevedo A. Tinnitus treatment with memantine. Otolaryngol Head Neck Surg. 2008;138(4):492–6.
55. Atri A. Current and future treatments in Alzheimer's disease. Semin Neurol. 2019;39(2):227–40.
56. Lee SH, Kim SH, Noh YH, Choi BM, Noh GJ, Park WD, et al. Pharmacokinetics of Memantine after a single and multiple dose of Oral and patch administration in rats. Basic Clin Pharmacol Toxicol. 2016;118(2):122–7.
57. Browne CJ, Morley JW, Parsons CH. Tracking the expression of excitatory and inhibitory neurotransmission-related proteins and neuroplasticity markers after noise induced hearing loss. PLoS One. 2012;7(3):e33272.
58. Dong S, Rodger J, Mulders WH, Robertson D. Tonotopic changes in GABA receptor expression in Guinea pig inferior colliculus after partial unilateral hearing loss. Brain Res. 2010;1342:24–32.
59. Zou QZ, Shang XL. Effect of salicylate on the large GABAergic neurons in the inferior colliculus of rats. Acta Neurol Belg. 2012;112(4):367–74.
60. Butt S, Ashraf F, Porter LA, Zhang H. Sodium salicylate reduces the level of GABAB receptors in the rat's inferior colliculus. Neuroscience. 2016;316:41–52.
61. Bauer CA, Brozoski TJ, Holder TM, Caspary DM. Effects of chronic salicylate on GABAergic activity in rat inferior colliculus. Hear Res. 2000;147(1–2):175–82.
62. Hakami T. Neuropharmacology of antiseizure drugs. Neuropsychopharmacol Rep. 2021;41:336.
63. Urits I, Li N, Berardino K, Artounian KA, Bandi P, Jung JW, et al. The use of antineuropathic medications for the treatment of chronic pain. Best Pract Res Clin Anaesthesiol. 2020;34(3):493–506.
64. Bertrand S, Ng GY, Purisai MG, Wolfe SE, Severidt MW, Nouel D, et al. The anticonvulsant, antihyperalgesic agent gabapentin is an agonist at brain gamma-aminobutyric acid type B receptors negatively coupled to voltage-dependent calcium channels. J Pharmacol Exp Ther. 2001;298(1):15–24.
65. Ng GY, Bertrand S, Sullivan R, Ethier N, Wang J, Yergey J, et al. Gamma-aminobutyric acid type B receptors with specific heterodimer composition and postsynaptic actions in hippocampal neurons are targets of anticonvulsant gabapentin action. Mol Pharmacol. 2001;59(1):144–52.
66. Kukkar A, Bali A, Singh N, Jaggi AS. Implications and mechanism of action of gabapentin in neuropathic pain. Arch Pharm Res. 2013;36(3):237–51.
67. Suarez LM, Suarez F, Del Olmo N, Ruiz M, Gonzalez-Escalada JR, Solis JM. Presynaptic NMDA autoreceptors facilitate axon excitability: a new molecular target for the anticonvulsant gabapentin. Eur J Neurosci. 2005;21(1):197–209.
68. Zapp JJ. Gabapentin for the treatment of tinnitus: a case report. Ear Nose Throat J. 2001;80(2):114–6.
69. Bauer CA, Brozoski TJ. Assessing tinnitus and prospective tinnitus therapeutics using a psychophysical animal model. J Assoc Res Otolaryngol. 2001;2(1):54–64.

70. Bauer CA, Brozoski TJ. Effect of gabapentin on the sensation and impact of tinnitus. Laryngoscope. 2006;116(5):675–81.
71. Piccirillo JF, Finnell J, Vlahiotis A, Chole RA, Spitznagel EJ. Relief of idiopathic subjective tinnitus: is gabapentin effective? Arch Otolaryngol Head Neck Surg. 2007;133(4):390–7.
72. Witsell DL, Hannley MT, Stinnet S, Tucci DL. Treatment of tinnitus with gabapentin: a pilot study. Otol Neurotol. 2007;28(1):11–5.
73. Bakhshaee M, Ghasemi M, Azarpazhooh M, Khadivi E, Rezaei S, Shakeri M, et al. Gabapentin effectiveness on the sensation of subjective idiopathic tinnitus: a pilot study. Eur Arch Otorhinolaryngol. 2008;265(5):525–30.
74. Dehkordi MA, Abolbashari S, Taheri R, Einolghozati S. Efficacy of gabapentin on subjective idiopathic tinnitus: a randomized, double-blind, placebo-controlled trial. Ear Nose Throat J. 2011;90(4):150–8.
75. Sachais BA, Logue JN, Carey MS. Baclofen, a new antispastic drug. A controlled, multicenter trial in patients with multiple sclerosis. Arch Neurol. 1977;34(7):422–8.
76. Westerberg BD, Roberson JB, Stach BA. A double-blind placebo-controlled trial of baclofen in the treatment of tinnitus. Am J Otol. 1996;17:896–903.
77. Møller AR. A double-blind placebo-controlled trial of baclofen in the treatment of tinnitus. Am J Otol. 1997;18(2):268–9.
78. Terrence CF, Sax M, Fromm GH, Chang CH, Yoo CS. Effect of baclofen enantiomorphs on the spinal trigeminal nucleus and steric similarities of carbamazepine. Pharmacology. 1983;27(2):85–94.
79. Fromm GH, Shibuya T, Nakata M, Terrence CF. Effects of D-baclofen and L-baclofen on the trigeminal nucleus. Neuropharmacology. 1990;29(3):249–54.
80. Sawynok J, Dickson C. D-baclofen is an antagonist at baclofen receptors mediating antinociception in the spinal cord. Pharmacology. 1985;31(5):248–59.
81. Fromm GH, Terrence CF. Comparison of L-baclofen and racemic baclofen in trigeminal neuralgia. Neurology. 1987;37(11):1725–8.
82. Zheng Y, Vagal S, Hamilton E, Darlington CL, Smith PF. A dose-response analysis of the effects of L-baclofen on chronic tinnitus caused by acoustic trauma in rats Neuropharmacology. 2012;62(2):940–6.
83. Auffret M, Rolland B, Deheul S, Loche V, Hennaux C, Cottencin O, et al. Severe tinnitus induced by off-label baclofen. Ann Pharmacother. 2014;48(5):656–9.
84. Nguyen T, Alzahrani T, Biloba G. StatPearls. Treasure Island, FL: StatPearls Publishing LLC; 2021. StatPearls publishing copyright © 2021.
85. Ibrahim MA, Ramadan HH, Mohammed RN. Evidence that ginkgo Biloba could use in the influenza and coronavirus COVID-19 infections. J Basic Clin Physiol Pharmacol. 2021;32(3):131–43.
86. Chan PC, Xia Q, Fu PP. Ginkgo biloba leave extract: biological, medicinal, and toxicological effects. J Environ Sci Health C Environ Carcinog Ecotoxicol Rev. 2007;25(3):211–44.
87. Maclennan KM, Darlington CL, Smith PF. The CNS effects of Ginkgo biloba extracts and ginkgolide B. Prog Neurobiol. 2002;67(3):235–57.
88. Jastreboff PJ, Zhou S, Jastreboff MM, Kwapisz U, Gryczynska U. Attenuation of salicylate-induced tinnitus by Ginkgo biloba extract in rats. Audiol Neurootol. 1997;2(4):197–212.
89. Holgers KM, Axelsson A, Pringle I. Ginkgo biloba extract for the treatment of tinnitus. Audiology. 1994;33(2):85–92.
90. Drew S, Davies E. Effectiveness of Ginkgo biloba in treating tinnitus: double blind, placebo controlled trial. BMJ. 2001;322(7278):73.
91. Morgenstern C, Biermann E. The efficacy of ginkgo special extract EGb 761 in patients with tinnitus. Int J Clin Pharmacol Ther. 2002;40(5):188–97.
92. Rejai D, Sivakumar A, Balaji N. Ginkgo biloba does not benefit patients with tinnitus: a randomized placebo-controlled double-blind trial and meta-analysis of randomized trials. Clin Otolaryngol Allied Sci. 2004;29:226–31.
93. Ihl R, Bachinskaya N, Korczyn AD, Vakhapova V, Tribanek M, Hoerr R, et al. Efficacy and safety of a once-daily formulation of Ginkgo biloba extract EGb 761 in dementia with neuropsychiatric features: a randomized controlled trial. Int J Geriatr Psychiatry. 2011;26(11):1186–94.
94. Canis M, Olzowy B, Welz C, Suckfüll M, Stelter K. Simvastatin and Ginkgo biloba in the treatment of subacute tinnitus: a retrospective study of 94 patients. Am J Otolaryngol. 2011;32(1):19–23.
95. von Boetticher A. Ginkgo biloba extract in the treatment of tinnitus: a systematic review. Neuropsychiatr Dis Treat. 2011;7:441–7.
96. Tziridis K, Korn S, Ahlf S, Schulze H. Protective effects of Ginkgo biloba extract EGb 761 against noise trauma-induced hearing loss and tinnitus development. Neural Plast. 2014;2014:427298.
97. Krauss P, Tziridis K, Buerbank S, Schilling A, Schulze H. Therapeutic value of Ginkgo biloba extract EGb 761® in an animal model (Meriones unguiculatus) for noise trauma induced hearing loss and tinnitus. PLoS One. 2016;11(6):e0157574.
98. Han SS, Nam EC, Won JY, Lee KU, Chun W, Choi HK, et al. Clonazepam quiets tinnitus: a randomised crossover study with Ginkgo biloba. J Neurol Neurosurg Psychiatry. 2012;83(8):821–7.
99. Procházková K, Šejna I, Skutil J, Hahn A. Ginkgo biloba extract EGb 761(®) versus pentoxifylline in chronic tinnitus: a randomized, double-blind clinical trial. Int J Clin Pharm. 2018;40(5):1335–41.
100. Kaltenbach JA, Afman CE. Hyperactivity in the dorsal cochlear nucleus after intense sound exposure and its resemblance to tone-evoked activity: a physiological model for tinnitus. Hear Res. 2000;140:165–72.
101. Hoffmann HJ, Reed G. Epidemiology of tinnitus. In: Tinnitus: theory and management. Hamilton: B.C. Decker; 2004. p. 16–41.
102. Kraus KS, Canlon B. Neuronal connectivity and interactions between the auditory and limbic systems. Effects of noise and tinnitus. Hear Res. 2012;288(1–2):34–46.
103. Maudoux A, Lefebvre P, Cabay JE, Demertzi A, Vanhaudenhuyse A, Laureys S, et al. Connectivity graph analysis of the auditory resting state network in tinnitus. Brain Res. 2012;1485:10–21.
104. Rauschecker JP, Leaver AM, Muhlau M. Tuning out the noise: limbic-auditory interactions in tinnitus. Neuron. 2010;66(6):819–26.
105. Perreau A, Tyler R, Mancini PC. Programming a Cochlear implant for tinnitus suppression. J Am Acad Audiol. 2020;31(4):302–8.
106. Yin L, Chen X, Lu X, An Y, Zhang T, Yan J. An updated meta-analysis: repetitive transcranial magnetic stimulation for treating tinnitus. J Int Med Res. 2021;49(3):300060521999549.
107. Stegeman I, Velde HM, Robe P, Stokroos RJ, Smit AL. Tinnitus treatment by vagus nerve stimulation: a systematic review. PLoS One. 2021;16(3):e0247221.
108. Byun YJ, Lee JA, Nguyen SA, Rizk HG, Meyer TA, Lambert PR. Transcutaneous electrical nerve stimulation for treatment of tinnitus: a systematic review and meta-analysis. Otol Neurotol. 2020;41(7):e767–e75.
109. Deklerck AN, Marechal C, Pérez Fernández AM, Keppler H, Van Roost D, Dhooge IJM. Invasive neuromodulation as a treatment for tinnitus: a systematic review. Neuromodulation. 2020;23(4):451–62.
110. Conlon B, Langguth B, Hamilton C, Hughes S, Meade E, Connor CO, et al. Bimodal neuromodulation combining sound and tongue stimulation reduces tinnitus symptoms in a large randomized clinical study. Sci Transl Med. 2020;12(564):eabb2830.
111. Yuan T, Yadollahpour A, Salgado-Ramírez J, Robles-Camarillo D, Ortega-Palacios R. Transcranial direct current stimulation for the treatment of tinnitus: a review of clinical trials and mechanisms of action. BMC Neurosci. 2018;19(1):66.

112. Luo H, Zhang X, Nation J, Pace E, Lepczyk L, Zhang J. Tinnitus suppression by electrical stimulation of the rat dorsal cochlear nucleus. Neurosci Lett. 2012;522(1):16–20.
113. Zhang J, Zhang Y, Zhang X. Auditory cortex electrical stimulation suppresses tinnitus in rats. J Assoc Res Otolaryngol. 2011;12(2):185–201.
114. Yang H, Xiong H, Ou Y, Xu Y, Pang J, Lai L, et al. Effect of repetitive transcranial magnetic stimulation on auditory function following acoustic trauma. Neurol Sci. 2016;37(9):1511–6.
115. Soussi T, Otto SR. Effects of electrical brainstem stimulation on tinnitus. Acta Otolaryngol. 1994;114(2):135–40.
116. De Ridder D, Vanneste S, van der Loo E, Plazier M, Menovsky T, van de Heyning P. Burst stimulation of the auditory cortex: a new form of neurostimulation for noise-like tinnitus suppression. J Neurosurg. 2010;112(6):1289–94.
117. De Ridder D, De Mulder G, Walsh V, Muggleton N, Sunaert S, Møller A. Magnetic and electrical stimulation of the auditory cortex for intractable tinnitus. Case report. J Neurosurg. 2004;100(3):560–4.
118. Litré CF, Theret E, Tran H, Lévèque M, Portefaix C, Gierski F, et al. Surgical treatment by electrical stimulation of the auditory cortex for intractable tinnitus. Brain Stimul. 2009;2(3):132–7.
119. Vanneste S, Fregni F, De Ridder D. Head-to-head comparison of transcranial random noise stimulation, transcranial AC stimulation, and transcranial DC stimulation for tinnitus. Front Psych. 2013;4:158.
120. Yakunina N, Nam EC. Direct and transcutaneous Vagus nerve stimulation for treatment of tinnitus: a scoping review. Front Neurosci. 2021;15:680590.
121. Buell EP, Borland MS, Loerwald KW, Chandler C, Hays SA, Engineer CT, et al. Vagus nerve stimulation rate and duration determine whether sensory pairing produces neural plasticity. Neuroscience. 2019;406:290–9.
122. Koehler SD, Pradhan S, Manis PB, Shore SE. Somatosensory inputs modify auditory spike timing in dorsal cochlear nucleus principal cells. Eur J Neurosci. 2011;33(3):409–20.
123. Koehler SD, Shore SE. Stimulus-timing dependent multisensory plasticity in the Guinea pig dorsal cochlear nucleus. PLoS One. 2013;8(3):e59828.
124. Wu C, Martel DT, Shore SE. Transcutaneous induction of stimulus-timing-dependent plasticity in dorsal cochlear nucleus. Front Syst Neurosci. 2015;9:116.
125. Koehler SD, Shore SE. Stimulus timing-dependent plasticity in dorsal cochlear nucleus is altered in tinnitus. J Neurosci. 2013;33(50):19647–56.
126. Hamilton C, D'Arcy S, Pearlmutter BA, Crispino G, Lalor EC, Conlon BJ. An investigation of feasibility and safety of bi-modal stimulation for the treatment of tinnitus: an open-label pilot study. Neuromodulation. 2016;19(8):832–7.
127. Butt MF, Albusoda A, Farmer AD, Aziz Q. The anatomical basis for transcutaneous auricular vagus nerve stimulation. J Anat. 2020;236(4):588–611.
128. Yakunina N, Kim SS, Nam EC. BOLD fMRI effects of transcutaneous vagus nerve stimulation in patients with chronic tinnitus. PLoS One. 2018;13(11):e0207281.
129. Hyvärinen P, Yrttiaho S, Lehtimäki J, Ilmoniemi RJ, Mäkitie A, Ylikoski J, et al. Transcutaneous vagus nerve stimulation modulates tinnitus-related beta- and gamma-band activity. Ear Hear. 2015;36(3):e76–85.
130. Galazyuk A, Brozoski TJ. Animal models of tinnitus: a review. Otolaryngol Clin N Am. 2020;53:469.
131. von der Behrens W. Animal models of subjective tinnitus. Neural Plast. 2014;2014:741452.
132. Zheng Y, McPherson K, Smith PF. Effects of early and late treatment with L-baclofen on the development and maintenance of tinnitus caused by acoustic trauma in rats. Neuroscience. 2014;258:410–21.
133. Beukes EW, Manchaiah V, Allen PM, Andersson G, Baguley DM. Exploring tinnitus heterogeneity. Prog Brain Res. 2021;260:79–99.
134. Figueiredo RR, Rates MA, Azevedo AA, Oliveira PM, Navarro PB. Correlation analysis of hearing thresholds, validated questionnaires and psychoacoustic measurements in tinnitus patients. Braz J Otorhinolaryngol. 2010;76(4):522–6.
135. Nascimento IDP, Almeida AA, Diniz JJ, Martins ML, Freitas T, Rosa M. Tinnitus evaluation: relationship between pitch matching and loudness, visual analog scale and tinnitus handicap inventory. Braz J Otorhinolaryngol. 2019;85(5):611–6.
136. Risey J, Briner W, Guth PS, Norris CH. The superiority of the Goodwin procedure over the traditional procedure in measuring the loudness level of tinnitus. Ear Hear. 1989;10(5):318–22.
137. Rabau S, Cox T, Punte AK, Waelkens B, Gilles A, Wouters K, et al. Changes over time of psychoacoustic outcome measurements are not a substitute for subjective outcome measurements in acute tinnitus. Eur Arch Otorhinolaryngol. 2015;272(3):573–81.
138. Yamamoto Y, Tamagawa S, Tanioka K, Suzuki T, Hotomi M, Ukai S, et al. Subjective loudness using external noise reflects the loudness and distress of tinnitus: a cross-sectional study. Otol Neurotol. 2020;41(6):e655–e62.
139. Landgrebe M, Azevedo A, Baguley D, Bauer C, Cacace A, Coelho C, et al. Methodological aspects of clinical trials in tinnitus: a proposal for an international standard. J Psychosom Res. 2012;73(2):112–21.
140. Kang DW, Kim SS, Park DC, Kim SH, Yeo SG. Objective and measurable biomarkers in chronic subjective tinnitus. Int J Mol Sci. 2021;22(12):6619.
141. Haider HF, Hoare DJ, Ribeiro SF, Ribeiro D, Caria H, Trigueiros N, et al. Evidence for biological markers of tinnitus: a systematic review. Prog Brain Res. 2021;262:345–98.
142. Cardon E, Joossen I, Vermeersch H, Jacquemin L, Mertens G, Vanderveken OM, et al. Systematic review and meta-analysis of late auditory evoked potentials as a candidate biomarker in the assessment of tinnitus. PLoS One. 2020;15(12):e0243785.
143. Liu Y, Niu H, Zhu J, Zhao P, Yin H, Ding H, et al. Morphological neuroimaging biomarkers for tinnitus: evidence obtained by applying machine learning. Neural Plast. 2019;2019:1712342.
144. Simoes J, Neff P, Schoisswohl S, Bulla J, Schecklmann M, Harrison S, et al. Toward personalized tinnitus treatment: an exploratory study based on internet Crowdsensing. Front Public Health. 2019;7:157.
145. Olivares O, Dabritz JH, King A, Gottlieb E, Halsey C. Research into cancer metabolomics: towards a clinical metamorphosis. Semin Cell Dev Biol. 2015;43:52–64.
146. Li M, Wang X, Aa J, Qin W, Zha W, Ge Y, et al. GC/TOFMS analysis of metabolites in serum and urine reveals metabolic perturbation of TCA cycle in db/db mice involved in diabetic nephropathy. Am J Physiol Renal Physiol. 2013;304(11):F1317–24.
147. Sethi S, Brietzke E. Omics-based biomarkers: application of metabolomics in neuropsychiatric disorders. Int J Neuropsychopharmacol. 2016;19(3):pyv096.
148. Huang TL, Lin CC. Advances in biomarkers of major depressive disorder. Adv Clin Chem. 2015;68:177–204.
149. Rankin NJ, Preiss D, Welsh P, Burgess KEV, Nelson SM, Lawlor DA, et al. The emergence of proton nuclear magnetic resonance metabolomics in the cardiovascular arena as viewed from a clinical perspective. Atherosclerosis. 2014;237(1):287–300.

150. Graham SF, Chevallier OP, Elliott CT, Holscher C, Johnston J, McGuinness B, et al. Untargeted metabolomic analysis of human plasma indicates differentially affected polyamine and L-arginine metabolism in mild cognitive impairment subjects converting to Alzheimer's disease. PLoS One. 2015;10(3): e0119452.
151. Loeb JA. Identifying targets for preventing epilepsy using systems biology. Neurosci Lett. 2011;497(3):205–12.
152. Vreeker GCM, Vangangelt KMH, Bladergroen MR, Nicolardi S, Mesker WE, Wuhrer M, et al. Serum N-glycan profiles differ for various breast cancer subtypes. Glycoconj J. 2021;38(3):387–95.
153. Wang X, Zhang L, Sun W, Pei LL, Tian M, Liang J, et al. Changes of metabolites in acute ischemic stroke and its subtypes. Front Neurosci. 2020;14:580929.
154. Bredesen DE. Metabolic profiling distinguishes three subtypes of Alzheimer's disease. Aging (Albany NY). 2015;7(8):595–600.

Part V

Diagnosis and Assessment

Diagnosis and Flowchart

25

Berthold Langguth

Abstract

1. Tinnitus can be a symptom of a wide range of different underlying pathologies and be accompanied by many different comorbidities, indicating the need for comprehensive multidisciplinary diagnostic assessment.

2. Exact diagnosis is required in each patient in order to provide the best management of tinnitus.

3. It is especially important to identify patients
   (a) Who can be treated by specific interventions.
   (b) Those in which tinnitus is a symptom of a severe underlying disease.
   (c) Those patients who require immediate therapeutic action.

4. Basic diagnostics should include a detailed case history, assessment of tinnitus severity, clinical ear examination, and audiological measurement of hearing function.

5. For a considerable number of patients, these first diagnostic steps in combination with counseling will be sufficient.

6. Further diagnostic steps are indicated if the findings of basic diagnostics reveal
   (a) relevant subjective impairment,
   (b) acute tinnitus onset together with acute hearing loss,
   (c) posttraumatic,
   (d) acute pulsatile tinnitus, as these characteristics point to a potentially dangerous underlying condition (e.g., carotid dissection).

7. All diagnostic and therapeutic steps should be accompanied by empathic and insightful counseling.

8. The goal of therapeutic management is maximal relief from tinnitus complaints. This requires exact knowledge, which symptoms are perceived as bothersome by the individual patient.

B. Langguth (✉)
Department of Psychiatry and Psychotherapy, University of Regensburg, Bezirksklinikum, Regensburg, Germany
e-mail: Berthold.Langguth@medbo.de

W. Schlee et al. (eds.), *Textbook of Tinnitus*, https://doi.org/10.1007/978-3-031-35647-6_25

Graphical Abstract

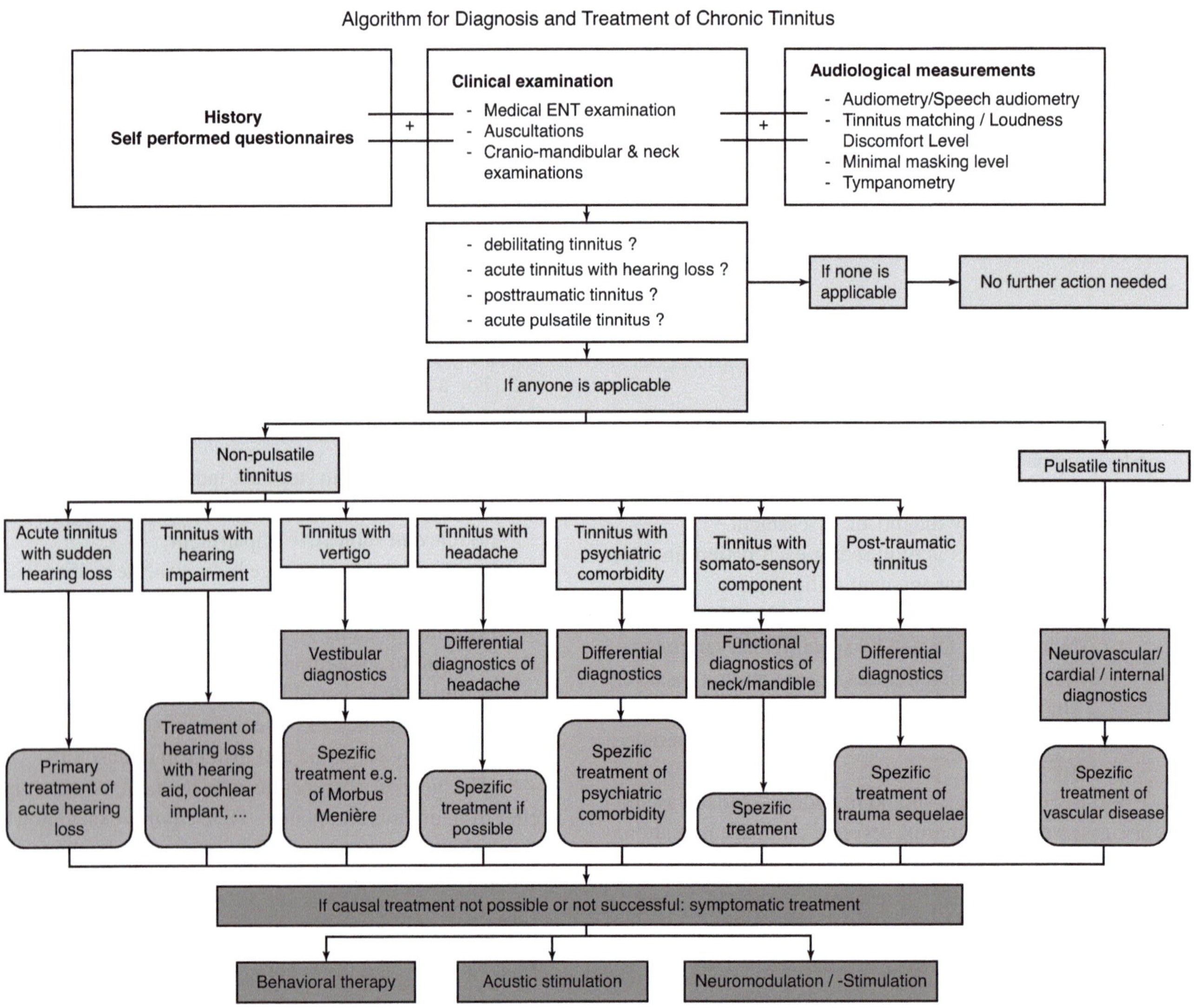

Introduction

Tinnitus is a highly heterogeneous condition. It can be experienced as a ringing, roaring, clicking, hissing, or buzzing. Tinnitus can start together with hearing loss but can also occur after neck trauma or during stressful life events. In some individuals, tinnitus is accompanied by insomnia, others have difficulty concentrating, and some complain about hyperacusis. Some individuals report that their tinnitus worsens by environmental sound; in others, the same sound may relieve their tinnitus. These clinical observations clearly show that tinnitus is not a single disease entity, but that there are many different forms of tinnitus, which are likely to vary in their pathophysiology and in their response to treatment interventions (see Chap. 7). This, in turn, implies that an exact differential diagnosis is of utmost importance in the management of tinnitus.

In the diagnostic assessment, it is important to identify those subforms of tinnitus, which can be treated causally [1] or highly efficiently [2] with specific interventions. These subforms of tinnitus require specific management or can benefit from specific treatment. Even if some of these conditions are relatively rare, considering the possibility of their occurrence is warranted because of the availability of specific treatment options.

Moreover, tinnitus can be the first symptom of potentially dangerous diseases, some of which may even become life-threatening if left undiagnosed and untreated (e.g., carotid dissection and vestibular schwannoma). Furthermore, tinnitus by itself may become life-threatening if accompanied by suicidal tendencies.

Therefore, each patient with tinnitus requires a careful and systematic diagnostic approach. Diagnostic assessment of tinnitus is challenging because multiple etiologies can result in the development of tinnitus. Even though hearing disorders are the most important risk factors for the development of tinnitus, other diseases such as brain tumors, neck injuries, temporomandibular dysfunction, or emotional disorders generally covered by other disciplines (e.g., neurology, psychiatry, orthopedics, dentistry, or neurosurgery) can be critically involved in the etiology or continuation of tinnitus. Therefore, the requirements of comprehensive tinnitus diagnosis and treatment can only be met by an integrated multidisciplinary approach.

In this chapter, a flowchart is presented to guide diagnosis and treatment of tinnitus based on currently available evidence (see Fig. 25.1). This flowchart has originally been developed in the framework of the Tinnitus Research Initiative (www.tinnituresearch.org) by a multidisciplinary and multinational group (ref TOT) and has been refined over time according to new evidence [3, 4].

A stepwise decision tree approach for tinnitus management is proposed, starting with basic diagnostic steps, which are recommended in all patients [5], and includes history taking for associated symptoms (for details, see also Chap. 26), a clinical examination (for details see Chap. 28), and audiological measurements (for details see Chap. 29). Depending on the findings of the first step, further diagnostic or therapeutic measures may or may not be necessary.

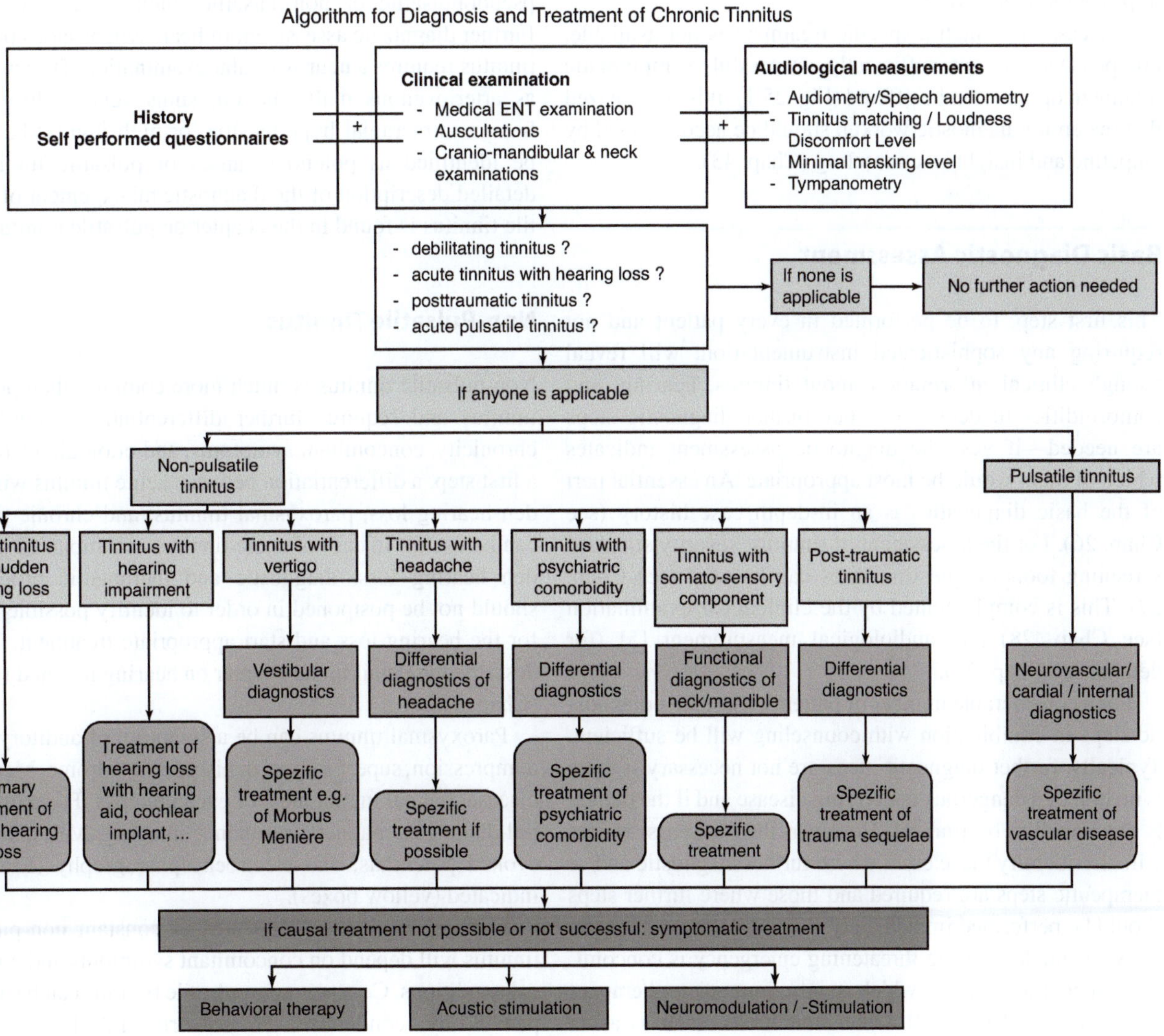

Fig. 25.1 Diagnostic and therapeutic algorithm

Further diagnostic steps are indicated if the findings of basic diagnostics reveal (1) relevant subjective impairment, (2) acute tinnitus onset together with acute hearing loss, (3) posttraumatic, or (4) acute pulsatile tinnitus, as these characteristics point to a potentially dangerous underlying condition (e.g., carotid dissection). Moreover, further diagnostic steps are recommended, if the tinnitus characteristics suggest that the patient suffers from objective tinnitus.

The second step consists of further diagnostic procedures depending on specific tinnitus features (e.g., pulsatile character) and depending on comorbidities. In some of these cases, a specific treatment is possible. One example is cases of tinnitus with unilateral deafness, where a cochlear implant is a potential causally oriented treatment option. In cases in which tinnitus is associated with a relevant comorbidity, treatment options for the comorbidity should be considered as well. For example, tinnitus can be a symptom of vestibular migraine. In this case, successful treatment of migraine can improve tinnitus as well.

For cases in which a specific treatment is not available, not possible, or not sufficiently successful, symptomatic treatment options can be offered (Fig. 25.1). It is emphasized that the entire diagnostic workup should be accompanied by empathic and insightful counseling (Chap. 43).

Basic Diagnostic Assessment

This first step, to be performed in every patient and not requiring any sophisticated instrumentation, will reveal enough clinical information about tinnitus, hearing, and comorbidities to decide whether further diagnostic steps are needed—if yes, the diagnostic assessment indicates which of them would be most appropriate. An essential part of the basic diagnostics is an in-depth case history (see Chap. 26). For the assessment of tinnitus, severity standard screening tools or questionnaires can be used (see Chap. 27). This is complemented by the clinical ear examination (see Chap. 28) and audiological measurement [5] (for details, see Chap. 29).

For a considerable number of patients, these first diagnostic steps in combination with counseling will be sufficient. Typically, further diagnostic steps are not necessary if there is no hint of a dangerous underlying disease and if the patient is not impaired by tinnitus. However, the basic assessment will also identify those cases where further diagnostic and/or therapeutic steps are required and those where further steps should be performed immediately.

An example of a life-threatening emergency is concomitant suicidal tendencies, which require immediate therapeutic action (see Chap. 42). Other conditions, such as acute tinnitus in combination with sudden hearing loss of recent onset, should also be treated as soon as possible (see Chap. 32). In conditions where a severe underlying disease cannot be excluded or when a patient is bothered by his tinnitus, further diagnostic steps are clearly indicated.

Further diagnostic procedures should be guided by specific clinical characteristics (Fig. 25.1). In a hierarchical diagnostic algorithm, the first differentiation should be between pulsatile vs. non-pulsatile tinnitus. This differentiation acknowledges the fundamental pathophysiological difference between these two forms of tinnitus.

Pulsatile Tinnitus

It is important to note that pulsatile refers to heart-synchronous or respiration-synchronous (venous hum) pulsatile tinnitus. Pulsatile tinnitus with a rhythm different from the heart rate or respiration rate should be classified here as pseudopulsatile or non-pulsatile tinnitus (see Chap. 40). Further diagnostic assessment of heart synchronous pulsatile tinnitus requires a neurovascular examination. Diseases such as arteriovenous malformation, sinus venous thrombosis, benign intracranial hypertension, or high jugular bulb may be identified as potential causes of pulsatile tinnitus. A detailed description of the diagnostic management of pulsatile tinnitus is found in the chapter on pulsatile tinnitus.

Non-Pulsatile Tinnitus

Non-pulsatile tinnitus is much more common than pulsatile tinnitus and requires further differentiation according to chronicity, concomitant symptoms, and etiologic factors. As a first step, a differentiation between acute tinnitus with sudden hearing loss, paroxysmal tinnitus, and chronic tinnitus can be useful. In case of acute tinnitus accompanied by sudden hearing loss, diagnostic and therapeutic procedures should not be postponed in order to identify possible causes for the hearing loss and start appropriate treatment. This is described in detail in the chapter on hearing loss and tinnitus (Chap. 32).

Paroxysmal tinnitus can be a symptom of auditory nerve compression, superior canal dehiscence syndrome, Ménière's disease, palatal myoclonus, or even epilepsy. For a differential diagnosis, magnetic resonance imaging (MRI), auditory evoked potentials, and electroencephalography (EEG) are indicated (yellow boxes).

Further diagnostic procedures of constant non-pulsatile tinnitus will depend on concomitant symptoms and etiological conditions. Constant non-pulsatile tinnitus can be accompanied by conductive or sensorineural hearing loss. Conductive hearing loss can be caused by otosclerosis, different forms of otitis, or Eustachian tube dysfunction. More information about tinnitus with conductive hearing loss is given in Chap. 32.

In case of sensorineural hearing loss, further diagnostic procedures are indicated for identifying the exact etiology. These can include magnetic resonance imaging (MRI) and auditory brainstem responses (ABR) (e.g., for excluding vestibular schwannoma) and also otoacoustic emissions for the assessment of outer hair cell function (see Chaps. 29 and 30).

Diagnostic assessment and therapeutic management of tinnitus occurring together with vertigo are indicative of specific pathologies such as Ménière's disease, superior canal dehiscence, or damage to the vestibulocochlear system. More details are found in Chap. 33.

If tinnitus presents with associated headache, increased intracranial pressure has to be excluded. Potential underlying pathologies such as space-occupying lesions (SOL), benign intracranial hypertension (BIH), disorders of cerebrospinal fluid (CSF) circulation, or craniocervical anomalies can be diagnosed by MRI (see Chap. 30). In specific cases, lumbar puncture and furosemide tests may help to determine whether reduced CSF pressure also alleviates tinnitus.

The co-occurrence of depression, anxiety, and insomnia with severe tinnitus has been frequently described. Immediate action is required when a patient reports acute suicidal thoughts. A detailed explanation of diagnostic procedures in case of psychiatric comorbidity is provided in Chap. 42.

When tinnitus is associated with neck or temporomandibular dysfunction or pain, a more detailed examination of these systems is recommended. Radiologic tests are indicated if structural alterations are suspected, whereas functional impairments can be best detected by physical examination performed by experienced dentists and physiotherapists. More details are presented in Chap. 31.

Specific diagnostic tests are indicated if tinnitus begins or worsens within 3 months after a traumatic event. It is important to note that a delay of several weeks between trauma and tinnitus onset does not exclude a potential etiologic relationship. Traumatic events may cause tinnitus in different ways. The indication for further diagnostic procedures depends on the trauma mechanism. Traumatic events that can cause tinnitus include noise, ear, head, neck, and also emotional trauma. In case of posttraumatic pulsatile tinnitus, the immediate diagnostic workup for vascular pathologies (especially carotid dissection) is mandatory. A detailed description of pathologies that can occur as a consequence of trauma and that may be involved in the generation of tinnitus is given in Chap. 38. This chapter also covers blast injuries, which occur especially in warfare and frequently cause tinnitus. Blast injuries are a particular diagnostic challenge since the tinnitus-inducing mechanisms may include noise, ear, head, neck, and emotional trauma.

Hyperacusis and phonophobia occur frequently together with tinnitus and require specific management, which is described in detail in Chap. 41.

Symptomatic Treatment

Symptomatic treatment should be considered in every patient who feels impaired by his tinnitus if specific causally oriented treatments are not available, not sufficiently effective, or not indicated for any other reason. Cognitive behavioral therapy (CBT) (see Chap. 44.) and auditory stimulation (see Chap. 46.) with counseling (see Chap. 43) are the most established treatment options. Auditory stimulation can be essentially differentiated in the use of sound for masking or partially masking tinnitus and in attempts to compensate for hearing deficits, e.g., by hearing aids. Also, specific forms of sound stimulation with a frequency composition according to the individual audiogram have been proposed. Tinnitus retraining therapy (TRT), a specific combination of auditory stimulation and counseling, is widely used and described in Chap. 47.

Pharmacotherapeutic options for the treatment of tinnitus are limited. However, even if there is currently no drug, which is approved by the US Food and Drug Administration (FDA) for the treatment of tinnitus, there are some promising results from clinical studies indicating the beneficial effects of specific drugs for subgroups of patients (see Chap. 48). Neuromodulatory approaches have been proposed very recently. Very promising results are available for transcranial magnetic stimulation (TMS) and bimodal stimulation. Neurobiofeedback, transcranial direct current stimulation (tDCS), cutaneous stimulation, and cortical electrical stimulation have also been investigated and shown some promise. A description of how these techniques are performed and which results have been obtained is given in the respective Chaps. 51, 52, 53 and 54.

In summary, a wide range of different pathologies can underlie tinnitus. The diagnostic challenge can best be met by a stepwise approach consisting of basic assessment procedures followed by more detailed diagnostic tests in selected patients. Here, important indications for further diagnostic steps and immediate treatment are summarized. If these diagnostic procedures do not reveal causally oriented treatment options or if results from such therapies are not satisfying, auditory stimulation, cognitive behavioral therapy, and neurostimulation are available as symptomatically oriented treatment options. This algorithm is based on currently available knowledge, and it is expected to evolve and be refined with time and criticism.

Acknowledgements
1. The algorithm for the diagnostic and therapeutic management of tinnitus patients has originally been developed in the framework of the Tinnitus Research Initiative (www.tinnituresearch.org) by a multidisciplinary (consisting of otolaryngologists, audiologists, neurologists, psychiatrists, psychotherapists, and a neurosurgeon) and multinational (Belgium, Brazil, France, Germany, Italy, New Zealand, and Spain) group (Biesinger Eberhard, Del Bo Luca, De Ridder Dirk, Goodey Ron, Herraiz Carlos, Kleinjung Tobias, Lainez Jose-Michel, Landgrebe Michael, Langguth Berthold, Paolino Michel, Questier Benjamin, Sanchez Tanit, and Searchfield Grant).

References

1. Van de Heyning P, Vermeire K, Diebl M, Nopp P, Anderson I, De Ridder D. Incapacitating unilateral tinnitus in single-sided deafness treated by cochlear implantation. Ann Otol Rhinol Laryngol. 2008;117(9):645–52.
2. Mardini MK. Ear-clicking "tinnitus" responding to carbamazepine. N Engl J Med. 1987;317(24):1542.
3. Langguth B, Kreuzer PM, Kleinjung T, De Ridder D. Tinnitus: causes and clinical management. Lancet Neurol. 2013;12(9):920–30.
4. Kreuzer PM, Vielsmeier V, Langguth B. Chronic tinnitus: an interdisciplinary challenge. Dtsch Arztebl Int. 2013;110(16):278–84.
5. Langguth B, Goodey R, Azevedo A, Bjorne A, Cacace A, Crocetti A, et al. Consensus for tinnitus patient assessment and treatment outcome measurement: tinnitus research initiative meeting, Regensburg, July 2006. Prog Brain Res. 2007;166:525–36.

26 Tinnitus History Taking

Berthold Langguth

Abstract

1. A detailed case history is required in all tinnitus patients in order to obtain the necessary information for differential diagnosis and therapeutic management.

2. Qualitative data are best being obtained through case history questionnaires or a structured interview.

3. A case history should contain information about the history and descriptive characteristics of the tinnitus, about potential risk factors for tinnitus development, about specific behavioral, social, interpersonal, and emotional consequences of tinnitus, about factors that may either exacerbate or reduce tinnitus severity.

4. Qualitative and quantitative assessment of tinnitus severity is relevant for both clinical management and research applications.

B. Langguth (✉)
Department of Psychiatry and Psychotherapy, University of Regensburg, Bezirksklinikum, Regensburg, Germany
e-mail: Berthold.Langguth@medbo.de

W. Schlee et al. (eds.), *Textbook of Tinnitus*, https://doi.org/10.1007/978-3-031-35647-6_26

Graphical Abstract

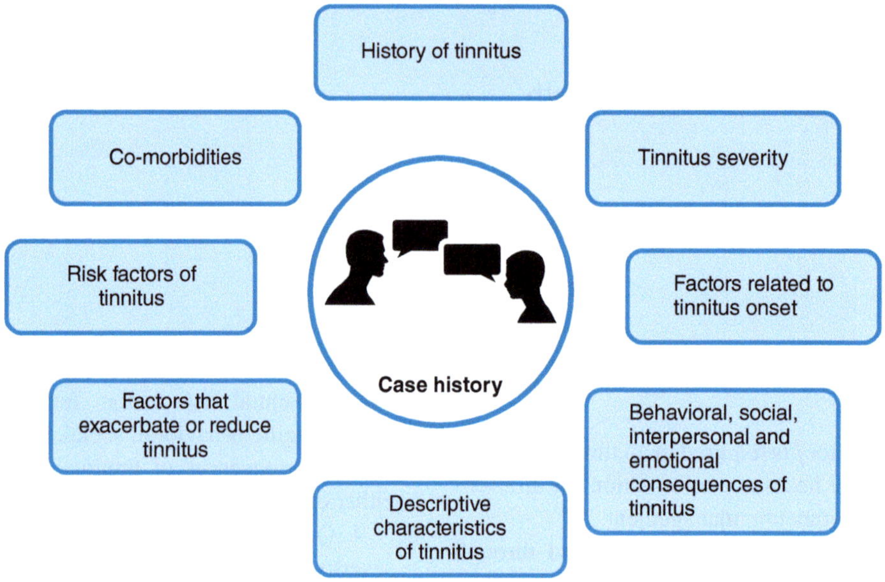

Introduction

Tinnitus has many forms and many characteristics. However, tinnitus is not readily apparent to others, and currently, no objective procedures are yet established for diagnosis of tinnitus. The assessment of the perceptual aspects of tinnitus depends almost entirely on the patient's report. You can only find out if a patient has tinnitus and what form of tinnitus he/she has by listening. The case history is of high importance for correct diagnosis in all areas of medicine; this is especially true for tinnitus, since it is fundamentally a self-report phenomenon. The subjective nature of tinnitus is not only a challenge in the clinical management of the individual with tinnitus, but also for research applications.

Therefore, in addition to an otologic (see Chap. 28) and audiologic assessment (see Chap. 29), a detailed case history is required in all tinnitus patients in order to obtain the necessary information for deciding about the therapeutic management. In many patients, a comprehensive diagnostic assessment including a detailed case history can be sufficient for tinnitus management. If a severe disorder (e.g., tumor or carotid dissection) can be excluded and the tinnitus is not perceived as a problem, no treatment is necessary. In all cases, the detailed case history represents also already the first therapeutic step, as the patient can share his experiences. He sees that his complaints are taken seriously and that the clinician is competent and caring, and understands the effects of tinnitus.

As the patient presents because of the tinnitus, it is useful to start the case history by asking the patient to describe his tinnitus from the onset. Was the onset gradual or immediate and were there any events associated with the onset? This can be acute hearing loss, noise trauma, an ear trauma, an ear infection, a general viral infection, neck pain or neck trauma, temporomandibular joint disorder, or stressful life events.

The next step is information about the time course of tinnitus. Did the tinnitus get worse or better over time? Was it fluctuating or constant? If there are fluctuations, is there any hint what can cause these fluctuations?

Then, the patient should be asked about the current perceptual characteristics of the tinnitus. What is the tinnitus laterality? Is the tinnitus tone- or noise-like or is it pulsating? It is important to provide information about influencing factors (e.g., reduction of tinnitus by environmental sound) and associated symptoms such as reduced sound tolerance, headache, and vertigo.

The loudness of tinnitus can be evaluated quantitatively, either by grading or by matching methods (see Chap. 29). In addition to details about the tinnitus percept, information about the perceived severity and the impact on an individual's life must also be assessed. Personality, comorbidities, or environmental circumstances contribute more to tinnitus-related distress, impairment, disability, and handicap than the perceptual characteristics of tinnitus [1, 2]. Therefore, the evaluation of the impact of tinnitus on a person's life needs to be multidimensional and take into account psychological and social factors. In this context, it is helpful to ask the patient what bothers most in relation to his tinnitus. This information is helpful because it provides an important information in which direction the treatment should be oriented.

An essential aspect is the information about tinnitus severity. This can range from "not impaired at all" to "completely impaired in all areas of life." Screening tools allow assessment of tinnitus severity based on a few questions, while numerous psychometrically validated questionnaires are available for quantitative assessment of tinnitus severity many. These questionnaires are helpful tools for quantifying the disabling and handicapping effects of tinnitus and provide insight into how the tinnitus sensation generates disability at the personal level and handicap at the societal level. Responses on these questionnaires can be summed, resulting in a total score or subscale scores. Based on the score, the tinnitus severity of an individual patient can be determined (e.g., in low, medium, moderate, or severe) (for more information, see Chap. 27).

If a patient is moderately or severely impaired, additional assessment by a psychologist or a psychiatrist may frequently be necessary. Psychological and psychiatric assessment involves the integration of information from multiple sources and tools, including clinical interview of the patient, rating scales, questionnaires, and observation of the patient's behavior during the interview. It is not only *what* the patients say, but also *how* they say it that is of relevance. Interviews with significant others or reports from previous therapists or physicians can provide further important information.

The clinician must also be aware that when people complain of tinnitus, other problems may be contributing to a negative emotional state. For example, a coexistent hearing impairment or hyperacusis, balance problems, pain, anxiety, or depression may contribute to the person's difficulties. Daily stressors or major life events may also have an impact on the person's ability to cope with the tinnitus, and patients may attribute their feelings of depression and anxiety incorrectly to the tinnitus. An aim of the initial assessment may also be to disentangle causal connections between tinnitus distress, other stressors, and negative emotional states.

Another important area of investigation concerns the risk of suicide. Rather than avoiding asking questions about suicide, the clinician should address this issue directly. Patients may consider suicide as a means to escape from tinnitus or it may be associated with a depressive disorder (for more detailed information, see Chap. 42). If results indicate the potential for self-harm, the clinician should refer the patient to a psychiatrist.

This chapter will provide guidance on taking a tinnitus of history to obtain all relevant information about a condition that is purely subjective in nature, namely a patient's tinnitus and its disabling and handicapping effects. This chapter should represent a practical reference for both clinicians and researchers. Also, the limitations of the different approaches will be discussed in order to allow the readers to select the most appropriate method for their specific clinical or research application.

Case History

A detailed history and primary source of descriptive data of the patient's tinnitus or tinnitus-related conditions can be obtained through the initial intake, either by a questionnaire or by structured interviews. The goal of the intake interview is to arrive at a thorough understanding of the nature of the tinnitus by exploring a broad range of inquiry, including causal, descriptive, and diagnostic variables. This information, together with otologic and audiologic assessment, forms the basis for further diagnostic and therapeutic management. In detail, a comprehensive clinical assessment should cover the following areas:

1. The history and descriptive characteristics of the tinnitus.
2. Specific behavioral, social, interpersonal, and emotional consequences of tinnitus.
3. Risk factors for tinnitus development or tinnitus maintenance.
4. Factors that may either exacerbate or reduce tinnitus severity.
5. Previous tinnitus treatments.
6. Relevant comorbidities.

This information can be obtained through interviews or self-report questionnaires or both. Many practitioners prefer questionnaires, as they offer advantages of standardized questions to provide reliable and complete information. Furthermore, they require less clinician time than interviews. Moreover, the questionnaires provide already a comprehensive documentation of the patient. Another advantage is their use in follow-up assessments of the patient's progress in order to monitor the effect of possible therapies. The comprehensive documentation of detailed patient information is clinically important and can be especially helpful in medico-legal cases.

For sure, there are also advantages of structured interviews. Relevant aspects can be explored in more detail and according to the patient's individual situation. Moreover, there might be clinical situations, which are only insufficiently reflected by a standardized questionnaire. An example is a patient with a long-lasting tinnitus, which got acutely worse. Most questionnaires might classify this case as either acute or chronic, but will not be suitable to reflect the situation as an acute exacerbation of a chronic condition.

Therefore, in clinical practice, intake questionnaires should be complemented by an interview to discuss ambiguous and individually relevant aspects in more detail. Moreover, the report in the patient's own words and the observation of the patient's behavior during the interview provides important additional information, as it is not only of relevance what the patient says, but also how he/she says it.

Several case history questionnaires have been published [3–6], but many clinicians and researchers have developed their own questionnaires in which they include those questions which they consider important and relevant. During a consensus workshop on tinnitus assessment in Regensburg in July 2006, an "items list" for tinnitus case history questionnaires (see Table 26.1) was compiled, which contains items common to most questionnaires currently in use and considered important by experts in the field. This list consists of 14 essential (level A) items and 21 highly desirable (level B) items. A case history questionnaire has also been developed as an example of how these items might be expressed (Tinnitus Sample Case History Questionnaire (TSCHQ), available in Czech, Dutch, English, French, German, Italian, Norwegian, Polish, Portuguese (European and Brazilian), Spanish, and Swedish languages at https://tinnitusresearch.net/index.php/for-researchers/resources).

Depending on their individual background, some clinicians will consider additional items as relevant (e.g., a clinician with physiotherapeutic experience will be more interested in detailed information about postural complaints). As an example, a recent initiative developed a new case history instrument with special emphasis on research questions [6].

The item list should therefore only be considered as a core list to which individual specializations can be added. In the following description, we want to give some examples of the relevance of the proposed items for further diagnostic or therapeutic procedures.

Demographic data, such as age, are of relevance since the causes of tinnitus are different in younger and older people. In elderly people, tinnitus is frequently associated with presbycusis [7]; other causal factors such as noise exposure or temporomandibular joint disorder may be more prominent in younger patients [8, 9]. A positive family history of tinnitus complaints can point to a genetic form of hearing loss as an underlying disorder. There is also increasing evidence that genetic factors may play a role for individual susceptibility to tinnitus as well [10–13] (see Chap. 5).

The duration of tinnitus is of high relevance for further diagnostic and therapeutic management. Whereas acute tinnitus, especially with abrupt onset, may be a sign of an acute dangerous disease, this is only very rarely the case in chronic tinnitus. Acute tinnitus also requires an entirely different therapeutic management than chronic tinnitus. The circumstances under which tinnitus started are also important (e.g., onset of tinnitus related to neck trauma needs a different diagnostic work-up than tinnitus that started during a stressful live event).

Table 26.1 Iteml s List for Case History Questionnaires **"Items list" for tinnitus case history questionnaires**

Items are ordered according to their level of significance	
Category "A" (= essential) in bold type.	
Background	
1	**Age**
2	**Gender**
3	Handedness
4	**Family history of tinnitus (parent, sibling, children)**
Tinnitus history	
5	**Initial onset. Time?**
6	**Initial onset. Mode? Gradual or abrupt?**
7	Initial onset. Associated events? Hearing change, acoustic trauma, otitis media,
Head trauma, whiplash, dental treatment, stress, other.	
8	**Pattern. Steady? Pulsatile? Other?**
9	**Site. Right ear? Left ear? Both ears? (Symmetrical?) Inside head?**
10	Intermittent or constant?
11	Fluctuant or non-fluctuant?
12	**Loudness. Scale 1–100. At worst and at best?**
13	Quality. Own words/give a list of choices.
14	Pure tone or noise? Uncertain/polyphonic?
15	Pitch. Very high? High? Medium? Low?
16	**Percentage of awake time aware of tinnitus?**
17	Percentage of awake time annoyed by tinnitus?
18	Previous tinnitus treatments (no, some, many)?
Modifying influences	
19	**Natural masking? Music, everyday sounds, other sounds?**
20	Aggravated by loud noise?
21	**Altered by head and neck movement or touching of head or upper limbs (specification of the respective movements)?**
22	Daytime nap. Worse? Better? No effect?
23	Effect of nocturnal sleep on daytime tinnitus?
24	Effect of stress?
25	Effect of medications? Which?
Related conditions	
26	**Hearing impairment?**
27	**Hearing aids (no, left ear, right ear, both ears; effect on tinnitus)?**
28	**Noise annoyance or intolerance?**
29	Noise-induced pain?
30	Headaches?
31	Vertigo/dizziness?
32	Temporomandibular disorder?
33	Neck pain?
34	Other pain syndromes?
35	Under treatment for psychiatric problems?

Among the sound characteristics reported by patients, the differentiation between pulsatile and non-pulsatile tinnitus is of greatest importance. In patients who describe pulsatile sounds, particularly if synchronous with the heartbeat, vascular origin should be suspected. Pulsatile tinnitus requires specific diagnostic procedures (see Chap. 40). Unilateral low-pitched tinnitus with low-frequency hearing loss in combination with intermittent vertigo attacks may indicate a diagnosis of Ménière's disease. Neurophysiological differences between tinnitus resembling "a pure tone" and "noise" have been suggested, and the response to specific therapeutic procedures may depend on this distinction [14, 15].

Tinnitus loudness can be assessed with numeric rating scales or visual analog scales and gives an estimate of the subjectively perceived loudness of the patient's tinnitus. The percentage of time patients are aware of their tinnitus varies enormously between "sometimes in quiet environments" and "always". There is also a difference between the time patients are aware of their tinnitus and the time they are annoyed by it. These factors are important for determining how intrusive the tinnitus may be in a specific patient.

Factors that improve or worsen tinnitus can be important predictors for treatment success (e.g., use of a sound generator if environmental sounds reduce tinnitus). Identifying therapies that have been tried, successfully or not, can also provide useful information for future treatment choices. In a recent large study that was based on a survey of 5017 patients, it could be shown that the response to a given treatment in the past predicts the response to other treatments [16].

When therapies in the past have failed, it should be asked exactly how the therapy had been performed. Possible reasons for failing could be an inadequate performance or insufficient duration of a given treatment.

There are several health disorders, which are frequently associated with tinnitus, such as hearing loss, hyperacusis, neck or temporomandibular joint disorders, vertigo, insomnia, headache, anxiety, or depression. These comorbidities may be a cause or consequence of tinnitus. In all cases, the co-occurrence of these disorders is of relevance for the therapeutic management. Irrespective of whether there is a causal relationship or not, successful treatment of tinnitus comorbidities can improve the patient's quality of life enormously. This, in turn, may also improve the patient's ability to cope with tinnitus, even if perceptual characteristics remain largely unchanged.

Although case history questionnaires are useful tools for obtaining information, they should not replace a thorough clinical intake interview. However, the use of a case history questionnaire can make the intake interview more efficient by providing an opportunity to discuss relevant items in detail. Patients should be encouraged to clarify questions when they are uncertain how to answer. In the discussion, patients can also describe aspects that are particularly important to them in their own words. Discussing the various items helps to establish a relationship between the clinician and patient. In this context, it is always helpful to ask patients what bothers them most about their tinnitus. This varies from patient to patient and has implications for the therapeutic management. If, for example, a patient suffers mainly from the lack of control, this can be addressed by cognitive behavioral therapy; if the main complaint is sleep disturbance, the treatment of the sleeping problem should be the main focus. Furthermore, the impact of tinnitus on the person's work, sleep (falling asleep, staying asleep), participation in enjoyable activities, social interaction (with friends, family, partner), and the general lifestyle has to be examined. Reactions to tinnitus can be very different, and it is the patient's reaction to tinnitus that causes problems, not the sound itself. In any case, this information should be communicated in a sensible way, since there action to tinnitus cannot be completely separated from the sound perception. However, in most cases of tinnitus there is currently no treatment available that can stop or clearly reduce the tinnitus sound. Therefore, the patient should understand that the reaction to tinnitus can be changed, even if the sound stays the same. If this message reaches the patient during the intake interview, a very important first step toward treatment has been achieved.

Assessment of Tinnitus-Related Impairment

Many people with tinnitus are neither bothered nor concerned about their tinnitus. There is also a group of patients who see a physician only because they are concerned that their tinnitus may be a sign of a serious ear or brain disease. Apart from those, all other people with tinnitus who seek medical attention are to some extent bothered by their tinnitus. However, there is a large variability in distress, from those who have learned to cope but would welcome some relief from the sound, to those who have severe problems with tinnitus in their daily lives. It has been repeatedly shown that the loudness or the pitch of the tinnitus sensation does not predict suffering [17]. Methods which directly quantify tinnitus distress, disability, and handicap are more appropriate for assessing the grade of suffering than tools which assess tinnitus loudness and pitch. Here, we present two screening tools, which allow an estimation of tinnitus severity based on a few questions, whereas for a more extensive, quantitative assessment of tinnitus severity several questionnaires are available (for details, see Chap. 27).

In the daily routine of an audiology or otolaryngology clinic, there is a high demand for fast and reliable classification instruments of tinnitus patients according to their severity. Here, a screening tool is presented which consists of three questions and allows screening for tinnitus severity in an objective and economic way [18]; Table 26.2).

Another possibility of a single, global measure of the impact of tinnitus on individuals is the following global item [19]:

Table 26.2 Scale for screening of Tinnitus Severity

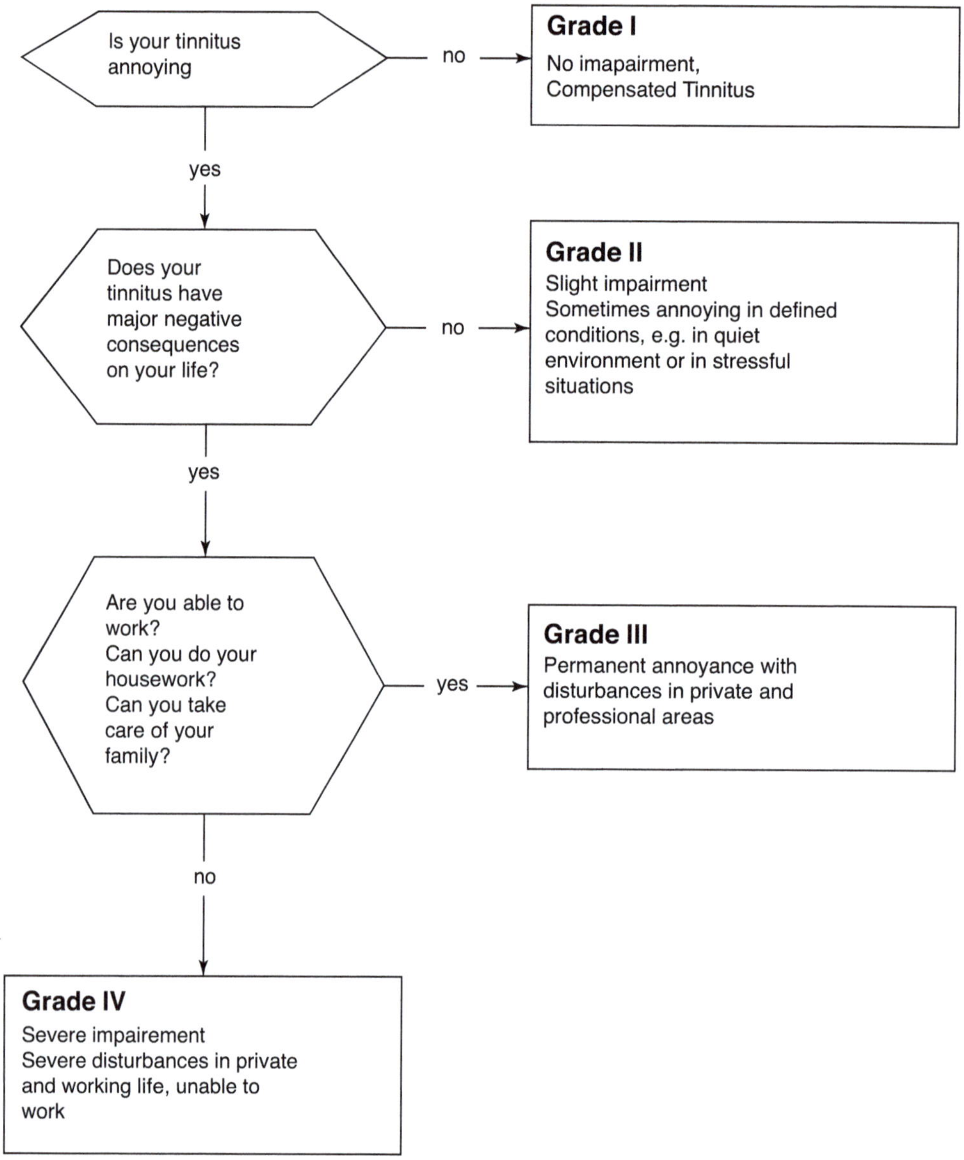

How much of a problem is your tinnitus?

Not a problem	0
A small problem	1
A moderate problem	2
A big problem	3
A very big problem	4

Preliminary data from the tinnitus clinic in Regensburg show that this 5-level response scale correlates highly with the score of the tinnitus questionnaire (see Fig. 26.1), indicating that it is a reliable, well-functioning global item for the screening of patients.

As mentioned above, the exact extent of the tinnitus case history also depends on the purpose. In most cases, the purpose is to provide a basis for individual patient management. However, a systematic case history is also a valuable resource for research because it provides standardized information that can be used to generate a clinical database. As an example, the TSCHQ is the mainstay of subtyping analyses using the TRI database [21–27] and has even been adopted for independent studies not involving the TRI database project [28, 29]. With increasing research applications of these clinical databases, the demand for more comprehensive information for scientific purposes emerged. Inspired by preceding projects and the importance of big data analyses for profiling tinnitus, a new research-oriented database [6] has been developed in the context of the European School for Interdisciplinary Tinnitus Research (ESIT) [30]. One of the

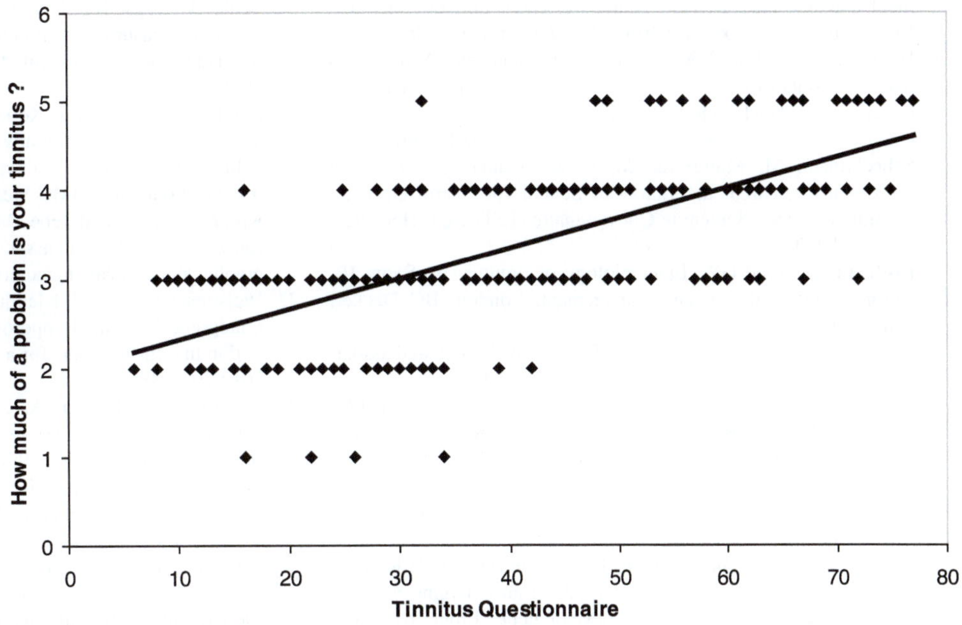

Fig. 26.1 Correlation between the screening question "How much of a problem is your tinnitus?" and the score in the Tinnitus Questionnaire [20] (*N*: 281; $r = 0.70$)

main objectives of this project is to further contribute to our understanding of tinnitus heterogeneity and to create a tinnitus profiling framework.

Tinnitus Diaries

Tinnitus diaries are self-report instruments that can be used to assess different aspects of tinnitus over time. As an example, tinnitus loudness, annoyance, mood, and stress can be assessed daily, and results can be displayed in a diagram. The information of such self-report diaries can be important for both the patient and the clinician.

A tinnitus diary can be an appropriate tool to examine changes of different tinnitus aspects over time, and correlations between intensity of tinnitus (e.g., loudness, annoyance) and different psycho-behavioral factors such as mood or stress. This allows, for example, the detection of triggers or of rhythmic changes over time. Such a protocol can reveal that mood and stress are correlated closer to tinnitus annoyance than loudness. By monitoring different parameters over a certain period of time, the patient can learn that it is not just the noise that bothers him, but other emotional, cognitive, and behavioral factors that influence tinnitus perception and reaction. Such self-report diaries are an established tool in the management of chronic pain and help patients to gain more control about the fluctuations of their tinnitus. These diaries are available as free apps (Track Your Tinnitus, TYT, Schlee) [20], and the generated data can also be used for research purposes [31–33] (for more information see Chap. 57).

Conclusion

There are different forms of tinnitus, which require specific management. The intake interview is of highest importance for obtaining comprehensive information about the patient's tinnitus in order to be able to make an exact diagnosis. Collected information from the interview, patient observation, self-report questionnaires, and tinnitus diaries should allow the clinician to get an idea of the nature of the tinnitus. In addition, this provides information about its time course, perceptual characteristics, comorbidities, the patient's difficulties, coping strategies, the impact of the tinnitus on his or her life, social relationships, and so on. Based on all this information, a specific treatment program may be developed, which is likely to be effective for an individual patient. Moreover, the information obtained by standardized Case History questionnaires and patient diaries can be aggregated in databases and used as a research tool for better understanding the heterogeneity of tinnitus.

References

1. Meikle MB, Vernon J, Johnson RM. The perceived severity of tinnitus. Some observations concerning a large population of tinnitus clinic patients. Otolaryngol Head Neck Surg. 1984;92(6):689–96.
2. Jakes SC, Hallam RS, Chambers C, Hinchcliffe R. A factor analytical study of tinnitus complaint behaviour. Audiology. 1985;24(3):195–206.
3. Stouffer JL, Tyler RS. Characterization of tinnitus by tinnitus patients. J Speech Hear Disord. 1990;55(3):439–53.
4. Langguth B, Goodey R, Azevedo A, Bjorne A, Cacace A, Crocetti A, et al. Consensus for tinnitus patient assessment and treat-

ment outcome measurement: tinnitus research initiative meeting, Regensburg, July 2006. Prog Brain Res. 2007;166:525–36.
5. Henry JA, Jastreboff MM, Jastreboff PJ, Schechter MA, Fausti SA. Assessment of patients for treatment with tinnitus retraining therapy. J Am Acad Audiol. 2002;13(10):523–44.
6. Genitsaridi E, Partyka M, Gallus S, Lopez-Escamez JA, Schecklmann M, Mielczarek M, et al. Standardised profiling for tinnitus research: the European School for Interdisciplinary Tinnitus Research Screening Questionnaire (ESIT-SQ). Hear Res. 2019;377:353–9.
7. Hoffman HJ, Reed GW. Epidemiology of tinnitus. In: Snow JB, editor. Tinnitus: theory and management. London: BC Decker; 2004. p. 16–41.
8. Coelho CB, Sanchez TG, Tyler RS. Tinnitus in children and associated risk factors. Prog Brain Res. 2007;166:179–91.
9. Vielsmeier V, Kleinjung T, Strutz J, Burgers R, Kreuzer PM, Langguth B. Tinnitus with temporomandibular joint disorders: a specific entity of tinnitus patients? Otolaryngol Head Neck Surg. 2011;145:748.
10. Sand PG, Langguth B, Kleinjung T, Eichhammer P. Genetics of chronic tinnitus. Prog Brain Res. 2007;166:159–68.
11. Lopez-Escamez JA, Bibas T, Cima RF, Van de Heyning P, Knipper M, Mazurek B, et al. Genetics of tinnitus: an emerging area for molecular diagnosis and drug development. Front Neurosci. 2016;10:377.
12. Cederroth CR, Trpchevska N, Langguth B. A new buzz for tinnitus-It's in the genes! JAMA Otolaryngol Head Neck Surg. 2020;146(11):1025–6.
13. Trpchevska N, Bulla J, Prada Hellberg M, Edvall NK, Lazar A, Mehraei G, et al. Sex-dependent aggregation of tinnitus in Swedish families. J Clin Med. 2020;9(12):3812.
14. Neff P, Zielonka L, Meyer M, Langguth B, Schecklmann M, Schlee W. Comparison of amplitude modulated sounds and pure tones at the tinnitus frequency: residual tinnitus suppression and stimulus evaluation. Trends Hear. 2019;23:2331216519833841.
15. De Ridder D, van der Loo E, Van der Kelen K, Menovsky T, Van de Heyning P, Moller A. Theta, alpha and beta burst transcranial magnetic stimulation: brain modulation in tinnitus. Int J Med Sci. 2007;4(5):237–41.
16. Simoes J, Neff P, Schoisswohl S, Bulla J, Schecklmann M, Harrison S, et al. Toward personalized tinnitus treatment: an exploratory study based on internet crowdsensing. Front Public Health. 2019;7:157.
17. Hiller W, Goebel G. Factors influencing tinnitus loudness and annoyance. Arch Otolaryngol Head Neck Surg. 2006;132(12):1323–30.
18. Biesinger E, Heiden C, Greimel V, Lendle T, Hoing R, Albegger K. Strategies in ambulatory treatment of tinnitus. HNO. 1998;46(2):157–69.
19. Meikle MB, Stewart BJ, Griest SE, Martin WH, Henry JA, Abrams HB, et al. Assessment of tinnitus: measurement of treatment outcomes. Prog Brain Res. 2007;166:511–21.
20. Schlee W, Pryss RC, Probst T, Schobel J, Bachmeier A, Reichert M, et al. Measuring the moment-to-moment variability of tinnitus: the TrackYourTinnitus smart phone app. Front Aging Neurosci. 2016;8:294.
21. Landgrebe M, Zeman F, Koller M, Eberl Y, Mohr M, Reiter J, et al. The tinnitus research initiative (TRI) database: a new approach for delineation of tinnitus subtypes and generation of predictors for treatment outcome. BMC Med Inform Decis Mak. 2010;10:42.
22. Kreuzer PM, Landgrebe M, Schecklmann M, Staudinger S, Langguth B. Trauma-associated tinnitus: audiological, demographic and clinical characteristics. PLoS One. 2012;7(9):e45599.
23. Vielsmeier V, Strutz J, Kleinjung T, Schecklmann M, Kreuzer PM, Landgrebe M, et al. Temporomandibular joint disorder complaints in tinnitus: further hints for a putative tinnitus subtype. PLoS One. 2012;7(6):e38887.
24. Vielsmeier V, Lehner A, Strutz J, Steffens T, Kreuzer PM, Schecklmann M, et al. The relevance of the high frequency audiometry in tinnitus patients with normal hearing in conventional pure-tone audiometry. Biomed Res Int. 2015;2015:302515.
25. Schecklmann M, Landgrebe M, Langguth B. Phenotypic characteristics of hyperacusis in tinnitus. PLoS One. 2014;9(1):e86944.
26. Langguth B, Hund V, Landgrebe M, Schecklmann M. Tinnitus patients with comorbid headaches: the influence of headache type and laterality on tinnitus characteristics. Front Neurol. 2017;8:440.
27. Langguth B, Landgrebe M, Schlee W, Schecklmann M, Vielsmeier V, Steffens T, et al. Different patterns of hearing loss among tinnitus patients: a latent class analysis of a large sample. Front Neurol. 2017;8:46.
28. Ward J, Vella C, Hoare DJ, Hall DA. Subtyping somatic tinnitus: a cross-sectional UK cohort study of demographic, clinical and audiological characteristics. PLoS One. 2015;10(5):e0126254.
29. Kojima T, Kanzaki S, Oishi N, Ogawa K. Clinical characteristics of patients with tinnitus evaluated with the tinnitus sample case history questionnaire in Japan: a case series. PLoS One. 2017;12(8):e0180609.
30. Schlee W, Hall DA, Canlon B, Cima RFF, de Kleine E, Hauck F, et al. Innovations in doctoral training and research on tinnitus: the European school on interdisciplinary tinnitus research (ESIT) perspective. Front Aging Neurosci. 2017;9:447.
31. Probst T, Pryss R, Langguth B, Schlee W. Emotion dynamics and tinnitus: daily life data from the "TrackYourTinnitus" application. Sci Rep. 2016;6:31166.
32. Probst T, Pryss RC, Langguth B, Rauschecker JP, Schobel J, Reichert M, et al. Does tinnitus depend on time-of-day? An ecological momentary assessment study with the "TrackYourTinnitus" application. Front Aging Neurosci. 2017;9:253.
33. Probst T, Pryss RC, Langguth B, Spiliopoulou M, Landgrebe M, Vesala M, et al. Outpatient tinnitus clinic, self-help web platform, or Mobile application to recruit tinnitus study samples? Front Aging Neurosci. 2017;9:113.

27 Tinnitus Questionnaires

Berthold Langguth and Annick Gilles

Abstract

Quantitative assessment of the different aspects of tinnitus is important for clinical management of tinnitus patients and essential for research applications.

Tinnitus is a subjective phenomenon, and there exist no established biomarkers. Assessment should include various aspects of tinnitus such as loudness, annoyance, distress, disability, and handicap.

A variety of validated questionnaires are available for quantifying tinnitus distress, disability, or handicap. Numeric rating scales and visual analog scales have been validated for the assessment of tinnitus loudness and annoyance.

In this chapter, we will discuss general requirements and psychometric properties of questionnaires and then present the most widely used instruments in detail. The selection of the questionnaire should be based on purpose (What should be assessed?), but also on psychometric data of the questionnaire and the availability of the questionnaire in a specific language.

B. Langguth (✉)
Department of Psychiatry and Psychotherapy, University of Regensburg, Bezirksklinikum, Regensburg, Germany
e-mail: Berthold.Langguth@medbo.de

A. Gilles
Faculty of Medicine and Health Sciences, Department of Translational Neuroscience, University of Antwerp, Wilrijk, Belgium

Department of Otorhinolaryngology and Head Neck Surgery, Antwerp University Hospital, Edegem, Belgium

Department of Education, Health and Social Work, University College Ghent, Ghent, Belgium
e-mail: Annick.Gilles@uza.be

W. Schlee et al. (eds.), *Textbook of Tinnitus*, https://doi.org/10.1007/978-3-031-35647-6_27

Graphical Abstract

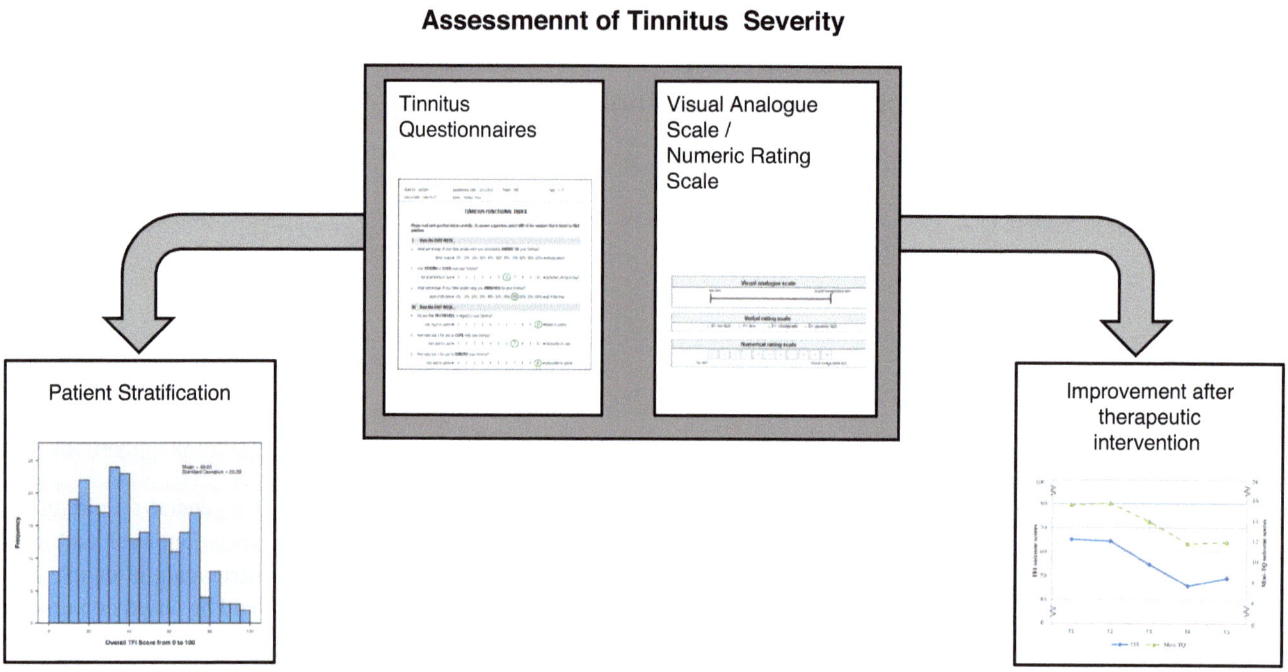

Highlights

- Quantitative assessment of tinnitus severity is relevant for both clinical management and research applications.
- Various validated questionnaires are available for quantifying tinnitus distress, disability, or handicap.
- The selection of the questionnaire should be based on purpose (what should be assessed?), but also on psychometric data of the questionnaire and the availability of the questionnaire in a specific language.
- Numeric rating scales and visual analog scales are easy applicable tools for quantifying different aspects of tinnitus (such as loudness or annoyance).

Introduction

Tinnitus is by definition a subjective percept, which can be associated with emotional distress, cognitive dysfunction, autonomic arousal, behavioral changes, and functional disability (see also Chap. 2).

Currently, no objective procedures are yet established for diagnosis or measuring tinnitus. The subjective nature of tinnitus is not only a challenge in the clinical management of the individual with tinnitus, but also for research applications. Various efforts have been made to establish valid and reliable assessment tools for both the tinnitus percept and the associated functional impairment.

Quantification of tinnitus-related impairment is highly important for clinical management. Many people with tinnitus are neither bothered nor concerned about their tinnitus. There is also a group of patients, who see a physician only because they are concerned that their tinnitus may be a sign of a serious ear or brain disease. Apart from those, all other people with tinnitus who seek medical attention are to some extent bothered by their tinnitus. However, there is a large variability in distress, ranging from those who have learned to cope but would welcome some relief from the sound, to those who have severe problems with tinnitus in their daily lives.

It has been repeatedly shown that the loudness or the pitch of the tinnitus sensation is only loosely associated with tinnitus distress [1–4]. Therefore, it is important to differentiate between methods for the assessment of tinnitus loudness and methods for the assessment of tinnitus distress and tinnitus-related handicap or disability. Methods which directly quantify tinnitus distress, disability, and handicap are more appropriate for assessing the amount of suffering.

Table 27.1 Questions to consider when performing an assessment

1 *What do I want to know?* > kind of information. (e.g., tinnitus characteristics, tinnitus-related impairments, comorbidity)
2 *Why do I want it to know?* > reason for evaluation. (e.g., for screening, treatment planning, measuring treatment outcome)
3 *How can I get the information?* > choice of appropriate assessment tools. (e.g., interview, rating scales, questionnaires, protocols)

Screening tools allow an estimation of tinnitus severity based on a few questions, whereas, for quantitative assessment of tinnitus severity, many psychometrically validated questionnaires are available. These questionnaires are helpful tools for quantifying disabling and handicapping effects of tinnitus, providing insight into how the tinnitus sensation generates a disability at a personal level and a handicap on the societal level. Responses on these questionnaires can be summed resulting in a total score or subscale scores. Based on the score, the tinnitus severity of an individual patient can be determined (e.g., in low, medium, moderate, or severe).

In the clinical assessment of tinnitus patients, the aims of the assessment (see Table 27.1) and the limitations of questionnaires have to be considered. Therefore, a comprehensive patient assessment should not rely solely on questionnaire scores, but requires the integration of information from multiple sources and tools, including in addition to questionnaires the clinical interview, and the observation of the patient's behavior during the interview [5]. It is not only *what* the patients say, but also *how* they say it that is of relevance. Sometimes interviews with significant others or reports from previous therapists or physicians provide further important information.

In addition to clinical applications, quantitative assessment by tinnitus questionnaires is an important tool for all kinds of different research applications.

In this chapter, we will review questionnaires and scales that are used for quantification of tinnitus and as outcome measurements for assessing the efficacy of therapeutic interventions (concerning standardized instrument for assessing the case history please refer to Chap. 26). It is our intent to provide a useful and practical reference both for clinicians and for researchers seeking information about the availability of different methods. Also, the limitations of the different methods will be discussed in order to allow the readers to select the most appropriate method for their specific clinical or research application (see Table 27.1).

Psychometric and Methodological Aspects

Different methodological aspects have to be considered in the use of quantitative measurement techniques (see also Table 27.2).

Table 27.2 Important aspects of questionnaire construction[a]

	Discriminative questionnaires	Evaluative questionnaires
Purpose	Quantitative diagnosis	Assessment of treatment outcome
1. Item selection	Responses of different patients or subjects should be heterogeneous (spread widely across the response continuum)	Lack of response heterogeneity is not a problem, may even improve an item's ability to show clear changes resulting from treatment
2. Item reduction	Items that most subjects answer the same are unable to reveal diagnostic differences and should be deleted	Delete any items that testing reveals are insensitive to change (regardless of whether they are sensitive to diagnostic differences)
3. Item response scaling	The chosen scaling should facilitate uniform interpretation by subjects (wording should not be ambiguous or confusing). Too much resolution may decrease subjects' response reliability	An items sensitivity to change is generally proportional to the number of response options it provides. Response scales should have high resolution (sufficient gradations) to register changes even if small
4. Test-retest reliability	Within-subject variance should be small, between-subject variance should be large and stable (reliability indicating stable individual differences)	Within-subject variance should be small when functional status remains constant, but show large changes in scores when functional status improves
5. Content validity	All or most of the important dimensions of the health problem should be addressed	Address only those dimensions capable of showing treatment-related change
6. Construct validity	Questionnaire scores should be highly correlated with well-established, comparable measures administered at that same time	Questionnaire scores after treatment should bear the predicted relationship to the same measures administered before treatment

[a] Modified from Meikle et al. 2007

Validity

First of all, one has to take into account which characteristic of tinnitus a questionnaire is targeting. Is a specific questionnaire assessing disability, handicap, or coping styles? In general, the validity of an instrument is reflected by its ability to yield "truthful," "correct," or "real" information (see also Fig. 27.1). Validation strategies include content validity, criterion-related validity, and construct validity. Content validity demonstrates to which extent the items of the scale reflect the characteristics to be measured, criterion-related validity measures how well the instrument correlates with a "gold standard," and construct validity reflects the degree to which an instrument purports to measure a theoretic construct of the characteristics to be assessed [7].

Fig. 27.1 Important steps in cross-cultural adaption of questionnaires (from [6])

Section 1. Preparation

- Adequate preparation can minimise the misuse of resources by reducing duplication of pre-existing questionnaires and by avoiding copyright infringement.
- Early communication with the source-language Questionnaire Developer can help to define the concepts underlying questionnaire items to reduce the risk of misinterpretation in later stages of translation and to highlight issues from past experiences.

Section 2. Translating the source language into the target language

- At least two bilingual translators should be briefed on the questionnaire, the health condition it measures and the translation requirements.
- Each translator should produce an independent forward translation, from the original source language to the target language.
- Discrepancies between the multiple independent translations should be reconciled and a single consolidated translation reported by a third independent team member.

Section 3. Translating the target language back into the source language

- At least one additional bilingual translator should independently produce a back translation from the target language back to the original source language.
- Discrepancies between the original source-language questionnaire and the back translation should be reported and resolved, including generating alternatives to consider in the next steps.

Section 4. Committee Review

- A multi-disciplinary team including at least one bilingual translator and a clinician should review the forward and back translation reports and agree on solutions to discrepancies to reach cross-cultural equivalence in the forward translation.
- If anything is changed this should undertake back translation in order to confirm equivalence.

Section 5. Field testing

- Cognitive debriefing and/or pilot testing should be conducted with the target audience to ensure that they understand the questions and that the questions are culturally appropriate.

Section 6. Reviewing and finalising the translation

- Final amendments to the questionnaire should use pilot data to ensure questions are correctly interpreted and culturally appropriate, before proofreading.
- A translation certification is issued to confirm the processes.
- A final report of the processes should be shared with the source-language Questionnaire Developer. As far as possible, the work should be disseminated to minimise duplication of translations into the same language.

Standardization and Norming

Can data assessed at place X at time X be compared to those at place Y and time Y?

Is a specific score high or low as compared to most other patients?

Standardization means that data are always assessed and performed in the same (i.e.) standardized way. Relevant issues can be whether a questionnaire is completed as an electronic version or as a paper version, or whether it is completed before or after the first consultation. Only a standardized way of assessment allows comparison across individuals, time, and clinical settings. Norming means obtaining information about the distribution of measures in a target population in the form of means, standard deviations, or percentiles. Normative data allow placement of the score of an individual in context of a target population.

Reliability

Does the tinnitus questionnaire have high test–retest reliability and stability?

Reliability describes the precision of the instrument and includes internal consistency but also reproducibility. Internal consistency reflects the inter-item consistency of a scale or subscales. It is expected that several items which assess the same construct (e.g., tinnitus handicap) correlate which each other. The statistical measure of this internal consistency is Cronbach's α.

Reproducibility can be differentiated in short- and long-term reproducibility. Short-term reproducibility may reflect effects of day-to-day fluctuations; long-term reproducibility describes stability over longer time intervals. This is of relevance when a questionnaire is used for evaluating effects of a specific intervention. If there is a lack of knowledge about the changes in a questionnaire score over time occurring without any treatment intervention, one cannot rely on uncontrolled observations of treatment effects. Documented changes in tinnitus scores may not be due to the treatment, per se, but rather to measurement error of the questionnaire used for assessing treatment outcome.

Responsiveness

Is the questionnaire sensitive for treatment-induced changes?

Responsiveness reflects the ability of a questionnaire to register changes following an individual's response to treatment intervention. This is especially required when an instrument is used as treatment outcome measure. This aspect of measurement instruments has also been characterized as evaluative [8, 9]. Variables which are stable over time and reflect, for example, the individual's personality are called *trait* parameters, whereas variables that reflect mainly the actual condition are called *state* variables.

From an evaluative questionnaire, one would expect that it samples mainly *state* variables that are likely to change under treatment. A large amount of change insensitive *trait*-variables are unable in detecting treatment effects and may even obscure them. In contrast, the inclusion of *trait* parameters can be useful for an instrument designed for diagnostic use (e.g., for discriminating between individuals with severe vs. mild tinnitus).

Another factor related to the responsiveness of a questionnaire is the number of response options for each item. A questionnaire which consists of items that can only be answered with two or three levels (e.g., yes and no) is, in general, less sensitive to changes than a questionnaire with 5 or more answer options per item. It should be noted that, apart from the Tinnitus Functional Index (TFI) [10], the currently available tinnitus questionnaires have not been specifically designed for evaluating treatment-related changes, but most of them have been used as outcome measures in clinical trials (for more detailed information about questionnaire construction, see also Table 27.2).

Minimal Clinical Important Improvement

Related to responsiveness is the question, which minimal changes of the questionnaire score are of clinical relevance. In a clinical study, a mean improvement of 2 points in a questionnaire with a total score of 100 may reach statistical significance, but this does not mean that 2-point improvement is also clinically significant and/or relevant to the patient. For the correct interpretation, which changes in outcome measurement instruments can be considered as clinically relevant, the concept of the minimal clinically important difference (MCID) has been introduced. Typically, the MCID is based on a combination of the statistical distribution of questionnaire scores (distribution based) and on the comparison of the score change with the subjective perceived improvement of patients (anchor-based).

Feasibility

Feasibility reflects the property of an instrument to be practically applicable in a real-world context. As an example, in order to be applicable in a high demanding clinical practice, tinnitus questionnaires should be brief and easy to administer, understand, score, and interpret.

Cultural and Language Bias

Questionnaires designed and tested in one population and language are not necessarily equally applicable in other languages. Moreover, questionnaires developed in one culture do not necessarily measure the same factors in another, even if the language is the same [11, 12]. Likewise, translation from one language to another can introduce changes in meaning and/or interpretation. One way of addressing these variations is to validate the questionnaire in each language and setting. This may lead to some items from the original questionnaire being moved into a different factor, or rejected as invalid. While this approach has merit in optimizing the questionnaire for a particular population there are at least two significant downsides: (1) considerable time is required to validate the questionnaire in each setting; and (2) cross-population comparisons become difficult. The latter of these two issues is most troublesome for researchers who might want to compare outcomes from two populations using the "same" questionnaire. For example, a questionnaire developed in the USA but optimized for New Zealand might omit questions [12]. If two treatments are compared between these countries and found to have the same questionnaire scores, it cannot be assumed that the treatments are equally effective because they actually do not ask the same questions. On the other hand, if the original questionnaire is used in its original form in both countries, cultural idiosyncrasies mean that they still measure different factors. This paradox is a limitation of questionnaires. Any "worldwide" standard should retain as many of its original items and factor structure when validated in different populations. Researchers should recognize the potential for population differences when using questionnaires.

Translation of Questionnaires

As mentioned above, the translation of questionnaires is far from trivial. Recently, a standard procedure for the translation of hearing-related questionnaires has been proposed to raise awareness about the inherent problems of the translation of questionnaires and to propose a good practice guide [6]. Six steps with 22 different items have been specified for creating a questionnaire that promotes equivalence to the original by accounting for any cultural differences (see Fig. 27.1). This procedure represents a gold standard for high-quality translation and cultural adaption of a questionnaire. However, the proposed procedure is demanding with respect to financial and human resources and may therefore not always be feasible.

Screening of Tinnitus Severity

In the daily routine of an audiological or otolaryngologic clinic, there is a high need for fast and reliable classification of tinnitus patients according to their severity. Those who suffer from tinnitus require an entirely different management than those who simply experience tinnitus, but are only slightly or not at all impaired by it. A validated screening question for the clinical context is the question "How much of a problem is your tinnitus?" with the answer options "Not a problem"(0), "A small problem" (1), "A moderate problem" (2), "A big problem" (3), or "A very big problem (4). This 5-level response scale correlates highly with the score of the tinnitus questionnaire (see Fig. 27.2), indicating that it is a reliable, well-functioning global question for screening patients [14].

Outcome Domains

In the last years, efforts were made to identify core outcome measures in tinnitus. This initiative was motivated by the question, which aspects of tinnitus are most relevant for patients and to develop specific outcome measurement instruments for assessing the effect of therapeutic interventions on the relevant domains.

For this purpose, critical and important tinnitus-related complaints ("outcome domains") were identified separately for three different therapeutic approaches, namely sound-based interventions, psychology-based interventions, and pharmacology-based interventions. A total of 719 international patients with tinnitus, healthcare professionals, clinical researchers, commercial representatives, and funders were recruited. Eligibility was primarily determined by experience of one of the three interventions of interest. Following recommended procedures for gaining consensus, three intervention-specific, three-round, Delphi surveys were delivered online. Each Delphi survey was followed by an in-person consensus meeting. Viewpoints and votes involved all stakeholder groups, with approximately a 1:1 ratio of patients to professionals. "Tinnitus intrusiveness" was voted in for all three interventions. For sound-based interventions, the minimum set included "ability to ignore," "concentration," "quality of sleep," and "sense of control." For psychology-based interventions, the minimum set included "acceptance of tinnitus," "mood," "negative thoughts and beliefs," and "sense of control." For pharmacology-based interventions, "tinnitus loudness" was the only, additional core outcome domain. In

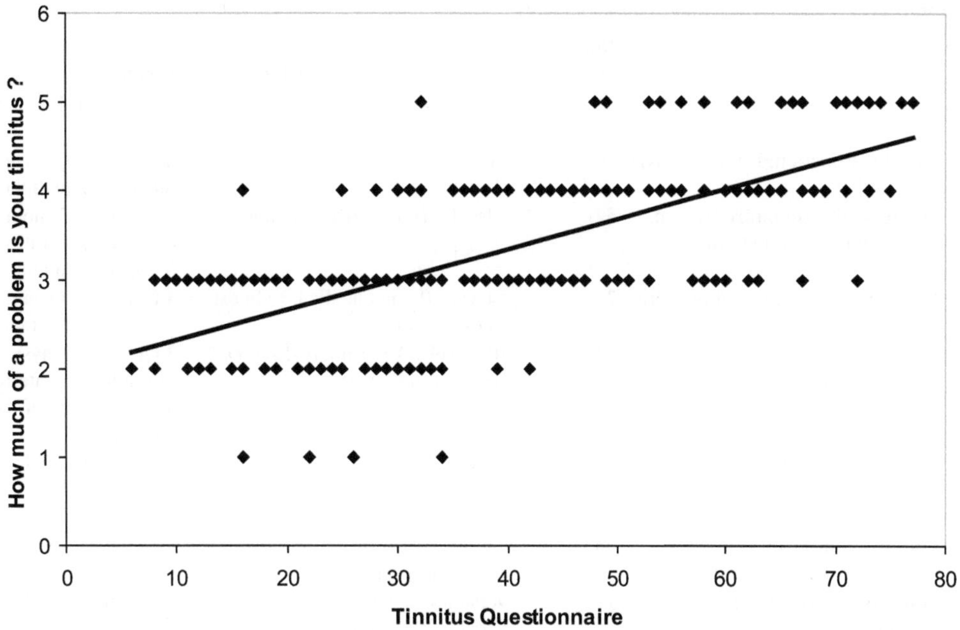

Fig. 27.2 Correlation between the screening question "How much of a problem is your tinnitus?" and the score in the Tinnitus Questionnaire [13] (*N*: 281; *r* = 0.70)

a second step, efforts will be made to identify how those outcome domains should best be measured. It has been proposed that the development of these intervention-specific standards might improve research quality, enhance clinical decision-making, and facilitate meta-analysis [6].

The identification of relevant core outcome domains for tinnitus interventions is, in principle, a valuable endeavor. Obviously, it is important that the outcome measurement instruments measure those aspects of tinnitus that are most relevant for patients. However, it should be noted that the approach has important limitations. First, it is questionable whether the participating patients are really representative for the international patient community, particularly, as cultural differences may play a relevant role in this context.

Second, there is the important epistemological question whether a domain can be clearly defined without the respective measurement method. As an example, tinnitus loudness can be measured by psychophysiological measures (e.g., minimal masking levels or loudness match) or by rating scales (visual analog scale or numeric rating scale). However, these two measures do not correlate high with each other. This means that tinnitus loudness measured by psychophysiological measurements and loudness measures by rating scales is not the same. But which of the two had the participants of the Delphi Survey in mind, when they voted? Similarly, the meaning of "tinnitus intrusiveness" is difficult to operationalize. A recent study compared the subscales of the Tinnitus Questionnaire and the Tinnitus Functional Index, which are both supposed to assess tinnitus intrusiveness. However, the subscales of these two questionnaires did not significantly correlate [15, 16].

Finally, there is the question, whether it is appropriate to identify different outcome domains depending on the investigated therapeutic approach. It seems much more reasonable that the same outcome measurement instruments are used for the various therapeutic approaches. This would enable a comprehensive comparison of the different therapeutic interventions and illustrate, which intervention can modify which domain. If for example the effect of psychological-based interventions on tinnitus loudness is not assessed, one will never know whether the intervention under study has an effect on this domain. However, from the perspective of the patient it would be highly desirable to know in advance which domains are influenced by a given intervention.

Tinnitus Questionnaires

Different questionnaires are available to assess specific aspects of patients with tinnitus (see Table 27.3). These questionnaires are score driven, which means the responses to single items are scored and then summed or averaged. Thus, total scores or subscale scores can be calculated.

There are specific questionnaires for assessing tinnitus-related cognitions (TCQ), coping styles (TCSQ), and fear of tinnitus (FTQ). The other questionnaires mainly aim to quantify tinnitus distress, disability, or handicap. Items of the different scales largely overlap. Accordingly, there is a relatively high correlation between the total scores of the different tinnitus severity and handicap questionnaires.

In addition to clinical applications, quantitative assessment by tinnitus questionnaires allows research applications.

Table 27.3 Quantitative Tinnitus questionnaires

	Number of items	Response options for each item	Factors
	25	3 levels: 4 = yes, 2 = sometimes, 0 = no	3 factors (1. Functional, 2. Emotional, 3. Catastrophic)
Tinnitus Functional Index Meikle et al. (2012)	**25**	11 levels	8 factors (cognitive, auditory, intrusive, sleep, relaxation, quality of life, emotional, sense of control)
Tinnitus Questionnaire Hallam, Jakes and Hinchcliffe (1988), Hallam (1996)	**52**	3 levels: True, partly true, not true	5 factors (1. Emotional distress, 2. Auditory perceptual difficulties, 3. Intrusiveness, 4 sleep disturbances, 5. Somatic complaints)
Tinnitus Reaction Questionnaire Wilson et al. (1991)	**26**	5 levels: 0 = not at all; 4 = almost all of the time	4 factors (1. General distress, 2. Interference, 3. Severity, 4. Avoidance)
Tinnitus Handicap Questionnaire Kuk et al. (1990)	**27**	101 levels: 0 = strongly disagree; 100 = strongly agree	3 factors (1. Physical, emotional, social consequences of tinnitus, 2. Interfering effects of tinnitus on the hearing ability of the patient, 3. The patient's view of tinnitus)
Subjective Tinnitus Severity Scale Halford and Anderson (1991)	**16**	2 levels: Yes and no	One-dimensional
Tinnitus Handicap/Support Scale Erlandsson et al. (1992)	**28**	5 levels: 1 = strongly disagree; 5 = strongly agree	3 factors (1. Perceived attitudes, 2. Social support, 3. Disability/ handicap)
Tinnitus Severity Index Meikle et al. (1995)	**12**	Version 1: 3 and 4 levels Version 2: 3–5 levels	One-dimensional
Tinnitus Beeinträchtigungs Fragebogen (TBF-12) Greimel et al. (2000)	**12**	3 levels: 4 = yes, 2 = sometimes, 0 = no	2 factors (1. Emotional-cognitive impairment, 2. Functional-communicative impairment)
Tinnitus cognitions questionnaire (Wilson and Henry 1998	**26**	5 levels; negative items: Never = 0, frequently = 4, positive items: Never = 4, frequently = 0	3 factors (1. Positive evaluation of tinnitus, 2. Hopelessness/despair. 3. Helplessness/victimization)
Tinnitus Coping Style Questionnaire Budd and Pugh (1996)	**33**	7 levels: Never = 1; always = 7	2 factors (1. Effective coping, 2. Maladaptive coping)
Fear of Tinnitus Questionnaire Fuller et al. (2019)	**17**	2 levels (yes and no)	3 factors

For example, tinnitus questionnaires have been successfully used for investigating the relationship between personality and psychopathology and their impact on tinnitus severity [17–19]. Furthermore, tinnitus questionnaires provide a method for researchers to quantify tinnitus severity as a criterion for subject selection. That is, self-report measures allow investigators to select only those patients indicating a certain degree of tinnitus severity to be included in a particular study. Minimum and maximum values of the individual's tinnitus score are defined in the research protocol as inclusion criteria, if it is expected that the treatment under study shows best effects in patients with specific tinnitus severity. Furthermore, self-report measures can be used to evaluate the effectiveness of a particular experimental treatment. There is general consensus that questionnaire scores are the best available measures of tinnitus consequence and should be used as primary outcome variables in randomized clinical trials for tinnitus treatment [20, 21].

Table 27.3 provides an overview of the most widely used quantitative tinnitus questionnaires in the English language. Figure 27.3 illustrates how much the various questionnaires have been used in the past [22]. In the following discussion, each of these questionnaires is presented in detail. A description of the questionnaire is followed by a short explanation of how the questionnaire is scored and interpreted. Psychometric characteristics of the questionnaire are presented, strengths and weaknesses of the instruments are discussed, and finally, it is indicated whether validated translations for the questionnaire are available.

Even if self-report questionnaires have been proven to be useful tools both in the clinical management of tinnitus and in research applications, some caution is advised in their use and interpretation. First, completing a questionnaire might not only measure specific aspects of a patient's tinnitus, but also influence the patient's tinnitus. Especially catastrophizing statements may induce or reinforce maladaptive coping strategies (e.g., statements about suicide). Also, statements such as, "I cannot sleep because of my tinnitus," may induce incorrect attributions. A patient who repeatedly reads such a statement, may become convinced that his insomnia may be caused by his tinnitus, which is not necessarily true and might result in incorrect beliefs such as, "as long as I have my tinnitus I will never be able to sleep well."

Second, it should be considered that self-report questionnaires can be subject to dissimulation or aggravation. Thus, just as a low score cannot exclude a significant impact of the

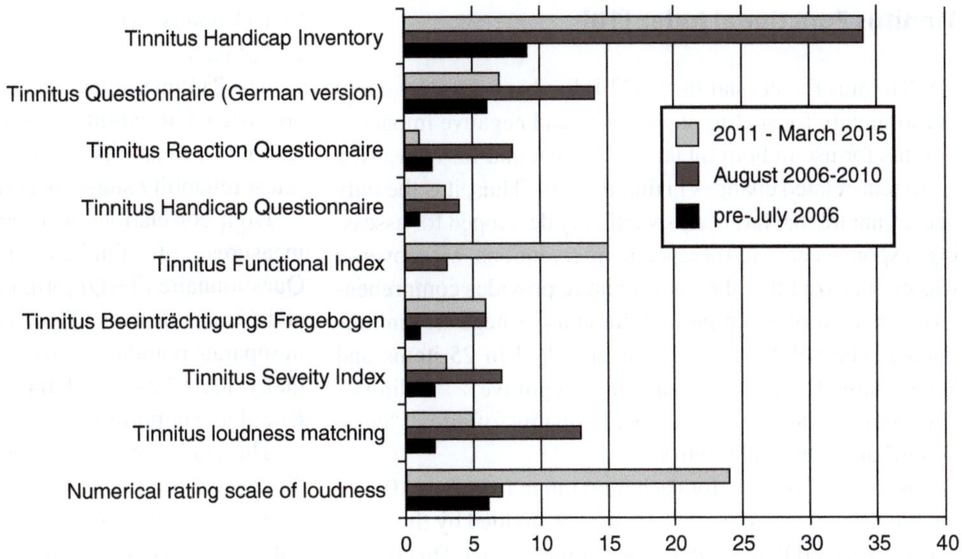

Fig. 27.3 Frequency of the use of the various questionnaires for tinnitus outcome measurement (from [22]

tinnitus on a patient's life, a high score is not proof of severe suffering either. Therefore, questionnaire results always have to be evaluated in the context of the clinical impression and the patient's tinnitus-related behavior. This is particularly relevant in a medicolegal context.

Tinnitus Handicap Inventory (THI) [23]

The 25-item Tinnitus Handicap Inventory consists of three subscales. The functional subscale (11 items) evaluates role limitations, the emotional subscale (nine items) reflects affective responses to tinnitus, and the catastrophic subscale (five items) probes the most severe reactions to tinnitus. However, the distinctness of the subscales has been questioned and the use of only the total score was recommended [24].

For each item of the inventory, the patient responds with "yes" (4 points), "sometimes" (2 points), or "no" (0 points). The responses are summed, with a total score ranging from 0 to 100 points. Higher scores represent greater perceived handicap. Handicap severity categories (0–16: no; 18–36: mild; 38–56: moderate; 58–100: severe) have been developed based on quartiles calculated for the total THI score [25].

The THI has very good internal consistency reliability (Cronbach's $\alpha = 0.93$) and high test–retest reliability for the total score ($r = 0.92$), as well as the subscales (ranging from 0.84 to 0.94). Test–retest reliability assessed, on average, 20 days after the initial administration was also high for the total score and the three subscales. A 95% confidence interval of 20 points for the total scale suggests that in an individual a difference of 20 points or more between pre- and post-treatment administration can be considered statistically significant. Convergent validity was assessed using the THQ, whereas construct validity was assessed using the Beck Depression Inventory, Modified Somatic Perception Questionnaire, symptom rating scales (e.g., sleep disturbance, annoyance), and perceived tinnitus pitch and loudness. High convergent validity with the TQ and the TFI has been demonstrated recently [14, 15, 24].

The THI is brief and easily administered and scored. It assesses the domains of function that are addressed by many available treatment interventions.

The test–retest data allow clinicians to judge effects of treatment interventions. Further data about retest stability over longer time intervals are desirable in order to evaluate changes in perceived handicap over the medium and long term.

The MCID has been determined by comparing treatment-related changes of the THI with the clinical global impression change scale. This evaluation revealed, that an improvement of at least 7 points of the THI score is needed, in order to be perceived as clinically relevant by the patients [26].

The THI is the most widely used tinnitus questionnaire, as evidenced by the number of citations [22]. Validated translations are published in many languages, including Spanish, French, German, Italian, Russian, Hebrew, Portuguese, Greek, Slovenian, Hungarian, Danish, Swedish, Norwegian, Korean, Chinese, Hindi, Urdi, Nepali, Malayalam, Thai, Philipino, Persian, Arabic, and Moroccan Arabic.

Because of its widespread use, the (additional) use of the THI has been recommended for all clinical studies in order to facilitate comparability between studies [21].

Tinnitus Functional Index [10]

The Tinnitus Functional Index (TFI) has been developed as a questionnaire for scaling the severity and negative impact of tinnitus for use in both intake assessment and for measuring treatment-related changes in tinnitus [10]. Thus, it is the only questionnaire that has been specifically developed for assessing responsiveness to therapeutic interventions. Moreover, it was emphasized that the questionnaire provides comprehensive coverage of all important domains of negative tinnitus impact. The validation procedure resulted in 25 items and eight subscales for the domains "cognitive," "auditory," "intrusive," "sleep," "relaxation," "quality of life," "emotional," and "sense of control."

The answer options for each item range from 0 to 10. For the total score, the sum of all answers is divided by the number of answered items and then multiplied by 10. This procedure results in a score between 0 and 100. The total score for the subscales can be calculated accordingly.

Psychometric properties of the TFI are very good with a Cronbach's alpha of 0.97 and test–retest reliability of 0.78. Also, the convergent validity (r = 0.86 with Tinnitus Handicap Inventory [THI]; r = 0.75 with visual analog scale [VAS]) and discriminant validity (r = 0.56 with Beck Depression Inventory-Primary Care [BDI-PC]) is good [10]. These data have been replicated in several independent samples. With respect to responsiveness, the TFI was successful at detecting improvement from the initial clinic visit to 3 months with moderate to large effect sizes and from initial to 6 months with large effect sizes. Effect sizes for the TFI were generally larger than those obtained for the VAS and THI. After careful evaluation, a 13-point reduction was proposed as criterion for the minimal clinically important difference (MCID) [10].

Validated translations of the TFI are available in Dutch, German, Italian, Chinese, Swedish, Polish, and Japanese.

Tinnitus Questionnaire (TQ) [27]

The 52-item Tinnitus Questionnaire (TQ) developed by Hallam and colleagues has been designed to measure several dimensions of patients' tinnitus complaints, namely emotional distress, auditory perceptual difficulties, and sleep disturbance. Questions relate either to the "noises" in the ear as the major cause of distress or reflect lack of coping skills.

Individuals indicate their level of agreement to each statement using one of three-response alternatives: true (2 points), partly true (1 point), or not true (0 points). Affirmative responses to an item (indicated by true) are identified as complaints about tinnitus, with the exception of items: 1, 7, 32, 40, 44, and 49, which are reverse-scored because they are considered positive statements. Possible scores range from 0 to 104 points, with higher scores reflecting greater tinnitus complaints.

The TQ instrument has been found to have high internal consistency reliability (Cronbach's α = 0.91–0.95) and high test–retest reliability (r = 0.91–0.94) [28, 29]. The high test–retest reliability suggests good stability over time.

High correlations were also found between the TQ and measures of tinnitus handicap (Tinnitus Handicap Questionnaire (THQ) [30], tinnitus handicap inventory [31], and tinnitus distress (TRQ) [13]). Factor analyses conducted in separate populations were consistent with the factors originally identified by Hallam and colleagues in the United Kingdom supporting the instrument's validity.

The TQ has been found to measure a number of different dimensions of tinnitus complaints and is a stable measure over time. In this connection, the TQ would be useful as an outcome measure in determining the effectiveness of treatment. The minimal clinical, important difference (MCID) of the TQ has been investigated in two studies [32, 33], which used a similar methodology, but different clinical samples and yielded different results.

One study was based on 757 patients from seven different centers in Germany who had received different forms of tinnitus treatment, including auditory stimulation, transcranial magnetic stimulation, behavioral therapy, and pharmacologic treatment. This analysis yielded an MCID of 5 points [32]. The other study was based on 202 patients from one center, who all received music therapy. This study revealed an MCID of 12 points [33]. Further research is needed to determine a universally accepted MCID for the TQ.

The TQ has been translated into German language and extensively validated [34, 35]. Factor analysis of the German translation of the TQ revealed that the dimensions of emotional and cognitive distress, intrusiveness, auditory perceptual difficulties, sleep disturbances, and somatic complaints can be differentiated [35]. This validation also resulted in a different scoring system, where some items were not used at all and others loaded in two factors, resulting in a maximum score of 84 points. Further translations in Dutch and French are based on the German version [36]. Also, a Chinese version of the TQ has been validated [37]. Also, a short version of the TQ has been validated, with a high correlation (r = 0.94) of the sum scores of the Mini-TQ and the TQ (Mini-TQ [14, 38],). The Mini-TQ is freely available in most European languages at https://www.tinnitus-liga.de/pages/sonstiges/aktionsleiste/tinnitus%2D%2D-test.php .

Tinnitus Reaction Questionnaire (TRQ) [13]

The Tinnitus Reaction Questionnaire has been developed for quantifying the psychological distress associated with tinnitus [13]. The 26 items of the TRQ relate to distress consequences such as anger, confusion, annoyance, helplessness, activity avoidance, and panic.

Each item on the TRQ is scored on a 5-point scale, ranging from 0 points to 4 points. The scores are summed with the total score ranging from 0 to 104 points, with higher scores reflecting greater distress.

The TRQ has high internal consistency reliability (Cronbach's $\alpha = 0.96$), as well as test–retest reliability ($r = 0.88$). Concerning construct validity, there are moderate-to-high correlations between the TRQ and clinician ratings and self-reported measures of anxiety and depression. A factor analysis revealed the factors general distress, interference, severity, and avoidance.

The TRQ represents an easy clinical tool for assessing tinnitus distress. However, no cut-off values for severity categories are available. High test–retest reliability period over a period ranging from 3 days to 3 weeks indicates short-term stability of the TRQ and its usefulness in quantifying treatment outcome, at least for short interventions. However, no data are available about what is considered a statistically significant or a clinical relevant change of the score. A French translation of the THQ has been validated [39] and compared with the English version, demonstrating only minor effects of language [40].

Tinnitus Handicap Questionnaire (THQ) [30]

The Tinnitus Handicap Questionnaire (THQ) also called "Iowa Tinnitus Handicap Questionnaire" is intended to be broad in scope but sensitive to patients' perceived degree of tinnitus handicap. By factor analysis, three factors have been differentiated. Factor 1 (15 items) reflects the physical, emotional, and social consequences of tinnitus; factor 2 (8 items) assesses the effects of tinnitus and hearing; and factor 3 (4 items) explores the patient's view on tinnitus.

For each item, the individual responds with a number between 0 and 100 indicating how much he or she disagrees (0 = strongly disagrees) or agrees (100 = strongly agrees) with the statement. After inverting scores obtained on items 25 and 26 by subtracting them from 100, mean scores can be calculated for the total or for each of the three factors. Higher scores indicate greater handicap.

The THQ demonstrated high internal consistency and reliability for the total scale (Cronbach's $\alpha = 0.95$), factor 1 (0.95), and factor 2 (0.88). Factor 3 yielded a low alpha (0.47), which may be due to the small number of items comprising this factor. A similar factor structure has been obtained in Australian [29] and New Zealand [41] samples.

Adequate construct validity of the THQ was documented by relative high correlations ($r > 0.50$) with perceived tinnitus loudness, life satisfaction, hearing threshold, depression, and general health status. High test–retest correlations have been obtained assessed over a 6-week period for the total score ($r = 0.89$), factor 1 ($r = 0.89$), and factor 2 ($r = 0.90$), whereas factor 3 yielded inadequate retest reliability ($r = 0.50$) [39]. Normative data for the THQ are available [29]. The percentile ranking allows determining severity for an individual patient relative to other patients with tinnitus. Comparison of the scores for Factor 1 (emotional and social effects) and Factor 2 (hearing) has been used to guide clinicians in treatment selection (high Factor 1—greater psychological management, high Factor 2—hearing aids [42]).

The 100-point response scale may be relatively sensitive for changes [41], but it may be somewhat problematic, especially for items, dealing with subjective strength of belief.

According to their authors, the THQ is among the most widely used questionnaires [43]. A French and a Persian translation of the THQ have been validated. Official, but unvalidated translations in various languages are available at https://medicine.uiowa.edu/oto/research/tinnitus-and-hyperacusis/tinnitus-questionnaires.

Tinnitus Activities Questionnaire

The Iowa Tinnitus Activities Questionnaire looks at the emotional aspect of tinnitus as well as problems that are associated with concentration, hearing, and sleep due to tinnitus. No psychometric data have been published. Unvalidated translations in many languages are available at https://medicine.uiowa.edu/oto/research/tinnitus-and-hyperacusis/tinnitus-questionnaires .

Tinnitus Severity Scale (TSS)

The Tinnitus Severity Scale (TSS) aims at quantifying individuals' cognitive and behavioral responses to tinnitus. The 15 items are categorized under the factors intrusiveness (four items), distress (six items), hearing loss (three items), sleep disturbance (one item), and medication (one item). Responses refer to the past week and range in score from 1 (no impact) to 4 (most impact). Each item is weighted from 1 to 3 points (total weight score = 39 points). The total score is calculated by multiplying each item's score by its weight and summing these products, resulting in a range between 39 points (39 weighting points × 1-point item score) to 156 points (39 weighting points × 4-point item score). The TSS has acceptable test–retest reliability ($r = 0.86$. No further psychometric data are available, limiting clinical and research applications.). There exists a validated Japanese translation of the TSS [44]. Further validated translations of the Scale into other languages are not published.

Subjective Tinnitus Severity Scale (STSS) [25]

The 16-item Subjective Tinnitus Severity Scale (STSS) was developed to provide a simple questionnaire to assess tinnitus severity. Each question is answered with either a "yes" or "no" response. Ten of the sixteen items earn a point if the response is "yes" (e.g., "Are you almost always aware of your tinnitus?"), whereas the other six items earn a point if the response is "no" (e.g., "When you are busy, do you quite often forget about your tinnitus?"), summing up to scores between 0 and 16 with higher scores reflecting greater overall severity. A Cronbach's α of 0.84 indicates high consistency reliability. The validity was established in a sample of 30 patients, where mean STSS scores were found to correlate highly with two independent clinical ratings of severity.

The STSS is extremely simple to administer and score. However, the lack of a classification scheme for the total score limits its diagnostic use. Furthermore, no data about test–retest reliability are available, limiting its applicability for measuring treatment outcome.

The original questionnaire is in the English language, validated translations in Dutch and French have been published.

Tinnitus Handicap/Support Scale (TH/SS) [45]

The 28-item Tinnitus Handicap/Support Scale (TH/SS) assesses the attitudes of significant others toward the person with tinnitus. Three factors were identified, including perceived attitudes or reactions of others (factor 1; 9 items), social support (factor 2; 10 items), and personal and social handicaps (factor 3; 9 items). Each statement on the scale is scored from 1 (strongly disagree) to 5 (strongly agree). The reliability of the TH/SS has not been examined. Construct validity of the TH/SS was assessed using a 10-item Tinnitus Severity Questionnaire (TSQ). This is the only questionnaire that has been designed to assess the influence of significant others in the overall management process, which can be helpful for counseling. The lack of retest reliability data limits both its clinical and scientific use.

The questionnaire is in English language and has not been validated in any other language.

The Tinnitus Severity Index

The Tinnitus Severity Index is a 12-item questionnaire which measures the effect of tinnitus on work and social activities and overall quality of life [46]. The 12 items of the TSI are totaled for a single severity index. This is one of the shorter tinnitus questionnaires that has been published. There have been 2 versions of the TSI, the original [46] using 3- and 4-point scales and a modified version using primarily a 5-point scale, with two 4-point questions and one 3-point question [47]. The TSI has had limited use outside of the US, but the original version has been normed in New Zealand as well [41]. The TSI has good internal consistency in both USA and NZ (Cronbach's α >0.87) populations. The TSI has been found to correlate to the subjective rating of tinnitus loudness but not hearing loss [41]. The TSI and THQ are correlated ($r = 0.77, p < 0.05$), suggesting that each questionnaire is measuring similar, but not exactly the same, elements of tinnitus [41]. The TSI scores have been shown to improve following comprehensive audiology-based tinnitus management programs [48], and use of SSRIs has improved scores [49].

The Tinnitus Handicap Questionnaire (Tinnitus Beeinträchtigungs Fragebogen; TBF-12)

Based on the Tinnitus Handicap Inventory (THI), a short version in German language has been developed and labeled TBF-12 [50] (or also THI-12). However, the correlation of the TBF-12 score and the THI score is rather low [14]. The final German version encompasses 12 items and distinguishes between the factors emotional-cognitive (items 3, 4, 6, 8, 10, 11 and 12) and functional-communicative impairments (items 1, 2, 5, 7, 9).

The internal consistency reliability of the TBF is high (Cronbach's $\alpha = 0.90$). The TBF-12 is easy to understand and administer, psychometrically robust, and well suitable as a screening instrument in primary care. In the context of a phase III trial, the questionnaire has been translated and linguistically evaluated in Spanish, Dutch, French, Portuguese, Czech, Spanish, Polish, and English, as well as African languages.

Tinnitus Cognitions Questionnaire (TCQ) [51]

In contrast to the scales assessing distress, disability, or handicap, the Tinnitus Cognitions Questionnaire (TCQ) focuses on the patient's reaction to tinnitus from a cognitive perspective. The 26 items assess positive and negative thoughts associated with tinnitus [61], especially important in the context of the psychological management of tinnitus. The TCQ consists of 13 negative items and 13 positive items, which are clearly separated. Each of the items is rated on a 5-point scale (0–4). The negative items (1–13) are scored 0–4, whereas the positive items (14–26) are reverse-scored, 4–0. The addition of the item scores reveals the total TCQ score, which can range from 0 to 104, with higher scores reflecting a tendency toward more negative and less positive thoughts in response to tinnitus.

The TCQ yielded both good test–retest reliability (r = 0.88) and internal consistency reliability (Cronbach's α = 0.91). A factor analysis revealed that the negative and positive cognitions represent independent factors. Construct and convergent validity was assessed between the TCQ-total, TCQ-positive, and TCQ-negative scores, as well as other measures of tinnitus-specific symptomatology (e.g., distress, handicap, complaint behavior), depression, automatic thoughts, and loss of control. The TCQ showed moderate correlations with other tinnitus-related measures (i.e., TRQ, THQ, and TQ), with the TCQ-negative subscale demonstrating higher correlations with each of the tinnitus- and non-tinnitus measures.

The TCQ is different from other questionnaires by focusing on cognitive responses in individuals with tinnitus. The information from the TCQ responses is especially useful in the context of cognitive-behavioral therapy for screening or stratifying patients, but also for outcome measurement. However, the latter requires data about test–retest reliability. It has to be considered that reporting about cognitions or thoughts may not be identical to engaging in these thoughts. No validated translations of the instrument have been published.

Tinnitus Coping Style Questionnaire (TCSQ) [52]

The Tinnitus Coping Style Questionnaire (TCSQ) is a 33-item scale developed to assess adaptive and coping strategies and consists of two factors [52]. Eighteen items comprise the maladaptive coping factor; the other 15 items comprise the effective coping subscale.

For each item, the patient indicates how frequently he/she employs each of the coping strategies on a 1 ("never") to 7 ("always") scale. Higher scores on the maladaptive coping subscale reflect poorer coping skills, whereas higher scores on the effective coping dimension are characterized by better acceptance of the tinnitus and use of a broad range of adaptive coping skills.

The internal consistency reliability values for the maladaptive coping and effectiveness coping subscales were 0.90 and 0.89, respectively. The two subscales were not significantly correlated (r = 0.13). Maladaptive coping strategies were significantly associated with measures of tinnitus severity, depression, and anxiety. In contrast, effective coping was not correlated with any of the tinnitus adjustment measures [52].

The TSCQ is specifically focused on coping strategies used by tinnitus sufferers. Information obtained with the TSCQ is fundamental in developing a cognitive-behavioral therapy program. After probing test–retest reliability of the instrument, the TSCQ might also be suitable for monitoring changes during cognitive-behavioral therapy.

Fear of Tinnitus Questionnaire (FTQ)

The Fear of Tinnitus Questionnaire (FTQ) is a brief, self-report measure of people's fears concerning potential cognitive, emotional, behavioral, and social consequences of living with tinnitus [53].

The FTQ has good internal reliability (α = 0.83, 95% confidence interval, 0.81–0.85) and test–retest reliability (average value intraclass correlation coefficient (ICC) = 0.92; 95% confidence interval, 0.89–0.95). Furthermore, the FTQ added statistically significant amounts of variance to models predicting tinnitus-related distress and interference in daily life [54]. There exists a validated Swedish translation of the FTQ [55].

Other Questionnaires

Beside tinnitus-related questionnaires, several other instruments referring to different comorbid conditions may be useful as part of a broad assessment of the patient and their problems. A large variety of self-report questionnaires are available for assessing depression, anxiety, sleep disorders, or health-related quality of life. A detailed description of these questionnaires is beyond the scope of this chapter. In general, these instruments are not necessary for basis assessment in every patient but may be helpful in specific cases.

Rating Scales

Rating scales (visual analog scales (VAS) or Likert type scales / numerical rating scales (NRS)) can be used for assessing different characteristics of tinnitus, such as loudness or annoyance. Examples for such scales are given in Fig. 27.4. Rating scales are easy to understand, but sometimes patients report difficulties because, generally, the maximum end of the scale is only very vaguely defined.

Apart from loudness and annoyance, other qualitative features of tinnitus can also be easily assessed with rating scales (e.g., intrusiveness or ability to ignore tinnitus). This can provide an opportunity to understand what the most important problem is for a given patient and may lead to the use of more individually tailored assessment monitoring tasks, such as tinnitus diaries or tinnitus protocols.

A big advantage of rating scales is that they are fast to perform and can be repeated easily, e.g., in the form of tinnitus protocols. Unfortunately, there are limited psychomet-

a

How loud to you perceive your tinnitus?

0 ------ 1 ------- 2 ------- 3 ------- 4 ------- 5 ------- 6

No tinnitus very loud

b

How loud do you perceive your tinnitus ?

0 ________________________________ 100

Fig. 27.4 Numeric rating scale (NRS) and visual analog scale (VAS) of loudness of tinnitus. Example for a numeric rating scale/Likert-like scale (**a**) and a visual analog scale (**b**) for assessment of subjectively perceived tinnitus loudness

ric data for visual analog and numeric rating scales. One recent study shows that in individuals with tinnitus who do not seek medical attention, rating scores are much lower than in those who seek help for their tinnitus [56].

Formal psychometric assessments of visual analog scales (VAS) for loudness and annoyance with a arrange from 0 to 100 revealed good test–retest reliability of 0.8 and 0.79, respectively. In terms of convergent validity, VAS loudness and VAS annoyance correlated well with the tinnitus questionnaire at all clinical visits (max $r = 0.67$, $p < 0.05$). MCID estimates clustered between 10 and 15 points [57].

Limitations

Questionnaires hold important limitations. First, almost all established questionnaires are self-report questionnaires and can be subject to dissimulation or aggravation occurring both consciously and unconsciously. Conscious aggravation can be relevant in a medicolegal context, whereas unconscious manipulation may occur as dissimulation of patients, who try to neglect their impairment.

A further potential confounding factor includes insufficient understanding or misunderstanding of the questions of the questionnaire or lack of attention during completion of the questionnaire. Moreover, comorbid conditions can influence the questionnaire score. As an example, answers to questions about communication difficulties are heavily influenced by comorbid hearing impairment.

It should also be considered that the relevance of the different aspects of tinnitus differs from patient to patient and may not be clearly reflected by a given questionnaire. As an example, an individual patient may be severely affected by concentration difficulties in the context of tinnitus. However, concentration impairment may only be reflected by a single item in the questionnaire and thus only minimally impact the total score of the questionnaire.

Finally, it should be noted that all questionnaires were validated in an adult population, consisting of cognitively unimpaired people with tinnitus. There exist no specifically validated instruments to assess tinnitus in children and young people or in cognitively impaired patients.

References

1. Meikle MB, Vernon J, Johnson RM. The perceived severity of tinnitus. Some observations concerning a large population of tinnitus clinic patients. Otolaryngol Head Neck Surg. 1984;92(6):689–96.
2. Jakes SC, Hallam RS, Chambers C, Hinchcliffe R. A factor analytical study of tinnitus complaint behaviour. Audiology. 1985;24(3):195–206.
3. Hiller W, Goebel G. Factors influencing tinnitus loudness and annoyance. Arch Otolaryngol Head Neck Surg. 2006;132(12):1323–30.
4. Rabau S, Cox T, Punte AK, Waelkens B, Gilles A, Wouters K, et al. Changes over time of psychoacoustic outcome measurements are not a substitute for subjective outcome measurements in acute tinnitus. Eur Arch Oto-Rhino-L. 2015;272(3):573–81.
5. Van de Heyning P, Gilles A, Rabau S, Van Rompaey V. Subjective tinnitus assessment and treatment in clinical practice: the necessity of personalized medicine. Curr Opin Otolaryngol Head Neck Surg. 2015;23(5):369–75.
6. Hall DA, Zaragoza Domingo S, Hamdache LZ, Manchaiah V, Thammaiah S, Evans C, et al. A good practice guide for translating and adapting hearing-related questionnaires for different languages and cultures. Int J Audiol. 2018;57(3):161–75.
7. Hyde ML. Reasonable psychometric standards for self-report outcome measures in audiological rehabilitation. Ear Hear. 2000;21(4 Suppl):24S–36S.
8. Kirshner B, Guyatt G. A methodological framework for assessing health indices. J Chronic Dis. 1985;38(1):27–36.
9. Meikle MB, Stewart BJ, Griest SE, Martin WH, Henry JA, Abrams HB, et al. Assessment of tinnitus: measurement of treatment outcomes. Prog Brain Res. 2007;166:511–21.
10. Meikle MB, Henry JA, Griest SE, Stewart BJ, Abrams HB, McArdle R, et al. The tinnitus functional index: development of a new clinical measure for chronic, intrusive tinnitus. Ear Hear. 2012;32(2):153–76.
11. Fackrell K, Hall DA, Barry JG, Hoare DJ. Performance of the tinnitus functional index as a diagnostic instrument in a UK clinical population. Hear Res. 2017;358:74.
12. Searchfield GD, Jerram C. Tinnitus assessment. Tinnitus discovery: Asia pacific tinnitus symposium. N Z Med J. 2010;123(1311):84.
13. Wilson PH, Henry J, Bowen M, Haralambous G. Tinnitus reaction questionnaire: psychometric properties of a measure of distress associated with tinnitus. J Speech Hear Res. 1991;34(1):197–201.
14. Zeman F, Koller M, Schecklmann M, Langguth B, Landgrebe M. Tinnitus assessment by means of standardized self-report questionnaires: psychometric properties of the tinnitus questionnaire (TQ), the tinnitus handicap inventory (THI), and their short versions in an international and multi-lingual sample. Health Qual Life Outcomes. 2012;10:128.

15. Boecking B, Brueggemann P, Kleinjung T, Mazurek B. All for one and one for all? - examining convergent validity and responsiveness of the German versions of the tinnitus questionnaire (TQ), tinnitus handicap inventory (THI), and tinnitus functional index (TFI). Front Psychol. 2021;12:596037.
16. Jacquemin L, Mertens G, Van de Heyning P, Vanderveken O, Topsakal V, De Hertogh W, et al. Sensitivity to change and convergent validity of the tinnitus functional index (TFI) and the tinnitus questionnaire (TQ): clinical and research perspectives. Hear Res. 2019;107796:107796.
17. Langguth B, Kleinjung T, Fischer B, Hajak G, Eichhammer P, Sand PG. Tinnitus severity, depression, and the big five personality traits. Prog Brain Res. 2007;166:221–5.
18. Milerova J, Anders M, Dvorak T, Sand PG, Koniger S, Langguth B. The influence of psychological factors on tinnitus severity. Gen Hosp Psychiatry. 2013;35(4):412–6.
19. Simoes JP, Neff PKA, Langguth B, Schlee W, Schecklmann M. The progression of chronic tinnitus over the years. Sci Rep. 2021;11(1):4162.
20. Dobie RA. A review of randomized clinical trials in tinnitus. Laryngoscope. 1999;109:1202–11.
21. Langguth B, Goodey R, Azevedo A, Bjorne A, Cacace A, Crocetti A, et al. Consensus for tinnitus patient assessment and treatment outcome measurement: tinnitus research initiative meeting, Regensburg, July 2006. Prog Brain Res. 2007;166:525–36.
22. Hall DA, Haider H, Szczepek AJ, Lau P, Rabau S, Jones-Diette J, et al. Systematic review of outcome domains and instruments used in clinical trials of tinnitus treatments in adults. Trials. 2016;17(1):270.
23. Newman CW, Jacobson GP, Spitzer JB. Development of the tinnitus handicap inventory. Arch Otolaryngol Head Neck Surg. 1996;122(2):143–8.
24. Baguley DM, Andersson G. Factor analysis of the tinnitus handicap inventory. Am J Audiol. 2003;12(1):31–4.
25. Halford JB, Anderson SD. Tinnitus severity measured by a subjective scale, audiometry and clinical judgement. J Laryngol Otol. 1991;105(2):89–93.
26. Zeman F, Koller M, Figueiredo R, Aazevedo A, Rates M, Coelho C, et al. Tinnitus handicap inventory for evaluating treatment effects: which changes are clinically relevant? Otolaryngol Head Neck Surg. 2011;145:282.
27. Hallam RS, Jakes SC, Hinchcliffe R. Cognitive variables in tinnitus annoyance. Br J Clin Psychol. 1988;27(Pt 3):213–22.
28. Hallam RS. Manual of the tinnitus questionnaire. London: The Psychological Corporation/Harcourt Brace; 1996.
29. Henry JL, Wilson PH. The psychometric properties of two measures of tinnitus complaint and handicap. Int Tinnitus J. 1998;4(2):114–21.
30. Kuk FK, Tyler RS, Russell D, Jordan H. The psychometric properties of a tinnitus handicap questionnaire. Ear Hear. 1990;11(6):434–45.
31. Baguley DM, Humphriss RL, Hodgson CA. Convergent validity of the tinnitus handicap inventory and the tinnitus questionnaire. J Laryngol Otol. 2000;114(11):840–3.
32. Adamchic I, Tass PA, Langguth B, Hauptmann C, Koller M, Schecklmann M, et al. Linking the tinnitus questionnaire and the subjective clinical global impression: which differences are clinically important? Health Qual Life Outcomes. 2012;10(1):79.
33. Hall DA, Mehta RL, Argstatter H. Interpreting the tinnitus questionnaire (German version): what individual differences are clinically important? Int J Audiol. 2018;57(7):553–7.
34. Goebel G, Hiller W. The tinnitus questionnaire. A standard instrument for grading the degree of tinnitus. Results of a multicenter study with the tinnitus questionnaire. HNO. 1994;42:166–72.
35. Hiller W, Goebel G. A psychometric study of complaints in chronic tinnitus. J Psychosom Res. 1992;36(4):337–48.
36. Meeus O, Blaivie C, Van de HP. Validation of the Dutch and the French version of the tinnitus questionnaire. B-ENT. 2007;3(Suppl 7):11–7.
37. Kam AC, Cheung AP, Chan PY, Leung EK, Wong TK, Tong MC, et al. Psychometric properties of a Chinese (Cantonese) version of the tinnitus questionnaire. Int J Audiol. 2009;48(8):568–75.
38. Hiller W, Goebel G. Rapid assessment of tinnitus-related psychological distress using the mini-TQ. Int J Audiol. 2004;43(10):600–4.
39. Meric C, Pham E, Chery-Croze S. Validation of French translation of the "tinnitus reaction questionnaire", Wilson et al. 1991. Encéphale. 1997;23(6):442–6.
40. Meric C, Pham E, Chery-Croze S. Validation assessment of a French version of the tinnitus reaction questionnaire: a comparison between data from English and French versions. J Speech Lang Hear Res. 2000;43(1):184–90.
41. Searchfield GD, Jerram C, Wise K, Raymond S. The impact of hearing loss on tinnitus severity. Aust N Z J Audiol. 2007;29:67–76.
42. Searchfield GD. Hearing aids and tinnitus. In: Tyler R, editor. Tinnitus treatment. New York: Thieme; 2007. p. 161–75.
43. Tyler RS, Oleson J, Noble W, Coelho C, Ji H. Clinical trials for tinnitus: study populations, designs, measurement variables, and data analysis. Prog Brain Res. 2007;166:499–509.
44. Wasano K, Kanzaki S, Sakashita T, Takahashi M, Inoue Y, Saito H, et al. A psychometric validation of the Japanese versions of new questionnaires on tinnitus (THI-12, TRS, TRSw, TSS, and TSSw). Acta Otolaryngol. 2013;133(5):491–8.
45. Erlandsson SI, Hallberg LR, Axelsson A. Psychological and audiological correlates of perceived tinnitus severity. Audiology. 1992;31(3):168–79.
46. Meikle MB, Griest S, Stewart BJ, Press LS. Measuring the negative impact of tinnitus: a brief severity index. Abstr Midwinter Res Meet Assoc Res Otolaryngol. 1995;18:167.
47. Folmer RL, Carroll JR. Long-term effectiveness of ear-level devices for tinnitus. Otolaryngol Head Neck Surg. 2006;134(1):132–7.
48. Henry JA, Schechter MA, Zaugg TL, Griest S, Jastreboff PJ, Vernon JA, et al. Outcomes of clinical trial: tinnitus masking versus tinnitus retraining therapy. J Am Acad Audiol. 2006;17(2):104–32.
49. Folmer RL, Shi YB. SSRI use by tinnitus patients: interactions between depression and tinnitus severity. Ear Nose Throat J. 2004;83(2):107–8, 10, 12.
50. Greimel KV, Leibetseder M, Unterrainer J, Albegger K. Can tinnitus be measured? Methods for assessment of tinnitus-specific disability and presentation of the tinnitus disability questionnaire. HNO. 1999;47(3):196–201.
51. Wilson PH, Henry JL. Tinnitus cognitions questionnaire: development and psychometric properties of a measure of dysfunctional cognitions associated with tinnitus. Int Tinnitus J. 1998;4(1):23–30.
52. Budd RJ, Pugh R. Tinnitus coping style and its relationship to tinnitus severity and emotional distress. J Psychosom Res. 1996;41(4):327–35.
53. Cima RF, Crombez G, Vlaeyen JW. Catastrophizing and fear of tinnitus predict quality of life in patients with chronic tinnitus. Ear Hear. 2011;32(5):634–41.
54. Fuller TE, Cima RFF, Van den Bussche E, Vlaeyen JWS. The fear of tinnitus questionnaire: toward a reliable and valid means of assessing fear in adults with tinnitus. Ear Hear. 2019;40(6):1467–77.
55. Muller K, Edvall NK, Idrizbegovic E, Huhn R, Cima R, Persson V, et al. Validation of online versions of tinnitus questionnaires translated into Swedish. Front Aging Neurosci. 2016;8:272.
56. Demeester K, van Wieringen A, Hendrickx JJ, Topsakal V, Fransen E, Van LL, et al. Prevalence of tinnitus and audiometric shape. B-ENT. 2007;3(Suppl 7):37–49.
57. Adamchic I, Langguth B, Hauptmann C, Tass PA. Psychometric evaluation of visual analog scale for the assessment of chronic tinnitus. Am J Audiol. 2012;21:215.

Clinical Otorhinolaryngological Assessment

28

Tobias Kleinjung and Alain Londero

Abstract

This chapter describes the tasks of the otolaryngologist when examining a patient with tinnitus. This is of great importance because the otolaryngologist is often the first point of contact for the patient. The detailed history and also the physical examination can provide the first clues to possible causes of tinnitus. Subsequently, the combination with the audiological examination can provide the basis for successful counseling. The otolaryngological examination is of particular importance in cases of objective tinnitus. Here, objectifiable findings can be obtained in otomicroscopy, such as pulsating movements of the tympanic membrane or middle-ear masses shining through the membrane. Last but not least, conditions such as chronic otitis media or otosclerosis, which in many cases are accompanied by tinnitus, can also be detected.

T. Kleinjung (✉)
Department of Otorhinolaryngology – Head and Neck Surgery, University Hospital Zurich, University of Zurich, Zurich, Switzerland
e-mail: tobias.kleinjung@usz.ch

A. Londero
Service ORL et CCF, Hôpital Européen Georges Pompidou, Assistance Publique—Hôpitaux de Paris, Faculté de Médecine Paris Descartes—Université de Paris, Paris, France

W. Schlee et al. (eds.), *Textbook of Tinnitus*, https://doi.org/10.1007/978-3-031-35647-6_28

Graphical Abstract

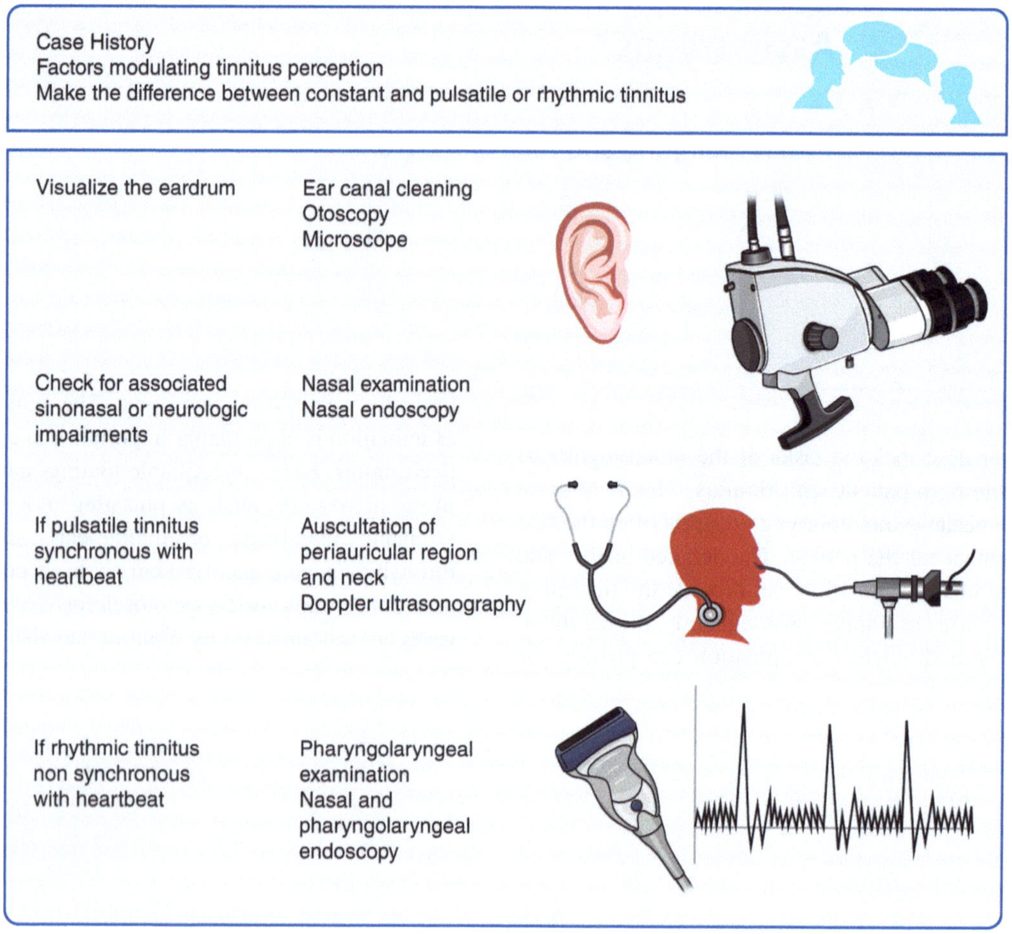

Highlights

- In most cases, tinnitus is the symptom of an underlying ENT (ear, nose, and throat) condition.
- ENT (syn. otorhinolaryngological) assessment is key to the identification of an ENT condition that might be accessible to medical or surgical curative interventions.
- This chapter describes the diagnostic procedures, which can be performed by the ENT specialist in an office setting.
- Special attention should be paid to all kinds of objective tinnitus, which can be caused by a vascular or muscular pathology.
- The combination of ENT clinical, audiological, and radiological findings will help to make the correct diagnosis and to provide a causally orientated treatment.

Introduction

Tinnitus is a symptom, and many disorders of the peripheral auditory system (external, middle, and inner ear, and auditory nerve) can cause both objective and subjective tinnitus [1–3] . The ear, nose, and throat (ENT) specialist is often the first port of call for patients with new-onset tinnitus, depending on the respective health system [4, 5]. This is why clinical guidelines highlight the importance of ENT clinical assessment as a prerequisite in tinnitus patients' management [6–8], the aim of which is to identify the ENT conditions that may have caused tinnitus. As a first step when taking the history of a patient with tinnitus, it is essential to enquire about previous or coexisting ENT conditions or treatments (i.e., congenital anomaly, trauma, infection, or surgery involving the ear). It is also important to check for the presence of audio-vestibular symptoms (i.e., hearing loss, vertigo and dizziness, sound sensitivity, sound distortion, aural fullness, earache, otorrhea) and other ENT related symptoms (i.e., sinus or nasal problems, headache, neck or facial pain, and facial nerve palsy). In addition, one should ask about factors that may modulate tinnitus perception, such as movements (jaws, head/neck, eyes, and limbs), sleep (night and nap), sound exposure, and stress. A form with structured questions to cover these topics would aid the collection of a comprehensive history for each patient [9, 10] (for more information about history taking, see also Chap. 26). The more commonly used methods in ENT clinical examination of a patient with tinnitus include ear canal and tympanic membrane inspection (otoscopy, otomicroscopy, and otoendoscopy), endoscopy of the nasopharynx, and auscultation of the peri-aural regions. Less frequently, other diagnostic methods such as a Doppler ultrasound examination of the neck vessels may be proposed in specialized ENT settings.

Otoscopy

A simple inspection of the external ear can reveal aural birth defects or surgical scars, which may be an indication of previous middle-ear surgery. The ear canal and eardrum can easily be visualized with an otoscope or a video-otoscope [11], while the examination of the external auditory canal and tympanic membrane is ideally performed using a microscope with up to 25× magnification. Normally, the external auditory canal is wide and the tympanic membrane is transparent. Cleaning the ear canal from cerumen debris and secretions (clotted blood, purulent discharge) often requires the use of micro-instruments (forceps, hooks, etc.) and when unavoidable suctioning. This noisy procedure [12] may be badly tolerated by tinnitus and hyperacusis patients and should therefore be thoroughly explained beforehand and immediately stopped in the case of intolerance [13]. Attention should be paid to bony exostoses[1] and tumors on the skin lining the ear canal [14]. The long process of the incus is often visible through the tympanic membrane in many cases, as well as the manubrium of the malleus with the umbo. Reddening of the tympanic membrane or increased vascular markings are indicative of acute otitis media. Otoscopy can detect fluid build-up in the tympanic cavity. Negative air pressure in the tympanic cavity causes retraction of the tympanic membrane and suggests Eustachian tube dysfunction. Perforations of the tympanic membrane indicate chronic otitis media. The presence of cholesteatoma[2] may cause the epitympanic perforation to be filled with keratin debris or granulation tissue. Foul-smelling otorrhea resulting from Pseudomonas aeruginosa infection is also characteristic of the presence of a cholesteatoma. In many cases, large tympanic membrane perforations permit inspection of the auditory ossicular chain and assessment of the tympanic mucosa. Otoscopy findings are usually normal in otosclerosis [15]. Schwartze's sign [3]is a rare finding, consisting of a pink blush of the mucosa near the promontory that can be seen through a translucent tympanic membrane. It is a sign of proliferation and dilation of blood vessels at the promontory and should be regarded as indicative of cochlear otosclerosis [16]. Rhythmic displacements of the tympanic membrane are present in a variety of pathologies also causing tinnitus [17]. When synchronous with the patient's respiration on forced nasal breathing, it is indicative of a patulous Eustachian tube [18]. Pulse synchronous movement of the tympanic membrane may indicate the presence of a glomus tumor [19]. This bluish-red tumor growing in a grape-like cluster may cause the tympanic membrane to bulge outward. In advanced cases, the tumor may also impinge into the external auditory canal. Rhythmic movements of the tympanic membrane are also noted in patients with palatal or middle ear myoclonus[4] [3]. Valsalva's maneuver and Toynbee's maneuver are clinical tests of Eustachian tube function. In Valsalva's maneuver, patients pinch their nose tightly between thumb and forefinger and then attempt to breathe out forcibly while keeping their mouth closed. An outward bulging tympanic membrane during a Valsalva's maneuver is an indication that the Eustachian tube functions normally and that air can reach the middle ear via the Eustachian tube. In Toynbee's maneuver, the patient is instructed to swallow, again with their nose pinched closed. This normally results in negative air pressure in the tympanic cavity that can be detected by otoscopy as an inward retraction of the tympanic mem-

[1]Exostosis: A cartilage-capped bony projection arising from any bone that develops from cartilage. From: Stedman's Electronic Medical Dictionary.

[2]Cholesteatoma: Squamous metaplasia or extension of squamous cell epithelium inward to line an expanding cystic cavity that may involve the middle ear or mastoid, erode surrounding bone, and become filled with a mass of keratinized squamous cell epithelial debris, usually resulting from chronic otitis media. The lesion often contains cholesterol clefts surrounded by inflammatory and foreign body giant cells, hence the name cholesteatoma. From: Stedman's Electronic Medical Dictionary.

[3]Schwartze's sign: A pink blush behind the tympanic membrane, sometimes seen in otosclerosis because of hyperemia of the mucous membrane around the promontory. First described by Schwartze in 1873. From: Dorland's Medical Dictionary.

[4]Myoclonus: One or a series of shock-like contractions of a group of muscles of variable regularity, synchrony, and symmetry, generally due to a central nervous system lesion. From:?

brane. An objective measure of Eustachian tube function can be obtained by tympanometry [20, 21] (see Chap. 29).

Endoscopy

Further examination of possible causes of dysfunction of the Eustachian tube can be done by examination of the nasal and pharyngeal structures using rigid or flexible endoscopes. Polypoid mucosal changes in the nasal cavity are indicative of chronic rhinosinusitis that may affect the function of the Eustachian tube. Attention should also be paid to the possible presence of space-occupying lesions in the nasopharynx that may obstruct the tubal orifice (hypertrophied lymphatic tissue and nasopharyngeal carcinomas). Many patients with a patulous Eustachian tube have a widening of the opening of the Eustachian tube in the nasopharynx [22, 23]. Biopsy of suspected space-occupying lesions should be done for histopathological examination. Objective tinnitus may be caused by myoclonus of the palatine muscles (the tensor and levator veli palatini). Twitching of these muscles can be observed by endoscopy [24].

Auscultation

Auscultation of the ear and neck vessels can be important in the diagnosis of objective tinnitus. A stethoscope can be used to detect signs of carotid artery stenosis, such as what may occur from atherosclerosis, vascular compression, and arteriovenous malformations. Dural arteriovenous fistulas murmur can be detected by auscultation of the upper neck and in the post-auricular region, and pressing down on the mastoid bone may interrupt the pulsatile tinnitus. The use of an electronic stethoscope is more sensitive than classic auscultation techniques. If a patient's tinnitus is affected by compression of the neck or from turning the head, it is a sign that tinnitus can be of venous origin. Such maneuvers would have no effect on pulsatile tinnitus of arterial origin [25]. Abnormal auscultatory findings require further clarification using Doppler ultrasound, MRI time-of-flight (ToF) angiography, or conventional angiography [26] (see also Chap. 30). Direct auscultation of the middle ear performed with a Toynbee tube inserted into the external auditory canal makes it possible to hear tinnitus that is caused by contractions of the stapedius or tensor tympani muscles of the middle ear [27].

Supplementary Radiological Diagnosis

Radiological examinations may be justified when otologic examinations are inconclusive regarding pathologies that may be involved in causing tinnitus [28, 29]. High-resolution computed tomography (CT) without contrast of the petrous portion of the temporal bones can be used to detect and examine structural bony changes of the external ear and its surroundings, the middle ear, and inner ear. MRI with or without Gadolinium contrast can be used to visualize a fluid-filled cochlea and the auditory vestibular nerves but also to discover vascular anomalies (ToF angiography). Detailed information regarding these techniques is provided in Chap. 30. In some countries (e.g., Germany), ultrasound techniques are part of an otologic examination. Doppler ultrasound allows visualization of carotid stenoses, arterial dissections, and arteriovenous malformations. Digital subtraction angiography is employed for the preoperative assessment of a glomus tumor, permitting identification of the main supplying vessel on the basis of the tumor blush. Interventional embolization of the supplying vessels during the same session prepares for efficient control of bleeding during subsequent surgical resection. Embolization or stenting is also used in terms of tinnitus therapy for dural AV fistulas or cerebral venous sinus abnormalities [30, 31] (see Chap. 30).

References

1. Nicolas-Puel C, Faulconbridge RL, Guitton M, Puel J-L, Mondain M, Uziel A. Characteristics of tinnitus and etiology of associated hearing loss: a study of 123 patients. Int Tinnitus J. 2002;8(1):37–44.
2. Mattox DE, Hudgins P. Algorithm for evaluation of pulsatile tinnitus. Acta Otolaryngol. 2008;128(4):427–31.
3. Park S-N, Bae S-C, Lee G-H, Song J, Park K-H, Jeon E, et al. Clinical characteristics and therapeutic response of objective tinnitus due to middle ear myoclonus: a large case series. Laryngoscope. 2013;123(10):2516–20.
4. Cima RFF, Kikidis D, Mazurek B, Haider H, Cederroth CR, Norena A, et al. Tinnitus healthcare: a survey revealing extensive variation in opinion and practices across Europe. BMJ Open. 2020;10(1):e029346.
5. Hall DA, Láinez MJ, Newman CW, Sanchez TG, Egler M, Tennigkeit F, et al. Treatment options for subjective tinnitus: self reports from a sample of general practitioners and ENT physicians within Europe and the USA. BMC Health Serv Res. 2011;11:302.
6. Lewis S, Chowdhury E, Stockdale D, Kennedy V. Assessment and management of tinnitus: summary of NICE guidance. BMJ. 2020;368:m976.
7. Cima RFF, Mazurek B, Haider H, Kikidis D, Lapira A, Noreña A, et al. A multidisciplinary European guideline for tinnitus: diagnostics, assessment, and treatment. HNO. 2019;67(1):10–42.
8. Tunkel DE, Bauer CA, Sun GH, Rosenfeld RM, Chandrasekhar SS, Cunningham ER, et al. Clinical practice guideline: tinnitus. Otolaryngol Head Neck Surg. 2014;151(2 Suppl):S1–40.
9. Genitsaridi E, Partyka M, Gallus S, Lopez-Escamez JA, Schecklmann M, Mielczarek M, et al. Standardised profiling for tinnitus research: the European School for Interdisciplinary Tinnitus Research Screening Questionnaire (ESIT-SQ). Hear Res. 2019;377:353–9.
10. Langguth B, Goodey R, Azevedo A, Bjorne A, Cacace A, Crocetti A, et al. Consensus for tinnitus patient assessment and treatment outcome measurement: tinnitus research initiative meeting, Regensburg, July 2006. Prog Brain Res. 2007;166:525–36.

11. Damery L, Lescanne E, Reffet K, Aussedat C, Bakhos D. Interest of video-otoscopy for the general practitioner. Eur Ann Otorhinolaryngol Head Neck Dis. 2019;136(1):13–7.
12. Young A, Reeve NH, Yang A, Kahane J, Cross C, Albanese A, et al. Sound levels with aural suctioning: effects of suction size, canal moisture, and distance from the eardrum. Laryngoscope Investig Otolaryngol. 2020;5(4):766–72.
13. Folmer RL, Shi BY. Chronic tinnitus resulting from cerumen removal procedures. Int Tinnitus J. 2004;10(1):42–6.
14. Ostrowski VB, Wiet RJ. Pathologic conditions of the external ear and auditory canal. Postgrad Med. 1996;100(3):223–8, 233–7.
15. Foster MF, Backous DD. Clinical evaluation of the patient with Otosclerosis. Otolaryngol Clin N Am. 2018;51(2):319–26.
16. Nakashima T, Sone M, Fujii H, Teranishi M, Yamamoto H, Otake H, et al. Blood flow to the promontory in cochlear otosclerosis. Clin Otolaryngol. 2006;31(2):110–5.
17. Nourollahian M, Irani S. Bilateral schwartze sign, decision-making for surgery. Iran J Otorhinolaryngol. 2013;25(73):263.
18. Luu K, Remillard A, Fandino M, Saxby A, Westerberg BD. Treatment effectiveness for symptoms of patulous Eustachian tube: a systematic review. Otol Neurotol. 2015;36(10):1593–600.
19. Sweeney AD, Carlson ML, Wanna GB, Bennett ML. Glomus tympanicum tumors. Otolaryngol Clin N Am. 2015;48(2):293–304.
20. Sayyid ZN, Thai A, Swanson A, Hosseini DK, Fitzgerald MB, Ma Y, et al. Rhythmic wave patterns on ambient pressure tympanometry in patients with objective tinnitus-associated pathologies. Otol Neurotol. 2020;41(3):e404–11.
21. Parsel SM, Unis GD, Souza SS, Bartley H, Bergeron JM, Master AN, et al. Interpretation of normal and abnormal tympanogram findings in Eustachian tube dysfunction. Otolaryngol Head Neck Surg. 2020;20:019459982096523.
22. Ward BK, Ashry Y, Poe DS. Patulous Eustachian tube dysfunction: patient demographics and comorbidities. Otol Neurotol. 2017;38(9):1362–9.
23. Grimmer JF, Poe DS. Update on Eustachian tube dysfunction and the patulous Eustachian tube. Curr Opin Otolaryngol Head Neck Surg. 2005;13(5):277–82.
24. Sinclair CF, Gurey LE, Blitzer A. Palatal myoclonus: algorithm for management with botulinum toxin based on clinical disease characteristics. Laryngoscope. 2014;124(5):1164–9.
25. Sismanis A. Pulsatile tinnitus: contemporary assessment and management. Curr Opin Otolaryngol Head Neck Surg. 2011;19(5):348–57.
26. Hofmann E, Behr R, Neumann-Haefelin T, Schwager K. Pulsatile tinnitus: imaging and differential diagnosis. Dtsch Arztebl Int. 2013;110(26):451–8.
27. Badia L, Parikh A, Brookes GB. Management of middle ear myoclonus. J Laryngol Otol. 1994;108(5):380–2.
28. Cunnane MB. Imaging of tinnitus. Neuroimaging Clin N Am. 2019;29(1):49–56.
29. Bathla G, Hegde A, Nagpal P, Agarwal A. Imaging in pulsatile tinnitus: case based review. JCIS. 2020;10:84.
30. Renieri L, Michelozzi C, Brinjikji W, Darcout J, Guenego A, Vukasinovic I, et al. PTA stent of Dural sinuses in brain DAVF: a report of 4 cases. Clin Neuroradiol. 2019;29(2):331–9.
31. Yang I-H, Pereira VM, Lenck S, Nicholson P, Orru E, Klostranec JM, et al. Endovascular treatment of debilitating tinnitus secondary to cerebral venous sinus abnormalities: a literature review and technical illustration. J Neurointerv Surg. 2019;11(8):841–6.

Audiological Assessment for Tinnitus

29

Giriraj S. Shekhawat, Karen Sparrow, and Lisa Callahan

Abstract

Comprehensive clinical assessment of tinnitus is foundation for getting a wholistic understanding about patients' tinnitus and planning a good management. Considering hearing loss is most commonly associated with tinnitus, hearing assessment should be integral part of tinnitus assessment battery. Along with comprehensive audiological assessment, it is also significant for the patient to undergo ENT evaluation to assess the presence and extent of medical involvement, and if needed, additional referrals should be arranged. This chapter focuses on the audiological assessment battery recommended for patients with tinnitus, such as detailed case history, otoscopy, pure tone audiometry, high-frequency audiometry, loudness discomfort level, speech audiometry, psychoacoustic measurement of tinnitus (pitch, loudness, minimum masking, residual inhibition) tympanometry and acoustic reflex testing, otoacoustic emissions, auditory brainstem response audiometry, and research assessments. Towards the end of this chapter, we have outlined a case study to supplement the clinical understanding.

G. S. Shekhawat (✉)
College of Education, Psychology, and Social Work, Flinders University, Adelaide, Australia

Ear Institute, University College London, London, UK

Tinnitus Research Initiative, Regensburg, Germany
e-mail: giriraj.shekhawat@flinders.edu.au

K. Sparrow · L. Callahan
College of Education, Psychology, and Social Work, Flinders University, Adelaide, Australia
e-mail: karen.sparrow@flinders.edu.au; lisa.callahan@flinders.edu.au

W. Schlee et al. (eds.), *Textbook of Tinnitus*, https://doi.org/10.1007/978-3-031-35647-6_29

Graphical Abstract

Audiological Assessment

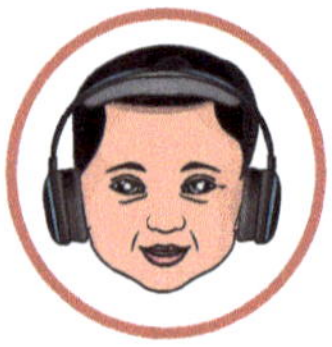

Examination	Abbreviation	Purpose
Pure Tone Audiometry	PTA	Hearing Function in the Standard Frequencies
High FrequencyAudiometry	HFA	Hearing Function in the High Frequency Range
Speech Audiometry		Speech Understanding
Tympanometry		Objective Test of Hearing Function
Acoustic Reflex Testing	AFT	Objective Test of Hearing Function
Otoacoustic Emissions	OAE	Objective Test of Hearing Function
Acoustic Brain Stem response	ABR	Objective Test of Hearing Function
Loudness Discomfort Level	LDL	Hyperacusis
Minimal Masking Level	MML	Tinnitus Loudness
Tinnitus Loudness Match	TLM	Tinnitus Loudness
Tinnitus Pitch Match	TPM	Tinnitus Pitch
Residual Inhibition	RI	Tinnitus Inhibition

Highlights

- Tinnitus is frequently associated with hearing loss.
- High-frequency audiometry (up to 16 KHz) is recommended to investigate the hearing status beyond conventional pure tone audiometry (up to 8 KHz).
- Warble tones/pulsed tones should be used instead of pure tones for assessing the hearing status of patients with tinnitus.
- Loudness Discomfort Level testing and Acoustic Reflex Threshold testing is not recommended in patients experience hyperacusis along with tinnitus.
- Tinnitus pitch is often matched to frequencies where hearing is impaired. Psychoacoustic measurements of tinnitus (pitch, loudness, and minimum masking levels) are advised for research and rehabilitation purposes.
- Tympanometry is not recommended in the presence of impacted wax or ruptured ear drum.
- Normal functioning outer ear and middle ear is prerequisite for conducting otoacoustic emissions, e.g., OAEs are not recommended in presence of outer/middle ear pathologies.
- The use of auditory brainstem response audiometry in the tinnitus diagnosis/outcome measure is debatable.

Abbreviations

2AFC	Two alternative forced choice
ABR	Auditory brainstem response
BOLD	Blood oxygen level dependent
CGI	Clinical global impression
dB	Decibel
DPOAE	Distortion product otoacoustic emission
EEG	Electroencephalography
fMRI	Functional magnetic resonance imaging
HFA	High-frequency audiometry
KHz	KiloHertz
LDL	Loudness discomfort level
MML	Minimum masking level
OAE	Otoacoustic emission
PI	Performance intensity.
PTA	Puretone audiometry
RI	Residual inhibition
SRT	Speech recognition threshold
TDCS	Transcranial direct current stimulation
TEOAE	Transient-evoked otoacoustic emission
TFI	Tinnitus Functional Index
THI	Tinnitus Handicap Inventory
TMJ	Temporomandibular joint
TQ	Tinnitus Questionnaire
TRQ	Tinnitus Reaction Questionnaire
TSCHQ	Tinnitus Sample Case History Questionnaire

TSI	Tinnitus Severity Index
TSNS	Tinnitus Severity Numeric Scale
VAS	Visual Analogue Scale

Introduction

Comprehensive clinical assessment of tinnitus is the foundation for a good management. Considering tinnitus is a multifaceted condition its assessment and management require a multidisciplinary team. There are several conditions which can trigger tinnitus such as obstruction in ear, hearing loss, head and neck trauma, temporomandibular joint disorders, traumatic brain injury, sinus and barometric trauma, and ototoxic drugs [1] and its assessment would require a careful medical and audiological assessment. Even if many etiologic factors can contribute to tinnitus, hearing loss is the most important risk factor. Therefore, in every patient with tinnitus, the hearing function should be tested. In this chapter, we will focus on the audiological assessment for tinnitus and the key factors one should be cognizant of when a patient presents with the primary complaint of tinnitus. Along with audiological assessment, it is also significant for the patient to undergo ENT evaluation (see also Chap. 28)—to assess the presence and extent of medical involvement and if needed additional referrals should be arranged.

Audiological Assessment

Case history: A thorough case history is essential to understand the clinically presented symptoms in detail to establish correct diagnosis and therapy [2]. It is fundamental for the clinician to establish strong rapport with patient and understand their primary concerns due to tinnitus. Key skills to develop strong professional relationship with patient and taking a good case history involves: listening, positive body language, eye contact, asking appropriate open-ended questions, and empathy [3]. The Tinnitus Sample Case History Questionnaire (TSCHQ) is a useful tool to get in-depth information. It is a standard questionnaire developed during the first Tinnitus Research Initiative meeting in 2006 [4]. It consists of 35 items (14 essential and 21 highly desirable) and assists in collecting in-depth information about participant's tinnitus (for more details, see also Chap. 26). For assessing tinnitus severity and tinnitus impact, there are several standardized tinnitus questionnaires available to offer valuable information about tinnitus and its impact such as Tinnitus Functional Index—TFI [5], Tinnitus Handicap Questionnaire—THQ [6], Tinnitus Handicap Inventory—THI [7], Tinnitus Severity Index—TSI [8], Tinnitus Reaction Questionnaire—TRQ [9], and Tinnitus Questionnaire—TQ [10] to name a few. Primary purpose of these questionnaires is to assess the impact of tinnitus and guiding the clinical decision-making towards management. There are several rating scales available to capture the overall tinnitus severity, its loudness, and annoyance such as Clinical Global Impression (CGI) [11], tinnitus severity numeric scale (TSNS) [12], and visual analogue scale [13] (see Chap. 27 for more information about tinnitus questionnaires and scales).

Otoscopy: Otoscopy is a clinical procedure used to assess the status of tympanic membrane (ear drum) and ear canal. In this procedure, an otoscope (a small device with focused light and magnifying glass) is inserted in the ear canal to check the status of outer ear (pinna), its adjoining areas, external auditory meatus, and tympanic membrane. Human ear canals produce wax called cerumen which protects from dust and foreign particles and has antibacterial properties. Due to the shape of ear canal, this wax is automatically excreted out of the canal; however, sometimes due to excessive wax production or accidentally pushing it while cleaning may result into blockage of ear canal and with time it can get impacted. Sometimes this impacted wax in the ear canal can be the cause of hearing impairment and tinnitus. Impacted wax can also interfere in audiological testing and require removal. Otoscopy is recommended before administrating any other audiological assessment (see also Chap. 28).

Puretone Audiometry (PTA) and High-Frequency Audiometry (HFA): Tinnitus is frequently associated with hearing loss [14]. This is commonly the result of some form of cochlear damage which is reflected in a hearing assessment [15, 16]. Pure tone threshold testing should be performed as an initial test for a patient presenting with tinnitus who may or may not be aware of some degree of hearing loss. During standard audiometry, frequencies from 250 Hz to 8 kHz are assessed [17]. In tinnitus patients with clinically normal hearing thresholds at the conventional audiometric frequencies, cochlear damage can be found through high-frequency audiometry, otoacoustic emissions, or other psychometric tests [18–21]. Hence, it is recommended to perform HFA.

High-frequency audiometry is performed in the range 10–16 kHz and can provide valuable information in the assessment of tinnitus [17, 22]. Roberts, Moffat, and Bosnyak (2006) reported that 25% of participants with tinnitus had hearing loss in the extended range despite normal hearing thresholds across the standard range to 8 kHz [23]. A study by Hyun et al. (2009) found that 66.7% of participants had normal hearing to 8 kHz but reduced hearing at one or more extended high frequencies (10, 12, 14, or 16 kHz) [24]. Furthermore, the pitch of the tinnitus has been frequently found to be within the range of the hearing loss [25]. Shekhawat et al. [26] looked at the audiological profile of 192 participants with tinnitus and revealed that the average hearing levels were normal in the low frequencies sloping to mild loss at 8 kHz, but moderate-to-severe hearing loss

SUBJECTIVE

Assessment	Considerations for clients with tinnitus
Case History	Include Tinnitus Case History Questionnaire (TSHQ)
Pure Tone Audiometry	Include high-frequency audiometry
Loudness Discomfort Level	Not recommended if client experiences hyperacusis
Speech Audiometry	Ensure appropriate language level
Psychoacoustic measures	Tinnitus pitch & loudness matching, minimum masking level and residual inhibition
Tinnitus Apps	Ensure the app is clinically validated before recommending

OBJECTIVE

Assessment	Considerations for clients with tinnitus
Otoscopy	As per guidelines
Tympanometry	Contraindications: perforation & impacted wax
Acoustic Reflex Testing	Not recommended if client experiences hyperacusis
Otoacoustic Emissions	Contraindication: middle ear pathology & impacted wax
Auditory Brainstem Response	As per guidelines
Neuroimaging (EEG & fMRI)	Used in research settings

Fig. 29.1 Audiological tests for tinnitus assessment

above 8 kHz (up to 16 kHz) [26] reflecting the significance of high-frequency testing in the tinnitus assessment battery [23, 24].

The following section provides key clinical strategies for PTA testing of the tinnitus client.

PTA instructions for the tinnitus patient should remain simple asking them to respond when they hear a tone / beep even if it is very soft. However, the clinician should avoid asking the patient to respond "even if they think they hear the tone stimulus" or "even if they are uncertain" as this may lead to over responding. It may be helpful/ reassuring for the patient to ask that they indicate if the tinnitus is making it difficult to hear a particular tone, so that adjustments can be implemented to make the testing easier for them.

PTA testing should be conducted using the modified Hughson Westlake threshold seeking procedure beginning at 1 kHz followed by 2–8 kHz (and above if testing extended high frequencies) and completing the audiogram with 500 Hz and 250 Hz. Interoctave frequencies should also be tested if the slope between adjacent frequencies is 20 dB or greater. Tinnitus patients are prone to greater variability in their test responses due to potential difficulties differentiating tinnitus and the test tones. Tinnitus is frequently of a high pitch and responses may become more variable as the frequency of the test tone increases. The clinician should be alert to time locking of the stimulus and response to be able to detect false-positive responses.

Before threshold seeking begins at each frequency, the clinician should ensure that they find an intensity level at which the patient gives a clear and confident response time locked to the signal. Speed of testing should be moderate. If too fast, false positives will be more difficult to distinguish from true responses and may lead to an unwarranted reduction in stimulus intensity. This in turn can lead to a cycle of testing under the client's threshold and inaccurate results. On the other hand, if testing is too slow, long gaps between stimuli may enhance patient uncertainty and over responding (Fig. 29.1).

If a false positive response is suspected, one practical strategy is to re-present the tone within a short time interval at the same intensity level. If the patient responds a second time, it may be considered a true response, or if not, the previous positive response should be considered as false positive. In this case, the stimulus intensity should be increased by 5 dB. If responses become variable, the frequencies at which this occurs should be noted. This will frequently occur

Fig. 29.2 Mark's hearing assessment

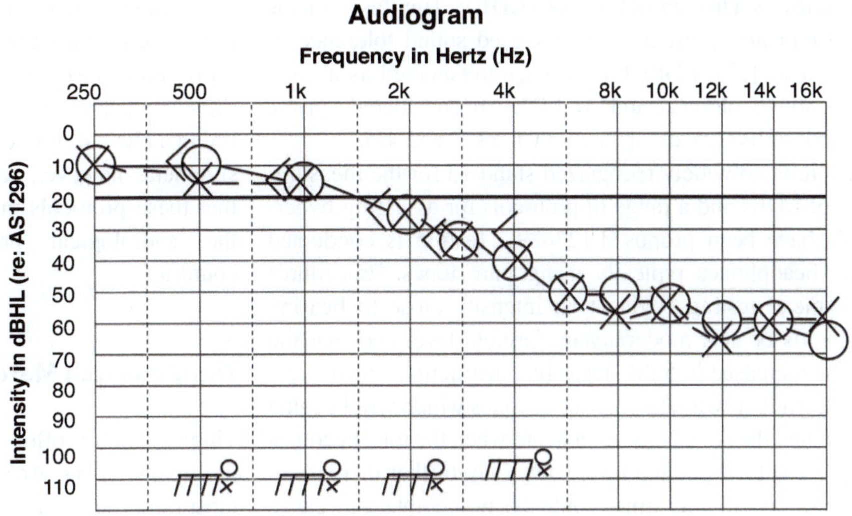

Modality	Right	Left
Air conduction - Earphones		
Unmasked	O	×
Masked	●	✖
Binaural - Sound field	□	
Bone Conduction - Mastoid		
Unmasked	<	>
Masked	[	]

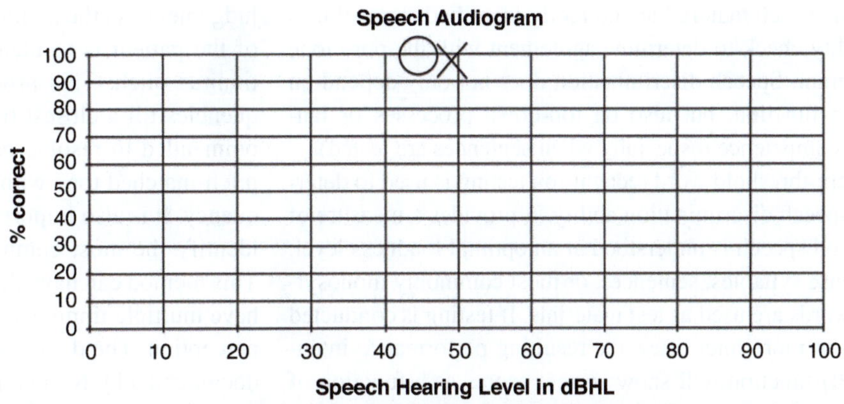

Ear	Otoscopy comment
R	Some soft wax in the ear canal, ear drum pearly and intact.
L	Some soft wax in the ear canal, ear drum pearly and intact.

close to the tinnitus pitch and this information may assist with subsequent tinnitus testing. The clinician should ask the patient whether they are having trouble distinguishing the tones due to the tinnitus. Warble tones or pulsed tones may be introduced at these frequencies. The patient should be informed of the change and reinstructed that the signal will be modified to make it easier for them to differentiate the stimulus tone and the tinnitus. In some instances, a warble tone may be more difficult to differentiate and a pulsed tone or manually pulse tone (the clinician presents two tones in close succession) may be more appropriate. An example for a pure tone audiometry report is given in Fig. 29.2.

Loudness Discomfort Level (LDL): Tinnitus patients may frequently present with decreased sound tolerance or hyperacusis [27]. LDLs have been implemented as a measure of sound tolerance and low LDLs are considered a prime indicator of hyperacusis (see also Chaps. 3 and 41).

There is no widely recognized standard for the measurement of LDLs and a range of protocols for assessing hyperacusis have been proposed [27–29]. Testing is conducted under headphones typically using pure tones. Procedures recommend testing begin at an intensity close to hearing thresholds or at a moderate/comfortable level and that the tone be increased in 5 dB steps. Test instructions make clear that the patient will hear a series of tones which will become louder, and they are asked to indicate when the tone becomes not just too loud but at a level where any further increase in loudness or stimulus time would be intolerable and cause discomfort.

While such protocols advise caution to avoid causing patient distress, others have recommended against the use of LDL measurements for tinnitus or hyperacusis patients [30]. The presentation of loud stimuli may be threatening to patients, cause an increase in anxiety about potential aggravation of the tinnitus, and potentially exacerbate the tinnitus and hyperacusis [30].

Speech Audiometry: Speech perception assessments are an important addition to the audiological test battery. Speech recognition thresholds (SRT) or the lowest level at which 50% of speech material are correctly identified are useful as a validity check to determine agreement with the pure tone audiogram. Speech discrimination does not only depend on hearing function, but also on top-down processes or language competence (especially when sentences are tested).

Supra-threshold word recognition testing is used to determine speech discrimination ability. It provides a measure of how well speech is understood at an optimal loudness level. Nonsense syllables, sentences, or most commonly monosyllabic words are used as test materials. If testing is conducted at two or more intensities, the resulting performance intensity (PI) function will show correct scores as a function of the presentation level. Individuals with a conductive or mild cochlear hearing loss will achieve close to a 100% score. However, maximum scores of less than 100% are expected for cochlear hearing losses of moderate or greater degree.

Speech discrimination scores can be used, in conjunction with the audiogram, as an effective basis for informational counselling about hearing status, how functional hearing difficulties relate to the test results and the potential fitting and benefits of amplification.

Psychoacoustic Measurement of Tinnitus: Psychoacoustic measurement of tinnitus, such as tinnitus pitch, tinnitus loudness, and minimum masking level (MML), is important part of clinical assessment test battery. These measurements can be helpful in offering management insights especially towards hearing aid programming for tinnitus and counselling. However, there is some debate about these being a reliable outcome measurement. We will be outlining a clinical protocol for pitch, loudness, and MML measurement; however, readers are encouraged to be mindful that these protocols may vary in clinical practice based on the audiological practice guidelines across various countries.

Tinnitus Pitch Matching

Tinnitus pitch is often matched to frequencies where hearing is impaired [31]. According to Shekhawat et al. [26], the most important audiometric predictor for tinnitus pitch is the frequency at which hearing threshold is approximately 50 dBHL. They hypothesize that this may reflect a transition from primarily Outer Hair Cell damage to lesions including Inner Hair Cells at these levels of hearing loss.

Two Alternative Forced Choice method (2AFC): Tinnitus pitch can be assessed using a 2 Alternative Forced Choice method (2AFC). In this method using an audiometer, several pairs of tones can be presented based on the configuration of audiogram and perceptual feedback from the patient about the pitch of tinnitus. The presentation level of these tones can be 10 to 15 dBSL to ensure ease of perceptual judgement. As the audiologist presents these tones, the role of the patient is to identify the tone which matches their tinnitus pitch. This process is repeated with various frequencies till a closest tinnitus pitch is identified. It is recommended to resolve octave confusion by comparing the pitch-matched tone with 1 octave above and below the frequency. It is also important to understand that the goal is to identify the most common pitch of the patient's tinnitus. This method can have limitations especially for people who have multiple tinnitus pitch/complex tones as their tinnitus perception. The data about test–retest reliability have been documented by Neff et al. 2019 [32].

Instructions: The instructions given to participants could be *"we want you to compare two sounds to your tinnitus. Indicate whether the first or second sound is closest to your tinnitus. Both sounds may not exactly match your tinnitus that is okay, we want to know which is most similar."* This could be repeated with the following instruction, *"we are now going to repeat this comparison, again indicate whether sound 1 or 2 is closest to your tinnitus"* [26].

Selection of test ear: It is recommended to choose ear with better hearing as the test ear if the tinnitus perception is equally loud on both sides or localized in the head. In case of unequal tinnitus loudness between the ears, the ear contralateral to the predominant or louder tinnitus should be the test ear. Exceptions to this rule are when contralateral ear has hearing loss in the severe to profound range, diplacusis, and cochlear dead regions (identified using TEN test or psychoacoustic tuning curves).

Tinnitus Loudness Matching

Method: Tinnitus loudness is measured at the frequency which is identified as tinnitus pitch. The audiometer dial is usually set at 5 dB steps during conventional hearing threshold measurement; however, for tinnitus loudness measurement, it can be changed to 1- or 2-dB steps. After that the first step is to identify the threshold of the patient at the tinnitus pitch, followed by which the tinnitus loudness is measured by presenting sound at the tinnitus pitch and gradually increasing its intensity till the patient indicates that the presented loudness is equal to that of their tinnitus. This measurement is usually repeated three times and the average of the three responses is taken as the loudness match.

Instructions

You will now hear a series of tones indicate when the sound is equally loud to your tinnitus. [26].

Selection of test ear: Test ear is selected using the same principles applied for tinnitus pitch matching. Usually, it is the contralateral ear to the tinnitus ear.

Minimum Masking Levels (MML)

Methods: MML is the minimum level of sound which can render the tinnitus inaudible. Measuring MML is similar to measuring the tinnitus loudness except in this case the patients are instructed to indicate the level at which their tinnitus is completely masked by the externally presented sounds instead of equal to it. In some cases, a "complete masking" of tinnitus is possible and in others its "partial masking" or "no masking." It is advised to mention this during the assessment. The first step for MML measurement is to identify the threshold of noise (narrow band noise) and then increase the intensity of the noise in 5 dB steps till the patient indicates the masking of tinnitus/patients' tolerance level is reached or the audiometric limit is reached. MML in sensation level is the difference between the masked level and threshold for that noise. Similar to loudness matching procedure, MML is repeated three times and the average of three trials is taken as the MML. It is recorded in sensation level (dBSL).

Instructions:

You will hear a hissing sound. Indicate each time you hear it, even if it is very quiet. The level of sound will gradually increase. Indicate when it covers your tinnitus. If the sound becomes uncomfortable indicate and it will be stopped [26].

Selection of test ear: The test ear is usually the side with the louder or predominant tinnitus; if there is no difference between the sides, each ear is tested separately.

Residual Inhibition (RI)

RI is defined as the phenomenon of tinnitus suppression following the offset of an auditory masker [33]. In a study by Vernon and Meikle (2003), out of 1451 research participants with tinnitus 88% have shown some form of RI [34]. Complete RI is described as the complete absence of tinnitus following the offset of masking and partial RI is the reduction of tinnitus loudness but not its complete absence. RI usually lasts for less than a minute and there are gaps in our understanding about the neurophysiological basis of this phenomenon. Efforts have been made to use therapeutic methods such as transcranial direct current stimulation (tDCS) to enhance RI [35]. In this pilot study, seven out of nine participants reported transient tinnitus suppression when sound stimulation was presented along with tDCS. Although more research is needed to understand RI and ways to extend the tinnitus suppression following acoustic stimulation, it is important to include RI in assessment test battery approach. RI assessment can give indications about the potential benefits a patient can get from sound therapy management options.

Tympanometry and Acoustic Reflex Testing

Both of these are standard tests used in the audiological test battery. They are objective tests confirming the findings of pure tone audiometry and giving additional information about the status of the middle ear.

Tympanometry

Tympanometry is a non-behavioural test which is used to assess the functioning of tympanic membrane and middle ear status. During this test, a small probe is placed in the ear canal which has three small openings: probe speaker (generates probe tone—220 Hz-65 dBHL), probe mic (records the sound pressure in ear canal), and air pump (change pressure from "positive" +200 mm/H_2O to "negative"–400 mm/H_2O). During the test, the amount of sound bouncing back from tympanic membrane at different air pressure levels is measured. It works on the principle that the physiologic middle ear is most efficient in passing sounds through when air

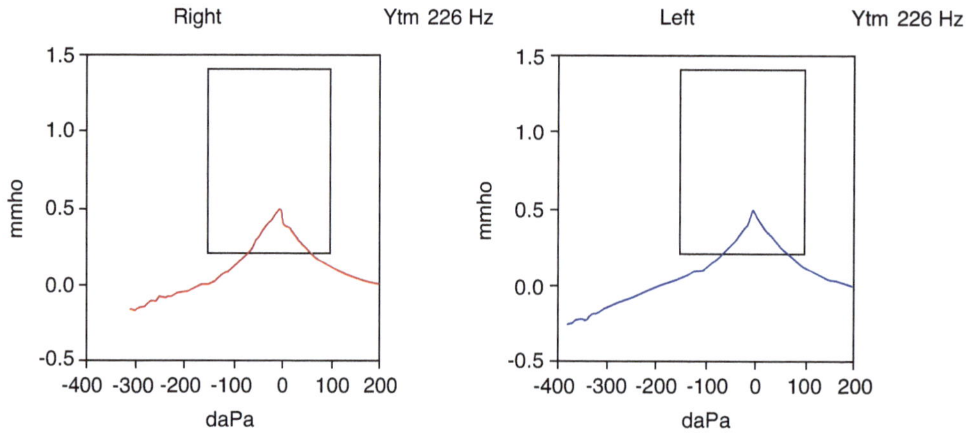

Fig. 29.3 Tympanogram

pressure is equal on both sides of the tympanic membrane which creates the least stiffness of the middle ear or most compliance. A tympanogram is a graphic display of tympanic membrane compliance as a function of pressure change in the ear canal. Different types of tympanograms are associated with various conditions [36]. The contraindication of this test is when the ear canal is occluded due to ear wax or ruptured tympanic membrane. An example of a tympanometry measurement is given in Fig. 29.3.

Acoustic Reflex Threshold (ART) Testing

During ART testing, the air pressure is kept at the normal room air pressure level and a sudden loud sound is presented in the ear which triggers the acoustic reflex resulting in the changing of the height of the static compliance of the tympanogram. Acoustic reflex arch engages with the outer ear, middle ear, cochlea, VIII cranial never, lower brain stem, V & VII cranial nerves terminating at the tensor tympani and stapedius muscles of the middle ear. In normal hearing individuals ART can be elicited at 90 dBHL. Acoustic reflex threshold is the lowest level of sound needed to generate a measurable change in middle ear compliance. The contraindication of this test is similar to that of tympanogram and additionally it is not recommended to conduct this test in patients with hyperacusis.

Otoacoustic Emissions (OAE)

OAEs are weak sound signals generated by outer hair cells (OHC) which can be measured in the ear canal [37]. OAE testing is a quick objective assessment which can help to reveal the status of OHCs in the inner ears. OAE testing is an important part of audiological test battery approach; however, its direct relevance in patients with tinnitus is questioned [38]. Normal functioning middle ear system is the prerequisite of the OAE testing, and hence, it cannot be performed in the presence of impacted wax, perforated tympanic membrane or middle ear pathologies. In clinical practice, two types of OAE testing are performed: transiently evoked OAE (TEOAE) and distortion product OAE (DPOAE).

In people with tinnitus, the presence of DPOAE decreases with increasing stimulus frequency. In a recent study, DPOAEs were present in 247 ears at 1 KHz, but only present in 11 ears at 8 KHz [26]. The percentage of abnormal DPOAEs increased with frequency, 23.29% had abnormal DPOAEs at 1 kHz, which doubled at 4 kHz (52.16%) and tripled at 8 kHz (77.08%) reflecting the dysfunctioning of OHCs especially at high frequencies. The majority of participants in this study (73%) matched their tinnitus pitch to 8 kHz and above, that is beyond frequencies associated with OHCs. This suggests that the damage to IHCs accompanying OHC dysfunction may be an important underlying factor or precursor for tinnitus generation.

Research study conducted by Elsaeid (2009) reported that 85% of tinnitus ears had abnormal TEOAEs, especially at 2, 4, and 8 kHz [39]. Granjeiro et al. (2008) found 70.2% and 68.4% of tinnitus participants showed abnormal TEOAEs and DPOAEs, respectively [40].

Auditory Brainstem Response (ABR) Audiometry

ABR is acoustically elicited signals representing the neural activation from VIII cranial nerve of cochlear nucleus up to the inferior colliculus [41]. ABR is a cost-effective, objective test used in clinical practice to diagnose hearing loss in infants, young children, functional hearing loss, and patients who are difficult to test behaviourally. It can facilitate differential diagnosis and identification of retro cochlear lesions, acoustic neuromas, and vestibular schwannomas [42]. ABR involves identifying waves I, III, & V absolute latency, amplitude, and inter-peak latencies and comparing it with normative data to infer the status of neural pathways involved in human hearing [43].

Although there is an increased research interest in using ABR for measuring auditory functioning in patients with tinnitus, its use for tinnitus diagnosis and/or as an outcome measure is debatable. A scoping review conducted by Milloy et al. 2017 [44] synthesized the ABR results from 1240 tinnitus patients and 664 controls revealing high level of heterogeneity between the results indicating the need for standardized ABR methods and need for greater stratification. The common consistent finding across the studies was the reduced amplitude and longer latency of wave I for people with tinnitus and normal hearing compared to matched controls.

Research Assessments: Assessments outlined here are not commonly used as part of audiological assessment battery. However, they are becoming increasingly popular and insightful during the research investigations such as neuroimaging (EEG, & fMRI) (see Chaps. 15 and 16.) and tinnitus apps (see Chap. 57).

Case Study

Mark is a retired 72-year-old man from Adelaide. Mark was referred to a community Audiology service by his general practitioner. Mark presented to his general practitioner with the complaint of a high-pitched ringing noise in both ears, which he had been noticing for the last few years. Mark reported that he felt the noise had been gradually increasing in volume since he started noticing it several years ago and that the noise was recently so loud that it was making it difficult for him to fall asleep at night. Mark also mentioned to his general practitioner that he had been exposed to loud noise while working with farm machinery in his 20s and 30s but had changed to working in a relatively quiet office at his local council for the remainder of his career. The audiologist undertook a standard tinnitus assessment battery, and the following results were obtained:

Results Summary

Mark's otoscopic examination did not reveal any evidence of outer or middle ear pathology in either ear. His tympanometry results further supported the otoscopy results and were indicative of normal middle ear function bilaterally. Mark's audiogram showed hearing within the normal range for low-frequency sounds, sloping to a mild-to-moderate, sensorineural hearing loss for the mid-, high, and very high-pitched sounds bilaterally. This is consistent with Mark's reported experience of his hearing loss and his history of loud noise exposure and the effects of aging. His tinnitus was pitch-matched to 6 kHz in both ears at 10 dB above threshold (10 dBSL), which is consistent with his degree and type of hearing loss. Mark's loudness discomfort levels were present between 105–110 dBHL between 500–4000 Hz. These are within the expected range for his degree and type of hearing loss and are not indicative of hyperacusis in addition to his experience of tinnitus. Mark's speech audiometry results indicate excellent speech discrimination scores with appropriate amplification in both ears, consistent with his degree and type of hearing loss. Mark's results indicate a typical presentation of tinnitus associated with damage to the sensorineural hearing mechanism, most likely due to loud noise exposure and the aging process. Further assessment with questionnaires that examine the impact of Mark's tinnitus on his quality of life would be beneficial in helping to plan appropriate counselling and management strategies for Mark.

Conclusion

Audiological assessment for tinnitus comprises of battery of tests, and they need to be interpreted in conjunction with each other instead of in isolation. Figure 29.1 summarizes the various subjective and objective tests used for tinnitus assessment and Fig. 29.4 outlines the key expert tips to keep in mind for tinnitus assessment. The present chapter is a guideline about the audiological assessment approach and is not a prescriptive direction. The procedure

Expert Tips

1. Audiological assessment should be a test battery approach
2. Test battery approach can vary based on national guidelines
3. Well structured assessment is integral for holistic tinnitus management

Fig. 29.4 Expert tips

and acceptable recommendations of these tests can vary across countries, and we strongly advise the readers to adhered to their national guidelines. A well-structured assessment can offer useful insights not only about the presenting symptoms of tinnitus but also towards its wholistic management as well.

References

1. Møller AR, Langguth B, DeRidder D, Kleinjung T. Textbook of tinnitus. Cham: Springer; 2010.
2. Van Thiel J, Kraan H, Van der Vleuten C. Reliability and feasibility of measuring medical interviewing skills: the revised Maastricht history-taking and advice checklist. Med Educ. 1991;25(3):224–9.
3. McCullagh M, Wright R. Good Practice. Student's book: communication skills in English for the medical practitioner. Cambridge: Cambridge University Press; 2008.
4. Langguth B, Goodey R, Azevedo A, Bjorne A, Cacace A, Crocetti A, et al. Consensus for tinnitus patient assessment and treatment outcome measurement: tinnitus research initiative meeting, Regensburg. Prog Brain Res. 2007;166:525–36.
5. Meikle MB, Henry JA, Griest SE, Stewart BJ, Abrams HB, McArdle R, et al. The tinnitus functional index: development of a new clinical measure for chronic intrusive tinnitus. Ear Hear. 2012;33:153–76.
6. Kuk FK, Tyler RS, Russell D, Jordan H. The psychometric properties of a tinnitus handicap questionnaire. Ear Hear. 1990;11:434–45.
7. Newman CW, Jacobson GP, Spitzer JB. Development of the tinnitus handicap inventory. Arch Otolaryngol Head Neck Surg. 1996;122:143–8.
8. Meikle MB, Griest SE, Stewart BJ, Press LS. Measuring the negative impact of tinnitus: a brief severity index. Abstr Assoc Res otolaryngol. 1995;18:167.
9. Wilson PH, Henry J, Bowen M, Haralambous G. Tinnitus reaction questionnaire: psychometric properties of a measure of distress associated with tinnitus. J Speech Hear Res. 1991;34:197–201.
10. Hallam RS, Jakes SC, Hinchcliffe R. Cognitive variables in tinnitus annoyance. Br J Clin Psychol. 1988;27:213–22.
11. Guy W. ECDEU assessment manual for psychopharmacology-revised (DHEW Publ no ADM 76–338). Rockville, MD: U.S. Department of Health, Education, and Welfare; 1976. p. 218–22.
12. The tinnitus research initiative. The tinnitus severity (numeric scale). Case report form University of Regensburg, Germany; 2009. p. 16,30,42,56,68,82 and 95.
13. Axelsson A, Coles R, Erlandsson S, Meikle M, Vernon J. Evaluation of tinnitus treatment: methodological aspects. J Audiol Med. 1993;2:141–50.
14. Lockwood AH, Salvi RJ, Coad ML, Towsley ML, Wack DS, Murphy BW. The functional neuroanatomy of tinnitus: evidence for limbic system links and neural plasticity. Neurology. 1998;50:114–20.
15. Nicolas-Puel C, Faulconbridge RL, Guitton M, Puel JL, Mondain M, Uziel A. Characteristics of tinnitus and etiology of associated hearing loss: a study of 123 patients. Int Tinnitus J. 2002;8:37–44.
16. Axelsson A, Ringdahl A. Tinnitus—a study of its prevalence and characteristics. Br J Audiol. 1989;23(1):53–62.
17. Laukli E, Mair IWS. High-frequency audiometry normative studies and preliminary experiences. Scand Audiol. 1985;14:151–8.
18. Schaette R, McAlpine D. Tinnitus with a normal audiogram: physiological evidence for hidden hearing loss and computational model. J Neurosci. 2011;31:13452–7.
19. Weisz N, Hartmann T, Dohrmann K, Schlee W, Norena A. High-frequency tinnitus without hearing loss does not mean absence of deafferentation. Hear Res. 2006;222(1–2):108–14.
20. Epp B, Hots J, Verhey JL, Schaette R. Increased intensity discrimination thresholds in tinnitus subjects with a normal audiogram. J Acoust Soc Am. 2012;132(3):EL196–201.
21. Gu JW, Herrmann BS, Levine RA, Melcher JR. Brainstem auditory evoked potentials suggest a role for the ventral cochlear nucleus in tinnitus. J Assoc Res Otolaryngol. 2012;13(6):819–33.
22. Masayuki S, Kimitaka K, Tomokazu K. Extended high-frequency ototoxicity induced by the first administration of cisplatin. Otolaryngol Head Neck Surg. 2000;122:828–33.
23. Roberts LE, Moffat G, Bosnyak DJ. Residual inhibition functions in relation to tinnitus spectra and auditory threshold shift. Acta Otolaryngol Suppl. 2006;126:27–33.
24. Shim HJ, Kim SK, Park CH, Lee SH, Yoon SW, Ki AR, et al. Hearing abilities at ultra-high frequency in patients with tinnitus. Clin Exp Otorhinolaryngol. 2009;2:169–74.
25. König O, Schaette R, Kempter R, Gross M. Course of hearing loss and occurrence of tinnitus. Hear Res. 2006;221:59–64.
26. Shekhawat GS, Searchfield GD, Stinear CM. The relationship between tinnitus pitch and hearing sensitivity. Eur Arch Otorhinolaryngol. 2014;271:41–8.
27. Jastreboff PJ, Jastreboff MM. Tinnitus and hyperacusis. In: Ballenger JJ, Snow JB, editors. Ballenger's otorhinolaryngology. 18th ed. Raleigh, NC: People's Medical Publishing House; 2016. p. 391–403.
28. Henry JA, Zaugg TL, Schechter MA. Clinical guide for audiologic tinnitus management II: treatment. Am J Audiol. 2005;14:49–70.
29. Tyler RS, Noble W, Coelho C, Haskell G, Bardia A. Tinnitus and hyperacusis. In: Katz J, Burkard R, Medwetsky L, Hood L, editors. Handbook of clinical audiology. 6th ed. Baltimore, MD: Lippincott Williams and Wilkins; 2009. p. 726–42.
30. Westcott M, Sanchez TG, Diges I, Saba C, Dineen R, McNeill C, et al. Tonic tensor tympani syndrome in tinnitus and hyperacusis patients: a multi-clinic prevalence study. Noise Health. 2013;15(63):117.
31. Norena A, Micheyl C, Chery-Croze S, Collet L. Psychoacoustic characterization of the tinnitus spectrum: implications for the underlying mechanisms of tinnitus. Audiol Neurootol. 2002;7:7.
32. Neff P, Langguth B, Schecklmann M, Hannemann R, Schlee W. Comparing three established methods for tinnitus pitch matching with respect to reliability, matching duration, and subjective satisfaction. Trends Hear. 2019;23:2331216519887247.
33. Feldmann H. Homolateral and contralateral masking of tinnitus by noise-bands and by pure tones. Int J Audiol. 1971;10:138–44.
34. Vernon JA, Meikle MB. Tinnitus: clinical measurement. Otolaryngol Clin N Am. 2003;36(2):293–305.

35. Shekhawat GS, Kobayashi K, Searchfield GD. Methodology for studying the transient effects of transcranial direct current stimulation combined with auditory residual inhibition on tinnitus. J Neurosci Methods. 2014;239:28. https://doi.org/10.1016/j.jneumeth.2014.09.025.
36. Jerger J. Clinical experience with impedance audiometry. Arch Otolaryngol. 1970;92(4):311–24.
37. Kemp DT. Otoacoustic emissions, their origin in cochlear function, and use. Br Med Bull. 2002;63(1):223–41.
38. Norton SJ, Schmidt AR, Stover LJ. Tinnitus and otoacoustic emissions: is there a link? Ear Hear. 1990;11(2):159–66.
39. Elsaeid MT. Evaluation of tinnitus patients with normal hearing sensitivity using TEOAEs and TEN test. Auris Nasus Larynx. 2009;36:633–6.
40. Granjeiro RC, Kehrle HM, Bezerra RL, Almeida VF, Sampaio ALL, Oliveira CA. Transient and distortion product evoked Otoacoustic emissions in normal hearing patients with and without tinnitus. Otolaryngol Head Neck Surg. 2008;138:502–6.
41. Melcher JR, Kiang NY. Generators of the brainstem auditory evoked potential in cat III: identified cell populations. Hear Res. 1996;93(1–2):52–71.
42. Rupa V, Job A, George M, Rajshekhar V. Cost-effective initial screening for vestibular schwannoma: auditory brainstem response or magnetic resonance imaging? Otolaryngol Head Neck Surg. 2003;128(6):823–8.
43. Verhulst S, Altoe A, Vasilkov V. Computational modeling of the human auditory periphery: auditory-nerve responses, evoked potentials and hearing loss. Hear Res. 2018;360:55–75.
44. Milloy V, Fournier P, Benoit D, Noreña A, Koravand A. Auditory brainstem responses in tinnitus: a review of who, how, and what? Front Aging Neurosci. 2017;9:237.

Clinical Neuroimaging in the Evaluation of Tinnitus

30

Bernhard Schuknecht and Tobias Kleinjung

Abstract

This chapter describes the imaging techniques used in neuroradiology to investigate patients with tinnitus in more detail. A radiological examination is not part of a routine evaluation, but is reserved for certain conditions. These may include cases of objective tinnitus, especially with pulse-synchronous sounds, in which vascular pathology is suspected. Another important point is the assessment of the middle ear and the cochlear and retrocochlear structures in cases of asymmetric hearing loss and tinnitus on the worse side. Mainly, techniques of computed tomography (CT) and magnetic resonance imaging (MRI) and MR angiography (MRA) are used. In addition to finding the underlying cause of the tinnitus, neuroradiological examination can then also point the way to adequate therapy. In some cases of pulsatile tinnitus, therapy of the tinnitus is possible with invasive neuroradiological techniques in the context of digital subtraction angiography (e.g. coiling, stenting and embolization).

B. Schuknecht (✉)
Medical Radiological Institute, Zurich, Switzerland
e-mail: bschuknecht@mri-roentgen.ch

T. Kleinjung
Department of Otorhinolaryngology—Head and Neck Surgery, University Hospital of Zurich, University of Zurich, Zurich, Switzerland
e-mail: tobias.kleinjung@usz.ch

W. Schlee et al. (eds.), *Textbook of Tinnitus*, https://doi.org/10.1007/978-3-031-35647-6_30

Graphical Abstract

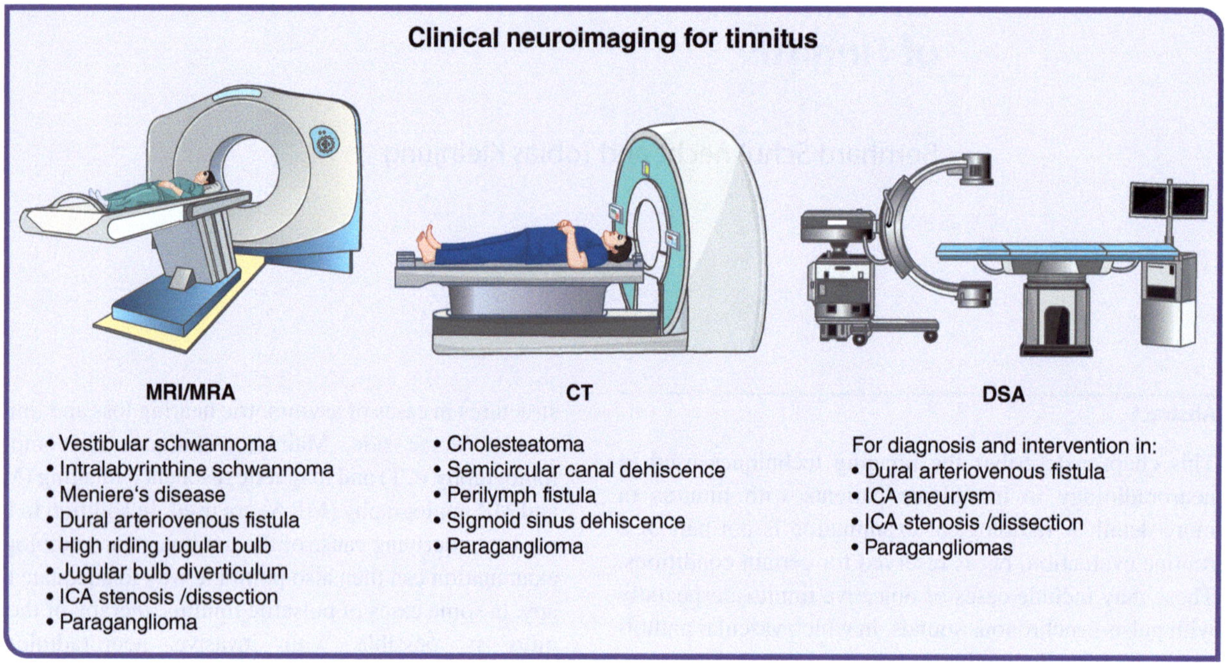

Abbreviations

AVF	Arteriovenous fistula
CCF	Carotid-cavernous fistula
CE	Contrast enhanced
CT	Computed tomography
CTA	Computed tomography angiography
DSA	Digital subtraction angiography
ECA	External carotid artery
FMD	Fibromuscular dysplasia
ICA	Internal carotid artery
IJV	Internal jugular vein
MRA	Magnetic resonance angiography
MRA	MR angiography
MRI	Magnetic resonance imaging
PG	Paraganglioma
SCCD	Superior semicircular canal dehiscence
TOF	Time of flight

Highlights

- Certain tinnitus cases require careful neuroradiological evaluation.
- The most important reasons for neuroradiological diagnostics are pulsatile tinnitus, unilateral tinnitus with ipsilateral sensorineural hearing loss and tinnitus in middle ear pathology.
- The principle modalities of investigation are magnetic resonance and computed tomography imaging of the temporal bones, possibly supplemented by appropriate MR angiography sequences for vascular imaging.
- Neuroradiologic imaging aims to confirm or rule out an underlying structural cause of the tinnitus.
- In the case of a detected structural lesion, adequate therapy can lead to complete elimination of the tinnitus.
- Some pathologies can be treated by interventional neuroradiological interventions by digital subtraction angiography (e.g. embolization or stenting).

Definitions

Tinnitus is defined as a sensation of sound in the absence of an external sound source.

Tinnitus is subjective when an external observer is not able to recall it. This is the case in the vast majority of subjects. It is termed objective, however, when it is audible usually by auscultation and in this situation often has a "pulsatile" character (Chap. 40).

Pulsatile tinnitus constitutes a rhythmic sound that is identical to or closely resembles the "pulse" of the patient. True pulsatile tinnitus may therefore vary according to the individual's heartrate. An additional characteristic of pulsatile tinnitus is the ability to attenuate the sound by manual compression of the common carotid or external carotid artery or the internal jugular vein. Pseudo-pulsatile could also be heard by an external observer in terms of an objective tinnitus, but has a non-rhythmic, clicking and salvo-like appearance. This term refers to those forms of tinnitus caused by pathological muscle contractions (e.g. spasms of middle ear or palatal muscles). Both entities, the vascular and muscle-related forms of tinnitus, may also be referred to as somatosounds.

Tinnitus can have a severe impact on the quality of life and sleep. Furthermore, it may indicate an underlying—rarely potentially life-threatening—cause. Therefore, a timely diagnosis is mandatory either confirming or more often excluding a treatable condition by neuroimaging [1]. Pulsatile tinnitus may have a vascular arterial, arteriovenous or venous cause or maybe of "nonvascular" origin [2, 3].

Though "true" pulsatile tinnitus represents less than 10% of manifestations, it offers a chance to detect an underlying pathology in 50% of patients by neuroimaging. With a cause identified in 42% [4] bilateral pulsatile tinnitus is less likely linked to a structural correlate.

Pre-Imaging Assessment

History, clinical assessment, otoscopy and audiometric testing are the first steps to evaluate a patient with pulsatile tinnitus prior to neuro-imaging (Chaps. 26, 28 and 29) [2].

Raised intracranial pressure, hypertension, thyrotoxicosis, pregnancy, anemia and atherosclerosis among many other causes may evoke pulsatile tinnitus (Chap. 40). Careful *history taking* is required therefore to reveal the character of tinnitus, its duration, triggering factors and accompanying symptoms such as headache or visual disturbance. If these conditions are satisfactory explanations and the tinnitus is responsive to subsequent targeted therapy, imaging evalation is not required.

Variations in character and intensity evoked by maneuvers such as rotation of the head, manual compression of the neck, retroauricular region, jugular vein or carotid artery may indicate a potential venous or arterial cause of the tinnitus. Auscultation of the mastoid and periauricular region is a means of designating tinnitus as both "objective" and "pulsatile" or non-pulsatile.

Otoscopy (including otomicroscopy and otoendoscopy) may attribute tinnitus to a potential temporal bone origin such as in tympanic or jugular paraganglioma, jugular bulb dehiscence or cholesteatoma (Chaps. 28 and 32).

Audiometry (Chap. 29) in conjunction with clinical findings not only distinguishes conductive and sensorineural hearing impairment but may also direct further investigations into a specific direction such as in otosclerosis (see Chap. 32) or Ménière's disease (Chap. 33).

Imaging Assessment

The role of imaging in patients with tinnitus is to detect or exclude a specific pathology that is treatable [4, 5]. Noninvasive identification of an underlying cause by imaging techniques is crucial for treatment decision making and for an estimate of the chance of cure [5, 6].

A structured imaging approach consists of examining the temporal bone, the head and neck and blood vessels as an "entity" [7]. The choice of imaging modality -ies depends on the type of tinnitus, associated symptoms and specific otoscopic and audiometric findings.

As an aid to choose the adequate technique, the principle specific advantages and disadvantages of the currently employed imaging techniques are addressed in Table 30.1.

The mainstay in the evaluation of tinnitus is magnetic resonance imaging (MRI) or computed tomography (CT). In general, lack of radiation and high soft tissue resolution are in favor for an MRI examination of the temporal bone and head. In contrast to MRI, CT depicts the bony anatomy and bone-related pathologies such as bone erosion with higher sensitivity, as is found in paragangliomas or otosclerosis.

Table 30.1 Common vascular causes of tinnitus

Arterial	Arteriovenous	Venous
ICA stenosis/dissection	Dural AVF transverse-sigmoid sinus	Jugular bulb—high riding
ICA fibromuscular dysplasia	Dural AVF carotid cavernous sinus	Jugular bulb—dehiscence
ICA aneurysm (petrous segment)	Dural AVF jugular foramen	Jugular bulb—diverticulum
Aberrant ICA?	Arteriovenous malformations	Transverse/sigmoid sinus stenosis
Stapedial artery?		Sigmoid sinus—diverticulum
		Sigmoid sinus—plate dehiscence
		Sigmoid sinus—diverticulum

MRI and CT therefore may provide complementary information once the bone is affected such as in bone plate dehiscence of the sigmoid sinus or jugular bulb.

Both MRI and CT are often supplemented by angiography of the specific modality [8, 9]. MR angiography, in conjunction with morphologic imaging, is indispensable to identify the lesions responsible for pulsatile tinnitus [10]. Time of flight (TOF) "MR angiography takes advantage of blood as an endogenous tracer". Only protons in motion due to blood flow generate signal, whereas the remainder of the tissue is "saturated", lacks magnetization and signal contribution. Inflow of signal works best in a horizontal plane perpendicular to the flow direction of vertically oriented vessels at the skull base. TOF MRA is suited to identify dural arteriovenous fistulas (AVF's), aneurysms, and arterial stenosis. The TOF technique provides high resolution arterial blood flow information but is less favorable to recognize venous flow and venous sinus stenosis.

Contrast enhanced MR angiography (CE MRA) produces a static image by acquisition of signal derived from intravenous administration of a contrast agent bolus (gadolinium) that fills the vessel lumina during the acquisition time of the sequence. This technique preferentially covers larger volumes such as the entire extra- and intracranial circulation usually in the coronal plane and enables detection of dural and venous sinus thrombosis as well.

Increasingly dynamic "time resolved" techniques 4D MRA [11] and 4D computed tomography angiography (CTA) [12] replace "static" MRA or CTA in order to noninvasively detect and evaluate the hemodynamics of dural AVF, aneurysms or vascular tumours (e.g. paragangliomas). The plane of acquisition is coronal and sagittal with subsecond (usually 0.8–0.9 s) time resolution. The high temporal resolution is achieved by using parallel imaging techniques and/or lowering spatial resolution. Despite its ability to maintain the spatial resolution, CTA entails radiation to the head and neck [12] and in addition is more demanding with respect to postprocessing.

The lack of radiation exposure therefore favors a combination of MRI and MRA initially and for follow –up examinations to assess treatment results [13].

Colour duplex sonography is a noninvasive technique that is suited to assess the vessel wall such as the plaque composition in internal carotid origin stenosis (B mode image). The mainstay, however, is to provide a spectral waveform with angle correction that is both sensitive and accurate regarding the velocity components assessed (systolic, enddiastolic and mean flow velocity). These enable quantification of stenoses and residual flow velocity in vessel dissection, indirect detection of extra- and intracranial fistulae, and follow-up evaluation after treatment of stenoses and arteriovenous fistulae. The major drawback that precludes widespread application is the dependence on the experience of the investigator.

Digital subtraction angiography (DSA) has undergone a change of paradigm from a diagnostic to a therapy-oriented modality. The first step still consists of confirmation of the previously obtained noninvasive information such as the vessel supply of a dural fistula, while the second step—either performed in the same session or in a separate subsequent procedure—is the endovascular therapy itself. Despite considerable progress in noninvasive techniques (e.g. MRI, MRA and CTA), DSA is regarded indispensable by most skull base surgeons and neurosurgeons as a diagnostic tool to specify vascular information and commonly combine with embolisation prior to any surgical treatment of a vascular lesion, e.g. a paraganglioma.

Limiting factors in applying certain modalities of the armamentarium of imaging techniques (colour Duplex ultrasound, MR/MRA, CT/CTA or DSA) are less often the non-availability of a modality, but the lack of familiarity with or the specific preference of a particular technique by the investigating neuroradiologist.

Pulsatile tinnitus can be differentiated into vascular and nonvascular causes.

Vascular abnormalities are distinguished into arterial, arteriovenous and venous (Table 30.2).

Arterial Vascular Abnormalities

Internal carotid artery (ICA) stenosis may cause pulsatile tinnitus once the vessel lumen is significantly narrowed to cause flow obstruction with resultant turbulence. Significant ICA origin stenosis (>70%), however, is a rare cause of pulsatile tinnitus given the distance of the carotid bifurcation to the skull base. In a series of 84 patients that comprised 45 patients with identified vascular causes, ICA stenosis was present in 13.3% (6/45 patients) [14]. It is mandatory therefore to scrutinize any patient with a carotid bifurcation or ICA origin stenosis for an additional high degree stenosis located in the upper cervical vessel segment or within the petrous portion. The carotid bifurcation is readily amenable to an ultrasound examination. However, CE MRA-, 4D MRA or CT-Angiography achieve a better delineation of the entire extra- and intracranial vasculature including the collateral circulation.

Fibromuscular dysplasia (FMD) is much less common than carotid atherosclerotic disease. FMD prevalence estimations range between 1% and 6.6%. Pulsatile tinnitus is a common manifestation in as much as 37.2% of affected patients. FMD is an idiopathic, segmentary, non-inflammatory and non-atherosclerotic disease that involves all layers of small to medium caliber arteries. Medial fibroplasia is the most common histologic type.

Table 30.2 Imaging techniques employed to assess pulsatile tinnitus

	Colour duplex	MRI morphologic sequences	MRA (TOF/4D MRA)
Advantages	Real-time hemodynamic info	Detection of tympanic paraganglioma	Hemodynamic info (4D-MRA)
	High sensitivity for low flow dural AVF	Detection of jugular, vagal, carotid PG	Vascular anatomic info TOF + 4D MRA
	Direct comparison ff endovascular tx	f-up assessment regarding size of PG	Detection of tympanic paraganglioma
	Pulsating lesions at carotid bifurcation	Lower cranial nerve involvement in PG	Detection of jugular, vagal, carotid PG
	Flow in fibromuscular dysplasia	Detection of endolymphatic sac pathology	Detection/location of dural sinus AVF
	Low-cost investigative procedure	Detection of vessel dissection	Drainage pattern in dural AVF
		Confirmation of cholesteatoma	Parent artery and/size of aneurysm
		Posterior fossa venous drainage anomalies	Venous sinus in Intracranial hypertension
		Intracranial hypertension	f-up prior and ff treatment
		Meniere disease (4 h delayed imaging)	
		Evaluation of tinnitus associated symptoms	
Disadvantages	Operator dependent technique	Technique dependent	Technique dependent
	Poor info regarding vessels involved	Time consuming at high spatial resolution	Time consuming at high spatial/time resolution
		Cost intensive	Cost intensive
		Claustrophobic patients	Claustrophobic patients
	Noncontrast CT of temporal bone	**CT angiography**	**Digital subtraction angiography**
Advantages	Detection of semicircular canal dehiscence	High temporal and spatial resolution	Combined diagnostic/therapeutic procedure
	Middle ear lesion w semicircular canal erosion	Combined bone and venous sinus info	High temporal and spatial resolution
	Detection of otosclerosis	Vessel wall plaque composition	Vessel morphology + hemodynamics
	Extent of tympanic + jugular PG	High accuracy for vessel stenosis	Highest accuracy for dural AVF
	Aberrant carotid/stapedial artery	Fast—extra-intracranial vessels	
	Jugular bulb, sigmoid sinus diverticulum		
	Endolymphatic duct/sac pathology		
Disadvantages	Most vascular causes unidentified	Radiation dose	Invasive
	Radiation exposure	Iodine containing contrast agent	Radiation dose
		Artifacts (teeth and skull base)	Iodine contrast agent
		No hemoynamic information	

CTA or MRA by TOF technique depict a "beads on a string" appearance which consists of alternating narrowing and dilatation of the vessel affected or tubular stenosis of a vessel segment that is usually in the upper cervical portion of the internal carotid and/or vertebral arteries. FMD additionally or rarely exclusively affects basal cerebral arteries [15].

Associated with FMD, a marked increase in the prevalence of vessel dissection (25.7%) and cerebral aneurysms formation (21.7%) was found in an US registry encompassing 12 centres [16]. To identify intracranial manifestations of FMD and a potential aneurysm, the cerebral arteries therefore need to be included into the imaging assessment.

Patients with acute **internal carotid artery dissection** may present by pulsatile tinnitus in 8.1–16% [17]. Carotid artery dissection commonly occur spontaneously by a tear in the intimal layer of the carotid artery and forms an intramural hematoma. This tear may happen spontaneously or may be caused by trauma [18, 19]. The intramural hematoma leads to narrowing and eventual formation of a thrombus. Traumatic dissection can be caused by either blunt or penetrating trauma. Blunt trauma typically involves a severe injury (car accident) with rapid deceleration and simultaneous hyperextension of the neck (whiplash), or it may follow minimal trauma (e.g. chiropractic manipulation as a classic example). The most common cause of spontaneous internal carotid artery dissection is "idiopathic", or rarely in the setting of a connective tissue disorder like FMD, Marfan syndrome or Ehlers-Danlos syndrome among others [20]. In a series of 63 patients with extracranial vessel dissection and pulsatile tinnitus, the ICA was affected in 49 patients (77.8%), the vertebral artery in nine (14.3%) and combined ICA and vertebral artery in five cases (7.9%) [21]. Pulsatile tinnitus is an independent predictor for excellent outcome regarding lack of stroke, vessel patency, or resolution of Horner's syndrome after three months.

Carotid artery dissection is associated with increased vessel tortuosity. Carotid dissection tends to involve the carotid foramen at the skull base where it is likely to transmit the sound to the cochlea (Fig. 30.1). The diagnosis has been facilitated by morphologic MR T1 noncontrast fat

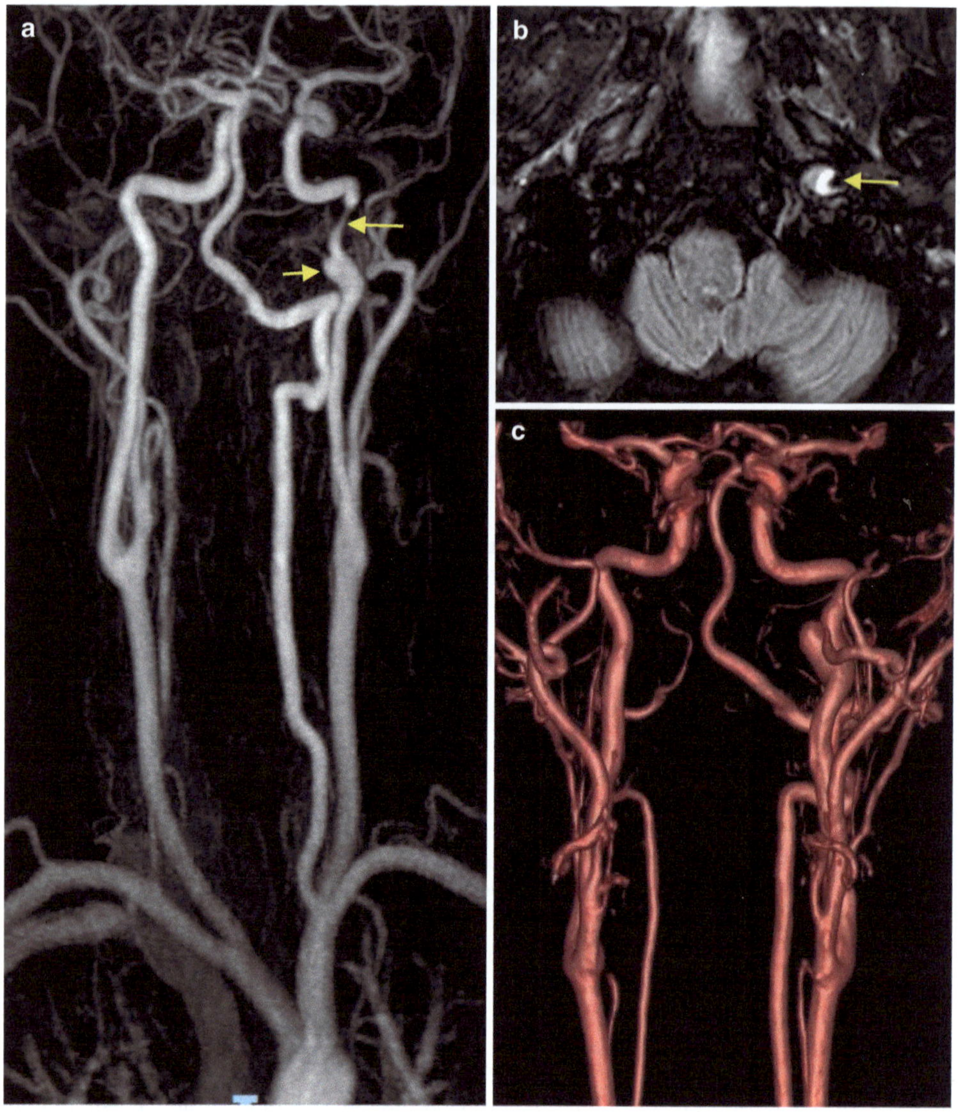

Fig. 30.1 (**a**–**c**) Internal carotid artery dissection. A 46-year-male with sudden onset left pulsatile tinnitus and Horner's syndrome CE MRA MIP- maximum intensity image (**a**) depicts high-degree left cervical ICA stenosis just below the carotid foramen and an adjacent proximal pseudoaneurysm (short arrow). Axial flair image (**b**) depicts the mural hematoma (arrow) and flow void of residual lumen (short arrow). On follow-up with CE MRA VR—volume rendering (**c**) at four months shows resolution of stenosis and slight progression of the size of the pseudoaneurysm (tinnitus had disappeared)

saturated sequences that depict the mural hematoma. Contrast enhanced MRA reveals the extent and degree of vessel stenosis. Colour duplex only shows indirect signs by reduction of peak systolic and enddiastolic velocities at the vessel origin. Dissection between the tunica intima and media is prone to lead to vessel occlusion and thus may not be associated with pulsatile tinnitus. Resolution of the mural hematoma by recanalisation over time may eliminate turbulence and thus attenuate or resolve the tinnitus as well.

Persistence or recurrence of tinnitus may be due to a **pseudoaneurysm** at the skull base, which is more prone to develop once the dissection extends between the media and adventitia. Therefore, MRI and MR-Angiography are recommended as follow-up examinations after three months. Stenting of persistent stenosis in conjunction with a pseudoaneurysm is a therapeutic option to eliminate persistent pulsatile tinnitus [22].

Aneurysm: Petrous segment carotid artery aneurysms are rare [23] and transmit sound caused by pulsations and turbulence to the adjacent cochlea. Because the carotid artery aneurysm usually is at least partially encased in bone, CTA is unsuited and the diagnosis is best established by MR-angiography either by TOF or CE MRA technique. This holds also true for a petrous segment internal carotid artery pseudoaneurysm and/or related stenosis. Endovascular treatment following diagnostic angiography with stenting or coil embolization is the preferred technique if treatment is required [23].

An **aberrant internal carotid artery** is a congenital anomaly and caused by failure of formation of the embryonic cervical ICA. The tympanic artery replaces the internal carotid artery. CTA, CE MRA or TOF MRA identify an aberrant ICA by a reduced caliber in comparison to the contralateral ICA. The aberrant vessel enters the middle ear cavity lateral to the promontory via an enlarged inferior tympanic

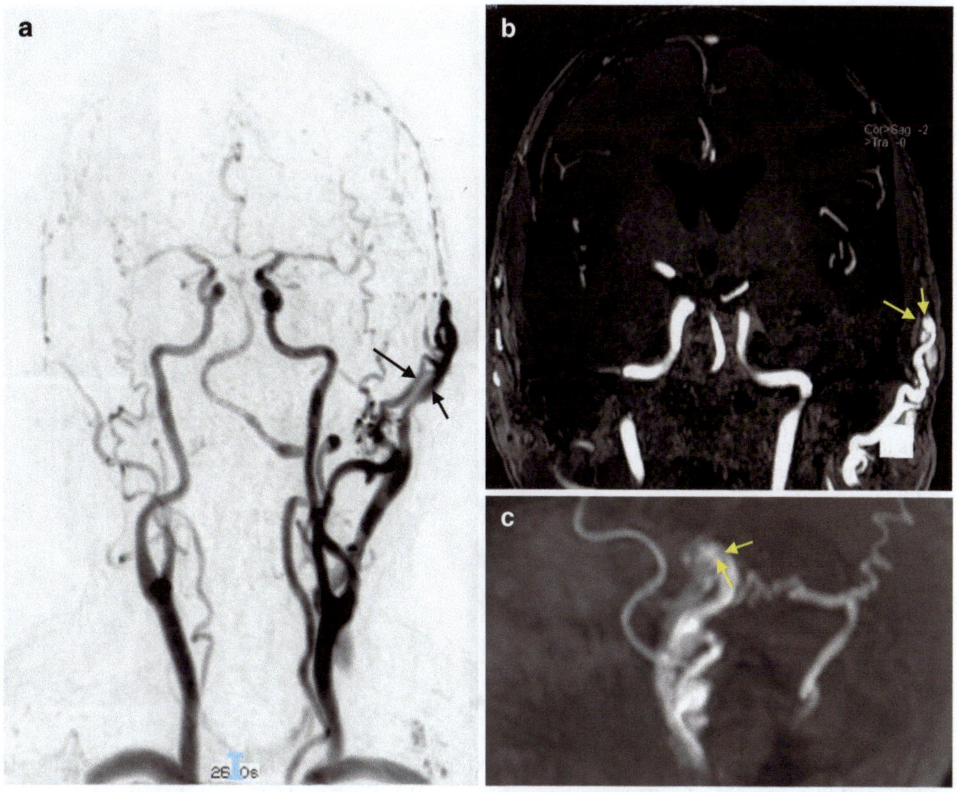

Fig. 30.2 (a–c) Arteriovenous fistula between the superficial temporal artery and retromandibular vein. An 80-year-old male with progressive pulsatile left tinnitus following a penetrating injury by a wood stick a year ago. Time-resolved (4D) MRA (**a**) depicts a fistula via the enlarged parietal branch of the left superior temporal artery (arrow) to the retromandibular vein (short arrow). The coronal reformat of the TOF MRA (**b**) and sagittal maximum intensity projection of TOF MRA (**c**) precisely identify the fistulous point (arrows)

canal. Temporal bone CT shows an elongated vascular structure posterior to the expected carotid foramen [9]. In some cases, an aberrant ICA may be visible as a white or reddish, pulsatile structure on otoscopy [24, 25].

A **persistent stapedial artery** may be associated with an aberrant internal carotid artery and is a congenital anomaly as well. It originates from the petrous segment of the genuine internal carotid artery, ascends along the promontory to course between the stapes crura. The persistent stapedial artery accompanies the tympanic portion of the facial nerve to continue as the middle meningeal artery. The foramen spinosum is missing.

A loop of the **anterior inferior cerebellar artery (AICA)** entering the internal auditory meatus is a common finding encountered in about 12.5% of temporal bones, e.g. at least one side [26]. The intrameatal AICA loop is occasionally considered being implicated in the etiology of pulsatile tinnitus in the context of a neurovascular compression syndrome [27] (Chap. 35). Neurovascular compression of the eighth cranial nerve might cause (paroxysmal) vertigo and (pulsatile) tinnitus. However, from a prominent perspective [28], "vascular loops… considered as a possible cause for otherwise unexplained otologic symptoms" are declared as one of the "myths in neurootology" and should be interpreted with major concern. A recent study, which compared ears that presented vascular loops with those that did not, found no association with neurotological manifestations such as tinnitus, hearing loss, or vertigo [26, 29].

Arteriovenous Pathologies

Extracranial arteriovenous fistulae are communications between an artery and the accompanying vein. Pulsatile tinnitus and/or a bruit on auscultation are common findings. The cervical vertebral artery is most often affected between the seventh and second vertebra followed by the atlas loop at the C1/2 level [30]. Venous drainage may involve spinal perimedullary, epidural or deep cervical veins.

External carotid artery fistulae may originate from the middle meningeal, superficial temporal, occipital, maxillary, and ascending pharyngeal arteries [31]. Contrary to vertebral artery fistulae, the most common etiology is trauma [32] (Fig. 30.2).

High flow in the vertebral arteries or external carotid artery branches renders colour duplex a sensitive and easily applicable screening tool when a bruit is present in the neck. A more objective assessment is *by noncontrast TOF* to depict the fistulous point and 4D MRA to ascertain the arterial and venous vessels involved.

Following preliminary TOF MRA, DSA is more specifically applied with a therapeutic intention to occlude the fistula in the same session using liquid embolic agents (glue) or coils. The diagnostic part of DSA needs to confirm or modify previously obtained noninvasive findings of a TOF or 4D MRA.

Carotid-Cavernous fistula (CCF) represent an abnormal communication between the cavernous sinus, the inter-

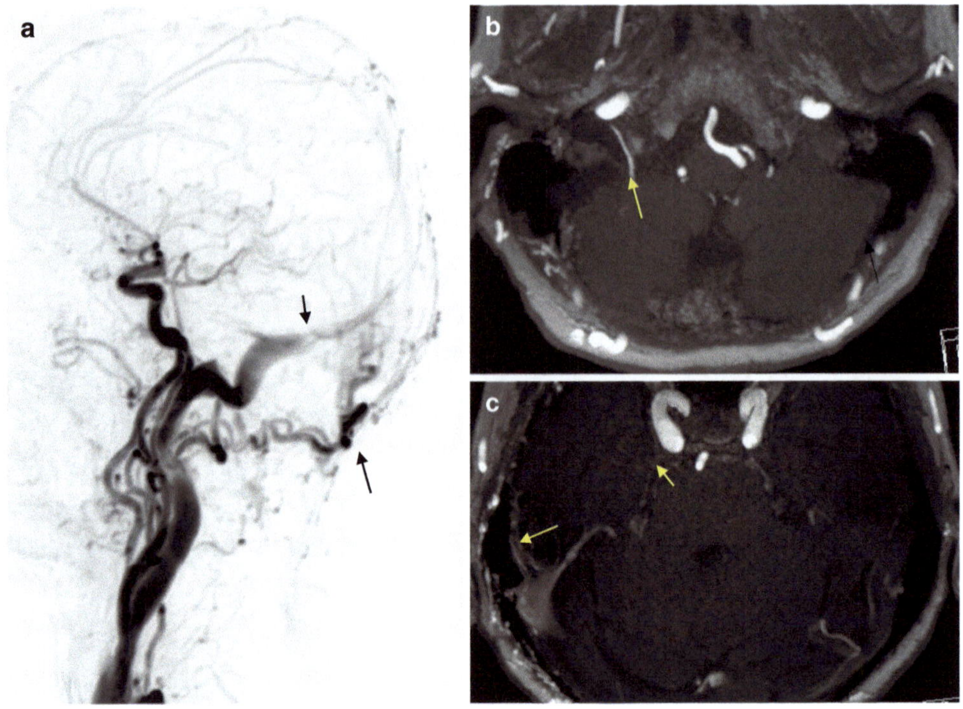

Fig. 30.3 (**a–c**) Dural transverse sigmoid sinus fistula. A 68-year-old-female with right pulsatile left tinnitus audible on retroauricular auscultation. Time-resolved (4D) MRA lateral projection (**a**) depicts a fistula derived from enlarged retroauricular and muscular branches of the occipital artery (arrow) and early filling of the sigmoid sinus (short arrow). No evidence of sinus or cortical venous reflux. TOF MRA axial source image (**b**) shows identical supply but additional meningeal contribution via the jugular foramen. Further supply (**c**) is identified to occur via the petrosquamosal artery (arrow) and tentorial branch of the ICA (short arrow)

nal carotid artery and/or branches of the external carotid artery (ECA), respectively. This entity represents the most common form of posttraumatic fistulas and can be seen in around 8% of skull base fractures affecting the middle cranial fossa [33]. CCFs are classified by the arterial system involved as proposed by Barrow et al. [34]. Type A are direct fistulas created between the ICA and the cavernous sinus, whereas types B to D are dural fistulas between meningeal branches of the ICA and the cavernous sinus (type B), meningeal branches of the ECA and the cavernous sinus (type C) or both (type D). Traumatic fistulae and ruptured cavernous segment internal carotid artery aneurysms cause high flow fistulae (type A), while type D is the most common type of a dural fistula. CCF constitute 10% of dural AVF. Pulsatile tinnitus is a common presentation in CCF fistulae. The pathways of venous drainage determine the clinical presentation [35]. In patients with a dural cavernous sinus fistula drainage via the superior and inferior petrosal sinus may cause pulsatile tinnitus while orbital drainage accounts for the more "classical" symptoms such as proptosis, chemosis, ophthalmoplegia or decreased visual acuity. A combination of noncontrast TOF MRA and time-resolved 4D MRA depict the presence, feeding arteries and drainage of dural carotid cavernous sinus fistulae. The first treatment option should be endovascular embolization with a combination of balloons, coils, stents, or liquid embolic agents depending on an arterial or venous approach [36].

Dural transverse/sigmoid sinus fistulae constitute pathologic communications between extracranial vessels involved in the arterial supply of the dura along the transverse and sigmoid sinus (Fig. 30.3). About 50% of dural AVFs involve the transverse and sigmoid sinus [26]. The most common presentation is pulsatile tinnitus. Pathologic recanalisation of a preceding sinus thrombosis with subsequent increased flow and enlargement of meningeal vessels is the most likely hypothesis for the origin of dural AVF's of any location. The formation of these thrombotic alterations might result from traumatic brain injury, infections, previous brain surgeries or tumors. Dural AVF of the transverse/sigmoid sinus maybe disclosed by colour duplex sonography due to increased flow within the occipital artery as a "marker" vessel. Despite its proximity to the temporal bone, pulsatile tinnitus is not universally present. An explanation is offered by differences in venous drainage included into the classification by Cognard et al. 1995 [37]. Type I represents antegrade flow within the main sinus involved, type II signifies reflux into other sinuses (IIa), cortical veins (IIb) or both (IIa + b). Type III consists of pure cortical venous drainage with venous ectasia in type IV and spinal drainage in type V. It is obvious that pulsatile tinnitus is more common in type I and II, while the risk of hemorrhage is increased in types that involve cortical venous drainage. TOF and 4D MRA (Fig. 30.3) are best suited to assess the often multipedicular arterial supply and the drainage pattern. Reduction in the intensity of pulsatile tinnitus and loss of tinnitus may indicate a shift in drainage from a venous sinus towards cortical venous drainage. This change in symptoms in a patient with a known dural AVF urgently indicates a new examination.

DSA is the ultimate technique to verify the presence of a dural AVF, to identify feeding arteries and classify the drain-

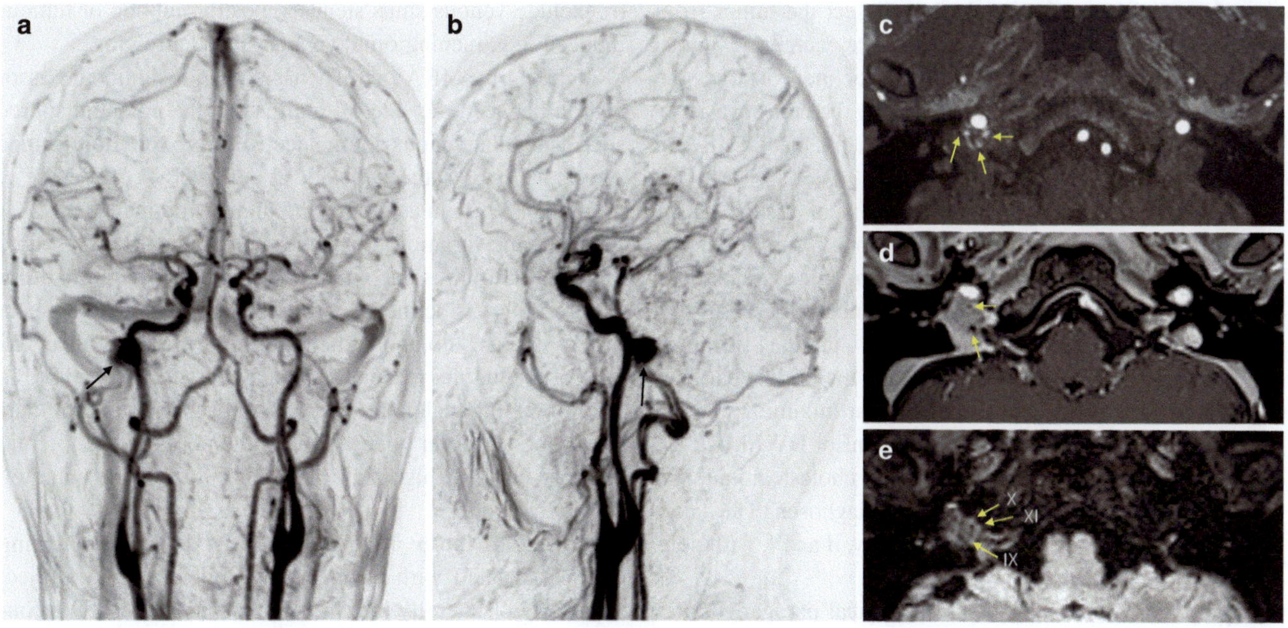

Fig. 30.4 (**a–e**) Jugular paraganglioma. A 46-year-old female with progressive pulsatile right sided tinnitus. 4D time-resolved MRA ap (**a**), lateral projection (**b**) depicts small hypervascular paraganglioma (arrow) posterior to ICA within the bulb of the patent jugular foramen. TOF MRA axial source image (**c**) reveals intratumoral vessels (short arrows). Some of them are visible as flow void on contrast enhanced axial T1 MR image at 0.5 mm (**d**). Neurographic sequence maximum intensity projection at 5 mm (**e**) enables visualization of cranial nerves IX–XI prior to surgery in relation to the tumour

age pattern. Patients who present with pulsatile tinnitus have a less aggressive clinical course with an estimated annual rate of intracerebral hemorrhage of 1.4–1.5% [38]. Despite the commonly annoying character of tinnitus, a patient with type I or IIa drainage harbours a less strict indication for endovascular treatment in comparison to a similar patient in whom cortical venous drainage signifies a life-threatening condition. Overall, about 92% of patients have complete resolution or marked improvement of pulsatile following endovascular treatment of dural AVFs [39].

Paragangliomas have in common an origin from neural crest cells associated with branchiomeric and autonomic ganglia and a high vascularisation from site-specific vessels. Depending on location, **paragangliomas** are classified as jugulo-tympanic, vagal or carotid. Carotid body tumours are the most common and present as a pulsating lesion at the carotid bifurcation followed by jugulotympanic paragangliomas (syn. Glomus tympanicum and glomus jugulare). The latter are characterized by the almost universal presence of pulsatile tinnitus and a typical otoscopic appearance. About 40% of paragangliomas are linked to genetic syndromes, most commonly mutations of the succinate dehydrogenase (SDH) enzyme. Multicentricity is expected to occur in 30–40% of these so-called "familial" paragangliomas and needs to be searched for by imaging.

Jugular foramen and tympanic paragangliomas require a contrast-enhanced MRI of the temporal bone (Fig. 30.4). High vascularization on MR morphologic sequences leads to a salt (punctate hemorrhages) and pepper (flow voids due to intratumoral vessels) appearance on T1 and T2 turbo spin echo sequences as a pathognomonic appearance of jugular, vagal and carotid paragangliomas. Tympanic tumours are smaller and therefore commonly lack this appearance.

Increasingly "neurographic MR sequences" are used to display the relation of the tumour to the course of cranial nerves IX-XII. Cranial nerve displacement versus encasement is a relevant distinction prior to potential surgery (Fig. 30.4).

The degree of vascularisation is displayed by high resolution TOF MRA. For tympanic paragangliomas arterial supply is via the inferior tympanic artery while jugular foramen tumours are primarily vascularized by the jugular branch of the ascending pharyngeal artery. In larger jugular paragangliomas, additional supply via external carotid and vertebral artery branches are identified non-invasively by a combination of TOF and 4D MRA.

However, 4D MRA needs to cover the head and neck-area to detect potential multicentricity, display the relation of the tumour to the carotid bifurcation (carotid body PG) and the posterior wall of the internal carotid artery (vagal PG) and the degree of jugular vein invasion (jugular PG). Proximity of paragangliomas to the internal carotid artery requires knowledge of the collateral supply via the anterior and posterior communicating arteries in case transient or permanent vessel occlusion maybe required to dissect the tumor from the vessel during surgery. Furthermore, cerebral venous drainage deserves attention as the tumor may obstruct the jugular vein. All this information may be non-invasively obtained by a combination of TOF MRA and by 4D MRA in carotid and vagal paragangliomas.

High-resolution CT depicts the extent of osseous invasion and, therefore, is an additional modality to verify the degree of bony invasion of jugulo-tympanic paragangliomas. CT also is ideal to provide a distinction between primary tympanic tumors and those jugular foramen paragangliomas that secondarily invade the middle ear cavity. CT also serves to identify middle ear inflammation and infection and in conjunction with a NonEpi DWI MRI, T1 and T2 sequences allows identifying cholesteatoma and cholesterol granuloma as alternative diagnoses. The latter two entities, however, manifest clinically, if at all, with non-pulsatile tinnitus.

Symptoms and management of cervical paragangliomas depend on their specific location and relation to adjacent vessels [40]. DSA is the final step to confirm the vessels involved and depict the venous drainage. The principal indication remaining for DSA is for the purpose of embolization to reduce blood supply when surgery is considered, or the tinnitus becomes unbearable. In cases where a surgical management is not possible, embolization of the paraganglioma might reduce the tumor growth [41].

Venous Causes

Intracranial hypertension is a condition of raised intracranial pressure associated with obesity commonly in women of childbearing age, vitamin A hypervitaminosis, high-dose tetracycline medication or is labelled as "idiopathic" if no cause is identified. Pulsatile tinnitus maybe a first sign of intracranial hypertension [42]. Associated symptoms consist of headache -at times posture related-, visual decline and papilledema and rarely VIth or VIIth cranial nerve palsy. An increased opening pressure of CSF (>200 mm) confirms diagnosis. Increased ICP is deemed secondary to elevated intra-abdominal, thoracic and subsequently cerebral venous pressure. Anatomic obstruction of the transverse venous sinuses is a common finding in idiopathic intracranial hypertension syndrome. Subsequent relief maybe achieved by stenting and dilatation of the venous segment involved. It is uncertain yet, whether venous sinus stenosis is the cause or resultant effect of the intracranial hypertension [43].

Suggestive MRI signs of benign intracranial hypertension include slit or small ventricles, flattening of the posterior aspect of the globe and empty sella. However, 4D MRA has replaced venous phase contrast angiography and is the technique of choice to rule out a causative dural fistula, confirm or exclude venous sinus stenosis, postthrombotic or tumour induced (e.g. meningioma) venous sinus narrowing.

Imaging by MRA or CTA has shown a significant association between the side of tinnitus and the potential source such as jugular venous dominance. **Jugular vein dominance** affects in 70–80% the right side as defined by a difference of more than 3 mm in caliber of the jugular foramen [12].

Anatomic variations that have been implicated as a source of pulsatile tinnitus encompass a **high riding jugular bulb**. "High riding" is defined as projection of the superior aspect of the jugular bulb above the basal turn of the cochlea. The bulb of the jugular foramen thus may exceed the level of the floor of the internal auditory canal to reach the superior margin of the temporal bone dorsal to the porus of the internal auditory canal. A high riding jugular bulb is more common on the right side.

A **jugular bulb diverticulum** is a focal outpouching often associated with a high riding bulb that may project superiorly or laterally into the middle ear. The osseous confines are intact. Paradoxically, jugular bulb diverticula are more likely to affect the left side [12]. A **dehiscent jugular bulb** is devoid of a bony covering and may display a variable degree of protrusion into the middle ear. This anomaly may be seen on otoscopy as a reddish mass shining through behind the tympanic membrane.

Further variations potentially related to pulsatile venous tinnitus consist of **sigmoid sinus dehiscence** and diverticulum formation. Sigmoid sinus dehiscence is a focal lack of compact bony covering to the adjacent mastoid, while a diverticum is an additional focal sigmoid sinus outpouching projecting into sinudural air cells. The prevalence of **sigmoid sinus diverticulum** in patients with pulsatile tinnitus was up to 20% of cases [12], compared to 1.2% [44] in asymptomatic individuals. The fact that the osseous contour of the jugular bulb and the sigmoid sinus are better identified by CT renders contrast enhanced CT the most suitable imaging technique to verify these anomalies [45]. An additional argument in favor of CT is a surgical transmastoid extraluminal approach aimed at "resurfacing" of the bony wall and insulating of the vascular segment by autologous or artificial material [46].

The **mastoid emissary vein** develops at the embryonic stage. By traversing the occipital bone behind the mastoid, the emissary vein connects the sigmoid sinus with the posterior auricular or occipital vein. Additional emissary veins are in midline position (occipital emissary vein) at the confluens sinuum (torcula) draining to the internal vertebral plexus and laterally behind the occipital condyle (posterior condylar veins) connecting to deep cervical veins. These emissary veins are valveless intra-extracranial venous communications that are easily identified by CTA [12]. Emissary veins function as drainage collaterals in case of sinus thrombosis, or fistulae and may pose an obstacle for a

Table 30.3 Non-vascular causes of tinnitus (preferred imaging modality)

Temporal bone lesions		Bone tumours		Miscellaneous	
Cholesteatoma	CT, MRI	Aneurysmal bone cyst	CT	Semicircular canal dehiscence	CT
Cholesterol granuloma	MRI	M. Paget	CT	Spontaneous tegmen defect	CT
Middle ear adenoma	CT, MRI	Fibrous dysplasia	CT	Patulous eustachian tube	MRI
Endolymphatic sac tumour	MRI			Perilymph fistula	CT
Meningioma	MRI			Vestibular schwannoma	MRI
Cavernous hemangioma	MRI				
Intralabyrinthine schwannoma	MRI				
Meniere's disease	MRI				

suboccipital surgical access. They are universally present and hardly relevant as an explanation of puls-synchronous tinnitus.

A spectrum of entities that has been associated with **non-pulsatile tinnitus** is summarized in Table 30.3.

Non-pulsatile tinnitus is most frequently related to inner ear disorders with subsequent sensorineural hearing loss like, noise exposure, presbycusis, ototoxicity, congenital abnormalities or systemic conditions. Unlike pulsatile tinnitus, potentially treatable causes are exceedingly rare. Consequently, most patients with non-pulsatile tinnitus do not reveal imaging abnormalities. Therefore, the "Clinical practice guideline" on tinnitus of the American Academy of Otolaryngology—Head and Neck Surgery recommends imaging only for patients whose tinnitus is unilateral, pulsatile, associated with asymmetric hearing loss, and/or additional neurologic symptoms [47].

In case of non-pulsatile tinnitus and when associated hearing loss is conductive, then temporal bone CT is preferred to identify otosclerosis, ossicular chain disruption, chronic otitis media (including cholesteatoma) or tympanosclerosis as potential causative middle ear findings. The clinical situation of asymmetric sensorineural hearing loss with concomitant non-pulsatile tinnitus in the worse hearing ear represents one of the most common reasons for MRI of the temporal bone. The primary goal is to find or exclude a structural abnormality in the labyrinth, the internal auditory canal, and the cerebellopontine angle region. The main pathologies found here are vestibular and intralabyrinthine schwannomas (Chap. 34), and rarely meningiomas [13]. A contrast-enhanced MRI examination with high spatial resolution (e.g. 0.25 to 0.5 mm) is the method of choice in order not to miss a small intralabyrinthine schwannoma or a small endolymphatic sac tumour.

Endolymphatic hydrops is considered a pathomechanism of Meniere's disease (Chap. 33). Thus, in cases of clinical suspicion (attacks of vertigo, low frequency sensorineural hearing loss, tinnitus, aural fulness), MRI can help to establish a definitive diagnosis of Meniere's disease. A 4 h delayed MRI after double dose of iv Gd administration by a particular Double inversion recovery sequence (3D real IR) or alternatively by an adapted FLAIR sequence has been developed to verify endolymphatic hydrops [48]. Further radiological studies could also contribute to differentiate different forms of Meniere's disease based on the radiological configuration of the vestibular aqueduct [49].

Superior semicircular canal dehiscence (SCCD) is present in 0.5% of cadaveric temporal bone studies and in another 1.4% a near dehiscence is present. It is considered a congenital anomaly; in 25%, both ears are affected. Patients may experience (pulsatile) tinnitus, symptoms of ear pressure, sound-induced vertigo ("Tullio phenomenon") and/or nystagmus, and bone conduction hyperacusis (pseudo-conductive hearing loss). However, commonly superior and less commonly posterior semicircular canal dehiscence (PCCD) are incidental findings. Temporal bone CT is the preferred imaging modality though high resolution MRI proved equally sensitive/for SCCD (100%) but less specific 96.5% for SCCD and 99.1% for PCCD [50].

Conclusion

The most common arterial pathologies causing pulsatile tinnitus consist of dural arteriovenous malformation, vessel dissections involving the skull base or aneurysms. Paragangliomas and idiopathic intracranial hypertension are additional common entities. Imaging needs to be focused on the temporal bone and cover the entire head and neck once additional symptoms such as headache and blurred vison, a bruit in the neck or a pulsating neck mass require extension of the examination. CT is required in case of bony involvement or detailed assessment of the temporal bone, ossicular chain and osseus contour of the labyrinth. MR with TOF, 4D MRA and CE technique is preferred over CTA due to its variability in application and lack of radiation.

The causal relationship of "tinnitus" and anatomic variations either arterial (e.g. aberrant internal carotid artery, stapedial artery) or venous (highriding/dehiscent jugular bulb, sigmoid sinus dehiscence, jugular or sigmoid sinus diverticum) or dehiscent semicircular canals have to be questioned as a relevant entity- unless vascular flow conditions or the ICP have changed due to an additional local or systemic process. In other words, the search for the true explanation of tinnitus in case of anatomic variants in particular on the venous side has to be continued by non-invasive imaging to definitely exclude an underlying causative treatable pathology.

References

1. Hofmann E, Nadjmi M, Ratzka M, Schuknecht B. Pulse synchronous vascular tinnitus: radiologic diagnosis and therapy. HNO. 1987;35(5):211–8.
2. Langguth B, Kreuzer PM, Kleinjung T, De Ridder D. Tinnitus: causes and clinical management. Lancet Neurol. 2013;12(9):920–30.
3. Abdalkader M, Nguyen TN, Norbash AM, Raz E, Shapiro M, Lenck S, et al. State of the art: venous causes of pulsatile tinnitus and diagnostic considerations guiding endovascular therapy. Radiology. 2021;300(1):2–16.
4. Hofmann E, Behr R, Neumann-Haefelin T, Schwager K. Pulsatile tinnitus: imaging and differential diagnosis. Dtsch Arztebl Int. 2013;110(26):451–8.
5. Pegge SAH, Steens SCA, Kunst HPM, Meijer FJA. Pulsatile tinnitus: differential diagnosis and radiological work-up. Curr Radiol Rep. 2017;5(1):5.
6. Tao AJ, Parikh NS, Patsalides A. The role of noninvasive imaging in the diagnostic workup for pulsatile tinnitus. Neuroradiol J. 2021;35:19714009211036696.
7. Vattoth S, Shah R, Cure JK. A compartment-based approach for the imaging evaluation of tinnitus. AJNR Am J Neuroradiol. 2010;31(2):211–8.
8. Cummins DD, Caton MT, Shah V, Meisel K, Glastonbury C, Amans MR. MRI and MR angiography evaluation of pulsatile tinnitus: a focused, physiology-based protocol. J Neuroimaging. 2021;32:253.
9. Madani G, Connor SE. Imaging in pulsatile tinnitus. Clin Radiol. 2009;64(3):319–28.
10. Dietz RR, Davis WL, Harnsberger HR, Jacobs JM, Blatter DD. MR imaging and MR angiography in the evaluation of pulsatile tinnitus. AJNR Am J Neuroradiol. 1994;15(5):879–89.
11. Wang Y, Kao E, Zhang Y, Tian B, Gong J, Faraji F, et al. Shape-appearance constrained segmentation and separation of vein and artery in pulsatile tinnitus patients based on MR angiography and flow MRI. Magn Reson Imaging. 2019;61:187–95.
12. Kumar R, Rice S, Lingam RK. Detecting causes of pulsatile tinnitus on CT arteriography-venography: a pictorial review. Eur J Radiol. 2021;139:109722.
13. Cunnane MB. Imaging of tinnitus. Neuroimaging Clin N Am. 2019;29(1):49–56.
14. Waldvogel D, Mattle HP, Sturzenegger M, Schroth G. Pulsatile tinnitus—a review of 84 patients. J Neurol. 1998;245(3):137–42.
15. Touze E, Oppenheim C, Trystram D, Nokam G, Pasquini M, Alamowitch S, et al. Fibromuscular dysplasia of cervical and intracranial arteries. Int J Stroke. 2010;5(4):296–305.
16. Kadian-Dodov D, Gornik HL, Gu X, Froehlich J, Bacharach JM, Chi YW, et al. Dissection and aneurysm in patients with fibromuscular dysplasia: findings from the U.S. registry for FMD. J Am Coll Cardiol. 2016;68(2):176–85.
17. Baumgartner RW, Arnold M, Baumgartner I, Mosso M, Gonner F, Studer A, et al. Carotid dissection with and without ischemic events: local symptoms and cerebral artery findings. Neurology. 2001;57(5):827–32.
18. Marciniec M, Sapko K, Kulczynski M, Popek-Marciniec S, Szczepanska-Szerej A, Rejdak K. Non-traumatic cervical artery dissection and ischemic stroke: a narrative review of recent research. Clin Neurol Neurosurg. 2019;187:105561.
19. Lleva P, Ahluwalia BS, Marks S, Sahni R, Tenner M, Risucci DA, et al. Traumatic and spontaneous carotid and vertebral artery dissection in a level 1 trauma center. J Clin Neurosci. 2012;19(8):1112–4.
20. Adham S, Billon C, Legrand A, Domigo V, Denarie N, Charpentier E, et al. Spontaneous cervical artery dissection in vascular Ehlers-Danlos syndrome: a cohort study. Stroke. 2021;52(5):1628–35.
21. Kellert L, Kloss M, Pezzini A, Debette S, Leys D, Caso V, et al. Prognostic significance of pulsatile tinnitus in cervical artery dissection. Eur J Neurol. 2016;23(7):1183–7.
22. Chen L, Chen L, Jiang Y, Hu F, He L, Zheng H. Pulsatile tinnitus was the only manifestation of internal carotid artery dissection. Neurol Sci. 2021;42(3):1221–2.
23. Kim SM, Kim CH, Lee CY. Petrous carotid aneurysm causing pulsatile tinnitus: case report and review of the literature. J Cerebrovasc Endovasc Neurosurg. 2018;20(1):35–9.
24. Endo K, Maruyama Y, Tsukatani T, Furukawa M. Aberrant internal carotid artery as a cause of objective pulsatile tinnitus. Auris Nasus Larynx. 2006;33(4):447–50.
25. Nicolay S, De Foer B, Bernaerts A, Van Dinther J, Parizel PM. Aberrant internal carotid artery presenting as a retrotympanic vascular mass. Acta Radiol Short Rep. 2014;3(10):2047981614553695.
26. Reisser C, Schuknecht HF. The anterior inferior cerebellar artery in the internal auditory canal. Laryngoscope. 1991;101(7 Pt 1):761–6.
27. Ramly NA, Roslenda AR, Suraya A, Asma A. Vascular loop in the cerebellopontine angle causing pulsatile tinnitus and headache: a case report. EXCLI J. 2014;13:192–6.
28. Schuknecht HF. Myths in neurotology. Am J Otol. 1992;13(2):124–6.
29. de Abreu JL, Kuniyoshi CH, Wolosker AB, Borri ML, Antunes A, Ota VK, et al. Vascular loops in the anterior inferior cerebellar artery, as identified by magnetic resonance imaging, and their relationship with otologic symptoms. Radiol Bras. 2016;49(5):300–4.
30. Breda MS, Amorim J, Rocha J, Dias L. Vertebro-vertebral fistula presenting as a pulsatile tinnitus. BMJ Case Rep. 2018;2018:2018.
31. Berenstein A, Scott J, Choi IS, Persky M. Percutaneous embolization of arteriovenous fistulas of the external carotid artery. AJNR Am J Neuroradiol. 1986;7(5):937–42.
32. Kreuzer PM, Landgrebe M, Vielsmeier V, Kleinjung T, De Ridder D, Langguth B. Trauma-associated tinnitus. J Head Trauma Rehabil. 2014;29(5):432–42.
33. Liang W, Xiaofeng Y, Weiguo L, Wusi Q, Gang S, Xuesheng Z. Traumatic carotid cavernous fistula accompanying basilar skull fracture: a study on the incidence of traumatic carotid cavernous fistula in the patients with basilar skull fracture and the prognostic analysis about traumatic carotid cavernous fistula. J Trauma. 2007;63(5):1014–20. discussion 20
34. Barrow DL, Spector RH, Braun IF, Landman JA, Tindall SC, Tindall GT. Classification and treatment of spontaneous carotid-cavernous sinus fistulas. J Neurosurg. 1985;62(2):248–56.
35. Williams ZR. Carotid-cavernous fistulae: a review of clinical presentation, therapeutic options, and visual prognosis. Int Ophthalmol Clin. 2018;58(2):271–94.
36. Gemmete JJ, Chaudhary N, Pandey A, Ansari S. Treatment of carotid cavernous fistulas. Curr Treat Options Neurol. 2010;12(1):43–53.
37. Cognard C, Gobin YP, Pierot L, Bailly AL, Houdart E, Casasco A, et al. Cerebral dural arteriovenous fistulas: clinical and angiographic correlation with a revised classification of venous drainage. Radiology. 1995;194(3):671–80.
38. Pingree GM, Fleming C, Reavey-Cantwell J, Coelho DH. Neurosurgical causes of pulsatile tinnitus: contemporary update. Neurosurgery. 2022;90(2):161–9.
39. An YH, Han S, Lee M, Rhee J, Kwon OK, Hwang G, et al. Dural arteriovenous fistula masquerading as pulsatile tinnitus: radiologic assessment and clinical implications. Sci Rep. 2016;6:36601.
40. Alkadhi H, Schuknecht B, Stoeckli SJ, Valavanis A. Evaluation of topography and vascularization of cervical paragangliomas by magnetic resonance imaging and color duplex sonography. Neuroradiology. 2002;44(1):83–90.
41. Yildiz E, Dahm V, Gstoettner W, Rossler K, Bauer B, Wressnegger A, et al. Long-term outcome and comparison of treatment modalities of temporal bone paragangliomas. Cancers (Basel). 2021;13(20):5083.

42. Sismanis A. Pulsatile tinnitus: contemporary assessment and management. Curr Opin Otolaryngol Head Neck Surg. 2011;19(5):348–57.
43. Lansley JA, Tucker W, Eriksen MR, Riordan-Eva P, Connor SEJ. Sigmoid sinus diverticulum, dehiscence, and venous sinus stenosis: potential causes of pulsatile tinnitus in patients with idiopathic intracranial hypertension? AJNR Am J Neuroradiol. 2017;38(9):1783–8.
44. Schoeff S, Nicholas B, Mukherjee S, Kesser BW. Imaging prevalence of sigmoid sinus dehiscence among patients with and without pulsatile tinnitus. Otolaryngol Head Neck Surg. 2014;150(5):841–6.
45. Friedmann DR, Eubig J, McGill M, Babb JS, Pramanik BK, Lalwani AK. Development of the jugular bulb: a radiologic study. Otol Neurotol. 2011;32(8):1389–95.
46. Eisenman DJ. Sinus wall reconstruction for sigmoid sinus diverticulum and dehiscence: a standardized surgical procedure for a range of radiographic findings. Otol Neurotol. 2011;32(7):1116–9.
47. Tunkel DE, Bauer CA, Sun GH, Rosenfeld RM, Chandrasekhar SS, Cunningham ER Jr, et al. Clinical practice guideline: tinnitus. Otolaryngol Head Neck Surg. 2014;151(2 Suppl):S1–S40.
48. Barath K, Schuknecht B, Naldi AM, Schrepfer T, Bockisch CJ, Hegemann SC. Detection and grading of endolymphatic hydrops in Meniere disease using MR imaging. AJNR Am J Neuroradiol. 2014;35(7):1387–92.
49. Bachinger D, Bruhlmann C, Honegger T, Michalopoulou E, Monge Naldi A, Wettstein VG, et al. Endotype-phenotype patterns in Meniere's disease based on gadolinium-enhanced MRI of the vestibular aqueduct. Front Neurol. 2019;10:303.
50. Browaeys P, Larson TL, Wong ML, Patel U. Can MRI replace CT in evaluating semicircular canal dehiscence? AJNR Am J Neuroradiol. 2013;34(7):1421–7.

31 Clinical Assessment of the Somatosensory System

Tanit Ganz Sanchez and Sarah Michiels

Abstract

Patients with somatosensory tinnitus have received growing attention. Researchers and clinicians have been identifying a group of specific characteristics in such patients that pose it as a subtype of subjective tinnitus.

Multiple interactions between the somatosensory and auditory systems have been studied so far, showing that different somatosensory stimuli can temporarily influence tinnitus perception, either by changing its loudness, pitch or location.

Such influence may be induced through muscle contractions of head and neck muscles, pressure of myofascial trigger points, tactile stimulation of the skin, among others.

Considering the importance of interdisciplinary management of tinnitus patients, health professionals involved with providing the first-line attendance for patients with tinnitus should differentiate this specific subgroup of subjects presenting somatosensory tinnitus.

This chapter will show the updated criteria for diagnosing somatosensory tinnitus from medical and audiological point of view, providing practical information to the professionals. Diagnosing it by means of specific information collected during history taking and physical examination is likely to optimize referral of such patients to therapeutic options focused on treating musculoskeletal disorders.

T. G. Sanchez (✉)
Otolaryngology Department, University of São Paulo Medical School, São Paulo, Brazil
e-mail: tanitsanchez@usp.br

S. Michiels
Musculoskeletal Rehabilitation, REVAL Rehabilitation Research Center, Faculty of Rehabilitation Sciences and Physiotherapy, Hasselt University, Diepenbeek, Belgium
e-mail: sarah.michiels@uhasselt.be

W. Schlee et al. (eds.), *Textbook of Tinnitus*, https://doi.org/10.1007/978-3-031-35647-6_31

Graphical Abstract

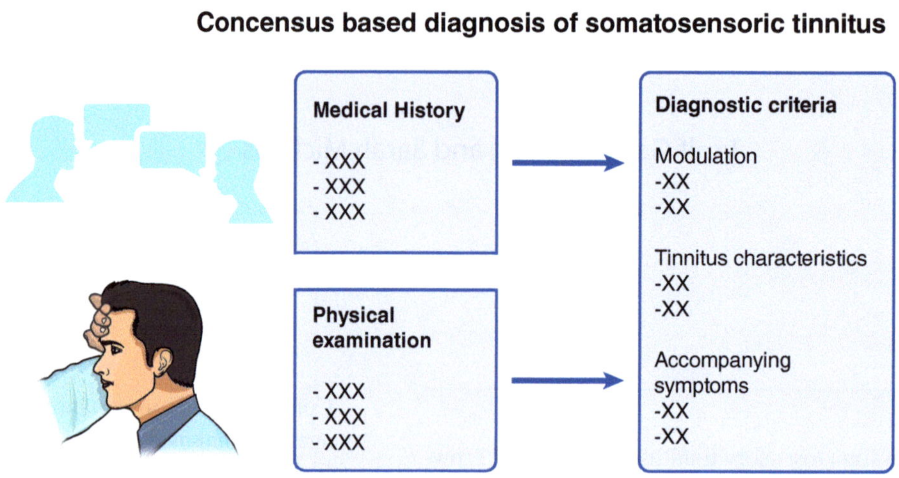

Highlights

- The understanding of the interactions between the somatosensory and auditory systems has been growing quickly, as different somatosensory stimuli can influence tinnitus loudness or pitch.
- Such influence may be detected through muscle contractions of head and neck muscles, pressure of myofascial trigger points, tactile stimulation of the skin, among others. This is the so-called somatosensory tinnitus, which is a subtype of subjective tinnitus.
- This chapter will discuss the diagnosis of somatosensory tinnitus from medical and audiological point of view, providing practical information to the professionals.

Interactions Between Somatosensory and Auditory Pathways

Most tinnitus cases are related to cochlear damages that trigger neural changes upwards in the central auditory system [1]. However, other systems than the auditory pathways may be involved in triggering or modulating tinnitus, such as the somatosensory, somatomotor and visual-motor systems.

Up to two thirds of patients notice that their tinnitus is somehow influenced by stimuli that are not related to sounds, such as forceful muscle contractions of head, neck and limbs [2–4], pressure of myofascial trigger points (MTP) [5], eye or orofacial movements [6–9], and cutaneous stimulation of the face and hands [6], among other stimuli. This chapter will focus on the influence that head and neck regions may exert on the auditory pathways.

The somatosensory system detects and allows the conscious perception of many experiences such as head and body position and movement, as well as temperature, touch (pressure, vibration) and pain (itch and tickle).

The primary receptor surface for the somatosensory system is spread in the skin, but also in muscles, tendons, fascia and joints. These structures relay sensations detected in the periphery of the body and convey them upwards through the spinal cord or cranial nerves, brainstem and thalamus to the sensory cortex in the parietal lobe [10].

There exist several interactions between the sensory and auditory pathways in the brain with the cochlear nucleus being the main structure to integrate afferent projections from the auditory nerve and those coming from the somatosensory system via trigeminal and dorsal column ganglia. From the cochlear nucleus, the information is further transmitted along the central auditory pathways (see details in Singer et al. 2013 [11] and Li et al. 2013 [12]).

The balance of integration between auditory and somatosensoric afferents may be disrupted in people with hearing damage. Animal studies have shown that a decrease of auditory input to the cochlear nucleus after cochlear damage results in upregulation of the influence of somatosensory inputs on neuronal activity in central auditory pathways [13, 14].

This increased influence of somatosensory input on central auditory pathways may be the neuronal correlate of the clinical observation that head or neck movements can modulate loudness and/or pitch of tinnitus. This modulation occurs in up to 2/3 of patients and may come from touching and moving the head, jaw or neck areas or by having increased muscle tension or restricted mobility in these regions.

This is known as somatosensory tinnitus (ST) which is a subtype of subjective tinnitus. In such cases, the altered somatosensory afference is able to cause or to modulate a given tinnitus perception.

A Timeline Optimization of the Diagnosis of Somatosensory Tinnitus (ST)

Typically, physicians (general practitioners, otolaryngologists, neurologists) and audiologists are the front-line professionals searched by the tinnitus patients, although a larger group of health professionals can contribute in clinical practice. Due to the involvement of jaw and neck in this subgroup of somatosensory tinnitus, rather than solely the auditory pathway, it is recommended that experienced dentists, physiotherapists and/or manual therapists (following regional differences) become also involved in the evaluation and treatment of such patients (see Chap. 37 about Treatment).

Despite the advances shown in literature, tinnitus remains seen as a non-treatable symptom and many professionals tell patients that "there is nothing to do" or that "you have to learn to live with it". Even if there exists no universally effective treatment for reducing tinnitus loudness, there is increasing consensus in the field that there exist different forms of tinnitus, which requires a more individualized treatment approach (see Chap. 7). Thus, it is worth to establish specific protocols for both diagnosis and treatment of ST, and this chapter provides a timeline for assessing such patients.

In the first edition of this 'Textbook of Tinnitus', Sanchez & Rocha, 2011, suggested a set of criteria based on patient's medical history to help diagnosing somatosensory tinnitus for diverse clinicians such as:

1. Evident history of head or neck trauma
2. Tinnitus associated with previous manipulation of teeth, jaw or cervical spine
3. Recurrent pain episodes of head, neck or shoulder girdle
4. Temporal coincidence between onset or increase of both pain and tinnitus
5. Increase of tinnitus during inadequate postures of resting, walking, working or sleeping
6. Intense bruxism periods during the day or night
7. Audiogram with symmetric pure tone thresholds in both ears (normal or abnormal) and unilateral or asymmetric tinnitus

An additional criterion is the presence of somatosensory modulation of tinnitus (immediate and temporary changes in loudness, pitch, or location that manifest during somatosensory stimulation in 65–80% of the patients [2, 5, 15–19]).

Recently, an effort has been made to establish consensus on diagnostic criteria for somatosensory tinnitus among experts worldwide to serve as a guideline for clinicians across all disciplines [20].

By conducting a systematic review of the literature, followed by a modified two-round Delphi survey and an in-person consensus meeting, the experts in ST agreed with the diagnostic criteria given by Sanchez & Rocha [16], and proposed a list of certain features that, when present, would strongly suggest a somatosensory influence on tinnitus but, when absent, would not rule out such influence (Tables 31.1, 31.2 and 31.3).

Later on, these criteria were further investigated in a group of 8221 patients with somatosensory and non-somatosensory tinnitus, in order to validate them empirically and identify their individual diagnostic value [21].

In general, the pre-test probability of somatosensory tinnitus diagnosis was 26%. However, this probability increased for each criterion that was present, and decreased with its absence, as shown below:

Table 31.1 Types of tinnitus modulation that strongly suggest somatosensory influence (adapted from Michiels et al. 2018 [20])

Criteria on tinnitus modulation Tinnitus modulation
• Evoked by voluntary movement of the head, neck and jaw
• Evoked by somatic maneuvers applied by professionals
• Evoked by pressure on myofascial trigger points

Table 31.2 Tinnitus characteristics that strongly suggest somatosensory influence (adapted from Michiels et al. 2018 [20])

Tinnitus characteristics
• Tinnitus and neck/jaw pain complaints appeared simultaneously
• Tinnitus and neck/jaw pain symptoms aggravate simultaneously
• Tinnitus is preceded by a head or neck trauma
• Tinnitus increases during bad postures
• Tinnitus pitch, loudness and/or location are reported to vary
• In case of unilateral tinnitus, audiogram does not show a correspondent hearing loss

Table 31.3 Accompanying symptoms that strongly suggest somatosensory influence of tinnitus (adapted from Michiels et al. 2018 [20])

Accompanying symptoms
• Frequent pain in the cervical spine, head or shoulder girdle
• Presence of tender myofascial trigger points
• Increased muscle tension in the suboccipital muscles
• Increased muscle tension in the extensor muscles of the cervical spine
• Temporomandibular disorders
• Teeth clenching or bruxism
• Dental diseases

The presence of:

(a) 'simultaneous increase of both tinnitus and neck / jaw pain' increased the probability of ST diagnosis to 79% (positive likelihood ratio + LR: 10.72).
(b) 'simultaneous onset' increased the probability to 69% (+LR: 6.29).
(c) 'influence of certain postures' increased the probability to 68% (+LR: 6.04).
(d) 'myofascial trigger points', 'head or neck trauma' and 'TMD diagnosis' increased the probability to just above 50%.

The absence of:

(a) 'neck pain' decreased the probability to 18% (−LR: 0.63).
(b) 'tension in the neck extensor muscles' decreased the probability to 19% (−LR: 0.63).

Interestingly, the presence of 'somatosensory modulation during voluntary movements' showed high specificity (82%) and low sensitivity (32%), but did not largely influence the probability of ST diagnosis (+LR: 1.81 and -LR: 0.82). Thus, the presence of somatosensory modulation (detailed below) should not be used as single criterion and its absence should not rule out ST diagnosis [21].

The presence of somatosensory modulation can be tested through different maneuvers, each one being sustained for 5 to 10 s in a silent environment, so as to ease the perception of changes in tinnitus parameters (loudness or pitch):

1. Maneuvers involving the temporomandibular joint (expected to increase the signals elicited by the tense muscles in the area innervated by the sensory part of the trigeminal nerve).
   (a) Active jaw movements (with and without resistance by the examiner): opening and closing, moving chin forward and backward, lateralizing chin to the right and left (Fig. 31.1).
   (b) Passive muscular palpation in order to search for myofascial trigger points (MTP) or tender points: masseter, temporalis and lateral pterygoid (Fig. 31.2).
   (c) Fatigue test (teeth closed with spatula between them in anterior, right and left positions during 1 min).
2. Maneuvers involving the neck:
   (a) Active neck movements (with and without resistance by the examiner): moving neck forward and backward, rotation to the right and left, and lateralization to the right and left (Figs. 31.3 and 31.4).
   (b) Passive muscular palpation in order to search for myofascial trigger points (MTP) or tender points: trapezius (upper fibers), sternocleidomastoid (sternal division), splenius capitis (near the mastoid process), and splenius cervicis. (Fig. 31.5).

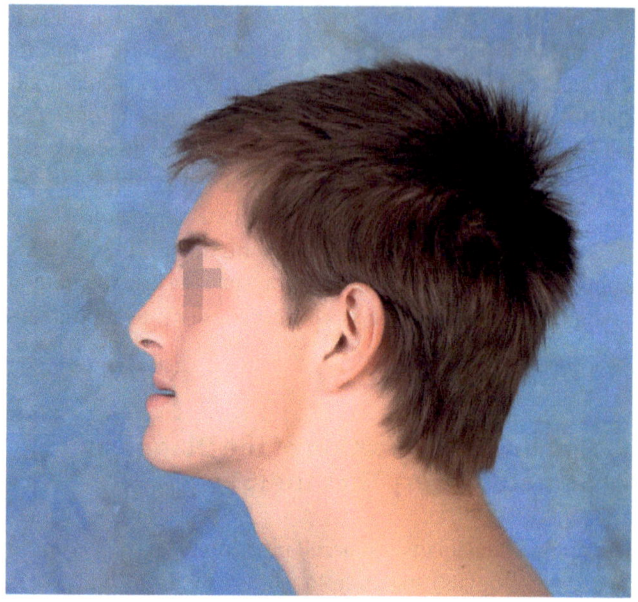

Fig. 31.1 Testing the presence of somatosensory modulation through an active jaw movement: moving chin forward (from Dr. Eberhard Biesinger)

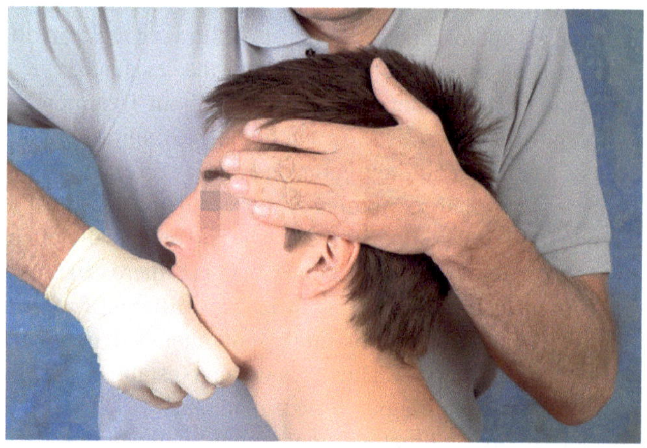

Fig. 31.2 Testing the presence of somatosensory modulation through passive muscular palpation in order to search for myofascial trigger points (from Dr. Eberhard Biesinger)

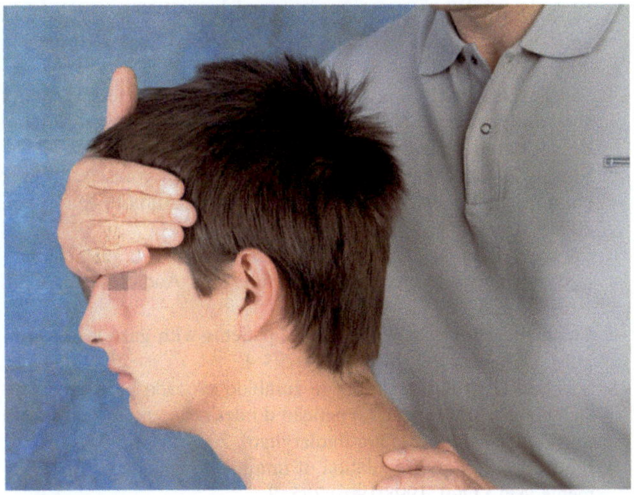

Fig. 31.3 Testing the presence of somatosensory modulation through an active neck movement with resistance by the examiner: moving neck forward (donated by Dr. Eberhard Biesinger)

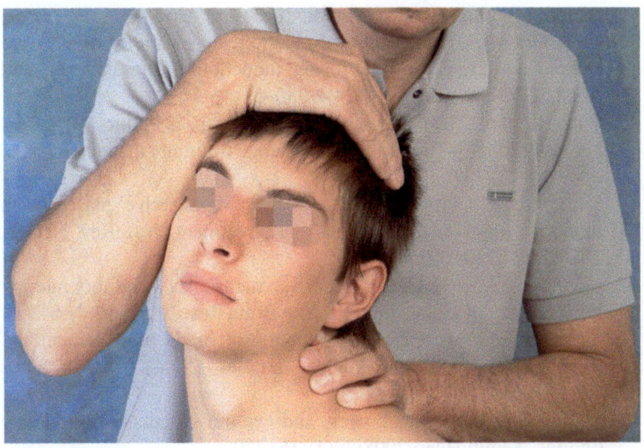

Fig. 31.4 Testing the presence of somatosensory modulation through an active neck movement with resistance by the examiner: rotating neck to the left (from Dr. Eberhard Biesinger)

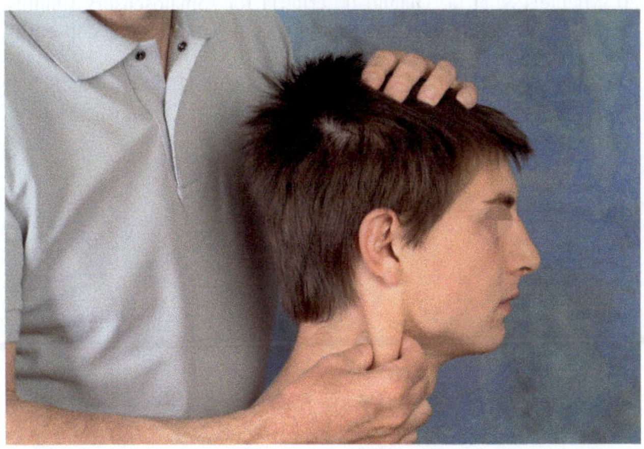

Fig. 31.5 Testing the presence of somatosensory modulation through passive muscular palpation to search for myofascial trigger points or tender points: sternocleidomastoid (from Dr. Eberhard Biesinger)

An Illustrated Case Report with Several Somatosensory Stimuli Over Tinnitus Loudness

More than one stimulus can trigger tinnitus modulation in the same subject. The patient reported below showed a complex and unique combination of somatosensory modulation, providing evidence for the multimodal nature of tinnitus generators (presented at II Meeting of Tinnitus Research Initiative).

"RTG, male, 54 years old, engineer, has noticed constant bilateral tinnitus 4 years before the appointment, worse on the left ear (Visual Analogue Scale = 10; Tinnitus Handicap Inventory = 62). Moreover, he complained of bilateral hearing loss (20 years), worse on the left ear. Previous complementary exams brought for the first visit included the following: (1) audiometry with bilateral sensorineural hearing loss, worse in the left ear. Tinnitus pitch was 12 kHz and loudness was detected due to the poor threshold at this frequency; (2) normal blood biochemistry; (3) temporal bone CT scan indicating bilateral non-dehiscent high jugular bulb; and (4) normal magnetic resonance imaging. Physical exam was normal, but his tinnitus presented a specific and repeatable pattern of temporary modulation with tactile stimulation of the head (Fig. 31.6):

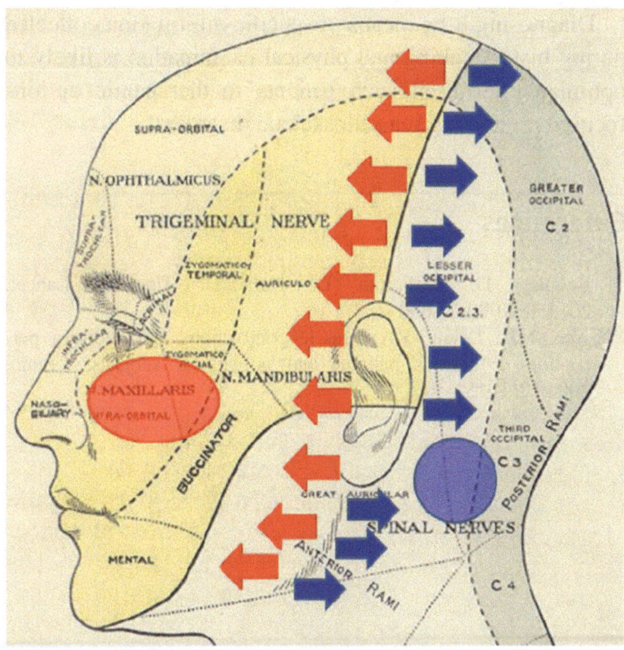

Fig. 31.6 Schematic distribution of diverse somatosensory modulation of tinnitus in a male patient. Red arrows represent areas where palpation evokes worsening of tinnitus; red oval represents area where palpation evokes the worst increase of tinnitus; blue arrows represent areas where palpation evokes reduction of tinnitus; and blue circle represents area where palpation evokes the maximum relief of tinnitus

- Slight worsening when he touched the left portion of his face in the corresponding area innervated by the three branches of trigeminal nerve, mainly in the maxillary branch. When the tactile stimulus was changed to pressuring the same region, he complained of a greater worsening as opposed to when he had merely touched it.
- Improvement with tactile stimuli in ipsilateral postauricular area following a similar pattern: a slight improvement during touching and a greater improvement after pressuring the region (VAS score decreased to 2).
- Modulation through muscular contractions: (a) improvement with head rotation to the right and left and (b) maximum opening of the mouth and clenching teeth produced bilateral improvement, and mandible lateralization to the right or to left improved only tinnitus contralateral to the maneuver.

Conclusions

Evidence has been pointing towards high prevalence of somatosensory tinnitus among tinnitus patients.

Considering the importance of interdisciplinary management of tinnitus patients, health professionals involved with providing the first-line attendance for patients with tinnitus should differentiate this specific subgroup of subjects presenting somatosensory tinnitus.

Diagnosing it by means of specific information collected during history taking and physical examination is likely to optimize referral of such patients to therapeutic options focused on treating musculoskeletal disorders.

References

1. Baguley D, McFerran D, Hall D. Tinnitus. Lancet. 2013;382(9904):1600–7.
2. Abel MD, Levine RA. Muscle contractions and auditory perception in tinnitus patients and nonclinical subjects. Cranio. 2004;22(3):181–91.
3. Sanchez TG, et al. The influence of voluntary muscle contractions upon the onset and modulation of tinnitus. Audiol Neuro Otol. 2002;7(6):370–5.
4. Sanchez TG, et al. Somatic modulation of tinnitus: test reliability and results after repetitive muscle contraction training. Ann Otol Rhinol Laryngol. 2007;116(1):30–5.
5. Rocha C, Sanchez TG, de Siqueira JTT. Myofascial trigger point: a possible way of modulating tinnitus. Audiol Neuro Otol. 2008;13(3):153–60.
6. Cacace AT, et al. Cutaneous-evoked tinnitus - I. phenomenology, psychophysics and functional imaging. Audiol Neuro Otol. 1999;4(5):247–57.
7. Coad ML, et al. Characteristics of patients with gaze-evoked tinnitus. Otol Neurotol. 2001;22(5):650–4.
8. Sanchez TP. MRB Abolição de zumbido evocado pela movimentação ocular por meio de repetição do deslocamento do olhar: um método inovador. Arq Otorhinolaryngol. 2007;11:451–3.
9. Pinchoff RJ, et al. Modulation of tinnitus by voluntary jaw movements. Am J Otol. 1998;19(6):785–9.
10. Kreutzer JS, Caplan B, et al. Somatosensory system. In: Kreutzer JS, Caplan B, et al., editors. Encyclopedia of clinical neuropsychology. New York, NY: Springer; 2011.
11. Singer W, et al. Noise-induced inner hair cell ribbon loss disturbs central arc mobilization: a novel molecular paradigm for understanding tinnitus. Mol Neurobiol. 2013;47(1):261–79.
12. Li S, Choi V, Tzounopoulos T. Pathogenic plasticity of Kv7.2/3 channel activity is essential for the induction of tinnitus. Proc Natl Acad Sci U S A. 2013;110(24):9980–5.
13. Wang H, et al. Plasticity at glycinergic synapses in dorsal cochlear nucleus of rats with behavioral evidence of tinnitus. Neuroscience. 2009;164(2):747–59.
14. Shore SE, Roberts LE, Langguth B. Maladaptive plasticity in tinnitus—triggers, mechanisms and treatment. Nat Rev Neurol. 2016;12(3):150–60.
15. Levine RA, Abel M, Cheng H. CNS somatosensory-auditory interactions elicit or modulate tinnitus. Exp Brain Res. 2003;153(4):643–8.
16. Sanchez TG, Rocha CB. Diagnosis and management of somatosensory tinnitus: review article. Clinics (Sao Paulo). 2011;66(6):1089–94.
17. Simmons R, et al. Head, neck, and eye movements that modulate tinnitus. Semin Hear. 2008;29(4):361–70.
18. Biesinger E, et al. Somatosensoric tinnitus. HNO. 2015;63(4):266–71.
19. Ward J, et al. Subtyping somatic tinnitus: a cross-sectional UK cohort study of demographic, clinical and audiological characteristics. PLoS One. 2015;10(5):e0126254.
20. Michiels S, et al. Diagnostic criteria for somatosensory tinnitus: a Delphi process and face-to-face meeting to establish consensus. Trends Hear. 2018;22:2331216518796403.
21. Michiels S, Cardon E, Gilles A, Goedhart H, Vesala M, Schlee W. Somatosensory tinnitus diagnosis. Part 1: Diagnostic value of existing criteria. Ear Hear. 2021;43(1):143.

Part VI

Management of Specific Forms of Tinnitus

Conductive and Sensorineural Hearing Loss

32

Tobias Kleinjung and Alain Londero

Abstract

Hearing loss is the symptom most commonly seen in association with tinnitus. According to the various models of tinnitus development, hearing loss also represents the crucial trigger mechanism for the development of tinnitus. Since different structures such as the outer ear, the middle ear and the inner ear are involved in the peripheral hearing process, a distinction is also made between conductive hearing loss, sensorineural hearing loss and retrocochlear hearing loss, depending on the localization of the pathology. This chapter highlights the main causes of conductive hearing loss and sensorineural hearing loss. A detailed clarification of the causes of hearing loss in tinnitus is important, as in many cases this also leads to specific therapies, which ideally will result in an improvement of hearing loss and tinnitus symptoms. In the case of middle ear hearing loss, these therapeutic approaches are primarily surgical in nature (tympanoplasty, stapes surgery), in the case of sensorineural hearing loss, the improvement is generally based on a prosthetic fitting with hearing aids or cochlear implants.

T. Kleinjung (✉)
Department of Otorhinolaryngology—Head and Neck Surgery, University Hospital of Zurich, University of Zurich, Zurich, Switzerland
e-mail: tobias.kleinjung@usz.ch

A. Londero
Service ORL et CCF, Hôpital Européen Georges Pompidou, Assistance Publique—Hôpitaux de Paris, Faculté de Médecine Paris Descartes—Université de Paris, Paris, France

W. Schlee et al. (eds.), *Textbook of Tinnitus*, https://doi.org/10.1007/978-3-031-35647-6_32

Graphical Abstract

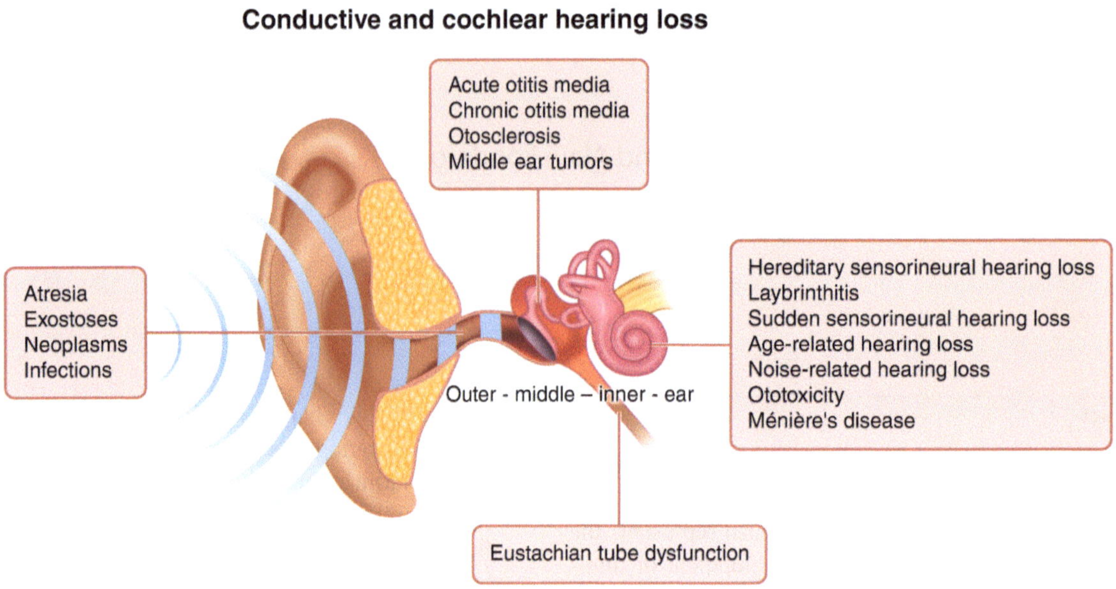

Abbreviations

AIED	Autoimmune inner ear disease
AOM	Acute otitis media
ET	Eustachian tube
ETD	Eustachian tube dysfunction
NSHL	Non-syndromic hearing loss
SHL	Syndromic hearing loss
SSNHL	Sudden sensorineural hearing loss

Highlights

- Hearing loss is the most frequent symptom associated with tinnitus.
- Most commonly the cause of a hearing loss is a lesion located in the peripheral auditory sensory organ: the ear.
- Conditions involving the external and middle ear generally induce a conductive hearing loss.
- Conditions involving the inner ear or the auditory nerve generally induce a sensorineural hearing loss.
- The accurate determination of the cause of the peripheral damage is relevant for tinnitus patients' management.
- Surgical restoration of hearing can improve tinnitus complaints in patients with tinnitus-associated hearing loss.
- New-onset tinnitus or worsening of a pre-existing tinnitus can occur as an unwanted side effect of middle-ear and inner-ear surgery.

Introduction

Even if not all patients displaying a hearing loss develop a subsequent tinnitus, it appears that the most frequent symptom associated with tinnitus is hearing loss [1]. Indeed, virtually any pathology involving the ear appears to have the capacity to cause both hearing loss and tinnitus. Further, tinnitus does not necessarily occur with the onset of hearing loss, but can also occur at any time later [2]. Moreover, a correlation has been demonstrated between the tinnitus pitch and the frequency range of hearing loss [3, 4] and the type of hearing loss [5, 6]. Even in persons with a perceived normal peripheral hearing and regular hearing thresholds in the standard audiogram between 125 and 8000 Hz changes in the ultrahigh frequency range can be measured and related to the development of tinnitus [7]. Another theory for the development of tinnitus in subjects with normal audiograms is the presence of "hidden hearing loss". This may be a consequence of noise exposure, which does not (yet) result in hair cell loss and thus not in an altered hearing threshold, but to a loss of synaptic connections between inner hair cells and auditory nerve fibers (spiral ganglion type I neurons) in the cochlea [8–12]. Clinically, this may be reflected by hearing difficulties in conditions of speech-in-noise.

This highlights the crucial role of lesions in the external, middle or inner ear for the emergence of tinnitus. Pathologies involving the external ear and middle ear generally lead to conductive hearing loss whereas lesions of the cochlea generally induce sensorineural hearing loss. Conductive hearing loss is due to an abnormal conduction of the sound waves through ear canal, eardrum or ossicles to the inner ear, in which the capacity to process the auditory input is preserved [13]. Sensorineural hearing loss is due to a dysfunction of the inner ear (inner and outer hair cells, first synapse with the auditory nerve) in which a sound wave passing normally though the external and middle ear is not converted to an appropriate nerve signal in the inner ear. These two types of hearing deficits may occur together in a variety of clinical situations (e.g. chronic otitis media may cause both conductive and sensorineural hearing loss). According to the currently most widely accepted pathophysiological models of tinnitus [14, 15] (see also Causes of Sensorineural Hearing Loss), chronic tinnitus cannot be sufficiently explained as a direct consequence of peripheral hearing loss. Tinnitus would rather be a consequence of a central maladaptive plasticity triggered by the sensory deprivation caused by these various forms of hearing loss (see Causes of Sensorineural Hearing Loss). Indeed, an unusually silent environment has been proven to induce a tinnitus percept [16, 17]. It has also been shown that reducing auditory input by wearing an earplug for a prolonged period of time can elicit a tinnitus [18]. The effect of conductive hearing loss would be analogous to the effect of wearing an earplug. It has also been suggested that long standing conductive hearing loss may have detrimental and long-term consequences on central auditory processing, especially when it occurs during critical periods of development in children [19]. On the other hand, the pathophysiological mechanisms explaining tinnitus associated with a sensorineural hearing loss may be even more complex, involving imbalances between inner and outer hair cells [20], and synaptic dysfunction [21]. In most cases, tinnitus that occurs together with hearing loss is subjective tinnitus. It is only rarely that an objective tinnitus, generally due to vascular turbulence, may be associated with hearing loss. In this case, the vascular lesion is located adjacent to the eardrum or the middle ear (e.g. intratympanic glomus tumor or extended glomus jugulare tumor) [22] (see Chap. 40).

Knowledge of the pathology of the hearing loss is significant, as appropriate therapy may also lead to improvement or even disappearance of tinnitus symptoms. Regarding treatment, the type of therapy depends on the type of hearing loss. In the case of sensorineural hearing loss, therapy usually involves instrumental techniques (hearing aid and cochlear implant). Many forms of conductive hearing loss, however, can be successfully treated by surgical interventions, leading to an improvement of hearing and potentially to a decrease or even disappearance of tinnitus.

Causes of Conductive Hearing Loss

Pathologies of the External Auditory Canal

Pathologies of the external auditory canal (or external acoustic meatus) leading to conductive hearing loss with subsequent tinnitus can be of a mechanical, inflammatory, or neoplastic nature. Genetic factors as well as exogenous noxious agents (e.g. thalidomide [23] or retinoid [24] embryopathy) may be involved in the development of auditory canal anomalies. Congenital changes resulting in partial occlusion or atresia of the external auditory canal cause hearing loss and possibly tinnitus. Severe forms may be accompanied by an auricular birth defect in addition to complete atresia of the external auditory canal. As syndromic components, external ear anomalies may occur in association with further dysmorphologies; for example, mid-facial dysplasia (mandibulofacial dysostosis, Treacher Collins syndrome [25]) or craniofacial dysostoses (Crouzon syndrome [26]). These anomalies may be accompanied by an additional anomaly of the middle ear that can be detected by high-resolution computed tomography [27]. Far more frequently, obstruction of the external auditory canal by wax is a mundane reason for the sudden onset of hearing loss and tinnitus. In addition, auditory canal blockage caused by inflammation (e.g. dermatitis, swimmer's otitis) may cause very painful swelling, redness, and discharge from the external auditory canal due to bacterial (Pseudomonas aeruginosa, Staphylococcus aureus) or, more rarely, fungal infection [28]. It is important to note that all procedures, especially suction, which aim to clear the ear canal of cerumen debris and secretions (wax, clotted blood, and purulent discharge) may induce tinnitus due to eardrum lesion or noise trauma [29, 30]. Neoplastic disorders leading to increasing stenosis and eventual occlusion of the external auditory canal may be benign or malignant. Exostoses[1] of the external auditory canal are benign new bone formations that occur with an incidence of 3–6% [31]. They may cause recurrent inflammation of the external ear canal with conductive hearing loss and transient tinnitus. Aside from constitutional factors, repeated thermal irritation of the external auditory canal by frequent contact with cold water (swimmer's ear and surfer's ear) has long been regarded as a predisposing factor [32]. Malignant neoplasms of the external auditory canal are far less common. These may arise from skin cells (basal cell carcinoma, squamous cell carcinoma,

[1]Exostosis: A cartilage-capped bony projection arising from any bone that develops from cartilage. Stedman's Electronic Medical Dictionary.

and malignant melanoma) or in the ceruminous glands (adenocarcinoma and adenoid cystic carcinoma) [33].

Surgery of the external auditory canal is required when space-occupying lesions either partially or completely block the external auditory canal and lead to conductive hearing loss [34]. This applies both to benign tumors, such as auditory canal exostoses, and to malignant tumors. If normal hearing is restored after uncomplicated healing, tinnitus that may have been present preoperatively can be expected to resolve partially or even completely.

Pathologies of the Middle Ear

Eustachian Tube Dysfunction

Pathologies of the middle ear leading to conductive hearing loss with subsequent tinnitus can be mechanical, inflammatory, traumatic or neoplastic in nature. Eustachian tube dysfunction (ETD) leads to impairment of the function of the middle ear [35]. Disturbances affecting the opening of the Eustachian tube (ET) are an important factor in the pathogenesis of many middle-ear conditions because the ventilation and drainage of the middle ear becomes dysfunctional [36]. The sequelae may include chronic mucoid otitis media (glue ear), recurrent acute otitis media, or chronic otitis media and eventually cholesteatoma. Eustachian tube opening dysfunction (ETD) may be caused by mechanical blockage of the tubal orifice in the nasopharynx (adenoids, tumor), by inflammatory swelling of the tubal mucosa, or by muscular insufficiency such as may occur in individuals with cleft palate [37, 38]. Conductive hearing loss, sometimes accompanied by tinnitus, may develop subsequent to ETD.

Myringotomy, followed by aspiration of fluid build-up in the middle ear and insertion of a small tube in the opening of the tympanic membrane, brings immediate relief of symptoms in cases of otitis media with effusion. This procedure may also result in remission of tinnitus along with a reduction of aural fullness and conductive hearing loss. Myringotomy, with or without tube insertion, can also positively influence the course of acute otitis media that does not respond favorably to pharmacological therapy [39]. In recent years, endoscopic balloon dilatation of the ET has become increasingly popular for the treatment of ETD [40]. This treatment approach is considered when ETD cannot be influenced in the long term by medication (topical or systemic decongestants and steroids) or by repeated myringotomies with or without tube insertions.

Conversely, patulous Eustachian tube is a relatively rare condition in which there is a permanently open connection between the middle ear and the nasopharynx through the Eustachian tube [41, 42]. This condition may entail a variety of symptoms, such as autophony (i.e. abnormal resonance of one's own voice and perception of one's own respiratory sounds), aural fullness and tinnitus. Reduced muscle tonus and weight loss are the main predisposing factors to the development of patulous Eustachian tube [43].

In addition to medical management, different surgical procedures which aim to close the abnormally open Eustachian tube have been proposed [44]. Several surgical methods have likewise been reported, including ventilation tube insertion, mass loading of the tympanic membrane, injection into the ET submucosa, shim surgery, plug surgery, ET reconstruction, and permanent ET closure [45].

Acute Otitis Media

Acute otitis media (AOM) is an inflammatory disease that often occurs secondary to rhinitis or pharyngitis. Common organisms that cause otitis media are Streptococci, Haemophilus influenzae, and Staphylococci [46]. The main symptoms are earache and hearing loss but tinnitus may occur as an additional symptom in many cases. The tinnitus may be objective, having a vascular origin, and may be perceived as a pulsatile pounding and/or buzzing sounds that are associated with the dilatation of vessels and high pulse amplitude of blood flow in the acute inflammatory stage. Antibiotics are the classical treatment of uncomplicated AOM in adults, and initial antibiotic choice is oriented to the most common causative pathogens. The antibiotics are usually administered systemically, but can also be added as ear drops if the tympanic membrane becomes perforated during the course of infection. Further therapy includes adequate pain management and decongestant medications.

Chronic Otitis Media

Chronic otitis media is an umbrella term that covers several different middle-ear pathologies. If the condition lasts several years, the extent of irreversible tissue destruction in the middle ear can differ substantially [47]. In addition to perforation of the eardrum and defects in the ossicular chain, enzymatic degradation processes associated with cholesteatoma[2] may occur and may lead to destructive erosion of the bony walls of the middle ear toward the cranial base. The common consequence of these pathologies is increasing conductive hearing loss with recurrent mucous or purulent discharge. Individuals for whom cholesteatoma causes erosion of the bony walls of the structures of the labyrinth may also have sensorineural hearing loss and even deafness because the pathologies have spread to the cochlea.

[2]Cholesteatoma: Squamous metaplasia or extension of squamous cell epithelium inward to line an expanding cystic cavity that may involve the middle ear or mastoid, erode surrounding bone, and become filled with a mass of keratinized squamous cell epithelial debris, usually resulting from chronic otitis media. The lesion often contains cholesterol clefts surrounded by inflammatory and foreign body giant cells, hence the name cholesteatoma. Stedman's Electronic Medical Dictionary.

Tympanoplasty

An impressive variety of surgical procedures has been proposed to treat chronic otitis media and improve hearing. "Tympanoplasty" is the general term used to describe such surgical procedures [48]. Tympanoplasty includes repair of the tympanic membrane after a perforation, inspection of the ossicular chain and, if necessary, its reconstruction by ossiculoplasty, and treatment of any inflammatory lesion that may be present in the different anatomical parts of the middle ear (atrium, attic) or petrous bone (mastoid). A full and comprehensive overview of tympanoplasty indications and techniques is beyond the scope of this chapter. Wullstein [49], however, categorizes five types of tympanoplasty dependent on the extent of reconstruction involved, and the first three of these will be presented briefly here. Tympanoplasty Type I involves the restoration of the perforated tympanic membrane by grafting; this procedure is done when the ossicular chain is intact. In Type II and III procedures, ossiculoplasty is an integral part of tympanoplasty. Tympanoplasty Type II is a procedure in which the patient's own auditory ossicles (parts of the incus or the head of the malleus), that is, organic material, are used for the reconstruction. In tympanoplasty Type III, alloplastic materials are used. The defective ossicles are repaired using synthetic prostheses that either replace the incus and are placed on the intact stapedial head (partial ossicular replacement prosthesis, PORP), or replace both the incus and stapedial suprastructure and are placed directly on the intact stapes footplate (total ossicular replacement prosthesis, TORP). Tympanoplasty Types IV and V no longer play a role in middle-ear surgery today. The techniques of tympanoplasty have an application in the treatment of chronic otitis media. In chronic mesotympanic otitis media (chronic suppurative otitis media), reconstruction of the sound conduction mechanism is necessary in 20–25% of cases. In cholesteatoma, 80% of patients require tympanoplasty Type III. Depending on the underlying pathology, the chosen tympanoplasty technique may be combined with procedures involving the external auditory canal (e.g. canalplasty) and mastoid (e.g. mastoidectomy). It should be noted that techniques of tympanoplasty are also used to correct malformations of the middle ear or to treat traumatic lesions of the eardrum and ossicular chain. Since the advent of microscopic middle-ear surgery in the 1950s, many tympanoplasty techniques have been described. The techniques differ in terms of the approach (e.g. transcanal, endaural, and retroauricular), in the graft material used for tympanic membrane replacement (e.g. temporalis fascia and cartilage), and in the design of the prosthesis and materials used (e.g. homologous incus, hydroxyapatite, gold, and titanium). There have been only few publications reporting results regarding the relief of preoperative tinnitus (Table 32.1). Nevertheless, those results available show that approximately 30% of patients who have had tympanoplasty are no longer aware of their tinnitus. In two of the four listed studies, complete remission of tinnitus was achieved [50, 51] in about a third of patients and more than 40% had partial remission; 4–8% became worse (Table 32.1). The assessment offered by Helms in an older study from 1981 [52] showed that approximately a third of patients became worse. The improvement in tinnitus symptoms after surgery may be attributed primarily to closure of the air-bone gap [53, 54]. Accordingly, Lima Ada et al. [51] found a strong correlation between postoperative hearing improvement and the reduction in tinnitus. It is reasonable to assume that there were other causes than the conductive hearing loss those patients who continued to suffer from the tinnitus percept despite showing adequate hearing improvement [55]. Kim et al. [56] demonstrated in their study that the degree of tinnitus improvement after tympanoplasty could be predicted by the pre-operative air-bone gap. They concluded that patients whose preoperative air-bone gap was less than 15 dB showed no improvement in postoperative tinnitus by means of a visual analog scale and a tinnitus questionnaire, whereas patients with more than 15 dB air-bone gap demonstrated significant tinnitus improvement in the respective measures.

Table 32.1 Effects of tympanoplasty on tinnitus

	n	Complete remission	Partial remission	No change	Worse
Baba et al. [50]	151	24.5%	41.7%	25.9%	7.9%
Helms [52]	59	33.3%	N/A	33.3%	33.3%
Lima Ada et al. [51]	23	34.8%	47.8%	13%	4.3%
Kim et al. [54]	28	N/A	50%	39.3%	10.7%

Otosclerosis

Otosclerosis is a frequently occurring otologic pathology [57] that is characterized by abnormal bone remodeling in the otic capsule that causes stapedial ankylosis, which in turn induces conductive hearing loss and tinnitus [58, 59]. Otosclerosis is responsible for 5–9% of all hearing losses and 18–22% of all conductive hearing losses [60]. The condition is encountered almost exclusively in Whites, very rarely occurring in Asians and almost never in Blacks [61]. The female-to-male ratio is approximately 2:1. The precise etiology remains unclear [59, 62]. Alongside genetic factors [63], the role of inflammatory processes (localized measles virus infection of the otic capsule) [64], endocrine factors [65], and immunological disease [66] have been considered in the etiopathogenesis. Independent of sex and age, tinnitus is a concomitant symptom in 65–91% of individuals with otosclerosis [58, 60, 67]. Tinnitus develops in many individuals with otosclerosis years before the onset of noticeable hearing loss, and sometimes persists despite an optimal hearing outcome from surgical management. Otosclerotic processes may spread to the cochlea and that may be responsible for persisting tinnitus. This condition, labeled "cochlear otosclerosis" by many authors, causes signs of sensorineural hearing loss [68]. It is also associated with changes in the stria vascularis, the organ of Corti and the spiral ligaments, as demonstrated in histopathology and radiology studies [69–72]. Even if it is a labyrinthine anomaly, one should note here that superior semi-circular canal dehiscence (or Minor's syndrome) may cause a conductive hearing loss associated with tinnitus, vertigo and auditory distortions [73]. Minor's syndrome is a differential diagnosis of otosclerosis [74] along with other much rarer cochlear lesions that may cause conductive hearing loss (endolymphatic hydrops or Menière's disease, enlarged vestibular aqueduct syndrome, gusher syndrome, cochlear dehiscence, Paget's disease) [75].

Table 32.2 Effects of stapes surgery on tinnitus

	n	Complete remission	Partial remission	No change	Worse
Ayache et al. [86]	48	56.3%	27.1%	12.5%	4.2%
Da Silva Lima [158]	23	39.1%	56.5%	4.4%	0%
Gersdorff et al. [60]	50	64%	16%	14%	6%
Oliveira [159]	19	52.6%	37%	10.4%	0%
Ramsay et al. [160]	268	48.2%	33.2%	7.8%	10.8%
Sakai et al. [87]	22	27%	41%	27%	5%
Sparano et al.	40	52.5%	32.5%	12.5%	2.5%
Szymanski et al. [161]	149	73%	17%	10%	0%
Ismi et al. [162]	69	50%	11%	39%	0%

Stapes Surgery

Conductive hearing loss and tinnitus are the main symptoms of otosclerosis. With the development of microscopic middle-ear surgery in the 1950s, surgical mobilization of the stapes in otosclerosis became the focal point of interest among middle-ear surgeons. In 1958, Shea performed the first stapedectomy, in which the stapes was replaced by prosthesis [76]. In the following years, the technique of stapedotomy evolved into a standard procedure, in which only the suprastructure of the stapes is removed, a perforation of the footplate is made, and a piston prosthesis is attached to the long process of the incus extending into the perforation of the stapes footplate (for review, see [77]). The introduction of laser surgery permitted "no-touch" perforation of the stapes footplate [78]. However, a recent review looking at the use of lasers in stapes surgery concludes that there is a slightly higher risk of tinnitus development when using lasers for footplate fenestration compared to conventional surgical techniques [79]. The main objective of stapes surgery is to improve hearing and, therefore, most studies published in this area focus on the hearing improvements achieved through the different techniques [80–82]. Hearing is improved in about 90% of patients and approximately 60% of patients have an air-bone gap of between 0 and 10 dB. No improvement in hearing occurs in approximately 8% of patients and a deterioration of hearing loss, including deafness, occurs in 2% of patients. Only few studies regarding the effect on tinnitus from stapes surgery have been published but recent data suggest that the improvement in quality of life is largely explained by the decrease of tinnitus perception [83]. Table 32.2 provides a summary of comparable studies conducted since 1990, in which partial remission, complete remission and no change to the tinnitus was reported. Generally, complete remission of tinnitus was achieved in approximately half of patients following stapes surgery, whereas another 30% reported partial improvement. Taken together, approximately 80% of those who had stapes surgery benefited from the operation in terms of tinnitus improvement. Most of the remaining patients reported no change, and fewer than 5% reported worsening of their tinnitus.

Many studies have shown tinnitus improvement to be independent of hearing improvement [84], but one older study by Glasgold et al. [85] showed a correlation between hearing improvement and tinnitus improvement. Ayache et al. [86] found no difference in reduction of tinnitus between stapedotomy and stapedectomy. In contrast, Sakai et al. [87] and Gersdorff et al. [60] noted better results after stapedotomy than with stapedectomy. No significant correlations between sex, tinnitus frequency, tinnitus duration, or extent of hearing loss and the effect on the tinnitus from stapes surgery were reported [86]. It is therefore unlikely that these factors would have prognostic value for stapes operation. It remains unclear whether the positive effect on the tinnitus after stapes surgery is due to the improvement in hearing or to other factors related to mobilization of the fixed footplate. The fact that many patients already experience an improvement in tinnitus immediately after surgery (i.e. in a state when the auditory canal is packed) favor the latter hypothesis. A recent review looking at the effect of stapes surgery on tinnitus concluded that in 254 cases evaluated with otosclerosis, tinnitus improved in 85% of cases and hearing improved in 93% of cases [84]. Thus, it seems justified to mention the highly probable effect of tinnitus improvement when counseling patients with otosclerosis before surgery.

Traumatic Lesions

There are three causes of traumatic lesions affecting the eardrum and the middle ear: direct mechanical or thermal injury, a pressure wave in the external auditory canal, or a fracture of the lateral skull base (petrous portion of the temporal bone). Depending on the extent of hearing loss, the possibility of a concomitant injury to the ossicular chain or the cochlea must also be considered. In case of fracture or displacement of the oval or round niche, a leakage of inner-ear liquid also called perilymph fistulae [88] may be present, inducing a variety of fluctuating symptoms such as vertigo, hearing loss, sound distortion and tinnitus [89]. Head trauma with concussion may also cause hearing loss and tinnitus as a consequence of labyrinthine concussion [90, 91] (Chap. 38). Medical management as well as the previously described surgical tympanoplasty I, II and III procedures are used to treat eardrum or ossicular traumatic lesions [92].

Tumors of the Middle Ear

Tumors affecting the middle ear are rare. The glomus tumor (synonyms: paraganglioma, chemodectoma) is one kind of benign tumor of the middle ear that displays destructive growth. Two locations of glomus tumors occur: glomus tympanicum tumors, which are limited to the middle ear, and glomus jugulare tumors, which are lesions that affect both the middle ear and the bulb of the jugular vein [22]. In histological terms, the tumors consist of non-chromaffin paraganglionic cells along the course of cranial nerves IX and X. The majority of glomus tumors occur in adulthood, with a genetic vulnerability and a female predominance [93]. Clinical diagnosis of glomus tumors is generally based on the symptom triad of conductive hearing loss, pulsatile tinnitus, and a red middle-ear tumor that can be seen through the eardrum using otoscopy [94]. In some patients, pulsatile objective tinnitus can be detected objectively by inserting a stethoscope or microphone in the external auditory canal. The sound is probably produced by the formation of microvascular shunts within the tumor mass [95]. With increasing tumor infiltration into the jugular foramen, additional deficits related to caudal cranial nerves IX-XI may become evident. The treatment of glomus tumors is usually surgical. A complete tumor removal leads to a complete cessation of the pulse synchronous tinnitus. However, in a case of extensive glomus tumors of the middle ear, a radical surgical removal of structures of the middle ear (ossicles) or even of the inner ear may be necessary. This then leads to a postoperative deterioration of hearing up to deafness (Chap. 40). Facial nerve schwannoma is another—very rare—benign tumor affecting the middle ear, characterized by slowly progressive facial paralysis as well as conductive hearing loss. Granulomatosis with polyangiitis[3] [96], Langerhans cell histiocytosis[4], and sarcoidosis[5] [97] are among the tumor-like lesions that potentially involve the middle ear and are also accompanied by tinnitus, in addition to conductive hearing loss. Malignant tumors that may involve the middle ear are squamous cell carcinoma and adenoid cystic carcinoma and adenomas.

Causes of Sensorineural Hearing Loss

The causal factors responsible for the development of sensorineural hearing loss can be many and varied. Aside from congenital factors (Chap. 5), the etiology may include infectious diseases, autoimmune diseases, toxic lesions, noise-related injury, traumatic damage (Chap. 38), age-induced changes (presbycusis) and sudden sensorineural hearing loss (syn. Sudden deafness). Furthermore, fluctuating (mostly low frequency) sensorineural hearing loss is one of the three signs of Menière's disease (Chap. 33). Depending on the cause, the form of sensorineural hearing loss can be different and have varying severity. All forms of hearing loss may be accompanied by tinnitus of varying intensity. The following section will examine those forms of sensorineural hearing loss that are not further discussed in dedicated chapters.

Sensorineural Hearing Loss of Genetic Origin

Impairment of hearing is the most common sensorineural pathology affecting humans. Approximately half of all cases

[3]Granulomatosis with polyangiitis (formerly called Wegener's disease): a disease, occurring mainly in the fourth and fifth decades, characterized by necrotizing granulomas and ulceration of the upper respiratory tract, with purulent rhinorrhea, nasal obstruction, and sometimes with otorrhea, hemoptysis, pulmonary infiltration and cavitation, and fever; exophthalmos, involvement of the larynx and pharynx, and glomerulonephritis may occur; the underlying condition is a vasculitis affecting small vessels, and is possibly due to an immune disorder. Stedman's Online Medical Dictionary.

[4]Langerhans cell histiocytosis: A set of closely related disorders unified by a common proliferating element, the Langerhans cell. Three overlapping clinical syndromes are recognized: a single site disease (eosinophilic granuloma), a multifocal unisystem process (Hand-Schuller-Christian syndrome), and a multifocal, multisystem histiocytosis (Letterer-Siwe syndrome). Formerly, this process was known as histiocytosis X. Stedman's Online Medical Dictionary.

[5]Sarcoidosis: A systemic granulomatous disease of unknown cause, especially involving the lungs with resulting interstitial fibrosis, but also involving lymph nodes, skin, liver, spleen, eyes, phalangeal bones, and parotid glands; granulomas are composed of epithelioid and multinucleated giant cells with little or no necrosis. Stedman's Online Medical Dictionary.

of prelingual hearing impairment have a genetic cause [98]. A distinction is made between genetic hearing loss occurring as a component of a specific (genetic) syndrome (30%) and non-syndromic hearing loss that occurs in the absence of any other genetic diseases or developmental anomalies [99]. Syndromic hearing loss (SHL) can be inherited in an autosomal dominant, autosomal recessive, or X-linked manner [100], and can be associated with developmental anomalies of the inner ear or petrous portion of the temporal bone, as is the case in Mondini[6] or Scheibe[7] dysplasia. Frequently, there is also a link with other organic disorders, such as thyroid disease (Pendred syndrome), renal dysfunction (Alport syndrome), or eye disease (Usher syndrome) [100]. Children with Down's syndrome are more likely to have congenital permanent inner ear hearing loss than the general population, in which the prevalence is 1.2–1.7 per 1000 live births in the US (2019). From their teens onward, subjects with Down's syndrome are likely to develop degenerative cochlear changes, and most will have significant hearing loss by the age of 40 [101]. Of non-syndromic hearing loss (NSHL), 80% have autosomal recessive, 18% an autosomal dominant, and 2% an X-linked or mitochondrial inheritance pattern [102]. In the majority, a single gene defect leads to the phenotypical development of hearing loss, which may not have its onset until later in life. In recent years, many gene loci and mutations have been described that are responsible for various forms of hearing loss. For example, known mutations affect the GJB2 gene, which codes for connexin-26, and the GJB6 gene, which codes for connexin-30 [103] (also Chap. 5).

Infections

Inflammation of the cochlea may develop simultaneously with acute or chronic otitis media when bacteria enter the cochlea through the round or oval window, or may develop together with meningitis when bacteria enter the cochlea and the vestibular apparatus via the internal auditory canal, the cochlear aqueduct, or the vestibular aqueduct. The resulting sensorineural hearing loss is commonly accompanied by tinnitus. Because of the involvement of the vestibular apparatus, the symptoms are often dominated by pronounced rotatory vertigo accompanied by nausea and vomiting. After meningitis, it is often the case that the cochlea is filled with bone (labyrinthitis ossificans or "white cochlea"), with complete obstruction of the membranous labyrinth [104]. The bacteria in borreliosis or syphilis can spread via blood to the inner ear. Many kinds of infections can cause damage to the cochlea or the inner ear as a whole [105]. Congenital rubella or cytomegalovirus infections are especially serious, and may lead to severe sensorineural hearing loss or deafness. Of the post-natal viral infections of the inner ear, epidemic parotitis (mumps) typically causes unilateral deafness without vestibular involvement. Herpes zoster oticus that is caused by re-infection with the varicella zoster virus can cause blisters in the external auditory canal and the pinna in addition to sensorineural hearing loss and tinnitus, vestibular symptoms, and facial nerve palsy. When the facial nerve is involved, the condition is known as Ramsey Hunt syndrome [106]. In addition to infection of the nerve sheaths, the symptoms may also be caused by secretion of toxins into the perilymph spaces of the inner ear [107].

Immunogenic Labyrinthitis

Sensorineural hearing loss may occur together with immunological diseases. This heterogeneous group of sensorineural hearing loss types falls under the heading "autoimmune inner ear disease" (AIED) [108]. Possible target structures for antibodies are the stria vascularis in the organ of Corti and the blood vessels supplying the inner ear. AIED is characterized by progressive, often fluctuating and usually bilateral sensorineural hearing loss with tinnitus and vertigo, and occurs more often in females [109]. The progression of hearing loss over time is too rapid to suggest presbycusis and too slow for a diagnosis of sudden deafness. AIED patients respond well to corticosteroids or immunosuppressant therapy [110]. Some patients with AIED present with a systemic autoimmune disease, such as granulomatosis with polyangiitis (formerly called Wegener's disease) (see Footnote 5), eosinophilic granulomatosis with polyangiitis (formerly called Churg Strauss syndrome), systemic lupus erythematosus [111], Cogan syndrome[8], or relapsing polychondritis[9] [112, 113]. As yet, there is no specific test battery

[6]Mondini dysplasia: Congenital anomaly of osseus and membranous otic labyrinth characterized by aplastic cochlea and deformity of the vestibule and semicircular canals with partial or complete loss of auditory and vestibular function may be associated with dilated vestibular aqueduct and spontaneous cerebrospinal fluid otorrhea resulting in meningitis. Stedman's Online Medical Dictionary.

[7]Scheibe dysplasia: Hearing impairment due to cochleosaccular dysplasia; usually autosomal recessive inheritance. Stedman's Online Medical Dictionary.

[8]Cogan syndrome: Typical Cogan syndrome is characterized by interstitial keratitis and vestibuloauditory dysfunction. There is generally a brief episode of inflammatory eye disease (interstitial keratitis) followed by bilateral audiovestibular symptoms. The interstitial keratitis usually occurs with sudden onset and is characterized by photophobia, lacrimation, and eye pain. The vestibuloauditory dysfunction is usually bilateral, presenting with tinnitus, sensorineural hearing loss, and acute episodes of vertigo.

[9]Relapsing polychondritis: A degenerative disease of cartilage producing a bizarre form of arthritis, with collapse of the ears, the cartilaginous portion of the nose, and the tracheobronchial tree; death may occur from chronic infection or suffocation because of loss of stability in the tracheobronchial tree; of autosomal origin. Stedman's Online Medical Dictionary.

that would unequivocally show the presence of an autoimmune reaction to structures of the inner ear. The recommendation is to use general laboratory tests (antinuclear antibodies, antineutrophil cytoplasmatic antibodies, anticochlear antibodies etc.) to screen for the presence of systemic signs in patients who are suspected of having an autoimmune disease [114, 115].

Age-Related Hearing Loss

Age-related hearing loss is the most common of all forms of hearing loss. It affects more than 40% of people over the age of 65 [116, 117]. Aside from physiological age-related processes, endogenous and exogenous factors such as hypoxia, exposure to loud noise, hypertension, hypercholesterolemia, or diabetes mellitus may cause or contribute to hearing loss in old age [118]. Consequently, excessive noise exposure and atherosclerosis contribute to the development of presbycusis in industrialized countries. The reported presence of tinnitus together with presbycusis varies between 8% and 72% [119]. The risk for the development of tinnitus rises with increasing age and with increasing noise exposure [120]. A recent review demonstrated that both age-related hearing loss and accompanying tinnitus affect mental health and psychological well-being [121]. This can further contribute to the development of cognitive decline, depression, anxiety and stress [122, 123].

Sudden Sensorineural Hearing Loss (Syn. Sudden Deafness)

The terms "sudden sensorineural hearing loss (SSNHL)" or "sudden deafness" refer to a sudden onset, usually unilateral, of cochlear hearing impairment of differing extents including complete deafness [124]. Thus, the term refers more to the description of a symptom rather than a classical diagnosis [125]. Since the terms in the narrow sense should be reserved for those forms of acute cochlear hearing loss for which an underlying cause is not identifiable, the addition of "idiopathic" may further specify the clinical picture of sudden sensorineural hearing loss ("idiopathic sudden deafness", "idiopathic sensorineural hearing loss"). There are different definitions to describe the extent of sensorineural hearing loss for which the term sudden sensorineural hearing loss can be used. The definition commonly used in the English-speaking world defines SSNHL as a hearing loss of at least 30 dB HL in three successive frequencies (125–8000 Hz) compared to the healthy opposite ear [126]. This hearing loss should have occurred in less than 72 h. In contrast, other definitions dispense with an exact specification of the extent of hearing loss in dB and classify in terms of frequency range into high-frequency, mid-frequency, low-frequency and pantonal sudden sensorineural hearing loss. The most common accompanying symptoms are tinnitus and a feeling of pressure in the respective ear (both in about 80% of cases). In 30% of patients, there is dizziness in addition to hearing loss, so that a vestibular dysfunction must be assumed in addition to the cochlear disorder. The mechanism of occurrence of SSNHL has not yet been clarified in detail. However, there are various models of how the hearing loss could occur. These theories are mainly based on animal experiments in which certain manipulations (e.g. noise trauma, reduced blood flow, application of aminoglycosides) were used to damage the inner ear including the hair cells in order to gain an understanding of the molecular mechanisms in the inner ear (Chap. 10). Ultimately, some evidence has been found for vascular, rheological, inflammatory, metabolic, mechanical, autoimmune, and genetic processes that may be involved in the development of SSNHL [127–132]. Presumably, all these various factors may interact. Finally, it has been shown that a pathological activation of a cellular stress reaction in the cochlear hair cells with release of oxygen and nitrogen radicals leads to damage of hair cells, thus causing subsequent sensorineural hearing loss [129].

Ototoxicity

More than 150 substances are known to potentially cause sensorineural hearing loss and/or tinnitus [133, 134]. Vertigo can occur as another known side effect. The effects can be either temporary or permanent. Furthermore, they can occur as a consequence of short-term or long-term treatment with the respective substance. The term ototoxicity has been introduced to describe such substances. The main ototoxic drugs belong to the classes of antibiotics (especially aminoglycosides, macrolides, and vancomycin), antimalarial drugs (quinine), anti-inflammatory drugs (salicylates andN-SAIDs), loop diuretics (ethacrynic acid andfurosemide) and antineoplastic drugs (platinum-containing chemotherapeutic agents) [135]. With platinum-containing substances, especially cisplatin and aminoglycosides, the hearing impairment is usually permanent, whereas with loop diuretics, macrolides and quinine the problem may disappear after discontinuation of the medication [136]. The main findings on the mechanism of injury with ototoxic drugs are based on animal experiments. The exact processes leading to damage in the stria vascularis, spiral ganglion cells, outer hair cells, and central auditory neurons will not be discussed here. This information can be found in relevant reviews [137–142]. In many clinical situations, especially in life-threatening tumor diseases or infections, there are often no alternatives to the ototoxic substances described above. Thus, the ototoxic risk is consciously accepted. In these situations, it is important to perform an individual monitoring of hearing function. Since the susceptibility and dose dependency for ototoxic side effects varies among individuals and cannot be predicted, it is important to detect damage to the auditory and vestibular organs at an early stage. It may then be possible to react with a dose adjustment or change to alternative medications. Since this is not always possible, the early administration of otoprotective medication has also become important in recent years. In this context, anti-oxidants such as N-acetylcysteine, amifostine, vitamin E, ebselen, lipoic acid or zinc come into consideration [136, 143, 144]. However, further well-designed studies are necessary before these drugs can be recommended for routine use in the various conditions. Intratympanic administration of the agents might help to protect from unwanted systemic side effects; for example, in terms of free radical scavengers which impair the cisplatin antitumor activity in vitro [136].

Noise-Related Hearing Loss

Depending on the extent of noise exposure (frequency, intensity, and duration), the subsequent hearing loss may be temporary or permanent [8]. The mildest form is the temporary threshold shift. In this case, hearing should return to normal within 1 week. Correspondingly, damage to the hair cells could not be proven in animal experiments. The next form is hidden hearing loss. Here, permanent losses are found in the synaptic connection between the cochlear hair cells and the auditory nerve. Here, too, the cochlear hair cells are not damaged. Hearing, however, shows an impairment in the understanding of speech under presence of disturbing environmental noise [145]. At the end of a prolonged noise exposure, the permanent threshold shift is a situation of permanent loss of neuronal connections and permanent hair cell damage. Depending on the extent and duration of noise exposure, the damage progresses from the outer hair cells to the inner hair cells. The hearing damage is reflected in a permanent change in the pure tone audiogram. Typically, the area of greatest vulnerability is found between 3 and 6 kHz [146]. However, it is important to emphasize that there is no linear relationship between the extent of noise exposure and the extent of hearing loss. As with age-related hearing loss, it depends on the interaction of extrinsic (noise and age) and intrinsic factors. The decisive intrinsic factors are genetic factors including sex, cortisol levels, and nutrition, among others [8].

In all forms, tinnitus may occur in addition to hearing impairment. This can be temporary (e.g. some hours of tinnitus perception after attending a loud music concert) or permanent. The latter would then be a sign for the existence of a hidden hearing loss or a measurable threshold change in the pure tone audiogram.

It should be mentioned here that an examination at the ear specialist with aspiration of material (e.g. wax) from the external auditory canal may well lead to considerable noise exposure. Depending on the closure of the aspirator by appropriate material, noise levels between 118 and 146 dB (A) were measured in a model [147]. According to a survey of patients in an ENT clinic, a number of respondents experienced post-interventional complaints in the form of hearing loss, tinnitus, and noise sensitivity [148]. The complaints were more frequent in patients with pathological ear structures (tympanic membrane perforation, mastoid cavity) than in normally configured ears. As a consequence of this study, the recommendation to the medical staff was to handle the intervention sensitively and to prepare the patients for a potential noise exposure, or to switch to alternative procedures in very sensitive patients [148]. It should also be mentioned that temporary or permanent threshold shift might also occur after all types of ear surgery. Possible causes of cochlear damage with subsequent development of tinnitus after ear surgery can be due to the drilling and suction noise, the direct contact of the drill and other instruments with the ossicles, or direct damage of the membranous labyrinth [148, 149].

As a consequence of the increasing knowledge of the damaging effects of noise exposure on the structures of the inner ear, prevention should be the first priority [150]. This has been acknowledged by the WHO, which has launched various campaigns to generate awareness of the problem in the population and to promote the use of noise reduction measures [151]. While guidelines for the wearing of adequate hearing protection for occupational noise exposure exist in many countries [152], measures for corresponding behavior in the leisure sector have only recently become increasingly introduced [153].

Therapy of Sensorineural Hearing Loss

In the case of sensorineural hearing loss and tinnitus, the treatment depends on acuity and the extent of the hearing loss. In the case of acute hearing disorders of the inner ear (sudden sensorineural hearing loss, noise trauma, and drug side effects), steroid application may be considered. According to a recent review paper, all types of steroid therapy are better than placebo in the treatment of acute sensorineural hearing loss [126, 135]; however, no international consensus on the dosage and form of application (systemic vs. local) has been agreed so far [154]. Therapeutic options for hair cell regeneration (stem cells, gene therapy, small molecules and drugs) or for the treatment of synaptopathy are currently the subject of intensive research [155], but a breakthrough with routine application is not expected in the near future. A challenge for these approaches is the need to achieve a sufficient drug concentration in the cochlea, which requires in many cases local administration (e.g. intratympanic application) [156, 157]. For further drug options in treating different forms of tinnitus with sensorineural hearing loss, refer Chap. 48.

In chronic hearing loss, the primary goal is the improvement of hearing by increasing auditory input to the brain. For this purpose, hearing aids or, in the case of almost complete hearing loss or deafness, cochlear implants are used for all forms of persistent hearing loss of a certain severity (refer Chap. 46).

Conclusion

Hearing loss is the most relevant risk factor for the development of tinnitus. Therefore, the diagnosis of an underlying hearing disorder is both important and relevant in the diagnosis and treatment of tinnitus. Taking a detailed case history is essential to get information about the possible cause of the hearing loss. On the one hand, informing the patient about the relationship between tinnitus and hearing loss is an important part of counseling and demystifies tinnitus. On the other hand, knowledge of the cause of the hearing loss provides possible implications for appropriate treatment for both hearing loss and tinnitus. An improvement in hearing can ultimately alleviate tinnitus symptoms. This can range from complete suppression to a substantial masking effect. However, it should be noted that in rare cases tinnitus may also occur as an unwanted side effect of surgical hearing improvement measures (middle-ear or ear canal surgery, cochlear implant).

References

1. Nicolas-Puel C, Faulconbridge RL, Guitton M, Puel J-L, Mondain M, Uziel A. Characteristics of tinnitus and etiology of associated hearing loss: a study of 123 patients. Int Tinnitus J. 2002;8(1):37–44.
2. Ukaegbe O, Ezeanolue B, Orji F. The influence of tinnitus on the audiometric threshold of sufferers. Int Arch Otorhinolaryngol. 2016;20(4):339–43.
3. Schecklmann M, Vielsmeier V, Steffens T, Landgrebe M, Langguth B, Kleinjung T. Relationship between audiometric slope and tinnitus pitch in tinnitus patients: insights into the mechanisms of tinnitus generation. PLoS One. 2012;7(4):e34878.
4. Norena A, Micheyl C, Chéry-Croze S, Collet L. Psychoacoustic characterization of the tinnitus spectrum: implications for the underlying mechanisms of tinnitus. Audiol Neurootol. 2002;7(6):358–69.
5. König O, Schaette R, Kempter R, Gross M. Course of hearing loss and occurrence of tinnitus. Hear Res. 2006;221(1–2):59–64.
6. Gollnast D, Tziridis K, Krauss P, Schilling A, Hoppe U, Schulze H. Analysis of audiometric differences of patients with and without tinnitus in a large clinical database. Front Neurol. 2017;8:31.
7. Vielsmeier V, Lehner A, Strutz J, Steffens T, Kreuzer PM, Schecklmann M, et al. The relevance of the high frequency audiometry in tinnitus patients with normal hearing in conventional pure-tone audiometry. Biomed Res Int. 2015;2015:302515, 1.
8. Hertzano R, Lipford EL, Depireux D. Noise. Otolaryngol Clin N Am. 2020;53(4):531–42.
9. Song Z, Wu Y, Tang D, Lu X, Qiao L, Wang J, et al. Tinnitus is associated with extended high-frequency hearing loss and hidden high-frequency damage in young patients. Otol Neurotol. 2020;42(3):377; [cited 2021 Mar 27]; Publish Ahead of Print. https://doi.org/10.1097/MAO.0000000000002983.
10. Kara E, Aydin K, Akbulut AA, et al. Assessment of hidden hearing loss in normal hearing individuals with and without tinnitus. Int Adv Otol. 2020;16(1):87–92.
11. Liberman MC. Noise-induced and age-related hearing loss: new perspectives and potential therapies. F1000Res. 2017;6:927.
12. Liberman MC, Kujawa SG. Cochlear synaptopathy in acquired sensorineural hearing loss: manifestations and mechanisms. Hear Res. 2017;349:138–47.
13. Davies RA. Audiometry and other hearing tests. Handb Clin Neurol. 2016;137:157–76.
14. Eggermont JJ, Roberts LE. The neuroscience of tinnitus: understanding abnormal and normal auditory perception. Front Syst Neurosci. 2012;6:53.
15. Noreña AJ. Revisiting the cochlear and central mechanisms of tinnitus and therapeutic approaches. Audiol Neurootol. 2015;20(Suppl 1):53–9.
16. Tucker DA, Phillips SL, Ruth RA, Clayton WA, Royster E, Todd AD. The effect of silence on tinnitus perception. Otolaryngol Head Neck Surg. 2005;132(1):20–4.
17. Knobel KAB, Sanchez TG. Influence of silence and attention on tinnitus perception. Otolaryngol Head Neck Surg. 2008;138(1):18–22.
18. Schaette R, Turtle C, Munro KJ. Reversible induction of phantom auditory sensations through simulated unilateral hearing loss. PLoS One. 2012;7(6):e35238.
19. Lauer AM, Dent ML, Sun W, Xu-Friedman MA. Effects of non-traumatic noise and conductive hearing loss on auditory system function. Neuroscience. 2019;407:182–91.
20. Tan CL, Lecluyse W, McFerran D, Meddis R. Tinnitus and patterns of hearing loss. JARO. 2013;14:275–82.
21. Knipper M, Van Dijk P, Nunes I, Rüttiger L, Zimmermann U. Advances in the neurobiology of hearing disorders: recent developments regarding the basis of tinnitus and hyperacusis. Prog Neurobiol. 2013;111:17–33.
22. Sweeney AD, Carlson ML, Wanna GB, Bennett ML. Glomus tympanicum tumors. Otolaryngol Clin N Am. 2015;48(2):293–304.
23. Takemori S, Tanaka Y, Suzuki JI. Thalidomide anomalies of the ear. Arch Otolaryngol. 1976;102(7):425–7.
24. Lee SM, Kim HM, Lee JS, Yoon CS, Park MS, Park KI, et al. A case of suspected isotretinoin-induced malformation in a baby of a mother who became pregnant one month after discontinuation of the drug. Yonsei Med J. 2009;50(3):445–7.
25. Aljerian A, Gilardino MS. Treacher Collins syndrome. Clin Plast Surg. 2019;46(2):197–205.
26. Orvidas LJ, Fabry LB, Diacova S, McDonald TJ. Hearing and otopathology in Crouzon syndrome. Laryngoscope. 1999;109(9):1372–5.
27. Yiin RSZ, Tang PH, Tan TY. Review of congenital inner ear abnormalities on CT temporal bone. Br J Radiol. 2011;84(1005):859–63.
28. Ostrowski VB, Wiet RJ. Pathologic conditions of the external ear and auditory canal. Postgrad Med. 1996;100(3):223–8, 233–7.
29. Folmer RL, Shi BY. Chronic tinnitus resulting from cerumen removal procedures. Int Tinnitus J. 2004;10(1):42–6.
30. Young A, Reeve NH, Yang A, Kahane J, Cross C, Albanese A, et al. Sound levels with aural suctioning: effects of suction size, canal moisture, and distance from the eardrum. Laryngoscope Investig Otolaryngol. 2020;5(4):766–72.

31. Attlmayr B, Smith IM. Prevalence of 'surfer's ear' in Cornish surfers. J Laryngol Otol. 2015;129(5):440–4.
32. Wang M-C, Liu C-Y, Shiao A-S, Wang T. Ear problems in swimmers. J Chin Med Assoc. 2005;68(8):347–52.
33. Ouaz K, Robier A, Lescanne E, Bobillier C, Morinière S, Bakhos D. Cancer of the external auditory canal. Eur Ann Otorhinolaryngol Head Neck Dis. 2013;130(4):175–82.
34. Spielmann PM, McKean S, White RD, Hussain SSM. Surgical management of external auditory canal lesions. J Laryngol Otol. 2013;127(3):246–51.
35. Ars B, Dirckx J. Eustachian tube function. Otolaryngol Clin N Am. 2016;49(5):1121–33.
36. Emmett SD, Kokesh J, Kaylie D. Chronic ear disease. Med Clin North Am. 2018;102(6):1063–79.
37. Karanth TK, Whittemore KR. Middle-ear disease in children with cleft palate. Auris Nasus Larynx. 2018;45(6):1143–51.
38. Timmermans K, Vander Poorten V, Desloovere C, Debruyne F. The middle ear of cleft palate patients in their early teens: a literature study and preliminary file study. B-ENT. 2006;2(Suppl 4):95–101.
39. Llewellyn A, Norman G, Harden M, Coatesworth A, Kimberling D, Schilder A, et al. Interventions for adult Eustachian tube dysfunction: a systematic review. Health Technol Assess. 2014;18(46):1–180, v–vi.
40. Froehlich MH, Le PT, Nguyen SA, McRackan TR, Rizk HG, Meyer TA. Eustachian tube balloon dilation: a systematic review and meta-analysis of treatment outcomes. Otolaryngol Head Neck Surg. 2020;163(5):870–82.
41. Bance M, Tysome JR, Smith ME. Patulous Eustachian tube (PET), a practical overview. World J Otorhinolaryngol Head Neck Surg. 2019;5(3):137–42.
42. Grimmer JF, Poe DS. Update on eustachian tube dysfunction and the patulous eustachian tube. Curr Opin Otolaryngol Head Neck Surg. 2005;13(5):277–82.
43. Poe DS. Diagnosis and management of the patulous eustachian tube. Otol Neurotol. 2007;28(5):668–77.
44. Luu K, Remillard A, Fandino M, Saxby A, Westerberg BD. Treatment effectiveness for symptoms of patulous Eustachian tube: a systematic review. Otol Neurotol. 2015;36(10):1593–600.
45. Ikeda R, Hidaka H, Kikuchi T, Ohta N, Kawase T, Katori Y, et al. Systematic review of surgical outcomes following repair of patulous Eustachian tube. Otol Neurotol. 2020;41(8):1012–20.
46. Pichichero ME. Otitis media. Pediatr Clin N Am. 2013;60(2):391–407.
47. Shirai N, Preciado D. Otitis media: what is new? Curr Opin Otolaryngol Head Neck Surg. 2019;27(6):495–8.
48. Brar S, Watters C, Winters R. Tympanoplasty. In: StatPearls. Treasure Island (FL): StatPearls Publishing; 2020; [cited 2021 Feb 20]. http://www.ncbi.nlm.nih.gov/books/NBK565863/.
49. Wullstein HL. Tympanoplasty: the fundamentals of the concept. Clin Otolaryngol Allied Sci. 1978;3(4):431–5.
50. Baba S, Yagi T, Fujikura T. Subjective evaluation and overall satisfaction after tympanoplasty for chronic simple suppurative otitis media. J Nippon Med Sch. 2004;71(1):17–24.
51. da Lima AS, Sanchez TG, Bonadia Moraes MF, Batezati Alves SC, Bento RF. The effect of timpanoplasty on tinnitus in patients with conductive hearing loss: a six month follow-up. Braz J Otorhinolaryngol. 2007;73(3):384–9.
52. Helms J. Tympanoplasty and tinnitus (author's transl). Laryngol Rhinol Otol (Stuttg). 1981;60(3):99–100.
53. Habesoglu M, Habesoglu TE, Karatas C, Tosun A, Gursel AO, Oysu C. Is there any predictor for tinnitus outcome in different types of otologic surgery? Eur Arch Otorhinolaryngol. 2013;270(8):2225–9.
54. Kim D-K, Park S-N, Kim MJ, Lee SY, Park K-H, Yeo SW. Tinnitus in patients with chronic otitis media before and after middle ear surgery. Eur Arch Otorhinolaryngol. 2011;268(10):1443–8.
55. Acikalin RM, Haci C, Altin F, Alimoglu Y. Is there any effect of anxiety and depression scores on the improvement of tinnitus after surgery in chronic otitis patients with tinnitus. Am J Otolaryngol. 2019;40(2):230–2.
56. Kim HC, Jang CH, Kim YY, Seong JY, Kang SH, Cho YB. Role of preoperative air-bone gap in tinnitus outcome after tympanoplasty for chronic otitis media with tinnitus. Braz J Otorhinolaryngol. 2018;84(2):173–7.
57. Crompton M, Cadge BA, Ziff JL, Mowat AJ, Nash R, Lavy JA, et al. The epidemiology of otosclerosis in a British cohort. Otol Neurotol. 2019;40(1):22–30.
58. Deggouj N, Castelein S, Gerard JM, Decat M, Gersdorff M. Tinnitus and otosclerosis. B-ENT. 2009;5(4):241–4.
59. Batson L, Rizzolo D. Otosclerosis: an update on diagnosis and treatment. JAAPA. 2017;30(2):17–22.
60. Gersdorff M, Nouwen J, Gilain C, Decat M, Betsch C. Tinnitus and otosclerosis. Eur Arch Otorhinolaryngol. 2000;257(6):314–6.
61. Altmann F, Glasgold A, Macduff JP. The incidence of otosclerosis as related to race and sex. Ann Otol Rhinol Laryngol. 1967;76(2):377–92.
62. Markou K, Goudakos J. An overview of the etiology of otosclerosis. Eur Arch Otorhinolaryngol. 2009;266(1):25–35.
63. Babcock TA, Liu XZ. Otosclerosis: from genetics to molecular biology. Otolaryngol Clin N Am. 2018;51(2):305–18.
64. Sagar PR, Shah P, Bollampally VC, Alhumaidi N, Malik BH. Otosclerosis and measles: Do measles have a role in Otosclerosis? A review article. Cureus. 2020;12(8):e9908.
65. Erdem D, Şevik Eliçora S, Güven B, Dinç AE. GPER-1 and sex-hormone levels in patients with otosclerosis. Am J Otolaryngol. 2020;41(3):102442.
66. Schrauwen I, Van Camp G. The etiology of otosclerosis: a combination of genes and environment. Laryngoscope. 2010;120(6):1195–202.
67. Gristwood RE, Venables WN. Otosclerosis and chronic tinnitus. Ann Otol Rhinol Laryngol. 2003;112(5):398–403.
68. Sobrinho PG, Oliveira CA, Venosa AR. Long-term follow-up of tinnitus in patients with otosclerosis after stapes surgery. Int Tinnitus J. 2004;10(2):197–201.
69. Doherty JK, Linthicum FH. Spiral ligament and stria vascularis changes in cochlear otosclerosis: effect on hearing level. Otol Neurotol. 2004;25(4):457–64.
70. Cureoglu S, Schachern PA, Ferlito A, Rinaldo A, Tsuprun V, Paparella MM. Otosclerosis: etiopathogenesis and histopathology. Am J Otolaryngol. 2006;27(5):334–40.
71. Redfors YD, Gröndahl HG, Hellgren J, Lindfors N, Nilsson I, Möller C. Otosclerosis: anatomy and pathology in the temporal bone assessed by multi-slice and cone-beam CT. Otol Neurotol. 2012;33(6):922–7.
72. Mafee MF, Valvassori GE, Deitch RL, Norouzi P, Henrikson GC, Capek V, et al. Use of CT in the evaluation of cochlear otosclerosis. Radiology. 1985;156(3):703–8.
73. Ward BK, Carey JP, Minor LB. Superior canal dehiscence syndrome: lessons from the first 20 years. Front Neurol. 2017;8:177.
74. Merchant SN, Rosowski JJ, McKenna MJ. Superior semicircular canal dehiscence mimicking otosclerotic hearing loss. In: Arnold W, Häusler R, editors. Advances in oto-rhino-laryngology. Basel: KARGER; 2007. p. 137–45; [cited 2021 Feb 20]. https://www.karger.com/Article/FullText/98790.
75. Scarpa A, Ralli M, Cassandro C, Gioacchini FM, et al. Inner-ear disorders presenting with air–bone gaps: a review. Int Adv Otol. 2020;16(1):111–6.
76. Shea JJ. Fenestration of the oval window. Ann Otol Rhinol Laryngol. 1958;67(4):932–51.
77. Nazarian R, McElveen JT, Eshraghi AA. History of otosclerosis and stapes surgery. Otolaryngol Clin N Am. 2018;51(2):275–90.
78. Wegner I, Kamalski DMA, Tange RA, Vincent R, Stegeman I, van der Heijden GJM, et al. Laser versus conventional fenestration in

stapedotomy for otosclerosis: a systematic review. Laryngoscope. 2014;124(7):1687–93.
79. Srivastava R, Cho W, Fergie N. The use of lasers in stapes surgery. Ear Nose Throat J. 2021;100(1_suppl):73S–6S, 73S.
80. Cheng HCS, Agrawal SK, Parnes LS. Stapedectomy versus stapedotomy. Otolaryngol Clin N Am. 2018;51(2):375–92.
81. Pauna HF, Pereira RC, Monsanto RC, Amaral MSA, Hyppolito MA. A comparison between endoscopic and microscopic approaches for stapes surgery: a systematic review. J Laryngol Otol. 2020;134(5):398–403.
82. Marchese MR, Paludetti G, De Corso E, Cianfrone F. Role of stapes surgery in improving hearing loss caused by otosclerosis. J Laryngol Otol. 2007;121(5):438–43.
83. Dziendziel B, Skarzynski H, Gos E, Skarzynski PH. Changes in hearing threshold and tinnitus severity after stapes surgery: which is more important to the patient's quality of life? ORL J Otorhinolaryngol Relat Spec. 2019;81(4):224–33.
84. Cavalcante AMG, de IMC S, Neves BJ, Oliveira CA, Bahmad F. Degree of tinnitus improvement with stapes surgery—a review. Braz J Otorhinolaryngol. 2018;84(4):514–8.
85. Glasgold A, Altmann F. The effect of stapes surgery on tinnitus in otosclerosis. Laryngoscope. 1966;76(9):1524–32.
86. Ayache D, Earally F, Elbaz P. Characteristics and postoperative course of tinnitus in otosclerosis. Otol Neurotol. 2003;24(1):48–51.
87. Sakai M, Sato M, Iida M, Ogata T, Ishida K. The effect on tinnitus of stapes surgery for otosclerosis. Rev Laryngol Otol Rhinol (Bord). 1995;116(1):27–30.
88. Sarna B, Abouzari M, Merna C, Jamshidi S, Saber T, Djalilian HR. Perilymphatic fistula: a review of classification, etiology, diagnosis, and treatment. Front Neurol. 2020;11:1046.
89. Deveze A, Matsuda H, Elziere M, Ikezono T. Diagnosis and treatment of perilymphatic fistula. Adv Otorhinolaryngol. 2018;81:133–45.
90. Folmer RL, Griest SE. Chronic tinnitus resulting from head or neck injuries. Laryngoscope. 2003;113(5):821–7.
91. Kreuzer PM, Landgrebe M, Schecklmann M, Staudinger S, Langguth B, TRI Database Study Group. Trauma-associated tinnitus: audiological, demographic and clinical characteristics. PLoS One. 2012;7(9):e45599.
92. Basson OJ, van Lierop AC. Conductive hearing loss after head trauma: review of ossicular pathology, management and outcomes. J Laryngol Otol. 2009;123(2):177–81.
93. Ikram A, Rehman A. Paraganglioma. In: StatPearls. Treasure Island (FL): StatPearls Publishing; 2020; [cited 2021 Feb 20]. http://www.ncbi.nlm.nih.gov/books/NBK549834/.
94. Williams MD. Paragangliomas of the head and neck: an overview from diagnosis to genetics. Head Neck Pathol. 2017;11(3):278–87.
95. Sismanis A. Pulsatile tinnitus: contemporary assessment and management. Curr Opin Otolaryngol Head Neck Surg. 2011;19(5):348–57.
96. Kloeck I, Crols R, De Belder T, Vandist V, Schmelzer B. Wegener's granulomatosis presenting as otomastoiditis. A case report. B-ENT. 2006;2(1):7–12.
97. Özdoğan A, Acioğlu E, Karaman E, Öz B, Müsellim B. A difficult case: sarcoidosis of the middle ear. Am J Otolaryngol. 2009;30(4):281–4.
98. Yang T, Guo L, Wang L, Yu X. Diagnosis, intervention, and prevention of genetic hearing loss. Adv Exp Med Biol. 2019;1130:73–92.
99. Smith RJH, Bale JF, White KR. Sensorineural hearing loss in children. Lancet. 2005;365(9462):879–90.
100. Bayazit YA, Yilmaz M. An overview of hereditary hearing loss. ORL J Otorhinolaryngol Relat Spec. 2006;68(2):57–63.
101. Bassett EC, Musso MF. Otolaryngologic management of down syndrome patients: what is new? Curr Opin Otolaryngol Head Neck Surg. 2017;25(6):493–7.
102. Bitner-Glindzicz M. Hereditary deafness and phenotyping in humans. Br Med Bull. 2002;63:73–94.
103. Nance WE. The genetics of deafness. Ment Retard Dev Disabil Res Rev. 2003;9(2):109–19.
104. Douglas SA, Sanli H, Gibson WPR. Meningitis resulting in hearing loss and labyrinthitis ossificans—does the causative organism matter? Cochlear Implants Int. 2008;9(2):90–6.
105. Cohen BE, Durstenfeld A, Roehm PC. Viral causes of hearing loss: a review for hearing health professionals. Trends Hear. 2014;18:2331216514541361.
106. Sweeney CJ, Gilden DH. Ramsay hunt syndrome. J Neurol Neurosurg Psychiatry. 2001;71(2):149–54.
107. Sugiura M, Naganawa S, Nakata S, Kojima S, Nakashima T. 3D-FLAIR MRI findings in a patient with Ramsay hunt syndrome. Acta Otolaryngol. 2007;127(5):547–9.
108. Das S, Bakshi SS, Seepana R. Demystifying autoimmune inner ear disease. Eur Arch Otorhinolaryngol. 2019;276(12):3267–74.
109. Ralli M, D'Aguanno V, Di Stadio A, De Virgilio A, Croce A, Longo L, et al. Audiovestibular symptoms in systemic autoimmune diseases. J Immunol Res. 2018;2018:5798103.
110. Strum D, Kim S, Shim T, Monfared A. An update on autoimmune inner ear disease: a systematic review of pharmacotherapy. Am J Otolaryngol. 2020;41(1):102310.
111. Rahne T, Plontke S, Keyßer G. Vasculitis and the ear: a literature review. Curr Opin Rheumatol. 2020;32(1):47–52.
112. Shamriz O, Tal Y, Gross M. Autoimmune inner ear disease: immune biomarkers, audiovestibular aspects, and therapeutic modalities of Cogan's syndrome. J Immunol Res. 2018;2018:1498640.
113. Bachor E, Blevins NH, Karmody C, Kühnel T. Otologic manifestations of relapsing polychondritis. Auris Nasus Larynx. 2006;33(2):135–41.
114. Ciorba A, Corazzi V, Bianchini C, Aimoni C, Pelucchi S, Skarżyński PH, et al. Autoimmune inner ear disease (AIED): A diagnostic challenge. Int J Immunopathol Pharmacol. 2018;32:2058738418808680.
115. Carlomagno A, Silveira G, Rebella M, Vola M, Danza A. The clinician faced with anticochlear antibodies: what to do with them? J Clin Rheumatol. 2018;24(3):113–5.
116. Cruickshanks KJ, Wiley TL, Tweed TS, Klein BE, Klein R, Mares-Perlman JA, et al. Prevalence of hearing loss in older adults in beaver dam, Wisconsin. The epidemiology of hearing loss study. Am J Epidemiol. 1998;148(9):879–86.
117. Roth TN, Hanebuth D, Probst R. Prevalence of age-related hearing loss in Europe: a review. Eur Arch Otorhinolaryngol. 2011;268(8):1101–7.
118. de LMBM F, Ramos Júnior AN, Mendes EP. Characterization of tinnitus in the elderly and its possible related disorders. Braz J Otorhinolaryngol. 2009;75(2):249–55.
119. McCormack A, Edmondson-Jones M, Somerset S, Hall D. A systematic review of the reporting of tinnitus prevalence and severity. Hear Res. 2016;337:70–9.
120. Ahmad N, Seidman M. Tinnitus in the older adult: epidemiology, pathophysiology and treatment options. Drugs Aging. 2004;21(5):297–305.
121. Jafari Z, Kolb BE, Mohajerani MH. Age-related hearing loss and tinnitus, dementia risk, and auditory amplification outcomes. Ageing Res Rev. 2019;56:100963.
122. Kim AS, Garcia Morales EE, Amjad H, Cotter VT, Lin FR, Lyketsos CG, et al. Association of hearing loss with neuropsychiatric symptoms in older adults with cognitive impairment. Am J Geriatr Psychiatry. 2020;29(6):544.
123. Lin FR, Ferrucci L, Metter EJ, An Y, Zonderman AB, Resnick SM. Hearing loss and cognition in the Baltimore longitudinal study of aging. Neuropsychology. 2011;25(6):763–70.
124. Schreiber BE, Agrup C, Haskard DO, Luxon LM. Sudden sensorineural hearing loss. Lancet. 2010;375(9721):1203–11.
125. Kleinjung T, Huber A. Der Hörsturz. Swiss Med Forum. 2016;16(48):1038; [cited 2021 Mar 28]. https://doi.emh.ch/smf.2016.02801.

126. Chandrasekhar SS, Tsai Do BS, Schwartz SR, Bontempo LJ, Faucett EA, Finestone SA, et al. Clinical practice guideline: sudden hearing loss (update). Otolaryngol Head Neck Surg. 2019;161(1_suppl):S1–45.
127. Veltri RW, Wilson WR, Sprinkle PM, Rodman SM, Kavesh DA. The implication of viruses in idiopathic sudden hearing loss: primary infection or reactivation of latent viruses? Otolaryngol Head Neck Surg. 1981;89(1):137–41.
128. Fusconi M, Chistolini A, Angelosanto N, Pignoloni P, Tombolini M, De Virgilio A, et al. Role of genetic and acquired prothrombotic risk factors in genesis of sudden sensorineural hearing loss. Audiol Neurotol. 2011;16(3):185–90.
129. Merchant SN, Adams JC, Nadol JB. Pathology and pathophysiology of idiopathic sudden sensorineural hearing loss. Otol Neurotol. 2005;26(2):151–60.
130. Corazzi V, Ciorba A, Bianchini C, Pelucchi S, Skarżyński PH, Hatzopoulos S. Genetic polymorphisms in sudden sensorineural hearing loss: an update. Ear Nose Throat J. 2020;100:337S.
131. Young Y-H. Contemporary review of the causes and differential diagnosis of sudden sensorineural hearing loss. Int J Audiol. 2020;59(4):243–53.
132. Greco A, Fusconi M, Gallo A, Marinelli C, Macri GF, De Vincentiis M. Sudden sensorineural hearing loss: an autoimmune disease? Autoimmun Rev. 2011;10(12):756–61.
133. Arslan E, Orzan E, Santarelli R. Global problem of drug-induced hearing loss. Ann N Y Acad Sci. 1999;884(1):1–14.
134. Cianfrone G, Pentangelo D, Cianfrone F, Mazzei F, Turchetta R, Orlando MP, et al. Pharmacological drugs inducing ototoxicity, vestibular symptoms and tinnitus: a reasoned and updated guide. Eur Rev Med Pharmacol Sci. 2011;15(6):601–36.
135. Kleinjung T, Langguth B. Pharmacotherapy of tinnitus. Curr Top Behav Neurosci. 2020;51:193. https://doi.org/10.1007/7854_2020_169; cited 2021 Mar 28].
136. Lanvers-Kaminsky C, Am Z-DA, Parfitt R, Ciarimboli G. Drug-induced ototoxicity: mechanisms, pharmacogenetics, and protective strategies. Clin Pharmacol Ther. 2017;101(4):491–500.
137. dos NAG S, Ferreira RS, dos Santos AC. Overview of cisplatin-induced neurotoxicity and ototoxicity, and the protective agents. Food Chem Toxicol. 2020;136:111079.
138. Kros CJ, Steyger PS. Aminoglycoside- and cisplatin-induced ototoxicity: mechanisms and otoprotective strategies. Cold Spring Harb Perspect Med. 2019;9(11):a033548.
139. Jiang M, Karasawa T, Steyger PS. Aminoglycoside-induced cochleotoxicity: a review. Front Cell Neurosci. 2017;11:308.
140. Ikeda AK, Prince AA, Chen JX, Lieu JEC, Shin JJ. Macrolide-associated sensorineural hearing loss: a systematic review: macrolide-associated SNHL. Laryngoscope. 2018;128(1):228–36.
141. Ding D, Liu H, Qi W, Jiang H, Li Y, Wu X, et al. Ototoxic effects and mechanisms of loop diuretics. J Otol. 2016;11(4):145–56.
142. Jung TT, Rhee CK, Lee CS, Park YS, Choi DC. Ototoxicity of salicylate, nonsteroidal antiinflammatory drugs, and quinine. Otolaryngol Clin N Am. 1993;26(5):791–810.
143. Pak JH, Kim Y, Yi J, Chung JW. Antioxidant therapy against oxidative damage of the inner ear: protection and preconditioning. Antioxidants. 2020;9(11):1076.
144. Kil J, Harruff EE, Longenecker RJ. Development of ebselen for the treatment of sensorineural hearing loss and tinnitus. Hear Res. 2021;108209:108209.
145. Wu PZ, Liberman LD, Bennett K, de Gruttola V, O'Malley JT, Liberman MC. Primary neural degeneration in the human cochlea: evidence for hidden hearing loss in the aging ear. Neuroscience. 2019;407:8–20.
146. Henderson D, Subramaniam M, Gratton MA, Saunders SS. Impact noise: the importance of level, duration, and repetition rate. J Acoust Soc Am. 1991;89(3):1350–7.
147. Luxenberger W, Lahousen T, Walch C. Suction-generated noise in an anatomic silicon ear model. Eur Arch Otorhinolaryngol. 2012;269(10):2291–3.
148. Addams-Williams J, Howarth A, Phillipps JJ. Microsuction aural toilet in ENT outpatients: a questionnaire to evaluate the patient experience. Eur Arch Otorhinolaryngol. 2010;267(12):1863–6.
149. Banakis Hartl RM, Mattingly JK, Greene NT, Farrell NF, Gubbels SP, Tollin DJ. Drill-induced cochlear injury during otologic surgery: intracochlear pressure evidence of acoustic trauma. Otol Neurotol. 2017;38(7):938–47.
150. Wang T-C, Chang T-Y, Tyler R, Lin Y-J, Liang W-M, Shau Y-W, et al. Noise induced hearing loss and tinnitus—new research developments and remaining gaps in disease assessment, treatment, and prevention. Brain Sci. 2020;10(10):732.
151. Chadha S, Cieza A. Promoting global action on hearing loss: world hearing day. Int J Audiol. 2017;56(3):145–7.
152. Tikka C, Verbeek JH, Kateman E, Morata TC, Dreschler WA, Ferrite S. Interventions to prevent occupational noise-induced hearing loss. Cochrane Database Syst Rev. 2017;7:CD006396.
153. Eichwald J, Scinicariello F, Telfer JL, Carroll YI. Use of personal hearing protection devices at loud athletic or entertainment events among adults—United States, 2018. MMWR Morb Mortal Wkly Rep. 2018;67(41):1151–5.
154. Ahmadzai N, Kilty S, Cheng W, Esmaeilisaraji L, Wolfe D, Bonaparte JP, et al. A systematic review and network meta-analysis of existing pharmacologic therapies in patients with idiopathic sudden sensorineural hearing loss. PLoS One. 2019;14(9):e0221713.
155. Diensthuber M, Stöver T. Strategies for a regenerative therapy of hearing loss. HNO. 2018;66(S1):39–46.
156. Kempfle JS. Endoscopic-assisted drug delivery for inner ear regeneration. Otolaryngol Clin N Am. 2021;54(1):189–200.
157. Nguyen K, Kempfle JS, Jung DH, McKenna CE. Recent advances in therapeutics and drug delivery for the treatment of inner ear diseases: a patent review (2011-2015). Expert Opin Ther Pat. 2017;27(2):191–202.
158. da Lima AS, Sanchez TG, Marcondes R, Bento RF. The effect of stapedotomy on tinnitus in patients with otospongiosis. Ear Nose Throat J. 2005;84(7):412–4.
159. Oliveira CA. How does stapes surgery influence severe disabling tinnitus in otosclerosis patients? Adv Otorhinolaryngol. 2007;65:343–7.
160. Ramsay H, Kärkkäinen J, Palva T. Success in surgery for otosclerosis: hearing improvement and other indicators. Am J Otolaryngol. 1997;18(1):23–8.
161. Szymański M, Gołabek W, Mills R. Effect of stapedectomy on subjective tinnitus. J Laryngol Otol. 2003;117(4):261–4.
162. Ismi O, Erdogan O, Yesilova M, Ozcan C, Ovla D, Gorur K. Does stapes surgery improve tinnitus in patients with otosclerosis? Braz J Otorhinolaryngol. 2017;83(5):568–73.

Meniere's Disease, a Set of Rare Disorders with Tinnitus

33

Patricia Perez-Carpena, Lidia Frejo, and Jose Antonio Lopez-Escamez

Abstract

Meniere's disease (MD) is a chronic inflammatory disorder of the inner ear, characterized by recurrent episodes of vertigo associated with tinnitus and fluctuating sensorineural hearing loss with a multifactorial origin. Most patients progress to chronic imbalance, moderate to severe hearing loss in the affected ear, and may develop persistent and disabling tinnitus. The disease usually begins in one ear with tinnitus and hearing loss, but can affect both ears, causing bilateral symptoms. The diagnosis of MD is based on clinical criteria defined by the Barany Society, and five clinical subgroups have been identified according to comorbidities such as migraine, autoimmunity, and autoinflammatory markers.

Genetic factors and the innate immune response seem to play a central role in the pathophysiology of the condition. Familial MD is found in 10% with dominant and recessive inheritance. It is associated with the accumulation of endolymph (endolymphatic hydrops, EH) in the cochlear duct and vestibular organs, according to human histopathological studies. However, EH is considered a late event in the pathophysiology of MD, which is associated with the development of the sensorineural hearing loss and the duration of the disease. The frequency of clinical episodes of vertigo is unpredictable, and therefore, biological markers of disease activity are necessary for therapeutic planning.

P. Perez-Carpena
Otology and Neurotology Group CTS 495, Department of Genomic Medicine, Centro de Genómica e Investigación Oncológica (GENyO) Pfizer-Universidad de Granada-Junta de Andalucía, Granada, Spain

Department of Otolaryngology, Hospital Universitario Virgen de las Nieves, Instituto de Investigación Biosanitaria, ibs.GRANADA, Granada, Spain

Sensorineural Pathology Programme, Centro de Investigación Biomédica en Red en Enfermedades Raras, Madrid, Spain

L. Frejo
Otology and Neurotology Group CTS 495, Department of Genomic Medicine, Centro de Genómica e Investigación Oncológica (GENyO) Pfizer-Universidad de Granada-Junta de Andalucía, Granada, Spain

Sensorineural Pathology Programme, Centro de Investigación Biomédica en Red en Enfermedades Raras, Madrid, Spain
e-mail: lidia.frejo@genyo.es

J. A. Lopez-Escamez (✉)
Otology and Neurotology Group CTS 495, Department of Genomic Medicine, Centro de Genómica e Investigación Oncológica (GENyO) Pfizer-Universidad de Granada-Junta de Andalucía, Granada, Spain

Department of Otolaryngology, Hospital Universitario Virgen de las Nieves, Instituto de Investigación Biosanitaria, ibs.GRANADA, Granada, Spain

Sensorineural Pathology Programme, Centro de Investigación Biomédica en Red en Enfermedades Raras, Madrid, Spain

Division of Otolaryngology, Department of Surgery, Universidad de Granada, Granada, Spain

Meniere's Disease Neuroscience Research Program, Faculty of Medicine & Health, School of Medical Sciences, The Kolling Institute, University of Sydney, Sydney, New South Wales, Australia
e-mail: jalopezescamez@ugr.es

W. Schlee et al. (eds.), *Textbook of Tinnitus*, https://doi.org/10.1007/978-3-031-35647-6_33

Graphical Abstract

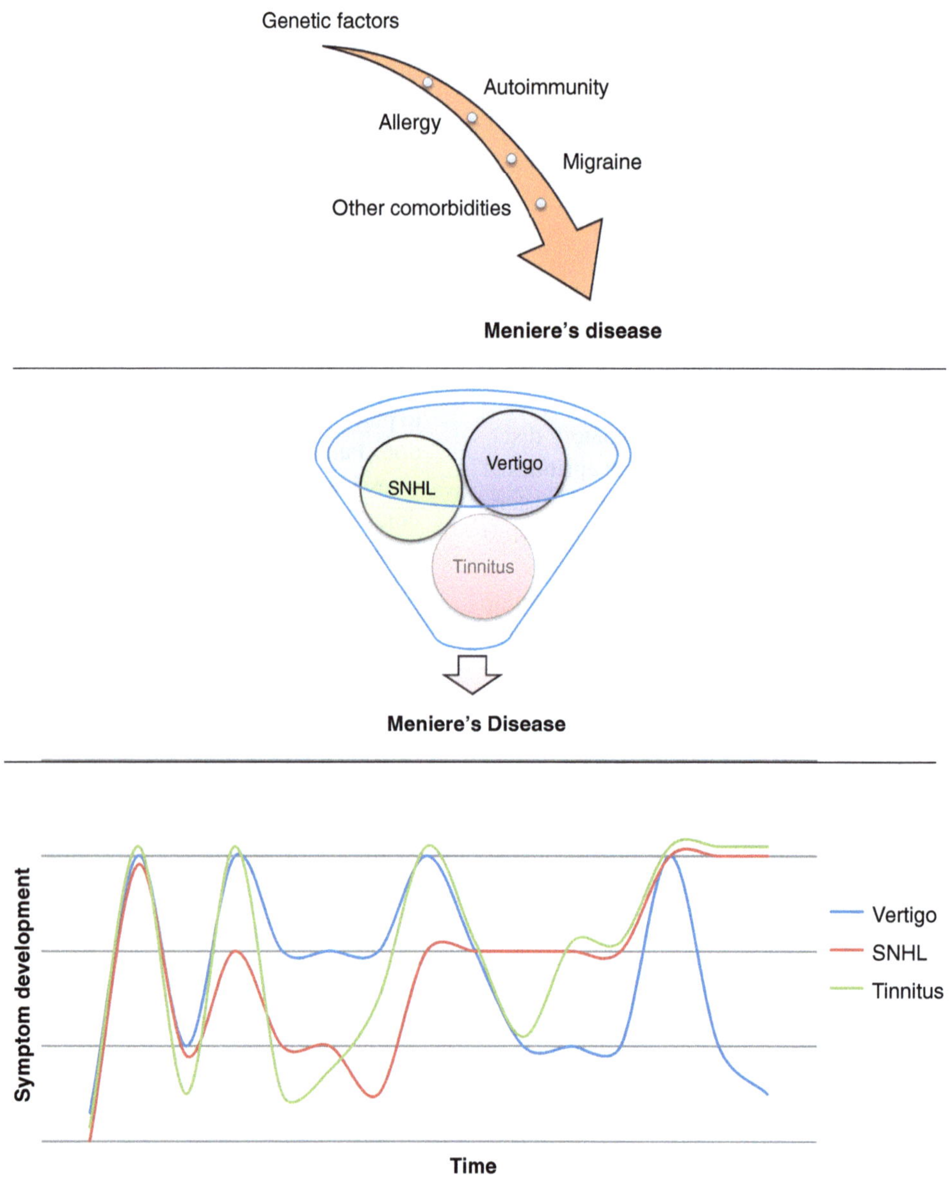

Highlights

- Ménière's disease is a set of rare disorders with a common phenotype defined by episodes of vertigo, tinnitus, ear fullness and sensorineural hearing loss.
- The pathological landmark of Meniere's disease is endolymphatic hydrops.
- Familial Meniere disease is observed in 10% of the cases with autosomal dominant and autosomal recessive patterns of inheritance.
- Tinnitus is a heterogeneous symptom in patients with Ménière's disease, which also suggests several potential mechanisms for tinnitus.
- Persistent tinnitus is commonly reported in advanced stages of Ménière's disease when cochlear damage leads to permanent hearing loss.

Introduction

In 1861, Prosper Ménière described a syndrome consisting of continuous or intermittent head noises accompanied by a decrease of hearing and intermittent attacks of vertigo, uncertain gait, and falling, accompanied by nausea, vomiting, and syncope [1]. The essence of Ménière's hypothesis was that the association of auditory and vestibular symptoms suggested the ear as the anatomic location of the disorder, in opposite to the central nervous system as previously thought.

Ménière's disease (MD) is an inner ear syndrome caused by a set of disorders affecting the inner ear and characterized by episodes of recurrent spontaneous vertigo, tinnitus, sensorineural hearing loss (SNHL), and aural fullness. It is a chronic, debilitating condition with an unpredictable course. Initially, it typically afflicts one ear (unilateral MD), but both ears can be involved in many patients (bilateral MD). In the first few years, the most disabling symptom is vertigo. Acute episodes usually occur repeatedly with a frequency of 5 to 10 crises per year, and they continue with remission stages of a variable duration of months to years [2, 3].

The condition is associated with endolymphatic hydrops (EH), which is caused by the accumulation of endolymph resulting in an enlargement of the endolymphatic space in the inner ear. The increase of the cochlear duct pressure may damage the stria vascularis, the organ of Corti, and other inner ear membranes at ultrastructural level by distorting its complex architecture. However, EH itself does not explain the attacks of vertigo, since histopathological studies have reported EH in individuals without MD symptoms [4].

Genetic factors and the immune response play an essential role in the pathophysiology of MD. The syndrome presents a strong familial aggregation and familial MD have been reported in 10% of cases, showing either an autosomal dominant [5] or autosomal recessive pattern of inheritance [6].

Epidemiological evidence supports genetic and immune factors in MD. In this regard, we can recall the finding of a higher prevalence in European population compared to others (Asian, Native American, and sub-Saharan), and the description of multiple families with MD and relatives with both SNHL and episodic vertigo showing incomplete penetrance and variable expressivity. These findings support an additive inheritance model of common and rare variants [7–10].

A higher prevalence of autoimmune disorders such as rheumatoid arthritis, systemic lupus erythematosus, autoimmune hypothyroidism, and psoriasis has been reported in MD [11, 12].

This has supported the hypothesis of an innate immune dysfunction in certain patients with MD [13]. An allelic variant has been identified in 6p21.33 (leading signal rs4947296) in patients with bilateral MD [14], but also with Graves' disease [15]. So, the description of genetic markers in certain MD patients results of special interest to define endophenotypes in MD [16].

The relationship between MD and both respiratory and food allergies has also been reported. Clinical improvement in MD patients with allergy has been observed after treatment of the allergy [17]. Several studies have reported a higher prevalence of migraine in MD [18], and a possible common etiology has been suggested [19, 20].

Based on that, we have reviewed the current knowledge on the pathophysiology and clinical management in MD, including MD studies published in the past 5 years, with a specific focus on tinnitus in MD.

Histology and Molecular Pathology

In 1938, Yamakawa in Japan [21] and Hallpike and Cairns in England [22] independently reported the finding of EH in temporal bones from patients with Ménière's syndrome. Hallpike and Cairns considered the hydrops as an essential morbid anatomy of a specific disease of the labyrinth. Other investigators described similar temporal bone findings over the next decade [23–27]. The hydrops seen in temporal bones was described as "idiopathic" since there was no obvious pathology in the temporal bones that could be considered causal.

Symptoms of MD originate in the inner ear and not in the eighth cranial nerve, brainstem, or other parts of the central nervous system. This is supported by the observation that labyrinthectomy results in immediate cessation of episodic vertigo and by histopathologic studies that have demonstrated EH and other pathologic changes in the inner ear (see below). Also, Thomsen and co-workers [28] found no discernible pathologic changes in the central nervous system that could account for symptoms in a post-mortem study of four cases with MD. Histopathological findings in MD are variable across different studies, suggesting that different mechanisms can lead to the development of EH.

Endolymphatic Hydrops

Endolymphatic hydrops is a consistent finding in MD [21–27, 29]. The hydrops principally involves the cochlear duct and saccule but can involve the utricle and ampullae of the semicircular canals (Fig. 33.1). This serves to distinguish the hydrops of MD from that seen in a variety of other ear pathologies, e.g., Mondini dysplasia, surgical trauma, temporal bone fracture, labyrinthitis, and syphilis [30, 31]. The walls of the membranous labyrinth may show areas of thinning, outpouching, and ruptures. In severe hydrops, distor-

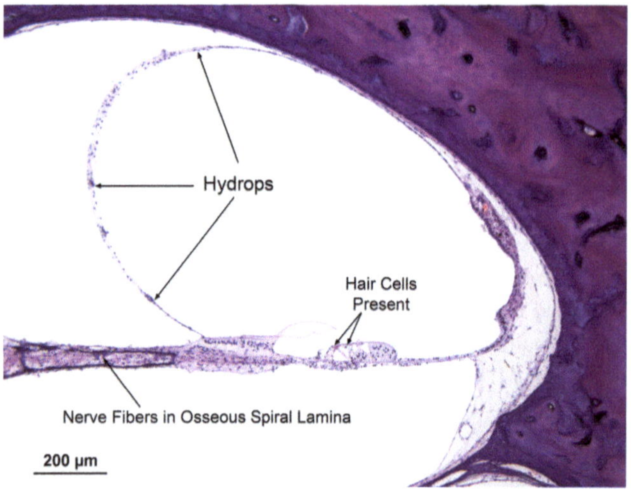

Fig. 33.1 Endolymphatic hydrops: Histological section of the cochlea (extracted from Lopez-Escamez JA, Morales C, Perez-Garrigues, Perez N (Eds.). Enfermedad de Meniere: desde las ciencias básicas a la medicina clínica. Ponencia Oficial Sociedad Española ORL. Euromedice. 2009. ISBN 978–84–96,727-76-2)

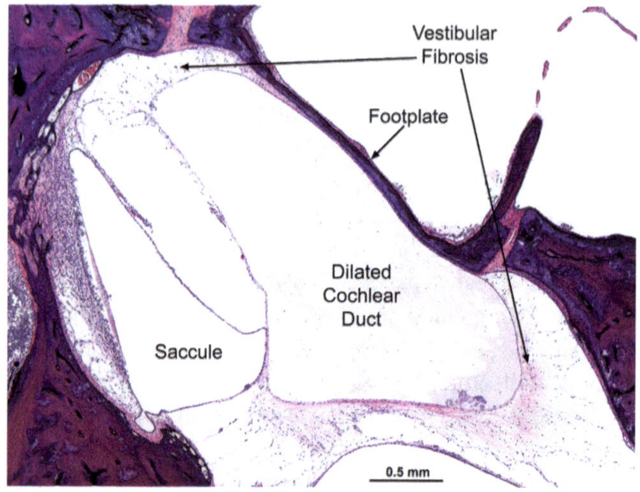

Fig. 33.2 Vestibular fibrosis: Histological section of the cochlea (extracted from Lopez-Escamez JA, Morales C, Perez-Garrigues, Perez N (Eds.). Enfermedad de Meniere: desde las ciencias básicas a la medicina clínica. Ponencia Oficial Sociedad Española ORL. Euromedice. 2009. ISBN 978–84–96,727-76-2)

tion and even collapse of the walls of the ampullae, utricle, and cochlear duct is observed. In some cases, papillary structures of uncertain significance have been observed within the ductus reuniens [29].

Vestibular Fibrosis

Proliferation of fibrous tissue within the vestibule is often observed (Fig. 33.2) which can result in the formation of a band of fibrous tissue between the under surface of the footplate and the utricle. This phenomenon is believed to be responsible for a positive Hennebert's sign (a positive "fistula sign without a fistula"), which is observed in about 30% of ears with MD [32].

Sensory Lesions

In most cases with MD, there is no significant loss of sensory hair cells in the cochlea [33], as determined by light microscopy (Fig. 33.1). In some patients believed to have advanced disease, permanent morphologic changes are observed under microscopic levels including loss of cochlear hair cells, atrophy of supporting cells in the organ of Corti, and distortion and atrophy of the tectorial membrane [33]. Using electron microscopy, Kimura et al. [34] and Nadol and Thornton [35] reported that significant pathological changes were present amongst surviving hair cells in the cochlea including fusion of cilia, disruption of cuticular bodies, and basal displacement of some outer hair cells with loss of contact with the tectorial membrane.

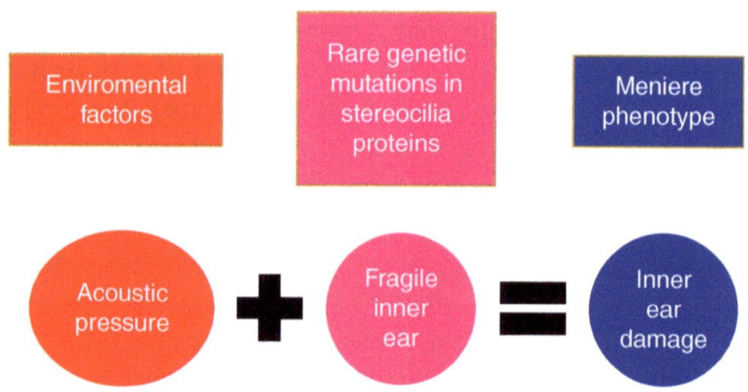

Fig. 33.3 Physiopathology of familial MD. We hypothesize that environmental factors such as sudden acoustic pressure in the cochlear duct in the carriers of rare genetic mutations in the proteins involved in the attachment of stereocilia among themselves or to the tectorial membrane such as otogelin (fragile organ od Corti) could induce a transient dysfunction leading to a permanent inner ear damage

The etiology of hearing loss, especially the fluctuating hearing loss, is not known. Because of the general lack of sensory cell lesions, we hypothesized that the increase of pressure associated with the hydrops in the cochlear duct may cause a detachment of the tectorial membrane from the hair cell stereocilia in the organ of Corti (Fig. 33.1), leading to a damage on the tip or ankle links, a loss of cohesiveness among stereocilia with a dysfunction in the opening of mechanotransduction channels that would explain the hearing loss (Fig. 33.3). This could be the case for autosomal recessive MD mediated by mutations in otogelin, a scaffolding protein involved in the cohesiveness among stereocilia and the tectorial membrane [6].

Vestibular sensory cells are generally present within the cristae and maculae when examined by light microscopy

[33, 36]. A detailed quantitative analysis of hair cell densities within the vestibular sense organs using Nomarski optics showed that type I hair cell densities were within the range for normative data, but there was a significant loss of type II hair cells for all three cristae and both maculae [37].

Neural Lesions

Neuronal cell counts of the spiral ganglion are normal in most patients. However, in about 10% of temporal bones, there is an isolated loss of cochlear neurons in the apex [33]. Loss of nerve fibers in the osseous spiral lamina has also been described [38]. At the ultrastructural level, Nadol and Thornton [35] showed a striking and statistically significant reduction in the number of afferent nerve endings and afferent synapses at the base of both inner and outer hair cells on the affected side in a case of unilateral MD. Scarpa's ganglion cell counts have been reported to be normal [36] or show significant loss [37].

The loss of spiral ganglion neurons can be the result of the lack of neurotrophins after cochlear damage. A burden analysis of rare missense variants in axonal guidance signaling genes such as *NTN4* or *NOX3* has been reported in patients with MD, suggesting an increased susceptibility to develop neural lesions [39].

Endolymphatic Sac and Vestibular Aqueduct

Hallpike and Cairns [22] observed a decrease in the amount of "loose" connective tissue around the endolymphatic sac in MD. However, they stated that this finding was not unique to MD and that they had also observed it in normal bones. Since then, many investigators have described pathologic changes such as hypoplasia of the vestibular aqueduct [40–42], hypoplasia of the endolymphatic sac [43] decreased vascularization of the sac [42], and perisaccular fibrosis [44] in cases with MD. In contrast, other studies [45–48] have shown that such findings are not a consistent feature of MD.

Pathophysiology and Mechanisms of Disease

Although the etiology of MD is still unknown, the main hypothesis considers MD as a multifactorial disorder. In fact, it seems that MD consists of a set of rare disorders with different etiologies, expressing a common phenotype [49].

Immune Response and Ménière's Disease

Different hypotheses have been proposed to explain the possible autoimmunity base related to MD including the appearance of cross-reactions with shared epitopes between inner ear proteins and microbial proteins, the development of damage related to constant high levels of cytokines and chemokines, or the presence of immunogenic factors that produce a persistent inflammatory response in the inner ear. Histological studies in animals discovered a large proliferation of cells of the immune system and an increase of fenestrated blood vessels in the inner ear, which supported the theory that the inner ear could have an immune function. Subsequent in vivo studies demonstrated the induction of antibodies production by the inner ear, providing further evidence that the endolymphatic sac has an immune response function [50]. Other studies have shown the presence of autoantigens against certain structures of the inner ear, in both patients with MD and autoimmune inner ear disease (AIED) [51].

Studies in animals have experimentally induced an immune-mediated EH after antigens and monoclonal antibodies exposure [52]. On the other hand, serum and blood studies in MD patients demonstrated the presence of antibodies against type II collagen, a connective tissue component present in the inner ear.

One of the immune response factors recently involved in MD is Fn14 (fibroblast growth factor-inducible 14; *Tnfrsf12a*), the receptor of the multifunctional cytokine tumor necrosis factor-like weak inducer of apoptosis (*Tnfsf12*; TWEAK), a member of the TNF superfamily involved in other autoimmune diseases, such as systemic lupus erythematosus or ulcerative colitis [53]. It has been discovered that one of its allelic variants (rs4947296) regulates the expression of multiple genes in the TWEAK/Fn14 pathway in peripheral blood mononuclear cells, leading to an inflammatory response mediated by NF-κβ in MD [54]. This variant has also been related to bilateral MD in the Spanish population, and it appears in up to 18% of patients with other autoimmune conditions. Multiple immunological factors could have an important etiological role in a subgroup of MD patients. Furthermore, studies on the use of glucocorticoids and other immunosuppressant in MD and the positive response after this treatment supports that autoimmunity could be the etiology in some MD patients [55].

Autoinflammatory diseases are caused by a hyperactive inflammatory response leading to an immune dysregulation, essentially mediated by IL-1β, type I IFN-mediated responses, and the transcription factor NFκB [56]. These diseases typically manifest themselves in the perinatal period, yet milder and later-onset forms are being diagnosed in the adulthood [57]. Some of these disorders have manifestations that mimic allergic and immunodeficiency disorders. Additionally, many of these diseases have SNHL as a symptom [56, 57], suggesting that potentially similar mechanisms of the molecular pathogenesis of hearing loss may exist.

AIED has overlapping audio-vestibular symptoms with MD. Patients with AIED show elevated levels of proinflammatory cytokines, such as TNFα and IL-1β resembling an autoinflammatory phenotype [58, 59]. Efforts are being made to increase the immunological disease continuum to involve monogenic and complex immune disorders that present both autoimmune and autoinflammatory indicators, where diseases such as AIED would fall [58]. Comparably to AIED, a subset of MD patients has shown overall elevated levels of proinflammatory cytokines, emphasizing IL-1β and TNFα expression [60–62].

Genetic Factors in Ménière's Disease

The genetic hypothesis of MD relies on facts like the variability of its prevalence according to the ethnic background, the familial aggregation studies, and the identification of some genes in familial MD with autosomal dominant and autosomal recessive inheritance. Several studies have demonstrated that 3–15% of patients have a relative with MD [63]. Most families have an autosomal dominant inheritance, with incomplete penetrance (about 60%); however, rare variants in *OTOG* gene have been reported in 6 families with MD with a compound heterozygous recessive pattern of inheritance [6]. The disorder usually develops at an earlier age in familial cases and tends to have more severe symptoms over generations, although in some families this statement could not be demonstrated. One study found one locus segregating the disease in four families on chromosome 14, near the COCH gene (DFNA9), although no mutations were found [64]. A second locus of the disease has been reported on chromosome 12p12.3 in a large Swedish family and several small family groups, though no pathogenic variants have been identified [65]. The genetic diagnosis of familial MD has been recently reviewed and 11 genes have been involved in the condition [66].

Sporadic MD has been related to many allelic variants, but these findings have not been replicated in an independent cohort, due to its heterogeneity.

According to this, MD could be considered an oligogenic disorder, as no gene is pathognomonic for MD. Furthermore, the description of a burden of rare missense variants in certain SNHL genes in sporadic cases through target sequencing panels supports the hypothesis that multiple genetic variants contribute to hearing loss in MD. These findings could help to clarify the genetic basis of MD in familial and sporadic cases [67, 68].

Migraine and Ménière's Disease

Many MD patients present headaches with migraine features associated or not with vertigo crises, and it has been suggested that these conditions could be part of the same process [19]. Moreover, a consistent higher prevalence of migraine in MD has been reported, particularly in women. Furthermore, there have been described cases of MD patients with associated vestibular migraine, suggesting a shared pathophysiology [69]. This observation could be explained if patients with the overlapping syndromes shared some common allelic variants with pleiotropic effects on the brain and the inner ear. There are some anatomical and clinical features to consider MD with migraine as an endophenotype of MD. A case-control study has found that patients with unilateral MD plus migraine have a reduced ipsilateral mastoid pneumatization, a shorter distance between the sigmoid sinus and the posterior wall of the external acoustic canal (anterior displacement of sigmoid sinus), an earlier age of onset, a higher frequency of vertigo attacks and a better hearing threshold [70, 71].

Allergy and Ménière's Disease

The first study where allergy and MD were related was published in 1923 [72]. The relationship between allergy and MD has been suggested in both food and environmental allergies [68]. Allergy is defined as a condition caused by hypersensitivity of the immune system to typically harmless substances in the environment, and as we commented previously, the greater susceptibility of the inner ear to certain aberrant immune reactions support this theory. Studies in animals have shown the presence of higher allergy markers associated with the development of endolymphatic hydrops after exposure to environmental antigens. In addition, another study showed a good clinical control of symptoms such as vertigo and tinnitus in MD patients who associated environmental or food allergy, after the prescription of a specific allergy treatment [73].

Other Comorbidities in Ménière's Disease

MD has also been related to other conditions such as BPPV, traumas, anatomical variability or psychological factors such as stress or anxiety. However, in the case of stress and anxiety, they are considered triggers of the attacks [74].

Clinical Variants in Ménière's Disease

MD patients have phenotypic heterogeneity [5], and it is difficult to characterize the outcome of the disease in its early stages. Even though the frequency of the spells of vertigo is typically greater during the earlier years [75–77], balance problems are observed during the course of the disease and may become severe if patients progress to a bilateral vestibular hypofunction [11, 78].

The epidemiological association of MD with migraine and several systemic autoimmune diseases (SAD), such as rheumatoid arthritis or psoriasis, sustains the hypothesis of an extended phenotype, beyond the audio-vestibular symptoms [12]. Although the diagnostic criteria for definite MD formulated by the Classification Committee of the Bárány Society in 2015 increase the accuracy in clinical diagnosis for MD, they do not reflect some comorbidities commonly observed in some patients such AD or migraine.

By using cluster analysis and clinical data from >1500 MD patients, several subgroups have been defined, according to four clinical predictors: delayed hydrops, history of Familial MD, migraine and history of SAD there were described 10 clinical subgroups of patients with MD (five Unilateral MD and five Bilateral MD) with strong potential etiological implications, and six of these subgroups were shared between UMD and BMD (type 3 FMD, type 4 MD with migraine and type 5 MD with SAD). These clinical variants observed in both UMD and BMD validate previous epidemiological studies, but they also indicate a separate role for genetics and autoimmunity as factors impacting the development of MD.

Clinical variants in Ménière's disease

Sporadic MD

Unilateral MD

Type 1 MD without migraine or autoimmune disorder (common MD)

Type 2 MD with previous SNHL (delayed MD)

Type 4 MD with migraine

Type 5 MD with autoimmune disorder

Bilateral MD

Type 1 MD with metachronic SNHL (common bilateral MD)

Type 2 MD with synchronic SNHL

Type 4 MD with migraine

Type 5 MD with autoimmune disorder

Familial MD (type 3)

Autosomal dominant (*COCH, DTNA, PRKCB, DPT, SEMA3D, MYO7A, TECTA*)

Autosomal recessive (*OTOG*)

Unilateral Ménière's Disease

Classical MD phenotype (or UMD type 1) is the most common clinical variant, and it includes sporadic patients without migraine or SAD. UMD type 2 is defined as delayed MD (previously known as delayed hydrops) and it is a rare condition. Most of patients are sporadic and do not have migraine. SAD is only observed in 10% of the patients, as expected in the general population. UMD type 3 includes all patients with FMD (described below). UMD type 4 is defined as sporadic cases plus migraine. This group might overlap with VM and it may share common pathophysiological mechanisms. Patients with MD can show migraine symptoms even during the attacks of vertigo [79], and this finding could make difficult the differential diagnosis of VM and MD [2, 80]. UMD type 5 could be considered as autoimmune MD, since all patients have another concurrent SAD and, all of them are sporadic without migraine.

Bilateral Ménière's Disease

Most patients start with SNHL in one ear, and it can appear in the other after several years (metachronic SNHL; 2–73% cases) [81, 82], but a substantial number of patients show simultaneous SNHL (synchronic SNHL). Therefore, bilateral involvement is a major concern for these individuals since the loss of vestibular function, and bilateral SNHL have significant influence in the health-related quality of life in them [83].

BMD type 1 is the most common clinical variant, and it includes metachronic MD patients. BMD type 2 has synchronic fluctuating bilateral SNHL. BMD type 3 includes all patients with familiar history of MD. BMD type 4 is associated with migraine in all cases, but they do not have familial history of MD. Like UMD type 4, this group may overlap with VM, and it might share common pathophysiological mechanisms. Finally, BMD type 5 could be considered as autoimmune MD, since all patients have another concomitant SAD. However, this group is heterogeneous and includes sporadic and familial patients, migraine and both synchronic and metachronic SNHL.

Familial Ménière's Disease

Although most MD patients are considered sporadic [70, 81], familial clustering has been reported in 8 to 9% of cases in European population [5], and in 6% of Korean population [84], which in addition supports a genetic impact to the disease [85].

FMD presents an autosomal dominant (AD) pattern of inheritance with incomplete penetrance and anticipation, showing an earlier onset compared to sporadic cases [86–88].The families may include patients with UMD or/and BMD, so epigenetic factors may influence uni- or bilateral involvement [5]. FMD can be subdivided in two subgroups (FMD with migraine and FMD without migraine). These findings confirm the early description of families with MD co-segregating migraine [89] and the more recent description of FMD without migraine [5, 90, 91] reflecting the genetic heterogeneity in FMD. Different whole-exome sequencing (WES)-based studies have identified several genes related to FMD. Single nucleotide variants (SNV) in *FAM136A*, *DTNA*,

PRKCB, SEMA3D, DPT, MYO7A, and TECTA genes were identified in four different families with AD inheritance with incomplete penetrance [8, 9, 63, 92, 93].

FMD may also show recessive inheritance. An enrichment of rare missense variants in the *OTOG* gene has been described in 46 families with MD, and six of them showed recessive compound heterozygous inheritance [6]. These findings support that several genes contribute to FMD, and it should be considered a rare polygenic disease.

Diagnosis of Ménière's Disease: Diagnostic Criteria

The Bárány Society has established an International Classification of Vestibular Disorders and promoted a consensus definition for several disorders, including MD. The diagnostic criteria were developed in a coordinated effort with the American Academy Otolaryngology-Head and Neck Surgery (AAO-HNS), the European Academy Otology and Neurotology, the Japan Society for Equilibrium Research, and the Korean Balance Society in 2015, considering two categories [94]:

Definition of Ménière's disease

Definite Meniere disease:

(a) Two or more spontaneous episodes of vertigo, lasting 20 minutes to 12 hours.
(b) Audiometrically documented low to medium frequency SNHL in one ear, defining the affected ear on at least one occasion before, during, or after one of the episodes of vertigo.
(c) Fluctuating aural symptoms (hearing, tinnitus, or fullness) in the affected ear.
(d) Not better accounted for by another vestibular diagnosis.

Probable Meniere disease:

(a) Two or more episodes of vertigo or dizziness, lasting 20 minutes to 24 hours.
(b) Fluctuating aural symptoms (hearing, tinnitus, or fullness) in the affected ear.
(c) Not better accounted for by another vestibular diagnosis.

Audiovestibular Examination in Ménière's Disease

The evaluation of hearing in patients with MD is essential to establish the diagnosis and during the follow-up [95]. Air and bone-conducted pure tone audiograms is the standard procedure to assess SNHL.

- Pure tone audiometry: This is the most useful test for MD diagnosis. A pure tone audiogram should be performed in all patients with an episodic vestibular syndrome. In MD, the demonstration of hearing fluctuations at low and medium frequencies during vertigo attacks is required for the diagnosis [96]. Likewise, to show this fluctuation, hearing thresholds must be tracked over time.
- Speech audiometry: For speech perception evaluation in patients with SNHL.
- Tympanometry: This test is applied for the evaluation of the middle ear status, and to rule out otitis media with effusion.
- Acoustic reflexes: This test evaluates the reflexive contraction of the stapes muscle and gives information about the vestibular and facial nerves' function.
- Otoacoustic emissions: This audiological test measures the sound generated from the outer hair cells of the cochlea and can be considered in selected patients with MD [95].
- Electrocochleography (ECoG): ECoG is an electrophysiological record of the cochlear function. It has variable sensitivity and specificity in patients with a clinical history consistent with MD [97–99].

In addition, a vestibular evaluation provides additional information during the diagnosis process and the follow-up. These tests help to confirm the vestibular hypofunction obtained after the first physical examination of the patient.

- Caloric tests: This is an objective test to demonstrate peripheral vestibular dysfunction. It is based on aural stimulation with different temperatures to evaluate horizontal semicircular canal function [100, 101], and it can confirm unilateral vestibular hypofunction in up to 75% of unilateral MD cases [102].
- Vestibular evoked myogenic potentials (VEMPs): This is a test that uses cervical or ocular muscles reflexes evoked by a loud noise in the ear or high-frequency vibration, which helps to evaluate the function of the saccule (cVEMP) and utricle (oVEMP) [103, 104]. Its role for MD diagnosis is so far unestablished (sensitivity: 50%; specificity: 49%) [105].

– Video head impulse test: This is an objective measure of the VOR for each semicircular canal. The VOR gain is used to track vestibular function during follow-up [101, 106].

MR Imaging in Ménière's Disease

The clinical utility of magnetic resonance imaging (MRI) for the diagnosis of MD is under debate. EH has been documented using three-dimensional fluid-attenuated inversion recovery (FLAIR) sequences. The use of intravenous gadolinium chelated-enhanced MRI allows visualization of EH [107]. In fact, the best way to assess EH on MRI is based in the inversion of the saccule-to-utricle area ratio, evaluated through a semi-quantitative grading method [108]. In patients with MD diagnostic criteria, the presence of EH in MRI is related to the hearing loss and probably with the duration of disease [109].

Although the visualization of EH has a high diagnostic value in patients with definite MD, it is important to remark the relatively high prevalence of EH in healthy individuals (31%) and other vestibular disorders such as vestibular migraine (28%) or vestibular schwannoma (26%). Endolymphatic hydrops is not a pathognomonic phenomenon, and detecting hydrops should not directly indicate a diagnosis of MD [110, 111].

Moreover, the most important factor to establish the diagnosis of MD is the temporal association of clinical signs and symptoms during the crises of the disease, such as the hearing fluctuation or tinnitus immediately before the vertigo attack. MRI is required for the exclusion of other diagnoses, according to the diagnostic criteria for MD.

Tinnitus in Ménière's Disease

There are two types of tinnitus in patients with MD, according to the clinical presentation:

(a) The tinnitus reported in one ear during the episode of vertigo that usually is a low-frequency noise of high loudness occurring immediately before the attack. This symptom is reported by most patients during the attacks. Although the mechanism is unknown, it is hypothesized that it is related to acute changes in the composition of the endolymph with random activation of the auditory afferents.
(b) The tinnitus reported out of the attacks being probably related to the inner ear damage causing a lack of trophic support in the nerve fibers when patients develop a persistent SNHL.

Tinnitus can be one of the most disabling symptoms in MD, together with vertigo episodes. Figure 33.4 shows the development of tinnitus through the evolution of the disease. In many cases, tinnitus is the initial symptom of the disease, and can precede the classical symptoms of hearing loss, vertigo, and aural fullness. As the disease evolves, the vertigo disappears, sometimes leaving a residual feeling of dizziness or unsteadiness as vestibular hypofunction ensues. In the advance stage, patients usually do not describe actual vertigo but more commonly feelings of imbalance. Meanwhile, the hearing loss becomes permanent and progresses with persistent tinnitus [112].

The tinnitus is commonly described as a low-frequency tone, and usually is a narrowband noise, described as a roaring or machine-like sound. At the beginning of the disease, tinnitus is intermittent and appears during the vertigo attacks in 83% of patients, disappearing after the acute crisis. As the disease evolves, tinnitus may become permanent, although changes in the tinnitus frequency or intensity can be perceived before or after the crisis. In general, patients mention that this change in its characteristics usually precedes and warns of the possibility of triggering a new vertigo crisis. In the last stages, when episodes of vertigo have disappeared, tinnitus becomes the predominant symptom, being the main cause of disability in MD, causing a significant deterioration in the perceived health-related quality of life [113].

A multicenter study described a psychoacoustic characterization of tinnitus in 100 MD patients, including an analysis of the impact of tinnitus in quality of life. This study observed that, although all MD patients reported tinnitus, it was permanent in 79% of them. Thirty-three patients reported to have a noise-like tinnitus (42%), 42 patients reported a single tonal tinnitus (53%), and four patients presented different tinnitus types. MD patients with tonal tinnitus present higher scores in Tinnitus Handicap Inventory (THI) compared with MD patients with noise-like tinnitus. There was a positive correlation between THI and Visual Analogue Scale (VAS), with a stronger association in patients with bilateral MD. Tinnitus extreme phenotype (TEP) in MD showed THI scores of 80 out of 100, with lower age of onset for both MD and tinnitus. In addition, annoyance in MD is associated with tonal type tinnitus and higher scores in THI and the Hospital Anxiety and Depression Scale (HADS), suggesting an association with anxiety and depression [114].

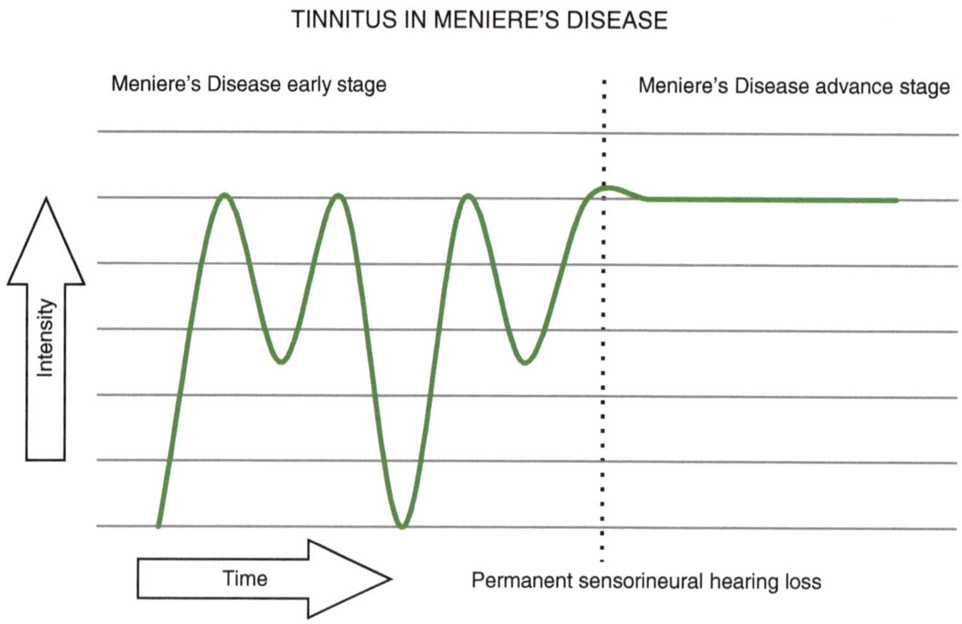

Fig. 33.4 Tinnitus behavior in MD. There are two types of tinnitus in MD: acute tinnitus occurring during the attacks of vertigo associated with transient hearing loss and persistent non-fluctuating tinnitus that usually develops when the hearing loss becomes permanent

Treatment

The treatment of MD should be personalized, according to the comorbid conditions of each patient. There is no single pill to fix symptoms for everybody since there is no etiological therapy. We currently treat symptoms: episodes of vertigo, hearing loss, and tinnitus. An excellent review has been recently published regarding the treatment of vertigo in MD [115]. Here, we will focus on the treatment of hearing loss and tinnitus.

Although therapeutic alternatives are limited, MD patients can benefit from different drug options. Corticosteroids have immunosuppressive, anti-inflammatory, and vasodilator effects, and also theoretical neuroprotective effects by the inhibition of lipid peroxidation and apoptosis [116, 117]. Also intratympanic corticosteroids have been classically administrated to obtain a more localized effect in the inner ear, and it has been considered as the first option since the side effects of intratympanic therapy associated with this therapy, like hearing loss, chronic symptoms of dizziness resulting from the fixed vestibular loss, or other adverse events, are very low [118–120]. Although both treatments are usually applied to control vertigo crises, they have also shown a positive effect on hearing thresholds, tinnitus annoyance and aural fullness, based in randomized control trials and systematic reviews [121, 122].

Ebselen (SPI-1005) is a promising drug that has been investigated in several clinical trials for hearing loss and is the first investigational new drug to advance to phase 3 in MD. This drug has demonstrated its effectiveness in studies in phase 2 for noise-induced hearing loss, and studies in ototoxicity and other neuroinflammatory diseases also showed early efficacy [123].

Hearing loss in MD presents a fluctuating course and the adaptation of hearing aids is difficult in the early stages of the disease. Some options can be offered in MD patients to improve speech recognition in noise, or to benefit from fluctuating hearing loss in the early stages, provided by hearing aids with multiple programs [124]. However, although the use of hearing aids in general population is recommended to improve the hearing loss and to relieve tinnitus, there is a lack of publications in this field. In more advanced stages of the disease, a cochlear implantation (CI) could be performed. The use of cochlear implants in MD can improve hearing, tinnitus, and vestibular function [125–127]. In addition, a review focusing on this topic has proven that CI is a good option with promising outcomes in terms of speech performances, regardless of the disease duration, uni- or bilaterality, age at implantation and stage of the disease [128].

In addition, and based on the effects of both CI and labyrinthectomy for hearing loss and vertigo, a recent study explored the option of performing both techniques simultaneously, with promising results for the improvement of sound localization, speech understanding and both tinnitus severity and quality of life [129]. According to these findings, a recent review demonstrated that CI with and without simultaneous labyrinthectomy appears as a viable treatment option for patients with MD, with high rates of tinnitus suppression and vertigo control, and similar postoperative speech perception outcomes to non-MD patients [130].

According to tinnitus in MD, these patients could also benefit from the general therapies that have shown effectiveness for tinnitus treatment, such as cognitive behavioral therapy (CBT).

References

1. Ménière P. Sur une forme de surdité grave dépendant d'une lésion de l'oreille interne. Gaz Méd de Paris. 1861;16(29)
2. Lopez-Escamez JA, et al. Diagnostic criteria for Menière's disease. J Vestib Res. 2015;25:1–7.
3. Espinosa Sanchez JM, et al. Menière's disease. In: LT FJM, editor. Handbook of clinical neurology, vol. 137. Amsterdam: Elsevier; 2016. p. 257–77.
4. Merchant SN, et al. Pathophysiology of Menière' syndrome are symptoms caused by endolymphatic hydrops? Otol Neurotol. 2005;26:74–81.
5. Requena T, et al. Familial clustering and genetic heterogeneity in Meniere's disease. Clin Genet. 2014;85(3):245–52.
6. Roman-Naranjo P, et al. Burden of rare variants in the OTOG gene in familial Meniere's disease. Ear Hear. 2020;41(6):1598–605.
7. Frejo L, et al. Genetics of vestibular disorders: pathophysiological insights. J Neurol. 2016;263(1):45–53.
8. Martín-Sierra C, et al. Variable expressivity and genetic heterogeneity involving DPT and SEMA3D genes in autosomal dominant familial Meniere's disease. Genetics. 2017;25(2):200–7.
9. Martín-Sierra C, et al. A novel missense variant in PRKCB segregates low-frequency hearing loss in an autosomal dominant family with Meniere's disease. Hum Mol Genet. 2016;25(16):3407–15.
10. Oberman B, et al. The aetiopathologies of Ménière's disease: a contemporary review. Acta Otorhinolaryngol Italica. 2017;37(4):250–63.
11. Gazquez I, et al. High prevalence of systemic autoimmune diseases in patients with Menière's disease. PLoS One. 2011;6(10):e26759.
12. Tyrrell JS, et al. Prevalence, associated factors, and comorbid conditions for Ménière's disease. Ear Hear. 2014;35(4):162–9.
13. Flook M, et al. Meniere's disease: genetics and the immune system. Curr Otorhinolaryngol Rep. 2018;5:1–8.
14. Frejo L, et al. Regulation of Fn14 receptor and NF-κB underlies inflammation in Meniere's disease. Front Immunol. 2017;8:1739.
15. Yuan F, et al. Genetic study of early-onset Graves' disease in the Chinese Han population. Clin Genet. 2018;93(1):103–10.
16. Penêda JF, et al. Immune-mediated inner ear disease: diagnostic and therapeutic approaches. Acta Otorrinolaringol Española. 2018;70:97.
17. Yang B, et al. The role of allergy in otologic disease. Otolaryngol Clin N Am. 2017;50(6):1091–101.
18. Ray J, et al. An epidemiological study to investigate the relationship between Meniere's disease and migraine. Clin Otolaryngol. 2016;41(6):707–10.
19. Ghavami Y, et al. Migraine features in patients with Meniere's disease. Laryngoscope. 2016;126(1):163–8.
20. Liu YF, et al. The intimate relationship between vestibular migraine and Meniere disease: a review of pathogenesis and presentation. Behav Neurol. 2016;2016:3182735.
21. Yamakawa K. Uber die pathologisch Veranderung bei einem Ménière-Kranken. J Otorhinolaryng Soc Japan. 1938;4:2310–2.
22. Hallpike C, et al. Observations on the pathology of Ménière's syndrome. J Laryngol Otol. 1938;53:625–55.
23. Nager F. Zur Histopathologie des Ohrschwindels. Pract Oto-Rhino-Laryngol. 1949;11:360–77.
24. Day K, et al. Hydrops of the labyrinth. Laryngoscope. 1949;59:213–27.
25. Cawthorne T. Ménière's disease. Ann Otol Rhinol Laryngol. 1947;56:18–38.
26. Altmann F, et al. Histological findings in Ménière's symptom complex. Ann Otol Rhinol Laryngol. 1943;52:52–80.
27. Lindsay J. Labyrinthine dropsy and Ménière's disease. Arch Otolaryngol. 1942;35:853–67.
28. Thomsen J, et al. Ménière's disease: peripheral or central origin. Acta Otolaryngol (Stockh) Suppl. 1984;406:46–51.
29. Schuknecht H. In: Press HU, editor. Pathology of the ear. Cambridge: Harvard University Press; 1974. p. 453–65.
30. Vasama J, et al. Ménière's disease and endolymphatic hydrops without Ménière's symptoms: temporal bone histopathology. Acta Otolaryngol. 1999;119(3):297–301.
31. Sperling N, et al. Symptomatic versus asymptomatic endolymphatic hydrops: a histopathologic comparison. Laryngoscope. 1993;103:277–85.
32. Nadol J. Positive Hennebert's sign in Ménière's disease. Arch Otolaryngol. 1977;103:524–30.
33. Schuknecht H. Pathology of the ear. Philadelphia, PA: Lea and Febiger; 1993.
34. Kimura R, et al. Electron microscopic observations in bilateral Ménière's disease. Ann Otol Rhinol Laryngol. 1976;85:791–801.
35. Nadol J, et al. Ultrastructural findings in a case of Ménière's disease. Ann Otol Rhinol Laryngol. 1987;96:449–54.
36. Richter E. Quantitative study of Scarpa's ganglion and vestibular sense organs in endolymphatic hydrops. Ann Otol Rhinol Laryngol. 1981;90:121–5.
37. Tsuji K, et al. Temporal bone studies of the human peripheral vestibular system: Meniere's disease. Ann Otol Rhinol Laryngol. 2000;109(181):26–31.
38. Spoendlin H, et al. Multicentre evaluation of the temporal bones obtained from a patient with suspected Menière's disease. Acta Otolaryngol Suppl. 1992;499:1–21.
39. Gallego-Martinez A, et al. Enrichment of damaging missense variants in genes related with axonal guidance signalling in sporadic Meniere's disease. J Med Genet. 2020;57(2):82–8.
40. Hebbar G, et al. Three-dimensional analysis of 61 human endolymphatic ducts and sacs in ears with and without Ménière's disease. Ann Otol Rhinol Laryngol. 1991;100:219–25.
41. Rizvi S, et al. Idiopathic endolymphatic hydrops and the vestibular aqueduct. Ann Otol. 1981;90:77–9.
42. Ikeda M, et al. Vascularity of endolymphatic sac in Ménière's disease: a histopathologic study. Ann Otol Rhinol Laryngol. 1985;94(118):6–10.
43. Eckhard A, et al. Inner ear pathologies impair sodium-regulated ion transport in Meniere's disease. Acta Neuropathol. 2019;137(2):343–57.
44. Ikeda M, et al. Endolymphatic duct and sac in patients with Ménière's disease: a temporal bone histopathologic study. Ann Otol Rhinol Laryngol. 1984;93:540–6.
45. Wackym P, et al. Re-evaluation of the role of the human endolymphatic sac in Ménière's disease. Otolaryngol Head Neck Surg. 1990;102:732–44.
46. Fraysse B, et al. Ménière's disease and endolymphatic hydrops: clinical-histopathological correlations. Ann Otol Rhinol Laryngol. 1980;89(Suppl 76):2–22.
47. Plantenga K, et al. The vestibular aqueduct and endolymphatic sac and duct in endolymphatic hydrops. Arch Otolaryngol. 1979;105:546–52.

48. Yuen S, et al. Vestibular aqueduct and endolymphatic duct in Ménière's disease. Arch Otolaryngol. 1972;96:553–5.
49. Gabriková D, et al. Familiar Meniere's disease restricted to 1.48 Mb on chromosome 12p12.3 by allelic and haplotype association. J Hum Genet. 2010;55:834–7.
50. Guild S, Guild SR. Observations upon the structure and normal contents of the ductus and saccus endolymphaticus in the guinea pig (Cavia cobaya). Am J Anat. 1927;39(102)
51. Cabrera S, et al. Intronic variants in the NFKB1 gene may influence hearing forecast in patients with unilateral sensorineural hearing loss in Meniere's disease. PLoS One. 2014;9(11)
52. Matsuoka H, et al. Induction of endolymphatic hydrops by directly infused monoclonal antibody against type II collagen CB11 peptide. Ann Otol Rhinol Laryngol. 2002;111(7 Pt 1):587–92.
53. Requena T, et al. Allelic variants in TLR10 gene may influence bilateral affectation and clinical course of Meniere's disease. Immunogenetics. 2013;65(5):345–55.
54. Gazquez I, et al. MICA-STR a.4 is associated with slower hearing loss progression in patients with Ménière's disease. Otol Neurotol. 2012;33(2):223–9.
55. Lopez-Escamez JA, et al. Association of a functional polymorphism of PTPN22 encoding a lymphoid protein phosphatase in bilateral Meniere's disease. Laryngoscope. 2010;120(1):103–7.
56. Broderick L. Hereditary autoinflammatory disorders: recognition and treatment. Immunol Allergy Clin N Am. 2019;39(1):13–29.
57. Martinez-Quiles N, et al. Updates on autoinflammatory diseases. Curr Opin Immunol. 2018;55:97–105.
58. Vambutas A, et al. AAO: autoimmune and autoinflammatory (disease) in otology: what is new in immune-mediated hearing loss. Laryngoscope Investig Otolaryngol. 2016;1(5):110–5.
59. Pathak S, et al. IL-1β is overexpressed and aberrantly regulated in corticosteroid nonresponders with autoimmune inner ear disease. J Immunol. 2011;186(3):1870–9.
60. Frejo L, et al. Proinflammatory cytokines and response to molds in mononuclear cells of patients with Meniere disease. Sci Rep. 2018;8(1):59.
61. Flook MFL, et al. Differential proinflammatory signature in vestibular migraine and Meniere disease. Front Immunol. 2019;10:1229.
62. Frejo L, et al. Cytokines and inflammation in Meniere disease. Clin Exp Otorhinolaryngol. 2022;15(1):49–59.
63. Requena T, et al. Identification of two novel mutations in FAM136A and DTNA genes in autosomal-dominant familial Meniere's disease. Hum Mol Genet. 2015;24(4):1119–26.
64. Gallego-Martinez A, et al. Excess of rare missense variants in hearing loss genes in sporadic Meniere disease. Front Genet. 2018;10:76.
65. Li Y-J, et al. Variants in the KCNE1 or KCNE3 gene and risk of Ménière's disease: a meta-analysis. J Vestib Res. 2016;25(5–6):211–8.
66. Escalera-Balsera A, et al. Systematic review of sequencing studies and gene expression profiling in familial Meniere disease. Genes (Basel). 2020;11(12):1414.
67. Gallego-Martinez A, et al. Genetic contribution to vestibular diseases. J Neurol. 2018;265(1):29–34.
68. Hietikko E, et al. Higher prevalence of autoimmune diseases and longer spells of vertigo in patients affected with familial Ménière's disease: a clinical comparison of familial and sporadic Ménière's disease. Am J Audiol. 2014;23(2):232–7.
69. Murofushi T, et al. Simultaneous presentation of definite vestibular migraine and definite Ménière's disease: overlapping syndrome of two diseases. Front Neurol. 2018;9:749.
70. Frejo L, et al. Extended phenotype and clinical subgroups in unilateral Meniere disease: a cross-sectional study with cluster analysis. Clin Otolaryngol. 2017;42(6):1172–80.
71. Diao T, et al. The clinical characteristics and anatomical variations in intractable unilateral Meniere's disease patients with and without migraine. J Vest Res. 2021;(in press).
72. Duke W. Ménière's syndrome caused by allergy. J Am Med Assoc. 1923;81(26):2179–81.
73. Ralli M, et al. Audiovestibular symptoms in systemic autoimmune diseases. J Immunol Res. 2018;19:5798103.
74. Kangasniemi E, et al. The theory of autoimmunity in Meniere's disease is lacking evidence. Auris Nasus Larynx. 2018;45(3):399–406.
75. Stahle J, et al. Long-term progression of Menière's disease. Am J Otol. 1989;10(3):170–3.
76. Belinchon A, et al. Evolution of symptoms in Ménière's disease. Audiol Neurootol. 2012;17(2):126–32.
77. Perez-Garrigues H, et al. Time course of episodes of definitive vertigo in Meniere's disease. Arch Otolaryngol Head Neck Surg. 2008;134(11):1149–54.
78. Huppert D, et al. Long-term course of Meniere's disease revisited. Acta Otolaryngol. 2010;130(6):644–51.
79. Lopez-Escamez JA, et al. Accompanying symptoms overlap during attacks in Meniere's disease and vestibular migraine. Front Neurol. 2014;5:265.
80. Lempert T, et al. Vestibular migraine: diagnostic criteria. Consensus document of the Bárány society and the international headache society. Acta Otorrinolaringol Espanola. 2013;64(6):428–33.
81. Frejo L, et al. Clinical subgroups in bilateral Meniere disease. Front Neurol. 2016;24(7):182.
82. House J, et al. Meniere's disease: prevalence of contralateral ear involvement. Otol Neurotol. 2006;27(3):355–61.
83. Lopez-Escamez J, et al. Impact of bilaterality and headache on health-related quality of life in Meniere's disease. Ann Otol Rhinol Laryngol. 2009;118(6):409–16.
84. Lee J, et al. Genetic aspects and clinical characteristics of familial Meniere's disease in a south Korean population. Laryngoscope. 2015;125(9):2175–80.
85. Roman-Naranjo P, et al. Genetics of vestibular syndromes. Curr Opin Neurol. 2018;31(1):105–10.
86. Birgerson L, et al. Familial Menière's disease: a genetic investigation. Am J Otol. 1987;8(4):323–6.
87. Klar J, et al. A Meniere's disease gene linked to chromosome 12p12.3. Am J Med Genet B Neuropsychiatr Genet. 2006;141B(5):463–7.
88. Morrison A, et al. Familial Ménière's disease: clinical and genetic aspects. J Laryngol Otol. 2009;123(1):29–37.
89. Oliveira C, et al. Occurrence of familial Meniere's syndrome and migraine in Brasília. Ann Otol Rhinol Laryngol. 2002;111(3 Pt 1):229–36.
90. Arweiler-Harbeck D, et al. Genetic aspects of familial Ménière's disease. Otol Neurotol. 2011;32(4):695–700.
91. Hietikko E, et al. Finnish familial Meniere disease is not linked to chromosome 12p12.3, and anticipation and cosegregation with migraine are not common findings. Genet Med. 2011;13(5):415–20.
92. Roman-Naranjo P, et al. Defective α-tectorin may involve tectorial membrane in familial Meniere disease. Clin Transl Med. 2022;12(6):e829.
93. Roman-Naranjo P, et al. Rare coding variants involving MYO7A and other genes encoding stereocilia link proteins in familial meniere disease. Hear Res. 2021;15:409.
94. Lopez-Escamez JA, et al. Diagnostic criteria for Menière's disease according to the classification Committee of the Bárány Society. HNO. 2017;65(11):887–93.
95. Sugihara EM, et al. Mastoid and inner ear measurements in patients with Menière's disease. Otol Neurotol. 2017;38(10):1484–9.

96. Hoa M, et al. Prognostic implications of and audiometric evidence for hearing fluctuation in Meniere's disease. Laryngoscope. 2015;125(12):S1–12.
97. Ziylan F, et al. Click stimulus Electrocochleography versus MRI with Intratympanic contrast in Ménière's disease: a systematic review. Otol Neurotol. 2016;37(5):421–7.
98. Lamounier P, et al. Electrocochleography for Ménière's disease: is it reliable? Braz J Otorhinolaryngol. 2014;80(6):527–32.
99. Hornibrook J. Tone burst Electrocochleography for the diagnosis of clinically certain Meniere's disease. Front Neurosci. 2017;11:301.
100. McMullen KP, et al. Correlation of objective audiometric and caloric function in Ménière's disease. Otolaryngol Head Neck Surg. 2017;156(5):912–6.
101. Cordero-Yanza JA, et al. Comparative study between the caloric vestibular and the video-head impulse tests in unilateral Menière's disease. Acta Otolaryngol. 2017;137(11):1178–82.
102. Wang H-M, et al. Analysis of auditory and vestibular function in patients with unilateral Menière's disease. Acta Otolaryngol. 2012;132:1246–51.
103. Maheu M, et al. The clinical utility of vestibular-evoked myogenic potentials in the diagnosis of Ménière's disease. Front Neurol. 2017;15(8):415.
104. Zhu Y, et al. Cervical VEMP threshold response curve in the identification of Ménière's disease. J Am Acad Audiol. 2014;25(3):278–88.
105. Jerin C, et al. Ocular vestibular evoked myogenic potential frequency tuning in certain Menière's disease. Hear Res. 2014;310:54–9.
106. Lee S-U, et al. Comparison of caloric and head-impulse tests during the attacks of Meniere's disease. Laryngoscope. 2017;127(3):702–8.
107. Naganawa S, et al. Visualization of endolymphatic hydrops with MR imaging in patients with Ménière's disease and related pathologies: current status of its methods and clinical significance. Jpn J Radiol. 2014;32(4):191–204.
108. Attyé A, et al. MRI of endolymphatic hydrops in patients with Meniere's disease: a case-controlled study with a simplified classification based on saccular morphology. Eur Radiol. 2016;27(8):3138–46.
109. Lopez-Escamez JA, et al. Systematic review of magnetic resonance imaging for diagnosis of Meniere disease. J Vest Res. 2018;29(2-3):121.
110. Lingam RKCS, Casselman JW, Beale T. MRI in otology: applications in cholesteatoma and Ménière's disease. Clin Radiol. 2018;73(1):35–44.
111. van der Lubbe MFJA, et al. The "hype" of hydrops in classifying vestibular disorders: a narrative review. J Neurol. 2020;267:197.
112. Lopez-Escamez JA, et al. Towards personalized medicine in Ménière's disease. F1000Res. 2018;7:F1000 Faculty Rev-295.
113. Manchaiah V, et al. Positive experiences associated with acquired hearing loss, Ménière's disease, and tinnitus: a review. Int J Audiol. 2015;54(1):1–10.
114. Perez-Carpena P, et al. A tinnitus symphony in 100 patients with Meniere's disease. Clin Otolaryngol. 2019;44:1176–80.
115. Espinosa-Sanchez J, et al. The pharmacological management of vertigo in Meniere disease. Expert Opin Pharmacother. 2020;21(14):1753–63.
116. Farhood Z, et al. The physiologic role of corticosteroids in Ménière's disease. Am J Otolaryngol. 2016;37(5):455–8.
117. Tassinari M, et al. Ménière's disease treatment: a patient-centered systematic review. Audiol Neurootol. 2015;20(3):153–65.
118. Chuang-Chuang A, et al. Are intratympanic corticosteroids effective for Ménière disease? Medwave. 2017;17(Suppl1)
119. McRackan TR, et al. Intratympanic dexamethasone as a symptomatic treatment for Ménière's disease. Otol Neurotol. 2014;35(9):1638–40.
120. Patel M. Intratympanic corticosteroids in Ménière's disease: a mini-review. J Otol. 2017;12(3):117–24.
121. Garduno-Anaya M, et al. Dexamethasone inner ear perfusion by intratympanic injection in unilateral Me'nie're's disease: a two-year prospective, placebo controlled, double-blind, randomized trial. Otolaryngol Head Neck Surg. 2005;133(2):285–94.
122. Phillips J, et al. Intratympanic steroids for Me'nie're's disease or syndrome. Cochrane Database Syst Rev. 2011;7:CD008514.
123. Kil J, et al. Development of Ebselen for the treatment of sensorineural hearing loss and tinnitus, hearing research. Hear Res. 2021;413:108209.
124. Valente M, et al. Problems and solutions for fitting amplification to patients with Ménière's disease. J Am Acad Audiol. 2006;17(1):6–15.
125. McNeill C, et al. Cochlear implant impedance fluctuation in Ménière's disease: a case study. Otol Neurotol. 2016;37(7):873–7.
126. McRackan TR, et al. Cochlear implantation in Ménière's disease patients. Otol Neurotol. 2014;35(3):421–5.
127. Mick P, et al. Cochlear implantation in patients with advanced Ménière's disease. Otol Neurotol. 2014;35(7):1172–8.
128. Kocharyan A, et al. Cochlear implantation in patients with Menière's disease: does disease activity affect the outcome? Otol Neurotol. 2020;41(9):1296–304.
129. Perkins E, et al. Simultaneous labyrinthectomy and cochlear implantation in unilateral Meniere's disease. Laryngoscope Investig Otolaryngol. 2018;3(3):255–30.
130. Villavisanis D, et al. Cochlear implantation in Meniere's disease: a systematic review and meta-analysis. Laryngoscope. 2021;131(8):1845–54.

Tinnitus and Vestibular Schwannoma

34

Dirk De Ridder and Tobias Kleinjung

Abstract

Vestibular schwannomas (VS) are associated with ipsilateral hearing loss (95%), tinnitus (70–80%), and disorders of balance (50%). However, unilateral hearing loss does not equate to a vestibular schwannoma. When an MRI scan is performed for unilateral hearing loss, in only 0.3% of patients, a VS is identified. Tinnitus is the principal symptom in 10% of VS patients, usually in very small or very large tumors, and is moderate to severe in 14% of individuals. It is mostly of high pitch.

Tinnitus improves when the cochlear nerve is transected, or hearing is saved during treatment. In general, microsurgery has better outcomes for tinnitus than stereotactic radiosurgery (SRS). This is likely related to the fact that after retrosigmoid and translabyrinthine, microsurgery tinnitus is often experienced as less troublesome than before the surgery.

D. De Ridder (✉)
Section of Neurosurgery, Department of Surgical Sciences, University of Otago, Dunedin, New Zealand
e-mail: dirk.deridder@otago.ac.nz

T. Kleinjung
Department of Otorhinolaryngology—Head and Neck Surgery, University Hospital of Zurich, University of Zurich, Zurich, Switzerland
e-mail: tobias.kleinjung@usz.ch

W. Schlee et al. (eds.), *Textbook of Tinnitus*, https://doi.org/10.1007/978-3-031-35647-6_34

Graphical Abstract

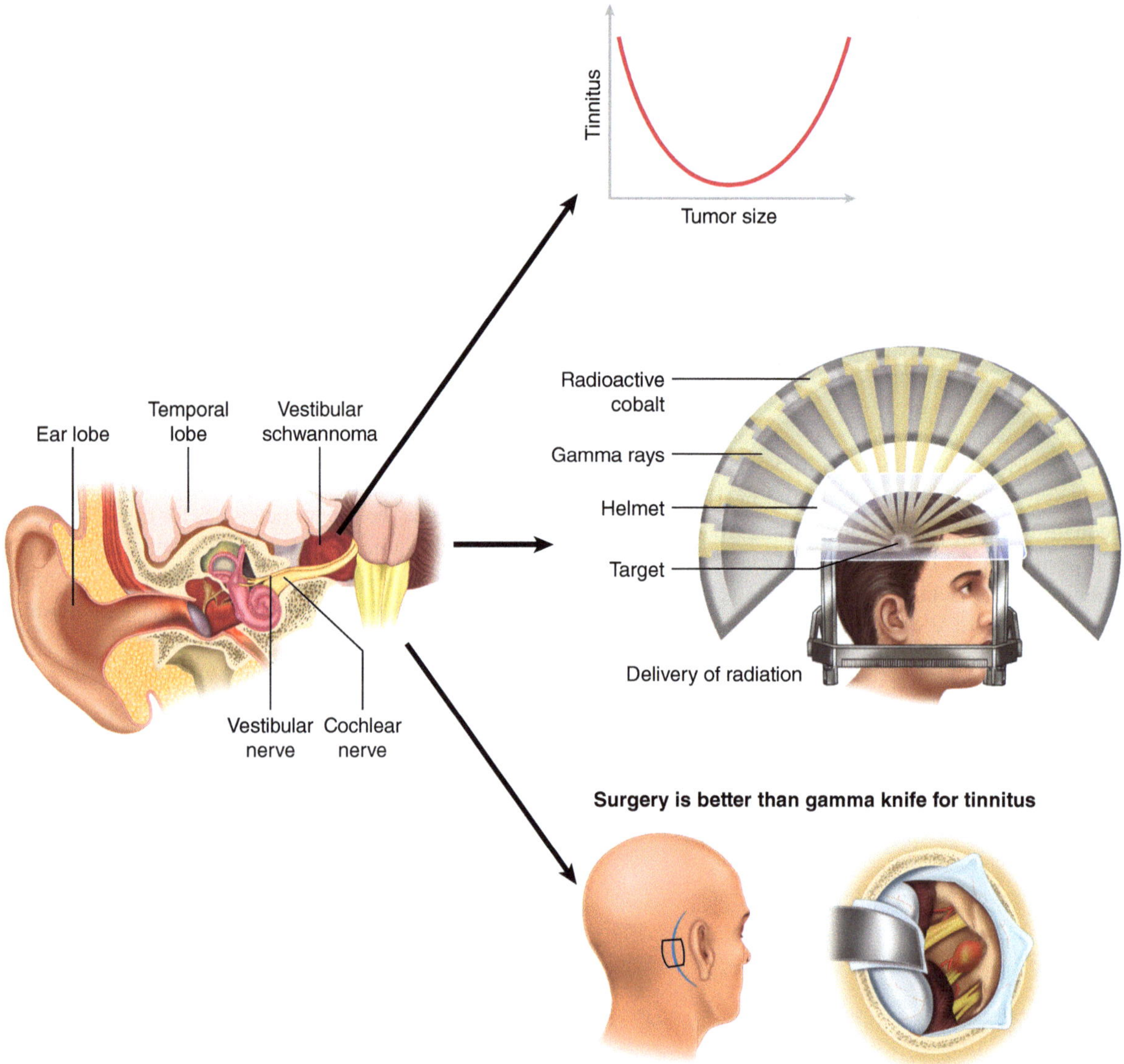

Abbreviations

Gy	Gray
ILS	Intralabyrinthine schwannoma
SRS	Stereotactic radiosurgery
THI	Tinnitus handicap inventory
VS	Vestibular schwannoma

Highlights

- Tinnitus is a common symptom in individuals with vestibular schwannoma (VS).
- MRI scan in unilateral hearing loss only detects vestibular schwannoma in 0.3% of patients.
- In 70–80% of cases, VS is ipsilateral to the tinnitus; it is the principal symptom in 10% and is moderate to severe in 14% of individuals.
- Tinnitus in VS is typically associated with hearing loss (95%) and disorders of balance (50%).
- Tinnitus in VS is mostly of high pitch.
- Tinnitus is the predominant symptom in very small and very large tumors.
- Tinnitus improves when the cochlear nerve is cut or hearing is saved during treatment.
- Microsurgery has better outcomes for tinnitus than stereotactic radiosurgery (SRS).
- After retrosigmoid and translabyrinthine, microsurgery tinnitus is often less troublesome than before the surgery.

Introduction

The name "acoustic neuroma" (correctly known as vestibular schwannoma, VS) is a misnomer because histologically the benign lesions derive from the neurilemma sheath, most commonly of the superior vestibular nerve and not the auditory nerve [1]. These tumors occur in two forms: 95% are unilateral, mostly presenting after the age of 50 and 5% occur bilaterally as a part of the signs of neurofibromatosis type 2, presenting at younger age (often before the age of 30) [2]. In neurofibromatosis type 1, unilateral VS are rare, with an incidence of about 2%. Bilateral VS are virtually nonexistent in neurofibromatosis type 1 [2].

The incidence of symptomatic VS is 3–5/100.000 [3], with 1.3/100.000 incidentally diagnosed tumors [3]. Postmortem studies indicate that the actual incidence is much higher (0.8%) [4] because many schwannoma remain asymptomatic.

Some epidemiological studies have found an association between the use of mobile phones and the incidence of VS [5–8], whereas other studies have not found such an association [9–11]. VS incidence has remained stable in the United States between 2004 and 2017, whereas mobile phone use has increased dramatically, arguing against an association [12]. Similarly, some epidemiological studies suggest an association between loud noise and VS [13].

The symptoms and signs of VS depend on the size of the lesion. When still intracanalicular, VS typically presents with a triad of symptoms: unilateral tinnitus (73%) [14], hearing loss (90–98%) [14–16], and balance problems (50%) [2]. The most common symptom is unilateral hearing loss [16], predominantly in high frequencies [2]. The hearing loss is progressive in most individuals with VS. Yet, when performing a MRI to exclude a VS in patients who present with unilateral hearing loss only results in detecting a VS in 0.3% of scanned people [17]. Sudden deafness occurs in 12% of people with a VS [18]. Yet, in patients with sudden sensorineural hearing loss, only 1.1% harbor a VS [19]. Low-frequency hearing loss occurs in individuals with large tumors [20]. In 7.7%, a VS is not associated with hearing loss [21]. These are most commonly small (1 cm) intracanalicular tumors [21]. In these patients, dizziness is the most common presenting symptom (60%), followed by headache (40%), visual changes (33%), and tinnitus (33%) [21]. In this context, it should be mentioned that incidental diagnoses of VS are consistently made in MRI examinations done for other reasons. These account for approximately 10% of all diagnosed VS [22]. Intralabyrinthine schwannomas (ILS) represent a special entity within schwannomas that can cause tinnitus [23]. These are rare tumors that may develop from the terminal schwann cells of the cochlear or vestibular nerves and may spread to the cochlea, vestibule, or semicircular canals [23]. ILS should be distinguished from the intracanalicular schwannomas described above, which develop primarily in the internal auditory canal and then progress per continuitatem toward the inner ear structures. With the improvement in imaging, ILS are now diagnosed more frequently [24]. Depending on the site of presentation, they may present with tinnitus, hearing loss, and/or vertigo. Following hearing loss, tinnitus is the second most common symptom of ILS at the time of diagnosis and is observed in approximately 70% of cases [25].

In VS, disequilibrium is more common than vertigo, and when disequilibrium is the first symptom, it seems to be correlated with rapidly growing tumors [26]. VS-related vertigo often occurs without nausea [15]. Tinnitus usually develops when the tumor is still intracanalicular [16], and is reported as the principal symptom in one of 10 patients who seek medical help [14]. Tinnitus is more common in small and large tumors than in medium-sized tumors [16] (Fig. 34.1).

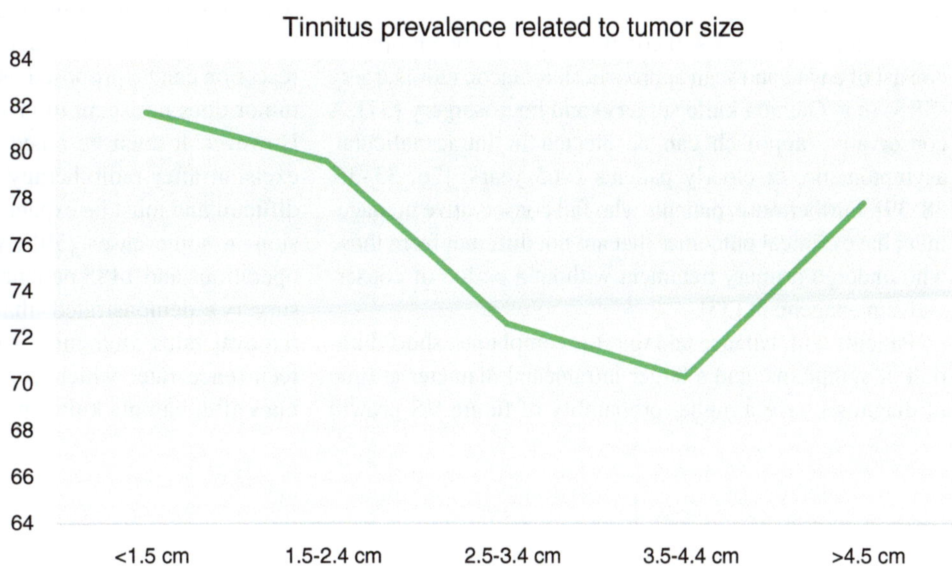

Fig. 34.1 Tinnitus percentage related to tumor size, based on [27]

Ongoing dizziness and headache are the strongest predictors of long-term quality-of-life reduction in patients with VS, while the impact of hearing loss, facial nerve function, and tinnitus are less by comparison [28].

When tumors extend into the cisternal space, hearing loss worsens and associated symptoms from compression of nearby cranial nerves may develop, such as facial numbness (in the midface area), facial palsy, otalgia, changes in taste, and, rarely, hoarseness or dysphagia. Compression of the brainstem and cerebellum can induce ataxia, diplopia, and other cerebellar signs. When a VS becomes very large, it obstructs the aqueduct causing collapse of the fourth ventricle leading to hydrocephalus and ultimately results in death if left untreated.

One-third of newly diagnosed VS will grow on follow-up of 1–3 years [29]. However, after 5 years, up to one-half will grow [29]. The only predictor for growth is growth in the first year [29]. If a VS growth is demonstrated by serial imaging, it usually continues to grow (63.9%). Only 30.6% arrest without treatment and 5.6–14% regress in size [30, 31]. In those who regress in size, tinnitus was observed in 47% and was stable or improved in the majority of cases [31]. Clinical factors such as hearing loss, vertigo, age, sex, and neither do tumor location nor tumor size [29].

The rate of growth of a VS is unpredictable, but the average growth is 0.7 [32] to 1 mm/year [33], with 92% growing less than 2 mm/year [33]. In about 60% of patients, the annual tumor growth rate is <1 mm/year; in about 30%, 1–3 mm/year; and in about 10%, ≥ 3 mm/year [34]. Intracanalicular tumors might grow slower than cisternal tumors [33], but this is not supported by all studies [34]. This might be related to the fact that growth rate is variable. In intracanalicular lesions, between 21.3% [35] and 70.6% [36] of patients demonstrate no tumor progression, but this variability signifies that potentially in as much as 76.6% of cases the tumor grows with resultant hearing loss [35]. Factors that may predict tumor growth of above 4 mm/year are cystic and hemorrhagic features in the tumor, and hormonal treatment [29].

Treatment for VS is still controversial. Treatment options consist of a wait and scan approach, stereotactic radiosurgery (SRS) (e.g. Gamma knife surgery) and microsurgery [37]. A conservative approach can be elected in intracanalicular, asymptomatic, or elderly patients (>65 years) [26, 33–36, 38, 39]. Furthermore, patients who fail conservative management have clinical outcomes that are not different from those who undergo primary treatment without a period of conservative management [33].

Patients with balance and tinnitus complaints, short duration of symptoms, and a larger intrameatal diameter at time of diagnosis have a higher probability of future VS growth [40]. Unsurprisingly, these patients with a short duration of hearing loss, balance disorders, as well as extracanalicular tumors, and cystic tumors, which grow faster, have a significantly higher chance of a change in treatment strategy [41].

Microsurgery is elected for large and giant tumors, as large VS are more difficult to control with SRS and liable to produce ataxia due to transient expansion post-irradiation [42]. However, in addition to growth rate, size, and location, clinical aspects also play a role in the decision for or against active therapy concepts. Here, in addition to age, the function of hearing plays a decisive role. Should there be an increasing hearing loss during a watch and scan strategy, especially when there is no longer any serviceable hearing in the affected ear, then it will be easier to decide in favor of therapy whether by surgery or SRS. Another consideration for certain tumors (especially smaller size, intracanalicular location) could be to plan the surgical therapy as long as a well-functioning hearing is still available. In this case, one would recommend a surgical technique with the highest possible chance of hearing preservation (e.g. transtemporal approach, see below).

For most small- and medium-sized VS, both microsurgery and SRS are valuable options. SRS, compared to surgical resection, seems to show superior outcomes for VS patients. A long-term tumor control rate of 94% after 5 years and 92.8% after 8 years [42] (transient facial palsy lower than 1%, and a probability of functional hearing preservation between 50 and 95%) can be achieved in experienced gamma knife centers treating large volumes of VS patients with state-of-the-art SRS [43]. Therefore, it has been suggested that unless a long-term follow-up examination indicates tumor progression at currently used radiation doses, SRS should be considered the best management strategy for the majority of VS patients [44, 45]. However, SRS does not arrest tumor growth in all patients: in 10% of patients who had SRS tumor progression continues [46]. A second SRS treatment can often arrest further growth [46, 47], but if it does not radical surgery results in facial nerve worsening in half of the patients [48] due to severe adhesions or changes of the facial nerve [49]. Partial or subtotal resection can be proposed when SRS fails since the residual tumor does not seem to grow after subtotal resection [49]. However, it must be noted that the conditions of surgical excision after radiotherapy may well be considered more difficult and must be expected to complicate complete excision in some cases [50]. A large study comparing 5005 operations and 1485 patients treated by SRS (gamma knife surgery) demonstrated that 96% of patients had total removal rates after microsurgical treatment, with a 1.8% recurrence rate, which compares favorably to recurrence rates after gamma knife surgery [51].

Based on these data, the following approach has been proposed: for lesions smaller than 2 cm, a conservative wait and scan approach; for growing lesions or lesions between 2 and 2.5 cm, either gamma knife or microsurgery; and for lesions bigger than 2.5 cm, microsurgery [37]. A combination of subtotal resection with adjunct SRS has been suggested as well to improve functional outcome in patients with VS that are larger than 4 cm [52, 53]. In summary, at experienced clinical centers, a team that includes otologists, neurosurgeons, and radiotherapists discusses the decision about a particular therapeutic approach for VS patients. In each decision, the individual structural and functional results of the diagnostic workup are taken into account.

Tinnitus and Vestibular Schwannoma

Tinnitus is a very common symptom in VS: between 45 and 80% of VS patients have tinnitus [2, 14–16, 27, 54–59]. It usually develops when the tumor is still intracanalicular [16], and is reported as the principal presenting symptom in one of 10 patients who seek medical help [14].

When tinnitus is the main presenting symptom, it seems to be perceived as severe [27]. The presence of tinnitus in VS is unrelated to patient age, gender, audiometric thresholds between 2000 and 4000 Hz, ipsilateral auditory brainstem response abnormalities, or caloric test abnormalities [27]. VS are most commonly associated with high-frequency hearing loss; the tinnitus is usually high pitched and localized to the tumor ear [2]. There is a correlation between the presence of tinnitus and the type of hearing loss with a tendency for patients without hearing loss to be less likely to experience tinnitus [27]. Greater age at the time of diagnosis seems to be associated with greater severity of the tinnitus. Abnormal caloric responses are also associated with a greater severity of tinnitus [27]. In ILS, about 10% of the affected patients with tinnitus might report on a pulsatile character of their tinnitus [25].

The presence of tinnitus is related to the tumor size [27]: it is more common when the tumor is small or when it is larger than 4.5 cm. This suggests that the tinnitus might be related to two different pathophysiological mechanisms, similarly to what has been described for microvascular compressions (see Chap. 35). The rate of tinnitus in vestibular schwannomas is higher in individuals with functional hearing than in deaf individuals [60, 61]. Deafness does not mean relief from tinnitus, and tinnitus persists in 46% of individuals who were deaf before the operation for vestibular schwannoma [60]. This may suggest that the tinnitus is initially caused by aberrant signal transmission in the auditory nerve [27], whereas at a later stage the tinnitus results from deafferentation, similarly to the tinnitus that occurs in connection with microvascular compressions.

Treatment Options for Tinnitus in Patients with Vestibular Schwannoma.

Conservative Treatment

It is uncertain if treating a small tumor leaves the patient with a better chance of obtaining relief from future tinnitus by observing it without treatment [37]. Between one-third [51] and one-half [62] of patients who are followed conservatively develop progressive hearing loss, which could result in more tinnitus. However, it is not known whether this is the case. If the decision has been made for a "watch and scan" approach and the tinnitus is highly distressing for the affected person, then all methods should be pursued that would also apply to affected persons without VS (e.g. hearing aid, CBT, etc.).

Microsurgery

After VS microneurosurgery, tinnitus disappears in 0–45%, becomes better in 16–17% of patients, while 30–83% do not experience any change, and 8–29% become worse [63–65]. Neither tumor size nor age at the time of the operation has an impact on the tinnitus that occurs after surgery [63]. Therefore, these factors cannot be used as predictors for who will improve, remain unchanged, or worsen postoperatively. Furthermore, there is no association between changes in the tinnitus and changes in the quality of life following surgical treatment of VS, suggesting that tinnitus may be of relatively minor importance in the overall quality of life of patients following microneurosurgery for VS [63]. If no tinnitus is perceived before surgery, almost 20–50% develop it afterwards [56, 66, 67].

Preoperative tinnitus is the strongest predictor of postoperative tinnitus [67]. In two-thirds (67.5%) of patients who have tinnitus preoperatively, the tinnitus remains after surgery, while the tinnitus disappears in only one-third (32.5%) of the operated patients [67]. In addition, postoperative hearing loss of non-functional hearing is reducing the risk of postoperative tinnitus [67]. At the same time, patients with no preoperative tinnitus but complete hearing loss had the lowest risk to suffer from postoperative tinnitus [67]. The attempt to achieve the best possible hearing preservation by means of certain surgical techniques has no influence on the postoperative tinnitus situation [54]. Therefore, due to the unclear prognosis, tinnitus cannot be used as a decision aid, neither for or against surgical intervention for a vestibular schwannoma nor for decision on specific surgical approaches [68].

The goal of all surgical methods is the total (or subtotal) removal of the vestibular schwannoma while preserving the function of the facial nerve and the (residual) hearing. This goal can be achieved in most cases due to microsurgical techniques with the use of surgical microscopes, endoscopes, intraoperative neuromonitoring (facial nerve and cochlear nerve) and in special cases, neuronavigational systems. Depending on the location and size of the tumor, as well as other factors (age, degree of hearing loss, and preference of the surgical team), different surgical approaches can be considered for the operation. Since the surgical removal of a VS is always accompanied by a complete loss of vestibular function on the affected side, it might be useful to accelerate the postoperative rehabilitation process by a targeted preoperative ablation of the vestibular function with gentamicin (so-called vestibular prehabilitation) [69, 70]. Furthermore, the use of transtympanic gentamycin can improve tinnitus [71] in up to 57% of patients with Meniere's disease, according to a systematic review [72]. But the transtympanic application of gentamycin does have a risk of inducing partial or complete hearing loss [71, 72], which can be prevented or limited by simultaneous application of dexamethasone [73].

At experienced centers, the operations are usually performed in collaboration between neurosurgeons and otologist ENT surgeons. The dominant approaches are the translabyrinthine approach through the inner ear and the retrosigmoid (suboccipital) approach.

For the translabyrinthine and retrosigmoid approaches, there are generally no limitations with respect to tumor size. Transtemporal tumor excision ("middle fossa approach") is only recommended for small tumor sizes of maximum 20 mm with a mostly intracanalicular location and a high chance of hearing preservation. Hearing preservation is only possible with transtemporal and retrosigmoid surgery, but has only proven to be useful in the case of residual hearing in the pure tone audiogram of more than 50 dB HL in average and additional speech discrimination for monosyllables of more than 50% [74]. If the cochlea and the cochlear nerve can be preserved during surgery, a cochlear implant (CI) can also be used after surgical therapy [75, 76]. The quality of life can be significantly improved by achieving binaural hearing and tinnitus suppression [77]. The prerequisite for a CI implantation is the demonstration of an intact nerve and sufficient evidence of fluid in the cochlea by means of a postoperative MRI scan. A positive promontory testing is prognostically favorable. In the case of an ILS, simultaneous cochlear implantation may also be considered in the course of tumor removal [78, 79]. A cochlear implant can also be given consideration after successful radiotherapy of a VS [80, 81]. Furthermore, many studies, including a meta-analysis have shown that a cochlear implant has a high chance of improving tinnitus [82, 83], also after resection of a VS [84]. For the most prominent approaches, the changes regarding tinnitus perception after therapy will be discussed in the following sections.

Retrosigmoid (Suboccipital) Resection

Tinnitus disappears in 20–62.5%, improves in 22–85%, remains unchanged in 10–35%, and worsens in 3.5–14% after tumor removal using the retrosigmoid approach [85–87]. Although the proportion of patients complaining of frequent tinnitus increases postoperatively, the number of patients who find the tinnitus troublesome decreases markedly [88]. There is no difference in tinnitus incidence whether the auditory nerve is resected or not during surgery [85]. If no tinnitus is present before surgery, it develops postoperatively in 8.5–10%, irrespective whether the auditory nerve was resected or not [85, 86]. Risk factors for developing tinnitus after microsurgery are sudden drops in perioperative blood pressure and hearing preservation surgery. A sudden drop in blood pressure during or after surgery is not only a negative prognostic factor for hearing preservation, but also for ipsilateral tinnitus in patients undergoing vestibular schwannoma surgery [89]. When attempting to achieve hearing preservation during removal of a VS in patients without preoperatively tinnitus, 85% develop tinnitus postoperatively compared to 31% of patients in operations where hearing preservation is not attempted in the translabyrinthine resection group [54]. However, a number of smaller studies seem to have opposite results: 50% of patients who had tinnitus preoperatively complained of it postoperatively, and only 8% developed tinnitus as a result of VS surgery which saved hearing [57]. These opposite results may be related to two important surgical outcomes: preservation of useful hearing and neurectomy of the eighth cranial nerve were main prognostic factors of tinnitus elimination. Preservation of cochlear nerve but loss of preoperative hearing is the main factor for tinnitus persistence and new onset tinnitus [90].

Translabyrinthine Resection

The tinnitus in individuals with VS is usually not bothersome [2, 27, 58, 59]. The tinnitus handicap and loudness improve after the translabyrinthine approach [91]. On an individual basis, the tinnitus handicap was worse in 6.5%, unchanged in 87%, and better in 6.5% [59]. There is a 35% risk for developing tinnitus when no preoperative tinnitus is present and a 15% chance that tinnitus disappears when present preoperatively with translabyrinthine surgery [58].

Patients who had a probable or definite nerve section had significantly lower postoperative tinnitus severity [92]. Based on these results, it may be suggested that patients with no tinnitus pre-operatively undergoing this form of surgery are unlikely to develop tinnitus after the operation, and if they do, it will not be severe enough to significantly affect their quality of life [93]. When asked what affects the post-operative quality of life, less than 4% of the patients mentioned tinnitus [94].

Translabyrinthine Versus Retrosigmoid Surgery for Tinnitus

Tinnitus prognosis in VS patients is better following translabyrinthine microsurgery relative to retrosigmoid microsurgery and is also better (independently) in patients with worse preoperative hearing. New-onset tinnitus was more likely to occur in patients with better preoperative hearing who underwent tumor removal via a translabyrinthine approach [95]. This is confirmed by a meta-analysis comparing translabyrinthine to retrosigmoid surgery for VS, demonstrating a lower rate of postoperative tinnitus in translabyrinthine surgery. However, it could not be excluded that this difference may have been due to a difference in the preoperative prevalence in the two surgical approaches [96].

Gamma Knife Surgery (SRS)

Tinnitus only changes or develops in few patients (4%) after SRS for VS [45, 97, 98]. Preoperative tinnitus does not seem to exacerbate on a group level, thus similar to microsurgery [99]. Also in patients with small VS and no hearing results from SRS and microsurgery are not significantly different with regards to tinnitus [100]. Some studies, however, do show less tinnitus in about 45% of patients who were treated with SRS [98, 101]. Whether hearing preservation in SRS is related to this is unknown. The overall serviceable hearing preservation rate is 71–77.8% at 3 years, 68.8% at 5 years, and 51.8% at 10 years [102, 103]. A similar functional hearing preservation at 3 years (80%) is seen in those patients with tinnitus as a first symptom [104]. The probability of preserving functional hearing is not only dependent of the presence of tinnitus as a first symptom. Hearing preservation is higher for smaller tumors in patients who have an initial symptom other than hearing decrease (91.1%), in patients younger than 50 years (83.7%), and in those treated with a dose to the cochlea of less than 4 Gy (90.9%) [102, 105]. Similar to microsurgical techniques, counseling regarding a prognosis for tinnitus after SRS is difficult [68]. Thus, this parameter should not be used as an aid in deciding for or against SRS.

Gamma Knife Surgery Versus Translabyrinthine Surgery

There is a higher rate of tinnitus improvement in translabyrinthine surgery (52%) than gamma knife treatment (16%) [106]. Gamma knife surgery has a significantly higher rate of tinnitus worsening (74%) than translabyrinthine surgery (11%) [106]. Tinnitus handicap inventory and VAS scores significantly decrease in translabyrinthine surgery in contrast to significant increases in gamma knife surgery [106].

Conclusion

Tinnitus is a common symptom in VS, but rarely distressing. In only 10% of patients, harboring a VS tinnitus is the principal symptom and in only 14% of these, the tinnitus is perceived as moderately to severely distressing. Using gamma knife (SRS) or translabyrinthine surgical removal does not alter the tinnitus at a group level, even though some individual patients may experience less tinnitus after the treatment. Retrosigmoid surgery seems to have an impact on the tinnitus, decreasing its severity, except when associated with surgery which saves hearing. Cochlear implantation might be an option for hearing restoration and tinnitus suppression in selected cases after surgical or radiosurgical treatment.

References

1. Eldridge R, Parry D. Vestibular schwannoma (acoustic neuroma). Consensus development conference. Neurosurgery. 1992;30(6):962–4.
2. Jackler R. Acoustic neuroma (vestibular schwannoma). In: Jackler R, Brackmann D, editors. Neurotology. St Louis: Mosby; 1994. p. 729–85.
3. Marinelli JP, et al. Global incidence of sporadic vestibular schwannoma: a systematic review. Otolaryngol Head Neck Surg. 2021;167:1945998211042006.
4. Leonard JR, Talbot ML. Asymptomatic acoustic neurilemoma. Arch Otolaryngol. 1970;91(2):117–24.
5. Ahlbom A, et al. Epidemiologic evidence on mobile phones and tumor risk: a review. Epidemiology. 2009;20(5):639–52.
6. Hardell L, et al. Meta-analysis of long-term mobile phone use and the association with brain tumours. Int J Oncol. 2008;32(5):1097–103.
7. Hardell L, et al. Vestibular schwannoma, tinnitus and cellular telephones. Neuroepidemiology. 2003;22(2):124–9.
8. Moon IS, et al. Association between vestibular schwannomas and mobile phone use. Tumour Biol. 2014;35(1):581–7.
9. Croft RJ, et al. Mobile phones and brain tumours: a review of epidemiological research. Australas Phys Eng Sci Med. 2008;31(4):255–67.
10. Momoli F, et al. Probabilistic multiple-bias modeling applied to the Canadian data from the interphone study of mobile phone use and risk of glioma, meningioma, acoustic neuroma, and parotid gland tumors. Am J Epidemiol. 2017;186(7):885–93.
11. Pettersson D, et al. Long-term mobile phone use and acoustic neuroma risk. Epidemiology. 2014;25(2):233–41.

12. Withrow DR, et al. Nonmalignant meningioma and vestibular schwannoma incidence trends in the United States, 2004-2017. Cancer. 2021;127(19):3579–90.
13. Hours M, et al. Can loud noise cause acoustic neuroma? Analysis of the INTERPHONE study in France. Occup Environ Med. 2009;66(7):480–6.
14. Moffat DA, et al. Clinical acumen and vestibular schwannoma. Am J Otol. 1998;19(1):82–7.
15. Kentala E, Pyykko I. Clinical picture of vestibular schwannoma. Auris Nasus Larynx. 2001;28(1):15–22.
16. Haapaniemi J, et al. Cochleovestibular symptoms related to the site of vestibular schwannoma. Acta Otolaryngol Suppl. 2000;543:14–6.
17. Saxby C, et al. The use of magnetic resonance imaging in the investigation of patients with unilateral non-pulsatile tinnitus without asymmetrical hearing loss. J Laryngol Otol. 2021;135(8):680–3.
18. Moffat DA, et al. Sudden deafness in vestibular schwannoma. J Laryngol Otol. 1994;108(2):116–9.
19. Yang W, et al. The prevalence and clinical characteristics of vestibular schwannoma among patients treated as sudden sensorineural hearing loss: a 10-year retrospective study in Southern China. Am J Otolaryngol. 2020;41(4):102452.
20. Nadol JB Jr, Diamond PF, Thornton AR. Correlation of hearing loss and radiologic dimensions of vestibular schwannomas (acoustic neuromas). Am J Otol. 1996;17(2):312–6.
21. Kellermeyer B, et al. Case series of vestibular schwannoma patients with no asymmetry in hearing. Am J Otolaryngol. 2021;42(5):103034.
22. Connor SEJ. Imaging of the vestibular schwannoma: diagnosis, monitoring, and treatment planning. Neuroimaging Clin N Am. 2021;31(4):451–71.
23. Choudhury B, Carlson ML, Jethanamest D. Intralabyrinthine schwannomas: disease presentation, tumor management, and hearing rehabilitation. J Neurol Surg B Skull Base. 2019;80(2):196–202.
24. Salzman KL, et al. Intralabyrinthine schwannomas: imaging diagnosis and classification. AJNR Am J Neuroradiol. 2012;33(1):104–9.
25. Dubernard X, et al. Clinical presentation of intralabyrinthine schwannomas: a multicenter study of 110 cases. Otol Neurotol. 2014;35(9):1641–9.
26. Malhotra PS, et al. Clinical, radiographic, and audiometric predictors in conservative management of vestibular schwannoma. Otol Neurotol. 2009;30(4):507–14.
27. Baguley DM, et al. The clinical characteristics of tinnitus in patients with vestibular schwannoma. Skull Base. 2006;16(2):49–58.
28. Carlson ML, et al. What drives quality of life in patients with sporadic vestibular schwannoma? Laryngoscope. 2015;125(7):1697–702.
29. Paldor I, Chen AS, Kaye AH. Growth rate of vestibular schwannoma. J Clin Neurosci. 2016;32:1–8.
30. Mick D, et al. Growing vestibular schwannomas: what happens next? Otol Neurotol. 2009;30(1):101–4.
31. Trau G, Venkatasamy A, Charpiot A. Vestibular schwannomas with spontaneous shrinkage: about 35 cases. Eur Arch Otorhinolaryngol. 2021;278:4235.
32. Battaglia A, Mastrodimos B, Cueva R. Comparison of growth patterns of acoustic neuromas with and without radiosurgery. Otol Neurotol. 2006;27(5):705–12.
33. Hajioff D, et al. Conservative management of vestibular schwannomas: third review of a 10-year prospective study. Clin Otolaryngol. 2008;33(3):255–9.
34. Bakkouri WE, et al. Conservative management of 386 cases of unilateral vestibular schwannoma: tumor growth and consequences for treatment. J Neurosurg. 2009;110(4):662–9.
35. Roche PH, et al. The wait and see strategy for intracanalicular vestibular schwannomas. Prog Neurol Surg. 2008;21:83–8.
36. Solares CA, Panizza B. Vestibular schwannoma: an understanding of growth should influence management decisions. Otol Neurotol. 2008;29(6):829–34.
37. Myrseth E, et al. Treatment of vestibular schwannomas. Why, when and how? Acta Neurochir. 2007;149(7):647–60; discussion 660.
38. Ferri GG, et al. Conservative management of vestibular schwannomas: an effective strategy. Laryngoscope. 2008;118(6):951–7.
39. Rosenberg SI. Natural history of acoustic neuromas. Laryngoscope. 2000;110(4):497–508.
40. Hentschel MA, et al. Development of a model to predict vestibular schwannoma growth: an opportunity to introduce new wait and scan strategies. Clin Otolaryngol. 2021;46(1):273–83.
41. Kleijwegt M, et al. Clinical predictors leading to change of initial conservative treatment of 836 vestibular schwannomas. J Neurol Surg B Skull Base. 2020;81(1):15–21.
42. Fukuoka S, et al. Gamma knife radiosurgery for vestibular schwannomas. Prog Neurol Surg. 2009;22:45–62.
43. Regis J, et al. Modern management of vestibular schwannomas. Prog Neurol Surg. 2007;20:129–41.
44. Pollock BE. Vestibular schwannoma management: an evidence-based comparison of stereotactic radiosurgery and microsurgical resection. Prog Neurol Surg. 2008;21:222–7.
45. Myrseth E, et al. Vestibular schwannoma: surgery or gamma knife radiosurgery? A prospective, nonrandomized study. Neurosurgery. 2009;64(4):654–61; discussion 661–3.
46. Liscak R, et al. Repeated treatment of vestibular schwannomas after gamma knife radiosurgery. Acta Neurochir. 2009;151(4):317–24; discussion 324.
47. Yomo S, et al. Repeat gamma knife surgery for regrowth of vestibular schwannomas. Neurosurgery. 2009;64(1):48–54; discussion 54–5.
48. Roche PH, et al. Surgical removal of vestibular schwannoma after failed gamma knife radiosurgery. Prog Neurol Surg. 2008;21:152–7.
49. Shuto T, et al. Microsurgery for vestibular schwannoma after gamma knife radiosurgery. Acta Neurochir. 2008;150(3):229–34; discussion 234.
50. Misra BK, Churi ON. Microsurgery of vestibular schwannoma post-radiosurgery. Neurol India. 2019;67(5):1274–8.
51. Yamakami I, et al. Conservative management, gamma-knife radiosurgery, and microsurgery for acoustic neurinomas: a systematic review of outcome and risk of three therapeutic options. Neurol Res. 2003;25(7):682–90.
52. Fuentes S, et al. Management of large vestibular schwannomas by combined surgical resection and gamma knife radiosurgery. Prog Neurol Surg. 2008;21:79–82.
53. Park CK, et al. Therapeutic strategy for large vestibular schwannomas. J Neuro-Oncol. 2006;77(2):167–71.
54. Kanzaki J, Satoh A, Kunihiro T. Does hearing preservation surgery for acoustic neuromas affect tinnitus? Skull Base Surg. 1999;9(3):169–76.
55. Humphriss RL, et al. Preoperative audiovestibular handicap in patients with vestibular schwannoma. Skull Base. 2006;16(4):193–9.
56. Levo H, Blomstedt G, Pyykko I. Tinnitus and vestibular schwannoma surgery. Acta Otolaryngol Suppl. 2000;543:28–9.
57. Catalano PJ, Post KD. Elimination of tinnitus following hearing preservation surgery for acoustic neuromas. Am J Otol. 1996;17(3):443–5.
58. Andersson G, et al. Tinnitus and translabyrinthine acoustic neuroma surgery. Audiol Neurootol. 1997;2(6):403–9.
59. Baguley DM, et al. Change in tinnitus handicap after translabyrinthine vestibular schwannoma excision. Otol Neurotol. 2005;26(5):1061–3.
60. Matthies C, Samii M. Management of 1000 vestibular schwannomas (acoustic neuromas): clinical presentation. Neurosurgery. 1997;40(1):1–9; discussion 9–10, 1.

61. Naros G, et al. Predictors of preoperative tinnitus in unilateral sporadic vestibular schwannoma. Front Neurol. 2017;8:378.
62. Smouha EE, et al. Conservative management of acoustic neuroma: a meta-analysis and proposed treatment algorithm. Laryngoscope. 2005;115(3):450–4.
63. Fahy C, Nikolopoulos TP, O'Donoghue GM. Acoustic neuroma surgery and tinnitus. Eur Arch Otorhinolaryngol. 2002;259(6):299–301.
64. Henrich DE, McCabe BF, Gantz BJ. Tinnitus and acoustic neuromas: analysis of the effect of surgical excision on postoperative tinnitus. Ear Nose Throat J. 1995;74(7):462–6.
65. Bell JR, et al. The persistence of tinnitus after acoustic neuroma surgery. Otolaryngol Head Neck Surg. 2016;155(2):317–23.
66. Berliner KI, et al. Acoustic tumors: effect of surgical removal on tinnitus. Am J Otol. 1992;13(1):13–7.
67. Trakolis L, et al. Postoperative tinnitus after vestibular schwannoma surgery depends on preoperative tinnitus and both pre- and postoperative hearing function. Front Neurol. 2018;9:136.
68. Juan JS, Basura GJ. Tinnitus management in lateral skull base lesions. J Neurol Surg B Skull Base. 2019;80(2):125–31.
69. Fellmann J, et al. Postural stability and handicap of dizziness after preoperative vestibular ablation and vestibular prehabilitation in patients undergoing vestibular schwannoma resection. J Vestib Res. 2021;32:49.
70. Tjernstrom F, et al. PREHAB vs. REHAB—presurgical treatment in vestibular schwannoma surgery enhances recovery of postural control better than postoperative rehabilitation: retrospective case series. J Vestib Res. 2018;27(5–6):313–25.
71. Shamas IU. Short term results of intra tympanic gentamicin and dexamethasone on hearing and tinnitus in Meniere's disease: a case control study. Int Tinnitus J. 2017;21(1):21–3.
72. Diamond C, et al. Systematic review of intratympanic gentamicin in Meniere's disease. J Otolaryngol. 2003;32(6):351–61.
73. Bae SH, et al. Effect of dexamethasone combination with gentamicin in chemical Labyrinthectomy on hearing preservation and vertigo control in patients with unilateral Meniere's disease: a randomized controlled clinical trial. J Clin Med. 2021;10(23):5581.
74. Schulz C, et al. Management of vestibular schwannomas. Laryngorhinootologie. 2018;97(12):875–96.
75. Tadokoro K, et al. Cochlear implantation in vestibular schwannoma: a systematic literature review. J Neurol Surg B Skull Base. 2021;82(6):643–51.
76. Patel EJ, et al. Cochlear implantation in sporadic vestibular schwannoma and other retrocochlear pathology: a case series. Otol Neurotol. 2021;42(4):e425–32.
77. Plontke SK, et al. Intralabyrinthine schwannomas : surgical management and hearing rehabilitation with cochlear implants. HNO. 2017;65(Suppl 2):136–48.
78. Pastor Gomis B, et al. Intralabyrinthine neurinoma: management, exeresis and auditory restoration with cochlear implant. Acta Otorrinolaringol Esp (Engl Ed). 2021;72(5):324–8.
79. Sudhoff H, et al. Quality control after intracochlear intralabyrinthine schwannoma resection and cochlear implantation. Brain Sci. 2021;11(9):1221.
80. Tian L, West N, Caye-Thomasen P. Cochlear implantation after radiotherapy of vestibular schwannomas. J Int Adv Otol. 2021;17(5):452–60.
81. Patel NS, et al. Cochlear implantation after radiosurgery for vestibular schwannoma. J Neurosurg. 2021;135(1):126–35.
82. Borges ALF, et al. Cochlear implant and tinnitus-a meta-analysis. Braz J Otorhinolaryngol. 2021;87(3):353–65.
83. Van de Heyning P, et al. Incapacitating unilateral tinnitus in single-sided deafness treated by cochlear implantation. Ann Otol Rhinol Laryngol. 2008;117(9):645–52.
84. Bartindale MR, Tadokoro KS, Kircher ML. Cochlear implantation in sporadic vestibular schwannoma: a systematic literature review. J Neurol Surg B Skull Base. 2019;80(6):632–9.
85. Kameda K, et al. Effect of tumor removal on tinnitus in patients with vestibular schwannoma. J Neurosurg. 2009;112(1):152.
86. Sardhara J, et al. Postoperative tinnitus after vestibular schwannoma surgery: a neglected entity. Neurol India. 2020;68(2):333–9.
87. Kohno M, et al. Prognosis of tinnitus after acoustic neuroma surgery—surgical management of postoperative tinnitus. World Neurosurg. 2014;81(2):357–67.
88. Rigby PL, et al. Acoustic neuroma surgery: outcome analysis of patient-perceived disability. Am J Otol. 1997;18(4):427–35.
89. Schaller BJ, et al. Difference in functional outcome of ipsilateral tinnitus after intraoperative occurrence of the trigemino-cardiac reflex in surgery for vestibular schwannomas. Acta Neurochir. 2008;150(2):157–60.
90. Chovanec M, et al. Does attempt at hearing preservation microsurgery of vestibular schwannoma affect postoperative tinnitus? Biomed Res Int. 2015;2015:783169.
91. Wang JJ, et al. Changes in tinnitus after vestibular schwannoma surgery. Sci Rep. 2019;9(1):1743.
92. Harcourt J, Thomsen J, Tos M. Translabyrinthine vestibular schwannoma surgery: postoperative tinnitus and cochlear nerve integrity. Auris Nasus Larynx. 1997;24(1):21–6.
93. Baguley DM, Moffat DA, Hardy DG. What is the effect of translabyrinthine acoustic schwannoma removal upon tinnitus? J Laryngol Otol. 1992;106(4):329–31.
94. Bateman N, et al. Impairments, disabilities, and handicaps after acoustic neuroma surgery. Clin Otolaryngol Allied Sci. 2000;25(1):62–5.
95. Zhang C, et al. Identification of factors associated with tinnitus outcomes following the microsurgical treatment of vestibular schwannoma patients. Acta Otolaryngol. 2021;141(4):334–9.
96. Jun W, et al. Comparison of translabyrinthine and retrosigmoid approach for treating vestibular schwannoma: a meta-analysis. Clin Neurol Neurosurg. 2020;196:105994.
97. Hempel JM, et al. Functional outcome after gamma knife treatment in vestibular schwannoma. Eur Arch Otorhinolaryngol. 2006;263(8):714–8.
98. Bertalanffy A, et al. Gamma knife radiosurgery of acoustic neurinomas. Acta Neurochir. 2001;143(7):689–95.
99. Karpinos M, et al. Treatment of acoustic neuroma: stereotactic radiosurgery vs. microsurgery. Int J Radiat Oncol Biol Phys. 2002;54(5):1410–21.
100. Coelho DH, et al. Small vestibular schwannomas with no hearing: comparison of functional outcomes in stereotactic radiosurgery and microsurgery. Laryngoscope. 2008;118(11):1909–16.
101. Niranjan A, et al. Dose reduction improves hearing preservation rates after intracanalicular acoustic tumor radiosurgery. Neurosurgery. 1999;45(4):753–62; discussion 762–5.
102. Johnson S, et al. Predicting hearing outcomes before primary radiosurgery for vestibular schwannomas. J Neurosurg. 2019:1–7.
103. Chopra R, et al. Long-term follow-up of acoustic schwannoma radiosurgery with marginal tumor doses of 12 to 13 Gy. Int J Radiat Oncol Biol Phys. 2007;68(3):845–51.
104. Regis J, et al. Hearing preservation in patients with unilateral vestibular schwannoma after gamma knife surgery. Prog Neurol Surg. 2008;21:142–51.
105. Tamura M, et al. Hearing preservation after gamma knife radiosurgery for vestibular schwannomas presenting with high-level hearing. Neurosurgery. 2009;64(2):289–96; discussion 296.
106. Park SH, et al. Change in tinnitus after treatment of vestibular schwannoma: microsurgery vs. gamma knife radiosurgery. Yonsei Med J. 2014;55(1):19–24.

Microvascular Compression of the Vestibulocochlear Nerve

35

Dirk De Ridder

Abstract

Microvascular contacts or compressions (MVC) of the vestibulocochlear nerve can result in tinnitus, both non-pulsatile and pulsatile tinnitus. For non-pulsatile tinnitus, the contact is most often located at the central nervous system segment, between the meatus and brainstem. For pulsatile tinnitus and typewriter tinnitus, the contact is at the intrameatal peripheral nervous system segment. The tinnitus is most commonly unilateral, presenting as intermittent paroxysms. Typically, in time more frequent bouts of tinnitus occur, which progressively last longer and longer. If a bilateral vascular compressions exist, the tinnitus alternates between left and right side. Associated symptoms are related to MVC of nearby nerves and include overt or cryptogenic hemifacial spasms, geniculate neuralgia, optokinetically induced short bouts of disabling positional vertigo, as well as hearing loss at the tinnitus frequency.

The diagnosis is made based on a typical history and confirmed by magnetic resonance imaging (MRI) anatomically, and auditory brainstem responses (ABR) functionally. MRI with constructive interference in steady state can visualize MVC of the auditory nerve and correlates with intraoperative findings. ABR correlates with disease progress and clinical symptoms. Tinnitus is causally related to a decrease in amplitude of peak II in the ipsilaterally elicited ABR. Furthermore, tinnitus frequency-specific hearing loss is causally related to prolongation of the ipsilateral interpeak latency I-III. Compensatory prolongation of interpeak latency III-V occurs contralaterally and is a sign of slowed signal transmission in the brainstem. Microvascular decompression should be performed before irreversible nerve damage is induced, before 4–5 years of tinnitus onset. Surgical outcomes are better if patients present with both tinnitus and vertigo. In patients with tinnitus only, 28% are cured and 45% improved, whereas in patients with both tinnitus and vertigo, 62% are cured and 23% improved.

D. De Ridder (✉)
Section of Neurosurgery, Department of Surgical Sciences, University of Otago, Dunedin, New Zealand
e-mail: dirk.deridder@otago.ac.nz

W. Schlee et al. (eds.), *Textbook of Tinnitus*, https://doi.org/10.1007/978-3-031-35647-6_35

Graphical Abstract

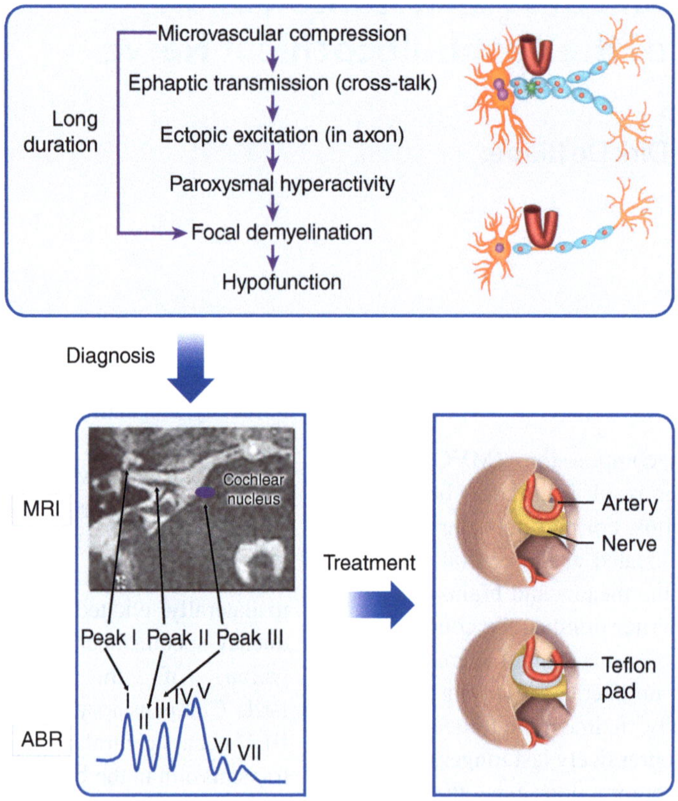

Abbreviations

AAO	American Academy of Otolaryngology
AAOO	American Academy of Ophthalmology and Otolaryngology
ABR	Auditory brainstem response
CISS	Constructive interference in steady state
CVCS	Cochleovestibular compression syndrome
ENT	Ear nose and throat
HFS	Hemifacial spasm
IPL	Interpeak latency
MRI	Magnetic resonance imaging
MVC	Microvascular compression
PNS	Peripheral nervous system

Highlights

- Microvascular contacts or compressions of the vestibulocochlear nerve can result in tinnitus.
- For non-pulsatile tinnitus, the contact most often is at the central nervous system segment.
- For pulsatile tinnitus and typewriter tinnitus, the contact is at the peripheral nervous system segment. The tinnitus is unilateral, and characterized by intermittent paroxysms of tinnitus.
  - A typical development consists of progressively more frequent bouts of tinnitus which last longer and longer.
  - If bilateral vascular compressions exist, the tinnitus alternates between left and right side, not simultaneous.
- Associated symptoms are related to associated contacts/compressions of nearby nerves and include overt or cryptogenic hemifacial spasms, geniculate neuralgia optokinetically induced short bouts of disabling positional vertigo, and tinnitus frequency specific hearing loss.
- Diagnosis is made by a typical history and confirmed by MRI.
- Auditory brainstem responses correlate with disease progress and clinical symptoms and can be used diagnostically.
  - Tinnitus is causally related to decrease in amplitude of peak II in the ipsilaterally elicited auditory brainstem response.
  - Tinnitus frequency-specific hearing loss is causally related to prolongation of the ipsilateral interpeak latency I-III.
  - Compensatory prolongation of interpeak latency III-V occurs contralaterally and is a sign of slowed signal transmission in the brainstem.

- Magnetic resonance imaging sequences with constructive interference in steady state can visualize vascular contacts/compressions of the auditory nerve and correlate with intraoperative findings.
- Microvascular decompression should be performed before irreversible nerve damage is induced, clinically before 4–5 years.
- Surgical outcomes are better if patients present with both tinnitus and vertigo.
  - In patients with tinnitus, only 28% are cured and 45% improved.
  - In patients with tinnitus and vertigo, 62% are cured and 23% improved.

Introduction

History

In 1875, Schulze reported the first case of microvascular compression, describing hemifacial spasm caused by an aneurysm of the vertebral artery, compressing the facial nerve [1]. In 1934, Dandy described the first case of trigeminal neuralgia secondary to a microvascular compression [2]. In the 1970s and 1980s, Jannetta popularized the concept and extended it to all other cranial nerves, proposing that an initial hyperactive phase is followed by a subsequent hypoactive phase [3, 4]. This included the vestibulocochlear nerve [5]. Aage and Margaretha Moller further elaborated on the pathophysiological mechanisms and surgical outcomes of microvascular compressions of the VIIIth cranial nerve, including developing ABR criteria, also investigating microvascular decompressions for tinnitus [6–15].

Definition

A blood vessel compressing a cranial nerve induces a nerve stimulation leading to a hyperactive cranial nerve syndrome [5, 8] with or without a loss of function (Fig. 35.1). It is diagnosed based on a typical clinical history, and is confirmed or excluded by MRI. The correlation between MRI and intraoperative findings is high, with a sensitivity of 96.7% and a specificity of 100% [16].

Primary and Secondary Microvascular Compressions

Microvascular compression can occur as such or can be induced based on a general lack of space in the posterior fossa such as seen in the Arnold-Chiari malformation [17–

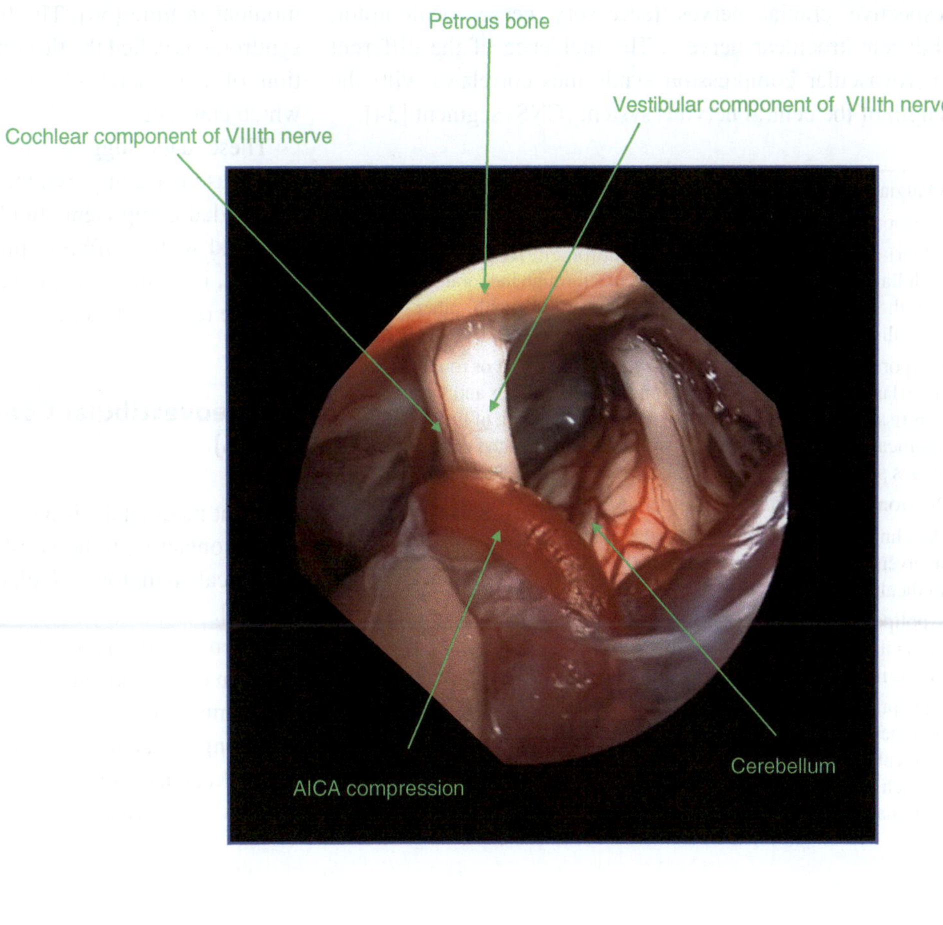

Fig. 35.1 Intraoperative picture of microvascular compression of the left vestibulocochlear nerve

19] or associated with space occupying lesions. This can result in a direct compression [20, 21], or indirect compression [22], but also contralaterally, possibly due to a decrease in intracranial space [23–27]. In Sindou's series [18] of 39 patients with Arnold-Chiari malformation, nine suffered from trigeminal neuralgia. After decompressing the foramen magnum, five of nine of these individuals got rid of their pain, whereas four persons required a second operation, consisting of a microvascular decompression. In his series of trigeminal neuralgias treated by microvascular decompression, the nerve was compressed between pons and petrous bone in 3.9% of people, due to the small size of the posterior fossa [28]. Removal of a tentorial meningioma can improve sudden hearing loss related to a microvascular compression of the vestibulocochlear nerve based on the same premises [22].

Characteristic Signs and Symptoms of Microvascular Compression

Examples of microvascular compression syndromes are trigeminal neuralgia, glossopharyngeal neuralgia, hemifacial spasm, disabling positional vertigo, tinnitus and otalgia[1][2][3][4][5][6][7][8]. Other clinical syndromes such as spasmodic torticollis [29], cyclic oculomotor spasm with paresis [30] or superior oblique myokymia [31, 32] and abducens spasm [33] may also be initiated by vascular compressions of the respective cranial nerves (accessory nerve, oculomotor, abducens trochlear nerves). The incidence of the different microvascular compression syndromes correlates with the length of the central nervous system (CNS) segment [34].

Microvascular compression (MVC) of cranial nerves usually occurs unilaterally and thus results in unilateral symptoms, [35–39] characterized by paroxysmal and intermittent spells of hyperactivity. The paroxysms typically become more frequent over time, the intermittent symptom-free periods become shorter and terminate in a constant dysfunction [40–42]. The symptoms of MVC can often be evoked by specific triggers [35, 40–42]. MVC syndromes are most common in late middle age (mean age 50 years) [35–39].

MVC of the vestibulocochlear nerve can cause any of the following paroxysmal symptoms depending on the place of compression: (disabling positional) vertigo [12], tinnitus [15, 43], hearing loss [44], paroxysmal otalgia with or without deep prosopalgia or feeling of pressure in the ear [45].

MVC rarely present bilaterally (1–12%) [37, 39, 46, 47], and if it does, the pain or spasm never occurs on both sides at the same time, but alternates. There usually is a delay between the onset of symptoms from one side and the development of symptoms of the other side [38, 48, 49], with only 2–3% of the bilateral cases starting simultaneously. Bilateral MVC is more common in familial cases [46, 48].

MVC syndromes that affect more than one cranial nerve occur rarely (incidence 2.8%), similar to bilateral MVCs [38]. The combination may occur on one side (1.5%) or bilaterally (1.3%) The mean age is higher than for unilateral symptoms, 63.2 years vs. 55.3 years, similarly to bilateral MVCs (61.4 years) [38]. If one blood vessel contacts two or more cranial nerves, symptoms do not develop at the same moment in time [50]. The best known double compression syndrome is called the tic convulsif, consisting of a combination of hemifacial spasm and trigeminal neuralgia [51], which can occur even bilaterally [50, 52].

These data suggest that if bilateral tinnitus is due to microvascular compression, it is expected that the left- and right-sided component should start at different moments in time and with a different pitch. Theoretically, true bilateral tinnitus, i.e. with same pitch, could occur if the compression is at the level of the cochlear nucleus.

Cochleovestibular Compression Syndrome (CVCS)

A recent meta-analysis has confirmed that blood vessels that are in contact with the vestibulocochlear nerve can result in otological symptoms, including hearing loss and tinnitus [53, 54].

Whereas initially, it was proposed that only vascular compression of the root entry zone of a cranial nerve could cause symptoms [55] it was later suggested that any vascular contact along the central nervous system segment (between the internal acoustic meatus and the brainstem) could result in tinnitus [34]. Vascular loops inside the internal acoustic

[1] Otalgia: Earache.

[2] Prosopalgia: Facial pain.

[3] Chiari malformation (Chiari II syndrome): Displacement of the medulla and cerebellar tonsils and vermis through the foramen magnum into the upper spinal canal; often associated with other cerebral anomalies.

[4] Corpora amylacea: One of a number of small ovoid or rounded, sometimes laminated, bodies resembling a grain of starch and found in nervous tissue, in the prostate, and in pulmonary alveoli; of little pathologic significance, and apparently derived from degenerated cells or proteinaceous secretions. Stedman's Electronic Medical Dictionary.

[5] Neuronitis: Inflammatory disorder of the neuron.

[6] Arachnoiditis: Inflammation of the arachnoid membrane often with involvement of the subjacent subarachnoid space. Stedman's Electronic Medical Dictionary.

[7] Apolipoprotein: The protein component of any lipoprotein complexes that is a normal constituent of plasma chylomicrons, HDL, LDL, and VLDL in humans. Stedman's Electronic Medical Dictionary.

[8] Ephaptic transmission: Related to an ephapse: A place where two or more nerve cell processes (axons and dendrites) touch without forming a typical synaptic contact; some form of neural transmission may occur at such nonsynaptic contact sites. Stedman's Electronic Medical Dictionary.

meatus along the morphologically more resistant peripheral nervous system segment however were described to produce either typewriter tinnitus [56] or pulsatile tinnitus [54, 57], but no non-pulsatile tinnitus, as confirmed by a systematic review and meta-analysis [53]. Typewriter tinnitus consists of paroxysms of tinnitus that is perceived as Morse code, machine gun-like staccato or typewriter sound and has been shown to be responsive to treatment with carbamazepine [56], analogous to trigeminal neuralgia.

Diagnostic Criteria of CVCS

Signs and Symptoms of the Cochleovestibular Compression Syndrome

Based on the analogy with other vascular compression syndromes, tinnitus caused by MVC would be expected to be unilateral and result in short lasting paroxysms with tinnitus free intervals becoming progressive shorter, ending in constant tinnitus. This kind of tinnitus would be expected to occur in middle-aged individuals and the tinnitus would not be expected to be associated with a flat hearing loss, as the typical MVC disorders, HFS, and TN are not associated with complete weakness or complete loss of sensation in the entire distribution of the cranial nerve. Persistent compression can result in changes in characteristics of the pain and sensory impairment [40]. In a similar fashion, long-standing HFS could result in facial palsy or Bell's palsy [58]. Similarly, chronic vestibular nerve compression can lead to hypofunctioning of the labyrinth, clinically expressed as gait instability [39].

Both parts of the vestibulocochlear nerve might be compressed at the same time, and symptoms from the vestibular nerve would be expected in individuals with tinnitus from MVC. A similar evolution is noted, with progressively more vertiginous spells and shorter symptom free periods [39, 42]. In contrast to Ménière's disease the spells are shorter lasting and have no aura and no postictal period. In a chronic stage, persistent instability is noted [39, 59].

It is of interest, however, that in Ryu's study, 73% of the patients with an MVC were diagnosed as having Ménière's disease [42]. The main electrophysiological difference between Ménière's disease and CVCS is that in Ménière's disease there are no abnormalities in peak II and interpeak latency (IPL) I-III of the auditory brainstem response (ABR) [13]. Two more nerves are in close relationship with the cochleovestibular nerve: the intermediate and the facial nerve. Vascular contact with the intermediate nerve is associated with geniculate neuralgia [36]. In the acute stage, intermittent paroxysmal bouts of otalgia occur; in a later stage, a deep dull hemifacial pain develops, known as prosopalgia [36].

Vascular contact with the root exit zone of the facial nerve can result in hemifacial spasm [60, 61] and concomitant contact with the cochleovestibular nerve can cause auditory signs including low frequency tinnitus and hearing loss [43, 62].

Characteristic Features of Tinnitus as a MVC Syndrome

Selection Criteria

1. Intermittent paroxysmal spells of tinnitus lasting only seconds
   (a) hearing loss at the tinnitus frequency
2. Associated ipsilateral symptoms from adjacent cranial nerves
   (a) cryptogenic or overt hemifacial spasms (facial nerve)
   (b) bouts of otalgia or feeling of pressure in the ear (intermediate nerve)
   (c) vertiginous spells: short lasting, optokinetically induced (vestibular nerve)
3. Positive MRI for vascular compression
4. Positive brainstem auditory evoked potential, using Møller's criteria

Classification of Cochleovestibular Compression Syndrome

It was proposed that CVCS can be classified into four different groups analogous to Ménière's disease. Ménière's disease is classified based on the American Academy of Ophthalmology and Otolaryngology's (AAOO), later replaced by the American Academy of Otolaryngology's (AAO) criteria [63, 64]. For tinnitus a similar classification can determine the certainty of the diagnosis of CVCS as the cause of tinnitus [45].

Possible CVCS: intermittent unilateral tinnitus spells without associated symptoms.

Probable CVCS: possible CVCS with associated symptoms: vertigo spells, ipsilateral cryptogenic or overt hemifacial spasm, ipsilateral pressure feeling in the ear or ipsilateral ear pain or deep dull hemifacial pain, ipsilateral frequency-specific hearing loss.

Definite CVCS: probable CVCS with abnormal ABR and/or abnormal MRI.

Certain CVCS: definite CVCS surgically proven.

Pathophysiology of the CVCS

Introduction

A cranial nerve has two parts, a central nervous system segment and a peripheral nervous system segment separated by a transition zone, known as the root entry or root exit zone (for sensory and motor nerves, respectively) or Obersteiner Redlich zone. The length of the CNS segment is different in every cranial nerve, with sensory fibers in general having a longer CNS segment than motor fibers of the cranial nerves [65]. For the VIIIth cranial nerve, the central nervous system segment encompasses the entire cisternal trajectory of the cochleovestibular nerve, with the root entry zone located at the entrance of the internal auditory canal, thus the root entry zone is located at the internal auditory meatus.

Functional Anatomy

The cochlear nerve contains approximately 30,000 axons [66], 90% of which are myelinated (type I), 10% of which are unmyelinated (type II) [67]. Myelinated nerve fibers represent the afferent neurons from the inner hair cells and the efferent neurons to the outer hair cells. Unmyelinated nerve fibers on the contrary represent the efferent neurons to the inner hair cells and the afferent neurons from the outer hair cells [67].

The average axon diameter of the PNS segment is fairly constant at ±3 μm [67] or 4.2 to 5.5 μm [68], suggesting conduction velocities of approximately 12 m/s [69] (11.6 PLUS_SPI −1.6 m/s). Whether differences exist in fiber spectrum, especially with regard to fiber diameter between apical and basal fibers in humans is still debated, it is not known whether a direct correlation exists between axonal diameters and tonotopy in humans, but it has been suggested [68].

The auditory system is tonotopically organized. This means that neurons sensitive to specific acoustic frequencies are topographically arranged in an orderly manner [70–73]. As the cochlea is tonotopically organized (Von Bekesy's place theory of pitch perception) as well as the cochlear nuclei, the inferior colliculus and the auditory cortex, the cochlear nerve has to be tonotopically organized as well [43] as shown in animal studies [74]. The cochlear nerve (as other cranial nerves) rotates as it travels through the auditory canal and cisternal segment in the subarachnoidal space towards the cochlear nucleus [75]. The tonotopy follows this rotation. This tonotopy has been demonstrated in the human as well, as in studies of microvascular decompressions of the vestibulocochlear nerve specific tinnitus pitches correlate with specific topographic locations of the compressions [43]. It has also been shown by means of a MRI technique, using 3D reconstructions of high resolution (0,6 mm slice thickness) heavily T2 weighted images (Constructive Interference in Steady State, CISS) [76], also known as virtual endoscopy [77].

Controversy of CVCS

Vascular loops in the cerebellopontine angle (CPA) and internal auditory meatus (IAM) are very common and should be regarded primarily as a normal variant [1, 53, 78]. The anterior inferior cerebellar artery (AICA) loops within the internal auditory meatus (IAM) in approximately 65% of post-mortem specimens, with most people being asymptomatic [79]. Other cadaveric studies have found similar occurrence rates with AICA loops outside the IAM in 19–40%, at the IAM in 33–56% and within the IAM in 25–27% [80]. In patients with tinnitus, the same frequency (65%) of intrameatal loops is found ipsilateral to the tinnitus [81]. Yet, on the contralateral side, 83% of loops were identified inside the IAM [81]. This has resulted in the concept that apart from the vascular compression, a second factor needs to be involved in order for the compression to become symptomatic.

Little is known what this second factor may be, but some information may be gained from trigeminal neuralgia, which commonly results from a vascular compression of the trigeminal nerve.

Learning from Trigeminal Neuralgia

Initially, it was hypothesized that herpes simplex in the trigeminal ganglion was the second factor. This was based on the clinical experience that Herpes Simplex Virus (HSV) reactivation, resulting in herpes labialis, occurs commonly after MVD surgery for trigeminal neuralgia [82, 83]. Herpes simplex reactivation occurs not only after microvascular decompression surgery, but also after balloon compression, glycerol neurolysis, surgical rhizotomy, and radiofrequency rhizotomy [84]. Cushing already noticed that after treatment of trigeminal neuralgia by removal of the trigeminal ganglion, herpes labialis reactivation occurred [85]. Latent HSV infection is detected in the trigeminal ganglia of 67% of individuals [86]. Since in trigeminal neuralgia, only 50% of patients harbor a latent HSV infection [83], the presence of herpes simplex may not be the required second factor or cause of trigeminal neuralgia. But instead herpes simplex reactivation may be a marker of altered trigeminal ganglion neuron function resulting from any kind of trigeminal nerve surgery [84].

DTI is a MRI technique that can evaluate the microstructure of a nerve via fractional anisotropy, radial diffusivity, mean diffusivity, and axial diffusivity. In asymptomatic vascular compressions of the trigeminal nerve, normal microstructure of the trigeminal nerve is identified using DTI measures. Thus, no demyelination, no axonal damage, no inflammation, and no edema is identified [87].

Symptomatic trigeminal neuralgia with vascular compression is characterized by disturbed microstructure of the trigeminal nerve, suggesting inflammation and edema which is not visible on gross imaging [88]. The same structural abnormalities are seen in trigeminal neuralgia without micro-

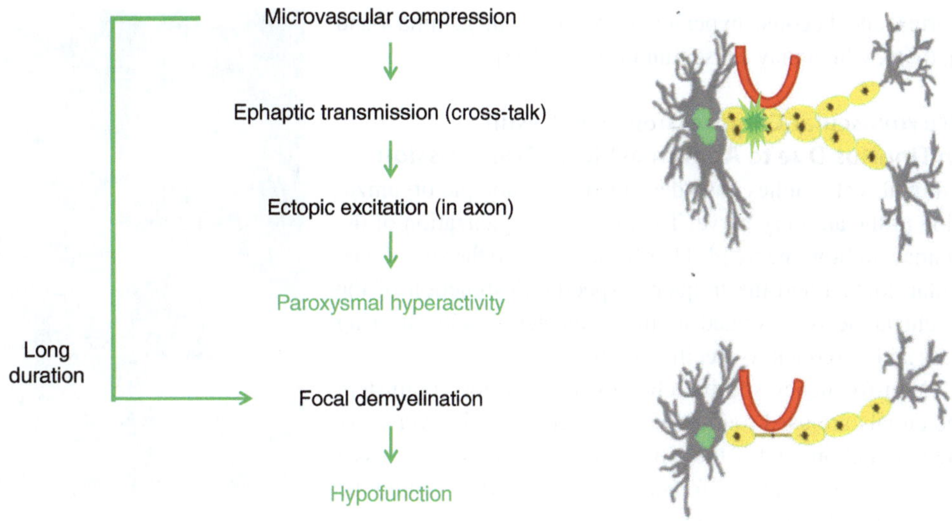

Fig. 35.2 Pathophysiological model of microvascular compression syndrome. Left image: microvascular compression leads to paroxysmal hyperactivity, i.e. typewriter tinnitus, via ephaptic transmission leading to ectopic excitation (top figure). In the long run the vascular compression can lead to nerve demyelination resulting in hypoactivity, i.e. hearing loss (lower figure). Right image: graphical depiction of ectopic axonal excitation (top figure), and nerve demyelination (lower figure)

vascular compressions [89] and in multiple sclerosis with trigeminal neuralgia [90]. The abnormal fractional anisotropy is independent of symptom duration, severity, and type of neurovascular conflict [91].

The abnormal fractional anisotropy, radial diffusivity, mean diffusivity, and axial diffusivity are only identified at the symptomatic side [92], and these structural abnormalities normalize after microvascular decompression surgery [93], associated with clinical improvement [93]. The preoperative axial diffusivity abnormality predicts the success of microvascular decompression surgery with 83.9% accuracy [94].

The structural abnormalities likely represent a neuroinflammatory state of the nerve and ganglion. This is in keeping with altered immune signaling molecules found in humans with trigeminal neuralgia. Higher cytokine levels of IL-1β, TNF-α, CCL2, IL-17A, IL-6, and CXCL8, as well as higher expression levels of chemokine receptors CCR1 (CD191), CR3 (CD11b), CCR2 (CD192), CXCR5 (CD185), and CCR5 (CD196) in the cells from saliva in patients with trigeminal neuralgia [95]. These higher levels of proinflammatory cytokines and chemokines are associated with lower growth factor levels of angiopoietin-2, bFGF, HGF, SCF, TGF-α, and VEGF [95]. Furthermore, there is a significant very high correlation between IL-6 concentration and severity of trigeminal neuralgia ($r = 0.943$) [96]. And similar results are found for hemifacial spasm, in which a very high correlation between IL6 and the severity of the hemifacial spasm is also identified ($r = 0.933$) [96].

MVC has been claimed to cause focal demyelination. In specimens obtained during microvascular decompression, surgery for trigeminal neuralgia axonopathy and axonal loss, demyelination, a range of less severe myelin abnormalities (dysmyelination), residual myelin debris, and the presence of excess collagen has been demonstrated [97–99]. No inflammatory cells are present at the compression site, but astrocyte processes are largely confined to the periphery of the lesion [99].

An ignition hypothesis of trigeminal neuralgia has been proposed [97, 100]. This model explains the major positive and negative symptoms of trigeminal neuralgia by axonopathy-induced changes in the electrical excitability of afferent axons in the trigeminal root and of neuronal somata in the trigeminal ganglion. The key pathophysiological changes include ephaptic transmission with associated cross-excitation among neighboring afferents leading to ectopic impulse discharge and after-discharges. The cross-excitation occurs predominantly in Aβ fibers, but also in Aδ, but not C fibers [101] (Fig. 35.2).

In summary, in trigeminal neuralgia, a neuroinflammatory state of the trigeminal nerve may render the nerve more sensitive for a vascular compression resulting in ephaptic transmission with cross-excitation, ectopic discharges, resulting in paroxysmal hyperactivity (Fig. 35.2).

Pathophysiological Model of CVCS

Similar hypotheses can be proposed for the pathology of MVC in general. Some of these concern the cranial nerve and some concern the respective nucleus. Hemifacial spasm has been studied extensively and evidence for hyperactivity in the facial motonucleus has been presented [60]. A former discarded hypothesis that blood vessels elongate and their brain "sags" with age has not received evidence [2, 5, 6, 102, 103]. It is not known if the formation of vascular loops in the posterior fossa that can come close to cranial nerve increases with age [103].

Focal demyelination, if it exists because of MVC, could cause ectopic excitation [6, 104–106]. Such ectopic excitation might cause dysfunction of the cochlear nerve most likely leading to a reorganization of the auditory nuclei in the auditory brainstem through activation of neural plasticity. Subsequently, the entire auditory tract including the auditory cortex and become hyperactive, resulting in gamma band activity, which may cause tinnitus [107, 108].

Microvascular Compressions Can Result in Tinnitus Due to Abnormal Signal Transmission

Animal (cat) studies have described the tonotopic organization of the auditory nerve. The tonotopic organization of the human auditory nerve [43] has been related to the site of vascular contact and the frequency-specific dysfunction of the cochlear nerve, revealed as the frequency-specific hearing loss and a frequency-specific tinnitus [43, 54].

Non-frequency-specific click evoked auditory brainstem potentials are used routinely in an attempt to discover early demyelination, and if the close contact with a blood vessel causes demyelination, frequency-specific ABR would be expected to be able to detect such focal demyelination.

The neural generators of the brain stem auditory evoked responses (ABR) in humans have been determined [70]. The generators of the ABR in humans are not the same as the generators of the ABR in animals, including in monkeys [70].

Peak I in humans is generated in the distal part of the cochlear nerve, peak II is generated in its central nervous system segment, peak III in the cochlear nuclei, peak IV in the superior olivary complex, peak V in the lateral lemniscus, and peak VI in the inferior colliculus (Fig. 35.3) [70].

The interpeak latency (IPL) I-II or I-III would therefore be expected to be increased. If the vascular compression occurs at the CNS segment [34], peak II would be expected to be affected. Evoked potentials in general are the result of synchronized firing pattern as a reaction to a sensory stimulus [70]. The more synchronized the nerves fire, the higher the summated amplitude will be. If MVC of the cochlear nerve causes functional impairment of some fibers, the temporal coherence of firing will decrease, resulting in a decrease of the amplitude of peak II. This hypothesis is supported by clinical findings that show a peak II decreases in individuals with tinnitus ipsilateral to microvascular compressions, with recurrence of peak II when surgical decompression is successful [45]. This suggests that the tinnitus is causally related to dysfunctional signal transmission at the site of compression in the initial stage of compression (Fig. 35.4).

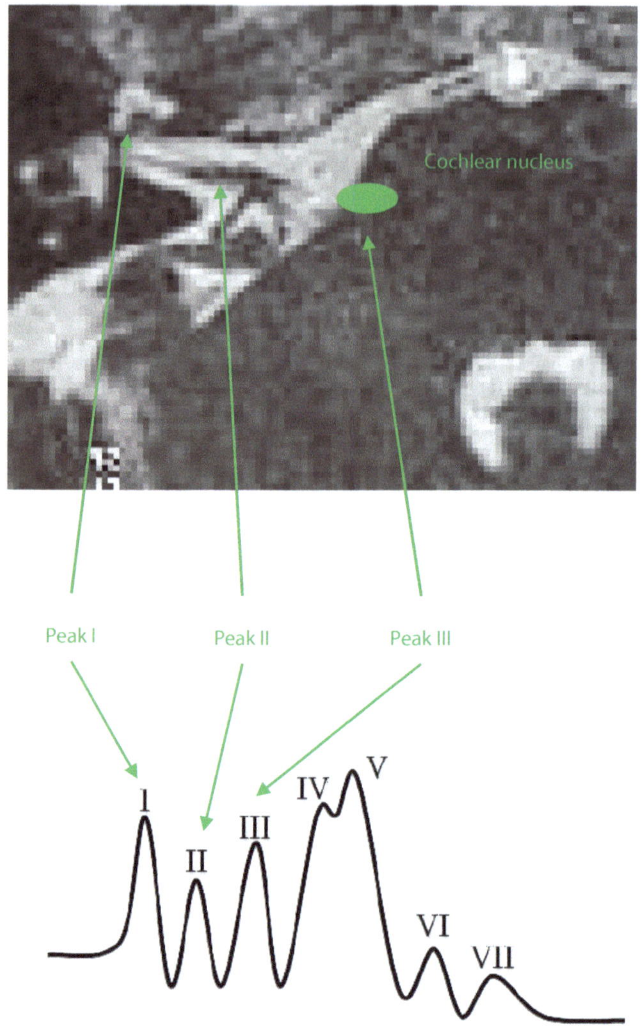

Fig. 35.3 Correlation between the anatomy and electrophysiology. Peak I of the auditory brainstem response (ABR) is generated by the cochlea, peak II by the cochlear nerve and peak III by the cochlear nucleus

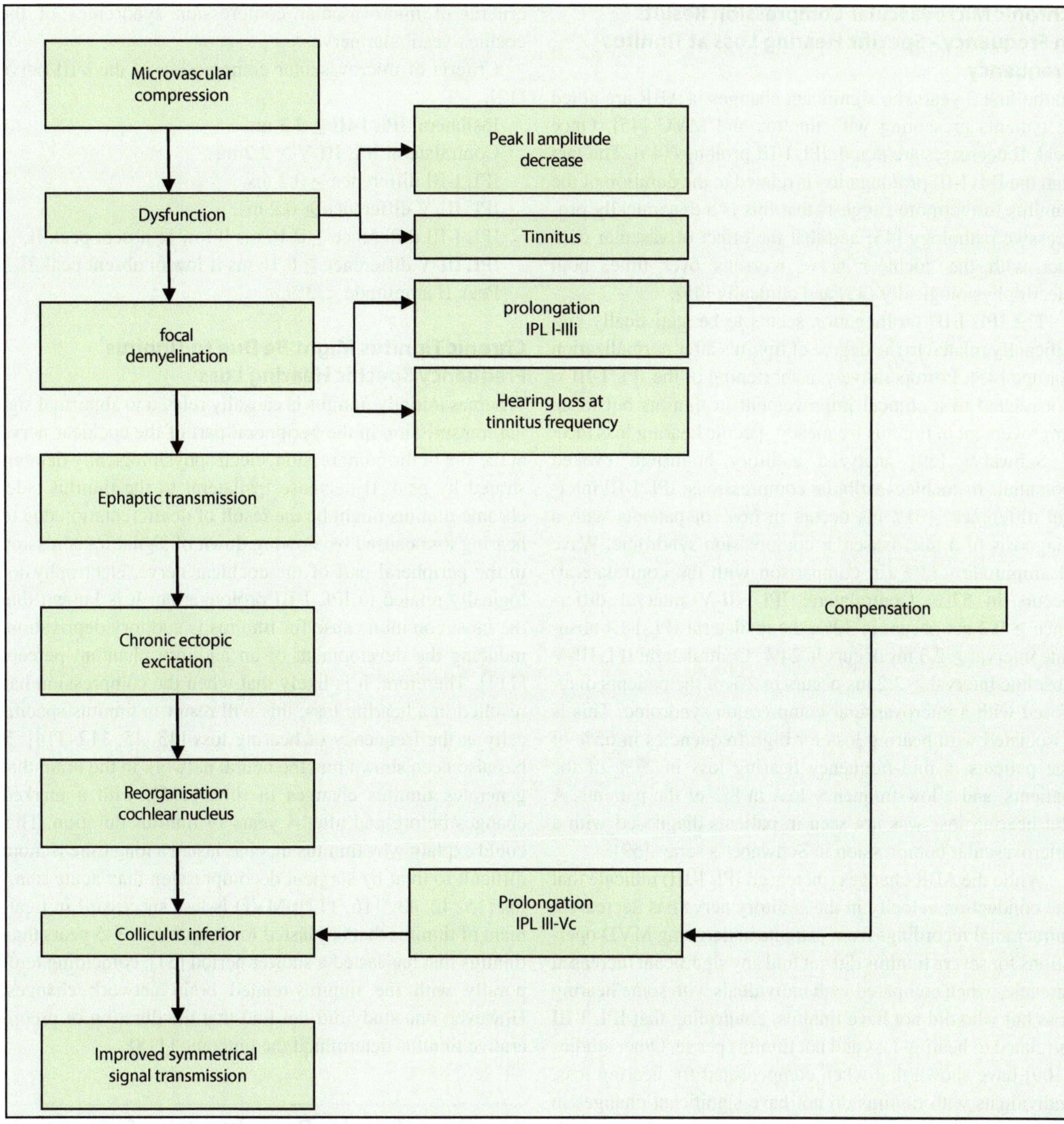

Fig. 35.4 Extended pathophysiological model of microvascular compression syndrome. When a blood vessel compresses a sensitized vestibulocochlear nerve (due to neuroinflammation) it can interfere with normal signal transmission. Whereas initially no electrophysiological changes occur, after 2 years, when enough fibers are involved, a decrease in the amplitude of peak II on the ABR develops. In time demyelination develops, slowing down signal transmission at the level of the compression resulting in an IPL I-III increase, associated with hearing loss at the tinnitus frequency. This signal transmission, slowing at the side of the compression is compensated by a contralateral slowing in the brainstem (contralateral IPL III-V prolongs). When hearing loss develops, the tinnitus might be related more to the deafferentation than ectopic discharges

Chronic Microvascular Compression Results in Frequency - Specific Hearing Loss at Tinnitus Frequency

In the first 2 years, no significant changes in ABR are noted in patients presenting with tinnitus and MVC [45]. Once peak II decreases are noted, IPL I-III prolongs [45]. The fact that the IPL I-III prolongation is related to the duration of the tinnitus furthermore suggests that this is a dynamically progressive pathology [45] and that the effect of vascular contact with the cochlear nerve worsens over time, both electrophysiologically [45] and clinically [45].

The IPL I-III prolongation seems to be statistically significantly related to the degree of tinnitus after normalization for age [45]. Postoperatively, a shortening of the IPL I-III is not related to a clinical improvement in tinnitus but to an improvement in tinnitus frequency specific hearing loss [45].

Schwaber [59] analyzed auditory brainstem evoked potentials in cochleovestibular compressions: IPL I-III interval difference $\geq$ 0.2 ms occurs in 66% of patients with a diagnosis of a microvascular compression syndrome. Wave II amplitude <33% (in comparison with the contralateral) occurs in 57%. Contralateral IPL III-V interval difference $\geq$ 0.2 ms occurs in 30%, the ipsilateral IPL I-III absolute interval $\geq$ 2.3 ms occurs in 24%. Contralateral IPL III-V absolute interval $\geq$ 2.2 ms occurs in 2% of the patients diagnosed with a microvascular compression syndrome. This is associated with hearing loss for high frequencies in 65% of the patients, a mid-frequency hearing loss in 27% of the patients, and a low-frequency loss in 8% of the patients. A flat hearing loss was not seen in patients diagnosed with a microvascular compression in Schwaber's series [59].

While the ABR changes (increased IPL I-III) indicate that the conduction velocity in the auditory nerve has decreased, intracranial recordings from patients undergoing MVD operations for severe tinnitus did not find any significant increased latencies when compared with individuals with some hearing loss but who did not have tinnitus, confirming that IPL I-III is related to hearing loss and not tinnitus per se. Other studies [109] have shown that when compensated for hearing loss, individuals with tinnitus do not have significant changes in auditory evoked potentials from the peripheral part (IPL I-III) of the ascending pathways but a slight change in the potentials recorded from the inferior colliculus.

Signals transmitted via the compressed nerve fibers arrive at the cochlear nuclei in delay (IPL I-III prolongs) in comparison to the contralateral input. Because auditory input arrives bilaterally, this slowing down of nerve conduction in the auditory nerve of the affected ear (ipsilateral IPL I-III) will be counterbalanced by slowing down the auditory signals coming from the contralateral ear [110]. As this slowing down can only occur in the brainstem, this will result in an increase in IPL III-V in the contralateral side. As such a pathophysiological explanation can be proposed for Møller's criteria of microvascular compression syndromes of the cochlea-vestibular nerve.

Criteria of microvascular compression of the VIII nerve [12].

Ipsilateral IPL I-III $\geq$ 2.3 ms.
Contralateral IPL III-V $\geq$ 2.2 ms.
IPL I-III difference $\geq$ 0.2 ms.
IPL III-V difference $\geq$ 0.2 ms.
IPL I-III difference $\geq$ 0.16 ms if low or absent peak II.
IPL III-V difference $\geq$ 0.16 ms if low or absent peak II.
Peak II amplitude <33%.

Chronic Tinnitus Might Be Due to Tinnitus Frequency Specific Hearing Loss

Whereas initially tinnitus is causally related to abnormal signal transmission in the peripheral part of the cochlear nerve at the site of the compression, electrophysiologically demonstrated by peak II decrease ipsilateral to the tinnitus side, chronic tinnitus might be the result of deafferentation due to hearing loss caused by slowing down of signal transmission in the peripheral part of the cochlear nerve, electrophysiologically related to IPL I-III prolongation. It is known that the most common cause for tinnitus is auditory deprivation, inducing the development of an auditory phantom percept [111]. Therefore, it is likely that when the compression has resulted in a hearing loss, this will result in tinnitus specifically at the frequency of hearing loss [43, 45, 112–114]. It has also been shown that the neural network in the brain that generates tinnitus changes in time [115], with a marked changes before and after 4 years of tinnitus duration. This could explain why tinnitus that has lasted a long time is more difficult to treat by surgical decompression than acute tinnitus [15, 42, 43, 116, 117]: MVD is less successful in treatment of tinnitus that has lasted for longer than 3–5 years than tinnitus that has lasted a shorter period [31], coinciding temporally with the tinnitus-related brain network changes. However, one study did not find that the duration of preoperative tinnitus determined the outcome [118].

Results of Vascular Decompression Surgery

Microvascular decompression surgery is a simple technique, in which a piece of teflon is interposed between the offending blood vessel, usually the anterior inferior cerebellar artery (AICA), and the vestibulocochlear nerve (VIIIth cranial nerve) via a retrosigmoid approach (Fig. 35.5). The cochlear component of the vestibulocochlear nerve is located inferiorly of the vestibular component, which faces the trigeminal nerve [43].

To date, there are no RCTs that investigate the outcome of microvascular decompression surgery of the vestibulocochlear nerve [1]. A systematic review has been performed

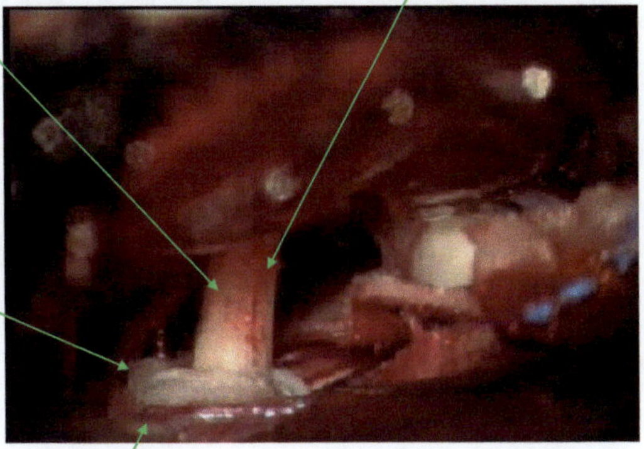

Fig. 35.5 Intraoperative picture of microvascular decompression of the left vestibulocochlear nerve

looking at outcomes following vestibulocochlear nerve decompression [119]. This review included 19 studies and a total of 545 patients [119]. Whereas vertigo improved in most patients (75–100%), tinnitus improvement was less obvious, and highly variable, ranging between 27.8 and 100% improvement. The 100% improvements were only noted in case reports. Hearing improved in 16% of the operated patients, while it deteriorated in 6.2%. A later review focusing on intrameatal vascular compressions concluded that microvascular decompression was successful for treating vertigo and tinnitus, but not for hearing loss [120].

A meta-analysis, involving 572 patients, demonstrated that microvascular decompression surgery can result in 28% complete relief for tinnitus, with 45% of patients improving without a complete relief, 25% of patients noting no change, and only 2% worsening [121]. In those patients who present with both tinnitus and vertigo, the success rates dramatically improved: 62% had complete relief, 23% improved, 11% experienced no change, and 4% worsened [121]. This is confirmed by another systematic review that showed 60% of patients who presented with tinnitus only improved [122].

Surgical Complications

Complications may result from the surgical approach. A systematic review and meta-analysis demonstrated that minor complications, such as transient facial weakness, transient abducens paresis, transient hearing loss, or CSF leak, were reported in 3% of patients and major complications such as permanent hearing loss, permanent facial palsy, or meningitis were recorded in 6% of patients [121]. The most common complication was permanent hearing deficit after surgery, occurring in 5% of patients. Overall, 11% of patients had complications following MVD. No strokes nor deaths were registered [121].

Conclusion

Microvascular decompression operations are more successful in treating tinnitus that has not lasted too long (less than 3–5 years). Outcomes of decompression surgery are also better if tinnitus presents with vertigo. In pure tinnitus, 28% of patients are cured and 45% improved, whereas in combined tinnitus plus vertigo 62% are cured and 23% improved. Worsening of tinnitus caused by MVD operations (2–4%) and other complications are rare but can be severe and life-threatening.

After a MVD operation, the hearing threshold of the frequency of the tinnitus may improve if IPL I-III normalizes and peak II reoccurs.

The following pathophysiological mechanism can be suggested for tinnitus (Fig. 35.6).

When a blood vessel comes into contact with the auditory part of a sensitized vestibulocochlear nerve (due to neuroinflammation), it can interfere with normal signal transmission. Initially, no electrophysiological changes can be retrieved. After 2 years, when enough fibers are involved, a decrease in the amplitude of peak II on the ABR develops. When the close contact with a blood vessel continues, signal transmission may slow down at the level of the compression resulting in an IPL I-III increase, associated with hearing loss at the tinnitus frequency. This signal transmission, slowing at the side of the compression, is compensated by a contralateral slowing in the brainstem (contralateral IPL III-V prolongs). When hearing loss develops, the tinnitus might be related more to the deafferentation than ectopic discharges. The deafferentation induces network changes in the brain

Tinnitus duration	Mechanism	ABR	Clinical
0-2 years	Vascular compression on nerve with neuroinflammation	No changes	Intermittent tinnitus?
>2 years	Disrupted signal transmission	Peak II amplitude decrease ipsilateral	Tinnitus
2-4 years	Demyelination	IPL I-III prolongation ipsilateral	Hearing loss at tinnitus frequency
>4 years	Compensation in brainstem	IPL III-V contralateral	?

Fig. 35.6 Summary of clinical tinnitus features and electrophysiology of microvascular compression of the vestibulocochlear nerve

based on neural plasticity and tinnitus at that stage has become a phantom percept. These tinnitus network changes alter in time, which might explain why surgical decompression has to be performed before 4 years in order to be successful.

References

1. Walijee H, et al. Microvascular compression of the vestibulocochlear nerve. Eur Arch Otorhinolaryngol. 2021;278(10):3625–31.
2. Dandy W. Concerning the cause of trigeminal neuralgia. Am J Surg. 1934;24:447–55.
3. Jannetta PJ. Microsurgery of cranial nerve cross-compression. Clin Neurosurg. 1979;26:607–15.
4. Jannetta PJ. Selection criteria for the treatment of cranial rhizopathies by microvascular decompression (honored guest lecture). Clin Neurosurg. 1997;44:69–77.
5. Jannetta PJ. Neurovascular cross-compression in patients with hyperactive dysfunction symptoms of the eighth cranial nerve. Surg Forum. 1975;26:467–9.
6. Moller AR. Vascular compression of cranial nerves: II: pathophysiology. Neurol Res. 1999;21(5):439–43.
7. Moller AR. The cranial nerve vascular compression syndrome: I. A review of treatment. Acta Neurochir (Wien). 1991;113(1–2):18–23.
8. Moller AR. The cranial nerve vascular compression syndrome: II. A review of pathophysiology. Acta Neurochir (Wien). 1991;113(1–2):24–30.
9. Moller AR. Is there a place for microvascular decompression? Acta Neurochir. 2005;147(9):921–3.
10. Moller AR, Moller MB. Microvascular decompression operations. Prog Brain Res. 2007;166:397–400.
11. Moller AR, et al. Compound action potentials recorded from the exposed eighth nerve in patients with intractable tinnitus. Laryngoscope. 1992;102(2):187–97.
12. Moller MB. Results of microvascular decompression of the eighth nerve as treatment for disabling positional vertigo. Ann Otol Rhinol Laryngol. 1990;99(9 Pt 1):724–9.
13. Moller MB. Controversy in Meniere's disease: results of microvascular decompression of the eighth nerve. Am J Otol. 1988;9(1):60–3.
14. Moller MB, Moller AR. Vascular compression syndrome of the eighth nerve. Clinical correlations and surgical findings. Neurol Clin. 1990;8(2):421–39.
15. Moller MB, et al. Vascular decompression surgery for severe tinnitus: selection criteria and results. Laryngoscope. 1993;103(4 Pt 1):421–7.
16. Leal PR, Froment JC, Sindou M. MRI sequences for detection of neurovascular conflicts in patients with trigeminal neuralgia and predictive value for characterization of the conflict (particularly degree of vascular compression). Neurochirurgie. 2010;56(1):43–9.
17. Rosetti P, et al. Arnold Chiari type I malformation presenting as a trigeminal neuralgia: case report. Neurosurgery. 1999;44(5):1122–3; discussion 1123–4.
18. Sindou M. Discussion on Arnold Chiari type I malformation presenting as a trigeminal neuralgia: case report. Neurosurgery. 1999;44(5):1123–4.
19. Kanpolat Y, et al. Chiari type I malformation presenting as glossopharyngeal neuralgia: case report. Neurosurgery. 2001;48(1):226–8.
20. Glocker FX, et al. Hemifacial spasm due to posterior fossa tumors: the impact of tumor location on electrophysiological findings. Clin Neurol Neurosurg. 1998;100(2):104–11.

21. Barker FG 2nd, et al. Long-term outcome after operation for trigeminal neuralgia in patients with posterior fossa tumors. J Neurosurg. 1996;84(5):818–25.
22. De Ridder D, et al. Remote tentorium meningioma causing sudden sensorineural deafness. Surg Neurol. 2008;70(3):312–7; discussion 318.
23. Matsuura N, Kondo A. Trigeminal neuralgia and hemifacial spasm as false localizing signs in patients with a contralateral mass of the posterior cranial fossa. Report of three cases. J Neurosurg. 1996;84(6):1067–71.
24. Cappabianca P, et al. Trigeminal neuralgia and contralateral mass. J Neurosurg. 1997;86(1):171–2.
25. Haddad FS, Taha JM. An unusual cause for trigeminal neuralgia: contralateral meningioma of the posterior fossa. Neurosurgery. 1990;26(6):1033–8.
26. Koenig M, Kalyan-Raman K, Sureka ON. Contralateral trigeminal nerve dysfunction as a false localizing sign in acoustic neuroma: a clinical and electrophysiological study. Neurosurgery. 1984;14(3):335–7.
27. Mase G, et al. Trigeminal neuralgia due to contralateral meningioma of the posterior cranial fossa. J Neurol Neurosurg Psychiatry. 1994;57(8):1010.
28. Sindou M, Howeidy T, Acevedo G. Anatomical observations during microvascular decompression for idiopathic trigeminal neuralgia (with correlations between topography of pain and site of the neurovascular conflict). Prospective study in a series of 579 patients. Acta Neurochir. 2002;144(1):1–12; discussion 12–3, 1.
29. Jho HD, Jannetta PJ. Microvascular decompression for spasmodic torticollis. Acta Neurochir. 1995;134(1–2):21–6.
30. Kommerell G, Mehdorn E, Ketelsen UP. Oculomotor paralysis with cyclic spasms; electromyographic and electron microscopic indications of chronic peripheral nerve irritation. Fortschr Ophthalmol. 1985;82(2):203–4.
31. Samii M, et al. Microvascular decompression for superior oblique myokymia: first experience. Case report. J Neurosurg. 1998;89(6):1020–4.
32. Scharwey K, et al. Remission of superior oblique myokymia after microvascular decompression. Ophthalmologica. 2000;214(6):426–8.
33. De Ridder D, Menovsky T. Neurovascular compression of the abducent nerve causing abducent palsy treated by microvascular decompression. Case report. J Neurosurg. 2007;107(6):1231–4.
34. De Ridder D, et al. Is the root entry/exit zone important in microvascular compression syndromes? Neurosurgery. 2002;51(2):427–33; discussion 433–4.
35. Resnick DK, et al. Microvascular decompression for glossopharyngeal neuralgia. Neurosurgery. 1995;36(1):64–8; discussion 68–9.
36. Lovely TJ, Jannetta PJ. Surgical management of geniculate neuralgia. Am J Otol. 1997;18(4):512–7.
37. Fukushima T. Microvascular decompression for hemifacial spasm: result in 2890 cases. In: Carter L, Spetzler R, Hamilton M, editors. Neurovascular surgery. New York, NY: McGraw Hill, Inc; 1995. p. 1133–45.
38. Kobata H, et al. Combined hyperactive dysfunction syndrome of the cranial nerves: trigeminal neuralgia, hemifacial spasm, and glossopharyngeal neuralgia: 11-year experience and review. Neurosurgery. 1998;43(6):1351–61; discussion 1361–2.
39. Moller MB, et al. Microvascular decompression of the eighth nerve in patients with disabling positional vertigo: selection criteria and operative results in 207 patients. Acta Neurochir. 1993;125(1–4):75–82.
40. Burchiel KJ, Slavin KV. On the natural history of trigeminal neuralgia. Neurosurgery. 2000;46(1):152–4; discussion 154–5.
41. Ehni G, Woltman H. Hemifacial spasm. Arch Neurol Psychiatr. 1945;53:205–11.
42. Ryu H, et al. Neurovascular compression syndrome of the eighth cranial nerve. What are the most reliable diagnostic signs? Acta Neurochir. 1998;140(12):1279–86.
43. De Ridder D, et al. Functional anatomy of the human cochlear nerve and its role in microvascular decompressions for tinnitus. Neurosurgery. 2004;54(2):381–8; discussion 388–90.
44. Okamura T, et al. Microvascular decompression for cochlear symptoms. J Neurosurg. 2000;93(3):421–6.
45. De Ridder D, et al. Tinnitus in vascular conflict of the eighth cranial nerve: a surgical pathophysiological approach to ABR changes. Prog Brain Res. 2007;166:401–11.
46. Pollack IF, Jannetta PJ, Bissonette DJ. Bilateral trigeminal neuralgia: a 14-year experience with microvascular decompression. J Neurosurg. 1988;68(4):559–65.
47. Rushton JG, Stevens JC, Miller RH. Glossopharyngeal (vagoglossopharyngeal) neuralgia: a study of 217 cases. Arch Neurol. 1981;38(4):201–5.
48. Tacconi L, Miles JB. Bilateral trigeminal neuralgia: a therapeutic dilemma. Br J Neurosurg. 2000;14(1):33–9.
49. Brisman R. Bilateral trigeminal neuralgia. J Neurosurg. 1987;67(1):44–8.
50. Fonoff ET, et al. Neurovascular compression in painful tic convulsif. Acta Neurochir. 2009;151(8):989–93.
51. Cook BR, Jannetta PJ. Tic convulsif: results in 11 cases treated with microvascular decompression of the fifth and seventh cranial nerves. J Neurosurg. 1984;61(5):949–51.
52. Felicio AC, et al. Bilateral hemifacial spasm and trigeminal neuralgia: a unique form of painful tic convulsif. Mov Disord. 2007;22(2):285–6.
53. Chadha NK, Weiner GM. Vascular loops causing otological symptoms: a systematic review and meta-analysis. Clin Otolaryngol. 2008;33(1):5–11.
54. Nowe V, et al. Does the location of a vascular loop in the cerebellopontine angle explain pulsatile and non-pulsatile tinnitus? Eur Radiol. 2004;14(12):2282–9.
55. Jannetta PJ. Observations on the etiology of trigeminal neuralgia, hemifacial spasm, acoustic nerve dysfunction and glossopharyngeal neuralgia. Definitive microsurgical treatment and results in 117 patients. Neurochirurgia (Stuttg). 1977;20(5):145–54.
56. Levine RA. Typewriter tinnitus: a carbamazepine-responsive syndrome related to auditory nerve vascular compression. ORL J Otorhinolaryngol Relat Spec. 2006;68(1):43–6; discussion 46–7.
57. De Ridder D, et al. Pulsatile tinnitus and the intrameatal vascular loop: why do we not hear our carotids? Neurosurgery. 2005;57(6):1213–7; discussion 1213–7.
58. Jannetta PJ, Bissonette DJ. Bell's palsy: a theory as to etiology. Observations in six patients. Laryngoscope. 1978;88(5):849–54.
59. Schwaber MK, Hall JW. Cochleovestibular nerve compression syndrome. I. Clinical features and audio vestibular findings. Laryngoscope. 1992;102(9):1020–9.
60. Moller AR. Pathophysiology of hemifacial spasm. Eur Arch Otorhinolaryngol. 1994:S78–81.
61. Moller AR, Jannetta PJ. Hemifacial spasm: results of electrophysiologic recording during microvascular decompression operations. Neurology. 1985;35(7):969–74.
62. Moller MB, Moller AR. Audiometric abnormalities in hemifacial spasm. Audiology. 1985;24(6):396–405.
63. CHE A-H. Committee on hearing and equilibrium guidelines for the diagnosis and evaluation of therapy in Meniere's disease. American Academy of otolaryngology-head and neck foundation, Inc. Otolaryngol Head Neck Surg. 1995;113(3):181–5.
64. Beasley NJ, Jones NS. Meniere's disease: evolution of a definition. J Laryngol Otol. 1996;110(12):1107–13.
65. Hamlyn PJ. Neurovascular compression of the cranial nerves in neurological and systemic disease. Amsterdam: Elsevier; 1999.

66. Spoendlin H, Schrott A. The spiral ganglion and the innervation of the human organ of Corti. Acta Otolaryngol. 1988;105(5–6):403–10.
67. Spoendlin H, Schrott A. Quantitative evaluation of the human cochlear nerve. Acta Otolaryngol Suppl. 1990;470:61–9; discussion 69-70.
68. Felix H, et al. Morphometric analysis of the cochlear nerve in man. Acta Otolaryngol. 1992;112(2):284–7.
69. Nguyen BH, Javel E, Levine SC. Physiologic identification of eighth nerve subdivisions: direct recordings with bipolar and monopolar electrodes. Am J Otol. 1999;20(4):522–34.
70. Moller AR. Hearing: its physiology and pathophysiology. 1st ed. San Diego: Academic Press; 2000.
71. Bear M, Connors BW, Paradiso M. Neuroscience: exploring the brain. 2nd ed. Baltimore: Lippincott Williams and Wilkins; 2001. p. 349–95.
72. Purves D, et al. Neuroscience. 1st ed. Sunderland: Sinauer Associates; 1997. p. 223–44.
73. Shepherd G. Neurobiology. 3rd ed. New York, NY: Oxford University Press; 1994.
74. Sando I. The anatomical interrelationships of the cochlear nerve fibers. Acta Otolaryng (Stockh). 1965;59:417–36.
75. Silverstein H, et al. The unrecognized rotation of the vestibular and cochlear nerves from the labyrinth to the brain stem: its implications to surgery of the eighth cranial nerve. Otolaryngol Head Neck Surg. 1986;95:543–9.
76. Casselman JW, et al. Constructive interference in steady state-3DFT MR imaging of the inner ear and cerebellopontine angle. AJNR Am J Neuroradiol. 1993;14(1):47–57.
77. Nowe V, et al. High-resolution virtual MR endoscopy of the cerebellopontine angle. AJR Am J Roentgenol. 2004;182(2):379–84.
78. Makins A, et al. Is there a correlation between vascular loops and unilateral auditory symptoms? Laryngoscope. 1998;108:1739–42.
79. Herzog JA, Bailey S, Meyer J. Vascular loops of the internal auditory canal: a diagnostic dilemma. Am J Otol. 1997;18(1):26–31.
80. McDermott AL, et al. Anterior inferior cerebellar artery syndrome: fact or fiction. Clin Otolaryngol Allied Sci. 2003;28(2):75–80.
81. Gultekin S, et al. Vascular loops at the cerebellopontine angle: is there a correlation with tinnitus? AJNR Am J Neuroradiol. 2008;29(9):1746–9.
82. Berra LV, et al. Herpes simplex reactivation after surgical treatment of trigeminal neuralgia: a retrospective cohort study. World Neurosurg. 2019;127:e16–21.
83. Pazin GJ, Ho M, Jannetta PJ. Reactivation of herpes simplex virus after decompression of the trigeminal nerve root. J Infect Dis. 1978;138(3):405–9.
84. Tenser RB. Occurrence of herpes simplex virus reactivation suggests a mechanism of trigeminal neuralgia surgical efficacy. World Neurosurg. 2015;84(2):279–82.
85. Cushing H. The surgical aspects of major neuralgia of the trigeminal nerve: a report of twenty cases of operation on the gasserian ganglion with anatomic and physiologic notes on the consequences of its removal. JAMA. 1905;44:1002–8
86. Croen KD, et al. Latent herpes simplex virus in human trigeminal ganglia. Detection of an immediate early gene "anti-sense" transcript by in situ hybridization. N Engl J Med. 1987;317(23):1427–32.
87. Lin W, Chen YL, Zhang QW. Vascular compression of the trigeminal nerve in asymptomatic individuals: a voxel-wise analysis of axial and radial diffusivity. Acta Neurochir. 2014;156(3):577–80.
88. DeSouza DD, Hodaie M, Davis KD. Diffusion imaging in trigeminal neuralgia reveals abnormal trigeminal nerve and brain white matter. Pain. 2014;155(9):1905–6.
89. Neetu S, et al. Microstructural abnormalities of the trigeminal nerve by diffusion-tensor imaging in trigeminal neuralgia without neurovascular compression. Neuroradiol J. 2016;29(1):13–8.
90. Chen DQ, et al. Diffusivity signatures characterize trigeminal neuralgia associated with multiple sclerosis. Mult Scler. 2016;22(1):51–63.
91. Lutz J, et al. Microstructural alterations in trigeminal neuralgia determined by diffusion tensor imaging are independent of symptom duration, severity, and type of neurovascular conflict. J Neurosurg. 2016;124(3):823–30.
92. Fujiwara S, et al. High-resolution diffusion tensor imaging for the detection of diffusion abnormalities in the trigeminal nerves of patients with trigeminal neuralgia caused by neurovascular compression. J Neuroimaging. 2011;21(2):e102–8.
93. DeSouza DD, Davis KD, Hodaie M. Reversal of insular and microstructural nerve abnormalities following effective surgical treatment for trigeminal neuralgia. Pain. 2015;156(6):1112–23.
94. Chao SH, et al. Correlation between brain circuit segregation and obesity. Behav Brain Res. 2018;337:218–27.
95. Patil S, Testarelli L. Assessment of growth factors, cytokines, and cellular markers in saliva of patients with trigeminal neuralgia. Molecules. 2021;26(10):2964.
96. Liu MX, et al. A correlative analysis between inflammatory cytokines and trigeminal neuralgia or hemifacial spasm. Neurol Res. 2019;41(4):335–40.
97. Devor M, Govrin-Lippmann R, Rappaport ZH. Mechanism of trigeminal neuralgia: an ultrastructural analysis of trigeminal root specimens obtained during microvascular decompression surgery. J Neurosurg. 2002;96(3):532–43.
98. Rappaport ZH, Govrin-Lippmann R, Devor M. An electron-microscopic analysis of biopsy samples of the trigeminal root taken during microvascular decompressive surgery. Stereotact Funct Neurosurg. 1997;68(1–4 Pt 1):182–6.
99. Hilton DA, et al. Pathological findings associated with trigeminal neuralgia caused by vascular compression. Neurosurgery. 1994;35(2):299–303; discussion 303.
100. Devor M, Amir R, Rappaport ZH. Pathophysiology of trigeminal neuralgia: the ignition hypothesis. Clin J Pain. 2002;18(1):4–13.
101. Amir R, Devor M. Axonal cross-excitation in nerve-end neuromas: comparison of A- and C-fibers. J Neurophysiol. 1992;68(4):1160–6.
102. Jannetta PJ. Hemifacial spasm: treatment by posterior fossa surgery. J Neurol Neurosurg Psychiatry. 1983;46(5):465–6.
103. Wilkins RH. Neurovascular compression syndromes. Neurol Clin. 1985;3(2):359–72.
104. Love S, Coakham HB. Trigeminal neuralgia: pathology and pathogenesis. Brain. 2001;124(Pt 12):2347–60.
105. Eidelman BH, et al. Vascular compression, hemifacial spasm, and multiple cranial neuropathy. Neurology. 1985;35(5):712–6.
106. Schwaber M. Vascular compression syndromes. In: Jackler R, Brackmann D, editors. Neurotology. St Louis: Mosby; 1994. p. 881–903.
107. van der Loo E, et al. Tinnitus intensity dependent gamma oscillations of the contralateral auditory cortex. PLoS One. 2009;4(10):e7396.
108. Weisz N, et al. The neural code of auditory phantom perception. J Neurosci. 2007;27(6):1479–84.
109. Møller AR, et al. Compound action potentials recorded from the exposed eighth nerve in patients with intractable tinnitus. Laryngoscope. 1992;102:187–97.
110. De Ridder D, et al. Vascular compression of the cochlear nerve and tinnitus: a pathophysiological investigation. Acta Neurochir. 2012;154(5):807–13.
111. Jastreboff PJ. Phantom auditory perception (tinnitus): mechanisms of generation and perception. Neurosci Res. 1990;8(4):221–54.
112. De Ridder D. Modulation of brain functions in tinnitus. Neuromodulation. 2004;7(2):146.

113. De Ridder D, et al. Frequency specific hearing improvement in microvascular decompression of the cochlear nerve. Acta Neurochir. 2005;147(5):495–501; discusssion 501.
114. Norena A, et al. Psychoacoustic characterization of the tinnitus spectrum: implications for the underlying mechanisms of tinnitus. Audiol Neurootol. 2002;7(6):358–69.
115. Schlee W, et al. Abnormal resting-state cortical coupling in chronic tinnitus. BMC Neurosci. 2009;10:11.
116. Jannetta P. Outcome after microvascular decompression for typical trigeminal neuralgia, hemifacial spasm, tinnitus, disabling positional vertigo, and glossopharyngeal neuralgia. In: Grady S, editor. Clinical neurosurgery. Baltimore: Williams and Wilkins; 1997. p. 331–84.
117. Brookes GB. Vascular-decompression surgery for severe tinnitus. Am J Otol. 1996;17(4):569–76.
118. Guevara N, et al. Microvascular decompression of cochlear nerve for tinnitus incapacity: pre-surgical data, surgical analyses and long-term follow-up of 15 patients. Eur Arch Otorhinolaryngol. 2008;265(4):397–401.
119. Yap L, Pothula VB, Lesser T. Microvascular decompression of cochleovestibular nerve. Eur Arch Otorhinolaryngol. 2008;265(8):861–9.
120. Esposito G, et al. Cochleovestibular nerve compression syndrome caused by Intrameatal anterior inferior cerebellar artery loop: synthesis of best evidence for clinical decisions. World Neurosurg. 2016;96:556–61.
121. van den Berge MJC, et al. Microvascular decompression of the cochleovestibular nerve for treatment of tinnitus and vertigo: a systematic review and meta-analysis of individual patient data. J Neurosurg. 2017;127(3):588–601.
122. Nash B, Carlson ML, Van Gompel JJ. Microvascular decompression for tinnitus: systematic review. J Neurosurg. 2017;126(4):1148–57.

Tinnitus and Cerebrovascular Diseases

36

Anna Piera, Alejandro Ponz, and Jose Miguel Láinez

Abstract

This chapter discusses cerebrovascular diseases as the cause of tinnitus as well as the underlying mechanisms, the diagnostic approach, and the treatment options, when possible.

Abbreviations

CTA	Computed tomography angiotomography
CVD	Cerebrovascular disease
DAVF	Dural arteriovenous fistula
GJT	Glomus jugulare tumor
HJB	High jugular bulb
ICA	Internal carotid artery
MRA	Magnetic resonance angiography
PT	Pulsatile tinnitus

Highlights

- Both objective and subjective tinnitus can be caused by cerebrovascular diseases.
- Pulsatile tinnitus can be caused by various vascular abnormalities and deserves a thorough evaluation because failure in detecting and treating some conditions can potentially lead to fatal consequences.
- In rare cases, ischemic cerebral or cochlear lesions can cause tinnitus.

A. Piera · A. Ponz
Department of Neurology, Hospital Clínico Universitario, Universidad Católica de Valencia, Valencia, Spain
e-mail: ponz_ale@gva.es

J. M. Láinez (✉)
Department of Neurology, University Clinic Hospital, Catholic University of Valencia, Valencia, Spain
e-mail: miguel.lainez@sen.es

Introduction

Based on its origin, tinnitus can be divided into two broad groups: objective and subjective tinnitus.

Objective tinnitus is caused when a sound generated inside the body reaches the ear due to its conduction through body tissues [1]. The frequent sources of objective tinnitus are turbulent blood flow inside an artery or involuntary muscle contractions. Distinctly, and unlike subjective tinnitus, an observer using a stethoscope or even a person listening to the individual at a close distance may be able to hear that sound.

Subjective tinnitus includes a broad group of sensations caused by abnormal neural activity in the nervous system, which is not elicited by sound activation of sensory cells in the cochlea. Pathophysiologically, subjective tinnitus shows similarities with central neuropathic pain and phantom limb syndrome [2, 3].

Based on a patient's perceived sound quality, tinnitus can also be classified as either pulsatile or nonpulsatile.

Most causes of tinnitus are subjective and nonpulsatile, with the auditory perception being present without an external stimulus. In these conditions, structural imaging is typically unremarkable. Nevertheless, nonpulsatile tinnitus can also be associated with treatable conditions of the central nervous system (CNS) such as stroke, demyelinating diseases, or tumors affecting the eighth cranial nerve [4].

Pulsatile tinnitus (PT) is often secondary to an identifiable vascular abnormality, acquired or congenital, which produces a physical sound that is perceived by the inner ear and that typically localizes to one side due to its usual unilateral origin. When of arterial origin, the perceived sound is typically synchronous with the patient's pulse. Pulsatile tinnitus is less common than is nonpulsatile tinnitus, accounting for less than 10% of tinnitus cases. It should be considered that in many cases with pulsatile tinnitus, no vascular abnormalities can be identified. This is especially the case for bilateral PT, in which a vascular origin can only be identified in extremely rare cases. Thus, bilateral PT is more likely of a nonvascular origin, e.g., anemia or an increased sensitivity to

W. Schlee et al. (eds.), *Textbook of Tinnitus*, https://doi.org/10.1007/978-3-031-35647-6_36

the perception of body sounds. In many cases, PT occurs together with nonpulsatile tinnitus; the patient describes a pulsatile component in addition to a nonpulsatile tinnitus component (for more information about PT, see also Chap. 40).

Neuroradiological imaging plays an important role in the diagnostic assessment of PT, in order to identify the underlying vascular abnormalities. The identification of these abnormalities is the basis for specific treatment [5] (for more information, see Chap. 30).

Cerebrovascular diseases, as well as other central nervous system (CNS) disorders, can occasionally be accompanied by tinnitus. However, it is extremely rare that tinnitus occurs in isolation as the only symptom of these disorders. In most cases, when tinnitus is caused by cerebrovascular or other CNS disorders, it is accompanied by other neurological or vascular symptoms. This is true for both cerebrovascular diseases, which typically cause objective tinnitus (e.g., PT in a carotid-cavernous fistula), and CNS disorders, which cause subjective tinnitus, such as those from ischemia of the inferior colliculus that can activate the subcortical auditory pathways and thereby cause tinnitus [6].

A bidirectional relation between tinnitus and cerebrovascular diseases can also be considered, as, based on a large case–control study performed in Taiwan, tinnitus has recently been identified as a risk factor or a clinical indicator of ischemic disease in young and middle-aged patients [7].

Pulsatile Tinnitus

PT due to a vascular cause can be generated by two possible pathophysiological mechanisms. First and most established, turbulent blood flow may generate a noise that, when close to the skull base or the inner ear, can be directly perceived by the auditory system. Examples of these are focal vascular stenosis or other conditions, leading to an increased local blood flow. In other instances, PT may be generated by the amplification of normal blood flow sounds at the skull base, what can occur as a consequence of inner ear changes, abnormal bone sound conduction, or loss of normal masking capacities [8, 9].

PT is perceived by an individual as pulsations or rhythmic variations in the tinnitus intensity synchronous with the heartbeat. PT can also be divided into subjective and objective.

Objective PT that is strongly associated with heartbeat is more likely caused by the turbulent blood flow inside the arteries or veins of the head or neck adjacent to the ear as well as on the surface or inside the head. This type of tinnitus can be described very differently by the patients but characteristically include a lower-pitched thumping or a booming sound. Objective pulsatile or rhythmic tinnitus can also be caused by respiration and be heard as a blowing sound coincidental with respiration. Tinnitus that sounds like a clicking rhythmic sound can be caused by muscle contractions in the head, such as those from muscles in the palate or in the middle ear [4, 8, 9].

Numerous causes of PT have been described in the literature, the frequency of which can vary broadly between individual reports. However, the most commonly identified causes of PT include atherosclerotic disease with arterial stenosis, vascular anatomical variants, benign intracranial hypertension, and vascular tumors of the skull base. A cause of PT can be identified in up to 70% of cases if a thorough study is performed. An underlying cause of PT is more likely to be found when the symptom is unilateral, compared to bilateral, and objective [9].

Vascular PT can in turn be divided into arterial, arteriovenous, or venous. However, not all forms of pulsatile tinnitus are of a vascular origin. Nonvascular cases include palatal, tensor tympani and stapedial myoclonus, chronic middle ear disease, dehiscent semicircular canal, patulous eustachian tube, or certain drugs. PT of a nonvascular origin is typically not synchronous with the heartbeat.

Patients with heart-synchronous PT require a thorough neurovascular evaluation to identify the cause of their tinnitus. Vascular imaging techniques must be employed to determine the origin and site of the lesion (see Chap. 30). Anyway, there are many forms of PT in which no identifiable cause can be detected (idiopathic PT). This can be caused by failure to properly interpret imaging studies or by missing trouble spots that may be either tangled in other structures or hidden by bones or other tissues. A clinical interview is crucial to identify this type of tinnitus. Many published studies describe different methods for treating objective tinnitus, but treatment will logically vary according to its origin [9, 10].

Objective Arterial Pulsatile Tinnitus: Differential Diagnosis

Many different pathologies of the cerebrovascular system have been reported as the cause of PT. Some are listed below.

Arteriosclerotic Disease

Stenoses of the carotid or the subclavian arteries are typical causes of PT, ipsilateral or contralateral to the side of tinnitus. Often, the intensity or the appearance of tinnitus is not related to the degree of stenosis [11]. Arteriosclerotic plaques are one of the most common causes of arterial stenosis in the head and neck and should be considered in elderly patients, particularly in those with vascular risk factors. Tinnitus may be generated from turbulent blood flow at the site of stenosis or, conversely, from compensatory increased blood flow in a cervical artery secondary to arteriosclerotic occlusion of another vessel. Tinnitus may occur because of stenosis located in any segment of the internal carotid artery (ICA), from the carotid bifurcation to the intracranial carotid siphon, and from stenosis involving the subclavian or vertebrobasilar system. Doppler ultrasonography (US) is a useful technique to identify these potential causes of pulsatile tinnitus. More advanced imaging techniques like magnetic resonance angiography (MRA) should be performed to evaluate the complete arterial system. If the stenosis of the cervical artery is causing neurological symptoms, then endarterectomy or angioplasty with stenting may be indicated. Even if such interventions can also relieve tinnitus [12, 13], the indication for the interventions is typically not the tinnitus but the reduction of the risk for thromboembolic brain lesions.

Arterial Dissection

PT rarely occurs together with cervicocephalic arterial dissection. A dissection consists of a tear in the intima of an artery, which allows blood to dissect into the vessel wall. Dissections can be either traumatic or spontaneous and commonly involve the cervical ICAs and distal intracranial vertebral arteries [14]. A minority of patients presenting with a cervical arterial dissection may have an underlying connective tissue disorder, which predisposes to intimal tearing. Acute dissections may produce PT by generating turbulent blood flow, either secondary to vessel narrowing from the mural hematoma or from the formation of a dissecting pseudoaneurysm [15]. In arterial dissection, tinnitus may occur together with ischemia, caused by carotid stenosis or by distal embolization of thrombotic material; other possible associated signs and symptoms include Horner's syndrome, neck and facial pain, and subarachnoid hemorrhage when the dissection reaches intracranial segments of the artery. Dissection of the vertebral artery may cause vertigo and other signs and symptoms if ischemia is produced in distal arterial territories. Angiography is essential if there is a high degree of suspicion of such pathologies, and delay in diagnosis should be avoided. Treatment of cervical arterial dissections is focused on preventing artery-to-artery embolism secondary to thrombus formation at the site of injury, with antiplatelet or anticoagulant therapy. Unless there are no conclusive data in the literature to recommend the use of anticoagulation over antiplatelet therapy, anticoagulation is usually preferred, especially when an associated intraluminal thrombus is detected under imaging techniques. If a significant arterial stenosis associated with the dissection remains, then stenting can be offered to maintain patency of the vessel [16].

Aberrant Internal Carotid Artery and Other Morphological Abnormalities

Anatomical variants involving arteries at the skull base are another potential source of PT. ICA morphological abnormalities that can present with PT are mainly tortuosities (having many turns and twists) and coiling of the artery. A common condition found is an aberrant ICA that appears to deviate from its normal anteromedial course through the petrous carotid canal to extend laterally into the middle ear. This variant is believed to arise when the cervical portion of the ICA fails to develop normally or regresses, giving place to two embryonic vessels, namely, the inferior tympanic and the caroticotympanic arteries, thus reconstituting the ICA at the level of the missing segment. Thus, an aberrant ICA follows a similar course of the inferior tympanic artery and should be identified before any middle ear surgery, as, during an otologic examination, it can appear as a vascular pulsatile structure located behind the tympanic membrane and should not be manipulated so as to prevent the catastrophic consequences of an inadvertent biopsy [17, 18].

Fibromuscular Dysplasia of the Cervical Arteries

Fibromuscular dysplasia is a segmental, non-atheromatous vasculopathy affecting medium-sized arteries, which typically, but not exclusively, affects middle-aged women. This condition typically involves the renal and cervical arteries. These vessels often display a characteristic beaded appearance with multifocal irregularities derived from abnormal sequential vessel dilatation and narrowing. Then, PT often occurs in the context of arterial stenosis and secondary turbulent blood flow [19]. Although most of the cases of fibromuscular dysplasia are asymptomatic, some patients may experience PT, headache, vertigo, transient ischemic attack, and stroke. These patients usually have a good prognosis and can be either not treated or treated with antiplatelet therapy. Only in case of symptomatic stenosis or stroke recurrence is there an indication for more aggressive treatment with angioplasty plus stenting or anticoagulation [20, 21].

Arteriovenous Fistulas (AVFs)

Tinnitus is a common symptom in individuals with intracranial arteriovenous fistulas (AVFs) (see Fig. 36.1) [22]. The occurrence of tinnitus is related to the location of the fistula and the location of the arteries feeding the fistula. Moreover, the tinnitus depends on the size of the lesion and the degree

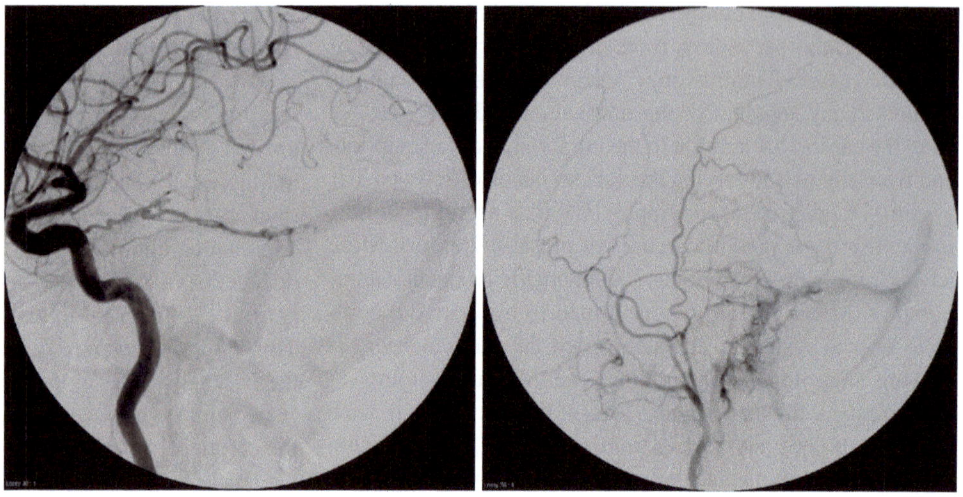

Fig. 36.1 A dural arteriovenous fistula with feeding arteries arising from the internal carotid artery (ICA) (left) and, as numerous tiny connections, from the external carotid artery (ECA) (right) draining into the sigmoid sinus

of the associated arteriovenous shunting. Dural arteriovenous fistulas (DAVFs) arising in the region of the transverse and sigmoid sinuses are a typical cause of vascular PT, whereas other vascular malformations like direct carotid-cavernous fistulas are less frequently involved [23]. DAVFs represent 10% of intracranial vascular malformations and are believed to be acquired lesions. DAVFs can produce intolerable PT, but the most important fact is that an accurate and prompt diagnosis is needed due to the increased risk of rupture and intracranial hemorrhage with possible fatal consequences. MRA can help identify a DAVF, but the gold-standard technique to characterize DAVF is a complete catheter angiography. Once a DAVF is diagnosed, a multidisciplinary approach is needed to determine the best treatment: surgical, endovascular, or stereotactic radiosurgery that is either applied alone or in combination [24–26].

Aneurysms

Cerebral aneurysms are rarely a cause of PT, but petrous carotid aneurysms and other intracranial aneurysms that cause tinnitus represent serious conditions (see Fig. 36.2). PT may be a symptom of compression when the aneurysm is located near auditory structures. Hemorrhage secondary to an aneurysm rupture can produce tinnitus as an acute symptom additionally to other serious symptoms directly related to the subarachnoid hemorrhage [27–29].

Vertebrobasilar and Carotid Dolichoectasia

Dolichoectasia is an angiopathy characterized by dilatation, elongation, and tortuosity of the brain arteries. Most frequently, the vertebral and basilar arteries are involved, whereas involvement of both the vertebrobasilar and carotid systems is rare [30, 31]. Magnetic resonance angiography (MRA) imaging or computed tomography angiography (CTA) can show the characteristic tortuosity of these arteries and even occasionally confirm a local compression of the cranial portion of the vestibulocochlear nerve [32].

Persistent Trigeminal Arteries

Persistent trigeminal arteries are rare and represent a remnant of the fetal carotid–basilar circulation. They typically extend from the internal carotid artery to the basilar artery. In rare instances, a persistent trigeminal artery is associated with a carotid-cavernous fistula. Patients with this condition may have PT in addition to other symptoms such as proptosis, eye pain, conjunctival injection, diplopia, and decreased visual acuity [33].

Subclavian Steal Syndrome

This syndrome is characterized by a subclavian artery stenosis located proximal to the origin of the vertebral artery. In this case, the subclavian artery steals blood from the vertebral artery that reverses its flow to supply the arm during exertion, resulting in vertebrobasilar insufficiency. As the vertebrobasilar arterial system feeds both the peripheral and central auditory and vestibular systems, symptoms such as dizziness, recurrent vertigo, hearing loss, and tinnitus may occur in the subclavian steal syndrome [34].

Internal Auditory Canal Vascular Loops

A vascular loop entering the internal auditory meatus can cause PT. Normally, the wall of the internal auditory meatus prevents vibrations of an artery from reaching the cochlea, but structural changes in the internal acoustic meatus or the

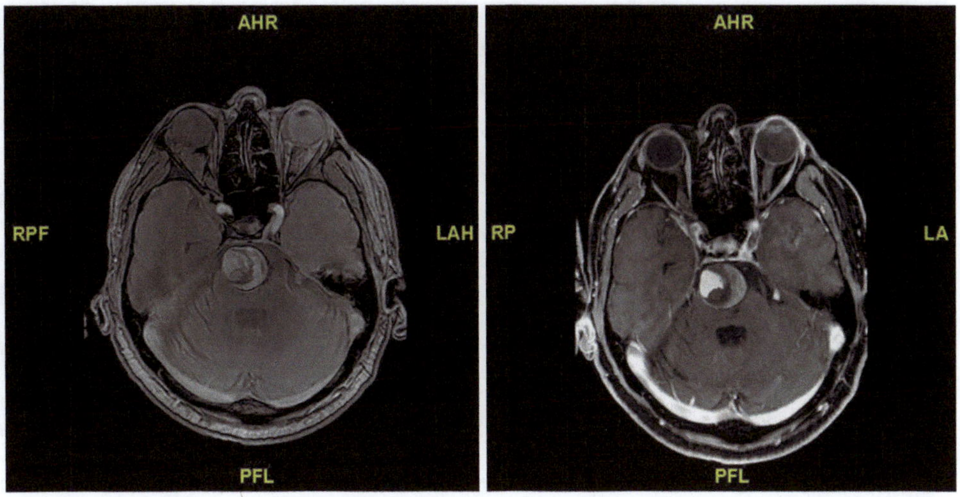

Fig. 36.2 Magnetic resonance imaging (MRI). Three-dimensional time-of-flight (3D-TOF) (left) and gadolinium (Gd)-enhanced T1 (right) sequences of a partially thrombosed giant basilar artery aneurysm with compressive effect on the brain stem and a close anatomical relation with the right auditory canal

pericarotid area can cause tinnitus. De Ridder et al. reported results of surgical insulation of the carotid artery in four patients, interpositioning a Teflon felt between the arterial loop and the cochlea, preventing arterial pulsations to be transmitted to the bone by a dampening effect of the pericarotid venous plexus, and eliminating this form of tinnitus in three of them [17].

The Proatlantal Intersegmental Artery

Primitive carotid–vertebral and carotid–basilar anastomoses are formed early during human embryogenesis at approximately 24 days. From cephalic to caudal direction, these anastomoses are cranial extensions of the primitive internal carotid, trigeminal, otic, hypoglossal, and proatlantal intersegmental arteries. The proatlantal intersegmental artery maintains the posterior circulation until the vertebral arteries are fully developed, between the seventh and eighth gestational weeks. Normal and abnormal morphofunctional aspects of the prenatal and postnatal forms of the proatlantal intersegmental artery have been described. When the proatlantal intersegmental artery fails to obliterate, it can produce symptoms affecting the function of the vertebrobasilar structures, such as hearing loss, tinnitus, and dizziness. In some individuals, these arteries do not present noticeable symptoms and are only found incidentally [35, 36].

Brainstem Telangiectasias

Unless not strictly arterial, here, we will discuss capillary telangiectasia, a dilation of small or terminal vessels, often found incidentally on magnetic resonance imaging due to its usual asymptomatic nature. Unless there is little evidence that such a lesion is responsible for any symptoms at all, it has occasionally been associated with minor neurological symptoms. In some reports, telangiectasia has been related to tinnitus and sensorineural hearing loss [37]. In such individuals, the auditory brainstem responses (ABRs) may show abnormalities regarding waves III and IV. Another possible sign is an asymmetry in optokinetic nystagmus that can be present in some individuals [38]. However, in most cases, the causal relationship is doubtful.

Objective Venous Pulsatile Tinnitus: Differential Diagnosis

Glomus Jugulare Tumors

Glomus jugulare tumors are benign and slow-growing lesions that can be locally aggressive because of their proximity to the lower cranial nerves and major vascular structures (see Fig. 36.3). These lesions are known causes of pulsatile tinnitus and other symptoms by their compression of the nerves at the skull base. Surgical resection is often difficult, and the possibilities of radiosurgery alone are limited. An individualized approach and experienced multidisciplinary teams are recommended. A combination of surgery, endovascular treatment, and gamma knife surgery has shown good results in some reports [39].

High Jugular Bulbs

A jugular bulb is normally surrounded by a bony layer in the jugular fossa. It is considered a high jugular bulb (HJB) when it is anatomically above the inferior surface of the bonny annulus, extending into the middle ear or located above the basal turn of the cochlea. The HJB is a frequent cause of objective pulsatile tinnitus. It may be dehiscent or

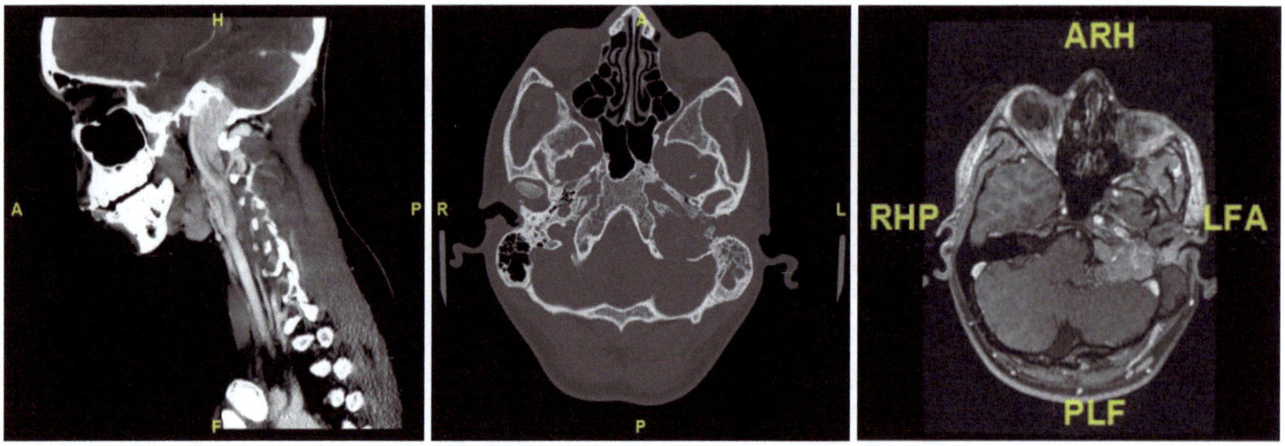

Fig. 36.3 A large left glomus jugulare occupying the left jugular foramen, eroding the petrous portion of the temporal bone and extending to the external auditory canal

aberrant. Techniques using endovascular management and surgery using ligation and embolization have been described to relieve this abnormality [40].

The Sigmoid or Jugular Diverticulum

Jugular bulb diverticulum is a rare condition. It has been reported that unilateral auditory symptoms may accompany this disorder, although it is more frequently asymptomatic. Some individuals with this condition are referred to clinics of neuro-otology with symptoms of unilateral sensorineural hearing loss and tinnitus. Tomographic venography is a useful tool to diagnose the condition [41]. Different endovascular techniques have been proposed as a possible effective therapeutic approach in selected patients [42, 43].

Condylar Vein Abnormalities

One of the most important venous foramina of the human skull is the condylar canal. This structure is described as the most stable and permanent venous emissary, with a prevalence of nearly 100%. It has been reported that patients with a dural arteriovenous fistula to the anterior condylar vein may show symptoms related to an unusual venous drainage. Pulsatile tinnitus may be the symptom of alarm for abnormalities of the jugular venous system [44].

Venous Angioma of the Posterior Fossa

A venous angioma can cause tinnitus by affecting the auditory pathway and the structures of the inner ear, similar to brainstem telangiectasias and other vascular malformations of the brainstem and other posterior fossa locations [32].

Sinus Thrombosis

Dural and deep sinus system thrombosis commonly present with headache and a variety of neurological symptoms that will depend on the location and the extension of the thrombosis and the surrounding edema or infarct. Dural sinus thrombosis may cause tinnitus accompanied with headache in some individuals, more commonly if the course is subacute. In sigmoid sinus thrombosis, the complaint is commonly unilateral, including head pain with ipsilateral PT [45].

Cerebrovascular Diseases with Subjective Tinnitus

Some cerebrovascular disorders can cause PT by affecting the auditory system at different levels. For example, a brain ischemic infarct involving the interior colliculus can produce acute or subacute tinnitus and even chronic subjective non-pulsatile tinnitus as a sequela, by its effect on the auditory pathway [46, 47]. However, cerebral ischemia or cerebral bleeding is an extremely rare cause of tinnitus. Whether ischemic lesions of the cochlea may contribute to the development of some forms of sudden hearing loss and subsequent tinnitus is still a matter of debate [48].

Interestingly, ischemic brain lesions can also suppress tinnitus. It has been reported that in a patient with tinnitus and Parkinson's disease, a lesion at the junction of the head and body of the caudate nucleus silenced bilateral tinnitus. Based on this observation, this area has been proposed as a target for deep brain stimulation for the treatment of tinnitus [49] (see also Chap. 53).

References

1. Moller AR. Pathophysiology of tinnitus. In: Sismanis A, editor. Otolaryngologic clinics of North America. Amsterdam: WB Saunders; 2003. p. 249–66.
2. Moller AR. Different forms of tinnitus. In: Chapter 2, textbook of tinnitus. New York, NY: Springer Link; 2011.
3. Shulman A, Goldstein B, Strashun AM. Central nervous system neurodegeneration and tinnitus: a clinical experience part II: translational neurovascular theory of neurodegenerative CNS disease and tinnitus. Int Tinnitus J. 2008;14(1):43–51.
4. Liess BD, Lollar KW, Christiansen SG, Vaslow D. Pulsatile tinnitus: a harbinger of a greater ill? Head Neck. 2009;31(2):269–73.
5. Hofmann E, Behr R, Neumann-Haefelin T, Schwager K. Pulsatile tinnitus: imaging and differential diagnosis. Dtsch Arztebl Int. 2013;110(26):451–8.
6. Lockwood AH, Salvi RJ, Burkard RF. Tinnitus. N Engl J Med. 2002;347(12):904–10.
7. Huang Y-S, Koo M, Chen J-C, Hwang J-H. The association between tinnitus and the risk of ischemic cerebrovascular disease in young and middle-aged patients: a secondary case-control analysis of a nationwide, population based health claim database. PLoS One. 2017;12(11):e0187474.
8. Sismanis A. Pulsatile tinnitus: contemporary assessment and management. Curr Opin Otolaryngol Head Neck Surg. 2011;19:348–57.
9. Miller TR, Serulle Y, Gandhi D. Arterial abnormalities leading to tinnitus. Neuroimaging Clin N Am. 2016;26(2):227–36.
10. Vattoh S, Shah R, Cure JK. A compartment-based approach for the imaging evaluation in tinnitus. AJNR Am J Neuroradiol. 2010;31(2):211–8.
11. Daneshi A, Hadizadeh H, Mahmoudian S, Sahebjam S, Jalesi A. Pulsatile tinnitus and carotid artery atherosclerosis. Int Tinnitus J. 2004;10(2):161–4.
12. Kirkby-Bott J, Gibbs HH. Carotid endarterectomy relieves pulsatile tinnitus associated with severe ipsilateral carotid stenosis. Eur J Vasc Endovasc Surg. 2004;27(6):651–3.
13. Sonmez G, Basekim CC, Ozturk E, Gungor A, Kizilkaya E. Imaging of pulsatile tinnitus: a review of 74 patients. Clin Imaging. 2007;31(2):102–8.
14. Pelkonen O, Tikkakoski T, Luotonen J, Sotaniemi K. Pulsatile tinnitus as a symptom of cervicocephalic arterial dissection. J Laryngol Otol. 2004;118(3):193–8.
15. Debette S, Leys D. Cervical-artery dissections: predisposing factors, diagnosis, and outcome. Lancet Neurol. 2009;8(7):668–78.
16. Cervical Artery Dissection in Stroke Study Trial Investigators. Antiplatelet therapy vs anticoagulation in cervical artery dissection: rationale and design of the cervical artery dissection in stroke study (CADISS). Int J Stroke. 2007;2(4):292–6.
17. De Ridder D, De Ridder L, Nowé V, Thierens H, Van De Heyning P, Moller A. Pulsatile tinnitus and the intrameatal vascular loop: why do we not hear our carotids? Neurosurgery. 2005;57(6):1213–7.
18. Chadha NK, Weiner GM. Vascular loops causing otological symptoms: a systematic review and meta-analysis. Clin Otolaryngol. 2008;33(1):5–11.
19. Foyt D, Carfrae MJ, Rapoport R. Fibromuscular displasia of the internal carotid artery causing pulsatile tinnitus. Otolaryngol Head Neck Surg. 2006;134(4):701–2.
20. Olin JW, Pierce M. Contemporary management of fibromuscular dysplasia. Curr Opin Cardiol. 2008;23(6):527–36.
21. Raj RK, Gandhi RT, Katzen BT. Fibromuscular displasia-related carotid pseudoaneurysm and pulsatile tinnitus. J Vasc Interv Radiol. 2012;23(12):1657.
22. Yeh SJ, Tsai LK, Jeng JS. Clinical and carotid ultrasonographic features of intracranial dural arteriovenous fistulas in patients with and without pulsatile tinnitus. J Neuroimaging. 2009;20:354.
23. Gandhi D, Chen J, Pearl M, et al. Intracranial dural arteriovenous fistulas: classification, imaging findings, and treatment. AJNR Am J Neuroradiol. 2012;33(6):1007–13.
24. Mehall CJ, Willner HI, LaRouere MJ. Pulsatile tinnitus associated with laterally placed sigmoid sinus. AJNR Am J Neuroradiol. 1995;16(4Suppl):905–7.
25. Noguchi K, Melhem ER, Kanazawa T, et al. Intracranial dural arteriovenous fistulas: evaluation with combined 3D time-of-flight MR angiography and MR angiography and MR digital substraction angiography. AJR Am J Roentgenol. 2004;182(1):183–90.
26. Jozef C. Carotid-cavernous fistula from the perspective of an ophtalmologist. A Review. Cesk Slov Oftalmol. 2020;1:1–8.
27. Depauw P, Caekebeke J, Vanhoenacker P. Objective pulsatile tinnitus caused by intrapetrous dissecting aneurysms. Clin Neurol Neurosurg. 2001;103(3):197–9.
28. Moonis G, Hwang CJ, Ahmed T, Weigele JB, Hurst RW. Otologic manifestations of petrous carotid aneurysms. AJNR Am J Neuroradiol. 2005;26(6):1324–7.
29. Austin JR, Maceri DR. Anterior communicating artery aneurysm presenting as pulsatile tinnitus. ORL J Otorhinolaryngol Relat Spec. 1993;55(1):54–7.
30. Titlic M, Tonkic A, Jukic I, Buca A, Kolic K, Batinic T. Tinnitus caused by vertebrobasilar dolichoectasia. Bratisl Lek Listy. 2007;108(10–11):455–7.
31. Herraiz C, Aparicio JM. Diagnostic clues in pulsatile tinnitus. Acta Otorrinolaringol Esp. 2007;58:426–33.
32. Kang M, Escott E. Imaging of tinnitus. Otolaryngol Clin N Am. 2008;41:179–93.
33. Ali S, Radaiedeh MM, Shaibani A, Russell EJ, Walker MT. Persistent trigeminal artery terminating in the posterior inferior cerebellar artery: case report. Neurosurgery. 2008;62(3):E746–8.
34. Psillas G, Kekes G, Constantidis J, Triaridis S, Vital V. Subclavian steal síndrome: neurotological manifestations. Acta Otorhinolaryngol Ital. 2007;27(1):33–7.
35. Vasovic L, Arsic S, Vlajkovic S, Jovanovic I, Jovanovic P, Ugrenovic P, Ugrenovic S, Andjelovic Z. Otic artery: a review of normal and pathological features. Med Sci Monit. 2010;16(5):RA101–9.
36. Li TH, Lan MY, Liu JS, Tseng YL, Wu HS, Chang YY. Type II proatlantal intersegmental artery associated with objective pulsatile tinnitus. Neurology. 2008;71(4):295–6.
37. De Carpentier J, Lynch N, Fisher A, et al. MR imaged neurovascular relationships at the cerebellopontine angle. Clin Otolryngol Allied Sci. 1996;21(4):312–6.
38. Scaglione C, Salvi F, Riguzzi P, Vergelli M, Tassinari CA, Mascalchi M. Symptomatic unruptured capillary telangiectasia of the brain stem: report of three cases and review of the literature. J Neurol Neurosurg Psychiatry. 2001;71(3):390–3.
39. Ramina R, Maniglia JJ, Ferrandes YB, Paschoal JR, Pfeilsticker LN, Neto MC, Borges G. Jugular foramen tumors: diagnosis and treatment. Neurosurg Focus. 2004;17(2):E5.
40. Yoon BN, Lee TH, Kong SK, Chon KM, Goh EK. Management of high jugular bulb with tinnitus transvenous stent-assisted coil embolization. Otolaryngol Head Neck Surg. 2008;139(5):740–1.
41. Bush ML, Jones RO, Given C. The value of CT venography in the diagnosis of jugular bulb diverticulum: a series of 3 cases. Ear Nose Throat J. 2009;88(4):E4–7.
42. Cuellar H, Maiti T, Patra DP, et al. Endovascular treatment of pulsatile tinnitus by sigmoid sinus aneurysm: technical note and review of the literature. World Neurosurg. 2018;113:238–43.
43. Drescher F, Maus V, Weber W, Fischer S. Pulsatile tinnitus due to an aneurysmatic diverticulum of the jugular bulb treated with the woven EndoBridge device. Interv Neuroradiol. 2020;26:235–8.
44. Raghuram K, Curé JK, Harnsberger HR. Condylar jugular diverticulum. J Comput Assist Tomogr. 2009;33(2):309–11.

45. Sigari F, Blair E, Redleaf M. Headache with unilateral pulsatile tinnitus in women can signal dural sinus thrombosis. Ann Otol Rhinol Laryngol. 2006;115(9):686–9.
46. Szirmai A. Cochleo vestibular dysfunction caused by cerebrovascular diseases. Int Tinnitus J. 2005;11(1):63–5.
47. Lee H. Sudden deaffness related to posterior circulation infarction in the territory of the nonanterior cerebellar artery: frequency, origin and vascular topographical pattern. Eur Neurol. 2008;59(6):302–6.
48. Lee H, Sohn SI, Jung DK, Cho YW, Lim JG, Yi SD, Lee SR, Sohn CH, Baloh RW. Sudden deafness and anterior inferior cerebellar artery infarction. Stroke. 2002;33:2807–12.
49. Larson PL, Cheung SW. A stroke of silence: tinnitus suppression following placement of a deep brain stimulation electrode with infarction in area. J Neurosurg. 2013;118:192–4.

Cervical and Masticatory Somatosensory System

37

Sarah Michiels and Tanit Ganz Sanchez

Abstract

Tinnitus can be influenced by altered somatosensory input from the cervical spine or temporomandibular area. Once this influence is diagnosed, treatment can be directed by a multidisciplinary team to the cervical spine, masticatory system, or dental area.

Several studies have been published more consistently about somatosensory tinnitus approaches. Most of them include techniques that are mainly applied by a physiotherapist, a chiropractor, or an osteopath because the rationale for using these techniques in such patients is to normalize the altered somatosensory input produced by increased muscle tension or restricted movement in the upper cervical spine or temporomandibular joint. Specific techniques may decrease muscle tension and increase mobility and stability, thus restoring somatosensory input and decreasing tinnitus perception.

The choice of specific techniques mostly depends on the dysfunction that is diagnosed in each patient. Therefore, somatosensory tinnitus management should be seen as a patient-centered therapy that should be tailored to the specific patient's needs.

In this chapter, we will discuss different approaches to treating somatosensory tinnitus, shedding light on the state of the art in treatments targeted at treating temporomandibular and cervical spine disorders.

S. Michiels (✉)
REVAL Rehabilitation Research Center, Faculty of Rehabilitation Sciences and Physiotherapy, Hasselt University, Diepenbeek, Belgium
e-mail: sarah.michiels@uhasselt.be

T. G. Sanchez
Otolaryngology Department, University of São Paulo Medical School, São Paulo, Brazil

W. Schlee et al. (eds.), *Textbook of Tinnitus*, https://doi.org/10.1007/978-3-031-35647-6_37

Graphical Abstract

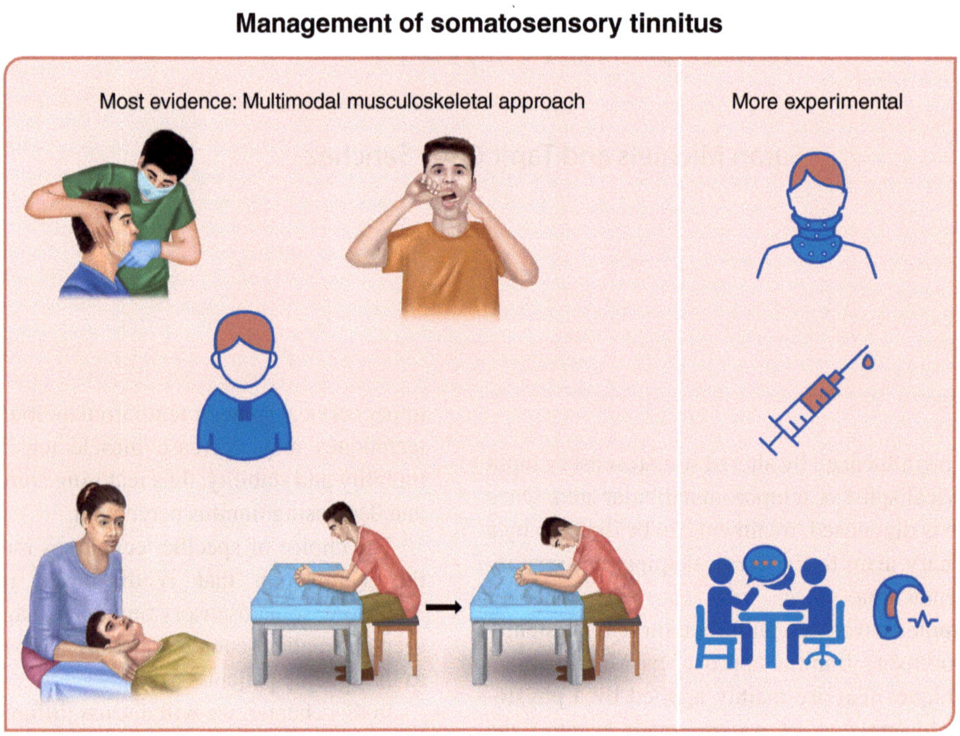

Highlights
- Patient-centered multimodal musculoskeletal treatment can decrease tinnitus severity and loudness.
- Other treatment options have been proposed but need further study.

Introduction

As discussed in Chap. 31, tinnitus can be influenced by altered somatosensory input from the cervical spine or temporomandibular area. Up to two-thirds of patients with tinnitus notice that their tinnitus is somehow influenced by stimuli that are not related to sounds, such as forceful muscle contractions of the head, neck, and limbs [1–3], pressure of myofascial trigger points (MTPs) [4], eye or orofacial movements [5–8], and cutaneous stimulation of the face and hands [5], among other stimuli. In these cases of so-called somatosensory tinnitus, the source of altered somatosensory input should be identified, so treatment can be directed to the cervical spine, masticatory system, or dental area. In the first edition of the *Textbook of Tinnitus* [9], a series of techniques have been suggested. The effectiveness of these techniques in tinnitus reduction, however, was mostly anecdotical, but, since then, several studies have been published on the topic. In this chapter, we will discuss the different approaches to treating somatosensory tinnitus, which have been studied since the previous publication of the *Textbook of Tinnitus* in 2011.

Musculoskeletal Treatment

Most somatosensory tinnitus approaches are based on techniques that are mainly applied by physiotherapists, chiropractors, or osteopaths, depending on regional differences. The main rationale for using these techniques in patients with somatosensory tinnitus is to normalize somatosensory input. In patients with somatosensory tinnitus, this somatosensory afference is often altered by increased muscle tension or restricted movement in the upper cervical spine or temporomandibular joint. Specific techniques are then used to decrease muscle tension and increase mobility and stability, so somatosensory afference will be restored and tinnitus perception might decrease.

The choice of specific techniques will largely depend on the dysfunction that is found in an individual patient. Therefore, somatosensory tinnitus management should be seen as a patient-centered therapy that should be tailored to the specific patient's needs.

State-of-the-Art Cervical Spine Treatment

For cervical spine treatment, clinical practice guidelines [10, 11] advise a combination of techniques to restore cervical spine function and reduce pain complaints. Primarily, counseling techniques are used to improve the patient's knowledge about his/her neck pain and to advise the patient toward good posture and movement habits. Additionally, exercises are recommended to improve the strength, coordination, and endurance of the stabilizing neck muscles, namely, the deep neck flexor muscles (the longus capitis and longus colli muscles) and the deep neck extensor muscles (the rectus capitis posterior minor and major and the obliquus inferior and superior muscles). Training these small muscles, which are located close to the vertebrae, will not only increase cervical spine stability but will also result in long-term reduction of excessive tension in the larger, more superficially located muscles (the upper trapezius, levator scapulae, and sternocleidomastoid muscles) that are often involved in somatosensory tinnitus.

In addition to the core content of counseling and exercises, other techniques can be added depending on the neck dysfunctions that are most prominent in an individual patient. As such, manual mobilizations or manipulations can be used to improve cervical spine mobility when needed. Other techniques, such as ischemic pressure or dry needling to deactivate myofascial trigger points,[1] can also be included in this approach, as long as they are used to support the effect of the core content.

Dry needling has the same goal of relaxing the trigger point but is a more invasive procedure. It involves multiple advances of a needle (mostly acupuncture needles are used) into the muscle at the region of the trigger point. Much like any injection technique, the physician should aim to elicit a local twitch response, reproduction of the patient's symptomatology, and relief of muscle tension [12].

[1]A myofascial trigger point is a hyperirritable spot, usually within a taut band of skeletal muscle, which is painful on compression and can give rise to characteristic referred pain, motor dysfunction, and autonomic phenomena [12]. One noninvasive way of treating these myofascial trigger points is the application of ischemic pressure. For this procedure, the therapist will first locate the trigger point and will then apply pressure to the point with increasing resistance and maintain this pressure until the therapist feels a relief of tension.

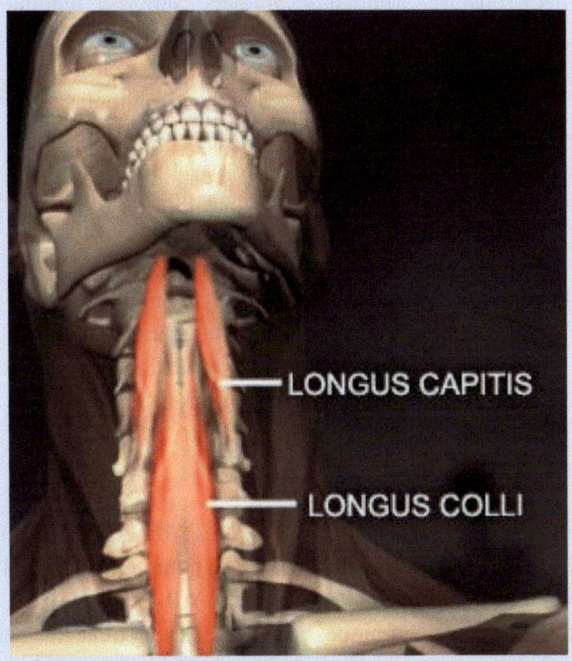

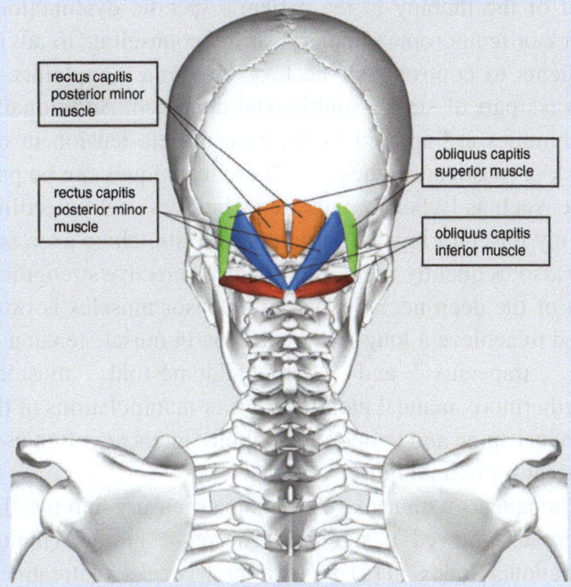

State-of-the-Art Temporomandibular Disorder Treatment

Based on the results of three systematic reviews [13–15], a combination of exercises and manual techniques is found to be effective in the treatment of temporomandibular disorders (TMDs). Exercises comprise passive and active stretching of the masticatory muscles and postural exercises to improve the head and neck posture. Manual techniques comprise manual mandibular traction or translation and myofascial release techniques of the masticatory muscles. Apart from local treatment of the temporomandibular area, adding cervical spine mobilizations and exercises is recommended when clinical investigations show additional dysfunctions in the cervical spine.

Apart from the combination of exercises and manual techniques, TMD treatment should also include counseling to address the underlying causes of TMD. Often advice on oral habits (bruxism, biting nails, chewing gum, etc.), stress reduction, and sleep hygiene will be added. In case of nighttime bruxism, occlusal splint therapy can be added.

In the previous years, five studies [16–20] were published that investigated such a "patient-centered multimodal musculoskeletal approach." All studies used a combination of techniques and exercises to treat the neck and jaw region according to the current state-of-the-art treatments as described above and tailored the exact content of the therapy to the patient's specific dysfunctions. Neck or temporomandibular disorder counseling, to advise patients to control their neck or jaw pain complaints, is always part of such a multimodal approach. Additionally, techniques are applied to decrease muscle tension in the neck or masticatory muscles. These techniques can be passive, such as ischemic pressure techniques or dry needling on myofascial trigger points, but active stretching exercises are also frequently used. Additionally, selective strengthening of the deep neck flexor and extensor muscles is often used to achieve a long-term reduction in muscle tension of the trapezius and sternocleidomastoid muscles. Furthermore, manual mobilizations or manipulations of the cervical spine and temporomandibular joints are often used to treat limited mobility.

In patients with neck-related somatosensory tinnitus, this approach showed a significant decrease in the Tinnitus Functional Index (TFI) score after 6 weeks of treatment ($p = 0.04$) [18] and a significant decrease in the visual analogue scale (VAS) score for tinnitus loudness ($p = 0.01$) after a maximum of 12 treatment sessions [19]. Patients who indicated a positive evolution after treatment on the global perceived effect scale showed an average decrease of 12 points on the TFI immediately after treatment and 17 points after follow-up [18]. Patients who did not perceive a positive evolution of their tinnitus showed an average increase of one point after treatment and two points after follow-up [18]. Additional analysis showed that patients whose tinnitus increased during episodes of neck pain or certain postures and patients with low-pitched tinnitus were more likely to benefit from this type of treatment [21].

In patients with primary temporomandibular disorders, the multimodal approach showed a significant and clinically relevant decrease of an average of 14 points in the TFI score after 9 weeks of treatment in 80 patients ($p < 0.001$) [20]. Similar results were found in 2 other studies, showing a significant decrease in VAS loudness (−13 points on average, $p < 0.001$), VAS annoyance (−15 points on average, $p < 0.001$), and Tinnitus Handicap Inventory (THI) (−15 points on average, $p < 0.001$) in 31 patients [16] and a significant decrease in VAS severity (average change: −2 points after treatment, −3 points after 3 months of follow-up, and −4 points after 6 months of follow-up, $p < 0.001$) in 61 patients [17].

Apart from the multimodal approach, specific musculoskeletal techniques have also been studied as single treatment options for somatosensory tinnitus [22–25].

Atan et al. [22] investigated the effect of Kinesio Tape application on the sternocleidomastoid, upper trapezius, and levator scapulae muscles in 15 patients with neck-related somatosensory tinnitus. Kinesio Tape is a type of elastic tape that is applied to decrease muscle tension or provide proprioceptive input. The use of this tape on all three muscles resulted in an average decrease in the THI score of 13.06 points ($p = 0.001$).

Three other studies used "myofascial trigger point deactivation" techniques as a way to decrease muscle tension. Rocha et al. [25] treated 37 patients with somatosensory tinnitus using ischemic pressure to deactivate the myofascial trigger points. They showed a significant decrease in THI and VAS annoyance after five sessions ($p < 0.001$).

Two other studies investigated dry needling, a technique that uses acupuncture needles for myofascial trigger point deactivation. Both studies showed good effects of dry needling on Numerical Rating Scale (NRS) scores for tinnitus severity [23], NRS for tinnitus loudness [26], and THI [26] in two cases of neck-related somatosensory tinnitus.

Finally, Wu et al. [24] showed a decrease of 44 points on the THI after "deep neck flexor exercises" in one case of neck-related somatosensory tinnitus.

Other Management Techniques

Apart from the studies on musculoskeletal management of somatosensory tinnitus, other techniques to normalize somatosensory afference have been investigated. Some of them have not been repeated in the literature, so the effect needs to be confirmed in larger controlled studies, before general use can be recommended.

Cervical Collars

One case study showed positive effects of intermittent cervical collar (individually adapted collars, Basko Healthcare Med Surg Innov Ltd., Lancaster, UK) application (15–30 min, 3–5 times a day), with complete tinnitus remission within 4 weeks [27]. This remission lasted for 5 months. Afterward, the tinnitus slightly resurged occasionally but disappeared again after short-term application of the cervical collar (15 min once every 2–4 weeks).

Injections

In 2005, one study reported the use of subcutaneous "botulinum toxin type A injections" around the ear for tinnitus treatment [28]. Botulinum toxin type A was subcutaneously injected into three sites around the ear: 1 cm above the superior aspect of the auricle, 1 cm behind the superior aspect of the auricle (2 o'clock position for the left ear and 10 o'clock position for the right ear), and 1 cm behind the inferior aspect of the auricle (5 o'clock position for the left ear and 7 o'clock position for the right ear), making certain to stay above the mastoid tip. This study showed a significant decrease in the average THI scores from baseline to 4 months after the injection in a group of 26 patients. No significant decrease was found in the group receiving a placebo injection. The authors indicated that further research was necessary to confirm these results. Unfortunately, no additional studies have been published on the topic in the meantime.

Another study, used a "cervical epidural steroid injection" to reduce tinnitus intensity to 75% in one patient [29]. This effect persisted for 5 weeks; thereafter, tinnitus intensity gradually increased again and returned to baseline after another 9 weeks.

In patients with temporomandibular disorders (TMDs) and tinnitus, one study showed positive results of lidocaine injections in the lateral pterygoid muscle [30]. On an average, 63% of their 39 participants experienced tinnitus relief 3–5 min after the injection, but the tinnitus returned after the anesthetics wore off [30].

Bimodal Stimulation Treatment (See Chap. 54)

Contrary to most techniques that have been suggested for the management of somatosensory tinnitus, Marks et al. [31] proposed a technique to influence the medullary connection between the auditory and somatosensory pathways in a more direct manner. The combination of auditory and electrical somatosensory stimulation showed a significant reduction in the TFI score in a group of 20 patients with unilateral pure-tone tinnitus that could be modulated by one or more somatic maneuvers. Additional studies are needed to confirm these results and to investigate the effect of this treatment in a less restricted sample of patients with somatosensory tinnitus.

Tinnitus Retraining Therapy (TRT)

Apart from the therapy options that are directed at normalizing somatosensory input or influencing the medullary auditory–somatosensory connection, one study investigated the effect of tinnitus retraining therapy (TRT) (see Chap. 47) in patients with somatosensory tinnitus [32]. Patients underwent a 3-month TRT protocol, including daily use of white noise generators with or without amplifications, combined with four structured counseling sessions. An average decrease in the THI score of 34.95 points was found ($p < 0.05$).

It must, however, be noted that patients were included in this study based on their ability to modulate their tinnitus by somatic maneuvers and the presence of facial dysesthesia. Patients with a diagnosis of temporomandibular disorders, however, were excluded from the study. This may raise questions about the diagnosis of somatosensory tinnitus in the patients included in this study. However, it remains interesting for future research to investigate whether patients with a clear somatosensory tinnitus diagnosis also react well to TRT treatment.

Is There a Cure?

Although we remain careful, we present a different perspective based on the fact that tinnitus patients want to be cured, but no randomized clinical trials with different approaches have shown this outcome yet. This specific point seems to favor many professionals worldwide to wrongfully believe that "there is nothing to do" or that "you have to learn to live with it." Considering these points, Sanchez et al. [33] published a systematic collection of 80 patients who reached a status of long-lasting total remission of tinnitus. By finding and interviewing ex-tinnitus sufferers who consider themselves cured, the authors selected subjects with any etiology of tinnitus that had been daily present for at least 3 months and has not been perceived anymore for at least the past 6 months, even in silence and paying attention to it [33].

Although it was not the aim of the study, we noticed that the total sample ($n = 80$) contains a small number of cases with somatosensory tinnitus ($n = 6$; 7.5%). This may reflect the fact that the majority of participants were referred to the research by otolaryngologists and audiologists. The duration of tinnitus ranged from 6 to 36 months, and the extent of total remission varied from 6 to 480 months when they entered the study.

Such patients attributed their total remission to physiotherapy, osteopathy, or chiropractic care ($n = 5$) and to cyclobenzaprine ($n = 1$), which is a centrally acting muscle relaxant with some evidence in the literature [34, 35] (see

Chap. 48). Further analysis has not revealed defined patterns for age, gender, localization, type of sound, or degree of annoyance when subjects with somatosensory tinnitus were compared to other etiologies of tinnitus of the total sample.

It is expected that this information does not have the same scientific strength as those generated by randomized clinical trials. However, it may point toward the fact that long-term total remission of tinnitus exists for patients with somatosensory tinnitus (among other etiologies) and that future clinical trials may be redirected to observe this so far unpredictable condition.

Multidisciplinary Treatment

Since the 1990s, scientists have described the possible influence of somatosensory input from the cervical spine and temporomandibular area on tinnitus complaints [8, 36]. In 1999, Levine first published a hypothesis for this tinnitus subtype, which he called somatic (or somatosensory) tinnitus (ST) [37]. In those early days, ST was described as a subtype of tinnitus. Through the years and with evolving knowledge, however, the idea of the existence of different tinnitus subtypes, based on their etiology, is increasingly being abandoned. Nowadays, tinnitus experts agree that in most patients, tinnitus has a multifactorial origin with a multitude of potential influencing factors [38–40]. In the light of this evolution, the treatment of somatosensory tinnitus should also include treatment of the other influencing factors of a patient's tinnitus. In the clinic, treatment of the cervical spine or temporomandibular disorders is often combined with psychological treatment to address excessive stress or anxiety, two factors that not only influence the tinnitus but also influence the neck and/or jaw dysfunction. In other patients, with severe hearing loss apart from a somatosensory influence on the tinnitus, it is also important to treat the hearing loss. This will lead to a more tailor-made approach for each patient.

Conclusions

Somatosensory tinnitus can be successfully treated using a variety of techniques. Currently, musculoskeletal treatment of the cervical spine and temporomandibular area has the highest level of evidence. Other techniques have been suggested but need further investigation in large randomized controlled trials (RCTs). Mostly, somatosensory tinnitus treatment shows a decrease in tinnitus severity or loudness, but, in rare cases, a total remission of the tinnitus is achieved. In individual clinical situations, it is important to keep in mind that the somatosensory influence is often only one of several influencing factors of a patient's tinnitus. As such, specific somatosensory tinnitus treatment should often be combined with, for instance, psychological or audiological treatment in a multidisciplinary approach.

A Case Report

A 55-year-old man was complaining of bilateral, nonpulsatile tinnitus for the past 12 months. The tinnitus started soon after a whiplash trauma in January 2020. Initially, the patient perceived a noise-like tinnitus, but, at the start of the treatment, it sounded more like a beep. At the first consult, the patient scored 60 points on the Tinnitus Functional Index (TFI) and 64/100 on the visual analogue scale for tinnitus loudness. Audiometry showed bilateral normal hearing. Neck complaints scored 20 points on the Neck Bournemouth Questionnaire (NBQ), indicating a substantial neck complaint. Signs of anxiety or depression were absent, based on the Hospital Anxiety and Depression scores. The patient also complained about some hyperacusis but remained just below the threshold of 28 points on the Hyperacusis Questionnaire. Specific somatosensory tinnitus questions showed that tinnitus and neck pain originated in the same time frame, immediately after the whiplash trauma. The patient was not sure whether the pain and tinnitus complaints increased and decreased simultaneously. Additionally, the patient is known to clench his teeth frequently, but no jaw pain was present. The patient's tinnitus could not be modulated during voluntary movements, pressure on myofascial trigger points or somatic maneuver testing. A clinical cervical spine examination showed normal mobility of the cervical spine but decreased extension mobility at the cervicothoracic junction. Muscle palpation showed increased tension in the upper trapezius, levator scapulae, and sternocleidomastoid muscles, including the presence of active myofascial trigger points. Strength and coordination testing of the deep neck flexor and extensor muscles and the shoulder-stabilizing muscles indicated decreased strength and coordination difficulties in all three muscle groups. These findings correspond to the patient's neck complaints during activities that require looking up (such as painting a ceiling) or activities in four-point kneeling (such as DIY tiling).

The following combination of treatment modalities was used:

- Extensive explanation about the abovementioned cervical spine dysfunctions and their influence on the patient's daily activities, combined with advice to temporarily adjust these daily activities to the current loadability of the cervical structures
- Extensive explanation on how the present cervical spine dysfunctions can influence the tinnitus and what can be expected during and after therapy

- Myofascial trigger point deactivation techniques of the upper trapezius, levator scapulae, and sternocleidomastoid muscles
- Progressive exercises to improve the strength and coordination of the deep neck flexor muscles (Figs. 37.1, 37.2, and 37.3)

The patient was treated by the musculoskeletal physiotherapist once a week and performed daily home exercises based on the abovementioned protocol. After the fifth treatment session, the patient indicated an improvement in both neck and tinnitus complaints on TFI and NBQ.

Results after treatment

After a 9-week physiotherapy program, including daily home exercises and a weekly in-clinic visit, the patient scored 45 points on the TFI (15 points decrease) and 10 points on the NBQ. Neck complaints had decreased to a level where the patient only perceived increased muscle tension and neck pain after high load activities. During these episodes, he noticed that his tinnitus also increases. In general, his tinnitus decreased to a level that did not constantly bother him anymore. It was agreed to extend the exercise program in order to further increase the coordination, strength, and endurance of his neck muscles using more challenging exercises adjusted to his high-load daily activities.

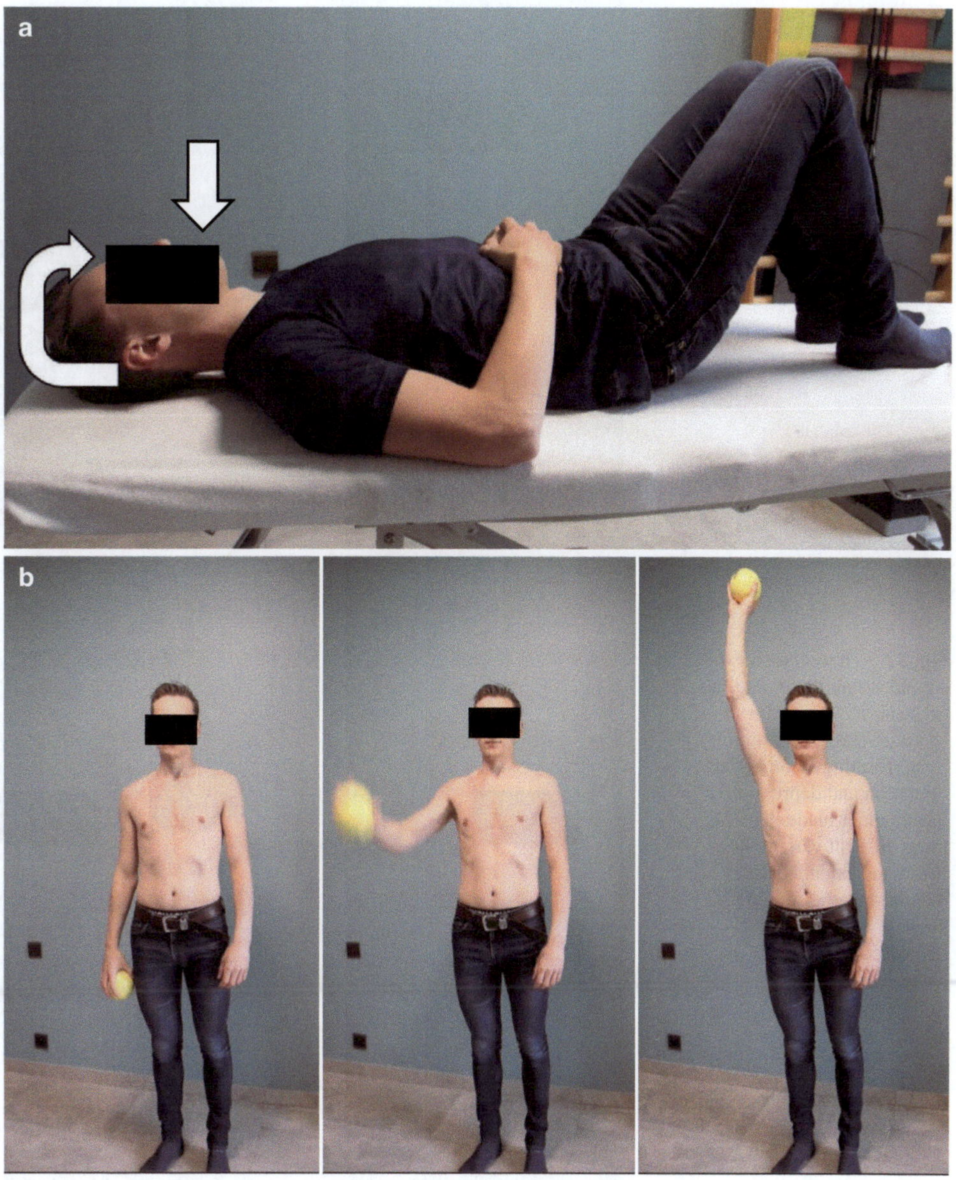

Fig. 37.1 Exercises for the deep neck flexor muscles. (**a**) Easiest exercise: activation of the deep neck flexors by performing a high cervical nodding movement without activation of the sternocleidomastoid muscles. (**b**) More functional exercise: lifting a weight while maintaining a slight high cervical flexion nod

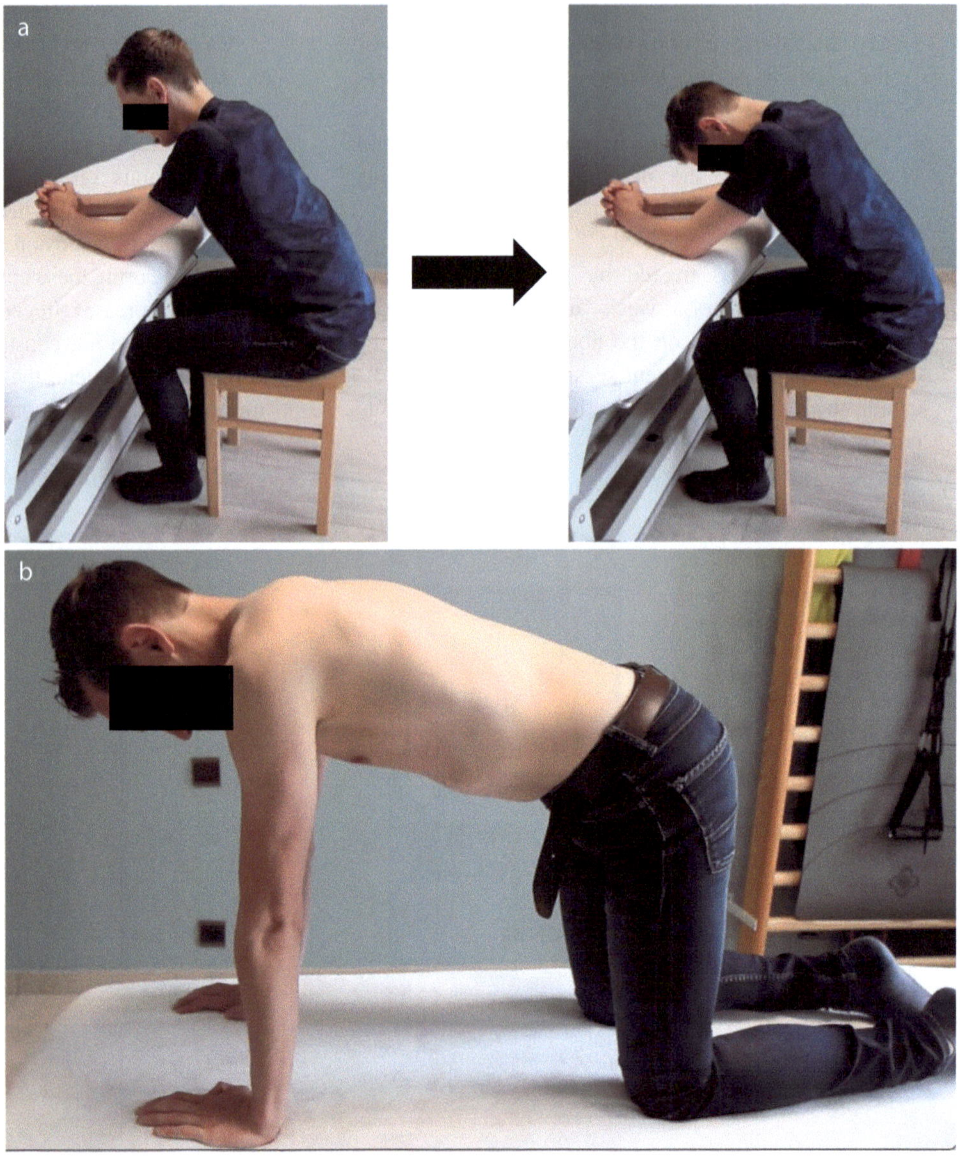

Fig. 37.2 Exercises for the deep neck extensor muscles. (**a**) Easiest exercise:, activation of the deep neck extensor muscles by performing a controlled flexion of the neck and afterward returning to the starting position. (**b**) The same exercise in a more challenging starting position

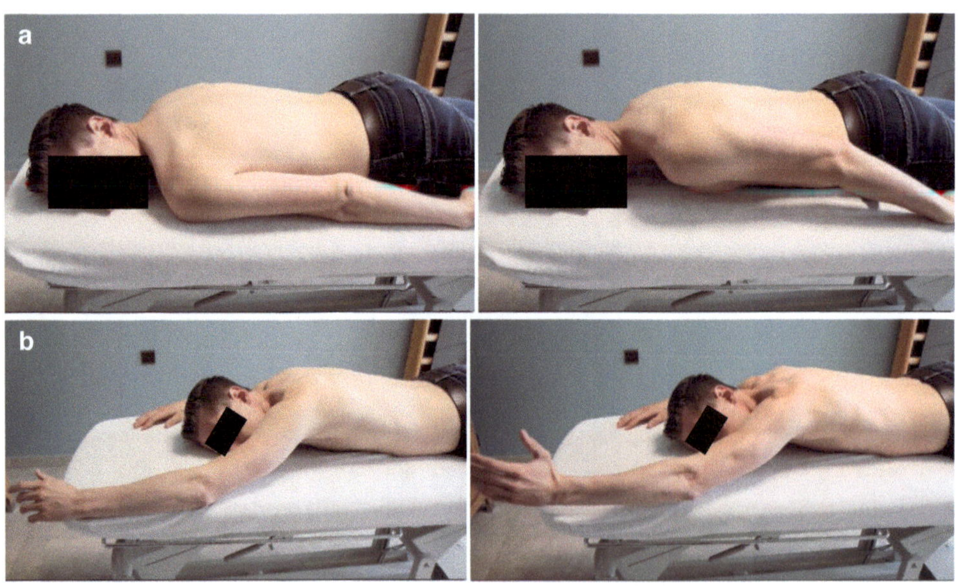

Fig. 37.3 Exercises for the shoulder-stabilizing muscles. (**a**) Easiest exercise for the shoulder-stabilizing muscles by performing a combined retraction and depression of the shoulder blade. (**b**) A more difficult variant, now lifting the extended arm while maintaining the shoulder blade in a retracted and depressed position

References

1. Abel MD, Levine RA. Muscle contractions and auditory perception in tinnitus patients and nonclinical subjects. Cranio. 2004;22(3):181–91.
2. Sanchez TG, Guerra GCY, Lorenzi MC, Brandao AL, Bento RF. The influence of voluntary muscle contractions upon the onset and modulation of tinnitus. Audiol Neurootol. 2002;7(6):370–5.
3. Sanchez TG, Da Silva LA, Brandão AL, Lorenzi MC, Bento RF. Somatic modulation of tinnitus: test reliability and results after repetitive muscle contraction training. Ann Otol Rhinol Laryngol. 2007;116(1):30–5.
4. Rocha C, Sanchez TG, de Siqueira JTT. Myofascial trigger point: a possible way of modulating tinnitus. Audiol Neurootol. 2008;13(3):153–60.
5. Cacace AT, Cousins JP, Parnes SM, Semenoff D, Holmes T, McFarland DJ, et al. Cutaneous-evoked tinnitus - I. Phenomenology, psychophysics and functional imaging. Audiol Neurootol. 1999;4(5):247–57.
6. Coad ML, Lockwood A, Salvi R, Burkard R. Characteristics of patients with gaze-evoked tinnitus. Otol Neurotol. 2001;22(5):650–4.
7. Sanchez TP. MRB Abolição de zumbido evocado pela movimentação ocular por meio de repetição do deslocamento do olhar: um método inovador. Arq Otorhinolaryngol. 2007;11:451–3.
8. Pinchoff RJ, Burkard RF, Salvi RJ, Coad ML, Lockwood AH. Modulation of tinnitus by voluntary jaw movements. Am J Otol. 1998;19(6):785–9.
9. Sanchez TG, Rocha B, Carina. Treatment of somatosensory tinnitus. In: Møller AR, Langguth B, Ridder D, Dirk KT, editors. Textbook of tinnitus. Berlin: Springer; 2011.
10. Cohen SP, Hooten WM. Advances in the diagnosis and management of neck pain. BMJ. 2017;358:j3221.
11. Cote P, Wong JJ, Sutton D, Shearer HM, Mior S, Randhawa K, et al. Management of neck pain and associated disorders: a clinical practice guideline from the Ontario Protocol for Traffic Injury Management (OPTIMa) Collaboration. Eur Spine J. 2016;25(7):2000–22.
12. Lavelle ED, Lavelle W, Smith HS. Myofascial trigger points. Med Clin North Am. 2007;91(2):229–39.
13. Martins WR, Blasczyk JC, Furlan A, de Oliveira M, Lagoa Goncalves KF, Bonini-Rocha AC, Dugailly PM, et al. Efficacy of musculoskeletal manual approach in the treatment of temporomandibular joint disorder: a systematic review with meta-analysis. Man Ther. 2016;21:10–7.
14. Armijo-Olivo S, Pitance L, Singh V, Neto F, Thie N, Michelotti A. Effectiveness of manual therapy and therapeutic exercise for temporomandibular disorders: systematic review and meta-analysis. Phys Ther. 2016;96(1):9–25.
15. Calixtre LB, Moreira RF, Franchini GH, Alburquerque-Sendin F, Oliveira AB. Manual therapy for the management of pain and limited range of motion in subjects with signs and symptoms of temporomandibular disorder: a systematic review of randomised controlled trials. J Oral Rehabil. 2015;42(11):847–61.
16. Côté C, Baril I, Morency C, Montminy S, Couture M, Leblond J, et al. Long-term effects of a multimodal physiotherapy program on the severity of somatosensory tinnitus and identification of clinical indicators predicting favorable outcomes of the program. J Am Acad Audiol. 2019;30(8):720–30.
17. Delgado de la Serna P, Plaza-Manzano G, Cleland J, Fernández-de-Las-Peñas C, Martín-Casas P, Díaz-Arribas MJ. Effects of cervico-mandibular manual therapy in patients with temporomandibular pain disorders and associated somatic tinnitus: a randomized clinical trial. Pain Med. 2020;21(3):613–24.
18. Michiels S, Van de Heyning P, Truijen S, Hallemans A, De Hertogh W. Does multi-modal cervical physical therapy improve tinnitus in patients with cervicogenic somatic tinnitus? Man Ther. 2016;26:125–31.
19. Oostendorp RA, Bakker I, Elvers H, Mikolajewska E, Michiels S, De Hertogh W, et al. Cervicogenic somatosensory tinnitus: an indication for manual therapy plus education? Part 2: a pilot study. Man Ther. 2016;23:106–13.
20. Van der Wal A, Michiels S, Van de Heyning P, Braem M, Visscher C, Topsakal V, et al. Treatment of somatosensory tinnitus: a randomized controlled trial studying the effect of orofacial treatment as part of a multidisciplinary program. J Clin Med. 2020;9(3):705.
21. Michiels S, Van de Heyning P, Truijen S, Hallemans A, De Hertogh W. Prognostic indicators for decrease in tinnitus severity after cervical physical therapy in patients with cervicogenic somatic tinnitus. Musculoskel Sci Pract. 2017;29:33–7.
22. Atan T, Atan D, Özel S. Effectiveness of kinesio taping in the treatment of somatosensory tinnitus: a randomized controlled trial. Complement Ther Clin Pract. 2020;39:101100.
23. Sajadi S, Forogh B, ZoghAli M. Cervical trigger point acupuncture for treatment of somatic tinnitus. J Acupunct Meridian Stud. 2019;12(6):197–200.
24. Wu D, Ham D, Rosedale R. Physiotherapy assessment and treatment of chronic subjective tinnitus using mechanical diagnosis and therapy: a case report. J Man Manip Ther. 2020;28(2):119–26.
25. Rocha CB, Sanchez TG. Efficacy of myofascial trigger point deactivation for tinnitus control. Braz J Otorhinolaryngol. 2012;78(6):21–6.
26. Womack A, Butts R, Dunning J. Dry needling as a novel intervention for cervicogenic somatosensory tinnitus: a case study. Physiother Theory Pract. 2020;38(9):1319–27.
27. Bechter K, Wieland M, Hamann GF. Chronic cervicogenic tinnitus rapidly resolved by intermittent use of cervical collar. Front Psychiatry. 2016;7:43.
28. Stidham KR, Solomon PH, Roberson JB. Evaluation of botulinum toxin A in treatment of tinnitus. Otolaryngol Head Neck Surg. 2005;132(6):883–9.
29. McCormick ZL, Walega DR. Cervical epidural steroid injection for refractory somatic tinnitus. Pain Pract. 2015;15(2):e28–33.
30. Bjorne A. Assessment of temporomandibular and cervical spine disorders in tinnitus patients. Prog Brain Res. 2007;166:215–9.
31. Marks KL, Martel DT, Wu C, Basura GJ, Roberts LE, Schvartz-Leyzac KC, et al. Auditory-somatosensory bimodal stimulation desynchronizes brain circuitry to reduce tinnitus in guinea pigs and humans. Sci Transl Med. 2018;10(422):eaal3175.
32. Ostermann K, Lurquin P, Horoi M, Cotton P, Herve V, Thill MP. Somatic tinnitus prevalence and treatment with tinnitus retraining therapy. B-ENT. 2016;12(1):59–65.
33. Sanchez TG, Valim CCA, Schlee W. Long-lasting total remission of tinnitus: a systematic collection of cases. Prog Brain Res. 2021;260:269–82.
34. Lobarinas E, Blair C, Spankovich C, Le Prell C. Partial to complete suppression of unilateral noise-induced tinnitus in rats after cyclobenzaprine treatment. J Assoc Res Otolaryngol. 2015;16(2):263–72.
35. Vanneste S, Figueiredo R, De Ridder D. Treatment of tinnitus with cyclobenzaprine: an open-label study. Int J Clin Pharmacol Ther. 2012;50(5):338–44.

36. Hiller W, Janca A, Burke KC. Association between tinnitus and somatoform disorders. J Psychosom Res. 1997;43(6):613–24.
37. Levine RA. Somatic (craniocervical) tinnitus and the dorsal cochlear nucleus hypothesis. Am J Otolaryngol. 1999;20(6):351–62.
38. Michiels S, Ganz Sanchez T, Oron Y, Gilles A, Haider HF, Erlandsson S, et al. Diagnostic criteria for somatosensory tinnitus: a delphi process and face-to-face meeting to establish consensus. Trends Hear. 2018;22:2331216518796403.
39. Van de Heyning P, Gilles A, Rabau S, Van Rompaey V. Subjective tinnitus assessment and treatment in clinical practice: the necessity of personalized medicine. Curr Opin Otolaryngol Head Neck Surg. 2015;23(5):369–75.
40. Cederroth CR, Gallus S, Hall DA, Kleinjung T, Langguth B, Maruotti A, et al. Editorial: towards an understanding of tinnitus heterogeneity. Front Aging Neurosci. 2019;11:53.

Trauma-Associated Tinnitus

38

Dirk De Ridder

Abstract

- Trauma-associated tinnitus can be both non-pulsatile and pulsatile.
- Trauma-associated non-pulsatile tinnitus can result from a trauma to the ear, neck, or head. Trauma to the ear includes temporal bone fracture, labyrinthine concussion, ossicular chain disruption (OChD), perilymphatic fistula, barotrauma, or noise trauma.
- Trauma-associated tinnitus is associated with more distress and depression.
- Trauma-associated pulsatile tinnitus is related to vascular lesions. Trauma-associated carotid dissection (CD), arteriovenous (AV) fistulas, or carotid-cavernous fistulas (CCFs) can cause pulsatile tinnitus.
- Trauma-associated stress disorder is associated with more severe tinnitus.
- The cause of trauma-associated non-pulsatile and pulsatile tinnitus may be a sign of a life-threatening disease, which may be treatable.

D. De Ridder (✉)
Section of Neurosurgery, Department of Surgical Sciences,
University of Otago, Dunedin, New Zealand
e-mail: dirk.deridder@otago.ac.nz

W. Schlee et al. (eds.), *Textbook of Tinnitus*, https://doi.org/10.1007/978-3-031-35647-6_38

Graphical Abstract

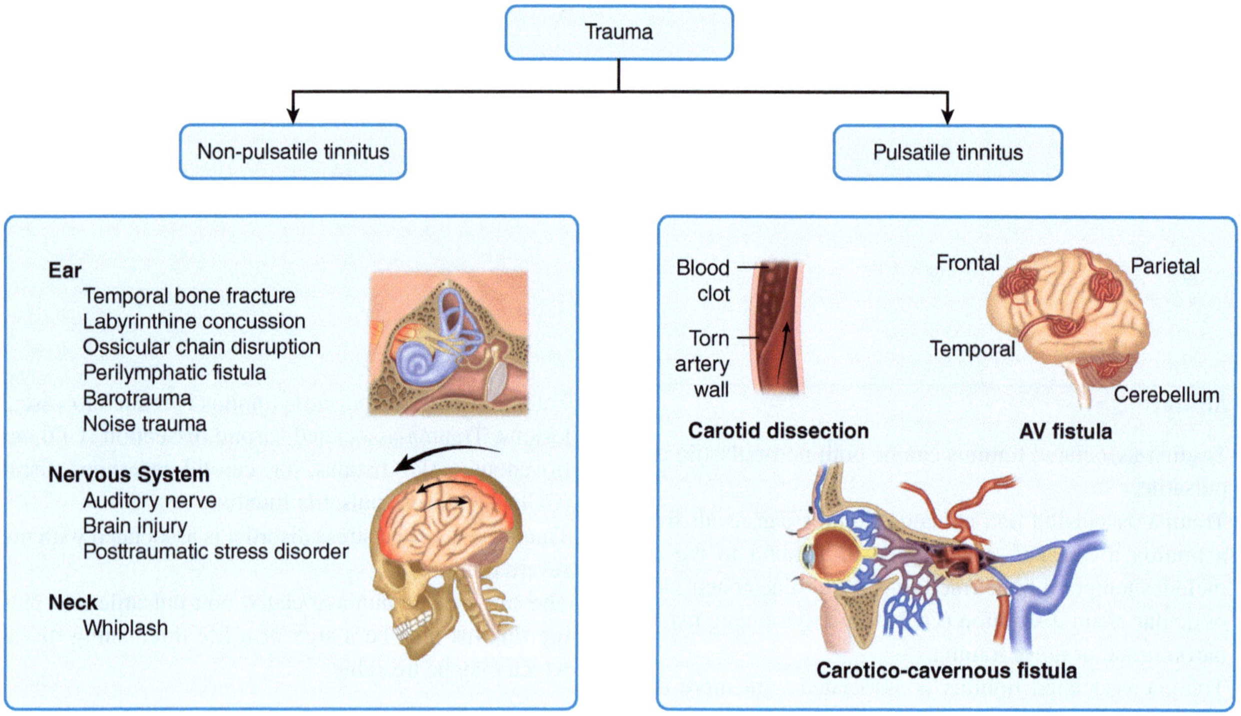

Abbreviations

AV	Arteriovenous
AVM	Arteriovenous malformation
CCF	Carotid-cavernous fistula
CD	Carotid dissection
CSF	Cerebrospinal fluid
MVC	Microvascular compression
OChD	Ossicular chain disruption
PTSD	Post-traumatic stress disorder
TBI	Traumatic brain injury

Introduction

Tinnitus often arises after or is associated with a trauma to the head, especially to the ear [1]. Mechanical, pressure-, noise-, or stress-related trauma can cause tinnitus. Trauma-associated tinnitus can be either non-pulsatile or pulsatile.

Noise-related trauma is the most common cause of tinnitus (and hearing loss). Louder noise results in more tinnitus [2]. In Germany and Belgium, exposure to leisure noise results in intermittent tinnitus among young adults in 60% and 68.5% of the cases, respectively [2, 3]. In addition, 89.5% of students exposed to loud music develop transient tinnitus [4].

Head [5] and neck injuries [6] are common causes of tinnitus [7, 8]. Tinnitus develops in up to 53% of individuals suffering from traumatic brain injuries (TBIs) and in up to 87% patients with hyperacusis (intolerance to sudden or loud noise) [8]. A total of 5–10% of patients presenting at specialized tinnitus centers describe that their tinnitus is associated with a trauma [7, 9].

Non-pulsatile tinnitus in head injuries can be due to injuries to the ear or the brain. Injuries to the ear may consist of petrous bone fractures, ossicular chain disruption (OChD) and perilymphatic fistulas, and barotraumas and noise trauma. Trauma-associated injuries to the auditory nerve and brain injuries can cause tinnitus as well. About 10–15% of whiplash injuries develop a whiplash syndrome consisting of persistent tinnitus combined with one or more of the following symptoms: headache, vertigo, instability, nausea, and hearing loss [10] (Table 38.1).

Patients suffering from trauma-associated tinnitus suffer from a higher mental burden than do tinnitus patients presenting with phantom perceptions based on other or unknown etiological factors, as trauma-associated tinnitus is associated with higher distress and depression levels, reflected by

Table 38.1 Causes of trauma-associated tinnitus

1. Non-pulsatile tinnitus
(a) Ear
• Temporal bone fracture
• Labyrinthine concussion
• Ossicular chain disruption
• Perilymphatic fistula
• Barotrauma
• Noise trauma
(b) Nervous system
• Auditory nerve
• Brain injury
(c) Trauma-associated stress disorder
(d) Neck
2. Pulsatile tinnitus
(a) Carotid dissection
(b) AV fistula
(c) Carotid-cavernous fistula

the higher scores in questionnaires such as the Tinnitus Questionnaire (TQ), the Tinnitus Handicap Inventory (THI), and Beck Depression Inventory (BDI) compared to tinnitus patients without trauma at tinnitus onset [9]. This is especially the case for patients with whiplash and head trauma [9]. Patients with trauma-associated noise-related tinnitus experience hyperacusis more frequently, are younger, have longer tinnitus duration, and are more frequently of the male gender [9].

Pulsatile Tinnitus

Trauma-associated pulsatile tinnitus can be the result of a carotid dissection (CD), arteriovenous (AV) fistulas, or carotid-cavernous fistulas (CCFs).

Carotid dissection (CD) Traumatic carotid dissections occur in approximately 1% of all individuals who have had blunt traumatic injury [11]. Pulsatile tinnitus is experienced in 16–27% of carotid dissections at the side of the dissection and can be the only symptom [12]. CD is asymptomatic in less than 10%, whereas more than 90% of individuals with CD develop carotid territory ischemia and/or local signs and symptoms on the side of dissection. Signs and symptoms from the side of dissection include head (65–68%), facial (34–53%), or neck pain (9–26%), Horner's syndrome[1] (28–41%), and cranial nerve palsy (8–16%), in particular of the hypoglossal nerve. The facial nerve may also be involved: dysgeusia[2] mainly results from the involvement of the chorda tympani (0.5–7.0%) or the glossopharyngeal nerve. A metal-like taste is typical for chorda tympani lesions. Transient paresis of the oculo motor (III, IV, and VI) nerves and the trigeminal nerve have been observed. In three-fourth of the carotid dissections, an ischemic event occurs, which includes ischemic stroke in 80–84%, transient ischemic attack in 15–16%, amaurosis fugax[3] in 3%, neuropathy in 4%, and retinal infarct in 1% [13].

Trauma-associated AV fistulas often result in an audible bruit, thus causing objective tinnitus or pulsatile (subjective tinnitus) tinnitus [14–16]. AV fistulas can develop after days, weeks, or even years [17]. The incidence at the middle meningeal artery in head injuries is 1.8% [15]. However, they can also occur along the superior sagittal sinus [16], the posterior auricular artery–internal jugular vein [14], the vertebral artery–vertebral plexus [17], the sigmoid and transverse sinuses [17], or even the scalp [17]. The middle meningeal artery fistula to the sphenoparietal sinus is often the result of linear fractures and most common in elderly people who have an adherent dura [15]. The sinus fistulas developing after trauma are often the result of a venous thrombosis [18–20], similar to the non-traumatic variant of AV fistulas. Treatment consists of embolization [18, 19] and, if this fails, surgical excision.

The most common trauma-associated fistulas are the carotid-cavernous fistulas (CCFs). They are divided in the more common high- and rare low-flow fistulas. In 3.8% of traumatic skull base fractures, a traumatic carotid-cavernous fistula is seen, especially in middle fossa fractures, where up to 8.3% develop a CCF [21]. These are characterized by pulsatile tinnitus, pulsating exophthalmia,[4] chemosis,[5] and visual deficit of the afflicted side [17]. The commonly used treatment is predominantly endovascular.

[1]Horner's syndrome: Ipsilateral myosis, ptosis, and facial anhydrosis; usually unilateral and due to an ipsilateral lesion of the cervical sympathetic chain or its central pathway; an ominous sign when it accompanies an ipsilateral traumatic brachial plexopathy because it usually indicates an avulsion of the C8 and T1 primary roots from the spinal cord. From Stedman's Electronic Medical Dictionary.

[2]Dysgeusia: Distortion or perversion in the perception of a tastant. An unpleasant perception may occur when a normally pleasant taste is present or the perception may occur when no tastant is present (gustatory hallucination). From Stedman's Electronic Medical Dictionary.

[3]Amaurosis fugax: A transient blindness that may result from a transient ischemia resulting from carotid artery insufficiency or retinal artery embolus or to centrifugal force (visual blackout in flight). From Stedman's Electronic Medical Dictionary.

[4]Exophthalmos: Protrusion of one or both eyeballs; can be congenital and familial, or due to pathology, such as a retroorbital tumor (usually unilateral) or thyroid disease (usually bilateral). From Stedman's Electronic Medical Dictionary.

[5]Chemosis: Edema of the bulbar conjunctiva, forming a swelling around the cornea. From Stedman's Electronic Medical Dictionary.

Non-pulsatile Trauma-Associated Tinnitus

Ear

Temporal Bone Fractures

In people who suffer a temporal bone fracture, 44% of patients present with balance problems, 56% with hypoacusis, 50–56% with tinnitus, and 15% with facial paralysis. In 75–80% of patients, the cochleovestibular sequelae are described as disabling [13, 22].

The common causes of temporal bone fractures are road accidents, falls, beatings, and gunshot wounds [23–25]. A total of 44% of temporal bone fractures occur after a motor vehicle accident [24]. Head trauma occurs in 75% of traffic accidents, and, in 5% of these, a petrous bone fracture is noted [26]. Of all head injuries hospitalized, 9% have a skull fracture and 2% of all these have temporal bone fractures [24]. Three kinds of fractures are noted after a substantial trauma to the temporal region: transverse, longitudinal, and mixed fractures. The most common fracture is the longitudinal fracture (82%) [23], characterized by visible laceration and fracture line of the external ear canal. A lateral impact to the head can cause tympanic membrane perforation or blood in the middle ear cavity with an ossicular chain disruption in about half of the patients [23]. Facial paralysis occurs in 3% [27]. Hearing loss is predominately conductive but may have a sensorineural component as well. Cerebrospinal fluid (CSF) leaks occur in 36% of patients with longitudinal temporal bone fractures [27].

Transverse fractures (11%) [23] resulting from an antero-posterior impact have a higher rate of sensorineural hearing loss (53%) [28], vertigo [28], and facial paralysis (63%) [23]. Tinnitus develops in 41% of transverse fractures [28]. CSF leaks occur in 25% of patients with transverse fractures [27]. Mixed fractures occur in 7% [23] of the traumata. Some head injuries can severely damage the auditory nerve, and can even sever the nerve, causing deafness and sometimes tinnitus.

Sometimes, a temporal bone fracture is associated with a labyrinthine concussion, even contralaterally [29].

Labyrinthine Concussion

Labyrinthine concussion may occur after less serious blows to the head [30], on the side of the trauma or sometimes on the opposite side [31]. Tinnitus, dizziness and vertigo, and high-frequency sensorineural hearing loss (4000–8000 Hz) are particularly common [32]. High frequencies are more vulnerable to trauma than are low frequencies, but recovery (32%) is obtained mainly in low frequencies [33]. In some individuals, onset may be delayed for several days [30]. Tinnitus improves in 39% of patients, but dizziness rarely improves [33]. Concomitant conductive hearing loss may occur from disruption of the ossicular chain or from bleeding into the middle ear cavity [32]. A blow to the mastoid or occiput may damage labyrinth membranes [30], causing the symptoms, as has been suggested by animal experiments [34, 35].

Ossicular Chain Disruption

Ossicular chain disruption (OChD) may occur without rupture of the eardrum or a temporal bone fracture and result in conductive hearing loss and tinnitus. Traffic accidents are the most common cause of OChD [36]. A total of 22% of the OChD cases are associated with a temporal bone fracture [36], and OChD occurs in 15% of temporal bone fractures [37]. There is often a long delay between the injury and treatment (an average of 5.7 years) [36]. The most common disruption is the incudostapedial joint followed by the incudomalleolar joint [23]. The stapes is the most commonly fractured followed by the malleus, with the incus almost never [23]. There is no literature available on tinnitus in trauma-associated ossicular chain disruption specifically, but any hearing loss may cause tinnitus because it activates neural plasticity. Treatment consists of ossicular chain reconstruction if symptoms persist after 2–3 months of recovery or disappearance of blood in the middle ear cavity.

Perilymphatic Fistulas

A perilymphatic fistula results from disruption of the membranes of the labyrinth most often at the round or oval window [30]. In half of the patients, barotraumas such as blowing the nose, lifting heavy goods, diving, and landing in an airplane are the cause [38]; in about 40%, a trauma is the cause [39].

The most prominent symptoms are tinnitus (61–76%), sudden or fluctuating hearing loss (83–93%), vertigo and dizziness (77–91%), and aural fullness (31%) [38, 40]. Subjective positive signs (i.e. vertigo and nystagmus induced by pressure changes in the external ear canal or with coughing or straining [30]) of the fistula are present in 71% of these patients [38], also known as Valsalva-induced vertigo.

Treatment consists of bed rest with the head elevated and prevention of straining. Analogous to cerebrospinal fluid leaks after lumbar punctures or intradural surgery, autologous intratympanic blood patches have been successfully performed to treat (presumed) perilymphatic fistulas [41]. Surgical packing of both cochlear windows with soft tissue grafts has also been carried out [30, 38–40]. If the symptoms persist, a ventriculoperitoneal shunt can be inserted [42, 43]. In general, vestibular symptoms show better improvement than do auditory symptoms [30, 38–40]. After surgical treatment, hearing recovers in 90%, a rapid disappearance of vertigo is noted in 89.9%, a loss of tinnitus in 45%, and, in 27%, an improvement is seen in tinnitus [44].

Barotraumas

A barotrauma to the ear may occur, for example, during descent from a high altitude or during ascent from underwater diving. Middle ear barotraumas are extremely common in commercial aircrew members, especially in those with repeated upper airway infections: 85% of Finish aircrew personnel have suffered from barotraumas, requiring medication or surgical treatments [45]. It is equally prevalent in commercial divers, with 81% of divers reporting a barotrauma that required treatment [45]. It is usually associated with sudden severe ear pain [30]. The cause is that the eustachian tube fails to equilibrate the pressure in the middle ear cavity to that of the increasing atmospheric pressures [46]. It causes inward displacement of the tympanic membrane, increased blood flow and swelling with fluid oozing into the middle ear cavity, sometimes even blood [30], which may lead to hearing loss and tinnitus [47]. In severe situations, it can cause rupture of the eardrum and ossicular chain disruption and even rupture of the round window, causing a perilymphatic fistula [46].

Blast injuries are special forms of combined barotrauma and noise trauma, resulting in hearing loss (55–72%) and tinnitus (66–88%) in most individuals who are exposed to large explosions; in 41%, both tinnitus and hearing loss occur [48–50]. Other symptoms include ear pain (41%) and distortion of sounds (28%) [49]. Two-thirds have a perforation of the eardrum, often on both sides (70%) [50]. In three-quarters of the people, the perforation heals spontaneously [50, 51]. Blast injuries can cause peripheral and central auditory system damage. The mechanical damage to the peripheral auditory system is caused by blast pressure waves transmitted directly through the ear canal. The damage to the central auditory system can be caused by blast wave impacts on the head or traumatic brain injury directly, or indirectly as a consequence of the peripheral auditory system damage [52, 53].

Treatment of barotraumas is conservative, but when ossicular chain disruption has occurred and a perilymphatic fistula is present, the treatment may be surgical.

Noise Trauma

There is a significant correlation between a history of exposure to noise trauma and high-pitched "whistling" tinnitus, and such tinnitus is significantly correlated with high-frequency hearing loss [54]. The frequency of tinnitus on pitch matching is the same as the worst frequency for hearing [55], most often at 4000 Hz [56]. The effect of exposure to noise on hearing loss has been well-studied but the relationship with tinnitus has only be studied to a lesser extent.

The prevalence of tinnitus in noise-exposed workers is 24% [57], significantly higher than that in the general population [58]. It has also been shown that noise-induced hearing loss usually has a steep slope, which is a risk factor for tinnitus prevalence and intensity [59, 60]. Furthermore, the more pronounced the hearing loss, the more discomfort the tinnitus generates [61] and the louder it is perceived [60]. Patients presenting with noise-induced tinnitus are mainly male and on average are 10 years younger than other tinnitus patients, suffering from bilateral high-pitched "whistling" tinnitus, correlated with their high-frequency hearing loss [54, 62]. Between 50 and 70% of young people who expose themselves to loud recreational noise have temporarily experienced tinnitus [63, 64]. After noise exposure by attending a concert, 20% of people develop transient hearing loss and tinnitus, and 13% perceive tinnitus for more than 3 months. Based on a systematic review, it has been calculated that 58.2% of young people exceed the recommended maximum daily noise dose, especially due to overexposure via personal listening devices (PLDs) [65]. Indeed, an iPod at maximal volume for 30 min causes transient threshold shift for <1 week [66]. Consequently, the use of a PLD is related to hearing loss in 9.6% of children, adolescents, and young adults, as shown by a meta-analysis [67]. Furthermore, the use of a PLD is related to transient tinnitus in 38.8% (8–69%) and permanent tinnitus in 2.2% of children, adolescents, and young adults [67].

Whereas noise exposure in young people is rising due to PLD use, noise exposure in professional musicians is even more pronounced. Rock musicians have 63% prevalence of hearing loss [68], and 20–26% experience tinnitus, which tends to be not bothersome [68, 69]. When wearing hearing protection, hearing loss does not develop [70]. In classical musicians, 32–50% have 15 dB hearing loss [68, 71], at the ear closest to the noise exposure, for example, the left ear for right-handed string players, and the hearing loss increases with age. Disc jockeys (DJs) are also prone to develop hearing loss and tinnitus: 70% have hearing loss and 74% tinnitus [72]. They develop hearing loss both at high and low frequencies and have tinnitus of the same sound spectra [73]. In up to 75% of DJs, tinnitus develops [73].

Cervical Spine Injuries

Whiplash Associated Tinnitus

A total of 10–15% of individuals who have suffered a whiplash injury develop symptoms such as tinnitus, deafness, and vertigo [10, 74, 75]. It has been hypothesized that tinnitus might develop because of the somatosensory influences on the dorsal cochlear nucleus [76] or narrowing and tearing in the auditory radiation in both hemispheres [77], analogous to what has been described in traumatic brain injuries [78]. As whiplash and traumatic brain injury coincide, it is not always easy to determine whether whiplash-associated tinnitus is cervicogenic or cerebrogenic. It is possible that tinnitus does not develop immediately after an injury but within several weeks. Even though this has not been described in detail in tinnitus, due to its pathophysiological and clinical analogy with pain [79–86], it is likely that tinnitus with a delayed onset might be underestimated. After stroke, almost 50% (13/27) of patients develop pain with a delay of 1 month and 10% with a delay of 2 or more years [87]. Similarly, after a spinal cord injury due to trauma or other causes, 26% of patients develop delayed pain, sometimes up to 6–7 months [88]. In phantom pain, this is also well-recognized. In 10–33% of patients, the onset of phantom pain starts 1 year after the amputation, and individual cases with 13-, 25-, and 30-year delays have been described [87]. This delayed onset is accompanied by neuroimmune activation and *N*-methyl-D-aspartate (NMDA)-dependent central sensitization of spinal nociceptive circuits [89]. (See also Chap. 31.)

Neuropsychological Disorders

Post-traumatic Stress Disorder

Post-traumatic stress disorder (PTSD) is an anxiety disorder caused by exposure to terrifying events. It is often accompanied by tinnitus. In Australian veterans with PTSD, over half report hearing loss or tinnitus and 43% report both [90]. The same is found in US veterans. Furthermore, those patients with PTSD rate their tinnitus as severe (29.4%) or extremely severe (18.7%). Thus, the prevalence of severe tinnitus in individuals with PTSD is much higher even than that in noise-exposed workers (24%) [57].The same is seen in refugees: 50% of Cambodian refugees suffer from tinnitus [91], and the prevalence of PTSD in these individuals is significantly higher than among individuals who do not have tinnitus. Of those patients who seek help for their tinnitus at a Veterans Tinnitus Clinic, 34% have PTSD [92]. It is not known whether it is the increased vigilance that causes the tinnitus.

Medicolegal Aspects

The onset of tinnitus in the context of a traumatic event is frequently an issue of medical expert opinions, in which the question of whether a trauma is causally related to the development of tinnitus should be answered.

The answer to this question is complex, as tinnitus in many cases has a multifactorial origin. Thus, the relevance of both the traumatic event and that of additional non-trauma-associated factors have to be considered.

Frequently, immediate tinnitus onset after trauma and trauma-induced hearing loss are considered as preconditions for the recognition of tinnitus as the consequence of an accident. This notion, however, is not consistent with the current knowledge about trauma-induced tinnitus. First, several trauma aspects can cause tinnitus without causing hearing loss (e.g., whiplash, head trauma, or emotional trauma); second, cochlear damage can occur, which is not detectable in the standard audiogram; and, third, tinnitus could develop with a delay of days to weeks after the trauma.

Thus, the assessment of whether a trauma is decisively causally related to development of tinnitus requires the consideration of all potential mechanisms by which trauma can cause tinnitus and should take into account that some of these mechanisms involve neuroplastic processes, which may require time to develop.

Summary

Tinnitus can be both non-pulsatile and pulsatile after a trauma. Non-pulsatile tinnitus is a common symptom after head and neck injuries, after noise trauma, barotrauma, and in PTSD. Some of the causes involved (e.g., ossicular chain disruption, perilymphatic fistula) can be successfully treated. Trauma-associated pulsatile tinnitus can be a sign of life-threatening disorders such as carotid-cavernous fistulas, arteriovenous malformations (AVMs), and carotid dissections.

References

1. Kreuzer PM, et al. Trauma-associated tinnitus. J Head Trauma Rehabil. 2014;29(5):432–42.
2. Weilnhammer V, et al. Exposure to leisure noise and intermittent tinnitus among young adults in Bavaria: longitudinal data from a prospective cohort study. Int J Audiol. 2021;61:1–8.
3. Degeest S, et al. Epidemiology and risk factors for tinnitus after leisure noise exposure in Flemish young adults. Int J Audiol. 2017;56(2):121–9.
4. Gilles A, et al. Prevalence of leisure noise-induced tinnitus and the attitude toward noise in university students. Otol Neurotol. 2012;33(6):899–906.
5. Sindhusake D, et al. Factors predicting severity of tinnitus: a population-based assessment. J Am Acad Audiol. 2004;15(4):269–80.
6. Sindhusake D, et al. Prevalence and characteristics of tinnitus in older adults: the Blue Mountains Hearing Study. Int J Audiol. 2003;42(5):289–94.
7. Folmer RL, Griest SE. Chronic tinnitus resulting from head or neck injuries. Laryngoscope. 2003;113(5):821–7.
8. Jury MA, Flynn MC. Auditory and vestibular sequelae to traumatic brain injury: a pilot study. N Z Med J. 2001;114(1134):286–8.
9. Kreuzer PM, et al. Trauma-associated tinnitus: audiological, demographic and clinical characteristics. PLoS One. 2012;7(9):e45599.
10. Claussen CF, Claussen E. Neurootological contributions to the diagnostic follow-up after whiplash injuries. Acta Otolaryngol Suppl. 1995;520(Pt 1):53–6.
11. Redekop GJ. Extracranial carotid and vertebral artery dissection: a review. Can J Neurol Sci. 2008;35(2):146–52.
12. Chen L, et al. Pulsatile tinnitus was the only manifestation of internal carotid artery dissection. Neurol Sci. 2021;42(3):1221–2.

13. Baumgartner RW, Bogousslavsky J. Clinical manifestations of carotid dissection. Front Neurol Neurosci. 2005;20:70–6.
14. Chae SW, et al. Tinnitus caused by traumatic posterior auricular artery--internal jugular vein fistula. J Laryngol Otol. 2001;115(4):313–5.
15. Freckmann N, Sartor K, Herrmann HD. Traumatic arteriovenous fistulae of the middle meningeal artery and neighbouring veins or dural sinuses. Acta Neurochir. 1981;55(3–4):273–81.
16. Fukai J, et al. Transarterial intravenous coil embolization of dural arteriovenous fistula involving the superior sagittal sinus. Surg Neurol. 2001;55(6):353–8.
17. D'Alise M, Caetano C, Batjer H. Vascular complications of head injury. In: Batjer H, editor. Cerebrovascular disease. Philadelphia: Lippincott-Raven; 1997.
18. Bishop FS, et al. Endovascular balloon angioplasty for treatment of posttraumatic venous sinus thrombosis. Case Rep J Neurosurg. 2009;111(1):17–21.
19. Kuether TA, et al. Endovascular treatment of traumatic dural sinus thrombosis: case report. Neurosurgery. 1998;42(5):1163–6; discussion 1166–7.
20. Zhao X, et al. Basilar skull fracture: a risk factor for transverse/sigmoid venous sinus obstruction. J Neurotrauma. 2008;25(2):104–11.
21. Liang W, et al. Traumatic carotid cavernous fistula accompanying basilar skull fracture: a study on the incidence of traumatic carotid cavernous fistula in the patients with basilar skull fracture and the prognostic analysis about traumatic carotid cavernous fistula. J Trauma. 2007;63(5):1014–20; discussion 1020.
22. Montava M, et al. Temporal bone fractures: sequelae and their impact on quality of life. Am J Otolaryngol. 2015;36(3):364–70.
23. Wysocki J. Cadaveric dissections based on observations of injuries to the temporal bone structures following head trauma. Skull Base. 2005;15(2):99–106; discussion 106–7.
24. Cannon CR, Jahrsdoerfer RA. Temporal bone fractures. Review of 90 cases. Arch Otolaryngol. 1983;109(5):285–8.
25. Brodie HA, Thompson TC. Management of complications from 820 temporal bone fractures. Am J Otol. 1997;18(2):188–97.
26. Granier M. et al. [Mild head trauma: complications and acousticovestibular sequelae]. Rev Stomatol Chir Maxillofac. 2006;107(4):253–63.
27. Chen J, et al. Temporal bone fracture and its complications. Chin J Traumatol. 2001;4(2):106–9.
28. Heid L, et al. Vertigo, dizziness, and tinnitus after otobasal fractures. Int Tinnitus J. 2004;10(1):94–100.
29. Villarreal IM, et al. Contralateral cochlear labyrinthine concussion without temporal bone fracture: unusual posttraumatic consequence. Case Rep Otolaryngol. 2016;2016:2123182.
30. Baloh RW. Dizziness, hearing loss and tinnitus, vol. 29. Philadelphia: F.A. Davis; 1998. p. 250.
31. Ulug T, Ulubil SA. Contralateral labyrinthine concussion in temporal bone fractures. J Otolaryngol. 2006;35(6):380–3.
32. Davies RA, Luxon LM. Dizziness following head injury: a neuro-otological study. J Neurol. 1995;242(4):222–30.
33. Choi MS, et al. Clinical characteristics of labyrinthine concussion. Korean J Audiol. 2013;17(1):13–7.
34. Schuknecht HF. Deafness following blows to the head: a clinical and experimental study. Trans Am Acad Ophthalmol Otolaryngol. 1951;55:407–17.
35. Schuknecht HF, Neff WD, Perlman HB. An experimental study of auditory damage following blows to the head. Ann Otol Rhinol Laryngol. 1951;60(2):273–89.
36. Yetiser S, et al. Traumatic ossicular dislocations: etiology and management. Am J Otolaryngol. 2008;29(1):31–6.
37. Wennmo C, Spandow O. Fractures of the temporal bone--chain incongruencies. Am J Otolaryngol. 1993;14(1):38–42.
38. Goto F, et al. Perilymph fistula--45 case analysis. Auris Nasus Larynx. 2001;28(1):29–33.
39. Fitzgerald DC. Persistent dizziness following head trauma and perilymphatic fistula. Arch Phys Med Rehabil. 1995;76(11):1017–20.
40. Glasscock ME III, et al. Traumatic perilymphatic fistula: how long can symptoms persist? A follow-up report. Am J Otol. 1992;13(4):333–8.
41. Foster PK. Autologous intratympanic blood patch for presumed perilymphatic fistulas. J Laryngol Otol. 2016;130(12):1158–61.
42. Lollis SS, et al. Ventriculoperitoneal shunt insertion for the treatment of refractory perilymphatic fistula. J Neurosurg. 2006;105(1):1–5.
43. Weider DJ, Roberts DW, Phillips J. Ventriculoperitoneal shunt as treatment for perilymphatic fistula: a report of six cases. Int Tinnitus J. 2005;11(2):137–45.
44. Morvan JB, et al. [Diagnosis and treatment of post-traumatic perilymphatic fistula: report of 16 cases]. Rev Laryngol Otol Rhinol (Bord). 2012;133(4–5):171–6.
45. Lindfors OH, et al. Middle ear barotraumas in commercial aircrew. Aerosp Med Hum Perform. 2021;92(3):182–9.
46. Mirza S, Richardson H. Otic barotrauma from air travel. J Laryngol Otol. 2005;119(5):366–70.
47. Becker GD, Parell GJ. Barotrauma of the ears and sinuses after scuba diving. Eur Arch Otorhinolaryngol. 2001;258(4):159–63.
48. Persaud R, et al. Otological trauma resulting from the Soho Nail Bomb in London, April 1999. Clin Otolaryngol Allied Sci. 2003;28(3):203–6.
49. Mrena R, et al. Otologic consequences of blast exposure: a Finnish case study of a shopping mall bomb explosion. Acta Otolaryngol. 2004;124(8):946–52.
50. Tungsinmunkong S, et al. Blast injury of the ears: the experience from Yala Hospital, Southern Thailand. J Med Assoc Thai. 2007;90(12):2662–8.
51. Kronenberg J, Ben-Shoshan J, Wolf M. Perforated tympanic membrane after blast injury. Am J Otol. 1993;14(1):92–4.
52. Jiang S, et al. Prevention of blast-induced auditory injury using 3D printed helmet and hearing protection device - a preliminary study on biomechanical modeling and animal. Mil Med. 2021;186(Suppl 1):537–45.
53. Shao N, et al. Central and peripheral auditory abnormalities in chinchilla animal model of blast-injury. Hear Res. 2021;407:108273.
54. Nicolas-Puel C, et al. Characteristics of tinnitus in a population of 555 patients: specificities of tinnitus induced by noise trauma. Int Tinnitus J. 2006;12(1):64–70.
55. Axelsson A, Prasher D. Tinnitus induced by occupational and leisure noise. Noise Health. 2000;2(8):47–54.
56. Cooper JC, Owen JH. Audiologic profile of noise-induced hearing loss. Arch Otolaryngol. 1976;102(3):148–50.
57. Phoon WH, Lee HS, Chia SE. Tinnitus in noise-exposed workers. Occup Med (Lond). 1993;43(1):35–8.
58. Axelsson A, Ringdahl A. Tinnitus--a study of its prevalence and characteristics. Br J Audiol. 1989;23(1):53–62.
59. Konig O, et al. Course of hearing loss and occurrence of tinnitus. Hear Res. 2006;221(1–2):59–64.
60. Demeester K, et al. Prevalence of tinnitus and audiometric shape. B-ENT. 2007;3(Suppl 7):37–49.
61. Dias A, Cordeiro R. Association between hearing loss level and degree of discomfort introduced by tinnitus in workers exposed to noise. Braz J Otorhinolaryngol. 2008;74(6):876–83.
62. Steinmetz LG, et al. The characteristics of tinnitus in workers exposed to noise. Braz J Otorhinolaryngol. 2009;75(1):7–14.
63. Quintanilla-Dieck Mde L, Artunduaga MA, Eavey RD. Intentional exposure to loud music: the second MTV.com survey reveals an opportunity to educate. J Pediatr. 2009;155(4):550–5.
64. Zocoli AM, et al. Brazilian young adults and noise: attitudes, habits, and audiological characteristics. Int J Audiol. 2009;48(10):692–9.
65. Jiang W, et al. Daily music exposure dose and hearing problems using personal listening devices in adolescents and young adults: a systematic review. Int J Audiol. 2016;55(4):197–205.

66. Gopal KV, et al. Risk assessment of recreational noise-induced hearing loss from exposure through a Personal Audio System-iPod Touch. J Am Acad Audiol. 2019;30(7):619–33.
67. le Clercq CMP, et al. Music-induced hearing loss in children, adolescents, and young adults: a systematic review and meta-analysis. Otol Neurotol. 2016;37(9):1208–16.
68. Di Stadio A, et al. Hearing loss, tinnitus, hyperacusis, and diplacusis in professional musicians: a systematic review. Int J Environ Res Public Health. 2018;15(10):15.
69. Stormer CC, et al. Hearing loss and tinnitus in rock musicians: a Norwegian survey. Noise Health. 2015;17(79):411–21.
70. Schmuziger N, Patscheke J, Probst R. Hearing in nonprofessional pop/rock musicians. Ear Hear. 2006;27(4):321–30.
71. Emmerich E, Rudel L, Richter F. Is the audiologic status of professional musicians a reflection of the noise exposure in classical orchestral music? Eur Arch Otorhinolaryngol. 2008;265(7):753–8.
72. Bray A, Szymanski M, Mills R. Noise induced hearing loss in dance music disc jockeys and an examination of sound levels in nightclubs. J Laryngol Otol. 2004;118(2):123–8.
73. Potier M, et al. The risks of amplified music for disc-jockeys working in nightclubs. Ear Hear. 2009;30:291.
74. Tranter RM, Graham JR. A review of the otological aspects of whiplash injury. J Forensic Legal Med. 2009;16(2):53–5.
75. Claussen C, Constantinescu L. Tinnitus in whiplash injury. Int Tinnitus J. 1995;1(2):105–14.
76. Levine RA. Somatic (craniocervical) tinnitus and the dorsal cochlear nucleus hypothesis. Am J Otolaryngol. 1999;20(6):351–62.
77. Lee SJ, et al. Diagnosis of tinnitus due to auditory radiation injury following whiplash injury: a case study. Diagnostics (Basel). 2019;10(1):10.
78. Jang SH, Bae CH, Seo JP. Injury of auditory radiation and sensorineural hearing loss from mild traumatic brain injury. Brain Inj. 2019;33(2):249–52.
79. De Ridder D, Van de Heyning P. The Darwinian plasticity hypothesis for tinnitus and pain. Prog Brain Res. 2007;166:55–60.
80. De Ridder D, Vanneste S. The Bayesian brain in imbalance: medial, lateral and descending pathways in tinnitus and pain: a perspective. Prog Brain Res. 2021;262:309–34.
81. Llinas RR, et al. Thalamocortical dysrhythmia: a neurological and neuropsychiatric syndrome characterized by magnetoencephalography. Proc Natl Acad Sci U S A. 1999;96(26):15222–7.
82. Moller AR. Similarities between severe tinnitus and chronic pain. J Am Acad Audiol. 2000;11(3):115–24.
83. Moller AR. Similarities between chronic pain and tinnitus. Am J Otol. 1997;18(5):577–85.
84. Tonndorf J. The analogy between tinnitus and pain: a suggestion for a physiological basis of chronic tinnitus. Hear Res. 1987;28(2–3):271–5.
85. Vanneste S, Song JJ, De Ridder D. Thalamocortical dysrhythmia detected by machine learning. Nat Commun. 2018;9(1):1103.
86. De Ridder D, et al. Phantom percepts: tinnitus and pain as persisting aversive memory networks. Proc Natl Acad Sci U S A. 2011;108(20):8075–80.
87. Schott GD. Delayed onset and resolution of pain: some observations and implications. Brain. 2001;124(Pt 6):1067–76.
88. Tasker RR, DeCarvalho GT, Dolan EJ. Intractable pain of spinal cord origin: clinical features and implications for surgery. J Neurosurg. 1992;77(3):373–8.
89. Vega-Avelaira D, et al. The emergence of adolescent onset pain hypersensitivity following neonatal nerve injury. Mol Pain. 2012;8:30.
90. Terhaag S, et al. A longitudinal exploration of self-reported hearing loss, tinnitus and PTSD treatment outcomes in Australian veterans. Psychosom Med. 2021;83:863.
91. Hinton DE, et al. Tinnitus among Cambodian refugees: relationship to PTSD severity. J Trauma Stress. 2006;19(4):541–6.
92. Fagelson MA. The association between tinnitus and posttraumatic stress disorder. Am J Audiol. 2007;16(2):107–17.

Tinnitus in Children and Adolescents

39

Susanne S. Nemholt and David M. Baguley

Abstract

Childhood tinnitus remains an under-researched topic area, though clinical and research interest in increasing. The literature indicates that childhood experiences of tinnitus are broadly as common as they are in adults and that in some cases it can be severe. There is an urgent need for age-appropriate and validated assessment and outcome measure tools to support progress in this important area of tinnitus.

David M. Baguley has died before the publication of this book.

S. S. Nemholt (✉)
Kommunikationscentret, The Social Division in the Capital Region of Denmark, Hellerup, Denmark
e-mail: susanne.nemholt@regionh.dk

D. M. Baguley (Deceased)
NIHR Biomedical Research Centre, School of Medicine, University of Nottingham, Nottingham, UK

Mental Health and Clinical Neurosciences, School of Medicine, University of Nottingham, Nottingham, UK

Nottingham Audiology Services, Nottingham University Hospitals, Nottingham, UK

W. Schlee et al. (eds.), *Textbook of Tinnitus*, https://doi.org/10.1007/978-3-031-35647-6_39

Graphical Abstract

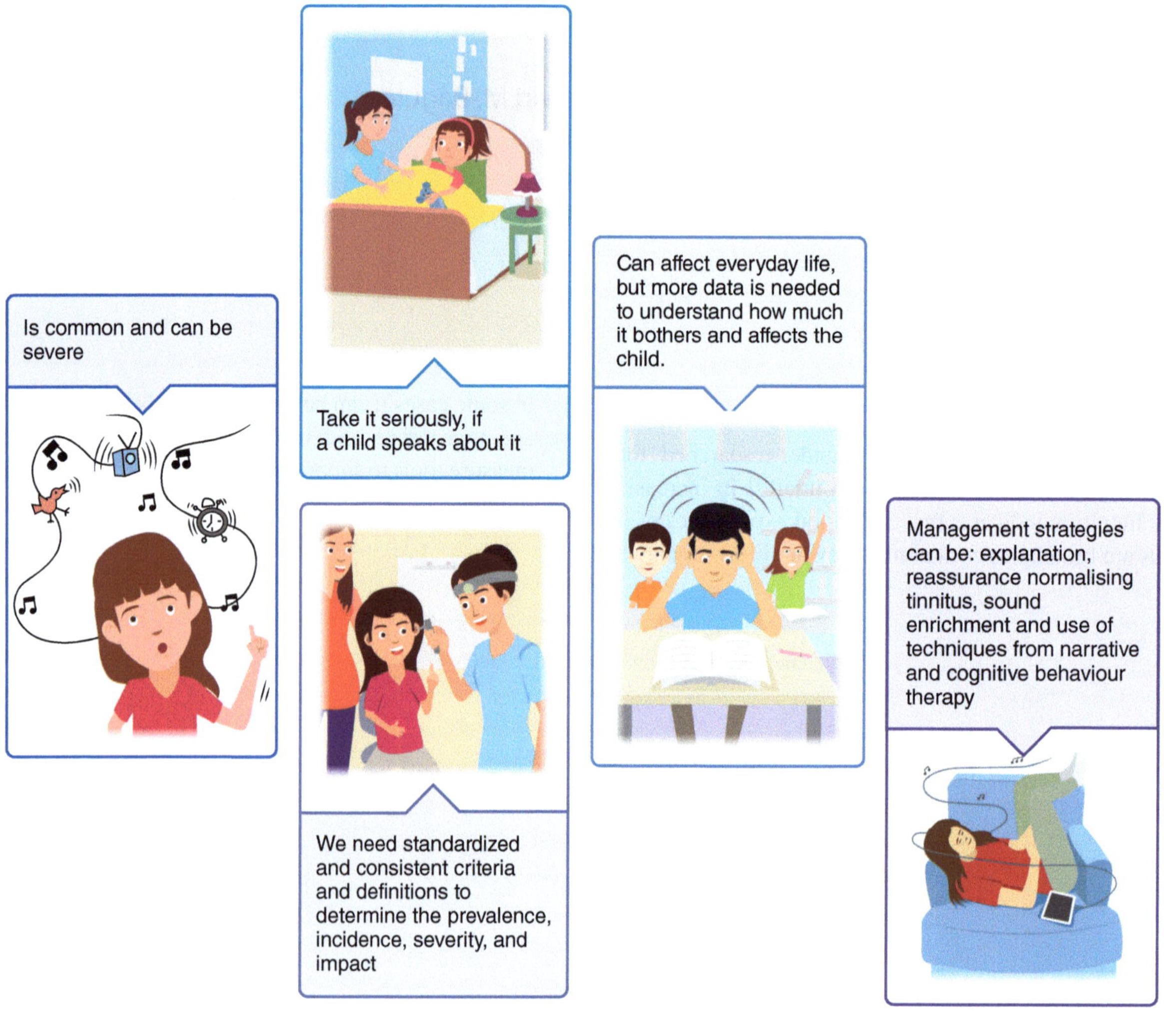

Abbreviations

ADHD Attention-deficit hyperactivity disorder
BSA British Society of Audiology
CF Cystic fibrosis
CI Cochlear implant
ENT Ear–nose–throat
GP General practitioner
MRI Magnetic resonance imaging
NIT Noise-induced tinnitus
ST Spontaneous tinnitus
UK United Kingdom
US United States
VAS Visual Analogue Scale

Highlights

- Tinnitus is a common experience for children, although methodological differences make studies difficult to compare.
- A set of standardized and consistent criteria are needed to robustly determine the prevalence, incidence, severity, and impact of tinnitus in childhood.
- More data are needed to understand how much it bothers and affects the child.
- If children speak about tinnitus, then clinicians need to take it seriously.
- Some researchers suggest that the prevalence figures in children are underestimated due to communication difficulties, whereas others argue that children overreport tinnitus, when asked, to satisfy the interviewer.

Introduction

Although there has been long-standing and substantial interest in tinnitus in adults, it is only recently that the tinnitus experiences of children and young people have been considered. As such, the existing literature is sparse is characterized by highly variable (and often imprecise) research designs and a lack of consistency in the definitions and outcome measures used [1]. In this chapter, we survey that which is known about tinnitus in childhood (used from this point on to also include young people), to delineate the important unanswered research questions.

Aetiology and Epidemiology

Over the years, there has been some debate as to what extent epidemiological data for the prevalence of childhood tinnitus can be relied upon, and concerns have been raised [2, 3] that there is a risk of both over- and underestimations of childhood tinnitus prevalence. Children are not likely to spontaneously report tinnitus [4, 5], and investigating tinnitus is seldom a part of routine paediatric otolaryngological practice [6]. Unfortunately, there is no standardized diagnostic tool for experience and severity of tinnitus, and there has been no consensus on a tinnitus definition among the epidemiological studies conducted in children and adults. Neither has there been agreement on how to formulate appropriate questions to determine its prevalence and severity [7, 8].

Definitions of Tinnitus

The primary challenge for studies investigating the prevalence of tinnitus lies in defining the tinnitus. Diverse definitions of tinnitus are applied across studies, e.g. "noises in your ears" [9, 10], "permanent tinnitus" [11, 12], tinnitus defined as a sound lasting for more than 5 min or exclusion of noise-induced tinnitus (NIT) (for example, [13–15]), and many studies do not provide a clear tinnitus definition (for example, [11, 16, 17]).

The lack of standardized diagnostic tools, and of agreement on how to formulate appropriate questions to uncover prevalence and severity [8, 18], makes it difficult to compare results across studies. Although there is no single agreed-upon definition of tinnitus, there are differences in the way that children are questioned about how any tinnitus sensation is noticeable [6, 19, 20], thus making comparison across studies impossible.

Table 39.1 provides a summary of the relevant studies, with specifics on the research questions used to define tinnitus in each study. The exact wording of the questions regarding tinnitus varied across studies from 1972 with a trend of development from a rather broad definition ("noise in the ears") moving towards more specific definitions such as duration of sound.

Table 39.1 Examples of research questions used to define tinnitus in childhood prevalence studies

Question asked (Reference)
Noises in your ears
"Do any of you get noises in your ears?"
It was explained that tinnitus does not include any of the sounds produced by hearing aids or coming from the child's surroundings [16].
The original set of questions was asked: "Do any of you get noises in your ears?"
It was explained that tinnitus does not include any of the sounds produced by hearing aids or coming from the child's surroundings [9].
Each child was asked whether he or she had noises in his or her ears.
If the child reported tinnitus, then he or she was asked to describe it. As a general rule, only children who were able to describe the noise were included in the tinnitus group [21].
Each child was asked whether he or she had noises in his or her ears [4].
"Have you ever heard a sound in your ear in the past year (a low buzzing, buzzing, humming, or machine-like sound, etc.)?" [22].
Ringing in your ears or sense of sounds not caused by external/environmental factors
Die Probanden wurden zunächst direkt gefragt: "Tritt bei Ihnen Ohrensausen auf oder nehmen Sie Geräusche wahr, die nicht von aussen oder der Umgebung verursacht werden?" [13]
Translated to English, the subjects were asked directly: "Do you have ringing in the ears or do you perceive sounds that are not caused by external or the environment?"
Noises in your ears such as ringing, buzzing or clicks
"Do you have any noises in your ears, such as ringing, buzzing or clicks? If so, how would you describe them?" [10]
"When you are not wearing your hearing aid, do you get noises, such as ringing, buzzing or clicks, in your ears?" If yes, a Tinnitus Questionnaire was used [23].
From the tinnitus protocol [24], it was assessed (a) whether they have any noise in their ears and (b) whether they are able to describe it [3].
Noises in your ears or head
"Do you sometimes hear noises in your head or ears?" [25]
"Have you ever had noises in your head or ears?" "Nowadays, do you hear noises in your head or ears? (1) Describe these noises" [26].
Each child was then interviewed and asked if they heard noises in their ears or head. It was explained to the children that these were not noises from their hearing aids or from outside but noises coming from their ears [2].
"Do you hear a noise inside your ears/head?" [27]
Noises in your ears or head without any known cause
"Do you hear any noise in your ears or in your head without any known cause?" [28]
"Do you ever get noises in your ears (not associated with noise exposure)?" [29]

(continued)

Table 39.1 (continued)

Question asked (Reference)
Tinnitus-like sound
Each child (accompanied by their parent) was asked about whether they had ever perceived tinnitus-like sounds [30]
"Do you hear tinnitus, whistles, or squeaks as you are falling asleep or when it is quiet in your room?" [22]
Sound in your ears without first having listened to loud music
1. "After listening to loud music or other loud sounds/noise, have you afterwards heard a ringing, buzzing or other sort of noise in your ears, even if the loud music or noise has been turned off?"
2. "Have you heard a ringing, buzzing or other sort of noise in your ears, without first having listened to loud music or other loud sounds?" [31]
1. "After listening to loud music or other loud sounds/noise, have you afterwards heard a sound in your ears even if the loud music or noise has been turned off (noise-induced tinnitus, permanent or temporary)?"
2. "Have you heard a sound in your ears without first having listened to loud music or other loud sounds (tinnitus, permanent or temporary without being induced by noise)?" [32]
Q1: "After listening to loud music or other loud sounds or noise, have you noticed that your hearing is worse (temporary hearing threshold shift)?"
Q2: "After listening to loud music or other loud sounds or noise, have you heard any ringing, buzzing or other sort of sound in your ear even after that the loud music or noise has been turned off (noise-induced tinnitus)?"
Q3: "Have you heard a ringing, buzzing or other sort of sound in your ears without first having listened to loud music or other loud sounds (spontaneous tinnitus)?" [33]
Q1: "After listening to loud music or other loud sounds or noise, have you heard any sort of sounds in your head or ear even after that the loud music or noise has been turned off?"
Q2: "Do you ever get noise in your head or ear without first having listened to loud music or other sounds?" [34]
Permanent tinnitus (buzzing or ringing)
1. "Do you have permanent tinnitus continuously 24 h a day?"
2. "How often have you had peeps or buzzing ears for 24 h or longer after attending concerts, discotheques, etc.?" [11]
1. "Do you have permanent tinnitus (buzzing or ringing) in your ears all the time?"
2. "Have you ever had temporary tinnitus continuing for 24 h or longer?" [35]
1. "Do you constantly perceive tinnitus (a laymen's term of "ringing in the ears" in the English language was used)?"
2. A numeric rating scale for loudness going from 0 (no tinnitus) to 10 (extremely loud, cannot possibly be louder) was used to evaluate temporary tinnitus [36]
Time frame (within a defined period)
"Within the past 6 months, have you experienced any noise such as ringing, buzzing, hissing, or any other sort of sound in your ear or your head that had no apparent cause?" [15]
"Within the past year, did you ever hear a sound (buzzing, hissing, ringing, humming, roaring, machinery noise) originating in your ear?" [17]
Participants were asked if they had heard ringing, buzzing, roaring or hissing sounds without any external acoustic source within the last year [37].
Tinnitus definition question including bothersome
"In the past 12 months, have you been bothered by ringing, roaring, or buzzing in your ears or head that lasts for 5 min or more (chronic tinnitus = more than 3 months)?" [14]

Different Types of Study Designs and Populations

Childhood tinnitus prevalence data are often presented in relation to a specific context, e.g. tinnitus in the general paediatric population, tinnitus among children with normal hearing or tinnitus in children with hearing impairment. Age, gender, the question used to identify tinnitus, and distinguishing between tinnitus sensation and tinnitus distress are also well-known methodological challenges when it comes to understanding the high degree of variety among estimates of the prevalence of childhood tinnitus. Table 39.2 shows some of the different designs, study populations and data collection used in epidemiological studies.

As illustrated in Table 39.2, many prevalence studies have been performed in school populations, but clinical settings and general population-based studies have also been undertaken. Some of the school-based studies are based on random samples of the study population in a given age range; others are performed on a specific study population, e.g. at schools of the deaf/hearing impaired [2, 16, 23, 28, 30]. Some studies are performed at ear–nose–throat (ENT)/audiology clinics [3, 21], whereas others are based on a representative sample from the background population [13, 14, 17, 37].

The majority of the studies are from the European region. In 2018, a study from Nigeria was published [39]. Although data from a non-first world nation are most welcome, the omission of the index tinnitus question from this publication limits the extent to which the results can be meaningfully interpreted.

Table 39.2 Study characteristics

Author (by date)	Place	Design (type of study)	Study temporality	Setting	Study population: Number of participants (females, if stated)	Age: Min–max age	Method to establish the hearing status	Data collection for tinnitus/ hyperacusis
Nodar [10]	United States	Cross-sectional	Prospective	General population (school)	2084	10–18	Audiometric screening	Questionnaire
Graham [16]	England	Cross-sectional	Retrospective	General population (school for HI children)	74	12–18	School records	Interview Questionnaire
Graham [9]	England	Cross-sectional	Retrospective	General population (school for HI children and school for the deaf)	158	12–18	From school records For the children with tinnitus present: otoscopy, audiometry, loudness discomfort levels, impedance and stapedius reflex thresholds	Interview Questionnaire
Mills and Cherry [21]	England	Cross-sectional	Prospective	Clinical (ENT/ audiology clinics; children with middle ear disease)	66 (34)	4–15	Clinical and audiometric data were recorded	Interview
				Clinical (ENT/ audiology clinics or schools; children with sensorineural hearing loss)	44 (12)	4–17		
Mills et al. [4]	England	Cross-sectional	Prospective	General population (routine school and community medical examination)	93 (39)	5–16	Otoscopy audiometry	Interview
Drukier [23]	United States	Cross-sectional	Prospective	General population (school for HI children)	331	6–18	Children with tinnitus underwent tympanometry and were only included as having tinnitus, if they passed the test	Questionnaire
Nagel and Drexel [13]	Germany	Cross-sectional	Prospective	General population (representative sample from the background population)	30	10	Audiometry	Interview
Viani [2]	England	Cross-sectional	Retrospective	General population (school for HI children)	102 (34)	6–17	Otoscopy Audiometry Tympanometry	Interview
Stouffer [25]	Canada	Cross-sectional	Retrospective	General population (school)	140	7–11 (NH) 7–11 (HI)	Audiometry Tympanometry	Interview
Holgers [31]	Sweden	Cross-sectional	Retrospective	General population (school)	964 (470)	7	Audiometry Tympanometry	Interview
Widen and Erlandsson [35]	Sweden	Cross-sectional	Retrospective	General population (school)	1285 (665)	13–19	Self-reported	Questionnaire
Holgers and Juul [32]	Sweden	Cross-sectional	Retrospective	General population (school)	274 (139)	9–16	Audiometry	Questionnaire
Aksoy et al. [26]	Turkey	Cross-sectional	Retrospective	General population (school)	1020 (Not stated)	6–16	Otoscopy Tympanometry Audiometry (only for those who reported tinnitus)	Questionnaire

(continued)

Table 39.2 (continued)

Author (by date)	Place	Design (type of study)	Study temporality	Setting	Study population: Number of participants (females, if stated)	Age Min–max age	Method to establish the hearing status	Data collection for tinnitus/ hyperacusis
Coelho et al. [27]	Brazil	Cross-sectional	Prospective	General population (school)	487 (229)	5–12	Otoscopy, tympanometry, audiometry, loudness discomfort levels	Questionnaire (parents) Interview (child)
Savastano [3]	Italy	Cross-sectional	Retrospective	Clinical (children who attended the ENT department (not just for a specific otologic problem)	1100 (368)	6–16	Otoscopy Tympanometry Audiometry	Interview
Celik et al. [28]	Turkey	Cross-sectional	Retrospective	General population (school (HI children))	500 (216)	6–18	Otoscopy Audiometry	Questionnaire
Chadha et al. [30]	Canada	Cross-sectional	Retrospective	General population (school (children with CI))	40 (18)	3–15	None (children with CI)	Interview (child with parents)
Juul et al. [33]	Sweden	Cross-sectional	Retrospective	General population (school)	756 (366)	7	Audiometry	Questionnaire
Gilles et al. [36]	Belgium	Cross-sectional	Retrospective	General population (high school)	3842 (2035)	14–18	None	Questionnaire
Landalv et al. [11]	Sweden	Cross-sectional	Retrospective	General population (upper secondary school)	240	15–19	Self-perception of hearing loss after attending clubs, discotheques, concerts etc.	Questionnaire
Mahboubi et al. [14]	United States	Cross-sectional	Retrospective	General population (representative sample from the background population)	3520	12–19	Otoscopy, tympanometry and audiometry	Questionnaire
Park et al. [37].	Korea	Cross-sectional	Retrospective	General population (representative sample from the background population)	3047 (1453)	12–19	Tympanometry and audiometry	Questionnaire
Park et al. [17]	Korea	Cross-sectional	Retrospective	General population (representative sample from the background population)	2213	12–18	Tympanometry and audiometry	Questionnaire
Piotrowska et al. [15]	Poland	Cross-sectional	Retrospective	General population (school)	7281 (3544) 7918 (4038)	7 12	Audiometry	Questionnaire Questionnaire
Humphriss et al. [29]	England	Cross-sectional	Prospective	Ongoing epidemiological cohort	7092 (3611)	11	Audiometry	Questionnaire
Nemholt et al. [34]	Denmark	Cross-sectional	Prospective	General population (school)	501 (275)	10–17	Otoscopy, tympanometry and audiometry	Questionnaire
Rhee et al. [22]	South Korea	Cross-sectional	Prospective	General population (school)	1593 (789)	12–13 15–16	Audiometry	Questionnaire
Raj-Koziak et al. [38]	Poland	Cross-sectional	Retrospective	General population (school)	43.064 (21.917)	11–13	Audiometry	Questionnaire

HI Hearing Impaired; *NH* Normal Hearing; *CI* Cochlear Implant. Data updated from Rosing et al. [1]

Estimates of the Prevalence of Tinnitus

Prevalence of childhood tinnitus in the literature varies according to definitions, questions used to assess the prevalence of tinnitus severity, age and whether the numbers are presented from the children with tinnitus or from the whole population (Table 39.3). Data from a systematic review [1] indicate that it is extremely difficult to compare prevalence results across studies. The prevalence estimates of tinnitus range from 4.7% to 46% in the general paediatric population and among children with normal hearing and from 23.5% to 62.2% in the population of children with hearing loss. Reported prevalence ranged from 6% to 41.9% when children with hearing loss and normal hearing were both included [1]. Similar findings in adults, presented in a systematic review [40], reported the prevalence of tinnitus in the range from 5.1% to 42.7% and the prevalence of bothersome tinnitus in the range from 3.0% to 30.9%.

Table 39.3 Prevalence of tinnitus in children

Author (by date within group)	Prevalence	Prevalence linked to				Severity description (percentage)
		Normal hearing	Hearing impaired	Noise induced	Gender *female*	
Tinnitus in the general paediatric population and among children with normal hearing						
Mills et al. [4]	29%					Bothered (*33. 3%)
Nagel and Drexel [13]	*27%					
Widen and Erlandsson [35]	8.8%			*21.6%		
Holgers and Juul [32]	* 46.0% (Q2)			52.9% (Q1)	35.6% *56.8%* Noise induced: 47.4% *58.2%*	Troublesome (*49.2%)
Aksoy et al. [26]	15.1%				54.5% *45.5%*	Bothersome (39%)
Gilles et al. [36]	* 18.3% (permanent)			*74.9% (temporary)	20% *17%* (permanent)	
Landalv et al. [11]	5.4% (permanent)			36.8%		Always worried (*30.8%)
Mahboubiet al. [14]	*7.5% * 4.7% (chronic)					Severe = a big problem (1.7%)
Park et al. [17]	* 17.6%					Severe in daily life (15.7%)
Park et al. [37]	* 17.7%				* 15.4% *20.3%*	Severe discomfort (*0.6%)
Humphriss et al [29]	28.1% (any)					Bothersome (4.4%)
Nemholt et al [34]	66.9% (any)			35.7%		Bothersome (34.6%)
Rhee et al. [22]	46% (any)				38.9% *53.7%*	Severe (9.1%)
Tinnitus in mixed - study population (children with hearing loss and normal hearing)						
Nodar [10]	* 15.2%	13.3%	58.6%			
Stouffer [25]		6% – 13%	24% – 29%			
Holgers [31]	12.4%	13%	8.8%	2.5%	47.5% *52.5%*	
Coelho et al. [27]	39%	37.7%	44.7%	*9.7%	36.0% *42.4%*	Bother (*44.7%)

Tab. 39.3 (continued)

Savastano [3]	34%	76.4%	23.5%		34,0% *34.0%*	More severely worried (4.8%) Always bothered (*12.0%)
Juul et al. [33]	41.9% (any)	40.8%	58%	23.9%		
Piotrowska et al. [15]	6% (age 7 and age 12)	1.5% (age 7) 0.8% (age 12)	*2.4% (age 7) *1.0% (age 12)			
Tinnitus in children with hearing impairment						
Graham [16]	62.2%		62.2%			Severely worried (*13%)
Graham [9]	49.4%		49.4%			Worried all the time (11%)
Mills and Cherry [21]	43.9% 29.5%		43.9% 29.5%			Bothered (*23.8%)
Drukier [23]	30%		30%		22% *40%*	Worried very much (*22%)
Viani [2]	23.5%		23.5%		23.5% *23.5%*	Occasionally concerned (*33.3%)
Celik et al. [28]	33.4%		33.4%		21.8% *34.7%*	Bothersome (All the time) (13.2%)
Chadha et al. [30]	38%		38%		40.9% *33.3%*	Any impact on quality -of-life (*20%)

(Hatched cells:) The prevalence was not investigated in the particular study

* Numbers calculated from the published data
Data updated from Rosing et al. [1]

Data updated from Rosing et al. [1]
[a] Numbers calculated from published data

In 2020, a large population-based Polish study on 43.064 children aged 11–13 years was published. Data were collected during a 5-year period [38] with an assessment of the prevalence of tinnitus as a secondary goal. In a questionnaire, parents were asked, "Does your child complain of tinnitus in their ears/head when in quiet?" Likewise, the child was asked, "Do you hear tinnitus, whistles, or squeaks as you are falling asleep or when it is quiet in your room?" The child was considered having tinnitus if both questions had a positive response. Overall, 3.1% of the children reported tinnitus, 3.0% of children with normal hearing and 9.0% of the children with hearing loss.

Risk Factors

Factors like age, gender, hearing status, and noise exposure have been linked to tinnitus as a possible way of explaining the variance in the prevalence numbers. A systematic review of the risk factors of paediatric tinnitus concluded that older-aged adolescents, females, and those with hearing loss may have a higher risk of tinnitus. Noise exposure and smoking in adolescents may represent especially important risk factors in paediatric tinnitus [41]. A retrospective chart review of electronic medical records of a tertiary paediatric hospital included 248 children aged 1–19 years of age with any diagnosis of tinnitus in their review. They found that age, normal hearing, noise exposure, history of trauma, and a psychiatric diagnosis in adolescence are factors associated with tinnitus [42].

Age

Comparing the prevalence of tinnitus as a function of age indicates a relatively low prevalence in the early and late teens and a higher prevalence in the mid-teens for the mixed-study population [3, 10]. In the population of children with hearing loss, findings reported an increase in tinnitus with age [2, 23, 28]. A study by Baguley et al. [43] investigated childhood tinnitus referred to four European tinnitus expert clinics. The mean age at referral was 13.8% (6–18 years) and only six cases (7%) were aged under 10 years.

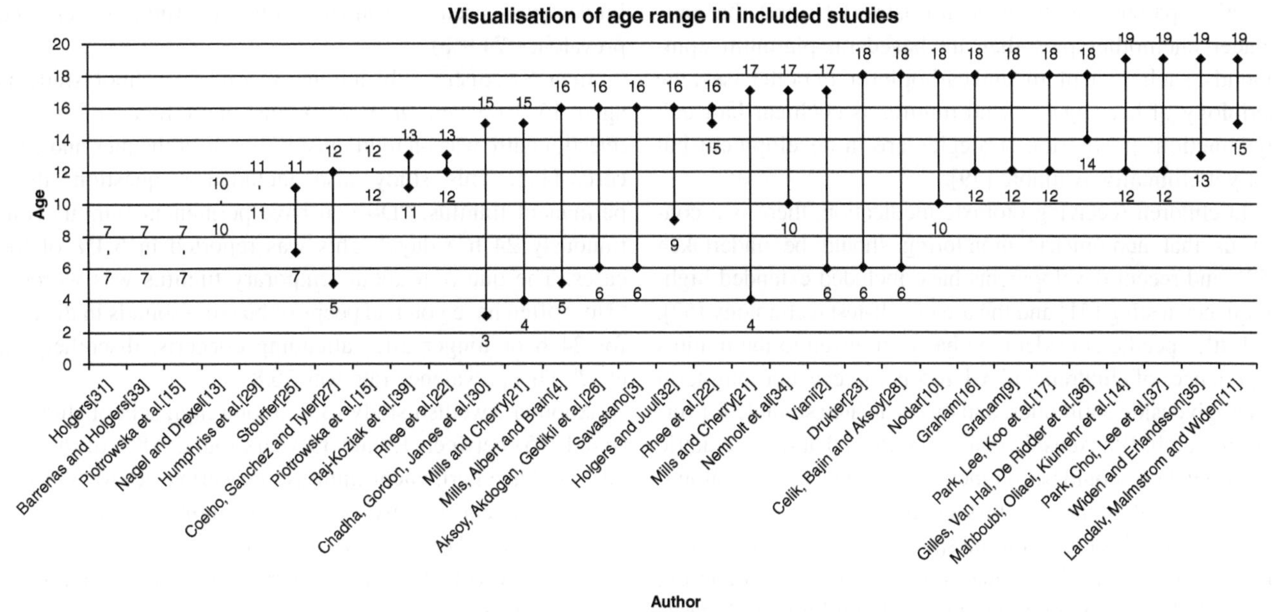

Fig. 39.1 The age distribution from studies presented in Tables 39.2 and 39.3. (Updated from Rosing et al. [1])

A possible explanation could be that children under a certain age are unable to understand and provide reliable answers to the research question, especially if the wording is too complex with many parameters [44]. Figure 39.1 shows the age distribution from studies presented in Tables 39.2 and 39.3.

Gender

Prevalence data indicate a slightly higher rate in females (17–56.8%) than in males (15.4–54.5%), as illustrated in Table 39.2. Some studies present prevalence linked to gender from the total number of children (for example, [2, 3, 27, 28, 32, 36]), whereas other studies present prevalence among the total number of children with tinnitus (for example, [26, 31]). Some studies do not provide information on how they calculated the prevalence linked to gender [23, 37]. All these factors considered together make comparison across studies difficult.

Hyperacusis

Tinnitus is often accompanied by hyperacusis. An English study among 7092 children aged 11 years were asked if they "ever experience over-sensitivity or distress to particular sounds?" and found that 9.6% (21/218) of the children with significant tinnitus (sound lasting more than seconds and being bothered by it) also had hyperacusis [29].

A study in Brazil studied 506 children aged 5–12 years and asked "Are you bothered by any kind of sound or noise?" They reported that 1.6% ($n = 8$) of all the children had both tinnitus and hyperacusis, 8.1% of those with tinnitus ($n = 99$) [27].

A Danish study investigated tinnitus and hyperacusis among 501 children between 10 and 16 years of age, asking the question "Are everyday sounds ever too loud for you?" The authors found that 18.8% (63 of the 335 children with tinnitus) also had hyperacusis. The presence of hyperacusis was significantly higher in children with spontaneous tinnitus (ST) (noise in your head or ears without first having listened to loud music or other sounds) [34].

Cochlear Implants

An important study by Chadha et al. [30] was performed on children with cochlear implants and, to date, is the only detailed exploration of tinnitus in this population. The authors looked at 40 children between 3 and 15 years of age and found that 38% (15/40) "ever had perceived tinnitus-like sounds". The severity, defined as "any impact on quality-of-life", was reported by 20% (3/15) of those with tinnitus. Although many adults with cochlear implant (CI) report that device use is beneficial for their tinnitus [45], there is a substantial residual impact, which can lead to insomnia [46, 47], depression, and to difficulties with Cochlear Implant tuning [48]. Tinnitus experiences in paediatric Cochlear Implant users is an under-researched area and is worthy of serious consideration.

Ototoxicity

Another specific population of substantial importance is that of children and young people who develop tinnitus (either with or without hearing loss) as a result of ototoxic medication. The two main categories of drugs that can be associated with tinnitus are aminoglycoside antibiotics (often when administered repeatedly and in substantial doses in patients with cystic fibrosis—CF) and the anti-cancer chemotherapies that are based on platinum compounds, such as cisplatin and carboplatin. In both cases, the aetiology of hearing loss and tinnitus is cochlear hair cell dysfunction: prevention strategies are in development but not yet clinically available [49].

In children receiving ototoxic medication, there is a consensus that audiometric monitoring should be undertaken [50], and recent developments have included extended high-frequency testing [51] and the use of self-test technology [52].

Little specific consideration has been given to the tinnitus experiences of children with CF receiving repeat or long-term aminoglycoside antibiotics, and this is an area suitable for further research. Blankenship et al. [51] noted that the paediatric CF population should be routinely asked about tinnitus, alongside enquiry about hearing loss and imbalance.

A growing literature on the specific tinnitus experiences of children undergoing cancer chemotherapy is becoming available [53]. New data include epidemiology, with cases reporting tinnitus three times as often as sibling controls [52]. Factors such as young age, cumulative dose, combined platinum-based chemotherapy and irradiation increase the incidence of tinnitus [54], but, in some children with cancer, tinnitus is reported without many or sometimes any of these factors, and some psychological issues may be at work [52]. Longitudinal studies indicate that tinnitus may be persistent and chronic [55] and may be burdensome into adulthood [54].

Noise Exposure

Noise exposure is a known risk factor for developing both tinnitus and hearing loss [18]. As a consequence, temporary tinnitus can be associated with a temporary threshold shift, following noise exposure [56]. A systematic review and meta-analysis providing an overview of music-induced hearing loss and its symptoms in children concluded that most studies reported no significant association between pure-tone air thresholds. In addition, exposure to loud music, significant changes in hearing thresholds and otoacoustic emissions, and a high tinnitus prevalence may suggest an association between music exposure and hearing loss in children [57]. It would be logical to assume that the prevalence of noise-induced tinnitus increases with age, as a consequence of loud music exposure in teens and adolescents compared with younger children.

A Flemish high school study among students aged 14–18 years (*n* = 3892) used a self-administered questionnaire to investigate permanent and temporary tinnitus [36]. Permanent tinnitus evaluated by a yes/no question, "Do you constantly perceive tinnitus?", was reported by 18.3% of the students. A numeric rating scale for loudness going from 0 (no tinnitus) to 10 (extremely loud, cannot possibly be louder) was used to evaluate temporary tinnitus (reported prevalence 74.9%).

In a Swedish study among secondary school students aged 15–19 years (*n* = 242), the main focus of a self-questionnaire was on loud music from discotheques and concerts [11]. This study also included a question about permanent tinnitus: "Do you have permanent tinnitus continuously 24 h a day?" This was reported in 5.4% of the cases. The question about temporary tinnitus was worded: "How often have you had peeps or buzzing sounds in the ears for 24 h or longer after attending concerts, discotheques, etc.?" This prevalence rate was 36.8%.

Another Swedish study [35] among high school students (*n* = 1285) between 13 and 19 years found 8.8% of the students to have permanent tinnitus, answering yes to "Do you have permanent tinnitus (buzzing or ringing in your ears all the time?" and 21.6% reported temporary tinnitus answering yes to "Have you ever had temporary tinnitus continuing for 24 h or longer?"

One Danish and three Swedish studies have examined the prevalence of noise-induced tinnitus (NIT) and spontaneous tinnitus (ST) using almost similar prevalence questions with different populations and age groups [31–34]. NIT was defined as sound present after listening to loud music or other loud sounds, and ST was sound present without having listened to loud music or other loud sounds. The studies identified a prevalence of NIT within the range of 2.5% (*n* = 24 out of 964 children aged 7 years) [31] to 52.9% (*n* = 145 out of 274 children aged 9–16 years) [32].

Two of the studies included a measure of bothersome tinnitus. Holgers et al. [32] found 22.6% (*n* = 62) of all the children (*n* = 274) to be annoyed by tinnitus sometimes or more often. This equals 49.2% of the children with tinnitus (*n* = 126). Nemholt et al. [34] found that although bothersome tinnitus was reported in 34.6% (*n* = 116) of children with any tinnitus, 23.2% of all the children (*n* = 501), only 8 of them (2.4%) were seriously bothered by it. However, children with NIT were more bothered by their tinnitus than were children with ST, and children who experienced their tinnitus all the time were also more bothered. The study had a presumption that the prevalence of NIT would increase with age, as a consequence of increased exposure to loud music among teens compared to younger children. However, this hypothesis could not be confirmed, possibly because there were too few children in each age group.

In general, NIT studies indicate that children above 12 years are more likely to develop noise-induced tinnitus than are children younger than 12 years. However, the reported differences in phrasing the question and the diversity in recall period in the research question can influence the prevalence estimates heavily and challenge the comparison across studies.

Tinnitus Severity

The challenge of getting an overview of children with tinnitus is further complicated by the fact that there is a substantial difference between "perceiving" a tinnitus sound and being "bothered" by the sound. A cross-sectional study among teenagers aged between 12 and 19 years in the United States (n = 3.520) [14] provided two definitions of bothersome tinnitus and thereby different prevalence numbers according to the definition. The presence of tinnitus was defined as being bothered by ringing, roaring or buzzing in your ears or head that lasts for 5 min or more (reported prevalence of 7.5%), and the condition was defined as chronic if it had lasted 3 months or more (reported prevalence of 4.7%).

In a systematic review [1], 16 studies had attempted to determine the severity of tinnitus and found that between 0.6% [37] and 49.2% [32] were bothered by their tinnitus. The question regarding troublesome tinnitus used different words for description, such as bothersome, uncomfortable, worried, and concerned. So, although prevalence studies show that tinnitus is a fairly common experience for children, it is still unclear how much it bothers and affects the child [19].

Given the lack of consistent evidence in this area, the classification "clinically significant tinnitus" defined as noises lasting more than seconds and being bothersome (either slightly or severely) has been suggested [29]. The study estimated the prevalence of clinically significant tinnitus as 3.1% among children aged 11 years. The same classification was used and reported by Nemholt et al. [34], who estimated the prevalence of clinically significant tinnitus as 15.6% among children aged 10–16 years examined for NIT and ST. The different format of the tinnitus questions used in the two studies as well as the different age groups may explain the different findings.

Comorbidity

Holgers and Juul [32] suggested that children with tinnitus have a higher rate of associated psychological difficulties, including anxiety and depression. They found that 32% of their young patients scored above the cut-off level for possible/probable clinical emotional/anxiety disorder for adolescents and 14.5% scored above the cut-off level for possible/probable clinical depression. No gender differences in depressive disorders were seen, but more girls (49%) than boys (26%) had anxiety disorders. No difference in the duration of tinnitus in children with or without anxiety disorders were reported, but children with depressive disorders had experienced tinnitus for a period of 24 months as compared to 17 months in the group without depression.

Kim et al. [58] found that scores for trait anxiety and depressive mood were higher among adolescents with tinnitus in their study and suggested that about one-third of adolescents experience tinnitus, which may be related to psycho-emotional factors.

Summary of Prevalence Data

- Data on prevalence vary considerably according to study design, study population, and the research questions posed.
- There is currently neither an internationally recognized standard definition for tinnitus nor a unique internationally recognized classification of these diagnoses. This raises additional difficulties in comparing results across studies.
- Study design and the study population need to be closely linked, and the tinnitus questions asked must reflect the age of the child.
- While the literature is variable, a consensus exists that tinnitus does exist among children and can be severe.
- The lack of consistency among studies indicates the necessity of examining the epidemiology of tinnitus in children and adolescents with a set of standardized criteria.

Clinical Characteristics

Studies have found that children rarely complain of tinnitus spontaneously [4, 5], and only a few children are seen at established tinnitus clinics [43]. In 2009, 88 cases of children were referred to 4 specialist European University Hospital Clinics, which accepted paediatric tinnitus referrals [43]. The number of children with tinnitus represented less than 1% of the total number of patients seen by the four services. A Danish study showed that only a small number of children with tinnitus and/or hyperacusis were seen at ear–nose–throat clinics or specialized services [59]. It could be that the children are seen at the general practitioner (GP) level, not being referred at all, or that just not that many children are bothered to a degree where they need help. There is currently limited knowledge on this subject, but studies have shown some possible explanations. Nodar [10] found that children rarely complain about tinnitus spontaneously and that when they do, there is probably a significant pathological cause. Kentish et al. [60] found that the children studied developed independent coping strategies to deal with tinnitus sound. Parents and general practitioners (GPs) may think that nothing can be accomplished by seeking clinical support [43]. Furthermore, a survey on UK GPs regarding their practice in adults with tinnitus showed that GPs with an interest in or experience of ear–nose–throat (ENT) were less likely to refer patients onwards and were more likely to assess for "red flags" such as pulsatile tinnitus [61].

Little is known about the subjective characteristics of childhood tinnitus. Even in adults, techniques such as tinnitus pitch and/or intensity masking are viewed as unreliable and highly subjective [62]. So, this will be even more the case for children. The descriptors that children use for tinnitus will often pertain to things with which they are familiar [19] and may well be highly age- and culture-specific as a result. Some practitioners use drawing as a technique to unlock a child's lived experience [19, 63], but care should be taken with interpretation.

Tinnitus-Related Problems in Children

There is limited literature available considering the effects of tinnitus on the health and well-being of children [5]. A study on 24 children aged 7–17 years attending a psychological clinic because of tinnitus showed that insomnia, anxiety and worry, and listening and attention problems were the main issues reported by the children [60]. In all, 71% of the children had developed coping strategies to deal with tinnitus before their first meeting. Specific concerns about tinnitus were reported by more than half of the children, and the parents shared these worries.

Another study on 25 children aged 6–16 years, interviewed during a consultation at a tinnitus department, showed that the biggest impacts on daily areal were on falling asleep, sleeping, and during lessons or studying at home. In some cases (24%), tinnitus caused worry and anxiety [64]. A recent scoping review has found that children with tinnitus experiences have a wide range of problems with a detrimental impact on their lives and well-being, which has been assessed to affect their learning and development [65]. To support development of a questionnaire measure of tinnitus in children, one of the purposes of the scoping review was to catalogue tinnitus problems reported in children in the literature. The main tinnitus-related problems observed in or reported by children are listed in Table 39.4.

Table 39.4 Tinnitus-related problems in children

Physical health
• Sleep difficulties (getting to sleep and waking at night)
• Headache, dizziness, ear pain, physical discomfort, tension in the neck/jaw
• Feeling of blocked ears, changes in appetite
Cognitive health
• General concentration and attention difficulties
• Concentration problems at school
Hearing and listening
• General hearing and listening difficulties
• Hearing and listening problems at school
Emotional health
• Negative emotions (annoyed, bothered, disturbed, anxious, worried, distressed, frightened, depressed)
• Fears and concerns about tinnitus
Quality of life
• Negative impact on quality of life
• Disruption of leisure and physical activities
• Disruption of school/learning activities
• Problems with social life
Feeling different/isolated
• Social isolation
• Feeling unable to talk to others about tinnitus
• Feeling different to everyone else

Data summarized from Smith et al. [65]

According to Kentish [19], questions about the occurrence, frequency, and duration of tinnitus must be matched to the child's cognitive and language level and carefully worded. In general, young children especially are likely to provide answers even when they do not understand the questions because they feel pressure to please the interviewer [66]. It is recommended to pre-test the question-and-answer process with a small number of respondents using cognitive interviews or focus group interviews [44]. This process will review whether it is necessary to revise items to increase understanding. Likewise, it is recommended to conduct a small-scale pilot test of a revised instrument with full procedures in the field as a final check before actual data collection. A pilot test of the methods with participants who are similar in age and share other characteristics of the study population will help refine instructions and question wordings and design.

The most important aspects of designing a questionnaire about tinnitus in children lie in phrasing questions so that they are age-relevant, making sure that the children understand the words used and asking about something that the child can remember. Younger children should be asked about the present rather than the past. Questions should be tested in a pilot study and reframed if necessary. It is also important to reflect on the tester–participant relationship.

Diagnostic Criteria

Diagnostics and Pathology

When a child presents at an otology or audiology unit, care needs to be taken to undertake sufficient investigation to exclude pathology and disease but not to burden or alarm the child and parents. Additionally, assessment should guide rehabilitation of treatment pathways. The Practice Guidance from the British Society of Audiology (BSA) [67] indicates that childhood tinnitus patients should only be seen within paediatric clinical settings and by paediatric audiologists, but, in some health economies and contexts, this may not be possible. Whatever the context, a careful history in childhood language is needed [5], to ascertain the lived experience of the patients, but also information from the parents about the presence of any of the major risk factors. Age-appropriate hearing assessment is needed, with care to adjust the technique when it appears that tinnitus may be interfering with the test results. Tympanometry can be regarded as standard, but care is needed with stapedial reflex testing in children with reduced sound tolerance. Loudness discomfort testing should be avoided unless absolutely necessary. Indications for magnetic resonance imaging (MRI) will be guided by local protocols, though these may have been designed with adults in mind rather than children.

Information about the incidence of otologic pathology in the paediatric tinnitus patient population is sparse. Martin and Snashall [68] reported on a series of 42 children who had presented to their specialist audiology unit with a complaint of tinnitus. Within that group, there were several with diagnoses such as juvenile Meniere's disease, noise-induced hearing loss, and a brainstem tumour. This was a highly selective group, however, and the only meaningful indication that can be taken at the present time is that otologic pathology is possible in this population.

A more recent study of otologic diagnoses in children presenting with tinnitus has been undertaken by Chan et al. [69], involving 180 patients (mean age 11.5 years). Definite diagnoses were identified in 53% of cases and generally involved childhood ear disease, though there were cases of head injury and ototoxicity. There were no cases of intracranial space-occupying lesions. More data are needed in this area to assess the risk of significant pathology in a childhood tinnitus population.

Interviewing Children

It has been suggested that difficulties in interviewing children may lead to inconsistency in responses [25]. Different approaches towards collecting reliable answers have been presented in prevalence studies. This could include explaining questions if they were unanswered or not understood [10] or using individual structural interviews, followed by a brief information about tinnitus and noise, and their influence on hearing function [31], or using a protocol of study for tinnitus in childhood [24] in which the child is tested for issues like capacity to describe tinnitus and annoyance degree [3].

Various methodological reflections and approaches have also been reported by researchers to collect reliable answers from younger children. These include making sure that the child understood the question, communication at the child's level, and re-explanation if necessary [2, 4, 21, 25, 27, 28, 70]. Despite these attempts to determine whether a child's response is reliable or not, it does not seem to be straightforward "how" to approach and succeed with this important issue. As earlier mentioned, the authors of the "Tinnitus in Children Practice Guidance" recommend that children should be seen by professionals trained in paediatrics and explains that such professionals are able to determine whether a child's response is reliable or not [71]. Unfortunately, no specific recommendations on how this is done are mentioned.

Proposed Possible Reasons as to Why Tinnitus is Under- or Overreported

- Children tend to worry less about themselves than do adults and are more distracted by their external environment and, e.g. while playing, may forget about tinnitus.
- Routinely asking a child about noises in their ears can potentially lead to overreporting of tinnitus because children are quick to give positive replies to direct questions.
- Children may assume that the noises are a normal part of life.
- Children under a certain age are unable to understand and give reliable answers.

Treatment Options

Tinnitus Assessment and Management

At present, there are no standard measures for assessment and management for tinnitus suitable and tested for children. However, in 2015, the Paediatric Audiology Interest Group of the British Society of Audiology developed "Tinnitus in children: Practice Guidance" for working with children with tinnitus. It is recommended that children should be managed in appropriate paediatric settings instead of being an add-on to tinnitus clinics for adults and that the healthcare professionals involved should have appropriate paediatric skills and knowledge of care pathways relevant to the paediatric population [19, 67]. In clinical practice, if a child ever mentions tinnitus, we should take notice of it and ask them open-ended questions like "is there anything else about your ears bothering you?" The BSA Guidance recommends that children attending an audiology service are routinely asked about noises in their ears [67]. Concerns have been raised that this could lead to overreporting of tinnitus and that children will self-report severe tinnitus [29].

Another clinical approach recommended by the BSA Guidance could be to look for "soft signs" to identify whether a child has tinnitus. Soft signs can be a pattern of variable audiograms, signs of anxiety or avoidance strategies when it comes to testing, unexplained dislike of hearing aids, dislike or distrust of one ear, perception that hearing is worse in one ear, reports of listening difficulties in noise and quiet, reports of difficulties in a specific lesson in school, avoidance of noisy or quiet situations, sleep difficulties, etc. [67].

Kentish et al. found that parents can be more concerned about tinnitus than their child and hold their own set of concerns. They recommended that information about the level of impact and distress associated with tinnitus should be gathered from parents and the child individually [60].

With regard to management strategies, the BSA Guidance [67] highlights that a good explanation of tinnitus forms the basis of all management plans. Reassurance, normalizing tinnitus, and help/support to develop a sense of control is important as is explaining tinnitus to children and parents. This can be done using the Child Friendly Tinnitus Model (see below), which, according to the Practice Guidance, has been found to be helpful in explaining tinnitus distress to parents as well. Use of hearing aids and sound enrichment as well as cognitive behavioural therapy and narrative therapy are also recommended approaches.

A recent evaluation of paediatric tinnitus services at the UK National Health Service audiology departments has found that nearly all services use the most BSA Guidance-recommended assessment and treatments [72]. The most widely used practices were the assessment of tinnitus history, hearing difficulties, current coping strategies, and factors that affect the child's tinnitus. Looking into treatment approaches, explanation and advice-giving were used most widely, with widespread use of hearing aids and non-wearable sound enrichment as well. Less widely used were the assessment of mental health and the use of psychological treatment approaches: cognitive behavioural therapy, mindfulness, and narrative therapy.

The Child-Friendly Tinnitus Model

The Child Friendly Tinnitus Model [73] is a modified pictorial version of the Psychological Model of Tinnitus by McKenna et al. [74] and is used as a framework for both information gathering and for counselling children and parents about tinnitus [19] (see Fig. 39.2). A traffic light represents the central auditory filtering system in the brain, which determines whether sounds reach conscious awareness or not. "Important sounds" are described as sounds that alert us to danger and sounds that interest us. Important sounds are given the green light, whereas not important sounds and sounds that we do not need to become consciously aware of are given the red light. Once the sounds reach conscious awareness, they can become linked to thoughts and a feeling of danger. Thereby, the emotional system can stimulate the autonomic nervous system, which, in this model, is symbolized as an alarm clock. This clock goes off when we feel endangered and makes us ready for fight or flight. Our thoughts, feelings, and body alarm can together affect the way that the traffic lights work. The child-friendly version has added a "worry" box to represent external stresses, such as exams, bullying, or other difficulties. These external stresses also have an impact on the system [19, 73]. No studies have yet investigated the treatment outcomes for children with tinnitus using the Practice Guidance and the Child-Friendly Tinnitus Model.

Narrative Therapy

Narrative techniques have been found to be useful in clinical practice treating children with tinnitus [63]. These are a way of paying attention to the child's story about tinnitus, to the meanings, beliefs, and mentions that children and their families have about tinnitus. Through drawing, play, and discussion, their view of tinnitus can be unrolled. Externalization is a narrative technique that can help children separate themselves from their problems ("the problem is the problem").

Treatment

Even though a number of strategies are used to treat children with bothersome tinnitus in clinical practice, little research has been conducted to evaluate their usefulness [65, 75]. A recent published systematic review on the effect of treatment of subjective tinnitus in children has included 6 studies of a total of 4447 studies for analysis and data extraction but could not determine effectiveness due to the high risk of bias of the included studies. Moreover, it was not possible to draw conclusions on long-term effects due to brief follow-up periods [76].

The main intervention techniques found in a study on interventions used for Danish children with tinnitus were counselling (including explanation), sound therapy (bedside/in ear), cognitive therapy, and educational assessment and school input [59]. Aside from these techniques that have also been reported by other studies [13, 60], this survey additionally identified use of the neurophysiological model, a Danish version of the Tinnitus Handicap Inventory and coping strategies. The study also found that intervention methods corresponding with the Danish guidelines for tinnitus management in adults [77] were used in 16% of the cases.

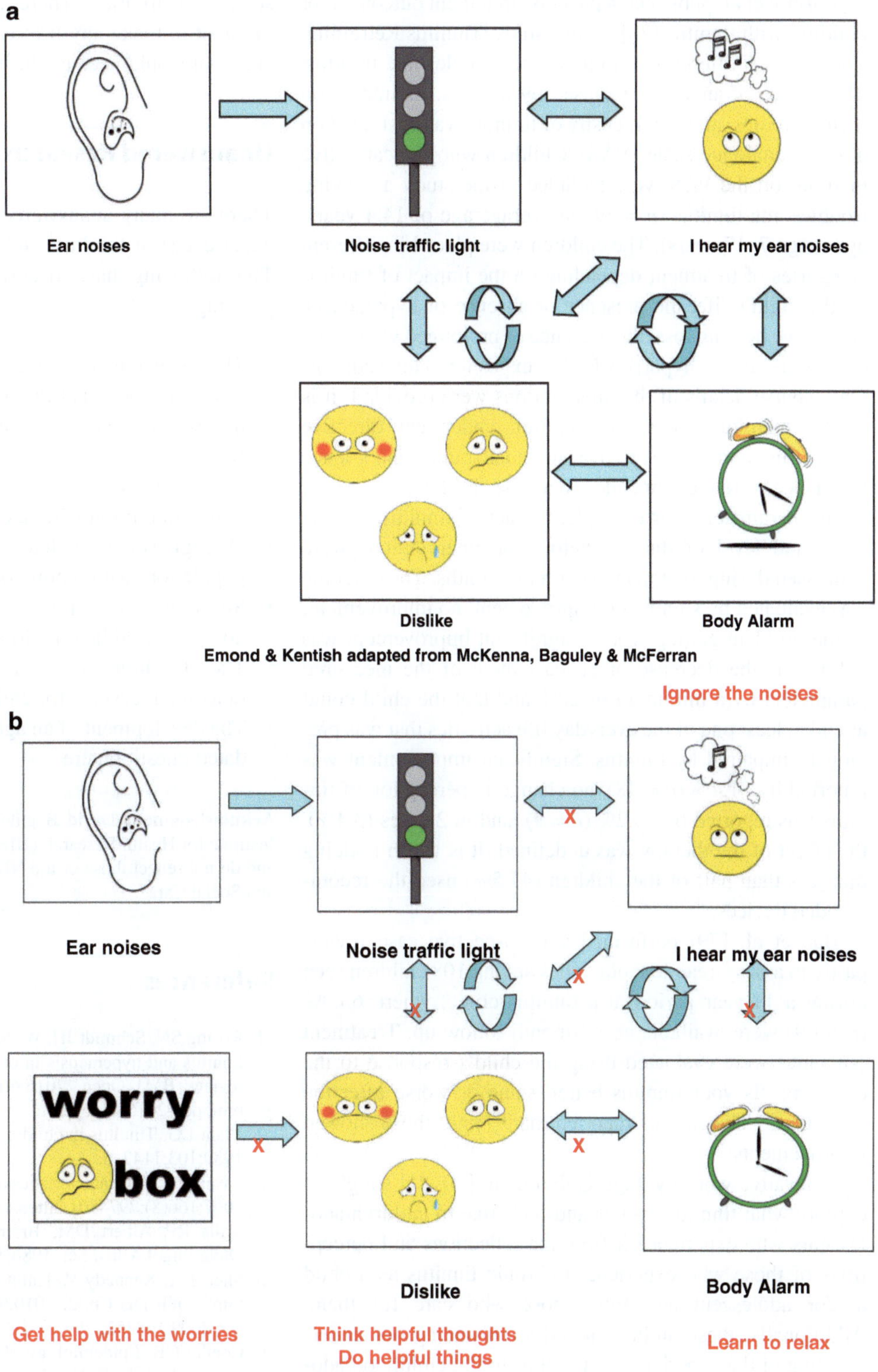

Fig. 39.2 (**a**, **b**) The Child-Friendly Tinnitus Model to understand tinnitus. (Figure from Emond and Kentish [73] (with permission))

Bartnik et al. published a paper on treatment outcomes for children with tinnitus [78]. In this study, Tinnitus Retraining Therapy was offered to children with troublesome tinnitus. The degree of annoyance caused by tinnitus, its impact on their activities, and the intensity of tinnitus was evaluated on a visual analogue scale (VAS). Children who indicated five or more on the VAS were included in the study as having troublesome tinnitus ($n = 59$, an average age of 14.4 years, age range 7–17 years). The children were placed in different categories of treatment depending on the impact of tinnitus on the child's life, the presence or absence of hyperacusis, subjective hearing loss, the presence of prolonged worsening of tinnitus, and/or hyperacusis after exposure to loud sounds. Only sparse details of the interventions were provided; it is briefly mentioned that the children underwent directive counselling and enriched environmental sounds and silence avoidance were recommended to all the children.

Six parameters (for example, impact of tinnitus, annoyance, and level of distress before the intervention) were addressed during treatment and after 6 months. The outcome was evaluated by significant improvement, no improvement, or the problem getting worse. Significant improvement was defined as the decrease of at least three of the measured parameters by a minimum of 20% and that the child could attend at least one of the everyday life activities that was previously impaired by tinnitus. Significant improvement was reported by 81.4% ($n = 48$), no change in perception of tinnitus was reported by 15.2% ($n = 9$), and in 2 cases (3.4%), the effect of the therapy was undefined. It is worth noticing that less than half of the children (47.5%) used the recommended devices.

Bae et al. [79] performed a retrospective case review partly to assess treatment outcomes among 108 children seen during a 11-year period at a tinnitus clinic, where 63.9% ($n = 69$) were available at a 3-month follow-up. Treatment outcomes were evaluated using the child's response to the question: "Is your tinnitus better, same or worse after the treatment?" The authors reported that 97% of those showed improvements.

Innovative work by Tegg-Quinn et al. [80, 81] sought to explore what tinnitus sounds and feels like to children/adolescents who experience it from the reflections and perceptions of those who experienced chronic tinnitus as a child and/or adolescent and from those who care for them. Additionally, these authors aimed at enhancing our understanding of the experience of tinnitus during childhood/adolescence and build a conceptual framework, which describes it. The complexity of the data gleaned in this study reinforces the view that childhood tinnitus experiences are heterogeneous and labile. One area that is missing in the literature is any suggestion of acute drug treatment for tinnitus in children. Another area of future interest could be potential associations with attention-deficit hyperactivity disorder (ADHD) and autism, as has been observed with hyperacusis and other sound sensitivities. There is insufficient evidence at the moment to make any firm conclusion, but this is clearly an area that would need exploring in the future.

Unanswered Research Questions

There are many unanswered questions regarding childhood experiences of tinnitus, and research in this area is sparse. The following have occurred to the chapter authors as pressing:

- The involvement of young people with troublesome tinnitus and their families in the identification of research questions, research design, and implementation
- Robust determination of the epidemiology and natural history of paediatric tinnitus—for which a clear and consistent definition will be essential
- Otologic studies to determine the pathophysiology in this population, with reports of treatment outcomes
- Study of specific populations, including ototoxicity, and noise-induced hearing loss
- The development of age-appropriate, patient-reported outcome measures for childhood tinnitus
- The development of an age-appropriate standardized validated questionnaire

Acknowledgment David Baguley is supported by the UK National Institute for Health Research (NIHR), but his views herein are his own and do not reflect those of the NIHR or the UK Department of Health and Social Care.

References

1. Rosing SN, Schmidt JH, Wedderkopp N, Baguley D. Prevalence of tinnitus and hyperacusis in children and adolescents: a systematic review. BMJ Open. 2016;6(6):e010596. https://doi.org/10.1136/bmjopen-2015-010596.
2. Viani LG. Tinnitus in children with hearing loss. J Laryngol Otol. 1989;103:1142–5.
3. Savastano M. Characteristics of tinnitus in childhood. Eur J Pediatr. 2007;166(8):797–801. https://doi.org/10.1007/s00431-006-0320-z.
4. Mills RP, Albert DM, Brain CE. Tinnitus in childhood. Clin Otolaryngol Allied Sci. 1986;11(6):431–4.
5. Shetye A, Kennedy V. Tinnitus in children: an uncommon symptom? Arch Dis Child. 2010;95(8):645–8. https://doi.org/10.1136/adc.2009.168252.
6. Coelho CB. Epidemiology of tinnitus in children. In: Møller AR, Langguth B, DeRidder D, Kleinjung T, editors. Textbook of tinnitus. Berlin: Springer; 2011. p. 39–45.
7. Baguley D, Andersson G, McKenna L, McFerran D. Tinnitus, a multidisciplinary approach. 2nd ed. Chichester, West Sussex: John Wiley & Sons, Ltd.; 2013.
8. Henry JA, Dennis KC, Schechter MA. General review of tinnitus: prevalence, mechanisms, effects, and management. J Speech Lang Hear Res. 2005;48(5):1204–35. https://doi.org/10.1044/1092-4388(2005/084).
9. Graham JM. Tinnitus in children with hearing loss. Ciba Found Symp. 1981;85:172–92.

10. Nodar R. Tinnitus aurium in school age children: A survey. J Auditory Res. 1972;12:133–5.
11. Landalv D, Malmstrom L, Widen SE. Adolescents' reported hearing symptoms and attitudes toward loud music. Noise Health. 2013;15(66):347–54. https://doi.org/10.4103/1463-1741.116584.
12. Widen SE, Erlandsson SI. The influence of socio-economic status on adolescent attitude to social noise and hearing protection. Noise Health. 2004;7(25):59–70.
13. Nagel D, Drexel MK. [Epidemiologic studies of tinnitus aurium]. Auris Nasus Larynx. 1989;16(Suppl 1):S23–31.
14. Mahboubi H, Oliaei S, Kiumehr S, Dwabe S, Djalilian HR. The prevalence and characteristics of tinnitus in the youth population of the United States. Laryngoscope. 2013;123(8):2001–8. https://doi.org/10.1002/lary.24015.
15. Piotrowska A, Raj-Koziak D, Lorens A, Skarzynski H. Tinnitus reported by children aged 7 and 12 years. Int J Pediatr Otorhinolaryngol. 2015;79(8):1346–50.
16. Graham J. Paediatric tinnitus. J Laryngol Otol Suppl. 1981;85(Suppl):117–20.
17. Park KH, Lee SH, Koo JW, Park HY, Lee KY, Choi YS, et al. Prevalence and associated factors of tinnitus: data from the Korean National Health and Nutrition Examination Survey 2009-2011. J Epidemiol. 2014;24(5):417–26.
18. Baguley D, McFerran D, Hall D. Tinnitus. Lancet. 2013;382(9904):1600–7. https://doi.org/10.1016/s0140-6736(13)60142-7.
19. Kentish RC. Manging tinnitus in childhood. In: Baguley D, Fagelson M, editors. Tinnitus: clinical and research perspectives. San Diego, CA: Plural Publishing, Inc.; 2016. p. xi, 364 pages, illustrations.
20. Nemholt S, Schmidt J, Wedderkopp N, Baguley D. Prevalence of tinnitus and/or hyperacusis in children and adolescents: study protocol for a systematic review. BMJ Open. 2015;5(1):e006649.
21. Mills RP, Cherry JR. Subjective tinnitus in children with otological disorders. Int J Pediatr Otorhinolaryngol. 1984;7(1):21–7.
22. Rhee J, Lee D, Suh MW, Lee JH, Hong YC, Oh SH, et al. Prevalence, associated factors, and comorbidities of tinnitus in adolescents. PLoS One. 2020;15(7):e0236723. https://doi.org/10.1371/journal.pone.0236723.
23. Drukier GS. The prevalence and characteristics of tinnitus with profound sensori-neural hearing impairment. Am Ann Deaf. 1989;134(4):260–4.
24. Savastano M. A protocol of study for tinnitus in childhood. Int J Pediatr Otorhinolaryngol. 2002;64(1):23–7.
25. Stouffer J, Tyler R, Booth J, Buckrell B. Tinnitus in normal-hearing and hearing-impaired children. In: Proceedings of the fourth international tinnitus seminar, Bordeaux, France, August 27–30. Kugler Publications; 1991.
26. Aksoy S, Akdogan O, Gedikli Y, Belgin E. The extent and levels of tinnitus in children of central Ankara. Int J Pediatr Otorhinolaryngol. 2007;71(2):263–8. https://doi.org/10.1016/j.ijporl.2006.10.008.
27. Coelho CB, Sanchez TG, Tyler RS. Tinnitus in children and associated risk factors. Prog Brain Res. 2007;166:179–91. https://doi.org/10.1016/s0079-6123(07)66016-6.
28. Celik N, Bajin MD, S. A. Tinnitus incidence and characteristics in children with hearing loss. J Int Adv Otol. 2009;5(3):365–9.
29. Humphriss R, Hall AJ, Baguley D. Prevalence and characteristics of spontaneous tinnitus in 11-year-old children. Int J Audiol. 2016;55(3):142–8. https://doi.org/10.3109/14992027.2015.1120890.
30. Chadha NK, Gordon KA, James AL, Papsin BC. Tinnitus is prevalent in children with cochlear implants. Int J Pediatr Otorhinolaryngol. 2009;73(5):671–5. https://doi.org/10.1016/j.ijporl.2008.12.032.
31. Holgers KM. Tinnitus in 7-year-old children. Eur J Pediatr. 2003;162(4):276–8. https://doi.org/10.1007/s00431-003-1183-1.
32. Holgers KM, Juul J. The suffering of tinnitus in childhood and adolescence. Int J Audiol. 2006;45(5):267–72. https://doi.org/10.1080/14992020500485668.
33. Juul J, Barrenas ML, Holgers KM. Tinnitus and hearing in 7-year-old children. Arch Dis Child. 2012;97(1):28–30. https://doi.org/10.1136/archdischild-2011-300270.
34. Nemholt S, Schmidt JH, Wedderkopp N, Baguley DM. A cross-sectional study of the prevalence and factors associated with tinnitus and/or hyperacusis in children. Ear Hear. 2020;41(2):344–55. https://doi.org/10.1097/aud.0000000000000759.
35. Widen SE, Erlandsson SI. Self-reported tinnitus and noise sensitivity among adolescents in Sweden. Noise Health. 2004;7(25):29–40.
36. Gilles A, Van Hal G, De Ridder D, Wouters K, Van de Heyning P. Epidemiology of noise-induced tinnitus and the attitudes and beliefs towards noise and hearing protection in adolescents. PLoS One. 2013;8(7):e70297. https://doi.org/10.1371/journal.pone.0070297.
37. Park B, Choi HG, Lee HJ, An SY, Kim SW, Lee JS, et al. Analysis of the prevalence of and risk factors for tinnitus in a young population. Otol Neurotol. 2014;35(7):1218–22. https://doi.org/10.1097/mao.0000000000000472.
38. Raj-Koziak D, Gos E, Swierniak W, Skarzynski H, Skarzynski PH. Prevalence of tinnitus in a sample of 43,064 children in Warsaw, Poland. Int J Audiol. 2020;60:614. https://doi.org/10.1080/14992027.2020.1849829.
39. Adegbiji WA, Olajide GT, Olubi O, Aluko AA, Olajuyin AO, Eletta PA, et al. Characteristics and management of childhood tinnitus in a developing country. Int Tinnitus J. 2018;22(1):66–71. https://doi.org/10.5935/0946-5448.20180011.
40. McCormack A, Edmondson-Jones M, Somerset S, Hall D. A systematic review of the reporting of tinnitus prevalence and severity. Hear Res. 2016;337:70–9. https://doi.org/10.1016/j.heares.2016.05.009.
41. Lee DY, Kim YH. Risk factors of pediatric tinnitus: systematic review and meta-analysis. Laryngoscope. 2018;128(6):1462–8. https://doi.org/10.1002/lary.26924.
42. Levi J, Basa K, Wong K, Morlet T, O'Reilly R. Cofactors of pediatric tinnitus: a look at the whole picture. Clin Pediatr (Phila). 2019;58(3):320–7. https://doi.org/10.1177/0009922818816426.
43. Baguley DM, Bartnik G, Kleinjung T, Savastano M, Hough EA. Troublesome tinnitus in childhood and adolescence: data from expert centres. Int J Pediatr Otorhinolaryngol. 2013;77(2):248–51. https://doi.org/10.1016/j.ijporl.2012.11.009.
44. Coyle K, Russel L, Shields J, Tanaka B. Collecting data from children aged 9-13; 2007.
45. Assouly KKS, van Heteren JAA, Stokroos RJ, Stegeman I, Smit AL. Cochlear implantation for patients with tinnitus - a systematic review. Prog Brain Res. 2021;260:27–50. https://doi.org/10.1016/bs.pbr.2020.06.013.
46. Pierzycki RH, Edmondson-Jones M, Dawes P, Munro KJ, Moore DR, Kitterick PT. Tinnitus and sleep difficulties after cochlear implantation. Ear Hear. 2016;37(6):e402–8. https://doi.org/10.1097/aud.0000000000000341.
47. Pierzycki RH, Kitterick PT. Insomnia, anxiety and depression in adult cochlear implant users with tinnitus. Ear Hear. 2020;42(1):235–43. https://doi.org/10.1097/aud.0000000000000900.
48. Pierzycki RH, Corner C, Fielden CA, Kitterick PT. Effects of tinnitus on cochlear implant programming. Trends Hear. 2019;23:2331216519836624. https://doi.org/10.1177/2331216519836624.
49. van As JW, van den Berg H, van Dalen EC. Medical interventions for the prevention of platinum-induced hearing loss in children with cancer. Cochrane Database Syst Rev. 2019;5(5):CD009219. https://doi.org/10.1002/14651858.CD009219.pub5.

50. Clemens E, van den Heuvel-Eibrink MM, Mulder RL, Kremer LCM, Hudson MM, Skinner R, et al. Recommendations for ototoxicity surveillance for childhood, adolescent, and young adult cancer survivors: a report from the International Late Effects of Childhood Cancer Guideline Harmonization Group in collaboration with the PanCare Consortium. Lancet Oncol. 2019;20(1):e29–41. https://doi.org/10.1016/s1470-2045(18)30858-1.
51. Blankenship CM, Hunter LL, Feeney MP, Cox M, Bittinger L, Garinis AC, et al. Functional impacts of aminoglycoside treatment on speech perception and extended high-frequency hearing loss in a pediatric cystic fibrosis cohort. Am J Audiol. 2021;30:834. https://doi.org/10.1044/2020_aja-20-00059.
52. Vijayasingam A, Frost E, Wilkins J, Gillen L, Premachandra P, McLaren K, et al. Tablet and web-based audiometry to screen for hearing loss in adults with cystic fibrosis. Thorax. 2020;75(8):632–9. https://doi.org/10.1136/thoraxjnl-2019-214177.
53. Meijer AJM, Fiocco MF, Janssens GO, Clemens E, Tissing WJE, Loonen JJ, et al. Risk factors associated with tinnitus in 2948 Dutch survivors of childhood cancer: a Dutch LATER questionnaire study. Neurooncol Adv. 2020;2(1):vdaa122. https://doi.org/10.1093/noajnl/vdaa122.
54. Meijer AJM, Clemens E, Hoetink AE, van Grotel M, van den Heuvel-Eibrink MM. Tinnitus during and after childhood cancer: a systematic review. Crit Rev Oncol Hematol. 2019;135:1–7. https://doi.org/10.1016/j.critrevonc.2019.01.004.
55. Weiss A, Sommer G, Kasteler R, Scheinemann K, Grotzer M, Kompis M, et al. Long-term auditory complications after childhood cancer: a report from the Swiss Childhood Cancer Survivor Study. Pediatr Blood Cancer. 2017;64(2):364–73. https://doi.org/10.1002/pbc.26212.
56. Baguley D. Mechanisms of tinnitus. Br Med Bull. 2002;63:195–212.
57. le Clercq CMP, van Ingen G, Ruytjens L, van der Schroeff MP. Music-induced hearing loss in children, adolescents, and young adults: a systematic review and meta-analysis. Otol Neurotol. 2016;37(9):1208–16. https://doi.org/10.1097/MAO.0000000000001163.
58. Kim SY, Jeon YJ, Lee JY, Kim YH. Characteristics of tinnitus in adolescents and association with psychoemotional factors. Laryngoscope. 2017;127(9):2113–9. https://doi.org/10.1002/lary.26334.
59. Rosing SN, Kapandais A, Schmidt J, Baguley D. Demographic data, referral patterns and interventions used for children and adolescents with tinnitus and hyperacusis in Denmark. Int J Pediatr Otorhinolaryngol. 2016;89:112–20. https://doi.org/10.1016/j.ijporl.2016.07.036.
60. Kentish RC, Crocker SR, McKenna L. Children's experience of tinnitus: a preliminary survey of children presenting to a psychology department. Br J Audiol. 2000;34(6):335–40.
61. El-Shunnar SK, Hoare DJ, Smith S, Gander PE, Kang S, Fackrell K, et al. Primary care for tinnitus: practice and opinion among GPs in England. J Eval Clin Pract. 2011;17(4):684–92. https://doi.org/10.1111/j.1365-2753.2011.01696.x.
62. Bartnik G. Managing tinnitus in adults: audiological strategies. In: Baguley D, Fagelson M, editors. Tinnitus: clinical and research perspectives. San Diego: Plural Publishing, Incorporated; 2015. p. 287–308.
63. Kentish RC, Crocker SR. Scary monsters and waterfalls: tinnitus narrative therapy for children. In: Tyler RS, editor. Tinnitus treatment: clinical protocols. New York: Thieme Medical Publishers, Incorporated; 2005. p. 217–29.
64. Raj-Koziak D, Bieńkowska K, Gos E, Włodarczyk E, Skarżyński H, Skarżyński PH. Audiological and psychological profiles of children with tinnitus. Hear Balance Commun. 2020;18(2):90–7. https://doi.org/10.1080/21695717.2019.1692590.
65. Smith H, Fackrell K, Kennedy V, Barry J, Partridge L, Hoare DJ. A scoping review to catalogue tinnitus problems in children. Int J Pediatr Otorhinolaryngol. 2019;122:141–51. https://doi.org/10.1016/j.ijporl.2019.04.006.
66. Weller D, Hobbs SD, Goodman GS. Challenges and innovations in research on childhood. In: Melton G, Ben-Arieh A, Cashmore J, Goodman GS, Worley NK, editors. The SAGE handbook of child research. London: SAGE Publications Ltd.; 2014. p. 363–70. https://doi.org/10.4135/9781446294758. http://sk.sagepub.com/reference/handbook-of-research-with-children.
67. Audiology BSo. Tinnitus in children: practice guidance; 2015.
68. Martin K, Snashall S. Children presenting with tinnitus: a retrospective study. Br J Audiol. 1994;28(2):111–5.
69. Chan KH, Jensen EL, Gao D. Pediatric tinnitus: a clinical perspective. Laryngoscope. 2018;128(3):727–31. https://doi.org/10.1002/lary.26851.
70. Båsjö S, Möller C, Widén S, Jutengren G, Kähäri K. Hearing thresholds, tinnitus, and headphone listening habits in nine-year-old children. Int J Audiol. 2016;55:587. https://doi.org/10.1080/14992027.2016.1190871.
71. Kennedy V, Kentish RC, Benton C, Munro C, Phillips J, Rogers C, et al. Paediatric tinnitus: the unmet clinical need. Int J Audiol. 2016;55:599. https://doi.org/10.1080/14992027.2016.1190467.
72. Smith H, Fackrell K, Kennedy V, Barry JG, Broomhead E, Hoare DJ. An evaluation of paediatric tinnitus services in UK National Health Service audiology departments. BMC Health Serv Res. 2020;20(1):214–1. https://doi.org/10.1186/s12913-020-5040-y.
73. Emond A, Kentish RC. Tinnitus counselling with children. Audacity. 2013;2:26–9.
74. McKenna L, Baguley D, McFerran D. Living with tinnitus and hyperacusis, vol Book, Whole. London: Sheldon; 2010.
75. Kentish RC. Tinnitus in children: practice guidance. Reading: British Society of Audiology; 2015.
76. Dullaart MJ, Kip M, Smit AL, Stegeman I. Treatment of tinnitus in children—a systematic review. Front Neurol. 2021;12:726803. https://doi.org/10.3389/fneur.2021.726803.
77. Danske Tale H-S. Vejledning for udredning af tinnitus og hyperakusis. Vejledninger i udredning Vol 1. S.l. Danske Tale-Høre-Synsinstitutioner: eksp. Center for Hjælpemidler og Kommunikation; 2007. p. 139 sider.
78. Bartnik G, Stepien A, Raj-Koziak D, Fabijanska A, Niedzialek I, Skarzynski H. Troublesome tinnitus in children: epidemiology, audiological profile, and preliminary results of treatment. Int J Pediatr. 2012;2012:945356. https://doi.org/10.1155/2012/945356.
79. Bae S-C, Park S-N, Park J-M, Kim M, Yeo S-W, Park S-Y. Childhood tinnitus: clinical characteristics and treatment. Am J Otolaryngol. 2014;35(2):207–10. https://doi.org/10.1016/j.amjoto.2013.10.003.
80. Tegg-Quinn S, Bennett RJ, Brennan-Jones CG, Barabash S, Mulders WHAM, Eikelboom RH. Reflections and perceptions of chronic tinnitus during childhood and adolescence. Int J Pediatr Otorhinolaryngol. 2020;138:110258. https://doi.org/10.1016/j.ijporl.2020.110258.
81. Tegg-Quinn S, Eikelboom RH, Brennan-Jones CG, Barabash S, Mulders WHAM, Bennett RJ. Reducing the impact of tinnitus on children and adolescents' lives: a mixed-methods concept mapping study. Int J Pediatr. 2021;2021:1–11. https://doi.org/10.1155/2021/5534192.

Pulsatile Tinnitus

40

Jae-Jin Song and Dirk De Ridder

Abstract

Pulsatile tinnitus (PT) is characterized by an auditory perception of pulse-synchronous sound. An alteration in the vascular hemodynamics causing turbulent flow, a vibration of a dehiscent vascular wall, or third window lesions are potential mechanisms of PT. Vascular PT can be subdivided into arterial, arteriovenous, and venous lesions. When the patient complains of psychoacoustic characteristics of PT, detailed physical examination and audiological evaluation complemented by etiology-targeted laboratory tests can provide diagnostic clues. Moreover, radiological evaluations such as brain magnetic resonance imaging (MRI) with angiography, temporal bone high-resolution computed tomography (CT), Doppler ultrasonography, and classical transfemoral cerebral angiography are recommended. Of various pathologies causing PT, dehiscence or diverticulum of the sigmoid sinus or jugular bulb is the most common cause that can be cured by surgical or interventional treatments. In addition, benign intracranial hypertension (BIH) is a common cause of PT. Although 15–50% of patients present with no definite diagnosis even after a meticulous diagnostic workup, the identification of the causal vascular pathology is vital for the optimal treatment of PT because successful surgical or interventional management is available in many cases.

J.-J. Song (✉)
Department of Otorhinolaryngology-Head & Neck Surgery, Seoul National University Bundang Hospital,
Seongnam, Republic of Korea
e-mail: jjsong96@snubh.org

D. De Ridder
Section of Neurosurgery, Department of Surgical Sciences,
University of Otago, Dunedin, New Zealand
e-mail: dirk.deridder@otago.ac.nz

W. Schlee et al. (eds.), *Textbook of Tinnitus*, https://doi.org/10.1007/978-3-031-35647-6_40

Graphical Abstract

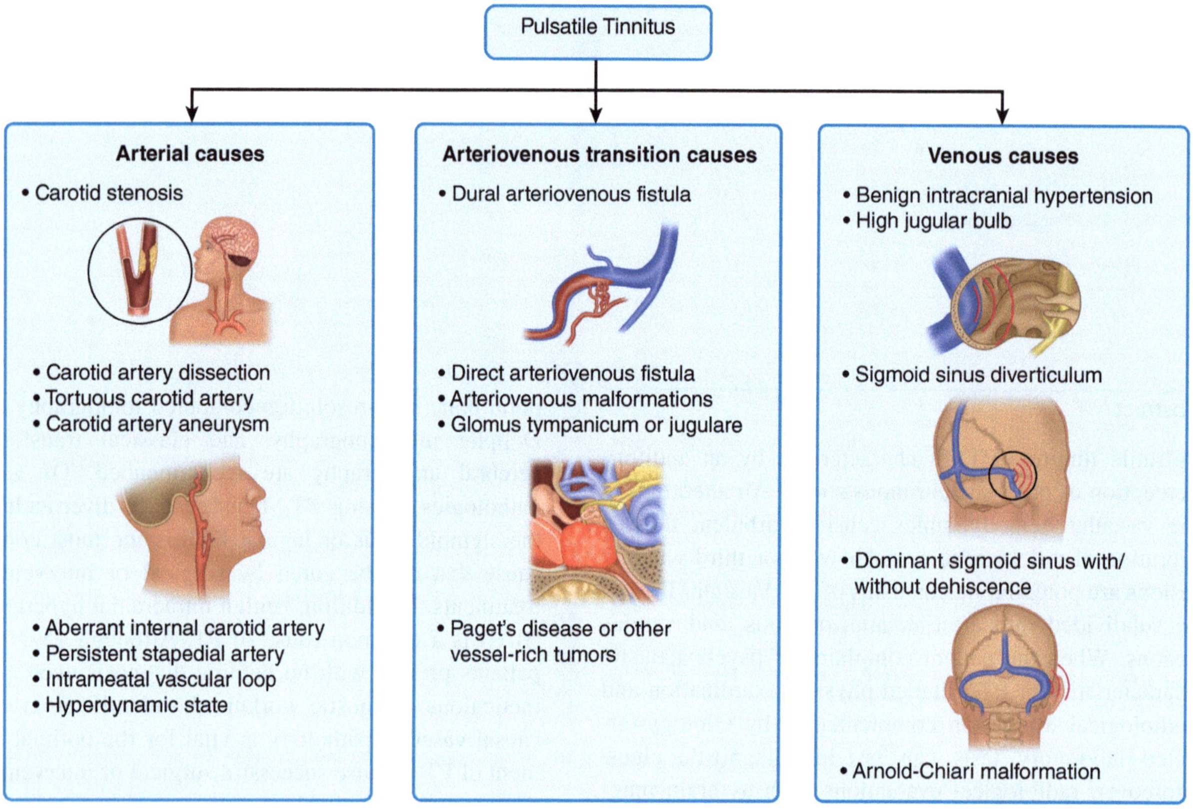

Abbreviations

AV	Arteriovenous
AVF	Arteriovenous fistula
AVM	Arteriovenous malformation
BIH	Benign intracranial hypertension
CSF	Cerebrospinal fluid
CT	Computed tomography
dAVF	Dural Arteriovenous fistula
DSA	Digital subtraction angiography
DSSD	Dominant sigmoid sinus with/without dehiscence
ICA	Internal carotid artery
LFHL	Low-frequency hearing loss
MRI	Magnetic resonance imaging
PT	Pulsatile tinnitus
SCDS	Semicircular canal dehiscence syndrome

Highlights

- Pulsatile tinnitus, in general, is not related to the pathology of the auditory system.
- Three types of vascular origins of pulsatile tinnitus exist: arterial, arteriovenous, and venous.
- The main causes of pulsatile tinnitus are related to aberrant/ectopic, stenosis, or other pathologies of the blood vessels, either arterial or venous.
  - Brain MRI with angiography, temporal bone high-resolution CT, Doppler ultrasonography, and classical transfemoral cerebral angiography are radiological diagnostic tools for pulsatile tinnitus.
- Dehiscence/diverticulum of the sigmoid sinus is a common surgically correctable cause of pulsatile tinnitus.
- Benign intracranial hypertension is a common cause of pulsatile tinnitus.
- In 15–50% of patients, no cause can be found for the pulsations.
- Pseudo-pulsatile tinnitus groups a number of muscle-related tinnitus types mimicking pulsatile tinnitus.

Introduction

Tinnitus can be subdivided in two entirely different entities: pulsatile and nonpulsatile tinnitus [1–3]. While nonpulsatile tinnitus, a far more common type of tinnitus encountered in outpatient clinics, is presumed to be caused by peripheral deafferentation-induced functional changes in the ascending auditory pathway, including the auditory and nonauditory cortices [4, 5] (see sections "Causes of Pulsatile Tinnitus" and "Diagnostic Workup in Subjects Presenting with Pulsatile Tinnitus"), pulsatile tinnitus (PT) represents only 4–10% of all types of tinnitus [6–8] and is mostly characterized by a perception of heartbeat-synchronous sound. PT is frequently equated with "objective tinnitus," since some cases of PT can be verified by an examiner [9, 10]. Objective tinnitus that is generated by muscle sounds due to myoclonus of the middle ear muscles or the palatal muscles may be termed "pseudo-pulsatile." This subgroup of PT is characterized by nonrhythmic salvo-like clicks that can be perceived in the affected ear. However, considering that only 20% of all PT cases are objectively detected by physicians [11], most cases of PT remain subjective, and, thus, PT is not equal to objectifiable tinnitus. In the remainder of this chapter, the term "PT" will be used to refer to all forms of tinnitus that are vascular in origin, whereas the term "pseudo-pulsatile" will be applied to those forms of tinnitus that are caused by pathological muscle contractions. Pulsatile tinnitus and pseudo-pulsatile tinnitus have been jointly called somatosounds, i.e., sounds that are generated by the body, and are picked up by the auditory system [12].

PT is characterized by an auditory perception of pulse-synchronous sound. It can be caused by pathologically altered blood flow in vessels in immediate or relatively close proximity to the ear. Major arteries supplying the brain (i.e., the common carotid artery or the internal carotid artery (ICA)) and major draining veins (the internal jugular vein, sigmoid sinus, or transverse sinus) may be involved in the perception of PT. Conversely, small vessels in the immediate proximity to the peripheral auditory structures can cause vibrations transmitted directly or via bone conduction or through the cerebrospinal fluid (CSF) (persistent stapedial artery) [13] or hypervascular tumors arising from blood vessels (glomus tympanicum or glomus jugulare tumors).

There are three potential mechanisms by which vascular wall anomalies may cause PT: (1) An alteration in the vascular hemodynamics may cause turbulent blood flow and lead to sound transmission [14, 15]. Examples of this PT would be vascular stenosis due to atherosclerosis or venous diverticulum. (2) A vibration of a dehiscent vascular wall even in the absence of turbulent flow may occur [16, 17]. Examples of this PT would be dehiscence of the bony wall of the sigmoid sinus or jugular bulb. (3) An abnormal sound perception may occur due to third window lesions in the inner ear [18, 19]. Identification of the causative vascular pathology and etiology-specific management are vital for the optimal treatment of PT patients because successful surgical or interventional management is available. In 50–85% of patients, a cause can be found for the auditory perceived pulsations [2, 20].

Causes of Pulsatile Tinnitus

Depending on the underlying vessels involved, the causes of PT can be subdivided into arterial, venous, or arteriovenous origins. Other causes such as superior semicircular canal dehiscence or pseudo-PT due to muscle contraction near the cochlea cannot be assigned to these three vascular origins (for an overview, see Table 40.1). Data on the incidence rates of these vascular origin entities vary markedly among authors [7] probably because radiologically abnormal-looking vascular structures cannot always be confirmed as a pathognomonic sign of PT. This will be further discussed in the "Radiological Evaluations" section below.

Arterial Causes

Carotid Stenosis

Carotid stenosis is a common cause [1–3] of arterial PT. The most common cause is atherosclerotic disease [21, 22].

Table 40.1 Causes of pulsatile tinnitus

Location	Causative lesions
Arterial	Carotid stenosis
	Carotid or vertebral artery dissection
	Carotid artery aneurysm
	Aberrant internal carotid artery
	Persistent stapedial artery
	Intrameatal vascular loop
	Benign intracranial hypertension
	Hyperdynamic state (anemia, thyrotoxicosis, pregnancy, etc.)
Arteriovenous transition	Dural arteriovenous fistula
	Direct arteriovenous fistula (i.e., carotid-cavernous)
	Arteriovenous malformations
	Glomus tympanicum or jugulare
	Paget's disease or other vessel-rich tumors
Venous	Benign intracranial hypertension
	High jugular bulb with/without dehiscence
	Sigmoid sinus diverticulum
	Dominant sigmoid sinus with/without dehiscence
	Arnold-Chiari malformation
Others	Semicircular canal dehiscence syndrome
	Pseudo-pulsatile tinnitus

Higher-grade carotid stenosis can result in turbulent blood flow that may give rise to PT as the initial manifestation of disease [22]. Moreover, complete occlusion of the carotid artery may present with contralateral PT because this results in compensatory flow acceleration in the carotid vessel on the opposite side [7]. Similarly, a hypoplastic basilar artery can result in a compensatory hyperdynamic flow in both carotid arteries, clinically presenting as bilateral arterial pulse-synchronous tinnitus [23].

PT due to carotid stenosis typically disappears when compressing the ipsilateral, internal, or common carotid artery. The diagnosis can be confirmed by Doppler sonography, magnetic resonance imaging (MRI), computed tomography (CT), or classical angiography. Treatment of the extracranial carotid artery stenosis includes endovascular stenting, dilation, or carotid endarterectomy. Carotid endarterectomy for PT has been reported to be effective in reducing or abolishing tinnitus in more than 90%. Proximal lesions lend themselves to carotid endarterectomy, whereas distal lesions have been treated by stenting [24]. For the rarer intracranial carotid artery stenosis, ligation of the symptomatic carotid artery after a balloon occlusion test or dilation and stenting of the intracranial portion of the carotid artery has been introduced. Overall, almost 70% of patients with carotid stenosis are cured by intervention, and up to 90% of these patients experience immediately abated symptoms [24].

A stenotic subclavian artery can also generate a treatable form of arterial PT [25]. Reversal of blood flow in an aberrant occipital artery can also cause PT, and this condition can also be treated by stenting [26]. Additionally, hyperdynamic flow in the internal carotid artery can present with PT, as seen in basilar artery atresia with predominant flow in both carotids [23].

Carotid Artery Dissection

Cervical carotid dissection is a relatively common condition. Most dissections may arise spontaneously or as a consequence of activities that cause a sudden stretch of the pharyngeal portion of the carotid artery. Traumatic carotid dissections occur in 1% of all patients with blunt injury [27]. The symptom triad of carotid artery dissection comprises acute head and neck pain, Horner's syndrome, and PT. Others may present with transient or persistent brain ischemia. Strokes are due to the migration of thrombus material originating from the dissected arterial lumen, resulting in an embolism of the intracranial arteries, most often the middle cerebral artery [28]. While less than 10% of the patients are asymptomatic, more than 90% of patients with carotid dissection present with local signs and symptoms on the side of dissection such as headache (65–68%), facial pain (34–53%), or neck pain (9–26%) as well as Horner's syndrome (28–41%) and cranial nerve palsy (8–16%). The hypoglossal nerve is most commonly involved, but the facial nerve, ocular motor nerves (III, IV, and VI), and trigeminal nerve may also be involved. An ischemic event such as ischemic stroke, transient ischemic attack, or ischemic optic neuropathy occurs in about 75% of subjects with carotid dissection [29].

The treatment of dissections in the territory supplied by the internal carotid or vertebral artery depends on the extent of the vascular pathology and the accompanying clinical features. Treatment includes anticoagulants or antiplatelet agents, and healing occurs within 3–6 months with a resolution of stenosis in 90% of patients and recanalization of occlusions in as many as 50% [27]. Endovascular interventions or open neurovascular surgery are also indicated in some cases.

Tortuous Carotid Artery

Turbulent blood flow can also be caused by a tortuous siphon-like extracranial internal carotid artery, leading to highly distressing ipsilateral heartbeat-synchronous pulsatile tinnitus [30]. Considering that a tortuous carotid is relatively common, it is important to know whether the tortuous artery is causing the PT. Using an intra-arterial balloon dilatation resulting in a transient, reversible, vascular occlusion distal to the siphon-like anomaly should diagnostically reduce the arterial pulsations. Subsequently, surgery can performed using Teflon as an external construct to straighten the siphon-like anomaly [30].

Carotid Artery Aneurysm

Aneurysms of the petrous carotid artery can lead to PT [31–35]. This may be caused by the aneurysm obliterating the pericarotid venous plexus, allowing the arterial pulsations to be directly transmitted to the cochlea and resulting in the perception of the arterial pulsations. However, this is not the only mechanism involved, as aneurysms of the anterior communicating artery are also related to PT [36]. Notably, PT due to aneurysms of the internal carotid artery or its branches are relatively rare [37]. A suggested mechanism of this phenomenon is the dampening effect of a peri-carotid venous plexus [23, 38].

Aberrant Internal Carotid Artery

Aberrant internal carotid arteries have also been implicated in arterial PT [16]. It is generally accepted that an aberrant internal carotid artery creates a collateral pathway resulting from agenesis of the first embryonic segment of the internal carotid artery. Instead, the inferior tympanic artery (a branch of the ascending pharyngeal artery) enlarges, communicates with the caroticotympanic artery, and resumes the usual course of the internal carotid artery in the horizontal portion of the petrous carotid canal. The aberrant carotid artery may be dehiscent and visible through the tympanic membrane as it courses through the middle ear [39].

Successful surgical treatments, including separation of the tympanic membrane from the aberrant internal carotid artery [40] or reinforcement of the dehiscent carotid canal using a piece of tragal cartilage under a microscope or an endoscope [41, 42], have been reported for the treatment of PT in subjects with an aberrant internal carotid artery.

Persistent Stapedial Artery

A persistent stapedial artery is a rare vascular anomaly, with an estimated prevalence of 0.02–0.5% [43]. It is a normal fetal artery that ordinarily disappears before birth. If it persists after birth, it can cause PT. The persistent stapedial artery runs through the obturator foramen between the crura of the stapes and across the promontory in the middle ear, leaving the middle ear to run along the tympanic portion of the facial nerve canal near the geniculate fossa. The two most common symptoms of the persistent stapedial artery are conductive hearing loss and PT. While conductive hearing loss may result from ossicular dampening caused by the traversing persistent stapedial artery or by a concomitant malformation of the stapes suprastructure [44], PT may develop due to sound transmission to the cochlea and potentially by transmission of pulsations via the stapes, where the persistent stapedial artery may abut the stapedial crura [44]. A recent systemic review has indicated that PT subsided after transection of the persistent stapedial artery [45].

Intrameatal Vascular Loop

Microvascular compressions of the cochlear nerve can cause incapacitating pulsatile or non-PT [46, 47] (see Chap. 35). Studies have shown that abnormal vascular loops around the internal auditory canal are encountered far more often in patients with PT than in patients with nonpulsatile tinnitus [48, 49]. Pathophysiologically, the sharp turn of the vascular loop in the triangular internal auditory canal creates a turbulence and thus creates concentrically irradiating sound waves. The internal auditory canal has a cave or funnel effect guiding the sound wave toward its end—the top of the triangle where the cochlea is located. The sounds waves at the CSF–bone interface are transferred to the cochlea via bone conduction, and, thus, one can perceive pulsatile tinnitus. However, physicians should keep in mind that unrelated nonpulsatile tinnitus is present in the majority of cases in which microvascular compression is detected by MRI scans. Instead, typewriter tinnitus, characterized by paroxysmal and clustered attacks of “staccato” sounds and excellent responses to carbamazepine treatment, presents in most cases of microvascular compression of the auditory nerve by the anterior inferior cerebellar artery [50, 51]. This is similar to other disorders of microvascular compressions of the cranial nerve roots, such as trigeminal neuralgia, hemifacial spasm, and vestibular paroxysmia. The diagnosis of microvascular compression in individuals with tinnitus is based on the clinical feature, auditory brainstem responses, MRI findings suggesting neurovascular compression, and clinical responses to carbamazepine [50–55]. However, if the vascular loop extends into the internal auditory meatus, it can cause arterial pulse-synchronous tinnitus via CSF/bone conduction [23, 49]. As in cases of typewriter tinnitus managed by microvascular decompression [56], placement of a Teflon felt between the vascular loop and the nerve (microvascular decompression) can abolish PT due to intrameatal vascular loops [23].

In a similar manner, an aberrant artery that crosses the mastoid may result in PT. Pulsations are transmitted via the bone conduction route due to the direct contact of the vascular and mastoid surface and are treated by ligation of the aberrant artery [57].

Hyperdynamic State (Anemia, Thyrotoxicosis, Pregnancy, Etc.)

PT can even be perceived in subjects without vascular pathologies in cases of a hyperdynamic blood flow, as in anemia, thyrotoxicosis, high blood pressure, or pregnancy. Anemia has been suggested to be an important cause of nonvascular PT as early as the 1970s [58]. In a recent study, the initial hemoglobin level of subjects with PT has been found to be significantly higher than those with nonpulsatile tinnitus [59]. Moreover, differences between initial and posttreatment hemoglobin levels were significantly associated with a subjective improvement with regard to PT [59]. The hyperdynamic blood flow may also result from arterial hypertension [60]. Thyrotoxicosis or pregnancy can also present with PT due to increased cardiac output [7, 61], and a correction of these underlying medical conditions can abate the symptom.

Arteriovenous Transition Causes

The patient experiences pulse-synchronous tinnitus with various arteriovenous transition etiologies. In subjects with arteriovenous etiologies, a presumed diagnosis can frequently be made during the physical examination at the outpatient clinic. Moreover, the pulsatile sound can be objectively detected by the examiner by auscultation in subjects with arteriovenous etiologies with an above-average chance [7].

Dural Arteriovenous Fistula (dAVF)

An intracranial dural arteriovenous fistula (dAVF) is one of the most common causes of arteriovenous pulse-synchronous tinnitus [31, 32]. A dAVF indicates an abnormal direct connection between the dural arteries and dural veins or a venous sinus, accounting for 10–15% of intracranial arteriovenous malformations (AVMs) [62, 63]. The etiopathogenesis ranges from postinfectious complications (e.g., after mastoiditis +/– sinus vein thrombosis) to post-traumatic changes (e.g., after a skull fracture) to complications after surgical interventions with craniotomy and opening of the dura. PT is often the sole initial symptom of a dAVF, but a high index of suspicion and an appropriate evaluation are essential. In a recent single center study, 30 of 220 patients (13.6%) who were diagnosed with a dAVF have presented with only PT as their initial symptom [64]. In this case series, the transverse–sigmoid sinus junction (70.0%) was the most common site, followed by the hypoglossal canal (10.0%) and the middle cranial fossa (6.7%) on radiological evaluation [64]. It is noteworthy that a dAVF of the transverse–sigmoid sinus can be suspected by auscultation of the mastoid area, and, thus, physicians should not forget to include auscultation of the mastoid area when evaluating subjects with PT at outpatient clinics. Cross-sectional images using contrast-enhanced temporal bone computed tomography and brain MRI with angiography provide useful information for the diagnosis of a dAVF, but, for a complete characterization and classification of a dAVF, classic transfemoral cerebral angiography should be performed [65]. In the same session, transarterial embolization (coils, glue, adhesives) of the fistula can cure or abate PT in more than 90% of the patients with a dAVF [64]. Moreover, studies on stereotactic radiosurgery have reported relatively good outcomes, with a complete occlusion rate of 44–87% without major complications [65, 66]. If intractable with endovascular or radiosurgical treatment, surgical excision of the dAVF and dura can be proposed [67–69]. The cure rate of surgical elimination of the dAVF has been reported to be nearly 100%, but the risk of transient and permanent morbidity remains up to 10% [65, 70].

Direct Arteriovenous Fistula (I.E., Carotid-Cavernous Fistula)

Sagittal sinus arteriovenous fistulas (AVFs) [71] and carotid-cavernous fistulas can generate PT as well, which disappears after embolization or gamma knife surgery. Either a spontaneous [72] or a post-traumatic [73] carotid-cavernous fistula can present with PT. When properly diagnosed, endovascular treatment with coiling of the cavernous sinus in combination with application of an embolic agent can ameliorate PT in most cases. In this regard, physicians should always evaluate any combined ophthalmological symptoms such as bulging eyes, deteriorating vision, and other signs or symptoms of cranial nerve palsy in subjects with PT to rule out carotid-cavernous fistulas.

Arteriovenous Malformations

Arteriovenous malformations (AVMs) are generally congenital. There are two types of AVMs with regard to the flow rate: fast-flowing and slow-flowing [74]. Most of the fast-flowing lesions are arteriovenous fistulas, whereas slow-flow AVMs are produced by venous, capillary, or lymphatic lesions [74]. Rare examples of AVMs associated with PT have been described in areas such as the external auditory canal and auricle [38, 75, 76], hypoglossal canal [77], and even the parotid gland [78]. The most common symptoms are pulsation of the mass or PT (51.2%), bleeding (41.5%), and pain (29.3%) [79]. The management options for AVMs include observation, embolization, mass excision, or resection of the involved area [76].

Glomus Tympanicum or Glomus Jugulare Tumors

Glomus tumors, also known as paragangliomas, are usually benign space-occupying lesions arising from an autonomic ganglion in direct proximity to the vessels and nerves. Glomus jugulare tumors originating from the parasympathetic ganglion in the jugular fossa and glomus tympanicum tumors arising from the cochlear promontory along the course of Jacobson's nerve are both characterized by the typical initial symptoms of unilateral hearing loss and PT. In particular, glomus tympanicum most commonly presents with PT (50–80%) and hearing loss (30–60%) [80]. Non-contrast computed tomography supported by temporal bone MRI and/or angiography of the temporal bone is critical to distinguish glomus tympanicum from glomus jugulare tumors and aids operative planning [80]. In contrast to visceral paragangliomas, head and neck paragangliomas are rarely (<4%) secretory [81, 82]. On otoendoscopic or otomicroscopic examination, glomus tympanicum tumors are always observed with a reddish, vascular-appearing mass in the inferior aspect of the mesotympanum. Glomus jugulare tumors, however, can only be observed through the tympanic membrane if the tumor grows into the tympanic cavity. In cases in which the tumor reaches the tympanic membrane, a pulse-synchronous movement of the eardrum can be observed.

Glomus tympanicum tumors presenting with PT and/or hearing loss can be removed via microscopic [83] or endoscopic [84, 85] surgical approaches. Approximately 40% of glomus jugulare tumors were reported to grow at an average of 0.9 mm per year, and no significant change in cranial nerve function was seen for most patients during more than 5 years of follow-up period. Treatment options are either a "wait-and-scan" policy or embolization and surgery [81]. If the tinnitus is incapacitating, then the embolization with surgery option can be helpful in terms of complete abolition of the tinnitus. Moreover, irradiation can reduce the vascularity responsible for the PT. In a recent report with a relatively large case series, management of glomus jugulare tumors with a conservative approach has been safe and effective with a low rate of new lower cranial nerve deficit [82]. However, the therapy with regard to an active or passive approach depends on various criteria, such as the tumor size, the dynamics of tumor growth, the age and general health of the patient, and the expected rehabilitation ability of the patient.

Paget's Disease or Other Vessel-Rich Tumors

Subjects with Paget's disease can present with PT when the temporal bone is involved [86, 87]. The presence of PT may reflect the presence of vascular channels and shunts that are created in the remodeled, hypervascular bone [87].

Other vessel-rich tumors of the petrous bone or skull base such as plasmacytoma [88], hemangiopericytoma [89], neuroendocrine carcinoma [90], and giant cell tumor [91] are also known to present with PT. Neurotological surgical management or combined chemoradiation are treatment options for these tumors.

Venous Causes

PT due to venous causes are often not pulse-synchronous. Triggering of venous PT may depend on several factors: respiratory rate, venous pulsations, and the transmission of nearby arterial flow sounds to the veins [6, 38]. One major difference compared with arterial or arteriovenous PT is that venous PT can be temporarily abated while compressing the affected side of the neck (causing transient occlusion of the internal jugular vein) or rotating the neck to the affected side. With the use of an ultrasound device, the compression of the vein can also be checked visually. If there are no other venous anomalies elsewhere, then venous PT tends to be perceived more on the right than on the left side because the right venous system generally develops as dominant [92–94].

Benign Intracranial Hypertension (BIH)

Benign intracranial hypertension (BIH), also known as pseudotumor cerebri or idiopathic intracranial hypertension [95], is another possible cause of PT. While some researchers have reported that 40% of the individuals they studied with PT were diagnosed with BIH [2] and about 60% of all patients with BIH report PT [96], others found that only 2% of the individuals with BIH had PT [16]. BIH afflicts young, overweight women almost exclusively [95, 97]. Clinical symptoms include arterial PT, venous hum, headache, and blurred vision. Patients with BIH can also present with ear fullness, low-frequency hearing loss (LFHL), and vertigo [1, 2, 95]. Uniquely, PT presents unilaterally in 80% of cases and can be the only symptom of BIH [2]. PT may become more prominent by maneuvers raising intracranial pressure such as the Valsalva maneuver, bending over, or coughing but may disappear temporarily by compressing the ipsilateral jugular vein. About half of all individuals with BIH may present with pseudo-low-frequency sensorineural hearing loss due to the masking effect of the pulsatile sound [98].

Ocular fundoscopy to evaluate the presence of papilledema [95, 97], and MRI with angiography to rule out empty sella as a result of pressure-induced prolapse of CSF-filled arachnoid through the diaphragma sellae, can help with the diagnosis [2]. In particular, an empty sella in a patient with PT raises suspicion of BIH as a possible result of prolonged intracranial pressure elevation. Moreover, spontaneous cerebrospinal fluid leak should be considered a sign of possible intracranial hypertension and needs surgical repair when it occurs [99]. A diagnosis is usually confirmed by lumbar puncture (opening pressure >20 cm water). Treatment consists of weight loss, diuretics, or ventriculoperitoneal or lumboperitoneal shunting. Endovascular stenting for more severe narrowing of the transverse sinus has been successfully used as an interventional treatment modality [100]. The response rate to therapy with regard to PT is reported to be high, in particular by the use of invasive treatment modalities [100, 101].

High Jugular Bulb

A jugular bulb is a vascular structure connecting the sigmoid sinus and the internal jugular vein. The most common anatomic variation of the jugular bulb in the temporal bone is a high jugular bulb [102]. Although a high jugular bulb with/without dehiscence rarely presents with otologic symptoms, it is primarily of concern as a cause of PT. Focal turbulent flow in the jugular bulb caused by increased irregularity of, or asymmetry in, vessel diameter may lead to the disruption of local laminar flow, and this can be delivered to the cochlea directly or via bone conduction [103] (Fig. 40.1a). It has been reported that jugular bulb abnormality on the right side accounts for approximately 80% of all cases, and PT mostly presents on the right side [92, 103, 104]. When the high bulb is dehiscent, it can be seen as a bluish mass in the hypotympanum on otomicroscopy [103], in contrast to the reddish mass in the anterior middle ear, which suggests a dehiscent/aberrant carotid artery [105]. A high jugular bulb with/without dehiscence can be diagnosed by temporal bone CT imaging.

Transtympanic middle ear floor resurfacing using autologous materials such as bone dust, temporalis fascia, and tragal cartilage [106] or bone cement [103, 107] has been reported to be effective in controlling PT in subjects with a high jugular bulb with dehiscence (Fig. 40.1b). Transvenous stent-assisted coil embolization for a dehiscent high jugular bulb could also demonstrate successful results [108]. One thing surgeons should keep in mind is that a surgical repair of a high jugular bulb with dehiscence does not always guarantee successful control of PT because a high jugular bulb with/without dehiscence is asymptomatic in most cases as mentioned above. Therefore, before planning surgical/inter-

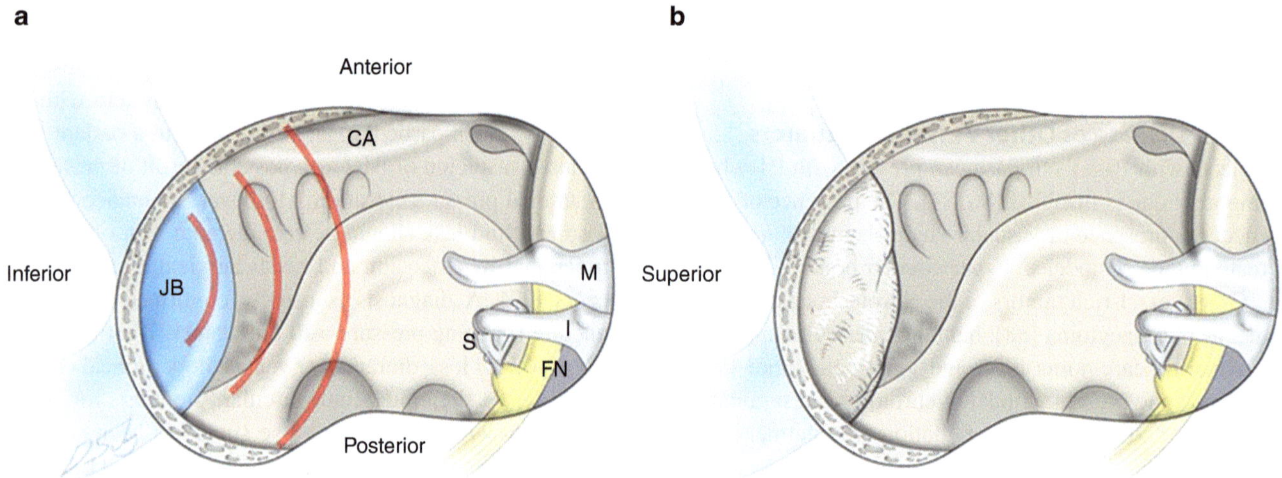

Fig. 40.1 A schematic illustration of the transtympanic jugular bulb resurfacing procedure. The tympanic membrane attached to the malleus is removed in this figure to better visualize the middle ear. (**a**) The middle ear cavity and the dehiscent portion of the jugular bulb are widely exposed via a transtympanic approach by elevating the tympanomeatal flap and then widening the tympanic annulus by drilling the posteroinferior meatal wall. (**b**) The dehiscent portion of the jugular bulb is first covered with a piece of temporalis muscle fascia and then extraluminal placement of bone cement is performed. *JB* jugular bulb, *CA* carotid artery, *M* malleus, *I* incus, *S* stapes, *FN* facial nerve

ventional treatment, a thorough clinical and radiological evaluation of the patient to rule out other possible causes of PT should be performed and treatment for the high jugular bulb should be decided only if it the jugular bulb is clinically and radiologically the cause of PT.

Sigmoid Sinus Diverticulum

Unilateral sigmoid sinus diverticulum has been reported to be found in 1.2% of asymptomatic subjects [8]; however, more than 20% of patients with PT of a clinically suspected venous origin had unilateral sigmoid sinus diverticulum confirmed by temporal bone computed tomographic angiography [8, 109]. Acute pressure erosion or congenital defect of the bony wall of the sigmoid sinus is unlikely because the sigmoid sinus is a low venous pressure system; additionally, in most cases reported, PT developed in the ear in late middle age [109–111]. When the diverticulum develops, focal vigorous turbulence of the blood flow may be generated (Fig. 40.2a, b, the cross-sectional view on the lower right side), and the sound energy from the turbulence may be conducted to the cochlea both via air and bone conduction through the adjacent bony structures or soft tissue. In most cases, sigmoid sinus diverticulum develops in a well-pneumatized mastoid cavity [110, 112].

To manage PT due to sigmoid sinus diverticulum, an external compression of the diverticulum and resurfacing of the bony wall via the transmastoid approach enable reduction of the diverticulum back to the surrounding normal sigmoid sinus and reinforce the bony wall of the venous sinus (Fig. 40.2c, d). Autologous material or bone cement is used and should lead to normalization of the focal turbulent flow [94, 112]. Due to the possibility of recurrence of the diverticulum, bone cement has been suggested to be advantageous over autologous material [94, 112]. In a recent case series, an intraoperative color-coded Doppler examination and extraluminal compression even under local anesthesia have shown successful symptom control rates in PT subjects with sigmoid sinus diverticulum [113]. Moreover, endovascular coiling for occlusion of the diverticulum successfully abates PT immediately after the procedure [114, 115].

Dominant Sigmoid Sinus with/Without Dehiscence (DSSD)

Along with sigmoid sinus diverticulum, a dominant sigmoid sinus with/without dehiscence (DSSD) is one of the most common identifiable vascular abnormalities causing vascular PT, occurring in approximately 18% of patients with PT [17, 111]. Therefore, DSSD and sigmoid sinus diverticulum may be the most common surgically correctable causes of PT. However, as in PT subjects with a high jugular bulb with/without dehiscence, a thorough investigation of other identifiable causes of PT should be conducted before deciding treatment options because asymptomatic DSSD can frequently be found and surgical management of non-pathognomonic DSSD cannot abate the symptom [116]. As in sigmoid sinus diverticulum, DSSD develops frequently on the right side. According to Poiseuille's law [117], an increased volumetric flow rate, indirectly proportional to the fourth power of the radius of the dominant venous system, may increase the likelihood of turbulent blood flow in the sigmoid sinus. In addition, an upstream stenosis has also

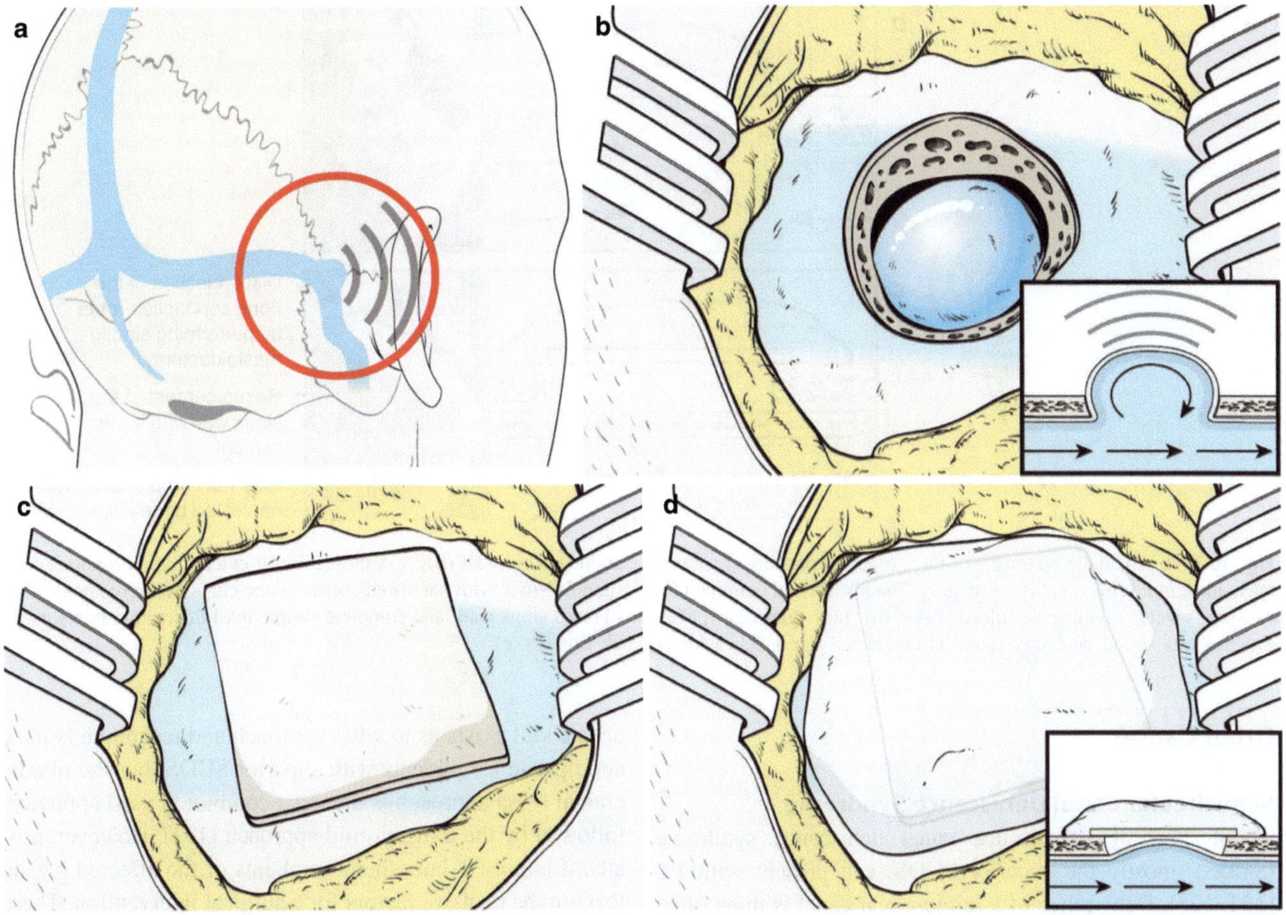

Fig. 40.2 Proposed pathophysiological mechanism of the development of a diverticulum and pulsatile tinnitus perception and symptom improvement after intervention in patients with sigmoid sinus diverticulum. (**a**) Development of a diverticulum usually in or adjacent to the region of the transverse–sigmoid sinus junction. (**b**) Surgically exposed diverticulum (bigger figure) and focal vigorous turbulence of the blood flow (the cross-sectional image on the lower right side) resulting in conduction of sound energy from the diverticulum to the middle ear through the adjacent bony structure or soft tissue. (**c**) External compression of the diverticulum with a harvested cortical bone chip and (**d**) resurfacing of the bony wall with bone cement, reducing the diverticulum back to the surrounding normal sigmoid sinus (SS) to abate focal turbulent flow

been suggested to be associated with the generation of PT in patients with DSSD [17], as the upstream stenosis-induced high jet flow may contribute to an increased irregularity or asymmetry of the sigmoid sinus. Hemodynamic change-induced turbulent flow may elicit the disruption of local laminar flow and continuous outward pressure, leading to focal dehiscence over the sigmoid sinus bony wall (Fig. 40.3a). A recent computational modeling study has supported this mechanism by demonstrating strong components of the rotational blood flow in the venous outflow tract in DSSD [118].

Surgical treatment by reshaping the sigmoid sinus itself and reinforcing the bony sigmoid sinus wall is the mainstay of treatment when the symptom is debilitating [94, 119] (Fig. 40.3b, c). As mentioned above, a relatively nonsignificant dominance of the ipsilesional sigmoid sinus should be ruled out to select appropriate surgical candidates. In addition, studies suggest that maintaining the normal diameter of the sigmoid sinus during surgery is imperative [120, 121] so as to not cause increased intracranial pressure-related postoperative complications. Therefore, the external compression of the sigmoid sinus using bone cement should be preceded by a thorough preoperative evaluation of the vascular anatomy to assess contralateral outflow and collateral flow [94].

Arnold-Chiari Malformation

The Arnold-Chiari malformation is a clinical entity in which there is a tonsillar herniation in the foramen magnum. A total of 7–10% of individuals with Arnold-Chiari malformations complain of either nonpulsatile or pulsatile tinnitus [122, 123]. PT most commonly consists of a venous hum, likely caused by raised intracranial pressure since it worsens on bending over and on Valsalva maneuvers. The pulsations disappear transiently on ipsilateral jugular vein compression. After surgical decompression of individuals with Arnold-Chiari malformations, PT often disappears [123].

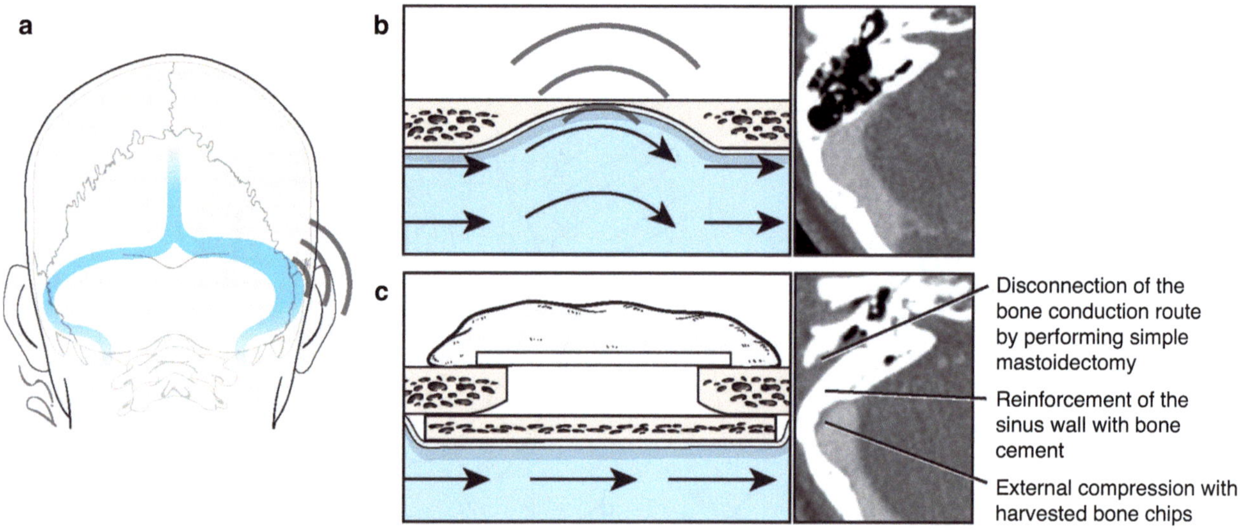

Fig. 40.3 A schematic summary of the surgical procedures of transmastoid sigmoid sinus-reshaping surgery. The ipsilesional dominant SS causing severe asymmetric blood flow (**a**) may generate pulse-synchronous sound, and this sound is conducted via a dehiscent or thinned bony wall (**b**). A combination of external compression of the sigmoid sinus with harvested cortical bone chips, reinforcement of the sigmoid sinus wall, and complete simple mastoidectomy quiets pulsatile tinnitus (**c**)

Other Causes

Semicircular Canal Dehiscence Syndrome

About 25% of semicircular canal dehiscence syndrome (SCDS), mostly the superior SCDS, can present with PT [124, 125]. Dehiscence of a semicircular canal is most often described for the superior canal [126], but posterior [127] and lateral [128] semicircular canal dehiscences have also been described. The most typical signs of canal dehiscence are autophony, ear fullness (94%) [129], and sound-induced vertigo (97%) (Tullio's phenomenon), followed by hyperacusis to somatosounds such as eye movements, head movements, and footsteps (39%). Pseudo-conductive hearing loss due to exaggerated bone conduction and impaired air conduction is also common. Most patients also suffer from chronic dizziness. In addition, most patients have sound- or Valsalva maneuver-evoked eye movements (oscillopsia) in the plane of the dehiscent canal. Tragal pressure evokes the nystagmus in 54% (Hennebert's sign), and one-fifth of patients show sound-evoked head movements. On laboratory examination, summating the potential to the action potential ratio measured by electrocochleography is significantly higher in the affected ear [130]. Both tympanometric examination and acoustic reflexes are normal. Cervical vestibular evoked myogenic potential (cVEMP) testing in patients with SCDS will often have responses with lower thresholds than in people without the syndrome. The definitive diagnosis is made by a high-resolution CT scan of the temporal bone. Treatment of symptomatic patients consists of surgical plugging (the better method) or resurfacing of the canal [125]. Considerable debate still exists as to what approach and technique is most appropriate for patients with superior SCDS, but the middle cranial fossa approach is the most commonly used approach, followed by the transmastoid approach [131]. However, usually, it is not PT but other complaints of the affected person that are the decisive factors for a surgical intervention. These are auditory hypersensitivity, disequilibrium, headache, and concentration difficulties [132].

Pseudo-Pulsatile Tinnitus

Several diseases such as palatal myoclonus [133], tensor tympani spasm [134, 135], stapedial muscle myoclonus [136], and a patulous eustachian tube [137] can cause non-vascular pulsatile tinnitus with a periodic nature. These pathologies generate neither arterial pulse-synchronous nor respiratory rate-synchronous tinnitus but tend to fluctuate in intensity (as in a stormy wind) or are perceived as rhythmic, salvo-like clicks.

The palatal myoclonus is often bilateral and caused by contractions of the peritubal muscles, especially the tensor veli palatini muscles [138]. It can be effectively treated by botulinum toxin injection into the peritubal muscles [139–141]. These injections can be administered under local spray anesthesia, ideally after palpation or even better under electromyographic control. The clinical effect can last up to 6 months. Therefore, repeated injections are usually necessary. Possible side effects are associated with movement disorders of the soft palate, which might cause hypernasality of the voice or nasal regurgitation of fluids during drinking [139–141].

Tensor tympani spasms and stapedial muscle contraction are called middle ear myoclonus. It generates rhythmic contractions (40–200 Hz) of the tympanic membrane synchronous with the rhythm of tinnitus. Middle ear myoclonus can be treated by sectioning of the tendons of both these muscles, resulting in an immediate improvement [140, 142, 143]. Alternatively, less invasive options are local administration of Botox to the respective muscles during tympanoscopy with soaked gel sponges. A systemic treatment for providing appropriate muscle relaxation is the administration of baclofen, carbamazepine, piracetam, orphenadrine, citrate, or benzodiazepines (clonazepam) [144]. However, this approach may be associated with significant side effects.

In subjects with a patulous eustachian tube and respiration-induced tinnitus, a systematic review with meta-analysis has demonstrated that intranasal corticosteroids are ineffective in chronic symptoms and the efficacy of nonsurgical options for patulous eustachian tube syndrome has yet to be determined [145]. Medical management improved subacute and chronic symptoms in 30–64% and 11–50% of cases, respectively [145]. However, different surgical procedures like mass loading of the tympanic membrane such as cartilage tympanoplasty, eustachian tube plugging, laser-assisted tuboplasty, and manipulation of eustachian tube musculature have been described [146]. A systematic review of surgical approaches for the management of a patulous eustachian tube demonstrates variable symptom improvement rates for the different treatments: ventilation tube insertion, 58%; mass loading of the tympanic membrane, 50%; eustachian tube injection, 47%; plug surgery, 81%; shim surgery, 62%; tuboplasty, 41%; and eustachian tube closure, 66% [147].

Newer techniques such as transpalatal eustachian tube augmentation in local and general anesthesia versus an augmentation with velotraction under general anesthesia have higher success rates with 100%, 80%, and 67%, respectively (after 6 months) [148].

Diagnostic Workup in Subjects Presenting with Pulsatile Tinnitus

As mentioned above, the identification of the causative vascular pathology and etiology-specific management are vital for the optimal treatment of PT patients because successful surgical or interventional management is available. Therefore, even during the first consultation at an outpatient clinic, meticulous history taking, physical examination, and requests for relevant audiological and radiological examination should be performed and the laboratory test results should be evaluated with care. Some tips that would be of help to diagnose the causative disease and select relevant treatment options will be described hereinafter.

Psychoacoustic Characteristics of Tinnitus

At first visit, physicians should ask whether the patient is perceiving "true" PT. When the patient describes the symptom as "pulsatile," the first question should be whether the sound is synchronous with the heartbeat or with radial pulse palpation. If the patient describes the "pulsatile sound" as respiration-synchronous, then pseudo-pulsatile tinnitus such as a patulous eustachian tube should be ruled out. If the sound is described as "very periodic and like clock ticking," then myoclonic tinnitus originating from the soft palate, eustachian tube, and tensor tympani and stapedius muscles of the middle ear should first be suspected and related physical examinations and laboratory tests should be performed.

Moreover, the psychoacoustic nature of the perceived pulsatile sound provides some clues for the tentative diagnosis. In other words, in most subjects with PT, low-frequency sounds are perceived [83, 119]. This has been objectively supported in recent studies using transcanal sound recording and spectrotemporal analysis (Fig. 40.4) by showing that the recorded signal was significantly stronger at low-frequency bands (125, 250, and 500 Hz) than those of normal controls [83, 119]. This is probably because high-frequency waves carry less energy than do low-frequency waves and are therefore reflected more easily than are the longer low-frequency waves. It is noteworthy that subjects with PT due to a dural arteriovenous fistula tend to perceive a mid-frequency "hissing" pulsatile sound that is different from the usual low-frequency PT presumably due to a relatively small amplitude and higher-frequency pulsatile sound coming from the relatively narrow fistula track [64]. Therefore, asking the perceived pitch of the pulsatile sound may give the physician a key to suspect a dural arteriovenous fistula.

Physical Examination and Audiological Evaluation

Where PT is suspected, otomicroscopy or otoendoscopy should be performed as a routine procedure to rule out any pulsating mass in the tympanic cavity. Arterial, arteriovenous, or venous causes such as an aberrant carotid artery, a persistent stapedial artery, glomus tympanicum or glomus jugulare tumors, and a high jugular bulb with dehiscence can be detected in this step. In particular, if a pulse-synchronous movement of the tympanic membrane is clearly detectable by the examiner, then the vascular lesion in the middle ear can be tentatively regarded as the pathognomonic lesion resulting in PT. As a supplementary investigation, the clinician must perform auscultation of the head and neck region to detect any audible flow sounds over the neck vessels, also including peri-auricular auscultation. In particular, vigorous

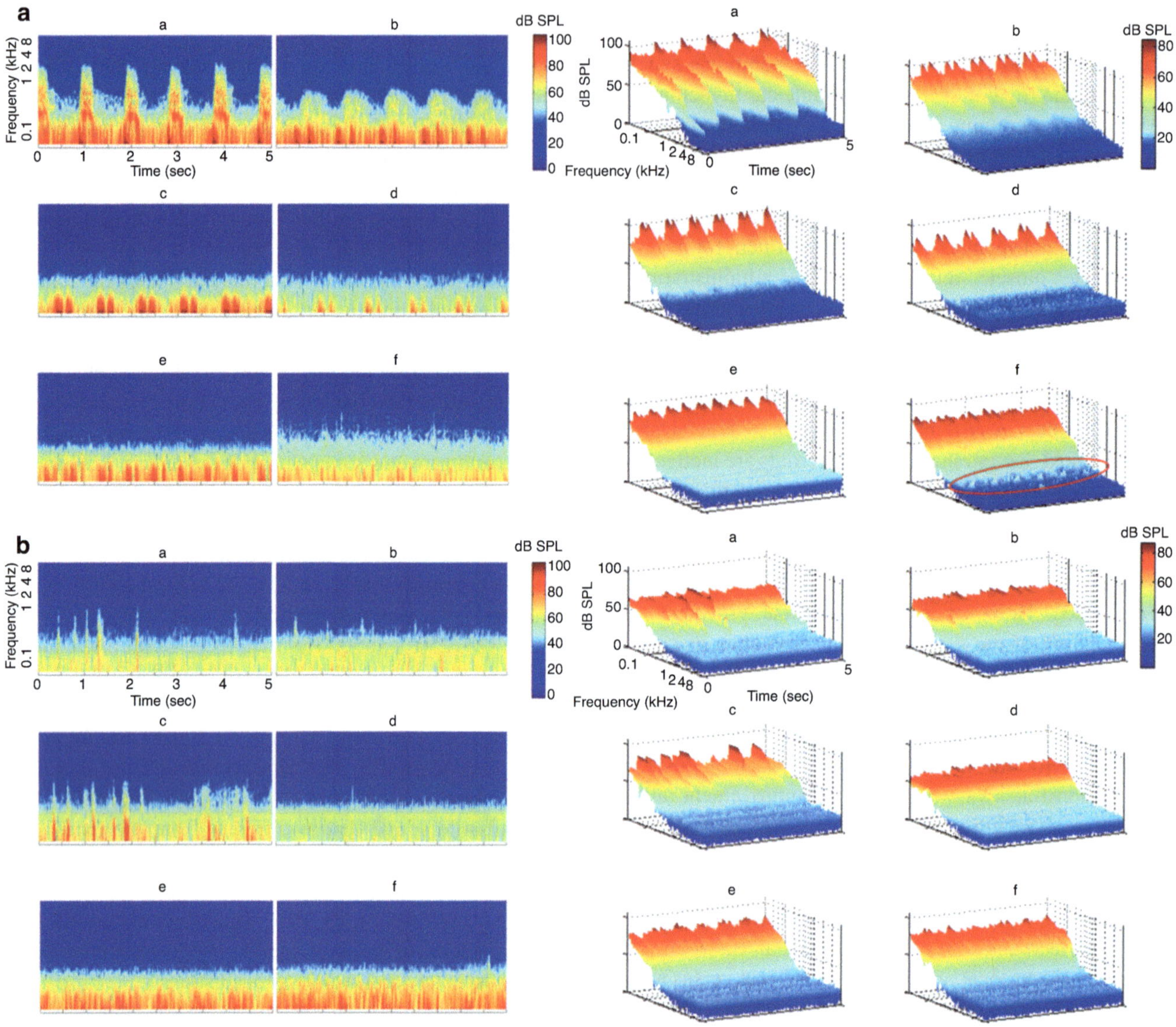

Fig. 40.4 (**a**) Each patients' recorded signals represented by two-dimensional spectrograms and three-dimensional waterfall diagrams. (a) The patient with an aberrant carotid artery; (b) the patient with jugular bulb dehiscence; (c) the patient with a glomus tympanicum; (d) the patient with sigmoid sinus diverticulum; (e) the patient with sigmoid sinus dehiscence; and (f) the patient with an arteriovenous fistula. (**b**) Each control subject's recorded signals represented by two-dimensional spectrograms and three-dimensional waterfall diagrams. There are no pulsatile sounds in the audible frequency range

pulse-synchronous sounds around the mastoid process area are highly indicative of the presence of a dural AVF, most frequently arising from the transverse or sigmoid sinus [64].

Manipulation of the cervical region is helpful to differentiate between an arterial and venous etiology for PT. For further information, readers are recommended to refer to a recent review article [7]. A temporary occlusion of the internal jugular vein by compressing over the sternocleidomastoid muscle may abate PT of an venous origin, whereas that of an arterial origin may not be affected. Moreover, PT of an venous origin may temporarily be abated by rotating the patient's neck to the side of PT because the ipsilateral internal jugular vein is collapsed at the level of the atlantoaxial joint of the cervical spine and thus the venous flow is hampered by rotating the neck to the tinnitus side [7]. From the same standpoint, venous PT is amplified by rotating the neck to the opposite side. To prevent possible serious complications such as severe bradycardia, hypotension, and dyspnea, strong compression of the neck to see the effect of internal carotid artery occlusion is not recommended. If at all, such manipulation should be performed while carefully monitoring the cardiovascular function.

At first visit, conventional pure-tone audiometry is recommended to be checked in all subjects with PT. In a recent study, more than 25% of the subjects with PT have presented with ipsilateral low-frequency hearing loss and this was significantly improved after surgical or interventional treatment [98, 149]. In addition, subjects with ipsilateral low-frequency hearing loss showed a higher rate of abnormal vascular structure as compared to those without hearing loss [98]. The authors coined the term "pseudo-low-frequency hearing loss" because the elevated low-frequency thresholds are not due to true hearing loss but due to the masking effect of the pulsatile sound. In this regard, the presence of pseudo-low-frequency hearing loss may indicate a higher possibility of discrete vascular abnormalities in subjects with PT. Additionally, a recent study has suggested that elimination of PT loudness and improvement of LFHL with manual compression over the ipsilateral neck during pure-tone audiometry may suggest the vascular origin of the PT [150]. Other helpful laboratory tests include blood tests to rule out the possible presence of anemia or thyrotoxicosis, and measurement of blood pressure and body mass index will be of additional help to the diagnosis. When benign intracranial hypertension is suspected, funduscopic examination to rule out papilledema and lumbar puncture to evaluate the opening pressure may be additionally needed.

Radiological Evaluations

Radiological evaluations should be performed after completing psychoacoustic evaluation, physical examination, and laboratory tests (see also Chap. 30). The basic radiological evaluation tool is a combination of temporal bone CT and brain MRI with angiography. By this basic evaluation, most clinical impressions obtained by psychoacoustic evaluation, physical examination, and laboratory tests can be further confirmed.

High-resolution temporal bone CT with/without contrast-enhanced scan is helpful in PT subjects due to lesions such as sigmoid sinus dehiscence/diverticulum, a high jugular bulb with dehiscence/diverticulum, an aberrant internal carotid artery, and glomus jugulare/tympanicum tumors. In addition, dehiscence of the ICA and semicircular canals can be found by performing a temporal bone CT scan.

By performing brain MRI with angiography, pathognomonic lesions such as dural arteriovenous fistulas, arteriovenous malformations, and vessel-rich tumors can be confirmed. In addition, vascular anomalies such as stenoses of the cervical or intracranial vessels, carotid dissections, aneurysms, diverticula, an aberrant internal carotid artery, or a high jugular bulb with dehiscence/diverticulum can be diagnosed by brain MRI with angiography. Additionally, intracranial changes following benign intracranial hypertension such as an empty sella or small ventricles or possible primary causes of intracranial hypertension such as venous sinus thromboses or brain tumors can be found by MRI.

Doppler ultrasonography of the neck vessels may be useful in PT subjects with suspicious atherosclerosis of the arteries supplying the brain. Recently, digital subtraction angiography (DSA) has not been frequently performed because brain MRI with angiography can replace most of the roles of DSA. However, digital subtraction angiography has important roles in the interventional embolization and stenting of different pathologies with PT. Such interventions may be used as definitive therapy (arteriovenous fistula, carotid-cavernous fistula) or as preparatory measures before surgical resections (glomus tumor) to reduce intraoperative bleeding [151]. Recently, four-dimensional DSA has been reported to be extremely useful in pretreatment planning and posttreatment follow-up of embolized brain dural arteriovenous fistulas or malformations [152, 153].

Conclusions

Pulsatile tinnitus can be subdivided into arterial, arteriovenous, and venous origins. Because successful surgical or interventional management is available in many cases, the identification of the causal vascular pathology and etiology-specific management are vital for the optimal treatment of pulsatile tinnitus patients. For a proper diagnosis of the causal pathology, thorough radiological evaluation and meticulous physical examination complemented by laboratory tests should be performed.

References

1. Sismanis A. Pulsatile tinnitus. Int Tinnitus J. 1997;3(1):39–40.
2. Sismanis A. Pulsatile tinnitus. A 15-year experience. Am J Otol. 1998;19(4):472–7.
3. Sismanis A. Pulsatile tinnitus. Otolaryngol Clin N Am. 2003;36(2):389–402, viii.
4. Vanneste S, Song JJ, De Ridder D. Thalamocortical dysrhythmia detected by machine learning. Nat Commun. 2018;9(1):1103.
5. Lee SY, Nam DW, Koo JW, De Ridder D, Vanneste S, Song JJ. No auditory experience, no tinnitus: lessons from subjects with congenital- and acquired single-sided deafness. Hear Res. 2017;354:9–15.
6. Liyanage SH, Singh A, Savundra P, Kalan A. Pulsatile tinnitus. J Laryngol Otol. 2006;120(2):93–7.
7. Hofmann E, Behr R, Neumann-Haefelin T, Schwager K. Pulsatile tinnitus: imaging and differential diagnosis. Dtsch Arztebl Int. 2013;110(26):451–8.
8. Schoeff S, Nicholas B, Mukherjee S, Kesser BW. Imaging prevalence of sigmoid sinus dehiscence among patients with and without pulsatile tinnitus. Otolaryngol Head Neck Surg. 2014;150(5):841–6.
9. Langguth B, Kreuzer PM, Kleinjung T, De Ridder D. Tinnitus: causes and clinical management. Lancet Neurol. 2013;12(9):920–30.

10. Elgoyhen AB, Langguth B, De Ridder D, Vanneste S. Tinnitus: perspectives from human neuroimaging. Nat Rev Neurosci. 2015;16(10):632–42.
11. Ahsan SF, Seidman M, Yaremchuk K. What is the best imaging modality in evaluating patients with unilateral pulsatile tinnitus? Laryngoscope. 2015;125(2):284–5.
12. Hazell JW. Tinnitus. II: surgical management of conditions associated with tinnitus and somatosounds. J Otolaryngol. 1990;19(1):6–10.
13. Silbergleit R, Quint DJ, Mehta BA, Patel SC, Metes JJ, Noujaim SE. The persistent stapedial artery. AJNR Am J Neuroradiol. 2000;21(3):572–7.
14. Sanchez TG, Murao M, de Medeiros I, Kii M, Bento RF, Caldas JG, et al. A new therapeutic procedure for treatment of objective venous pulsatile tinnitus. Int Tinnitus J. 2002;8(1):54–7.
15. Kao E, Kefayati S, Amans MR, Faraji F, Ballweber M, Halbach V, et al. Flow patterns in the jugular veins of pulsatile tinnitus patients. J Biomech. 2017;52:61–7.
16. Mattox DE, Hudgins P. Algorithm for evaluation of pulsatile tinnitus. Acta Otolaryngol. 2008;128(4):427–31.
17. Eisenman DJ, Raghavan P, Hertzano R, Morales R. Evaluation and treatment of pulsatile tinnitus associated with sigmoid sinus wall anomalies. Laryngoscope. 2018;128(Suppl 2):S1–13.
18. Wang JR, Parnes LS. Superior semicircular canal dehiscence associated with external, middle, and inner ear abnormalities. Laryngoscope. 2010;120(2):390–3.
19. Friedmann DR, Le BT, Pramanik BK, Lalwani AK. Clinical spectrum of patients with erosion of the inner ear by jugular bulb abnormalities. Laryngoscope. 2010;120(2):365–72.
20. Lynch P, Mitton T, Killeen DE, Kutz JW, Newcomer M. Diagnosing pulsatile tinnitus: a review of 251 patients. Otol Neurotol. 2022;43(1):128–36.
21. Sismanis A, Smoker WR. Pulsatile tinnitus: recent advances in diagnosis. Laryngoscope. 1994;104(6 Pt 1):681–8.
22. Sismanis A, Stamm MA, Sobel M. Objective tinnitus in patients with atherosclerotic carotid artery disease. Am J Otol. 1994;15(3):404–7.
23. De Ridder D, De Ridder L, Nowe V, Thierens H, Van de Heyning P, Moller A. Pulsatile tinnitus and the intrameatal vascular loop: why do we not hear our carotids? Neurosurgery. 2005;57(6):1213–7; discussion 7.
24. Singh DP, Forte AJ, Brewer MB, Nowygrod R. Bilateral carotid endarterectomy as treatment of vascular pulsatile tinnitus. J Vasc Surg. 2009;50(1):183–5.
25. Lehmann MF, Mounayer C, Benndorf G, Piotin M, Moret J. Pulsatile tinnitus: a symptom of chronic subclavian artery occlusion. AJNR Am J Neuroradiol. 2005;26(8):1960–3.
26. Cowley PO, Jones R, Tuch P, McAuliffe W. Pulsatile tinnitus from reversal of flow in an aberrant occipital artery: resolved after carotid artery stenting. AJNR Am J Neuroradiol. 2009;30(5):995–7.
27. Redekop GJ. Extracranial carotid and vertebral artery dissection: a review. Can J Neurol Sci. 2008;35(2):146–52.
28. Selim M, Caplan LR. Carotid artery dissection. Curr Treat Options Cardiovasc Med. 2004;6(3):249–53.
29. Baumgartner RW, Bogousslavsky J. Clinical manifestations of carotid dissection. Front Neurol Neurosci. 2005;20:70–6.
30. De Ridder D, Vanneste S, Menovsky T. Pulsatile tinnitus due to a tortuous siphon-like internal carotid artery successfully treated by arterial remodeling. Case Rep Otolaryngol. 2013;2013:938787.
31. Dietz RR, Davis WL, Harnsberger HR, Jacobs JM, Blatter DD. MR imaging and MR angiography in the evaluation of pulsatile tinnitus. AJNR Am J Neuroradiol. 1994;15(5):879–89.
32. Waldvogel D, Mattle HP, Sturzenegger M, Schroth G. Pulsatile tinnitus--a review of 84 patients. J Neurol. 1998;245(3):137–42.
33. Moonis G, Hwang CJ, Ahmed T, Weigele JB, Hurst RW. Otologic manifestations of petrous carotid aneurysms. AJNR Am J Neuroradiol. 2005;26(6):1324–7.
34. Liu JK, Gottfried ON, Amini A, Couldwell WT. Aneurysms of the petrous internal carotid artery: anatomy, origins, and treatment. Neurosurg Focus. 2004;17(5):E13.
35. Depauw P, Caekebeke J, Vanhoenacker P. Objective pulsatile tinnitus caused by intrapetrous dissecting aneurysm. Clin Neurol Neurosurg. 2001;103(3):197–9.
36. Austin JR, Maceri DR. Anterior communicating artery aneurysm presenting as pulsatile tinnitus. ORL J Otorhinolaryngol Relat Spec. 1993;55(1):54–7.
37. Zager EL, Shaver EG, Hurst RW, Flamm ES. Distal anterior inferior cerebellar artery aneurysms. Report of four cases. J Neurosurg. 2002;97(3):692–6.
38. De Ridder D. Pulsatile Tinnitus. In: Moller A, Langguth B, De Ridder D, Kleinjung T, editors. Textbook of tinnitus. New York: Springer; 2011. p. 467–75.
39. Weissman JL, Hirsch BE. Imaging of tinnitus: a review. Radiology. 2000;216(2):342–9.
40. Honkura Y, Hidaka H, Ohta J, Gorai S, Katori Y, Kobayashi T. Surgical treatment for the aberrant internal carotid artery in the middle ear with pulsatile tinnitus. Auris Nasus Larynx. 2014;41(2):215–8.
41. Moon IS, Lee WS. Images in clinical medicine. Internal carotid artery in the middle ear. N Engl J Med. 2014;371(4):e5.
42. Hashim ND, Jang SH, Moon IS. Endoscopic intervention of aberrant carotid artery in the middle ear. Otol Neurotol. 2021;42(1):e82–5.
43. Moreano EH, Paparella MM, Zelterman D, Goycoolea MV. Prevalence of facial canal dehiscence and of persistent stapedial artery in the human middle ear: a report of 1000 temporal bones. Laryngoscope. 1994;104(3 Pt 1):309–20.
44. LoVerde ZJ, Shlapak DP, Benson JC, Carlson ML, Lane JI. The many faces of persistent stapedial artery: CT findings and embryologic explanations. AJNR Am J Neuroradiol. 2021;42(1):160–6.
45. Goderie TPM, Alkhateeb WHF, Smit CF, Hensen EF. Surgical management of a persistent stapedial artery: a review. Otol Neurotol. 2017;38(6):788–91.
46. Ryu H, Yamamoto S, Sugiyama K, Nozue M. Neurovascular compression syndrome of the eighth cranial nerve. What are the most reliable diagnostic signs? Acta Neurochir. 1998;140(12):1279–86.
47. Ryu H, Yamamoto S, Sugiyama K, Uemura K, Nozue M. Neurovascular decompression of the eighth cranial nerve in patients with hemifacial spasm and incidental tinnitus: an alternative way to study tinnitus. J Neurosurg. 1998;88(2):232–6.
48. Chadha NK, Weiner GM. Vascular loops causing otological symptoms: a systematic review and meta-analysis. Clin Otolaryngol. 2008;33(1):5–11.
49. Nowe V, De Ridder D, Van de Heyning PH, Wang XL, Gielen J, Van Goethem J, et al. Does the location of a vascular loop in the cerebellopontine angle explain pulsatile and non-pulsatile tinnitus? Eur Radiol. 2004;14(12):2282–9.
50. Sunwoo W, Jeon YJ, Bae YJ, Jang JH, Koo JW, Song JJ. Typewriter tinnitus revisited: the typical symptoms and the initial response to carbamazepine are the most reliable diagnostic clues. Sci Rep. 2017;7(1):10615.
51. Bae YJ, Jeon YJ, Choi BS, Koo JW, Song JJ. The role of MRI in diagnosing neurovascular compression of the cochlear nerve resulting in typewriter tinnitus. AJNR Am J Neuroradiol. 2017;38(6):1212–7.
52. Moller MB, Moller AR, Jannetta PJ, Jho HD. Vascular decompression surgery for severe tinnitus: selection criteria and results. Laryngoscope. 1993;103(4 Pt 1):421–7.

53. Brookes GB. Vascular-decompression surgery for severe tinnitus. Am J Otol. 1996;17(4):569–76.
54. Ko Y, Park CW. Microvascular decompression for tinnitus. Stereotact Funct Neurosurg. 1997;68(1–4 Pt 1):266–9.
55. De Ridder D, Ryu H, Moller AR, Nowe V, Van de Heyning P, Verlooy J. Functional anatomy of the human cochlear nerve and its role in microvascular decompressions for tinnitus. Neurosurgery. 2004;54(2):381–8; discussion 8–90.
56. Mathiesen T, Brantberg K. Microvascular decompression for typewriter tinnitus-case report. Acta Neurochir. 2015;157(2):333–6.
57. Hsieh YL, Xu X, Guo P, Wang W. Pulsatile tinnitus caused by an aberrant artery running over the surface of mastoid bone. Auris Nasus Larynx. 2021;48(6):1181–8.
58. Cochran JH Jr, Kosmicki PW. Tinnitus as a presenting symptom in pernicious anemia. Ann Otol Rhinol Laryngol. 1979;88(2 Pt 1):297.
59. Sunwoo W, Lee DY, Lee JY, Lee M, Kang Y, Park MH, et al. Characteristics of tinnitus found in anemia patients and analysis of population-based survey. Auris Nasus Larynx. 2018;45(6):1152–8.
60. NICE. Evidence review for imaging to investigate the cause of pulsatile tinnitus: tinnitus: assessment and management: evidence review NICE evidence reviews collection. London; 2020.
61. Sismanis A. Pulsatile tinnitus: contemporary assessment and management. Curr Opin Otolaryngol Head Neck Surg. 2011;19(5):348–57.
62. Kwon BJ, Han MH, Kang HS, Chang KH. MR imaging findings of intracranial dural arteriovenous fistulas: relations with venous drainage patterns. AJNR Am J Neuroradiol. 2005;26(10):2500–7.
63. Newton TH, Cronqvist S. Involvement of dural arteries in intracranial arteriovenous malformations. Radiology. 1969;93(5):1071–8.
64. An YH, Han S, Lee M, Rhee J, Kwon OK, Hwang G, et al. Dural arteriovenous fistula masquerading as pulsatile tinnitus: radiologic assessment and clinical implications. Sci Rep. 2016;6:36601.
65. Gandhi D, Chen J, Pearl M, Huang J, Gemmete JJ, Kathuria S. Intracranial dural arteriovenous fistulas: classification, imaging findings, and treatment. AJNR Am J Neuroradiol. 2012;33(6):1007–13.
66. Kiyosue H, Hori Y, Okahara M, Tanoue S, Sagara Y, Matsumoto S, et al. Treatment of intracranial dural arteriovenous fistulas: current strategies based on location and hemodynamics, and alternative techniques of transcatheter embolization. Radiographics. 2004;24(6):1637–53.
67. Bavinzski G, Richling B, Killer M, Gruber A, Levy D. Evolution of different therapeutic strategies in the treatment of cranial dural arteriovenous fistulas--report of 30 cases. Acta Neurochir. 1996;138(2):132–8.
68. Steinberg GK, Chang SD, Levy RP, Marks MP, Frankel K, Marcellus M. Surgical resection of large incompletely treated intracranial arteriovenous malformations following stereotactic radiosurgery. J Neurosurg. 1996;84(6):920–8.
69. Awad I, Barrow D. Dural arteriovenous malformations. Park Ridge, IL: American Association Neurological Surgeons; 1993.
70. Wachter D, Hans F, Psychogios MN, Knauth M, Rohde V. Microsurgery can cure most intracranial dural arteriovenous fistulae of the sinus and non-sinus type. Neurosurg Rev. 2011;34(3):337–45; discussion 45.
71. Arat A, Inci S. Treatment of a superior sagittal sinus dural arteriovenous fistula with Onyx: technical case report. Neurosurgery. 2006;59(1 Suppl 1):ONSE169–70; discussion ONSE-70.
72. Sirakov SS, Kitov BD, Sirakova KS, Kehayov II. Spontaneous direct carotid-cavernous fistula in an elderly patient. Folia Med (Plovdiv). 2017;59(4):472–6.
73. Lerut B, De Vuyst C, Ghekiere J, Vanopdenbosch L, Kuhweide R. Post-traumatic pulsatile tinnitus: the hallmark of a direct carotico-cavernous fistula. J Laryngol Otol. 2007;121(11):1103–7.
74. Gupta R, Agrawal A. Arteriovenous malformation of external ear and temporal region: a case report. Int J Res Med Sci. 2015;3:3427–9.
75. Woo HJ, Song SY, Kim YD, Bai CH. Arteriovenous malformation of the external ear: a case report. Auris Nasus Larynx. 2008;35(4):556–8.
76. Kim SH, Han SH, Song Y, Park CS, Song JJ. Arteriovenous malformation of the external ear: a clinical assessment with a scoping review of the literature. Braz J Otorhinolaryngol. 2017;83(6):683–90.
77. Manabe S, Satoh K, Matsubara S, Satomi J, Hanaoka M, Nagahiro S. Characteristics, diagnosis and treatment of hypoglossal canal dural arteriovenous fistula: report of nine cases. Neuroradiology. 2008;50(8):715–21.
78. Chen MC, Chung WY, Luo CB, Wu HM. Arteriovenous malformation in the parotid region presenting as pulsatile tinnitus: a case report. Head Neck. 2009;32:NA.
79. Wu JK, Bisdorff A, Gelbert F, Enjolras O, Burrows PE, Mulliken JB. Auricular arteriovenous malformation: evaluation, management, and outcome. Plast Reconstr Surg. 2005;115(4):985–95.
80. Sweeney AD, Carlson ML, Wanna GB, Bennett ML. Glomus tympanicum tumors. Otolaryngol Clin N Am. 2015;48(2):293–304.
81. Wanna GB, Sweeney AD, Haynes DS, Carlson ML. Contemporary management of jugular paragangliomas. Otolaryngol Clin N Am. 2015;48(2):331–41.
82. Manzoor NF, Yancey KL, Aulino JM, Sherry AD, Khattab MH, Cmelak A, et al. Contemporary management of jugular paragangliomas with neural preservation. Otolaryngol Head Neck Surg. 2021;164(2):391–8.
83. Song JJ, An GS, Choi I, De Ridder D, Kim SY, Choi HS, et al. Objectification and differential diagnosis of vascular pulsatile tinnitus by transcanal sound recording and spectrotemporal analysis: a preliminary study. Otol Neurotol. 2016;37(6):613–20.
84. Kaul VF, Filip P, Schwam ZG, Wanna GB. Nuances in transcanal endoscopic surgical technique for glomus tympanicum tumors. Am J Otolaryngol. 2020;41(5):102562.
85. Killeen DE, Wick CC, Hunter JB, Rivas A, Wanna GB, Nogueira JF, et al. Endoscopic management of middle ear paragangliomas: a case series. Otol Neurotol. 2017;38(3):408–15.
86. Levine SB, Snow JB Jr. Pulsatile tinnitus. Laryngoscope. 1987;97(4):401–6.
87. Deep NL, Besch-Stokes JG, Lane JI, Driscoll CLW, Carlson ML. Paget's disease of the temporal bone: a single-institution contemporary review of 27 patients. Otol Neurotol. 2017;38(6):907–15.
88. Megerian CA, McKenna MJ, Nadol JB Jr. Non-paraganglioma jugular foramen lesions masquerading as glomus jugulare tumors. Am J Otol. 1995;16(1):94–8.
89. Hayenga HN, Bishop AJ, Wardak Z, Sen C, Mickey B. Intraspinal dissemination and local recurrence of an intracranial hemangiopericytoma. World Neurosurg. 2019;123:68–75.
90. Leonetti JP, Shirazi MA, Marzo S, Anderson D. Neuroendocrine carcinoma of the jugular foramen. Ear Nose Throat J. 2008;87(2):86, 8–91.
91. Akyigit A, Karlidag T, Sakallioglu O, Polat C, Keles E. Giant cell tumor of bone involving the temporomandibular joint and temporal bone. J Craniofac Surg. 2014;25(4):1397–9.
92. Friedmann DR, Eubig J, McGill M, Babb JS, Pramanik BK, Lalwani AK. Development of the jugular bulb: a radiologic study. Otol Neurotol. 2011;32(8):1389–95.
93. Alper F, Kantarci M, Dane S, Gumustekin K, Onbas O, Durur I. Importance of anatomical asymmetries of transverse sinuses: an MR venographic study. Cerebrovasc Dis. 2004;18(3):236–9.
94. Lee SY, Kim MK, Bae YJ, An GS, Lee K, Choi BY, et al. Longitudinal analysis of surgical outcome in subjects with pul-

satile tinnitus originating from the sigmoid sinus. Sci Rep. 2020;10(1):18194.
95. Jindal M, Hiam L, Raman A, Rejali D. Idiopathic intracranial hypertension in otolaryngology. Eur Arch Otorhinolaryngol. 2009;266(6):803–6.
96. Shaw GY, Million SK. Benign intracranial hypertension: a diagnostic dilemma. Case Rep Otolaryngol. 2012;2012:814696.
97. Donaldson JO. Pathogenesis of pseudotumor cerebri syndromes. Neurology. 1981;31(7):877–80.
98. Jeon HW, Kim SY, Choi BS, Bae YJ, Koo JW, Song JJ. Pseudo-low frequency hearing loss and its improvement after treatment may be objective signs of significant vascular pathology in patients with pulsatile tinnitus. Otol Neurotol. 2016;37(9):1344–9.
99. Schlosser RJ, Woodworth BA, Wilensky EM, Grady MS, Bolger WE. Spontaneous cerebrospinal fluid leaks: a variant of benign intracranial hypertension. Ann Otol Rhinol Laryngol. 2006;115(7):495–500.
100. Donnet A, Metellus P, Levrier O, Mekkaoui C, Fuentes S, Dufour H, et al. Endovascular treatment of idiopathic intracranial hypertension: clinical and radiologic outcome of 10 consecutive patients. Neurology. 2008;70(8):641–7.
101. Sismanis A. Otologic manifestations of benign intracranial hypertension syndrome: diagnosis and management. Laryngoscope. 1987;97(8 Pt 2 Suppl 42):1–17.
102. Friedmann DR, Eubig J, Winata LS, Pramanik BK, Merchant SN, Lalwani AK. Prevalence of jugular bulb abnormalities and resultant inner ear dehiscence: a histopathologic and radiologic study. Otolaryngol Head Neck Surg. 2012;147(4):750–6.
103. Lee S-Y, Song S-K, Park SJ, Park HG, Choi BY, Koo J-W, et al. Jugular bulb resurfacing with bone cement for patients with high dehiscent jugular bulb and ipsilateral pulsatile tinnitus. Otol Neurotol. 2019;40(2):192–9.
104. Weiss RL, Zahtz G, Goldofsky E, Parnes H, Shikowitz MJ. High jugular bulb and conductive hearing loss. Laryngoscope. 1997;107(3):321–7.
105. Jastreboff PJ, Gray CG, Mattox DE. Tinnitus and hyperacusis. In: Cummings CW, Frederickson JM, Harker LA, Krause CJ, Richardson MA, Schuller DE, editors. Otolaryngology, head & neck surgery. 3rd ed. St Louis: Mosby; 1998. p. 3198–222.
106. El-Begermy MA, Rabie AN. A novel surgical technique for management of tinnitus due to high dehiscent jugular bulb. Otolaryngol Head Neck Surg. 2010;142(4):576–81.
107. DeHart AN, Shaia WT, Coelho DH. Hydroxyapatite cement resurfacing the dehiscent jugular bulb: novel treatment for pulsatile tinnitus. Laryngoscope. 2018;128(5):1186–90.
108. Oh SJ, Kim D, Lee JI, Ko JK, Choi SW, Kong SK, et al. Transvenous stent-assisted coil embolization for management of dehiscent high jugular bulb with tinnitus and contralateral hypoplastic venous sinuses. Otol Neurotol. 2019;40(9):1253–9.
109. Otto KJ, Hudgins PA, Abdelkafy W, Mattox DE. Sigmoid sinus diverticulum: a new surgical approach to the correction of pulsatile tinnitus. Otol Neurotol. 2007;28(1):48–53.
110. Liu Z, Chen C, Wang Z, Gong S, Xian J, Wang Y, et al. Sigmoid sinus diverticulum and pulsatile tinnitus: analysis of CT scans from 15 cases. Acta Radiol. 2013;54(7):812–6.
111. Grewal AK, Kim HY, Comstock RH III, Berkowitz F, Kim HJ, Jay AK. Clinical presentation and imaging findings in patients with pulsatile tinnitus and sigmoid sinus diverticulum/dehiscence. Otol Neurotol. 2014;35(1):16–21.
112. Song JJ, Kim YJ, Kim SY, An YS, Kim K, Lee SY, et al. Sinus wall resurfacing for patients with temporal bone venous sinus diverticulum and ipsilateral pulsatile tinnitus. Neurosurgery. 2015;77(5):709–17.
113. Hsieh YL, Xu X, Hsieh YD, Hsieh YC, Wang D, Guo P, et al. Hydroacoustic analysis and extraluminal compression surgical insights of venous pulsatile tinnitus. Auris Nasus Larynx. 2021;48:852.
114. Mehanna R, Shaltoni H, Morsi H, Mawad M. Endovascular treatment of sigmoid sinus aneurysm presenting as devastating pulsatile tinnitus. A case report and review of literature. Interv Neuroradiol. 2010;16(4):451–4.
115. Park YH, Kwon HJ. Awake embolization of sigmoid sinus diverticulum causing pulsatile tinnitus: simultaneous confirmative diagnosis and treatment. Interv Neuroradiol. 2011;17(3):376–9.
116. Kim CS, Kim SY, Choi H, Koo JW, Yoo SY, An GS, et al. Transmastoid reshaping of the sigmoid sinus: preliminary study of a novel surgical method to quiet pulsatile tinnitus of an unrecognized vascular origin. J Neurosurg. 2016;125(2):441–9.
117. Sutera SP, Skalak R. The history of Poiseuille's law. Annu Rev Fluid Mech. 1993;25(1):1–20.
118. Amans MR, Haraldsson H, Kao E, Kefayati S, Meisel K, Khangura R, et al. MR venous flow in sigmoid sinus diverticulum. AJNR Am J Neuroradiol. 2018;39(11):2108–13.
119. Kim SH, An GS, Choi I, Koo JW, Lee K, Song JJ. Pre-treatment objective diagnosis and post-treatment outcome evaluation in patients with vascular pulsatile tinnitus using transcanal recording and spectro-temporal analysis. PLoS One. 2016;11(6):e0157722.
120. Zhaohui L, Cheng D, Xiao W, Xiaoyi H, Pengfei Z, Han L, et al. Association between idiopathic intracranial hypertension and sigmoid sinus dehiscence/diverticulum with pulsatile tinnitus: a retrospective imaging study. Neuroradiology. 2015;57(7):747–53.
121. Wee JH, Song JJ, Koo JW, Kim CS. Increased intracranial pressure after surgical treatment of pulsatile tinnitus from a prominent sigmoid sinus. Otol Neurotol. 2012;33(6):e41–2.
122. Paul KS, Lye RH, Strang FA, Dutton J, Arnold-Chiari malformation. Review of 71 cases. J Neurosurg. 1983;58(2):183–7.
123. Wiggs WJ Jr, Sismanis A, Laine FJ. Pulsatile tinnitus associated with congenital central nervous system malformations. Am J Otol. 1996;17(2):241–4.
124. Hillman TA, Kertesz TR, Hadley K, Shelton C. Reversible peripheral vestibulopathy: the treatment of superior canal dehiscence. Otolaryngol Head Neck Surg. 2006;134(3):431–6.
125. Minor LB. Clinical manifestations of superior semicircular canal dehiscence. Laryngoscope. 2005;115(10):1717–27.
126. Minor LB, Cremer PD, Carey JP, Della Santina CC, Streubel SO, Weg N. Symptoms and signs in superior canal dehiscence syndrome. Ann N Y Acad Sci. 2001;942:259–73.
127. Russo JE, Crowson MG, DeAngelo EJ, Belden CJ, Saunders JE. Posterior semicircular canal dehiscence: CT prevalence and clinical symptoms. Otol Neurotol. 2014;35(2):310–4.
128. Elmali M, Polat AV, Kucuk H, Atmaca S, Aksoy A. Semicircular canal dehiscence: frequency and distribution on temporal bone CT and its relationship with the clinical outcomes. Eur J Radiol. 2013;82(10):e606–9.
129. Zhou G, Gopen Q, Poe DS. Clinical and diagnostic characterization of canal dehiscence syndrome: a great otologic mimicker. Otol Neurotol. 2007;28(7):920–6.
130. Park JH, Lee SY, Song JJ, Choi BY, Koo JW. Electrocochleographic findings in superior canal dehiscence syndrome. Hear Res. 2015;323:61–7.
131. Walsh EM. Current management of superior semicircular canal dehiscence syndrome. Curr Opin Otolaryngol Head Neck Surg. 2020;28(5):340–5.
132. Mehta N, Arram E, Rouhani MJ, Dimitrov L, Ubhi HK, Khalil S, et al. Superior semi-circular canal dehiscence syndrome: quantifying the effectiveness of treatment from the patient's perspective. J Laryngol Otol. 2021;136(9):809–22.
133. MacKinnon DM. Objective tinnitus due to palatal myoclonus. J Laryngol Otol. 1968;82(4):369–74.
134. Badia L, Parikh A, Brookes GB. Management of middle ear myoclonus. J Laryngol Otol. 1994;108(5):380–2.
135. Zipfel TE, Kaza SR, Greene JS. Middle-ear myoclonus. J Laryngol Otol. 2000;114(3):207–9.

136. Golz A, Fradis M, Martzu D, Netzer A, Joachims HZ. Stapedius muscle myoclonus. Ann Otol Rhinol Laryngol. 2003;112(6):522–4.
137. Virtanen H. Objective tubal tinnitus: a report of two cases. J Laryngol Otol. 1983;97(9):857–62.
138. Salehi PP, Kasle D, Torabi SJ, Michaelides E, Hildrew DM. The etiology, pathogeneses, and treatment of objective tinnitus: unique case series and literature review. Am J Otolaryngol. 2019;40(4):594–7.
139. Penney SE, Bruce IA, Saeed SR. Botulinum toxin is effective and safe for palatal tremor: a report of five cases and a review of the literature. J Neurol. 2006;253(7):857–60.
140. Park JM, Kim WJ, Han JS, Park SY, Park SN. Management of palatal myoclonic tinnitus based on clinical characteristics: a large case series study. Acta Otolaryngol. 2020;140(7):553–7.
141. Sinclair CF, Gurey LE, Blitzer A. Palatal myoclonus: algorithm for management with botulinum toxin based on clinical disease characteristics. Laryngoscope. 2014;124(5):1164–9.
142. Park SN, Bae SC, Lee GH, Song JN, Park KH, Jeon EJ, et al. Clinical characteristics and therapeutic response of objective tinnitus due to middle ear myoclonus: a large case series. Laryngoscope. 2013;123(10):2516–20.
143. Kim DK, Park JM, Han JJ, Chung YM, Kim JM, Park SY, et al. Long-term effects of middle ear tendon resection on middle ear myoclonic tinnitus, hearing, and hyperacusis. Audiol Neurootol. 2017;22(6):343–9.
144. Bhimrao SK, Masterson L, Baguley D. Systematic review of management strategies for middle ear myoclonus. Otolaryngol Head Neck Surg. 2012;146(5):698–706.
145. Mehta NK, Ma C, Nguyen SA, McRackan TR, Meyer TA, Lambert PR. Medical management for eustachian tube dysfunction in adults: a systematic review and meta-analysis. Laryngoscope. 2021;132:849.
146. Luu K, Remillard A, Fandino M, Saxby A, Westerberg BD. Treatment effectiveness for symptoms of patulous eustachian tube: a systematic review. Otol Neurotol. 2015;36(10):1593–600.
147. Ikeda R, Hidaka H, Kikuchi T, Ohta N, Kawase T, Katori Y, et al. Systematic review of surgical outcomes following repair of patulous eustachian tube. Otol Neurotol. 2020;41(8):1012–20.
148. Sudhoff H, Ay N, Todt I, Sauzet O, Bernal-Sprekelsen M, Scholtz LU. A novel technique for patulous eustachian tube augmentation. Eur Arch Otorhinolaryngol. 2021;278(7):2219–24.
149. Ettyreddy AR, Shew MA, Durakovic N, Chole RA, Herzog J, Buchman CA, et al. Prevalence, surgical management, and audiologic impact of sigmoid sinus dehiscence causing pulsatile tinnitus. Otol Neurotol. 2021;42(1):82–91.
150. Lee SJ, Lee SY, Choi BY, Koo JW, Hong SH, Song JJ. Preoperative significance of ipsilateral manual neck compression in patients with pulsatile tinnitus secondary to sigmoid sinus dehiscences and diverticula. Front Neurol. 2022;13:869244.
151. Ashour R, Aziz-Sultan A. Preoperative tumor embolization. Neurosurg Clin N Am. 2014;25(3):607–17.
152. Kato N, Yuki I, Hataoka S, Dahmani C, Otani K, Abe Y, et al. 4D digital subtraction angiography for the temporal flow visualization of intracranial aneurysms and vascular malformations. J Stroke Cerebrovasc Dis. 2020;29(12):105327.
153. Dissaux B, Eugene F, Ognard J, Gauvrit JY, Gentric JC, Ferre JC. Assessment of 4D MR angiography at 3T compared with DSA for the follow-up of embolized brain dural arteriovenous fistula: a dual-center study. AJNR Am J Neuroradiol. 2021;42(2):340–6.

Hyperacusis and Tinnitus

41

Martin Schecklmann, Laure Jacquemin, and David M. Baguley

Abstract

One well-accepted definition of hyperacusis is that it is a general hypersensitivity or hyper-reactivity to sounds, which are well-tolerated by other people or by the person itself in the past. The major impact is on the level of the behavioural response, as patients with hyperacusis are likely to avoid loud sounds due to their subjective aversiveness, which again leads to avoidance of normal sounds as well because of the increased sensitization of their hearing system. For the assessment of hyperacusis, psychoacoustic measurements (uncomfortable loudness levels (ULLs)) and different questionnaires for the various psychological symptoms are available. Animal and human neuroscience studies of hyperacusis (in tinnitus) mostly affirm the prominent model of increased central neural gain (increased sensitization of the hearing system). This fits well with the most prominent treatment of desensitization to avoided sounds as implemented in psychology-based interventions such as cognitive behavioural therapy (CBT). This sounds like a success story. However, open issues are related to hyperacusis subtyping, overcoming the limited validity and small correlation of audiological measures and questionnaires, disentangling mechanisms of hyperacusis and tinnitus from those of other conditions, transferring neuroscience data to personalized treatment regimens and, overall, affirming the proposed concepts with experimental data. Thus, more research is needed, as can be seen in the available literature, which shows that hyperacusis is the smaller and later-born sibling of tinnitus.

David M. Baguley has died before the publication of this book.

M. Schecklmann (✉)
Department of Psychiatry and Psychotherapy, Interdisciplinary Tinnitus Clinic, University of Regensburg, Regensburg, Germany
e-mail: Martin.Schecklmann@medbo.de

L. Jacquemin
University Department of Otorhinolaryngology and Head & Neck Surgery, Antwerp University Hospital, Edegem, Belgium

Department of Translational Neurosciences, Faculty of Medicine and Health Sciences, University of Antwerp, Wilrijk, Belgium
e-mail: Laure.Jacquemin@uza.be

D. M. Baguley (Deceased)
Nottingham Biomedical Research Centre, National Institute for Health Research, Ropewalk House, Nottingham, UK

Hearing Sciences, Mental Health and Clinical Neurosciences, School of Medicine, University of Nottingham, Nottingham, UK

Nottingham University Hospitals NHS Trust, Nottingham, UK

W. Schlee et al. (eds.), *Textbook of Tinnitus*, https://doi.org/10.1007/978-3-031-35647-6_41

Graphical Abstract

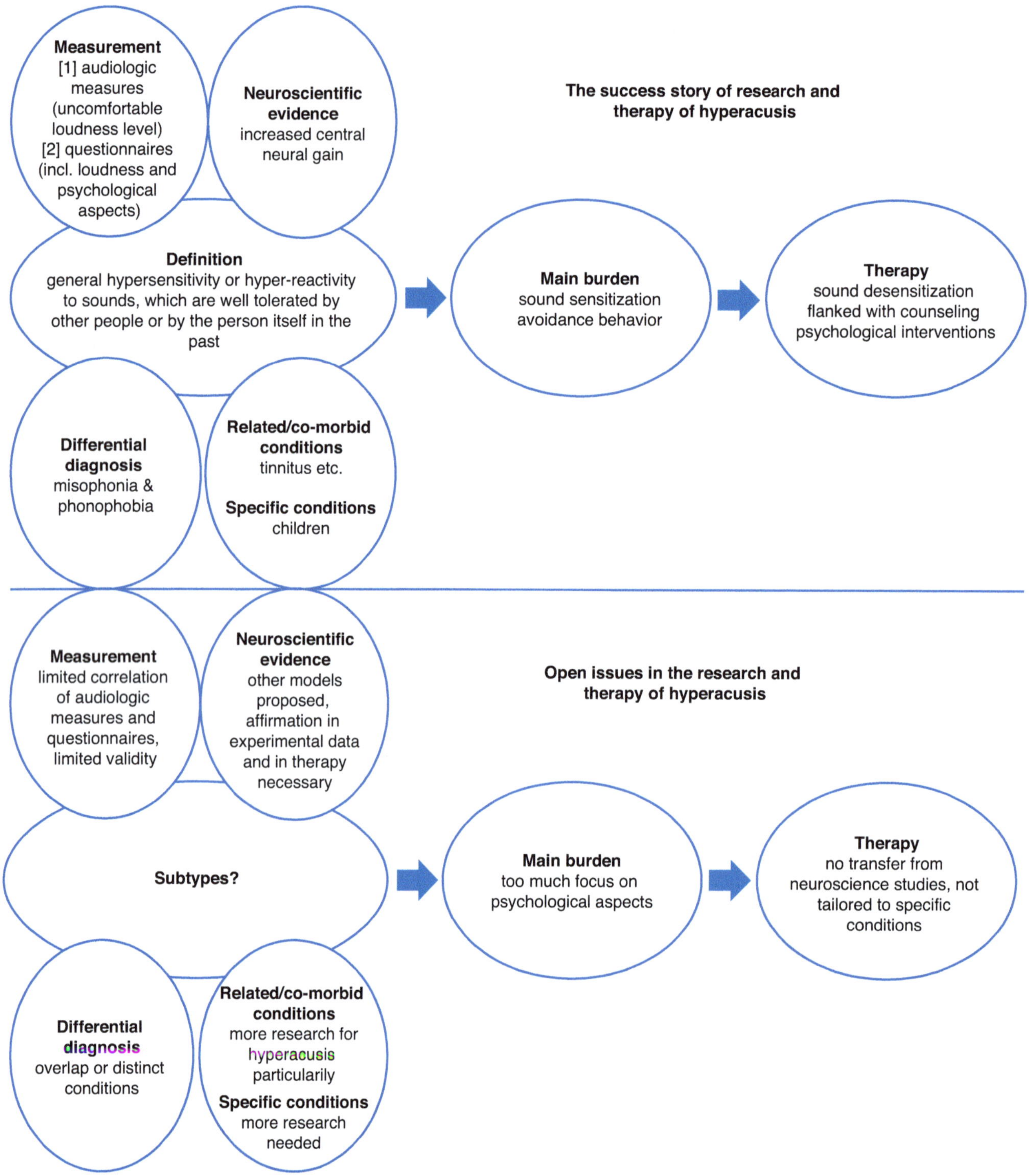

Highlights
- Hyperacusis is a general hypersensitivity or hyper-reactivity to sounds.
- The most prominent model is that of increased neural gain.
- Hyperacusis is subjectively measured with psychoacoustic measurements and questionnaires.
- Patients with hyperacusis may show dysfunctional avoidance of loud sounds, which can be treated with cognitive behavioural therapy with the aim of reducing the avoidance behaviour.
- Open issues are related to subtypes, comorbidities (especially tinnitus) and transfer of measurements and neuroscience data to therapy.
- Hyperacusis is neglected in research, in contrast to tinnitus.

Definitions, Commonalities and Divergences

Several definitions and terminologies have been published and are available for hyperacusis. Essentially, hyperacusis can be seen as a general hypersensitivity or hyper-reactivity to sounds, which are well-tolerated by other people or by the person itself in the past [1]. As it is defined as a "general" hypersensitivity to sounds, it does not include fear of specific sounds (which then is phonophobia), anger and/or disgust associated with the bodily noises of others (which then is misophonia) or abnormal loudness growth and discomfort to specific frequencies related to cochlear hearing loss (which then is recruitment) (for more information on the definition of hyperacusis and related disorders, see Chap. 3). Hyperacusis often involves an increased emotional or painful perception, with corresponding physiological arousal, and results in avoidance or protective behaviour. Hence, it is associated with increased attention to the auditory stimuli.

Hyperacusis is often comorbid with tinnitus, which is the perception of a sound in the absence of an external auditory source [2, 3]. More specifically, it has been shown that up to 79% of tinnitus patients report hyperacusis [4], but evidence is heterogeneous and also lower numbers have been published [5]. Until recently, these two conditions had been believed to have common underlying mechanisms and needed similar treatments, with attention primarily focused on tinnitus [1]. More specifically, both conditions are often associated with hearing dysfunction [6] and an increased incidence of depression, anxiety and stress [5]. Similar altered neural activities in auditory and non-auditory areas have been demonstrated in both conditions [7–9].

It has been suggested that hyperacusis is a precursive tinnitus state [10]. However, it may also be the consequence of decompensated tinnitus with increased attention to auditory perceptions. More specifically, some patients associate their tinnitus with sound exposure, as the tinnitus started after a noise trauma or they experienced tinnitus worsening after being in loud environments (which were not too loud per se). The latter can be considered in the context of "residual excitation". In a certain number of patients, presenting loud sounds (commonly, noise-like sounds) leads to an increase in tinnitus loudness [11] and is not associated with general hypersensitivity per se. Thus, it has to be determined whether this kind of hypersensitivity in patients with tinnitus is a different subtype of hyperacusis.

Despite the similarities between tinnitus and hyperacusis, Baguley and Hoare [5] called attention to the fact that these conditions should be approached as distinct phenomena that are markedly divergent ([2, 12]; see [13] for a review on hyperacusis). Hyperacusis is frequently experienced in both the ears, whereas tinnitus is often lateralized [14]. Furthermore, hyperacusis is rarely intermittent, in contrast to the fluctuating character of tinnitus [15]. While the perception of sounds is vivid and salient in hyperacusis patients, the tinnitus percept is formless or primitive [16]. Moreover, the ability to be modulated by somatic manipulations seems rare for hyperacusis but common for tinnitus [17]. Finally, contrary to tinnitus, the effectiveness of self-help for hyperacusis is unknown and might be highly limited [5, 18].

Basics, Facts and Science-Based Knowledge

A non-systematic literature review was conducted on 6 November 2020 on PubMed (National Center for Biotechnology Information, USA) using the search terms "tinnitus", "(hyperacusis OR hyperacousis) AND tinnitus" and "(hyperacusis OR hyperacousis) NOT tinnitus" to shed light on the publications of hyperacusis in the context of tinnitus. First, we focused on the frequency of publications. We found 13.724 hits for tinnitus, 947 for tinnitus, including hyperacusis, and 478 for hyperacusis, excluding tinnitus. This means that 10-fold more publications are available for tinnitus in contrast to hyperacusis (with or without tinnitus). The number of publications does not equal the frequency of comorbid hyperacusis in tinnitus, as hyperacusis may have a prevalence of up to 50% in chronic tinnitus [19, 20] or even higher [4]. About half of the publications in hyperacusis are related to tinnitus, and, again, these numbers do not fit with the reported prevalence rates of tinnitus in hyperacusis, which may be up to 90% [5]. Inspection of the number of publications dealing with either tinnitus or hyperacusis as the main issue (counting the number of publications using tinnitus or hyperacusis in the title of the publication) reveals that 156 papers investigated tinnitus, 41 used hyperacusis as the single main topic, 97 used both as the main issues and 175 mentioned both conditions but not in the title. In summary, hyperacusis can be seen as the smaller and later-born (first publication 1948) sibling of tinnitus (first publication 1888), and there is a need for more scientific and, as a result, clinical work on this specific condition that is highly comorbid with tinnitus.

The first edition of the *Textbook of Tinnitus* was released in 2010. If we repeat the literature research from above, 7568 literature hits could be found for tinnitus in 2010 (as a reminder, it was 13.724 in the year 2020), 153 for tinnitus and hyperacusis in 2010 in contrast to 469 hits for both conditions in 2020. This means an 1.8-fold increase of the publications on tinnitus and a 3.1-fold increase of the publications on hyperacusis, showing that research on hyperacusis is catching up. The smaller sibling grows taller.

Second, in addition to the number of publications in the field of hyperacusis and tinnitus, we also want to show the research topics with regard to hyperacusis in order to provide an overview of the orientation of this scientific field. This exploratory literature overview has the limitation that we focused on the title and abstract, thus ignoring the exact content of the papers.

We show the topics and the number of publications in Table 41.1 for publications dealing with hyperacusis alone

Table 41.1 An overview of the research topics based on a literature review at the end of 2020 divided into publications investigating hyperacusis without and with tinnitus

Number of hyperacusis studies without tinnitus	478	469	Number of hyperacusis studies with tinnitus
Specific syndromes: facial nerve conditions, genetic disorders, neurodegeneration syndromes, infectious diseases, neurological disorders and conditions, inner ear conditions, autoimmune disorders	98	32	Specific syndromes: facial nerve conditions, genetic disorders, neurological disorders and conditions, inner ear conditions, autoimmune disorders, other conditions
Superior canal dehiscence	23	13	Superior canal dehiscence
Association with pain: pain, migraine, headache, chronic pain, hypervigilance, fibromyalgia	63	4	Association with pain: pain threshold, migraine, headache, vestibular migraine
n/a		5	Temporomandibular joint disorder, somatosensory tinnitus
Vertigo,	8		n/a
Concussion, traumatic brain injury	10	7	Traumatic brain injury, blunt trauma, whiplash, head injury
Exposure to radioactive, chemical substances	3	1	Cobalt
Autism	21	1	Autism
Misophonia, phonophobia	7	11	Misophonia, phonophobia, diplacusis, polyacousis
n/a		6	Lidocaine, steroid, endogenous opioids, serotonin, valproate, menstrual cycle, hormones
Middle ear: middle ear reflexes, middle ear conditions (otosclerosis, ossicular chain dislocation, otitis media, cholesteatoma), stapedotomy, tympanoplasty, round and oval window surgery, eustachian tube	27	6	Middle ear: stapedial reflex, tonic tensor tympani syndrome, tympanic membrane displacement test, eustachian tube
Audiology: hearing aids, hearing, deafness, cochlear implant, hearing devices, uncomfortable loudness levels (ULLs), speech comprehension, otoacoustic emissions, recruitment, correlation of audiological measures with questionnaires, loudness growth functions, auditory brainstem responses, psychophysics, decruitment	127	80	Audiology and hearing conditions: speech in noise, discomfort during ULLs, speech comprehension, hidden hearing loss, auditory brain stem responses audiometry, optoacoustic emissions, gap detection, acoustic shock, noise exposure, low-level noise, acoustic trauma, acute hearing loss, age-related hearing loss, working environment, autoimmune hearing loss, earplug-induced, musicians, blast injury, musicians, music use
Children	6	17	Children
Mental health, personality, sleep, antidepressants, drug withdrawal, benzodiazepine dependence, pervasive refusal syndrome, childhood attention-deficit hyperactivity disorder (ADHD)	14	16	Mental health, insomnia, self-harm
Epidemiology, phenomenology, questionnaires, health literacy (Internet)	9	57	Aetiology, phenomenology of hyperacusis and/or tinnitus, clinical characteristics of tinnitus, cognition in tinnitus, tinnitus loudness, double tinnitus, healthcare cost of tinnitus, association with cardiovascular disease, association with or interaction between tinnitus and hyperacusis, samples of tinnitus and hyperacusis, questionnaires, health education, readability, eHealth, computational models
Neuroimaging, electroencephalography	4	13	Neuroimaging, electroencephalography, evoked potentials, magnetic resonance spectroscopy, magnetic resonance imaging

Table 41.1 (continued)

Number of hyperacusis studies without tinnitus	478	469	Number of hyperacusis studies with tinnitus
Studies in animals: salicylate-induced, noise-induced, mutant mice, deletion, drug-induced, lesion, rats, mice, cats, border collies, guinea pigs, horses	38	71	Studies in animals: aminoglycoside-induced, salicylate-induced, noise-induced, rats, mice, guinea pigs, cochlea, startle, manganese uptake, N-Methyl-D-aspartate blocker evoked potentials, electrophysiology, compound action potential, surgery, gap detection, drug therapy
n/a		33	Psychotherapy and related therapies: eye movement desensititazion and reprocessing, CBT, tinnitus retraining therapy (TRT), Internet-based counselling
Sound therapy	2	13	Sound therapy, trigeminal-auditory therapy, masker
n/a		5	Multi-modal therapies
n/a		6	Cochlear implant, cochlear labyrinthectomy, electrical promontory stimulation
n/a		2	Brain stimulation
n/a		3	Dietary supplements, zinc, antioxidants
n/a		2	Laser therapy, physiotherapeutic electric stimulation
Reviews, overviews, statements, summaries (including studies on animals)	11	65	Reviews, overviews, statements, summaries (including studies on animals)
Not assignable	7		

and with hyperacusis in combination with tinnitus. We categorized the publications by inspection of the title and when in doubt by inspection of the abstract. This table shows us that research on "hyperacusis without tinnitus" is focused on specific syndromes, whereas research on "hyperacusis in the context of tinnitus" has more substance with respect to aetiological studies (phenomenology, neuroscience and animal studies), therapy studies and review articles. A bulk of studies deal with middle ear issues and audiological measures. Little attention goes to specific topics, such as hyperacusis in children, and to mental health issues—although these issues are definitely not of lesser importance. Hence, whereas a large number of publications are related to the aetiology and phenomenology of hyperacusis in tinnitus patients, the number of publications on therapies is rather small. This imbalance is even higher in hyperacusis-only research. This relatively limited effort in the field of therapy may be due to the limited knowledge on the mechanisms of hyperacusis. This conclusion might motivate both clinicians and researchers to intentionally focus more on treatments in the future.

Animal Behavioural and Human Neuroscience Studies

In general, neuroscience research can be split into two fields: studies in animals and studies in humans. As can be seen from Table 41.1, the bulk of studies consider animals with respect to hyperacusis and tinnitus. Human neuroscience studies seem to be in the minority [21]. Animal studies focus on animal models of tinnitus and/or hyperacusis, i.e. animals receive a specific intervention (e.g. noise trauma), which is assumed to result in tinnitus and/or hyperacusis, and specific measurements (e.g. behavioural experiments) are considered to represent these conditions with sufficient validity. Typically, recordings are related to the measurements of single or small units of hair cells in the inner ear or neurons along the auditory pathway (see also Chap. 23). Humans, on the other hand, can be asked about their tinnitus/hyperacusis, and, typically, measurements are restricted to non-invasive recordings of a large assembly of co-active neurons. Recently, there have also been studies bridging the gap, e.g. brain activity in animals or brainstem recordings in implanted patients (deep brain stimulation). Nonetheless, each field has not only its advantages but also its limitations, and, as such, so far, there is no cure for tinnitus and hyperacusis.

In the field of human neuroscience, certain methods for measuring brain activity are used. Magnetic resonance imaging (MRI) mainly measures the grey matter brain structure with a resolution in the millimetre range. Diffusion tensor imaging records the white matter tracts. Functional MRI (fMRI) records brain activity via oxygenated blood in the brain. Functional near-infrared spectroscopy (fNIRS) is related to fMRI and measures oxygenated blood in skull-near areas via a non-magnetic technique. Similar to fMRI and NIRS, magneto- and electroencephalography measure the electrical activity of the brain via sensors placed on the skull of the subjects. Depending on the paradigm, resting state or task/stimulus-evoked activity can be recorded.

The most widely accepted neural mechanism for the generation of hyperacusis (in comorbid tinnitus) is an increase of central neural gain [5, 22] or, in other words, an increase in responsiveness of the auditory sensory system on the neural level [23] (see also Chap. 18). In brief, increased gain/responsiveness leads to tinnitus by increased spontaneous activity and hence to hyperacusis by an increased response to auditory stimuli. Where along the auditory pathway this adaptation, whether in association with or in the absence of cochlear pathology, takes place is not clear, but there is evidence from animal and human studies for changes in subcortical and cortical areas [23–25]. However, these data and studies lack adequate control conditions (animals with hearing damage but not with tinnitus/hyperacusis or humans without tinnitus/hyperacusis with comparable hearing loss) and heterogeneous definitions of hyperacusis are used [5]. To sum up, changes in neural gain occur after hearing loss and co-occur in tinnitus/hyperacusis, and it seems to be a necessary condition, but it is not clear whether increased neural gain is sufficient to explain tinnitus and/or hyperacusis [22]. Some considerations question this model [26]. Thus, alternative mechanisms are under debate to determine which of them take place along the auditory pathway [27, 28] up to specific brain networks, for example ("focused attention, resetting of sensory predictions, failure of sensory gating, altered sensory predictions, formation of pervasive memory traces and/or entry into global perceptual networks"; [22]).

The majority of the human studies just deal with either tinnitus or hyperacusis in isolation. There is a scarcity of work that tries to disentangle the neural effects of tinnitus from those of hyperacusis. Two fMRI studies potentially show some evidence for increased activity in the subcortical [29, 30] and cortical parts of the hearing pathway [30] in tinnitus patients with hyperacusis in contrast to patients without. One electroencephalogram (EEG) study found increased beta power in the dorsal anterior cingulate cortex and the orbitofrontal cortex, increased alpha power in the auditory cortex and increased connectivity for these areas for patients with tinnitus and hyperacusis in contrast to patients with tinnitus alone [9]. One case study could not disentangle EEG activity between one patient with tinnitus and one with hyperacusis, both without hearing loss [31]. This case report showed increased gamma activity in the auditory cortices in both patients. These findings represent only one example, showing more neuronal commonalities than differences between patients with tinnitus with and without hyperacusis. Findings of structural and functional changes of the auditory cortex and connected networks in patients with hyperacusis alone [8, 32–34] can also be found in patients with tinnitus [21, 35, 36], and, for some of these studies, it was not specified whether the tinnitus patients also experienced hyperacusis.

In the field of animal studies, measurements target functioning of the inner ear, single neurons and cell assemblies along the auditory pathway with several different methods. For details, we refer to review articles in the field of tinnitus [37, 38] (see also Chaps. 10, 11 and 23). Measurements are similar for tinnitus and hyperacusis, with the measures of tinnitus more related to steady (resting state) and hyperacusis to sound-evoked activity. However, such measurements alone are not specific to tinnitus or hyperacusis. A prerequisite in animal studies is how to measure hyperacusis. Hayes et al. provide a clear overview of measurement models of tinnitus and hyperacusis [39]. Tinnitus can be measured with behavioural paradigms of conditioned responses (training of animals to behave in a certain way for a specific sound condition and measurement of the change of behaviour as a measure for tinnitus after experimental induction of hearing loss; [40–46]) or using an inherent reflex, which is modulated by specific sound conditions (gap pre-pulse inhibition of the acoustic startle reflex; [47]). Experimental hyperacusis models are also conditioned behavioural models or based on the acoustic startle reflex [39]. To disentangle the phenomenon of tinnitus from that of hyperacusis, it is necessary to measure models for tinnitus and hyperacusis in the same samples by measuring the startle reflex and gap detection, respectively [48–50]. However, there are methodological ambiguities, e.g. gap detection data may be explained to some extent by mechanisms of noise sensitivity [51]. In addition, it is also questioned which experimental model measures which condition in general, and the problem of the validity of animal models of either tinnitus or hyperacusis is a matter of debate [37].

Animal studies show the same picture as does the human literature, in that there is limited work, which tries to disentangle tinnitus from hyperacusis. Thomas et al. could induce hyperacusis without tinnitus after 2 weeks of moderate sound exposure, followed by 1 week of exposure to 7-kHz tone pips, which was associated with an expansion of the 7-kHz frequency region in the primary auditory cortex [52]. Muca et al. showed manganese-enhanced magnetic resonance imaging-specific changes related to tinnitus (superior olivary complex and cochlear nucleus), noise sensitivity (inferior colliculus) and hearing loss in the specific brain nuclei [53]. Turner and Larsen showed that 12 months after noise exposure, tinnitus is more likely to occur in rats with low or modest noise trauma and hyperacusis is more likely to occur in high noise trauma [54].

To sum up, there is a substantial and urgent need for human and animal neuroscience studies, which try to disentangle the phenomenon of tinnitus from that of hyperacusis (and hearing loss), i.e. to measure tinnitus and hyperacusis in the same samples and to derive dependent variables from neuroscience methods with sufficient validity. Furthermore, neuroscience studies so far have shown a limited translation to management strategies to lower the suffering of patients.

Impact/Burden on the Patient

As hyperacusis affects the perception of everyday sounds, it is not surprising that it may heavily impact one's emotional well-being and quality of life. Factors associated with hyperacusis impact include comorbid hearing loss and both physical and mental health challenges [55]. Patients with hyperacusis might be easily awakened from sleep by sounds or have difficulties falling asleep due to annoyance with sounds in their environment or even anticipated sounds. In extreme cases, even touching the bedcover, for example, is highly distressing. Moreover, communication problems may occur in environments with background noise. Some patients report speech recognition problems in noise [56], which is related to the extent of their hyperacusis [57]. Patients with hyperacusis might also benefit from hearing aids to compensate for their hearing loss, but the fitting of hearing aids is a challenge as they perceive sound as uncomfortably loud in general. Therefore, audiologists might need to increase compression or decrease the maximum output level for these patients, which leads to suboptimal speech recognition performance [58]. Finally, patients with hyperacusis might avoid social, occupational and recreational activities and may wear hearing protection out of fear of discomfort and potential consequences of noise exposure [59, 60]. As such, a typical patient with hyperacusis will wear ear protection in public places (or at least always have them with him/her) or avoid traffic situations or household chores (e.g. vacuuming, use of the extractor). These avoidance behaviours are intuitive but can potentially lead to exacerbation of the symptoms [61]. Evidently, hyperacusis can lead to a highly substantial decrease in the quality of life.

As patients' experiences often differ, Tyler et al. [56] proposed a framework for subtypes of hyperacusis based on the defining feature of their experience, namely, loudness, annoyance, fear and pain hyperacusis. "Loudness hyperacusis" is present when moderately intense sounds are perceived as extremely loud. Sometimes sounds are not perceived as loud and still there is a negative emotional reaction involved. This is what the authors call "annoyance hyperacusis", but it could be argued this is a description of misophonia [62]. Similarly, "fear hyperacusis" could be seen as an alternative term for phonophobia. As such, it is important to disentangle hyperacusis from misophonia and phonophobia (see also Chap. 3). A differentiator might be general fear/discomfort vs. specific sounds. Finally, "pain hyperacusis" involves a pain experience (e.g. stabbing pain) in response to the sound levels lower than the pain limit of normal hearing. Although this subtyping might support diagnosis and management, it is important to differentiate hyperacusis from other conditions. Additionally, the categories proposed by Tyler et al. [56] cannot be mutually exclusive, and an individual patient may fit in several categories [63]. In a Delphi survey on the definition of hyperacusis [1], experiences of annoyance and fear were common features of hyperacusis but pain was not.

Measurement of Hyperacusis

For the assessment of hyperacusis, two main methods are available: on the one hand, psychoacoustic measurements, in which the loudness of sounds is evaluated, and, on the other hand, questionnaires for assessing the various symptoms of hyperacusis. The questionnaires include not only items for the loudness of sounds but also ask for psychological aspects. The correlation of both methods is only low-to-moderate. Thus, in sum, none of the single measurement methods are valid to measure hyperacusis objectively.

Audiology-Based/Psychoacoustic Measures

The field of audiology uses calibrated equipment to measure the functioning of the ears and the auditory pathways and determine whether the recorded values fall within a range of normal or distorted functioning. The measurements often involve answers of the patients. For quantifying hyperacusis, uncomfortable loudness levels (ULLs) can be determined [64, 65]. Another broadly equivalent term is "loudness discomfort levels (LDLs)". ULLs or LDLs are measured by presenting increasing sound volumes of different frequencies to determine when the patient judges the sounds as uncomfortable. It has to be distinguished from intolerable (so loud as it is not tolerable anymore), which has also been used in the literature. The patient responses can be dichotomous (comfortable vs. uncomfortable) [7], categorical (e.g. soft, comfortable, loud, uncomfortable loud) [66] or metrically scaled [67]. The two last mentioned methods allow the measurement of loudness growth functions (perceived loudness depending on the intensity of the sound). The sound stimulus used is usually a pure tone, but variations are also known, e.g. the use of modulated tones or noise [64], the use of several frequencies to obtain loudness functions [7] and the ratings of natural sounds [68]. The testing of different frequencies is insofar of interest as it might help disentangle hyperacusis (hypersensitivity to sounds not defined at specific frequencies) from recruitment phenomena (hypersensitivity to sounds with frequencies in the range of hearing loss) [69]. Certain ULL ranges are indicated as normal (ULL_{min} $\geq$77 dB HL [70]). However, the exact normative values are under debate as there are concerns about the reliability of ULLs [64, 71, 72]. In sum, hyperacusis is related to decreased ULLs; however, sensitivity and specificity are not high enough to assume sufficient validity of ULLs as a measure of hyperacusis. Nonetheless, this audiometric measure may support the clinical diagnosis of hyperacusis or provide information on therapy-induced change.

The low quality in criteria such as objectivity, reliability and validity may be related to the subjective nature of the ULL and the lack of standardization of the measurements. Limited validity is shown by only moderate correlations of ULLs with hyperacusis questionnaires. More objective measures such as middle ear reflexes or otoacoustic emissions reveal some associations with hyperacusis but were shown to be even less valid for measuring hyperacusis than ULLs [73–75].

Questionnaires

Hyperacusis is defined by phenomenological descriptions. Thus, besides interviewing the patients, standardized questionnaires are useful for the assessment of hyperacusis. These inventories assess both loudness sensitivity and related psychological aspects, e.g. annoyance or fear ([56]; see also the chapter "Burden/Impact on the Patient" above [76]) and aim to quantify the degree of suffering from hyperacusis. Four different questionnaires can be found in peer-reviewed journals and are reviewed below.

The "Hyperacusis Questionnaire (HQ)" is the most known and commonly used measure. It is available in English and in other languages such as Dutch, Italian and Turkish [77–79]. Data for internal consistency and cut-off values are available, but the latter is under discussion and there is some controversy in this regard. Fackrell et al. [80] have proposed a revised 10-item version of the HQ, but this has not yet been independently validated. Scientific re-evaluations could partly replicate the factor structure. Un-evaluated versions with a different number of items are available online, but great caution is advised regarding their use.

The *Geräuschüberempfindlichkeitsfragebogen* (*GÜF*) is a German inventory of which an unvalidated English translation was published [81, 82]. Information with respect to retest reliability, sensitivity/specificity and norm values are limited. Normative values are based on the inter-quartile range. External validation with two screening items for hyperacusis in the Tinnitus Sample Case History Questionnaire of the Tinnitus Research Initiative provide a hint for a cut-off score separating hyperacusis from normal hearing [83].

The "Multiple-Activity Scale for Hyperacusis (MASH)" was developed to assess the real-world impact of hyperacusis [4] and showed a good correlation with the HQ [77].

Recently, the "Inventory of Hyperacusis Symptoms (IHS)" has been published with items that were derived from the three afore-mentioned questionnaires [84]. All the available instruments have limitations. Reliability has only been assessed by measuring internal consistency and, except for the HQ test samples, was restricted to tinnitus patients with hyperacusis. Retest reliability or the sensitivity for measuring treatment effects is not clear. Practically all instruments assess not only loudness hyperacusis but also psychosocial aspects such as emotions (e.g. fear and annoyance), pain, arousal, quality of life and hearing aspects. The analysis of these facets of hyperacusis might help identify the individual needs for treatment and can thus be useful in clinical practice.

One aspect of questionnaire design that is rarely considered is that of readability (for details, see also the topic of health literacy in Chap. 43). This is important as if questionnaire items are incomprehensible to a patient, then the results will be invalid. Regarding hyperacusis questionnaires, each of the instruments described above requires a reading age above that, which is the standard for medical literature [85], and this will need to be taken into account in the design of future questionnaires.

Treatment of Hyperacusis

Treatments focused on decreasing hyperacusis-related distress are gathering pace, but evidence on the effectiveness of the different approaches available is limited. Most studies focus on patients with a secondary complaint of hyperacusis or with hyperacusis as part of a symptom set. As such, current management of hyperacusis often contains cognitive behavioural therapy (CBT) or tinnitus retraining therapy (TRT) (including sound therapy) in the modified form.

CBT

CBT is a well-established and popular psychological intervention [86], and its use in hyperacusis aims to alleviate anxiety by adapting dysfunctional cognitions and targeting safety-seeking behaviours. Breaking a vicious cycle, which is triggered by sound and adversely affects a patient's activities and mood, is at the heart of this therapy for hyperacusis (see [87] for a more detailed description of the vicious circle and this approach). Parts of the vicious circle are the sensation of a (loud) sound, dysfunctional cognitions ("this sound is harmful"), negative emotions (anxiety, worries), physiological reactions (startle reaction, activation of the sympathetic nerve system) and behavioural consequences (avoidance of potential loud situations). The avoidance of sounds lead to a decreased experience that sounds are not harmful, affirm the dysfunctional cognitions and strengthen the avoidance behaviour. The next loud sound might result in even stronger activation of this vicious circle, resulting in the worst case in mental disorders such as depression. In other words, CBT aims to alleviate the symptoms by identifying the thought process and modifying it with cognitive and behavioural methods. It helps in reducing the avoidance behaviour and aims for exposition of avoided situations.

There are little published data concerning the manualized conduction and effectiveness of CBT for hyperacusis. Manualized treatments are rarely available. In Germany, one module of a CBT manual for tinnitus deals with hyperacusis [88]. One of the first studies on this topic was a randomized controlled trial (RCT) published by Juris and colleagues in 2014. This RCT compared 6 sessions of CBT to a waiting list and included 62 patients with a primary complaint of hyperacusis who had presented to an ear–nose–throat (ENT) clinic. Although there was a general improvement for both groups, this improvement was significantly larger for the CBT group [89]. Hence, CBT for hyperacusis seemed promising. However, specialized psychological care is not easily accessible due to the general shortage of CBT therapists, high costs, long waiting lists, long distances and the perceived stigma of psychological treatments [90, 91]. Consequently, two studies were conducted on the effectiveness of audiologist-guided Internet-based CBT (iCBT) by Beukes et al. [92, 93]. Eight weeks of iCBT (primarily focused on tinnitus) was compared with face-to-face appointments without a CBT component (in the first study) or 8 weeks of monitoring (in the second study). The first study showed equal effectiveness in terms of change in the HQ, and the second study found a slightly greater improvement for the active group. It is important to note that these studies were focused on tinnitus relief, explaining the small differences found. Finally, a small retrospective study on audiologist-delivered CBT, analyzing the results of 14 patients with hyperacusis, demonstrated a significant decrease in HQ [94]. In sum, the limited evidence available on CBT for hyperacusis seems encouraging in reducing hyperacusis-related distress, but RCTs in patients with the primary complaint of hyperacusis and with active control groups are needed to assess the effectiveness of CBT for hyperacusis.

TRT

Directive counselling is applied in TRT in order to initiate habituation to intolerable sounds [95]. TRT was originally focused on tinnitus and later adapted with minor modifications to hyperacusis. The idea behind this therapy is that the brain can select and block unimportant stimuli from reaching awareness and hinder the reactions it would otherwise evoke. The founders of this therapy state that the negative associations with these sounds should be minimized to make this process possible [96]. TRT involves a form of psychoeducation on the mechanisms behind hyperacusis, so the patient realises the benign nature of his/her complaints and understands how habituation can be achieved. For example, the appropriate use of noise protection can be discussed. Next, sound therapy is applied to support this process using low-level, broadband noise generators in both the ears and table-top sound devices (e.g. smartphones).

Desensitization can be achieved by exposing patients to sounds. Sound therapy for hyperacusis can be conducted in two ways: (1) introducing the sound at a quiet and comfortable level and maintaining that intensity, which might "recalibrate" the auditory gain, or (2) introducing the sound at a quiet level and gradually increasing the intensity over time, similar to a graduated exposure program for desensitization [97]. Evidently, the sound used has to be neutral without evoking a negative reaction. With regard to the intensity level, the sound should be just audible but not too loud to avoid interference with speech recognition (see [98] for more details).

An RCT investigating the effects of noise generators and/or TRT counselling on loudness judgements in patients with bilateral sensorineural hearing losses and reduced dynamic ranges was conducted by Formby et al. [99]. The combination of both techniques was demonstrated to be the most successful approach, with an increase of minimal 10 dB in uncomfortable loudness for 82% of the patients in this group. Noreña et al. [100] offered an individualized acoustic signal, consisting of pure tones of different frequencies with the amplitude as a function of the audiogram, to eight participants with hyperacusis in a pilot study. This enriched auditory environment compensated for the decreased auditory input from hearing loss and reduced hyperacusis. While sound-based approaches have shown to be beneficial for some patients (see [101] for a review of the evidence), most published studies are case reports, reported changes have been modest and complete remission was rare. In our opinion, a combination of psychological (CBT, TRT) and sound therapy (with environmental sounds, hearing aids/implants; please note that exposition to sounds is inherent in the concepts of CBT and TRT) seems to be the most promising therapy option for most patients [5].

Other Treatments

The co-occurrence of hyperacusis with other medical conditions (see Chap. 3) leads to reports of changes in hyperacusis after treatments focused on another medical condition. For example, an association between hyperacusis and migraine was pointed out by Abouzari et al. [102], who found migraine-related symptoms in their cohort of patients with hyperacusis. This led them to conducting multi-modal migraine prophylaxis therapy, a therapy consisting of pharmacotherapy (e.g. nortriptyline) and counselling (focused on lifestyle/dietary modifications), in 25 patients. Their results were encouraging, as 88% reported subjective resolution of the symptoms after treatment, but replicating studies are warranted. With regard to pharmacotherapy in general, Baguley and Hoare [5] suggested that some form of analgesia might be effective in sound-evoked otalgia, but evidence for this is also missing. Medications are mostly prescribed to target comorbid anxiety or depression instead of the hyperacusis itself. Serotonergic medication as used in depression might be one future treatment option for hypersensitivity to sounds as some case reports have shown [103]. One possible link is the loudness dependence of the auditory evoked potentials, which is considered as a biomarker for central serotonergic functions [104]. In 2015, Silverstein et al. suggested minimally invasive surgery (i.e. round and oval window reinforcement), as there were reports of improvement in sound tolerance after surgery for superior semicircular canal dehiscence (SSCD) [105]. In a paper of 2020, the results of 47 adults with moderate-to-severe hyperacusis for at least 3 months who underwent this surgery were reported. Patients were excluded from this study if they had Meniere's disease, active middle ear disease, were pregnant or scored 11 or greater on a screening questionnaire for anxiety and depression (Hospital Anxiety and Depression Scale—HADS). An average improvement of 15 points on the HQ was demonstrated, which sustained in the long term (i.e. a mean follow-up of 2 years after surgery) [106]. Future research on this topic would benefit from replication by other surgeons as well as including a control group.

Special Needs in Children

As there is a high incidence of hyperacusis in developmental disorders (see Chap. 3), it is not surprising that hyperacusis is also a significant clinical concern in children with prevalence numbers reported to vary between 3.2 and 17.1% [107]. A study in the United Kingdom by Hall et al. [108] reported that 3.7% of 11-year-olds experience oversensitivity or distress to particular sounds, with male gender, higher maternal education level and readmission to hospital in the first 4 weeks of life being the risk factors [108]. Hence, hyperacusis also occurs in children with no other health concerns. Behavioural reactions, such as covering their ears, aggressiveness or crying, might indicate that sounds are troublesome to a child. While young children's parents might avoid certain situations for their children to avoid distress, older children might try to cope by themselves by avoiding noisy situations [109]. In both situations, social interactions and family functioning are disturbed.

Concerning assessment and treatment in this population, little evidence is available. As can be seen in the literature research (Table 41.1), most studies are dealing with hyperacusis and tinnitus, which means that the focus in rarely on hyperacusis. This results in clinical staff feeling unsupported and unprepared to help these patients. The child's parents can provide information on the child's situation during semi-structured interviews, but no validated questionnaires for a paediatric population are published. ULLs are often not conducted, which can be attributed to the unreliability of the measure and the distress it can cause [109]. Similarly, modification of the current treatment options for adults is proposed in the literature. However, details of the content or proven effectiveness are lacking.

With research on hyperacusis in adults being emergent, it is not surprising that there is little evidence on the assessment and the treatment of it in children. Nevertheless, paediatricians and paediatric audiologists and otologists see these children at their consultations and have no scientific support to help them. More research on this topic is highly valuable and urgently needed and should not only be restricted to comorbid tinnitus conditions, with a validated questionnaire and a tailored treatment protocol being the first steps to move forwards in this field.

Summary

A current overview of hyperacusis raises more questions than answers. Firm evidence regarding mechanisms is sparse, and although proposals around maladaptive central auditory gain are of great interest, experimental data are not yet available to confirm this.

Similarly, information about the epidemiology of hyperacusis is scant (see Chap. 3), and data on the impact of hyperacusis derive from studies of specific groups and populations, in particular of patients with a primary complaint of tinnitus. There is increasing scientific evidence for associations between hyperacusis and mental and physical health.

Treatment approaches for hyperacusis and evidence for them are highly limited (psychology-based therapies, sound stimulation, some specific but not yet well-evaluated medical/surgical approaches) and are often related to treatments for tinnitus or other diseases. From a clinical perspective, one important aspect is to lower the perceived distress. On the other hand, it is necessary to find out the exact aetiological mechanisms in order to develop specific therapies. Related pathologies such as recruitment have also only limited therapeutic solutions. As the above-provided literature review suggested, it is time to further intensify the work on hyperacusis (with or without tinnitus). Besides lowering the distress, it is also important to decrease or prevent avoidance behaviour. Thus, as a general conclusion (based on limited knowledge), the best suggestion for clinicians is the stepwise reduction of avoidance behaviour, desensitization to sounds and psychology-based treatments in highly distressed patients flanked by counselling in each case.

References

1. Adams B, Sereda M, Casey A, Byrom P, Stockdale D, Hoare DJ. A Delphi survey to determine a definition and description of hyperacusis by clinician consensus. Int J Audiol. 2020;1–7:607.
2. Baguley DM. Hyperacusis. J R Soc Med. 2003;96(12):582–5.
3. Jastreboff PJ. Phantom auditory perception (tinnitus): mechanisms of generation and perception. Neurosci Res. 1990;8(4):221–54.
4. Dauman R, Bouscau-Faure F. Assessment and amelioration of hyperacusis in tinnitus patients. Acta Otolaryngol. 2005;125(5):503–9.
5. Baguley DM, Hoare DJ. Hyperacusis: major research questions. HNO. 2018;66(5):358–63.
6. Nelson JJ, Chen K. The relationship of tinnitus, hyperacusis, and hearing loss. Ear Nose Throat J. 2004;83(7):472–6.
7. Hébert S, Fournier P, Noreña A. The auditory sensitivity is increased in tinnitus ears. J Neurosci. 2013;33(6):2356–64.
8. Hwang JH, Chou PH, Wu CW, Chen JH, Liu TC. Brain activation in patients with idiopathic hyperacusis. Am J Otolaryngol. 2009;30(6):432–4.
9. Song J-J, De Ridder D, Weisz N, Schlee W, Van de Heyning P, Vanneste S. Hyperacusis-associated pathological resting-state brain oscillations in the tinnitus brain: a hyperresponsiveness network with paradoxically inactive auditory cortex. Brain Struct Funct. 2014;219(3):1113–28.
10. Jastreboff PJ, Hazell JW. A neurophysiological approach to tinnitus: clinical implications. Br J Audiol. 1993;27(1):7–17.
11. Sedley W, Teki S, Kumar S, Barnes GR, Bamiou DE, Griffiths TD. Single-subject oscillatory gamma responses in tinnitus. Brain. 2012;135(10):3089–100.
12. Baguley D, McFerran D, Hall D. Tinnitus. Lancet. 2013;382(9904):1600–7.
13. Baguley DM. Reflections on the association between tinnitus and hyperacusis. In: Fagelson M, Baguley DM, editors. Hyperacusis and disorders of sound intolerance. San Diego: Plural Publishing; 2016. p. 181–90.
14. Stouffer JL, Tyler RS. Characterization of tinnitus by tinnitus patients. J Speech Hear Disord. 1990;55(3):439–53.
15. Henry JA, Galvez G, Turbin MB, Thielman EJ, McMillan GP, Istvan JA. Pilot study to evaluate ecological momentary assessment of tinnitus. Ear Hear. 2012;33(2):179.
16. Suzuki FAB, Suzuki FA, Onishi ET, Penido NO. Psychoacoustic classification of persistent tinnitus. Braz J Otorhinolaryngol. 2018;84(5):583–90.
17. Ward J, Vella C, Hoare DJ, Hall DA. Subtyping somatic tinnitus: a cross-sectional UK cohort study of demographic, clinical and audiological characteristics. PLoS One. 2015;10(5):e0126254.
18. Nyenhuis N, Golm D, Kröner-Herwig B. A systematic review and meta-analysis on the efficacy of self-help interventions in tinnitus. Cogn Behav Ther. 2013;42(2):159–69.
19. Schecklmann M, Landgrebe M, Langguth B, T. R. I. Database Study Group. Phenotypic characteristics of hyperacusis in tinnitus. PLoS One. 2014;9(1):e86944.
20. Cederroth CR, Lugo A, Edvall NK, Lazar A, Lopez-Escamez JA, Bulla J, et al. Association between hyperacusis and tinnitus. J Clin Med. 2020;9(8):2412.
21. Elgoyhen AB, Langguth B, De Ridder D, Vanneste S. Tinnitus: perspectives from human neuroimaging. Nat Rev Neurosci. 2015;16(10):632–42.
22. Sedley W. Tinnitus: does gain explain? Neuroscience. 2019;407:213–28.
23. Brotherton H, Plack CJ, Maslin M, Schaette R, Munro KJ. Pump up the volume: could excessive neural gain explain tinnitus and hyperacusis? Audiol Neurootol. 2015;20(4):273–82.
24. Auerbach BD, Rodrigues PV, Salvi RJ. Central gain control in tinnitus and hyperacusis. Front Neurol. 2014;5:206.
25. Roberts LE, Sanchez TG, Bruce IC. Tinnitus and hyperacusis: relationship, mechanisms, and initiating conditions. Hyperacusis and disorders of sound intolerance: clinical and research perspectives. San Diego, CA: Plural Publishing; 2018. p. 77–105.
26. Möhrle D, Hofmeier B, Amend M, Wolpert S, Ni K, Bing D, et al. Enhanced central neural gain compensates acoustic trauma-induced cochlear impairment, but unlikely correlates with tinnitus and hyperacusis. Neuroscience. 2019;407:146–69.
27. Eggermont JJ. Separate auditory pathways for the induction and maintenance of tinnitus and hyperacusis? Prog Brain Res. 2021;260:101–27.
28. Zeng FG. Tinnitus and hyperacusis: central noise, gain and variance. Curr Opin Physiol. 2020;18:123–9.
29. Gu JW, Halpin CF, Nam EC, Levine RA, Melcher JR. Tinnitus, diminished sound-level tolerance, and elevated auditory activity in humans with clinically normal hearing sensitivity. J Neurophysiol. 2010;104(6):3361–70.
30. Koops EA, van Dijk P. Hyperacusis in tinnitus patients relates to enlarged subcortical and cortical responses to sound except at the tinnitus frequency. Hear Res. 2021;401:108158.
31. Bae EB, Lee JH. Severe temporal hyper-activated states caused by noise in tinnitus and hyperacusis with normal hearing. J Audiol Otol. 2019;23(3):160–6.
32. Boucher O, Turgeon C, Champoux S, Ménard L, Rouleau I, Lassonde M, et al. Hyperacusis following unilateral damage to the insular cortex: a three-case report. Brain Res. 2015;1606:102–12.
33. Kliuchko M, Heinonen-Guzejev M, Vuust P, Tervaniemi M, Brattico E. A window into the brain mechanisms associated with noise sensitivity. Sci Rep. 2016;6(1):39236.
34. Mahoney CJ, Rohrer JD, Goll JC, Fox NC, Rossor MN, Warren JD. Structural neuroanatomy of tinnitus and hyperacusis in semantic dementia. J Neurol Neurosurg Psychiatry. 2011;82(11):1274–8.
35. Adjamian P, Hall DA, Palmer AR, Allan TW, Langers DR. Neuroanatomical abnormalities in chronic tinnitus in the human brain. Neurosci Biobehav Rev. 2014;45(100):119–33.
36. Knipper M, van Dijk P, Schulze H, Mazurek B, Krauss P, Scheper V, et al. The neural bases of tinnitus: lessons from deafness and cochlear implants. J Neurosci. 2020;40(38):7190.
37. Eggermont JJ. Hearing loss, hyperacusis, or tinnitus: what is modeled in animal research? Hear Res. 2013;295:140–9.
38. Eggermont JJ. Can animal models contribute to understanding tinnitus heterogeneity in humans? Front Aging Neurosci. 2016;8:265.
39. Hayes SH, Radziwon KE, Stolzberg DJ, Salvi RJ. Behavioral models of tinnitus and hyperacusis in animals. Front Neurol. 2014;5:179.
40. Jastreboff PJ, Brennan JF, Coleman JK, Sasaki CT. Phantom auditory sensation in rats: an animal model for tinnitus. Behav Neurosci. 1988;102(6):811–22.
41. Bauer CA, Brozoski TJ, Rojas R, Boley J, Wyder M. Behavioral model of chronic tinnitus in rats. Otolaryngol Head Neck Surg. 1999;121(4):457–62.
42. Heffner HE, Harrington IA. Tinnitus in hamsters following exposure to intense sound. Hear Res. 2002;170(1–2):83–95.
43. Rüttiger L, Ciuffani J, Zenner HP, Knipper M. A behavioral paradigm to judge acute sodium salicylate-induced sound experience in rats: a new approach for an animal model on tinnitus. Hear Res. 2003;180(1–2):39–50.
44. Lobarinas E, Sun W, Cushing R, Salvi R. A novel behavioral paradigm for assessing tinnitus using schedule-induced polydipsia avoidance conditioning (SIP-AC). Hear Res. 2004;190(1):109–14.
45. Sederholm F, Swedberg MD. Establishment of auditory discrimination and detection of tinnitus induced by salicylic acid and intense tone exposure in the rat. Brain Res. 2013;1510:48–62.

46. Stolzberg D, Hayes SH, Kashanian N, Radziwon K, Salvi RJ, Allman BL. A novel behavioral assay for the assessment of acute tinnitus in rats optimized for simultaneous recording of oscillatory neural activity. J Neurosci Methods. 2013;219(2):224–32.
47. Turner JG, Brozoski TJ, Bauer CA, Parrish JL, Myers K, Hughes LF, et al. Gap detection deficits in rats with tinnitus: a potential novel screening tool. Behav Neurosci. 2006;120(1):188–95.
48. Turner JG, Parrish J. Gap detection methods for assessing salicylate-induced tinnitus and hyperacusis in rats. Am J Audiol. 2008;17(2):S185–S92.
49. Rybalko N, Mitrovic D, Šuta D, Bureš Z, Popelář J, Syka J. Behavioral evaluation of auditory function abnormalities in adult rats with normal hearing thresholds that were exposed to noise during early development. Physiol Behav. 2019;210:112620.
50. Chen G, Lee C, Sandridge SA, Butler HM, Manzoor NF, Kaltenbach JA. Behavioral evidence for possible simultaneous induction of hyperacusis and tinnitus following intense sound exposure. J Assoc Res Otolaryngol. 2013;14(3):413–24.
51. Salloum RH, Sandridge S, Patton DJ, Stillitano G, Dawson G, Niforatos J, et al. Untangling the effects of tinnitus and hypersensitivity to sound (hyperacusis) in the gap detection test. Hear Res. 2016;331:92–100.
52. Thomas ME, Guercio GD, Drudik KM, de Villers-Sidani E. Evidence of hyperacusis in adult rats following non-traumatic sound exposure. Front Syst Neurosci. 2019;13:55.
53. Muca A, Standafer E, Apawu AK, Ahmad F, Ghoddoussi F, Hali M, et al. Tinnitus and temporary hearing loss result in differential noise-induced spatial reorganization of brain activity. Brain Struct Funct. 2018;223(5):2343–60.
54. Turner JG, Larsen D. Effects of noise exposure on development of tinnitus and hyperacusis: prevalence rates 12 months after exposure in middle-aged rats. Hear Res. 2016;334:30–6.
55. Smit AL, Stegeman I, Eikelboom RH, Baguley DM, Bennett RJ, Tegg-Quinn S, et al. Prevalence of hyperacusis and its relation to health: the Busselton Healthy Ageing Study. Laryngoscope. 2021;131(12):E2887–96.
56. Tyler RS, Pienkowski M, Roncancio ER, Jun HJ, Brozoski T, Dauman N, et al. A review of hyperacusis and future directions: part I. Definitions and manifestations. Am J Audiol. 2014;23(4):402–19.
57. Vielsmeier V, Kreuzer PM, Haubner F, Steffens T, Semmler PR, Kleinjung T, et al. Speech comprehension difficulties in chronic tinnitus and its relation to hyperacusis. Front Aging Neurosci. 2016;8:293.
58. Formby C, Hawley M, Sherlock L, Gold S, Segar A, Gmitter C, et al. Intervention for restricted dynamic range and reduced sound tolerance. J Acoust Soc Am. 2008;123(5):3717.
59. Blaesing L, Kroener-Herwig B. Self-reported and behavioral sound avoidance in tinnitus and hyperacusis subjects, and association with anxiety ratings. Int J Audiol. 2012;51(8):611–7.
60. Paulin J, Andersson L, Nordin S. Characteristics of hyperacusis in the general population. Noise Health. 2016;18(83):178–84.
61. Munro KJ, Turtle C, Schaette R. Plasticity and modified loudness following short-term unilateral deprivation: evidence of multiple gain mechanisms within the auditory system. J Acoust Soc Am. 2014;135(1):315–22.
62. Enzler F, Loriot C, Fournier P, Noreña AJ. A psychoacoustic test for misophonia assessment. Sci Rep. 2021;11(1):11044.
63. Fagelson M, Baguley DM. Disorders of sound tolerance: history and terminology. In: Fagelson M, Baguley DM, editors. Hyperacusis and disorders of sound intolerance. San Diego: Plural Publishing, Inc.; 2018. p. 3–14.
64. BSA BSoA. Recommended procedure determination of uncomfortable loudness levels; 2018.
65. Aazh H, Moore BCJ. Incidence of discomfort during pure-tone audiometry and measurement of uncomfortable loudness levels among people seeking help for tinnitus and/or hyperacusis. Am J Audiol. 2017;26(3):226–32.
66. Keidser G, Seymour J, Dillon H, Grant F, Byrne D. An efficient, adaptive method of measuring loudness growth functions. Scand Audiol. 1999;28(1):3–14.
67. Tyler RS, Noble WG, Coelho C, Haskell G, Bardia A. Tinnitus and hyperacusis. 6th ed. Philadelphia: Lippincott Williams & Wilkins; 2009. p. 726–42.
68. Enzler F, Fournier P, Norena AJ. A psychoacoustic test for diagnosing hyperacusis based on ratings of natural sounds. Hear Res. 2021;400:108124.
69. Schaaf H, Klofat B, Hesse G. [Hyperacusis, phonophobia, and recruitment. Abnormal deviations of hearing associated with hypersensitivity to sound]. HNO. 2003;51(12):1005–11.
70. Aazh H, Moore BCJ. Factors related to uncomfortable loudness levels for patients seen in a tinnitus and hyperacusis clinic. Int J Audiol. 2017;56(10):793–800.
71. Fackrell K, Hoare DJ. Scales and questionnaires of decresed sound tolerance. In: Fagelson M, Baguley DM, editors. Hyperacusis and disorders of sound intolerance. San Diego: Plural Publishing, Inc.; 2018. p. 43–60.
72. Stephens SD, Blegvad B, Krogh HJ. The value of some suprathreshold auditory measures. Scand Audiol. 1977;6(4):213–21.
73. Gordon AG. Abnormal middle ear muscle reflexes and audiosensitivity. Br J Audiol. 1986;20(2):95–9.
74. Downs DW, Crum MA. The hyperactive acoustic reflex. Four case studies. Arch Otolaryngol. 1980;106(7):401–4.
75. Saxena U, Singh BP, Kumar SBR, Chacko G, Bharath K. Acoustic reflexes in individuals having hyperacusis of the auditory origin. Indian J Otolaryngol Head Neck Surg. 2020;72(4):497–502.
76. Pienkowski M, Tyler RS, Roncancio ER, Jun HJ, Brozoski T, Dauman N, et al. A review of hyperacusis and future directions: part II. Measurement, mechanisms, and treatment. Am J Audiol. 2014;23(4):420–36.
77. Meeus OM, Spaepen M, Ridder DD, Heyning PH. Correlation between hyperacusis measurements in daily ENT practice. Int J Audiol. 2010;49(1):7–13.
78. Fioretti A, Tortorella F, Masedu F, Valenti M, Fusetti M, Pavaci S. Validity of the Italian version of Khalfa's questionnaire on hyperacusis. Acta Otorhinolaryngol Ital. 2015;35(2):110–5.
79. Erinc M, Derinsu U. Turkish adaptation of Khalfa Hyperacusis Questionnaire. Medeni Med J. 2020;35(2):142–50.
80. Fackrell K, Fearnley C, Hoare DJ, Sereda M. Hyperacusis questionnaire as a tool for measuring hypersensitivity to sound in a tinnitus research population. Biomed Res Int. 2015;2015:290425.
81. Bläsing L, Goebel G, Flötzinger U, Berthold A, Kröner-Herwig B. Hypersensitivity to sound in tinnitus patients: an analysis of a construct based on questionnaire and audiological data. Int J Audiol. 2010;49(7):518–26.
82. Nelting M, Rienhoff NK, Hesse G, Lamparter U. Die Erfassung des subjektiven Leidens unter Hyperakusis mit einem Selbstbeurteilungsbogen zur Geräuschüberempfindlichkeit (GÜF). Laryngorhinootologie. 2002;81(05):327–34.
83. Schecklmann M, Lehner A, Schlee W, Vielsmeier V, Landgrebe M, Langguth B. Validation of screening questions for hyperacusis in chronic tinnitus. Biomed Res Int. 2015;2015:191479.
84. Greenberg B, Carlos M. Psychometric properties and factor structure of a new scale to measure hyperacusis: introducing the inventory of hyperacusis symptoms. Ear Hear. 2018;39(5):1025–34.
85. Margol-Gromada M, Sereda M, Baguley DM. Readability assessment of self-report hyperacusis questionnaires. Int J Audiol. 2020;59(7):506–12.
86. Beck AT. Cognitive therapy and the emotional disorders. New York: Penguin Publishing Group; 1979.
87. Aazh H, Landgrebe M, Danesh AA, Moore BC. Cognitive behavioral therapy for alleviating the distress caused by tinnitus, hyper-

acusis and misophonia: current perspectives. Psychol Res Behav Manag. 2019;12:991–1002.
88. Weise C, Kleinstäuber M, Kaldo V, Andersson G. Mit Tinnitus leben lernen: Ein Manual für Therapeuten und Betroffene. Berlin: Springer; 2016.
89. Jüris L, Andersson G, Larsen HC, Ekselius L. Cognitive behaviour therapy for hyperacusis: a randomized controlled trial. Behav Res Ther. 2014;54:30–7.
90. Kobak KA, Craske MG, Rose RD, Wolitsky-Taylor K. Web-based therapist training on cognitive behavior therapy for anxiety disorders: a pilot study. Psychotherapy (Chic). 2013;50(2):235–47.
91. Webb CA, Rosso IM, Rauch SL. Internet-based cognitive-behavioral therapy for depression: current progress and future directions. Harv Rev Psychiatry. 2017;25(3):114–22.
92. Beukes EW, Andersson G, Allen PM, Manchaiah V, Baguley DM. Effectiveness of guided internet-based cognitive behavioral therapy vs face-to-face clinical care for treatment of tinnitus: a randomized clinical trial. JAMA Otolaryngol Head Neck Surg. 2018;144(12):1126–33.
93. Beukes EW, Baguley DM, Allen PM, Manchaiah V, Andersson G. Audiologist-guided internet-based cognitive behavior therapy for adults with tinnitus in the United Kingdom: a randomized controlled trial. Ear Hear. 2018;39(3):423–33.
94. Aazh H, Moore BCJ. Effectiveness of audiologist-delivered cognitive behavioral therapy for tinnitus and hyperacusis rehabilitation: outcomes for patients treated in routine practice. Am J Audiol. 2018;27(4):547–58.
95. Jastreboff PJ, Hazell JWP. Tinnitus retraining therapy (TRT): clinical implementation of the model. Tinnitus retraining therapy: implementing the neurophysiological model. Cambridge: Cambridge University Press; 2008.
96. Jastreboff PJ, Jastreboff MM. Tinnitus retraining therapy (TRT) as a method for treatment of tinnitus and hyperacusis patients. J Am Acad Audiol. 2000;11(3):162–77.
97. Hazell JWP, Sheldrake JB. Hyperacusis and tinnitus. Tinnitus. 1992;91:245–8.
98. Jastreboff PJ, Jastreboff MM. Treatments for decreased sound tolerance (hyperacusis and misophonia). Semin Hear. 2014;35(02):105–20.
99. Formby C, Hawley M, Sherlock LP, Gold S, Parton J, Brooks R, et al. Intervention for restricted dynamic range and reduced sound tolerance: clinical trial using a tinnitus retraining therapy protocol for hyperacusis. Proc Meetings Acoust. 2013;19(1):050083.
100. Noreña AJ, Chery-Croze S. Enriched acoustic environment rescales auditory sensitivity. Neuroreport. 2007;18(12):1251.
101. Pienkowski M. Rationale and efficacy of sound therapies for tinnitus and hyperacusis. Neuroscience. 2019;407:120–34.
102. Abouzari M, Tan D, Sarna B, Ghavami Y, Goshtasbi K, Parker EM, et al. Efficacy of multi-modal migraine prophylaxis therapy on hyperacusis patients. Ann Otol Rhinol Laryngol. 2020;129(5):421–7.
103. Gopal KV, Daly DM, Daniloff RG, Pennartz L. Effects of selective serotonin reuptake inhibitors on auditory processing: case study. J Am Acad Audiol. 2000;11(8):454–63.
104. Yoon S, Kim Y, Lee SH. Does the loudness dependence of auditory evoked potential predict response to selective serotonin reuptake inhibitors?: a meta-analysis. Clin Psychopharmacol Neurosci. 2021;19(2):254–61.
105. Silverstein H, Wu YH, Hagan S. Round and oval window reinforcement for the treatment of hyperacusis. Am J Otolaryngol. 2015;36(2):158–62.
106. Silverstein H, Kellermeyer B, Martinez U. Minimally invasive surgery for the treatment of hyperacusis: new technique and long term results. Am J Otolaryngol. 2020;41(1):102319.
107. Rosing SN, Schmidt JH, Wedderkopp N, Baguley DM. Prevalence of tinnitus and hyperacusis in children and adolescents: a systematic review. BMJ Open. 2016;6(6):e010596.
108. Hall AJ, Humphriss R, Baguley DM, Parker M, Steer CD. Prevalence and risk factors for reduced sound tolerance (hyperacusis) in children. Int J Audiol. 2016;55(3):135–41.
109. Potgieter I, Fackrell K, Kennedy V, Crunkhorn R, Hoare DJ. Hyperacusis in children: a scoping review. BMC Pediatr. 2020;20(1):319.

Tinnitus and Psychiatric Comorbidities

42

Berthold Langguth and Michael Landgrebe

Abstract

1. Tinnitus is often accompanied by psychiatric comorbidities, especially in its severe forms.
2. Many different comorbid psychiatric disorders have been reported in individuals with severe tinnitus, and among them are depression, anxiety, insomnia, somatoform disorders, psychosis, personality disorders, and body concept disorders.
3. The exact relationship between tinnitus and psychiatric disorders may vary from patient to patient. Psychiatric disorders may evolve as a consequence of tinnitus, may represent predisposing factors, may evolve together with tinnitus as the consequences of a third factor (e.g., trauma), or may just co-occur with tinnitus by coincidence.
4. Psychiatric comorbidities play a major role in creating the distress experienced by many individuals with tinnitus.
5. Similar brain areas are involved in the pathophysiology of tinnitus and affective disorders, which explains the close interrelationship between these two disorders.
6. The occurrence of hyperacusis and phonophobia in tinnitus patients is an indicator of a comorbid anxiety disorder
7. In patients with tinnitus and comorbid psychiatric disorders, both tinnitus and the psychiatric comorbidity should be specifically treated.
8. Treatment options include pharmacological (e.g., antidepressants) and psychotherapeutic (e.g., cognitive behavioral therapy) approaches.

B. Langguth (✉)
Department of Psychiatry and Psychotherapy, University of Regensburg, Bezirksklinikum, Regensburg, Germany
e-mail: Berthold.Langguth@medbo.de

M. Landgrebe
Department of Psychiatry, Psychosomatics and Psychotherapy, kbo-Lech-Mangfall-Hosptial Agatharied, Hausham, Germany
e-mail: Michael.Landgrebe@kbo.de

W. Schlee et al. (eds.), *Textbook of Tinnitus*, https://doi.org/10.1007/978-3-031-35647-6_42

Graphical Abstract

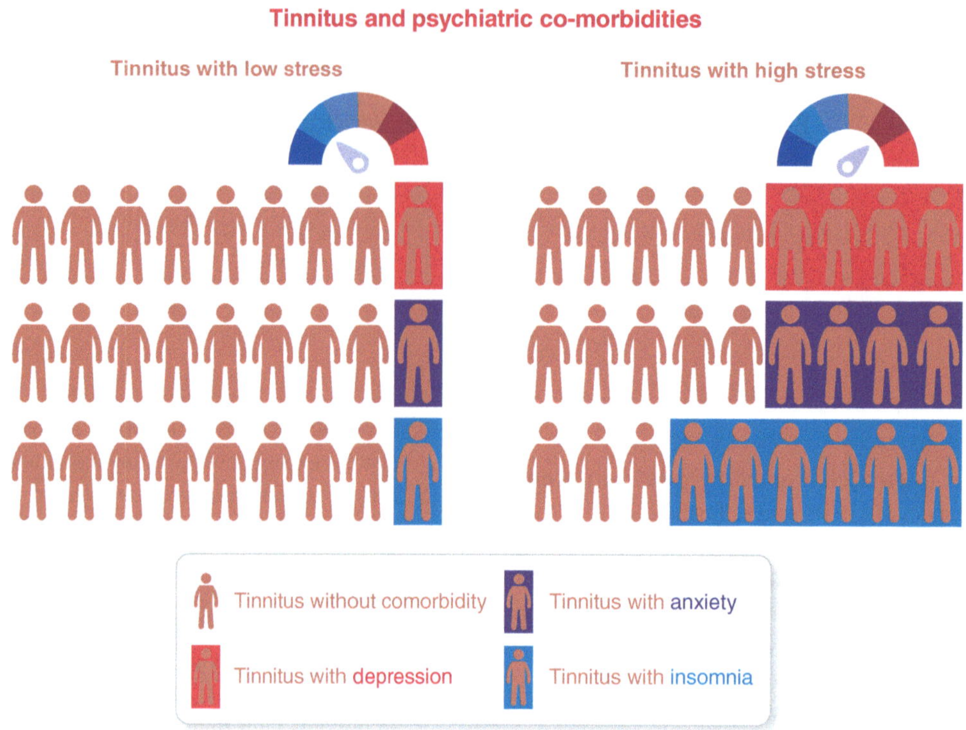

Introduction

Tinnitus, the perception of a phantom sound, is reported by up to 20% of the general population (see Chap. 4), but most of those who have tinnitus are not severely affected by it. Nevertheless, there is a group of individuals with tinnitus, who are severely suffering and sometimes even feel suicidal because of their tinnitus [1, 2].

In order to distinguish between these two conditions, it has been recently proposed to use the term "tinnitus" for the auditory percept and the term "tinnitus disorder" to describe tinnitus and the associated suffering [3] (see Chap. 2).

For the management of a patient with severely disabling tinnitus, it is important to identify what causes tinnitus-related distress and disability. Patients with high scores in tinnitus questionnaires such as the Tinnitus Handicap Inventory (THI) suffer much more frequently from psychiatric disorders than do those with low scores in the tinnitus questionnaires [4–6]. The most frequently reported psychiatric symptoms in this patient group are symptoms of depression and anxiety [5, 7]. The incidence of further psychiatric disorders such as post-traumatic stress disorder (PTSD) [8], somatoform disorder [9], psychosis [10], obsessive-compulsive disorder [11], or body image disorder [12] is also increased among individuals with tinnitus. Published studies agree that there is a high degree of correlation between severe tinnitus and symptoms of depression and anxiety, but the different studies vary with respect to the exact prevalence rates of psychiatric comorbidities. Differences in patient selection are presumably the main reason for this variability (e.g., population survey vs. primary care vs. highly specialized tinnitus centers [13, 14]). Differences in the used diagnostic criteria [3] also contribute to the variation in results.

When tinnitus is associated with suffering, the suffering is typically attributed to be a consequence of the individual's tinnitus. However, there is abundant evidence that personality traits as well as psychiatric disorders may represent the risk factors for the development of tinnitus and the course of tinnitus. Prospective studies have demonstrated that people who suffer from depression have an increased risk of developing tinnitus [15]. Traumatic life events might also increase the risk of developing tinnitus [8]. With respect to psychological traits, it could be demonstrated that patients who score high on neuroticism tend to suffer more from their tinnitus [16, 17]. Moreover, higher scores of neuroticism have been associated with an increase of tinnitus severity over time [18] and a higher impact of environmental stressors on tinnitus suffering [19].

Thus, the interplay between tinnitus and psychiatric symptoms is complex, and the exact relationship between tinnitus and psychiatric disorders may vary from patient to patient. In an individual patient, it can be difficult to differentiate whether tinnitus has caused a reactive psychiatric comorbidity, if a preexisting but compensated psychiatric disorder flares up due to the tinnitus, or whether a well-managed tinnitus reappears due to the onset of a psychiatric disease. Moreover, the co-occurrence of tinnitus and a psychiatric disorder may be the result of common risk factors (e.g., genetic predisposition, specific personality traits, critical life events) or a pure coincidence, as both tinnitus and psychiatric disorders are frequent disorders. In an individual case, the exact etiological relationship between tinnitus and co-occurring psychiatric disorders is frequently difficult to disentangle. Independently from the exact relationship with the patient's tinnitus, the psychiatric disorders that occur together with tinnitus should always be treated. Efficient treatment of the concurrent psychiatric disorder reduces the burden of disease and improves the quality of life of the tinnitus patient. Special emphasis must be placed on the emergency treatment of tinnitus patients who are suicidal. These patients must be referred to a psychiatrist or a psychotherapist for immediate diagnosis and treatment.

Moreover, assessment of a psychiatric comorbidity should not be restricted to chronic tinnitus, as affective disorders are also relevant in acute stages of tinnitus [20]. Therefore, psychiatric treatment should also be considered in acute tinnitus, since the amount of distress in the acute stage (<1-week duration) seems to predict the amount of suffering in the chronic situation [21].

In this chapter, we will discuss the co-occurrence of tinnitus and affective disorders from etiological and pathophysiological perspectives. Moreover, we will provide guidance for the diagnosis and therapeutic management of comorbid depression, anxiety, and suicidal ideation, as these are the most relevant psychiatric problems among tinnitus patients.

Detection of a Psychiatric Comorbidity in a Nonpsychiatric Setting

The majority of tinnitus patients do not show any signs of a psychiatric comorbidity, especially those who have mild forms of tinnitus, which are well-managed. However, if tinnitus patients suffer from depression or anxiety, it is important to recognize and treat these disorders.

In clinical practice, severely suffering tinnitus patients primarily seek medical help for their tinnitus and not for their depression or anxiety. Depending on the health-care system, patients with tinnitus present at their general practitioner, at an otorhinolaryngologist, or at an audiologist but rarely present primarily at a psychiatrist. Patients seek help because of their tinnitus; additional symptoms, which may be present, are only mentioned in passing. Most patients are reluctant to talk about affective symptoms such as mood disturbances or anxiety in a nonpsychiatric setting, and this increases the likelihood that these symptoms are overlooked, as has been shown in large survey studies. In practitioner offices, the correct diagnosis of major depression represents a substantial problem; patients with mild-to-moderate depression are particularly at the risk of being overlooked. For all clinicians who are caring for tinnitus patients but are not specialized in psychiatry, the following questions are relevant:

- What are the signs that a psychiatric comorbidity is likely when treating a patient with tinnitus?
- What are the reasonable screening instruments for psychiatric disorders?
- What should be done if comorbid psychiatric disorders are suspected?
- How should patients at a risk of suicide be managed?
- How can comorbid depression be treated?
- How can comorbid anxiety be treated?

Warning Signs of Potential Psychiatric Comorbidity

Most individuals with tinnitus do not suffer substantially and have little or no impairment of their quality of life. They are also typically able to work and are not restricted by their tinnitus in their everyday life. Some patients with tinnitus seek medical help because they are concerned that their tinnitus may be a sign of a dangerous disease such as a brain tumor. Information about the pathophysiology of tinnitus, counseling (see Chap. 43), a clinical and audiological examination of the ears, and, in case of suspicion, the exclusion of a vestibular schwannoma is sufficient (see Chaps. 28 and 29). In these cases, any psychiatric comorbidity appears to be unlikely. Severe and disabling tinnitus ("tinnitus disorder" according to the recently proposed classification [3]), however, is often accompanied by symptoms such as depressed mood and anxiety. Tinnitus severity can be either assessed by scales, which are easy to perform, or by validated questionnaires (see Chap. 27). Patients with grade III and IV (Table 42.1) or high scores in tinnitus questionnaires (i.e., a total score of more than 47 in the tinnitus questionnaire or of more than 56 in the Tinnitus Handicap Inventory) should be examined with focus on signs of depression or anxiety [14].

Table 42.1 Tinnitus grading according to Biesinger et al. [22]

Grade I	Tinnitus is well-compensated. No psychological strain.
Grade II	Tinnitus appears only in silence and is disturbing during periods of stress and pressure.
Grade III	Tinnitus continuously interferes in the private and professional areas. Emotional, cognitive, and physical disturbances occur.
Grade IV	Tinnitus leads to the complete decompensation in the private area; disability.

What Are the Reasonable Screening Instruments for Psychiatric Symptoms?

The most frequent symptoms of depression are depressed mood, loss of interest, and sleep disorders. However, in a nonpsychiatric setting, circumstances such as time limitations often do not allow an extensive interview to specifically explore all potential symptoms of depression or anxiety. Moreover, specific training and experience are required for assessing affective signs and should be carried out by a psychiatrist or psychologist. However, everybody who treats tinnitus patients should be familiar with the screening instruments for frequent psychiatric disorders, which are based on a few key questions and are easy to perform. For depression, the following two questions have been proposed:

1. During the past month, have you often been bothered by feeling down, depressed, or hopeless?
2. During the past month, have you often been bothered by little interest or pleasure in doing things? [23].

If the patient answers with "yes" to one of the both questions, then depression is likely and referral to a psychiatrist or psychologist should be made. Similar screening questions for anxiety disorders are used in standardized, semi-structured diagnostic interviews like the MINI International Neuropsychiatric Interview (M.I.N.I. [24]; see Table 42.2) and can be used for screening for anxiety disorders.

Table 42.2 Screening questions for different forms of anxiety disorders according to the MINI International Neuropsychiatric Interview (M.I.N.I.; [24])

Disorder	Screening question
Panic disorder	Have you, on more than one occasion, had spells or attacks when you suddenly felt anxious, frightened, uncomfortable or uneasy, even in situations where most people would not feel that way? Did the spells surge to a peak, within 10 min of starting?
Agoraphobia	Do you feel anxious or uneasy in places or situations where you might have a panic attack or panic-like symptoms, or where help might not be available or escape might be difficult: like being in a crowd, standing in a line (queue), when you are away from home or alone at home, or when crossing a bridge, travelling in a bus, train or car?
Social phobia	In the past month were you fearful or embarrassed being watched, being the focus of attention, or fearful of being humiliated? This includes things like speaking in public, eating in public or with others, writing while someone watches, or being in social situations.
Specific phobia	In the past month have you been bothered by recurrent thoughts, impulses, or images that were unwanted, distasteful, inappropriate, intrusive, or distressing (e.g., the idea that you were dirty, contaminated or had germs, or fear of contaminating others, or fear of harming someone even though you didn't want to, or fearing you would act on some impulse, or fear or superstitions that you would be responsible for things going wrong,) or obsessions with sexual thoughts, images or impulses, or hoarding, collecting, or religious obsessions.

What to Do If a Patient with Tinnitus Is Also Suspected to Have Depression and Anxiety

A patient who is suspected of suffering from depressive symptoms, anxiety, or any other psychiatric disorder should be referred to a psychiatrist for further diagnostic and therapeutic management. In clinical practice, this may sometimes be difficult, since patients may interpret the referral to a psychiatrist as a sign that they are not taken seriously or are considered to be "crazy." Thus, it frequently requires a careful explanation that tinnitus can cause a high amount of distress and that a comprehensive treatment concept will include approaches to both reducing tinnitus (e.g., hearing aids, noise generators, etc.) and the associated suffering (e.g., cognitive behavioral therapy, treatment of psychiatric comorbidities). Thus, the patient should understand that the treatment of psychiatric comorbidities is an important part of tinnitus treatment. This has to be explained to the patient, as, in most cases, the intuitive assumption of the patients is that their suffering can only be reduced by reducing or stopping the tinnitus percept. Frequently, it is helpful to explain the distinction between the perception of sound and the reaction to it. Moreover, it is easily understandable that anxiety and depression have an impact on the reaction to the tinnitus sound.

Additionally, a close collaboration with psychiatrists and psychologists, who are interested in tinnitus and have experience with the diagnosis and management of tinnitus patients, will make it easier for otologists or audiologists to refer their patients for psychiatric diagnosis and therapy.

How to Manage a Suicidal Patient?

It is rare that tinnitus patients are acutely suicidal. Nevertheless, in severely suffering tinnitus patients, potential suicidal ideations should always be explored and taken seriously, as suicidal ideations are life-threatening and are therefore an acute emergency.

The most important risk factor for suicide is depressive disorder, both in tinnitus patients [1, 25, 26] and in non-tinnitus patients. Further risk factors include male gender, elder age, and social isolation. Hence, a severely depressed mood, which cannot be modulated and is accompanied by social withdrawal, hopelessness, or even psychotic symptoms, is an important warning sign of a high risk of suicide.

Table 42.3 Screening questions and assessment of suicidality according to the MINI International Neuropsychiatric Interview (M.I.N.I.; [24])

Question	Score if "Yes"
Think you would be better off dead or wish you were dead?	1
Want to harm yourself?	2
Think about suicide?	6
Have a suicide plan?	10
Attempt suicide	10
In your lifetime: Did you ever make a suicide attempt	4

Current suicide risk: 1–5 points = low; 6–9 points = moderate; 10 or more points = high

If one suspects that a patient is at a risk of suicide, then the seriousness of the patient's suicidal thoughts should be evaluated by directly asking the patient about suicidal ideations or even asking if the patient has concrete plans of how to commit suicide. Discussing the issue of suicide with a patient does not increase the risk of them actually committing suicide. On the contrary, most patients feel relieved to have the opportunity to talk about their thoughts. Although there is no general rule on how to manage patients who are suicidal, one possible approach to this sensitive area is to first talk about passive suicidal ideas. This may be introduced by asking, for example, "In the past month, did you think that you would be better dead or wish you were dead?" Further screening questions to estimate the risk that the patient will actually commit suicide are provided in Table 42.3. If it becomes clear from the clinical interview that the patient is suffering from suicidal ideas, then the patient should be immediately referred to a psychiatrist. A patient with serious suicidal and concrete plans of how to commit suicide can be considered an emergency case and requires immediate referral to a psychiatrist or a psychiatric hospital.

Tinnitus and Depression

There is abundant evidence of an increased prevalence of depressive symptoms in individuals with tinnitus, especially in those with disabling tinnitus [14]. High correlation scores have also been reported between the results of tinnitus severity measures and depression scales [16, 27]. Thus, the occurrence of comorbid depression may explain to some extent why some individuals suffer severely from tinnitus, whereas other individuals are not bothered by it. Further studies have shown an additional role for specific personality traits such as anxiety, obsessiveness, or neuroticism [11, 17, 28]. Moreover, the personality factor neuroticism is related to an increase of tinnitus severity over time [18] or in the context of additional stressors [19].

However, it is important to note that all these findings are mainly derived from studies, which used self-report questionnaires for the assessment of depressive symptoms, not from structured interviews. This difference is important, since the presence of depressive symptoms does not automatically mean that a patient fulfills the diagnostic criteria for a depressive disorder. Depressive symptoms may be indicative of a depressive disorder, but they can also occur in the context of a large variety of other psychiatric disorders, such as bipolar disorders, personality disorders, anxiety disorders, dementia, or addiction, just to name a few. Therefore, further studies using structured interviews will be needed to exactly determine the prevalence of comorbid psychiatric disorders in tinnitus.

Diagnosis of Depression

As mentioned above, the two questions: "During the past month, have you often been bothered by feeling down, depressed, or hopeless?" and "During the past month, have you often been bothered by little interest or pleasure in doing things?" are useful to screen for depression. A more detailed screening instrument is the Mini International Neuropsychiatric Interview (M.I.N.I., [24])]. Depressive symptoms may occur in a variety of psychiatric diseases. Thus, the exact differential diagnosis is of importance, as it has important consequences for the therapeutic management. For example, depressive symptoms can occur in the context of a bipolar affective disorder or a post-traumatic stress disorder, which requires a different therapeutic management than does major depression. Thus, when screening questions suggest potential comorbid depression, a psychiatrist should be involved in further diagnostic assessment and therapeutic management.

The exact diagnostic classification may further depend on the classification system. The most widely used classification systems are the "Diagnostic and Statistical Manual of Mental Disorders" of the American Psychiatric Association (DSM-V) and the "International Classification of Diseases" (ICD-10) of the World Health Organization (WHO). The classification criteria for major depression (DSM-V) and depressive disorders (ICD-10) are displayed in Tables 42.4 and 42.5, respectively.

Interplay Between Tinnitus and Depression

As mentioned in the introduction to this chapter, various relationships between tinnitus and depression may occur: Depressive symptoms may develop as a reaction to tinnitus. Specific vulnerability factors such as anxiety or obsessive personality traits may contribute to the development of such

Table 42.4 The DSM-V criteria for major depression (American Psychiatric Association: Diagnostic and Statistical Manual of Mental Disorders 2013)

- At least five of the following symptoms have to have been present during the same 2-week period (and at least one of the symptoms must be either diminished interest/pleasure or depressed mood):
  - Depressed mood: For children and adolescents, this can also be an irritable mood
  - Diminished interest or loss of pleasure in almost all activities (anhedonia)
  - Significant weight change or appetite disturbance: For children, this can be failure to achieve the expected weight gain
  - Sleep disturbance (insomnia or hypersomnia)
  - Psychomotor agitation or retardation
  - Fatigue or loss of energy
  - Feelings of worthlessness
  - Diminished ability to think or concentrate; indecisiveness
  - Recurrent thoughts of death, recurrent suicidal ideation without a specific plan, or a suicide attempt or specific plan for committing suicide
- The symptoms cause significant distress or impairment in social, occupational, or other important areas of functioning
- The symptoms are not attributable to the physiological effects of a substance (e.g., a drug of abuse, a medication) or another medical condition
- The disturbance is not better explained by a persistent schizoaffective disorder, schizophrenia, a delusional disorder, or another specified or unspecified schizophrenia spectrum and other psychotic disorders
- There has never been a manic episode or a hypomanic episode

Table 42.5 ICD-10 criteria for a depressive episode [16]

1. General criteria for a depressive episode:
   (a) The depressive episode should last for at least 2 weeks
   (b) The episode is not attributable to psychoactive substance use or any organic mental disorder
2. The presence of at least two of the following symptoms:
   (a) Depressed mood to a degree that is definitively abnormal for the individual, present for most of the day and almost every day, largely uninfluenced by environmental circumstances, and sustained for at least 2 weeks
   (b) Marked loss of interest or ability to enjoy activities that were previously pleasurable
   (c) Decreased energy or increased fatigability
3. An additional symptom or symptoms from the following should be present, to give a total of at least four:
   (a) Loss of confidence and self-esteem and feelings of inferiority
   (b) Unreasonable feelings of self-reproaches or excessive and inappropriate guilt
   (c) Recurrent thoughts of death or suicide or any suicidal behavior
   (d) Complaints or evidence of diminished ability to concentrate or think, accompanied by indecisiveness or vacillation
   (e) Change in psychomotor activity, with agitation or inhibition
   (f) Sleep disturbances of any type
   (g) Changes in appetite (decrease or increase) with corresponding weight change
4. There may or may not be the somatic syndrome

depressive reactions. In other cases, in which tinnitus exists for a long time without causing any substantial distress, a depressive episode may lead to decompensation of the tinnitus with subsequent impairment in the quality of life. There is also the possibility that tinnitus and depressive symptoms are consequences of a third condition (e.g., traumatic event). Finally, tinnitus and depressive disorders may also co-occur incidentally since both are relatively frequent conditions. In clinical practice, the differential diagnosis of all relevant factors contributing to tinnitus distress is of importance, since all these factors may represent potential targets for treatment. As an example, let us consider a patient who complains about chronic tinnitus with variations of perceived distress, ranging from severe disturbances to none at all. Psychiatric exploration may reveal a comorbid seasonal affective disorder or a comorbid bipolar disorder, which explains the variations in tinnitus distress. In this case, the comorbid psychiatric condition should be specifically treated with the primary aim of mood stabilization, which, in turn, will lead to decreased variations of tinnitus-associated distress and impairment.

Pathophysiological Similarities Between Depression and Tinnitus

Pathophysiological models of tinnitus have claimed the involvement of the frontal and limbic brain regions. In his neurophysiological model of tinnitus (Chap. 20), Jastreboff hypothesized in detail that the prefrontal cortex may be the brain structure that integrates the sensory and emotional aspects of tinnitus and may be involved in the emotional and autonomic reaction to tinnitus [29]. The activation of the nonclassical (extralemniscal) ascending auditory pathways in some forms of tinnitus [30] (see Chap. 9) may explain the co-activation of the cortical association areas, limbic areas, and the autonomic nervous system. Recent neuroimaging studies (in nondepressed individuals with tinnitus) have confirmed the involvement of the prefrontal cortex, the subgenual cingulate cortex, and the amygdalohippocampal area in the pathophysiology of tinnitus (for a review, see [31] or Chap. 15). These brain areas are well-known as critical parts of brain networks, functionally altered in individuals with depressive disorders [32, 33]. Thus, imaging data suggest that the neuronal correlates of tinnitus and depression overlap in limbic networks, which provides a possible explanation for the co-occurrence of tinnitus and depressive symptoms.

In this context, an important role for the dorsal cochlear nucleus (DCN) has also been proposed [34]. There is increasing evidence from animal studies that the DCN is an important contributor to tinnitus. There are direct projections from the DCN to brainstem structures such as the locus coeruleus, reticular formation, and raphe nuclei, which are the principle sites for synthesis of serotonin and noradrenaline and are implicated in the control of attention and emotional responses. Thus, attentional and emotional disorders, such as anxiety and depression, commonly associated with tinnitus may result from an interplay between these nonauditory brainstem structures and the DCN.

Serotonergic dysfunction, believed to play an important role in the pathophysiology of depression, may also be involved in tinnitus generation [35, 36]. However, evidence for this hypothesis is scarce.

Finally, neuroendocrine alterations, such as a hypothalamic–pituitary–adrenal axis dysfunction, which are pathognomonic for stress-related disorders, such as depression or post-traumatic stress disorder (PTSD), have been described in tinnitus patients [37, 38], indicating another pathophysiological overlap between tinnitus and affective disorders. However, these findings should not be overstressed, as tinnitus patients differ only slightly from controls in physiological reactivity during stress tests, indicating relatively normal psychophysiological reactivity [39, 40].

Treatment Options for Depression

There are several reasons why patients with tinnitus and depression should be promptly and efficiently treated. Efficient treatment depends on the exact etiology of comorbid depressive symptoms. If diagnostic assessment reveals a major depression (see Table 42.4), then the standard treatment options include antidepressants and psychotherapy. There is a large variety of antidepressants available, which differ in their mechanisms of action and in their side effects. In addition, there are some antidepressants that specifically address specific symptoms of depression. For example, amitriptyline, trimipramine, mirtazapine, and agomelatine have sleep-inducing effects and are preferentially used in patients with insomnia. In contrast, venlafaxine, duloxetine, and bupropion exert an activating effect and are preferred in patients, who suffer from loss of energy. Thus, the choice of the best antidepressant is complex and depends on the patient's previous experience with specific drugs, the predominant symptom of depression, comorbidities, and the co-medication and the side effect profile of the specific drug. Cognitive behavioral therapy (CBT) has also been shown to be efficient in the treatment of depression (see Chap. 44). Very recently, online-based CBT, e.g., delivered via specific smartphone apps, has shown efficacy as well (see Chap. 57). Further non-pharmacological treatment options include light therapy, sleep deprivation, transcranial magnetic stimulation, or aerobic exercise.

Several antidepressants have been investigated for their use in tinnitus [41] (see Chap. 48). Two randomized double-blind placebo-controlled studies investigated the effects of antidepressants in patients with tinnitus and comorbid depression. The tricyclic nortriptyline significantly reduced depression scores, tinnitus disability scores, and tinnitus loudness relative to placebo [42]. The serotonin reuptake inhibitor sertraline was also significantly more effective than placebo in reducing tinnitus severity [43]. In both studies, reduction in tinnitus disability scores correlated highly with a reduction in depression scores, suggesting that antidepressants have beneficial results in depressed tinnitus patients but that this is mainly due to the antidepressant effect of the drug.

However, induction or worsening of tinnitus has also been reported in the context of treatment with antidepressants, both as a side effect of drugs such as phenelzine, amitriptyline, protriptyline, doxepin, imipramine, fluoxetine, trazadone, bupropion, and venlafaxine [44, 45]. Worsening of tinnitus has also been associated with withdrawal of antidepressants (venlafaxine and sertraline) [46]. Interestingly, transcranial magnetic stimulation of the dorsolateral prefrontal cortex, performed for the treatment of depression, has also been described to both improve tinnitus [47] and, in rare cases, exacerbate tinnitus [48]. This suggests that tinnitus can be generated or worsened by modulation of neural activity in the frontal cortex [49]. Thus, the complex interactions between antidepressant treatment and tinnitus may be explained by antidepressant-induced modulation of frontal cortex networks [50], which, in turn, may result in altered top-down control of activity in the central auditory pathways.

Tinnitus and Anxiety

Anxiety belongs to the most basic physiological emotions of human beings. It represents a biosocial signal contributing to the development of normal interpersonal relations and a risk-sensitive interaction with the environment. Anxiety is an indicator of thread and points to potential dangers. The subjective perception of anxiety and its related threads, however, is very much influenced by learning processes, which gradually leads to modified perceptions and cognitive evaluations of internal and external dangers. This, in turn, determines the individual's level of tolerated anxiety and shapes behavioral styles to recover safety. Hence, anxiety fulfills important physiological functions, which are essential for survival. In this respect, anxiety does not represent a pathological symptom. However, it gains clinical relevance in cases of too much or too little anxiety.

"Anxiety" and "fear" often occur together and their symptoms overlap, but these terms are not interchangeable. Fear relates to a known or understood threat, whereas anxiety follows from an unknown, expected, or poorly defined threat.

Patients with tinnitus and anxiety often also suffer from hyperacusis or phonophobia. Hyperacusis has been defined as lowered tolerance to ordinary environmental sounds or as a consistently exaggerated [51] or inappropriate response to sounds that are neither threatening nor uncomfortably loud to a typical person [52]. In phonophobia, specific sounds evoke negative emotions such as anxiety and fear. Phonophobia represents a form of a specific phobia (for more information about hyperacusis and phonophobia, please see Chap. 3).

Diagnosis and Classification of Anxiety Disorders

Anxiety as a symptom may be part of almost every psychiatric disease. When anxiety reaches an extraordinary level, it is subjectively perceived as unrealistic, causes a high burden, and impairs social functioning; it may be regarded as a disease, and the diagnosis of an anxiety disorder may be fulfilled. In general, anxiety always appears on different levels, i.e., an emotional, a cognitive (e.g., subjective beliefs regarding danger), a motor (e.g., behavioral attitudes like fight, fright, or flight), and an autonomic level (e.g., somatic reactions like tachycardia, stress hormone secretion, etc.). In the International Classification of Diseases (ICD-10) of the WHO, the diagnostic criteria for several anxiety disorders have been defined. These are phobic disorders (ICD-10: F40; e.g., agoraphobia, social, and specific phobias) and other anxiety disorders (ICD-10: F41; e.g., panic disorder, generalized anxiety disorder, anxiety and depression mixed). Phobic disorders are characterized by anxiety and fear occurring primarily in specific situations or in response to specific things, which are not normally dangerous to the individual (e.g., fear of public places, busses, etc., or fear of specific things, for example, spiders). In contrast, in the other anxiety disorders, symptoms occur independently of specific triggers. Both forms of anxiety disorders have in common that individuals try to avoid situations associated with anxiety. This, in turn, stabilizes symptoms because avoidance behavior prevents them from realizing that the anticipated danger is not real and hinders them from learning adaptive strategies.

Similar avoidance behavior is also found in tinnitus patients. Especially in people suffering from hyperacusis, phonophobia develops frequently and noise is avoided. However, the avoidance of sound is counterproductive, since there is clear evidence that reduced environmental sound increases phantom auditory perceptions like tinnitus [53]. Therefore, changing this dysfunctional avoidance behavior represents a major aim of cognitive behavioral therapy interventions, both for anxiety disorders and tinnitus.

Interplay Between Tinnitus and Anxiety Disorders

Epidemiological studies indicate that anxiety disorders are highly prevalent. However, due to diverging diagnostic criteria, prevalence rates vary substantially between studies. Lifetime prevalence rates range from about 1.2% for panic disorders up to 5% for specific phobias. The most frequent anxiety disorder seems to be social phobia, for which the lifetime prevalence rate of 13.3% has been reported [54]. Anxiety is even more frequent in individuals with tinnitus. Various studies reported that 19% up to 45% of tinnitus patients experience anxiety [7, 55, 56]. A recent study using an Internet-adapted version of the WHO short form of the Composite Diagnostic Interview (CIDI-SF [7]) has found 12-month prevalence rates of 60% for generalized anxiety disorder, 83% for specific phobia, 67% for social phobia, 58% for agoraphobia, and 21% for panic disorder in a self-selected population of tinnitus patients [13]. Although these data have to be interpreted with caution because of selection bias, because they have been collected by an Internet survey, and because verification of the diagnoses by a psychiatrist was not performed, this study, together with the others, indicates that anxiety is a common phenomenon among individuals with tinnitus. Its clinical relevance is further underlined by the fact that tinnitus severity and distress are linked to comorbid anxiety and depression [5], which is also very often a comorbid condition in anxiety disorders. Detection and diagnosis of anxiety symptoms in tinnitus patients therefore represents an important task for every health-care professional dealing with tinnitus patients. Especially in severe forms with substantial impairment of the quality of life, the probability of a comorbid psychiatric disorder like anxiety or depression is increased. In those cases, a detailed exploration for anxiety symptoms should be performed. Screening questions for different forms of anxiety disorders are displayed in Table 42.2. If these screening questions reveal hints of an anxiety disorder, then patients should be referred for further diagnosis and treatment to psychiatrists or psychotherapists.

Pathophysiological Similarities Between Anxiety Disorders and Tinnitus

The etiopathogenesis of anxiety symptoms is multifactorial. Anxiety patients are often characterized by some accentuated personality traits (e.g., introversion and neuroticism).

Other important factors are dysfunctional cognitive processes, anxiety sensitivity, and attentional bias. A behavioral consequence of these dysfunctional cognitions is biased perceptions of potential dangers, misinterpretation of physiological signs (like heartbeat) as signals of danger, and the feeling of being unable to control these symptoms. Many aspects of such dysfunctional cognitions are also frequently found in tinnitus patients, even if they do not suffer from anxiety symptoms. For example, being unable to control their tinnitus and the fear that the tinnitus will get worse are very often mentioned by tinnitus patients as one major reason to seek medical help. It is important to note that these fearful beliefs depend to a significant extent on the interaction and communication between patient and health-care providers. Medical doctors may trigger anxiety by exaggerating the risk of dangerous diseases, which may underlie tinnitus (e.g., brain tumors), and also by informing the patient that there is no help for their tinnitus and that they have to live with it. Therefore, how information about tinnitus—its pathophysiological basis and potential treatment options—is provided can be critical to how a patient learns to cope with tinnitus. Informing the patient in an empathic way and providing hope are important factors for preventing the development of anxiety (see Chap. 43). This is even more important since there is evidence that anticipatory processes and dysfunctional activation of a cortical distress network seem to play a role in the pathophysiology of tinnitus [57]. Cognitive behavioral treatment strategies in tinnitus patients focus on these dysfunctional cognitive and anticipatory processes and have been shown to be able to improve the quality of life in tinnitus patients [58].

On a neurobiological level, many different brain regions have been identified to be involved in the generation of arousal and anxiety. The arousal level is under the control of the brainstem nuclei, mainly the locus coeruleus. However, arousal alone is not equal to anxiety. Anxiety also depends on connoted emotions, which are generated within the limbic system and involves structures such as the amygdalae, hippocampus, septal nuclei, and the hypothalamus. Recent studies have pointed to a critical role of the amygdale in generation of anxiety, especially in the formation of emotional, anxiety-related memories. There is emerging evidence that the limbic system is also involved in the pathogenesis of tinnitus. A variety of studies have shown functional activations as well as structural alterations in limbic areas in individuals with tinnitus, pointing to a role of these structures in the pathogenesis of tinnitus [31]. This is further underlined by the fact that the severity of tinnitus is closely related to concurrent symptoms of anxiety and depression [59]. Just by treating these symptoms, the functional impairment of tinnitus patients may be improved [60].

In summary, anxiety is a frequent symptom, which may occur as a normal physiological phenomenon but also in the context of almost every somatic or psychiatric disorder. Anxiety is a common phenomenon in individuals with tinnitus, and the prevalence rates of anxiety disorders are extremely high. Furthermore, anxiety is often associated with depression. Neurobiology shows that tinnitus and both depression and anxiety share similar neural circuits, underlining the close interrelationship of these syndromes. Finally, tinnitus severity is associated with comorbid anxiety and depression, indicating the necessity to detect and treat these symptoms when treating patients with tinnitus.

Treatment Strategies

The principal treatment options for anxiety disorders are pharmacotherapy and psychotherapy. First-line pharmacological treatment options for anxiety disorders like panic disorder, social phobia, and generalized anxiety disorder are antidepressants, predominantly selective serotonin reuptake inhibitors (SSRIs), and combined serotonin and norepinephrine reuptake inhibitors (SNRIs; e.g., venlafaxine or duloxetine). Moreover, mirtazapine or tricyclic antidepressants may have beneficial effects.

The selection of an antidepressant for the individual patient may depend on the most prominent symptoms (e.g., agitation, lack of drive, or sleep problems), the side effect profile of the drug, concurrent other medical conditions, or the necessity of other medications, which may increase the risk of unfavorable drug–drug interactions. Therefore, it is advisable that pharmacological treatment is managed by a psychiatrist. Besides classical antidepressants, some other substances may sometimes have beneficial effects in the treatment of tinnitus patients with anxiety. For example, pregabalin, buspirone, and opipramol have all shown efficacy in the treatment of anxiety disorders and thus represent additional options for the treatment of anxiety disorders in tinnitus patients.

All mentioned drugs exert their anxiolytic effects after continuous treatment over weeks to months. In contrast, benzodiazepines have acute anxiolytic properties. Several pilot studies also suggest the beneficial effects of benzodiazepines on tinnitus (see Chap. 48). However, benzodiazepines are regarded to be addictive and, therefore, regular use over longer periods of time should be avoided. Tinnitus has also been reported to occur ore worsen after discontinuation of benzodiazepines [61]. Thus, the administration of benzodiazepines for the treatment of anxiety in tinnitus patients should be restricted to use as rescue medication. For this purpose, short-acting substances such as alprazolam should be preferred. Sometimes, just having this efficient rescue medication available gives the patient some form of control over his/her symptoms and reduces the fear of developing severe anxiety or panic attacks.

Psychotherapy is the other important treatment option, especially in patients with tinnitus who are severely affected and have psychological distress symptoms (see Chaps. 44 and 45). Cognitive behavioral therapy (CBT) aims at modifying dysfunctional cognitions and avoidance behavior in the context of tinnitus. There exist specific forms of CBT for tinnitus and for anxiety disorders. Whether CBT for an individual patient should focus primarily on the tinnitus or on his/her comorbid psychiatry disorders may depend on the patient's predominant symptoms. Besides classical face-to-face psychotherapy, nowadays, Internet-based psychotherapeutic approaches have been established for depression, anxiety, insomnia, and tinnitus [58, 62, 63].

Avoidance of unpleasant sounds represents a substantial problem in individuals who have hyperacusis and phonophobia in addition to their tinnitus. Both hyperacusis and phonophobia can be efficiently treated by cognitive behavioral therapy (see also Chaps. 3 and 44).

In summary, in patients with tinnitus and concurrent anxiety symptoms or anxiety disorder, a broad variety of pharmacological and psychotherapeutic treatment options can have a beneficial effect on both tinnitus and anxiety. Decisions for the best individual treatment require psychiatric experience and depend on individual symptoms that may be concomitant with other medical conditions depending on the individual patient's acceptance.

References

1. Lewis JE, Stephens SD, McKenna L. Tinnitus and suicide. Clin Otolaryngol Allied Sci. 1994;19(1):50–4.
2. Langguth B. A review of tinnitus symptoms beyond 'ringing in the ears': a call to action. CurrMed Res Opin. 2011;27(8):1635–43.
3. De Ridder D, Schlee W, Vanneste S, Londero A, Weisz N, Kleinjung T, et al. Tinnitus and tinnitus disorder: theoretical and operational definitions (an international multidisciplinary proposal). Prog Brain Res. 2021;260:1–25.
4. Henry JL, Wilson PH. Coping with tinnitus: two studies of psychological and audiological characteristics of patients with high and low tinnitus-related distress. Int Tinnitus J. 1995;1(2):85–92.
5. Zoger S, Svedlund J, Holgers KM. Relationship between tinnitus severity and psychiatric disorders. Psychosomatics. 2006;47(4):282–8.
6. Crocetti A, Forti S, Ambrosetti U, Bo LD. Questionnaires to evaluate anxiety and depressive levels in tinnitus patients. Otolaryngol Head Neck Surg. 2009;140(3):403–5.
7. Belli S, Belli H, Bahcebasi T, Ozcetin A, Alpay E, Ertem U. Assessment of psychopathological aspects and psychiatric comorbidities in patients affected by tinnitus. EurArch Otorhinolaryngol. 2008;265(3):279–85.
8. Fagelson MA. The association between tinnitus and posttraumatic stress disorder. Am J Audiol. 2007;16(2):107–17.
9. Hiller W, Janca A, Burke KC. Association between tinnitus and somatoform disorders. J Psychosom Res. 1997;43(6):613–24.
10. D'Amelio R, Delb W. Comorbidity of schizophrenic psychosis and tinnitus. A hitherto neglected theme in research and therapy. HNO. 2008;56(7):670–2.
11. Folmer RL, Griest SE, Martin WH. Obsessive-compulsiveness in a population of tinnitus patients. Int Tinnitus J. 2008;14(2):127–30.
12. Stuerz K, Lafenthaler M, Pfaffenberger N, Kopp M, Gutweniger S, Guenther V. Body image and body concept in patients with chronic tinnitus. Eur Arch Otorhinolaryngol. 2009;266(7):961–5.
13. Andersson G, Carlbring P, Kaldo V, Strom L. Screening of psychiatric disorders via the internet. A pilot study with tinnitus patients. Nord J Psychiatry. 2004;58(4):287–91.
14. Langguth B, Landgrebe M, Kleinjung T, Sand GP, Hajak G. Tinnitus and depression. World J Biol Psychiatry. 2011;12(7):489–500.
15. Hebert S, Canlon B, Hasson D. Emotional exhaustion as a predictor of tinnitus. Psychother Psychosom. 2012;81(5):324–6.
16. Langguth B, Kleinjung T, Fischer B, Hajak G, Eichhammer P, Sand PG. Tinnitus severity, depression, and the big five personality traits. Prog Brain Res. 2007;166:221–5.
17. Milerova J, Anders M, Dvorak T, Sand PG, Koniger S, Langguth B. The influence of psychological factors on tinnitus severity. Gen Hosp Psychiatry. 2013;35(4):412–6.
18. Simoes JP, Neff PKA, Langguth B, Schlee W, Schecklmann M. The progression of chronic tinnitus over the years. Sci Rep. 2021;11(1):4162.
19. Schlee W, Holleland S, Bulla J, Simoes J, Neff P, Schoisswohl S, et al. The effect of environmental stressors on tinnitus: a prospective longitudinal study on the impact of the COVID-19 pandemic. J Clin Med. 2020;9(9):2756.
20. Konzag TA, Rubler D, Bandemer-Greulich U, Frommer J, Fikentscher E. [Psychological comorbidity in subacute and chronic tinnitus outpatients]. Z Psychosom Med Psychother. 2005;51(3):247–60.
21. D'Amelio R, Archonti C, Scholz S, Falkai P, Plinkert PK, Delb W. [Psychological distress associated with acute tinnitus]. HNO. 2004;52(7):599–603.
22. https://pubmed.ncbi.nlm.nih.gov/9556716/.
23. Whooley MA, Simon GE. Managing depression in medical outpatients. N Engl J Med. 2000;343(26):1942–50.
24. Sheehan DV, Lecrubier Y, Sheehan KH, Amorim P, Janavs J, Weiller E, et al. The Mini-International Neuropsychiatric Interview (M.I.N.I.): the development and validation of a structured diagnostic psychiatric interview for DSM-IV and ICD-10. J Clin Psychiatry. 1998;59(Suppl 20):22–33; quiz 4–57.
25. Turner O, Windfuhr K, Kapur N. Suicide in deaf populations: a literature review. Ann Gen Psychiatry. 2007;6:26.
26. Jacobson GP, McCaslin DL. A search for evidence of a direct relationship between tinnitus and suicide. J Am Acad Audiol. 2001;12(10):493–6.
27. Robinson SK, McQuaid JR, Viirre ES, Betzig LL, Miller DL, Bailey KA, et al. Relationship of tinnitus questionnaires to depressive symptoms, quality of well-being, and internal focus. Int Tinnitus J. 2003;9(2):97–103.
28. Weber JH, Jagsch R, Hallas B. [The relationship between tinnitus, personality, and depression]. Z Psychosom Med Psychother. 2008;54(3):227–40.
29. Hazell JW, Jastreboff PJ. Tinnitus. I: auditory mechanisms: a model for tinnitus and hearing impairment. J Otolaryngol. 1990;19:1–5.
30. Moller AR. Pathophysiology of tinnitus. Otolaryngol Clin North Am. 2003;36:249–66.
31. Elgoyhen AB, Langguth B, De Ridder D, Vanneste S. Tinnitus: perspectives from human neuroimaging. Nat Rev Neurosci. 2015;16:632.
32. Drevets WC, Price JL, Furey ML. Brain structural and functional abnormalities in mood disorders: implications for neurocircuitry models of depression. Brain Struct Funct. 2008;213(1–2):93–118.
33. Mayberg HS. Limbic-cortical dysregulation: a proposed model of depression. J Neuropsychiatry Clin Neurosci. 1997;9:471–81.
34. Kaltenbach JA. The dorsal cochlear nucleus as a participant in the auditory, attentional and emotional components of tinnitus. Heart Res. 2006;216–217:224–34.

35. Simpson JJ, Davies WE. A review of evidence in support of a role for 5-HT in the perception of tinnitus. Heart Res. 2000;145:1–7.
36. Rauschecker JP, Leaver AM, Muhlau M. Tuning out the noise: limbic-auditory interactions in tinnitus. Neuron. 2010;66(6):819–26.
37. Hebert S, Lupien SJ. Salivary cortisol levels, subjective stress, and tinnitus intensity in tinnitus sufferers during noise exposure in the laboratory. Int J Hyg Environ Health. 2009;212(1):37–44.
38. Hebert S, Lupien SJ. The sound of stress: blunted cortisol reactivity to psychosocial stress in tinnitus sufferers. Neurosci Lett. 2007;411(2):138–42.
39. Heinecke K, Weise C, Schwarz K, Rief W. Physiological and psychological stress reactivity in chronic tinnitus. J Behav Med. 2008;31(3):179–88.
40. Betz LT, Muhlberger A, Langguth B, Schecklmann M. Stress reactivity in chronic tinnitus. Sci Rep. 2017;7:41521.
41. Baldo P, Doree C, Molin P, McFerran D, Cecco S. Antidepressants for patients with tinnitus. Cochrane Database Syst Rev. 2012;9:CD003853.
42. Sullivan M, Katon W, Russo J, Dobie R, Sakai C. A randomized trial of nortriptyline for severe chronic tinnitus. Effects on depression, disability, and tinnitus symptoms. Arch Intern Med. 1993;153(19):2251–9.
43. Zoger S, Svedlund J, Holgers KM. The effects of sertraline on severe tinnitus suffering--a randomized, double-blind, placebo-controlled study. J Clin Psychopharmacol. 2006;26(1):32–9.
44. Elgoyhen AB, Langguth B. Pharmacological approaches to the treatment of tinnitus. Drug Discov Today. 2010;15(7–8):300–5.
45. Elgoyhen AB, Langguth B, Nowak W, Schecklmann M, De Ridder D, Vanneste S. Identifying tinnitus-related genes based on a side-effect network analysis. CPT Pharmacometrics Syst Pharmacol. 2014;3:e97.
46. Robinson SK, Viirre ES, Stein MB. Antidepressant therapy in tinnitus. Heart Res. 2007;226(1–2):221–31.
47. Ciminelli P, Machado S, Palmeira M, Coutinho ESF, Sender D, Nardi AE. Dorsomedial prefrontal cortex repetitive transcranial magnetic stimulation for tinnitus: promising results of a blinded, randomized, sham-controlled study. Ear Hear. 2020;42(1):12–9.
48. Marcondes R, Fregni F, Pascual-Leone A. Tinnitus and brain activation: insights from transcranial magnetic stimulation. Ear Nose Throat J. 2006;85(4):233–8.
49. De Ridder D, Vanneste S, Plazier M, Menovsky T, van de Heyning P, Kovacs S, et al. Dorsolateral prefrontal cortex transcranial magnetic stimulation and electrode implant for intractable tinnitus. World Neurosurg. 2012;77(5–6):778–84.
50. Ishizaki J, Yamamoto H, Takahashi T, Takeda M, Yano M, Mimura M. Changes in regional cerebral blood flow following antidepressant treatment in late-life depression. Int J Geriatr Psychiatry. 2008;23(8):805–11.
51. Vernon JA. Pathophysiology of tinnitus: a special case--hyperacusis and a proposed treatment. Am J Otol. 1987;8(3):201–2.
52. Klein AJ, Armstrong BL, Greer MK, Brown FR III. Hyperacusis and otitis media in individuals with Williams syndrome. J Speech Hear Disord. 1990;55(2):339–44.
53. Del Bo L, Forti S, Ambrosetti U, Costanzo S, Mauro D, Ugazio G, et al. Tinnitus aurium in persons with normal hearing: 55 years later. Otolaryngol Head Neck Surg. 2008;139(3):391–4.
54. Kessler RC, Crum RM, Warner LA, Nelson CB, Schulenberg J, Anthony JC. Lifetime co-occurrence of DSM-III-R alcohol abuse and dependence with other psychiatric disorders in the National Comorbidity Survey. Arch Gen Psychiatry. 1997;54(4):313–21.
55. Marciano E, Carrabba L, Giannini P, Sementina C, Verde P, Bruno C, et al. Psychiatric comorbidity in a population of outpatients affected by tinnitus. Int J Audiol. 2003;42(1):4–9.
56. Zoger S, Svedlund J, Holgers KM. Psychiatric disorders in tinnitus patients without severe hearing impairment: 24 month follow-up of patients at an audiological clinic. Audiology. 2001;40(3):133–40.
57. Landgrebe M, Frick U, Hauser S, Hajak G, Langguth B. Association of tinnitus and electromagnetic hypersensitivity: hints for a shared pathophysiology? PLoS One. 2009;4(3):e5026.
58. Fuller T, Cima R, Langguth B, Mazurek B, Vlaeyen JW, Hoare DJ. Cognitive behavioural therapy for tinnitus. Cochrane Database Syst Rev. 2020;1:CD012614.
59. Holgers KM, Erlandsson SI, Barrenas ML. Predictive factors for the severity of tinnitus. Audiology. 2000;39(5):284–91.
60. Katon W, Sullivan M, Russo J, Dobie R, Sakai C. Depressive symptoms and measures of disability: a prospective study. J Affect Disord. 1993;27(4):245–54.
61. Busto U, Fornazzari L, Naranjo CA. Protracted tinnitus after discontinuation of long-term therapeutic use of benzodiazepines. J Clin Psychopharmacol. 1988;8(5):359–62.
62. Moshe I, Terhorst Y, Philippi P, Domhardt M, Cuijpers P, Cristea I, et al. Digital interventions for the treatment of depression: a meta-analytic review. Psychol Bull. 2021;147(8):749–86.
63. Yu H, Zhang Y, Liu Q, Yan R. Efficacy of online and face-to-face cognitive behavioral therapy in the treatment of neurological insomnia: a systematic review and meta-analysis. Ann Palliat Med. 2021;10(10):10684–96.

Part VII

Tinnitus Treatment

Tinnitus Counselling and Psychoeducation

43

Grant D. Searchfield, Martin Schecklmann, and Maria Kleinstaeuber

Abstract

Counselling is an essential component of almost all tinnitus therapies and is practiced in some form or another by most tinnitus clinicians. Tinnitus counselling is a professional relationship that empowers diverse individuals with tinnitus to accomplish their wellness goals. Tinnitus is a complex experience, making it a difficult condition to treat and to live with. Some of the difficulties that accompany tinnitus include high levels of emotional distress, sleep disruptions, and concentration and attention problems along with reduced life quality. Tinnitus counselling aims to reduce the negative impact that tinnitus has on patient's lives. Counselling helps identify treatment goals, barriers, and means to achieve these through conversation and empowering self-directed changes to thoughts and activities in daily life. To facilitate these goals, instruction and psychoeducation help individuals understand their tinnitus, so as to reduce the occurrence and level of distress. Providing patients with information in an educational way about what their tinnitus is, and what it is not, helps demystify the condition, which can reduce their suffering. This chapter will clarify the role of tinnitus counselling and describe the different counselling styles. The perspectives of different professionals in providing counselling, focusing on audiologists and psychologists, are discussed. A counselling framework (AREA: Attend, React, Explain, Adapt) is presented as an example of how clinicians can organize their tinnitus counselling. This chapter provides a toolbox of counselling components for clinicians to select from and apply according to their individual counselling style.

G. D. Searchfield (✉)
Audiology Section, School of Population Health, Faculty of Medical and Health Sciences, The University of Auckland, Auckland, New Zealand

Eisdell Moore Centre, The University of Auckland, Auckland, New Zealand

Centre for Brain Research, The University of Auckland, Auckland, New Zealand
e-mail: g.searchfield@auckland.ac.nz

M. Schecklmann
Department of Psychiatry and Psychotherapy, Interdisciplinary Tinnitus Clinic, University of Regensburg, Regensburg, Germany
e-mail: Martin.Schecklmann@medbo.de

M. Kleinstaeuber
Department of Psychology, Emma Eccles Jones College of Education and Human Services, Utah State University, Logan, UT, USA
e-mail: maria.kleinstaeuber@usu.edu

W. Schlee et al. (eds.), *Textbook of Tinnitus*, https://doi.org/10.1007/978-3-031-35647-6_43

Graphical Abstract

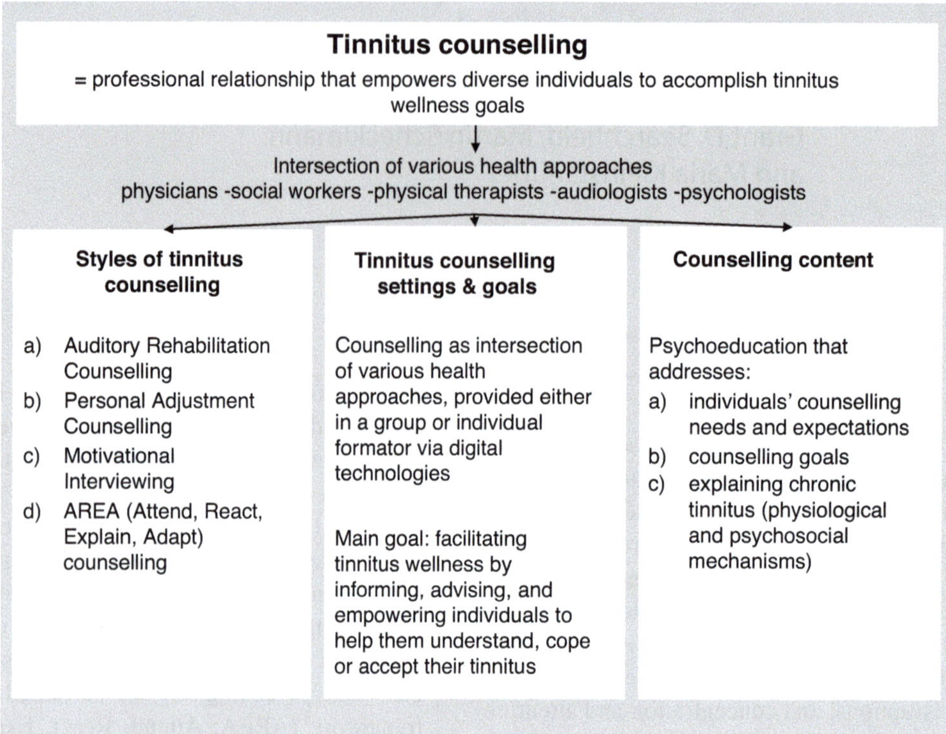

Highlights

- Tinnitus is a dysfunction of the auditory system for which a curing treatment has not yet been identified. For clinicians and patients, the treatment of chronic tinnitus has to focus on symptom management.
- Successful tinnitus management helps individuals with tinnitus to deal with symptom-related distress and impairment and to improve their quality of life.
- To engage individuals with tinnitus in symptom management, it is important that they understand the complexity of their symptoms. Tinnitus counselling is an important and effective approach to educate individuals with tinnitus about their symptoms and the role of psychosocial factors (e.g. negative symptom-related thoughts and emotions, sleep difficulties, high level of perceived stress) in perpetuating their symptoms.
- Counselling is an approach that can be applied by various disciplines involved in tinnitus management. A number of professionals provide counselling for tinnitus, including physicians, social workers, physical therapists, audiologists, and psychologists.
- Different styles of counselling exist, such as auditory rehabilitation counselling, personal adjustment counselling, motivational interviewing, or solution-focused counselling.
- The AREA (Attend, React, Explain, Adapt) model of affective adaptation helps people make sense of an event through avenues such as past experiences, for example. This model has been adapted for tinnitus counselling. It constitutes a holistic approach to tinnitus counselling that includes aspects of both motivational interviewing and solution-focused therapy.
- A central component of tinnitus counselling is psychoeducation that addresses topics such as individuals' counselling needs and expectations, setting counselling goals, and explaining chronic tinnitus, including its physiological and psychosocial mechanisms (e.g. role of stress, attention focusing, emotions and thoughts, self-efficacy, disturbed sleep).

Introduction

Counselling is not a single, simple construct; it constitutes a range of methods in which clinicians and patients communicate potential solutions to problems that the patient has identified. A consensus definition from the American Counselling Association is that: "Counselling is a professional relationship that empowers diverse individuals, families, and groups to accomplish mental health, wellness, education and career goals" ([1], p. 368). In the context of tinnitus, counselling can be defined as "the professional relationship that empowers diverse individuals to accomplish tinnitus wellness goals". There are several keywords in the definition that we will explore throughout this chapter: "professional" (who should provide counselling?), "relationship" (what is the nature of the relationship?), "empowers" (how can we assist patients towards solutions?), "diverse individuals" (what do individuals with tinnitus experience?), "accomplish tinnitus wellness" (what outcomes can we expect from counselling?) and "goals" (what are these? why are they important?).

Tinnitus counselling facilitates tinnitus wellness by informing, advising, and empowering individuals to help them understand, cope, or accept their tinnitus. Counselling may be the single most important component of the management of tinnitus [2] with virtually all treatment strategies using it in some form or another. Given its importance, it is critical that clinicians understand their tinnitus counselling capabilities; our aim is to support this goal. There are many topics and approaches within tinnitus counselling, and tinnitus counsellors include a wide range of professionals in medicine and rehabilitation. In this chapter, we discuss the different counselling styles (approaches/philosophies) provided by different professionals. In particular, we describe the different perspectives of psychologists and audiologists in counselling roles. Although this chapter focuses on counselling for tinnitus, the underlying counselling principles can be applied to other auditory conditions such as hyperacusis as well.

Tinnitus Is a Diverse Individual Experience: Why Counselling Is Needed

Tinnitus is the perception of sound in the absence of an external physical sound source. It is a highly heterogeneous experience; it can be heard as different sounds and appears to have different aetiologies and effects [3]. Tinnitus can range from being a slight nuisance through to a disorder that affects the quality of life. Approximately 20% of the population experiences persistent tinnitus, with 0.5–2% reporting tinnitus that produces sufficient annoyance to interfere with day-to-day activities [4–6]. Why some people have marked distress or handicap associated with their tinnitus while others do not is not always clear but may relate to comorbid anxiety and depression [7], stressful events and post-traumatic stress disorder [8], or dysfunctional coping strategies. Distressing tinnitus is associated with difficulty in concentrating, sleep disorder, anxiety, and depression [9]. Severe tinnitus is recognized as an outcome of a complex interaction between auditory and emotion neural processing, which is impacted by psychosocial context and experience [10]. The most common self-reported tinnitus complaints include its negative effects on lifestyle (93%), general health (5.6%), hearing (52.7%), emotional problems (69.4%), difficulties with the persistence of tinnitus (48.6%), poor concentration (33.3%), and, rarely, suicide (6.9%) [11]. There is limited evidence for treatments that aim to remove the tinnitus sound, consequently addressing the psychological aspects of tinnitus are critical for reducing disability. Counselling should be part of every intervention. If the role of psychological processes is ignored, then elimination strategies might be ineffective because dysfunctional coping strategies remain.

Counselling helps reduce patients' unhealthy thoughts, feelings, or actions towards tinnitus. Benefits may be achieved by discussion and providing written or web-based information about relaxation, attention towards tinnitus, and sleep. The manner and content of counselling should be tailored for the patient and reflect the clinician's background and knowledge, leading to a specific counselling style [12].

Counselling Styles: The Relationship

A number of professionals provide counselling for tinnitus, including physicians, social workers, physical therapists, audiologists, and psychologists. Physicians need to effectively communicate diagnoses and treatment plans. Audiologists and psychologists are two of the primary rehabilitation professionals in the tinnitus field. Counselling is practiced by each professional through different, though complimentary, lenses (Fig. 43.1). Each professional group may apply a different counselling style and focus on different content. Our discussion of the counselling style, content, and recommendations reflects the authors' world views and professional perspectives, as audiologists and psychologists. The amount, and possibly the type, of counselling undertaken by clinicians will reflect the professional scopes of practice in different countries.

Counselling is the cornerstone of psychological practice, and most counselling theories have arisen from psychology. Psychologists have a strong understanding of the mental health dimensions of tinnitus. Accordingly, psychologists apply counselling strategies in the context of multi-modal

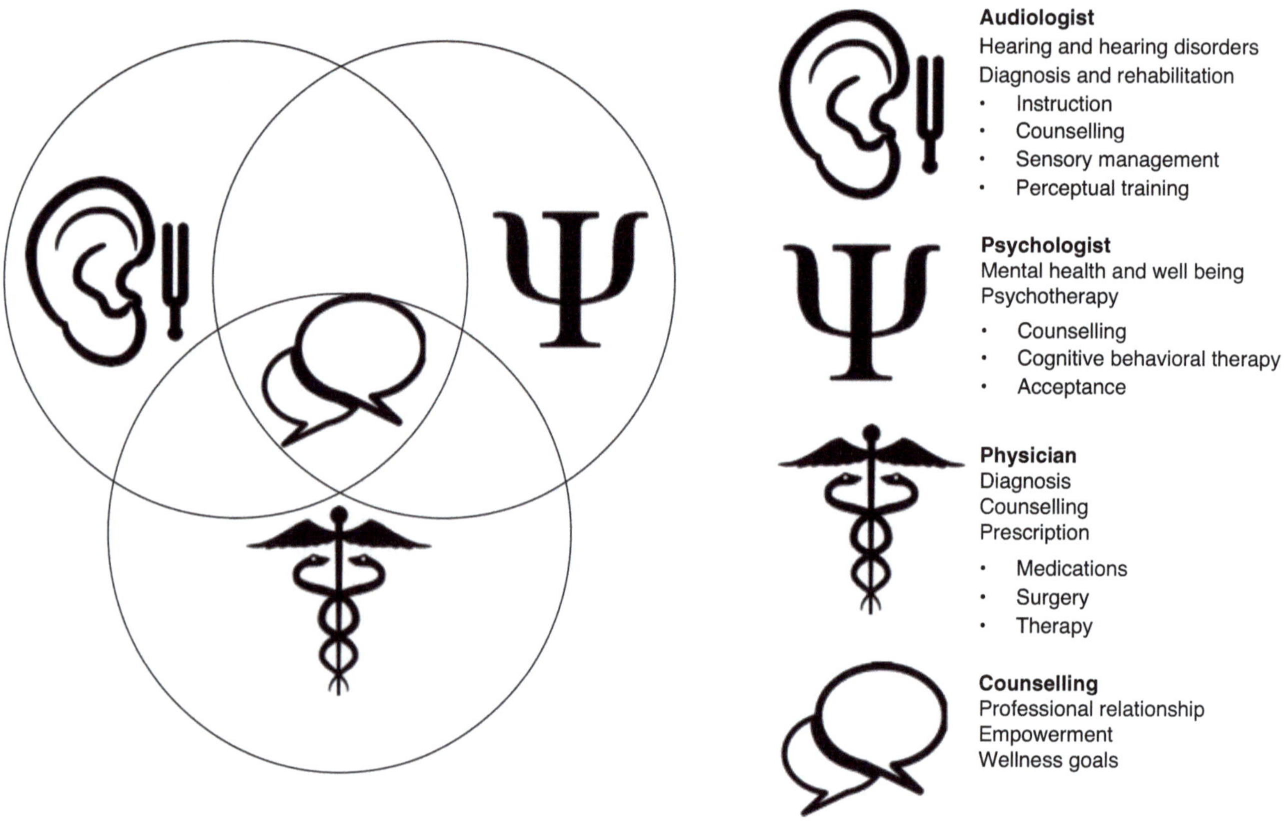

Fig. 43.1 Counselling as the intersection of various health approaches to tinnitus management. Counselling is a professional relationship that empowers individuals with tinnitus to accomplish their wellness goals. Each profession brings a different perspective to counselling. Audiology, psychology, and medicine are illustrated as examples of professions using counselling

psychological tinnitus management, mainly based on approaches of cognitive behavioural therapy (CBT) and/or acceptance and commitment therapy, to expand patients' health literacy about tinnitus, to develop with the patient an explanatory model of chronic tinnitus, and to introduce certain strategies of psychological symptom management (see Chap. xxx). Audiologists have strengths in the understanding of auditory perception and processing. The audiological treatment of tinnitus applies counselling to facilitate an understanding of hearing processes and disorders, including neurophysiology and psychosocial effects. Audiology counselling is geared towards mitigating the negative effects of hearing disorders. Tinnitus experts require knowledge across all these areas, as tinnitus is both an auditory perception and is associated with psychological distress. So, audiologists should familiarize themselves with general counselling skills and principles [12], whereas psychologists should seek continuing their education in hearing science. Good counselling is important irrespective of the professional background of therapists. Knowledge, training, and individual personality will determine the style of counselling [13]. Ethical adherence to the scope of practice will determine the content of counselling practice and when referrals to other professionals are appropriate.

There is no single gold-standard method of counselling. A tinnitus counsellor needs to be flexible in approach and match solutions to needs, an approach that is not easily summarized in a manual. A key point of this chapter is that clinicians can offer many different counselling solutions to tinnitus, but each clinician should discover and acknowledge their world views and counselling style. In addition, each patient has their own views, so a variety of approaches are necessary. Clark and English [12] suggest that awareness of social styles both of the clinician and the patient enable effective counselling. The diversity in the methods and backgrounds of clinicians is actually a strength of the tinnitus field, given the heterogeneity of the patient [3].

Auditory Rehabilitation Counselling

Boothroyd's (2007) model of auditory rehabilitation identifies four components of therapy: instruction, counselling, sensory management (e.g. hearing aids), and perceptual training [14]. Audiological counselling is not precisely defined but generally takes the form of a natural conversation with goals consistent with patient-centred care [12]. Rehabilitative audiology instruction and counselling tend to focus on the face-value hearing issues with traditionally limited emphasis on the affective components of hearing loss [12]. Audiologist-based counselling for tinnitus typically includes description of the tinnitus, instruction on basic ear and brain physiology, and suggestions on auditory strategies for disrupting the perception of tinnitus ("sound therapy") [15]. However, audiologists need to avoid the "content trap" in which diagnostic and neurophysiological outcomes are explained in great detail, but the patient is after something other than information [12, 16]. Another strength of audiology practice is needs assessment. It is essential to understand what patients want from therapy. Most audiologists will be familiar with the Client Oriented Scale of Improvement (COSI); a widely used tool to determine hearing needs for hearing aid fittings [17]. A tinnitus variation of the COSI—the Client Orientated Scale of Improvement in Tinnitus (COSIT, Searchfield [18])—enables the patient to identify specific situations, in which tinnitus is bothersome, e.g. "I want to be able to relax and not focus on my tinnitus after work", and the solutions and likelihood of success are discussed with the patient.

Audiology-based, psychology-informed counselling approaches have been introduced, which address affective components of the patients experience while maintaining the strengths of the audiological rehabilitation method [19, 20]. These audiological approaches borrow from several psychological traditions and include adjustment counselling [12, 20], motivational interviewing [21] and solution-focused therapy [16].

Personal Adjustment Counselling

Personal adjustment counselling, a patient-centred approach, helps patients identify and overcome emotional and social barriers to rehabilitation through support of learning, self-efficacy, and skill acquisition [20]. The Rogerian principles of congruence of self, unconditional positive regard, and empathic understanding [22] are the key components of this approach [12].

1. Congruence with self: The clinician needs to be open and authentic, avoiding a façade of professional elitism. This allows the patient to be at the centre of discussions, and it builds trust, e.g. "It sounds like your tinnitus is causing you a lot of frustration, I can only imagine what it's like for you at the moment, tell me some more about it..." It is important that the professional be knowledgeable in their area of specialty but demonstrates an understanding of the patient's problem in their language. The professional also needs to express their own belief in the chosen treatment plan [23].
2. Unconditional positive regard: The clinician should genuinely care about the patient, irrespective of gender, age, ethnicity, knowledge, beliefs, etc. This can help patients accept and take responsibility for themselves. Rather than correcting beliefs in an authoritarian way, e.g. "that's not true, don't worry", recognition of a patient's world views and beliefs aids in adjusting unhelpful views, e.g. "I understand why you are worried that you'll always have tinnitus as a problem, I've read lot of stories like that on the internet too, have you come across positive stories? What do you think about what people experience?...here is another source [webpage] with some different views, if you have a chance have a look and let's discuss next time we meet..."
3. Empathy:. Creation of a safe counselling environment in which the individuals' experiences are understood, e.g. "having the tinnitus 24/7 the way you explain must be very difficult"

Motivational Interviewing

Motivational interviewing attempts to promote patient motivation towards treatment goals and reduce barriers to change [24]. Client motivation is modified based on the perception of the value of implementing a plan, probability of success, and environmental barriers to change [25]. There are four main principles to motivational interviewing in rehabilitation counselling practice [24] with application to tinnitus (in italics).

1. Empathy: *As described for personal adjustment counselling.*
2. Roll with resistance: Calmly discuss rather than fight against the patient's views, e.g. "...you think there is a tumor causing your tinnitus, that must be a big worry, you know—it's actually quite a common concern but very rare, lets discuss the tests that have been done and why we aren't worried that this is the cause..."
3. Develop discrepancy: Gently explore differences between current and ideal behaviour in response to tinnitus, e.g. "you mentioned you frequently go into a quiet room to check your tinnitus, I understand you want to know if your tinnitus has changed, have you tried the exercises to focus on other sounds we talked about? That's an approach that you felt helped reduce the tinnitus, it's really the opposite of listening out to the tinnitus...do you think that would be a better habit?"
4. Support self-efficacy: Aid patients in gaining confidence and commitment to changes, e.g. "it's wonderful that you've found a yoga group you enjoy, that should help with your goals of relaxing and meeting new friends...so you have less focus on tinnitus, that must feel good—reaching that goal".

In patient interactions, the therapist uses open-ended questions to explore topics, namely, affirmation of patient beliefs and understandings as well as reflections; to maintain client-centred focus; and to provide summaries of motivational conflicts to link the topics discussed [24]. Motivation may be a common factor that can be used to unite many psychological theories [26].

Solution-Focused Counselling

Solution-focused counselling is the process of working with a patient to find solutions and taking small steps towards the patient's goals and future, rather than focusing on the problem and past [16, 27]. It attempts to build self-efficacy [27] and solutions that fit with the patients' world view [28]. The counsellor collaborates with the patient to identify their strengths and resources—what has helped in the past that can then be strengthened and applied more routinely [28].

Assumptions of solution-focused therapy based on Blair's study [16] with an example of application to tinnitus (in italics) are as follows:

1. Change is occurring all the time and world views can be modified. *Discover the patient's perspective of tinnitus and work with the patient to modify if negative.*
2. Small changes lead to larger changes. *Taking time to apply tinnitus therapy strategies on a regular basis rather than reaching ideal behaviour immediately.*
3. Patients are cooperating. *Cooperation needs to be viewed through the patients' lens of understanding the tinnitus. A solution based on patients' view aids collaboration and adopting solutions also known as "unconditional positive regard".*
4. Patients can solve their problems. *Solutions need to be tailored by the person with tinnitus, to implement strategies that will work for them, in their world.*
5. Meaning and experience are interactionally constructed. *Tinnitus conflicts with experience of sound requiring a new understanding of its meaning.*
6. Actions and descriptions are circular. *Once the reality of tinnitus is created, similar external views are sought and this reinforces beliefs, e.g. a patient is a member of tinnitus Internet forums with opinions consistent with own views; as an alternative, the patient is encouraged to seek science-based discussions.*
7. The meaning of the message is in the response received. *Patient's understanding of the information that is provided about tinnitus is more important than the detail and quantity of tinnitus information provided.*
8. Solutions involve others (e.g. family members, spouse or partner). *Significant others should be involved in the tinnitus therapy process to understand what goals are realistic and recognize the progress towards solutions and accommodations that others may need to make in this process.*

Counselling in Different Settings and the Role of Digital Health

This chapter, to this point, has focused on traditional counselling methods, with the assumption that most counselling occurs at a clinical office/consulting room with discussion between the clinician and tinnitus sufferer (potentially along with family or significant others). However, counselling can be provided in other ways, such as either in a group or in individual sessions, in a clinic or remotely via the Internet, and, sometimes, a mixture of methods can be applied. In some countries, the number of patients with tinnitus seeking appointments exceeds the number of therapy places. Group counselling may help this to some extent, and progressive treatments, for example, Progressive Tinnitus Management used in the United States Veteran Affairs hospitals, provide individualized treatment only if more cost-effective approaches, such as group education, are insufficient [29]. Group counselling allows for the presentation of information to more patients in less time, but it limits the one-on-one relationship between the patient and clinician [30]. Shared group experiences may help individuals realize that they are not alone [30, 31]. However, the observation of other group members' success may evoke envy or, on the other hand, failures may affirm the futility of tinnitus therapy [32].

The counselling chosen should also reflect the environment and resources available (i.e. physical location, types of patients, support networks, and referral options). A clinician in a small town may be required to undertake greater counselling across a broader scope of practice than a member of a multidisciplinary team in a large hospital.

Digital technologies may help fill the gap between demand and supply for tinnitus counselling and make resources available for more isolated clinicians, through self-directed Internet or app-based counselling [33]. It is easy to share information about the aspects of tinnitus on the Internet, in ways that can be undertaken independently of, or to enhance, clinic-based talk therapy (e.g. diagrams, animations, interactive text). Currently, this material is largely information-based and is not personalized. However, artificial intelligence may help in selection of patient-tailored information and include virtual clinicians. There is evidence that Internet-based CBT is effective [34]. A hope is that counselling provided at the optimal time, perhaps at an acute stage of tinnitus, will increase tinnitus wellness and may help avoid tinnitus chronification and decompensation [35].

Counselling Content

Thompson et al. have undertaken several studies examining the psychological management of tinnitus and an examination of what might be contained in a manualized form of therapy for audiologists ([36, 37], Table 43.1). There is considerable overlap in content, and the comparison illustrates the breadth of solutions practiced in psychology, which address cognition and thought processes, and the focus of audiology on information and situation-based solutions. Tinnitus counselling topics should be selected on the basis of need and be applied within the context of the clinician's profession and recognized scope of practice. Audiologists may be more comfortable describing audiological assessments and the pros and cons of hearing aids and communication strategies, whereas psychologists may find discussions of stress, attention, anxiety, and depression a more familiar territory.

Some topics identified in Table 43.1 may be discussed with patients as part of counselling, but the implementation may require referrals, as, therapeutically, they are components of CBT (for example, thought challenging). We believe that the majority of tinnitus participants will benefit from counselling regarding one or more topics from a "counselling toolbox" described below. Clinicians can choose topics based on perceived patient needs, as one choses items from a menu. The greatest difference between psychological and audiological counselling may be in how the counselling style is applied to content. Certain counselling content may also suit different approaches better than others, for example, content of counselling in tinnitus retraining therapy (TRT) (see Chap. xxxx) and tinnitus activities treatment (TAT) (see Chap. xxx) differs.

Table 43.1 A comparison of literature reviews of psychological therapies for tinnitus with a Delphi review of consensus content for tinnitus counselling by audiologists [36, 37]

Psychology review	Audiology Delphi	Concept examples
Tinnitus education	Tinnitus education	Auditory neuroscience information
Relaxation	Relaxation	Relaxation techniques/breathing exercises
Attention		Attention shifting/imagery
Psychoeducation	Psychoeducation	Psychological models
Treatment rationale	Treatment rationale	Treatment options and roles
Behavioural intervention	Behavioural intervention	Reduce negative thoughts
Evaluation	Evaluation	Tinnitus impact
Treatment planning	Treatment planning	Identify objectives
Sound enrichment	Sound enrichment	Avoid silence
Treatment reflection	Treatment reflection	Assess outcomes
Sleep hygiene	Sleep hygiene	Advise good sleep practice
Thought identification		Identify cognitive distortions
Thought challenging		Restructure thoughts
Comorbidity	Comorbidity	Discuss hearing/mental health
Relapse prevention	Relapse prevention	Risk factors and management
Mindfulness		Mindfulness meditation
Interpersonal skills		Social communication skills
Lifestyle advice	Lifestyle advice	General health and well-being
Common therapeutic skills	Common therapeutic skills	Rapport/empathy/active listening
Social comparison		Share experiences
Emotion	Emotion	Effect of tinnitus on emotion
Problem-solving		Identify smaller achievable goals
Acceptance and delusion		Accept experiences
Self-concept		Improve esteem/self-image
Worry time		Consider worries within a constrained time
	Support and resource signposting	Resource sharing

Counselling Toolbox

Tinnitus counselling content may be similar across professions but can be applied in ways suited to different world views. We have found that the following counselling items help most tinnitus patients.

- Assessing counselling needs
- Setting counselling goals and addressing expectations
- Explaining tinnitus and the importance of health literacy
- Psychoeducation: Psychosocial factors and tinnitus
- Role of stress
- Role of attention focusing in tinnitus
- Role of emotions and thoughts
- Self-efficacy
- Tinnitus and disturbed sleep
- Sound enrichment
- Maintenance and re-emergent tinnitus
- Interdisciplinary referral

Assessing Patients' Counselling Needs

To assess patients' counselling needs, we have to gain a better understanding of the individuals' experience of their tinnitus, the impact it has on their life, and their ability to cope [69]. Several well-validated, self-report instruments are available to help assess various domains of everyday life functioning in individuals with tinnitus. Commonly used instruments include the Tinnitus Functional Index (TFI) [38] and the Tinnitus Primary Function Questionnaire [39]. How well individuals accept ringing in their ear can be assessed with the Tinnitus Acceptance Questionnaire [40]. Dysfunctional beliefs associated with tinnitus can be assessed with the Tinnitus Cognitions Scale [41]. The Tinnitus Fear-Avoidance Cognitions and Behaviors Scale [42] is a validated tool to measure the avoidance beliefs and behaviours associated with tinnitus. Tinnitus can be associated with psychological problems such as anxiety and/or depression. It is appropriate in an initial assessment to determine the presence of these conditions that may impact a person's tinnitus. The Patient Health Questionnaire-9 (PHQ-9) [43] and the General Anxiety Disorder Scale-7 (GAD-7) [44] are reliable tools to assess symptoms of depression and anxiety, respectively. Completing such questionnaires aids in identifying patients for more in-depth psychological assessment.

Setting Counselling Goals

Goal setting is important in most patient-centred models and critical to solution-focused therapy. It help patients work towards, achieve, and maintain treatment success [45]. Enthusiasm to match performance to goals drives the increase in self-satisfaction [46]. Goal setting can positively impact an individual's performance through a self-regulatory process. These processes include enabling the individual to focus their attention, promote effort, and initiate task-related strategies [47]. The SMART goal approach—specific, measurable, achievable, realistic, and time-bound—can be used to assist the selection and setting of goals [48]. Clinicians need to help patients identify solutions to their difficulties and the areas they want to change and then facilitate the patient's selection and adoption of helpful strategies. In order for goal setting to be effective, they must be adequately difficult to motivate effort but not so difficult that they discourage an individual from achieving them [49–51]. Outcomes need to be quantifiable so as to provide a record of achievement (Locke and Latham [52]; Locke [51]). Short-term goals facilitate focusing on the task at hand and, as such, increase motivation and expectations [53], i.e. small changes, and successes, leading to larger changes [16]. As mentioned in audiological rehabilitation counselling, the COSIT is a useful tool to record and assess SMART goals. Patients identify up to five situations in which they want solutions, then they rank these in priority, and the clinician can then discuss solutions and realistic outcomes. The COSIT is a useful way of tracking progress towards achieving goals as well as setting them. At stages throughout the tinnitus rehabilitation process, the problems identified using the COSIT are re-examined and improvement in tinnitus in each situation is determined. Patients indicate the degree of change (1 = worse to 5 = much better) and the amount of annoyance caused by tinnitus after therapy (1 = almost always to 5 = hardly ever). If improvement is not shown, then appropriate steps can be undertaken to address the problem. When the initial goals are achieved, further goals and solutions can be explored.

Explaining Tinnitus and the Importance of Health Literacy

A recent meta-analysis has found that educational counselling alone has similar benefits to other psychological and combination therapies [54]. The more knowledgeable patients are, the better the health outcomes [55, 56].

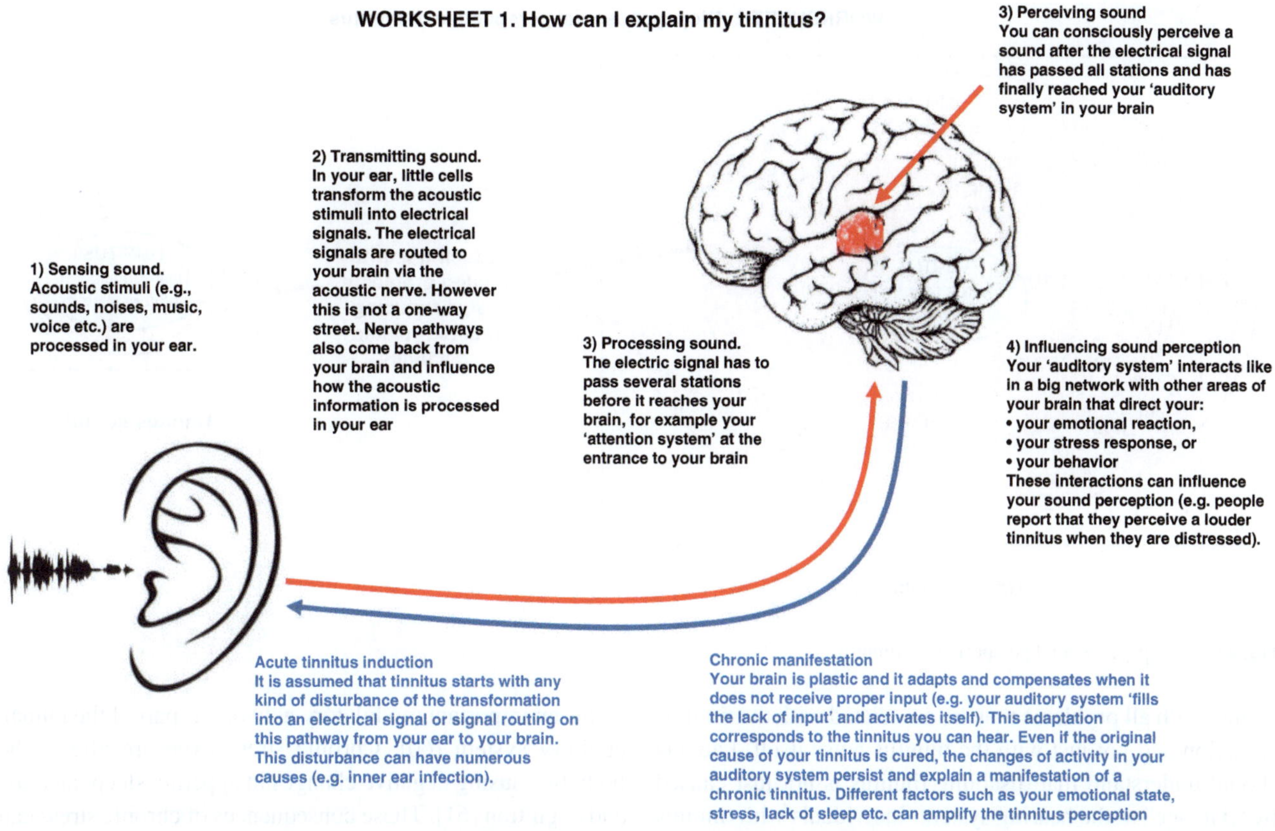

Fig. 43.2 How can I explain my tinnitus?

Instruction can sometimes be sufficient to address fears of the patient such that further counselling is not required. For individuals with tinnitus, it is important to be provided with a conceptual model to explain how a tinnitus sensation evolves and manifests as a chronic symptom. It is important that this conceptual model is plausible and simple. It does not need to be medically exact, but it has to make sense to the patient (Fig. 43.2). Typical topics include: tinnitus epidemiology, anatomy and physiology, the basis of hearing loss, tinnitus mechanisms, how the central nervous system works, and the transition from an acute to a chronic, disabling tinnitus.

Another task of counselling is to empower patients to take care of their well-being. A move towards this self-efficacy is to develop health literacy. Health literacy is the ability that individuals have to obtain, process, and understand the basic health information needed to make appropriate health decisions [57]. Many patients start their tinnitus journey by searching for treatments on the Internet. It is important that the patients know how to search for evidence-based solutions, avoiding misinformation. To facilitate this, tinnitus organizations, researchers, and clinicians need to develop readable material relevant to the patient's perspective [58]. Tinnitus patients need to be able to obtain and understand tinnitus information.

Psychoeducation: Psychosocial Factors and Tinnitus

Biopsychosocial perspectives of tinnitus as well as psychological and social concepts are presented alongside the biological (medical) aspects of the condition. Psychoeducation in the context of tinnitus counselling helps the patient with tinnitus to differentiate between tinnitus sensation and tinnitus distress. Engel described a biopsychosocial model of somatic conditions in the early 1980s [59]. Tinnitus involves, in addition to the auditory sensation, numerous other factors, such as the individual's personal experiences and behaviours, interactions with the social environment, or cultural factors, for example [10]. Explaining this model to patients can help them understand that coping with tinnitus involves

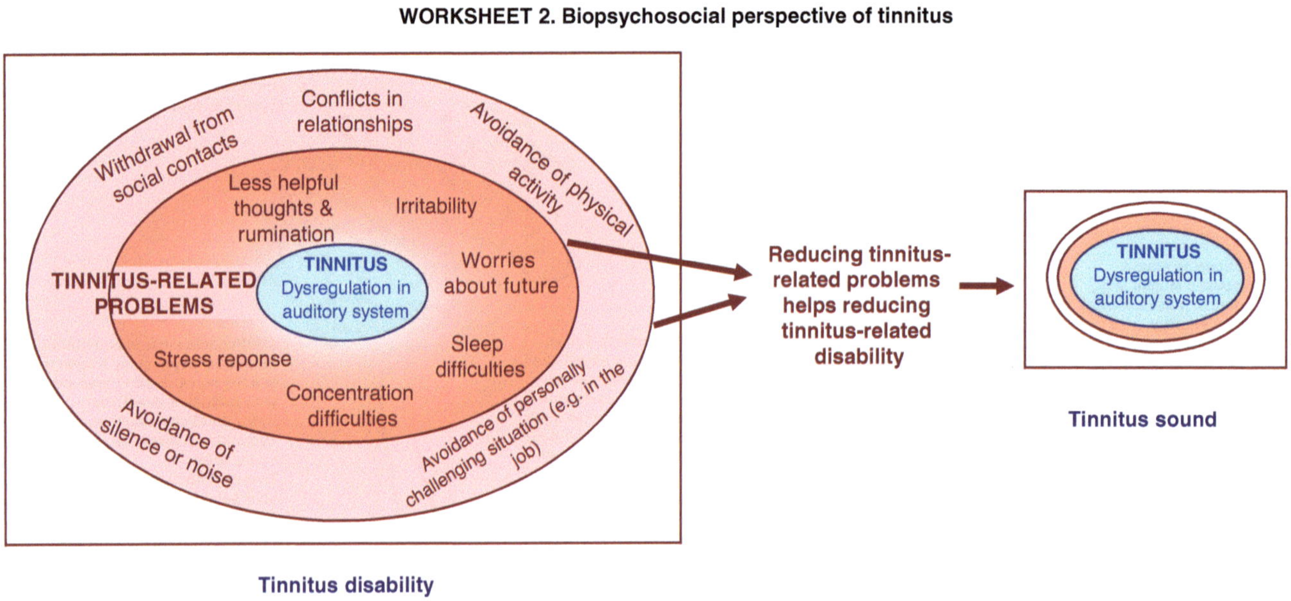

Fig. 43.3 Biopsychosocial perspective of tinnitus

coping with all problems that are associated with the tinnitus sensation and not just with the tinnitus noise itself. Patients should understand that disabling tinnitus is not just caused by "damage" to the hearing system. Individuals with tinnitus often want, even expect, that by identifying the "damage", it can be fixed. Counselling can help individuals understand that tinnitus is a complex phenomenon that involves the interaction of numerous processes in their brain and the rest of their body. Examples of this are a significant number of individuals in the general population report tinnitus, but 1–2% feel significantly disturbed; tinnitus loudness is not necessarily associated with tinnitus distress, and individuals with normal hearing and without tinnitus who, when left in a soundproof room, start hearing tinnitus-like sounds. Figure 43.3 provides some ideas of how these holistic concepts can be embedded in tinnitus counselling. In the following sections, we will discuss a selection of psychosocial, lifestyle factors that should be addressed, with psychoeducation, for almost every patient with chronic and distressing tinnitus.

The Role of Stress

There are various pathways of stress influencing the chronic manifestation of tinnitus, and these are not completely understood. Changes in the neurotransmitter metabolism as a consequence of chronic stress exposure are discussed as one of the main mechanisms. For example, stress negatively influences the serotonergic receptor function. Serotonin plays a crucial role in the development of tinnitus because it forms an important modulatory network as part of the human auditory system [60]. Chronic stress exposure affects the body by causing negative changes in appetite, sleep, anxiety, and cognition [61]. These consequences of chronic stress can perpetuate and amplify tinnitus [62]. Thus, it is important to educate patients about the role of stress in the tinnitus pathology.

Stress and tinnitus can be introduced by beginning with a discussion about the life-protecting function of the human stress response. Although our stress response is actually protective, it is not highly adaptive to forms of persistent stress that we experience in a modern society. Patients are often interested in understanding the stress system, including the function of the sympathetic and parasympathetic part of our autonomous nervous system. Introducing stress education with biomedical content can help build a therapeutic alliance, especially with those patients who understand their tinnitus solely as a biomedical phenomenon.

Introducing stress management as part of tinnitus counselling targets different goals. A long-term goal is to reduce tinnitus perpetuation and chronic stress response. Other important goals are to establish a balance between external or internal stressors (e.g. stressful external events, negative self-talk) and resilience and stress resistance (Fig. 43.4). The choice of a relaxation strategy is a highly individualized decision. Patients should be provided with resources and should be encouraged to practice different forms of relaxation strategies, giving each enough time to show effect though. Some individuals prefer more "physical" forms of relaxation (e.g. progressive muscle relaxation), other individuals prefer more "cognitive" relaxation strategies (e.g.

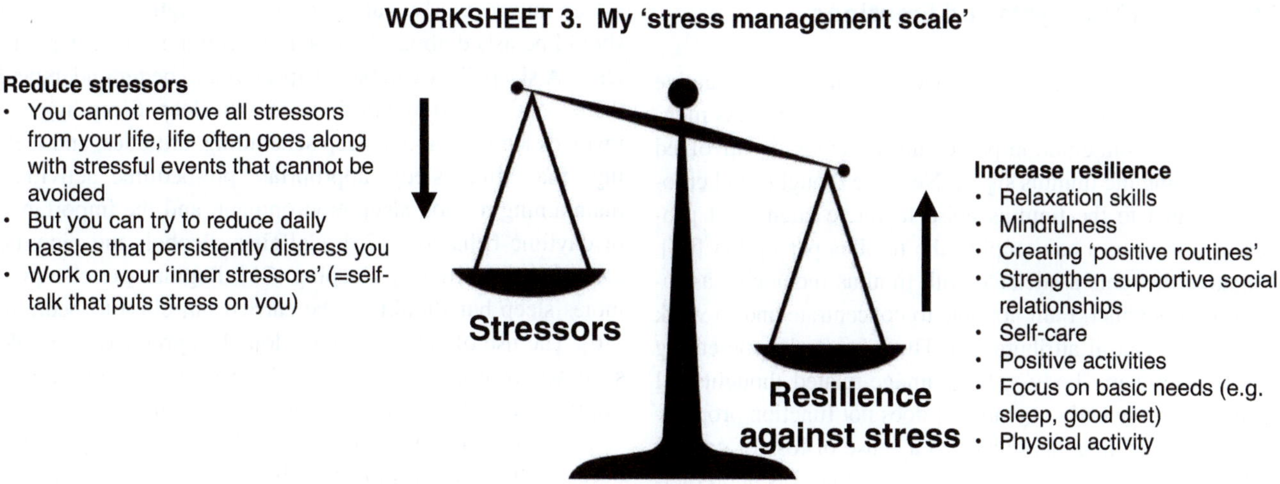

Fig. 43.4 My 'stress management scale'

positive imagery, mindfulness, and meditation). Numerous relaxation apps are available to help patients with the practice. Relaxation training is an important component of CBT (see Chap. 44).

Understanding the Role of Attention Focusing in Tinnitus

Attention appears to play an important role in tinnitus annoyance and maintenance. Tinnitus can often become a dominant feature in the sufferers' soundscape, consuming attentional resources and potentially affecting cognition [63, 64]. Psychoeducation can help patients better understand the role of their attention system in the development of chronic tinnitus. The basic principles of our attention system should be explained to patients. For example, "the human attention system functions like a 'filter'. It can filter out more or less important input. It is connected to the limbic system in the brain, which is responsible for processing emotions. Stimuli that are associated with negative emotions, including a bothering tinnitus, are more prone to activate our attention system. Focusing attention on the tinnitus can have amplifying effects on the ringing in the ear". Behavioural experiments that help patients "experience" the effect of attention focusing on their perceptions can be helpful (see example instruction in Table 43.2). The acquisition of attention control skills should allow patients to shift their attention to and from tinnitus [23, 65]. If the sufferer can learn the perceptual reality of tinnitus, it will be placed in its appropriate context [66], thus reducing the focus on tinnitus [10].

Table 43.2 How does attention influence our perception of sound and tinnitus?

1. Imagine you lie in your bed and sleep. What would be most likely to wake you up? The background noise of the fridge? A crying baby? Unfamiliar noises from outside? How do explain differences in how likely different sounds can wake you up?
Our attention system amplifies sounds that are unfamiliar or are associated with negative emotions.
Listen to but do not watch a movie: Listen to a movie with closed eyes and try to guess what happens just by listening to the sound scenery.
Listen for about 5 min to a piece of music and try to focus your attention on the melody of a certain musical instrument (e.g. focus on the drums and rhythm) What has happened to your tinnitus?
Sit in a park and close your eyes. Listen attentively to all sounds that appear in your environment. Try to recognize the sounds and the source of the sound and label it in your mind (e.g., dog barking, car passing, church bell).
What has happened to your tinnitus?
Listening intensively to a specific sound or acoustic stimulus can let other sounds (including a tinnitus) stay in the background
Read a newspaper article of a topic that you are especially interested in.
Get outside, sit in the grass for a while, and close your eyes. Touch the ground and objects surrounding you (e.g., grass, branches, leaves, flowers).
Take all spice jars out of your kitchen cabinet. Open them. Close your eyes and smell on each of the jars. Concentrate on the different smells and try recognize each spice.
Can you remember what you have heard during these experiments?
Shifting attention to certain senses (e.g. sense of touch or smell) or concentrating on certain cognitively demanding activities can let other sensations (e.g. sound) stay in the background.

The Role of Thoughts and Emotions

According to cognitive behavioural theories, negative thoughts can induce negative emotional states [67]. As mentioned earlier, our emotion-processing system is also involved in processing the tinnitus signal. Negative thoughts and emotions related to the tinnitus noise facilitate attentional processes that in turn can amplify the tinnitus perception [68]. Negative thoughts associated with tinnitus include catastrophizing thoughts ("I am not able to concentrate and to work anymore"), causal attributions ("There has to be something wrong within my body"), body image-related thoughts ("I cannot trust my body anymore, it does not function properly anymore"), or thoughts related to a sense of loss of control (e.g. "My tinnitus gets worse out of the blue. It is unpredictable"). There are also various emotional states associated with tinnitus, for example, some individuals experience sadness and grief about losing their quality of life and functioning, whereas others become anxious because of worries about their future. Other individuals get angry, irritable, or frustrated because they tend to see their tinnitus as a "scapegoat" for all their problems in life. Psychoeducation as a part of tinnitus counselling helps patients understand how cognitions and emotions can influence their tinnitus perception, for example, by explaining neurophysiological models [69]. For many individuals, just talking about the role of beliefs and identifying their problematic, tinnitus-amplifying beliefs can have recovering effects. For individuals who struggle with rigid cognitive schemata, cognitive behavioural strategies (CBT) and a referral to a clinical psychologist or a physician specializing in psychosomatic medicine are indicated.

Self-Efficacy

Self-efficacy in the context of tinnitus management is defined as "beliefs (i.e. confidence) individuals have in their capabilities to perform skills needed to accomplish a specific goal or behavior" [70], p. 424). Research in the treatment of various chronic health conditions, e.g. chronic pain, shows that self-efficacy beliefs play an important role in treatment outcomes and management of the condition [71]. Individuals with chronic health conditions develop self-efficacy in the management of their condition by developing a sense of control over their symptom(s). All strategies described in this toolbox have the goal to gain back control over the tinnitus and can contribute to strengthen the individual's self-efficacy.

Tinnitus and Disturbed Sleep

Improving their quality and ability to sleep is an extremely common goal for tinnitus sufferers [11, 72, 73]. Sleep problems associated with tinnitus may include difficulty falling asleep and regularly waking during the night [74]. Patients should be asked about their bedtime routines and sleep patterns. A sleep diary can be a helpful tool to better understand the patient's individual difficulties with sleep. Sleep hygiene involves learning about sleep scheduling, attitudes, and feelings that affect sleep, appropriate pre-bedtime activities, maintaining a good sleep environment, and the importance of daytime behaviour [75]. Caffeine, alcohol, and nicotine can result in difficulty sleeping [76]. Regular exercise promotes sleep but should not be carried out close to bedtime [76]. The use of sleep hygiene alone has produced variable success; however, when applied alongside with CBT, greater improvement in tinnitus symptoms have been observed [77].

Some tinnitus sufferers have difficulties falling asleep because they have ruminating thoughts, mostly worries. A helpful strategy can be journaling. Patients can keep a journal to write down all their less helpful and bothering thoughts and set aside a "worry time" during the day. During worry time, they actively reflect on their beliefs and challenge them with cognitive reappraisal strategies or try to solve the problems they worry about [78].

Sound Enrichment

Sound enrichment, a type of sound therapy, is the addition of background sound to otherwise quiet environments. The use of sound to manage or treat tinnitus can include use of recorded music through to complex hearing aids (see Chap. XXX). Sound is a tinnitus therapy tool used by audiologists and, to a lesser extent, by other professionals. There is debate about the merits of sound therapy above the counselling that accompanies it [79]. Sound may be valuable to provide tinnitus relief [80], partial masking [81], and as an aid to habituation [82]. Counselling for sound therapy should provide the rationale for use of the sound, the device selected, and likelihood of success. We believe that sound therapy should be viewed as an aid to therapy, as part of a holistic approach, and its use should match the goals of the patient.

Maintenance and Re-Emergent Tinnitus

The patient should be made aware that a previously compensated tinnitus may occasionally reappear and that this is not a reason to worry about a resurgence of problematic tinnitus. Normal life stress, anxieties, and life events could all trigger the re-emergence of tinnitus. Reassurance that the re-emerged tinnitus is likely a consequence of these life events should again reduce the salience of tinnitus. Changes in hearing could also trigger a resumption of tinnitus, such as exposure to a sudden loud noise (e.g. an alarm). It is not feasible to protect hearing against all these events, as they are usually random and unexpected, and, instead, anxiety and stress should be managed with the goal of reducing the risk of psychological shock accompanying noise [83]. Patients should be made aware of dangerous sounds and how to avoid further injury [84], but use of hearing protection should be limited to only when exposed to loud harmful sounds. Overprotection may result in auditory deprivation and hyperacusis. Counselling the progressive use of less protection may assist transition from dependence on hearing protection to more normal use.

Involving the patient in self-directed care (worksheets and online resources) helps develop self-efficacy and engagement in ongoing counselling, aimed towards the therapy goals [85], and maintaining gains achieved in counselling sessions. One of the primary benefits of using homework is that the techniques learned during the intervention are practiced outside the session [85]. As part of a continuity of care, clinicians should also be prepared for ongoing enquiries from patients, and, typically, these enquires seek reassurance. Mutually agreed processes for ongoing communication should establish when and how patients can contact the clinician (e.g. email, telephone, consultation). It is important to promote self-efficacy and responsibility for self-directed care, but an easy means for the parties to communicate is also needed.

Interdisciplinary Referrals

Irrespective of an individual clinicians' expertise and experience, there will be always be patients who will benefit from consultations with other professionals. This may take the form of medical referrals to otology, psychology services, hearing therapy or social workers (for community counselling), neurology (e.g. head injury), maxillofacial surgery (e.g. temporomandibular joint assessment), physiotherapy (for neck and back complaints), psychiatry (for management of medications) and audiologists (hearing aids and sound therapy), and neuroradiology (for imaging of the head and neck), amongst many other possibilities. Depending on the health system, i.e. urban or rural setting, government publicly funded or private, wealthy or developing country, the tinnitus clinician will have different expertise. In some settings, patients may pass through a multidisciplinary clinic, whereas in other situations, the patient may have to see "a-jack-of-all-trades" clinician. Building relationships with professionals of different disciplines is an essential part of developing a tinnitus clinic, no matter the setting. Explaining reasons for referrals, in a positive and non-alarmist manner, is a critical component of tinnitus counselling. Patients should understand the benefits of seeing the clinician being referred to and not fear the consequences or reasons for the referral (e.g. a common worry concerning medical referral is "that must mean a brain tumour!"). Patients often like the consistency of seeing the same clinician, so, when a referral is needed from the primary clinician to another for their expertise, reassurance that the clinician is not handing them off to someone else, i.e. "abandoning them", is important.

An Example of a Tinnitus Counselling Framework: AREA (Attend, React, Explain, Adapt)

Clinicians should choose a counselling framework based on their preferred counselling style, perspectives, and scope of practice. In this book, there are several frameworks for therapy that use different counselling styles, including tinnitus retraining therapy, tinnitus activities treatment, and cognitive behavioural therapy. AREA (Attend, React, Explain, Adapt) counselling is another framework that incorporates psychological and audiological knowledge, based on a psychosocial "ecological" model of tinnitus.

Wilson and Gilbert [86] proposed an AREA (Attend, React, Explain, Adapt) model of affective adaptation in which people make sense of an event through avenues such as past experiences, hypothetical alternatives, or existing knowledge paradigms. This model was adopted and modified for tinnitus in light of its concepts of affective adaptation shared with the psychosocial "ecological" model of tinnitus [10]. In this model, an emotional event initiates physiological arousal from the sympathetic system, which triggers antagonistic physiological processes from the parasympathetic system ("React), to consciously adapt a patient's needs to engage in other activities. Perception of the tinnitus is based on the evaluation of differences to previous experiences rather than absolute magnitudes [87]. Tinnitus has greater emotional impact when paid attention ("Attend"), and people attend more strongly—and emotionally—to self-relevant, unexplained events. If patients can explain and understand the experience ("Explain"), then adaptation ("Adapt") can occur with less attention and reduced emotional response to the tinnitus.

The tinnitus AREA counselling content is fairly holistic and includes aspects of both motivational interviewing and solution-focused therapy. The counselling session(s) begin with problem-free talk: how the patient is today, i.e. "how's life", before "what is your goal in attending our clinic", thus creating goals for the session and identifying solutions based around the ideal future [88], and "what is your ideal future—best outcome—.... if you had no tinnitus what would you do differently?" To assist patients in putting tinnitus in context, instructions on the ecological model, auditory system, and neurophysiology are provided. This centres on tinnitus as a component of everyday perception and engagement with our environment and the role of attention in promoting tinnitus perception due to its inconstancy with learned realities. A differentiating aspect of this model from counselling focused on neurophysiology is its acknowledgement of affect and conversations to address this: “How does your tinnitus make you feel?” Aligned with the solution-based focus [88] and a process of shared decision-making [89], the counselling draws heavily on the SMART goal setting using the COSIT tool to negotiate achievable, often incremental, patient goals. In a departure from a solely problem-solving process, the clinician does consider the aetiology and behavioural tests with neurophysiological correlates. Although many elements of tinnitus are “unexplained” [89], we have sufficient basis for clinical decision-making based on assessments (e.g. the audiogram and questionnaires), and grounding the patient in the knowledge that tinnitus is a perception, not imagined, is useful.

Each session is based on individual needs and incorporates instructions along with discussion; the topics typically covered include: Attend (attention-grabbing aspects of tinnitus, attention refocusing, Worksheet 4); React (tinnitus and stress, perceived threat, e.g. Worksheet 3); Explain (why understanding tinnitus is important, how we hear, biopsychological principles, e.g. Worksheets 1 and 2); and Adapt (meaning of adaptation, perceptual adaptation, affective adaptation, assistance through sound therapy, visualization and guided imagery, hearing and active listening, and brain/attention training).

Summary

Although there are different approaches to the management of tinnitus, fundamentally, the vital elements of a management approach include education and tools to manage the tinnitus and its effects. How these are addressed and provided to the patient varies considerably between programs and practices (due to resources, practitioner training, experience, and practicality of program delivery). Education alone can be a sufficient intervention for some patients [54, 65, 90, 91]. Due to the complexity and multiple factors that impact the emotional well-being of an individual, a multidisciplinary team approach is best when treating a patient with tinnitus [30, 92, 93]. All clinicians should be comfortable in providing counselling. However, circumstances will determine which professionals will be providing tinnitus counselling within different settings. The time spent with a patient will differ between counselling approaches and patient needs. There is no gold standard for the number or length of counselling sessions. A single counselling session of 60–90-min duration, when provided with homework tasks, may be the minimum amount of counselling required to be an effective intervention [94]. We encourage clinicians to embrace opportunities to improve their counselling [95] while at the same time recognizing the roots of their professional training so as to be mindful of where their, and others’, expertise lies.

References

1. Kaplan DM, Tarvydas VM, Gladding ST. 20/20: a vision for the future of counseling: the new consensus definition of counseling. J Couns Dev. 2014;92(3):366–72.
2. Coles RR, Hallam RS. Tinnitus and its management. Br Med Bull. 1987;43(4):983–98.
3. Cederroth CR, Gallus S, Hall DA, Kleinjung T, Langguth B, Maruotti A, et al. Towards an understanding of tinnitus heterogeneity. Front Aging Neurosci. 2019;11:53.
4. Coles R. Epidemiology of tinnitus (2). Demographic and clinical features. J Laryngol Otol. 1984;Suppl 2:195–202.
5. Cooper JC. Health and nutrition examination survey of 1971-75: part II. Tinnitus, subjective hearing loss, and well being. J Am Acad Audiol. 1994;5:37–43.
6. Udupi VA, Uppunda AK, Mohan KM, Alex J, Mahendra MH. The relationship of perceived severity of tinnitus with depression, anxiety, hearing status, age and gender in individuals with tinnitus. Int Tinnitus J. 2013;18(1):29–34.
7. Lindberg P, Scott B. The use and predictive value of psychological profiles in helpseeking and non-helpseeking tinnitus sufferers. In: Hazell JW, editor. Proceedings of the sixth international tinnitus seminar, Cambridge UK September 5th-9th 1999. London: The Tinnitus and Hyperacusis Centre; 1999. p. 114–7.
8. Fagelson MA. The association between tinnitus and posttraumatic stress disorder. Am J Audiol. 2007;16(2):107–17.
9. Baguley D, McFerran D, Hall D. Tinnitus. Lancet. 2013;382(9904):1600–7.
10. Searchfield GD. Tinnitus what and where: an ecological framework. Front Neurol. 2014;5:271.
11. Tyler RS, Baker LJ. Difficulties experienced by tinnitus sufferers. J Speech Hear Disord. 1983;48(2):150–4.
12. Clark JG, English KM. Counseling in audiologic practice. Boston: Pearson Education; 2004.
13. Heffler B, Sandell R. The role of learning style in choosing one’s therapeutic orientation. Psychother Res. 2009;19(3):283–92.
14. Boothroyd A. Adult aural rehabilitation: what is it and does it work? Trends Amplif. 2007;11(2):63–71.
15. Searchfield GD, Linford T, Durai M. Sound therapy and aural rehabilitation for tinnitus: a person centred therapy framework based on an ecological model of tinnitus. Disabil Rehabil. 2019;41(16):1966–73.
16. Blair JC. Principles of solution focused therapy and their application to audiology. Perspect Public Health Issues Relat Hear Balance. 2014;15(1):27–33.
17. Dillon H, James A, Ginis J. Client Oriented Scale of Improvement (COSI) and its relationship to several other measures of benefit and satisfaction provided by hearing aids. J Am Acad Audiol. 1997;8:27–43.
18. Searchfield GD. A client oriented scale of improvement in tinnitus for therapy goal planning and assessing outcomes. J Am Acad Audiol. 2019;30(4):327–37.
19. Cienkowski KM, Saunders GH. An examination of hearing aid counseling implemented by audiologists. Perspect Aural Rehabil Instrum. 2013;20(2):67–76.
20. Meibos A, Muñoz K, Twohig M. Counseling competencies in audiology: a modified delphi study. Am J Audiol. 2019;28(2):285–99.
21. Mcfarlane L-A. Motivational interviewing: practical strategies for speech-language pathologists and audiologists. Can J Speech Lang Pathol Audiol. 2012;36(1):8–16.
22. Rogers CR. The foundations of the person-centered approach. Education. 1979;100(2):98–107.
23. Tyler R, Noble W, Preece JP, Dunn CC, Witt SA. Psychological treatments for tinnitus. In: Snow JB, editor. Tinnitus: theory and management. Ontario: BC Decker; 2004. p. 314–25.

24. Wagner CC, McMahon BT. Motivational interviewing and rehabilitation counseling practice. Rehabil Couns Bull. 2004;47(3):152–61.
25. Roessler RT. Factors affecting client achievement of rehabilitation goals. J Appl Rehabil Couns. 1980;11(4):169–72.
26. Jensen MP, Nielson WR, Kerns RD. Toward the development of a motivational model of pain self-management. J Pain. 2003;4(9):477–92.
27. Simm R, Iddon J, Barker C. A community pain service solution-focused pain management programme: delivery and preliminary outcome data. Br J Pain. 2014;8(1):49–56.
28. Corcoran J, Pillai V. A review of the research on solution-focused therapy. Br J Soc Work. 2009;39(2):234–42.
29. Henry J, Zaugg T, Myers P, Kendall C. Progressive tinnitus management. Clinical handbook for audiologists appendixes, vol. 59. Long Beach, CA: VA Employee Education System; 2010. p. 97.
30. Newman CW, Sandridge SA. Incorporating group and individual sessions into a tinnitus management clinic. In: Tyler R, editor. Tinnitus treatment: clinical protocols. New York: Thieme Medical Publishers; 2005. p. 187–97.
31. McKenna L, Daniel H. The psychological management of tinnitus related insomnia. Tinnitus treatments. New York: Thieme; 2005.
32. Jakes S, Hallam R, McKenna L, Hinchcliffe R. Group cognitive therapy for medical patients: an application to tinnitus. Cogn Ther Res. 1992;16(1):67–82.
33. Gander PE, Hoare DJ, Collins L, Smith S, Hall DA. Tinnitus referral pathways within the National Health Service in England: a survey of their perceived effectiveness among audiology staff. BMC Health Serv Res. 2011;11(1):1–11.
34. Fuller T, Cima R, Langguth B, Mazurek B, Vlaeyen JW, Hoare DJ. Cognitive behavioural therapy for tinnitus. Cochrane Database of Systematic Reviews. 2020;1(1):CD012614.
35. Guitton MJ. Telemedicine in tinnitus: feasibility, advantages, limitations, and perspectives. ISRN Otolaryngol. 2013;2013:218265.
36. Thompson DM, Taylor J, Hall DA, Walker D-M, McMurran M, Casey A, et al. Patients' and clinicians' views of the psychological components of tinnitus treatment that could inform audiologists' usual care: a Delphi survey. Ear Hear. 2018;39(2):367.
37. Thompson DM, Hall DA, Walker D-M, Hoare DJ. Psychological therapy for people with tinnitus: a scoping review of treatment components. Ear Hear. 2017;38(2):149.
38. Meikle MB, Henry JA, Griest SE, Stewart BJ, Abrams HB, McArdle R, et al. The tinnitus functional index: development of a new clinical measure for chronic, intrusive tinnitus. Ear Hear. 2012;33(2):153–76. https://doi.org/10.1097/AUD.0b013e31822f67c0.
39. Tyler R, Ji H, Perreau A, Witt S, Noble W, Coelho C. Development and validation of the tinnitus primary function questionnaire. Am J Audiol. 2014;23(3):260–72.
40. Westin V, Hayes SC, Andersson G. Is it the sound or your relationship to it? The role of acceptance in predicting tinnitus impact. Behav Res Ther. 2008;46(12):1259–65.
41. Conrad I, Kleinstäuber M, Jasper K, Hiller W, Andersson G, Weise C. The role of dysfunctional cognitions in patients with chronic tinnitus. Ear Hear. 2015;36(5):e279–89.
42. Kleinstäuber M, Jasper K, Schweda I, Hiller W, Andersson G, Weise C. The role of fear-avoidance cognitions and behaviors in patients with chronic tinnitus. Cogn Behav Ther. 2013;42(2):84–99.
43. Kroenke K, Spitzer RL, Williams JB. The PHQ-9: validity of a brief depression severity measure. J Gen Intern Med. 2001;16(9):606–13.
44. Spitzer RL, Kroenke K, Williams JB, Löwe B. A brief measure for assessing generalized anxiety disorder: the GAD-7. Arch Intern Med. 2006;166(10):1092–7.
45. West RL, Thorn RM. Goal-setting, self-efficacy, and memory performance in older and younger adults. Exp Aging Res. 2001;27(1):41–65.
46. Bandura A, Cervone D. Differential engagement of self-reactive influences in cognitive motivation. Organ Behav Hum Decis Process. 1986;38(1):92–113.
47. Locke EA, Latham GP. A theory of goal setting & task performance. Hoboken: Prentice-Hall; 1990.
48. Swinton L. Project YOU part I: goal setting guide. http://www.uncommon-knowledge.co.uk/goal_setting/Goal_Setting_Guide.pdf. 2004. Accessed 13 Nov 2005.
49. Lee TW, Locke EA, Latham GP. Goal setting theory and job performance. In: Pervin LA, editor. Goal concepts in personality and social psychology. Mahwah: Lawrence Erlbaum Associates; 1989.
50. Bandura A. Self-regulation of motivation and action through internal standards and goal systems. In: Pervin LA, editor. Goal concepts in personality and social psychology. Hillsdale, NJ: Lawrence Erlbaum Associates; 1989. p. 19–85.
51. Locke EA. Toward a theory of task motivation and incentives. Organ Behav Huma Perform. 1968;3(2):157–89. http://www.elsevier.com/wps/find/journaldescriptioncws_home/622929/description#description.
52. Lee TW, Locke EA, Latham GP. Goal setting theory and job performance. In L. A. Pervin (Ed.), Goal concepts in personality and social psychology. Lawrence Erlbaum Associates, Inc. 1989: 291–326.
53. Manderlink G, Harackiewicz JM. Proximal versus distal goal setting and intrinsic motivation. J Pers Soc Psychol. 1984;47(4):918–28.
54. Xiang T, Zhong J, Lu T, Pu J-m, Liu L, Xiao Y, et al. Effect of educational counseling alone on people with tinnitus: meta-analysis of randomized controlled trials. Patient Educ Couns. 2020;103(1):44–54.
55. Lukens EP, McFarlane WR. Psychoeducation as evidence-based practice: considerations for practice, research, and policy. Brief Treat Crisis Interv. 2004;4(3):205–25.
56. Lucksted A, McFarlane W, Downing D, Dixon L. Recent developments in family psychoeducation as an evidence-based practice. J Marital Fam Ther. 2012;38(1):101–21.
57. Brach C, Harris LM. Healthy people 2030 health literacy definition tells organizations: make information and services easy to find, understand, and use. J Gen Intern Med. 2021;36(4):1084–5.
58. Manchaiah V, Dockens AL, Flagge A, Bellon-Harn M, Azios JH, Kelly-Campbell RJ, et al. Quality and readability of English-language Internet information for tinnitus. J Am Acad Audiol. 2019;30(1):31–40.
59. Engel GL. The clinical application of the biopsychosocial model. J Med Philos. 1981;6(2):101–24.
60. Simpson JJ, Davies WE. A review of evidence in support of a role for 5-HT in the perception of tinnitus. Hear Res. 2000;145(1–2):1–7.
61. Marin M-F, Lord C, Andrews J, Juster R-P, Sindi S, Arsenault-Lapierre G, et al. Chronic stress, cognitive functioning and mental health. Neurobiol Learn Mem. 2011;96(4):583–95.
62. Lu T, Li S, Ma Y, Lai D, Zhong J, Li G, et al. Positive correlation between tinnitus severity and poor sleep quality prior to tinnitus onset: a retrospective study. Psychiatric Q. 2020;91(2):379–88.
63. Tegg-Quinn S, Bennett RJ, Eikelboom RH, Baguley DM. The impact of tinnitus upon cognition in adults: a systematic review. Int J Audiol. 2016;55(10):533–40.
64. Mohamad N, Hoare DJ, Hall DA. The consequences of tinnitus and tinnitus severity on cognition: a review of the behavioural evidence. Hear Res. 2016;332:199–209.
65. Henry J, Wilson PH. The psychological management of tinnitus: comparison of a combined cognitive educational program, education alone and a waiting-list control. Int Tinnitus J. 1996;1:9–20.
66. Feldmann H. Tinnitus - reality or phantom. In: Aran JM, Dauman R, editors. Tinnitus 91: proceedings of the fourth international tinnitus seminar. Amsterdam: Kugler Publications; 1992.

67. Hallam R. Psychological approaches to the evaluation and management of tinnitus distress. In: Tinnitus. Edimburgh: Churcill-Livingstone; 1987. p. 156–75.
68. Jastreboff PJ, Hazell JW. A neurophysiological approach to tinnitus: clinical implications. Br J Audiol. 1993;27(1):7–17.
69. Tyler RS. Neurophysiological models, psychological models, and treatments for tinnitus. In: Tinnitus treatment: clinical protocols. Stuttgart: Thieme; 2006. p. 1–22.
70. Smith SL, Fagelson M. Development of the self-efficacy for tinnitus management questionnaire. J Am Acad Audiol. 2011;22(7):424–40.
71. Hayward R, Stynes S. Self-efficacy as a prognostic factor and treatment moderator in chronic musculoskeletal pain patients attending pain management programmes: a systematic review. Musculoskeletal Care. 2021;19(3):278–92.
72. Jakes SC, Hallam RS, Chambers C, Hinchcliffe R. A factor analytical study of tinnitus complaint behaviour. Audiology. 1985;24(3):195–206.
73. Axelsson A, Ringdahl A. Tinnitus: a study of its prevalence and characteristics. Br J Audiol. 1989;23(1):53–62.
74. Tyler R. Psychoacoustical measurement. In: Tyler R, editor. Handbook of tinnitus. San Diego: Singular Publications; 2000. p. 149–80.
75. Nau SD, Walsh JK. Sleep hygiene of insomnia patients. Sleep Hyg. 1983;12:268.
76. McKenna L, Daniel HC. Tinnitus-related insomnia treatment. In: Tyler R, editor. Tinnitus treatment: clinical protocols. New York: Thieme Medical Publishers; 2005. p. 81–95.
77. Harvey L, Inglis SJ, Espie CA. Insomniacs' reported use of CBT components and relationship to long-term clinical outcome. Behav Res Ther. 2002;40(1):75–83.
78. Nash J. Stress and diabetes: the use of "worry time" as a way of managing stress. J Diabetes Nurs. 2014;18:329–32.
79. Mckenna L, Irwin R. Sound therapy for tinnitus–sacred cow or idol worship?: an investigation of the evidence. Audiol Med. 2008;6(1):16–24.
80. Vernon J, Schleuning A. Tinnitus: a new management. Laryngoscope. 1978;88(3):413–9.
81. Tyler RS, Bentler RA. Tinnitus maskers and hearing aids for tinnitus. Seminars in hearing: Copyright© 1987. Stuttgart: Thieme Medical Publishers; 1987. p. 49–60.
82. Jastreboff PJ, Jastreboff MM. Tinnitus retraining therapy (TRT) as a method for treatment of tinnitus and hyperacusis patients. J Am Acad Audiol. 2000;11(3):162–77.
83. McFerran D, Baguley D. Acoustic shock. J Laryngol Otol. 2007;121(4):301–5.
84. Martin WH. Dangerous decibels: partnership for preventing noise-induced hearing loss and tinnitus in children. Semin Hear. 2008;29(1):102–10.
85. Kazantzis N, Lampropoulos GK. Reflecting on homework in psychotherapy: what can we conclude from research and experience? J Clin Psychol. 2002;58(5):577–85.
86. Wilson TD, Gilbert DT. Explaining away: a model of affective adaptation. Perspect Psychol Sci. 2008;3(5):370–86.
87. Searchfield GD, Kobayashi K, Sanders M. An adaptation level theory of tinnitus audibility. Front Syst Neurosci. 2012;6:46. https://doi.org/10.3389/fnsys.2012.00046.
88. Lethem J. Brief solution focused therapy. Child Adolesc Ment Health. 2002;7(4):189–92.
89. Pryce H, Hall A, Marks E, Culhane BA, Swift S, Straus J, et al. Shared decision-making in tinnitus care–an exploration of clinical encounters. Br J Health Psychol. 2018;23(3):630–45.
90. Kroner-Herwig B, Frenzel A, Fritsche G, Schilkowsky G, Esser G. The management of chronic tinnitus: comparison of an outpatient cognitive-behavioral group training to minimal-contact interventions. J Psychosom Res. 2003;54(4):381–9.
91. Laurikainen E, Johansson R, Akaan-Penttila E, Haapaniemi J. Treatment of severe tinnitus. Acta Otolaryngol Suppl (Stockh). 2000;543:77–8.
92. Andersson G, Baguley D, McKenna L, McFerran D. Tinnitus: a multidisciplinary approach. London: Whurr Publishers Ltd; 2005.
93. Cima RFF, Mazurek B, Haider H, Kikidis D, Lapira A, Noreña A, et al. A multidisciplinary European guideline for tinnitus: diagnostics, assessment, and treatment. HNO. 2019;67(1):10–42.
94. Searchfield GD, Boone M, Bensam J, Durai M, Hodgson S-A, Linford T, et al. A proof-of-concept study of the benefits of a single-session of tinnitus instruction and counselling with homework on tinnitus. Int J Audiol. 2020;59(5):374–82.
95. Searchfield GD, Fok C, Donaldson T, Durai M, Kleinstauber M, Linford T, et al. An evaluation of a continuing education workshop for audiologists on the assessment and management of tinnitus. J Contin Educ Health Prof. 2020;40(2):125–30. https://doi.org/10.1097/CEH.0000000000000285.

CBT for Tinnitus

44

Thomas Fuller and Derek J. Hoare

Abstract

Cognitive behavioural therapy (CBT) for tinnitus is a collective term for many psychotherapeutic techniques used in combination to address tinnitus-related distress and interference in daily life. In other words, CBT is not one "pure", discrete, standardised treatment, nor is the goal of CBT to remove or cure a person of their tinnitus. Immediately, this hints at the strengths and challenges associated with this multi-faceted psychological treatment. This chapter provides you, the reader, with an overview of why a psychological treatment such as CBT might be relevant and applicable to tinnitus distress, what it is, the evidence base underpinning it, and future directions in which CBT might develop.

T. Fuller (✉)
Clinical Psychological Science, Faculty of Psychology and Neuroscience, Maastricht University, Maastricht, The Netherlands
e-mail: Thomas.fuller@maastrichtuniversity.nl

D. J. Hoare
NIHR Nottingham Biomedical Research Centre, Hearing Sciences, Mental Health and Clinical Neurosciences, School of Medicine, University of Nottingham, Nottingham, UK
e-mail: Derek.Hoare@nottingham.ac.uk

W. Schlee et al. (eds.), *Textbook of Tinnitus*, https://doi.org/10.1007/978-3-031-35647-6_44

Graphical Abstract

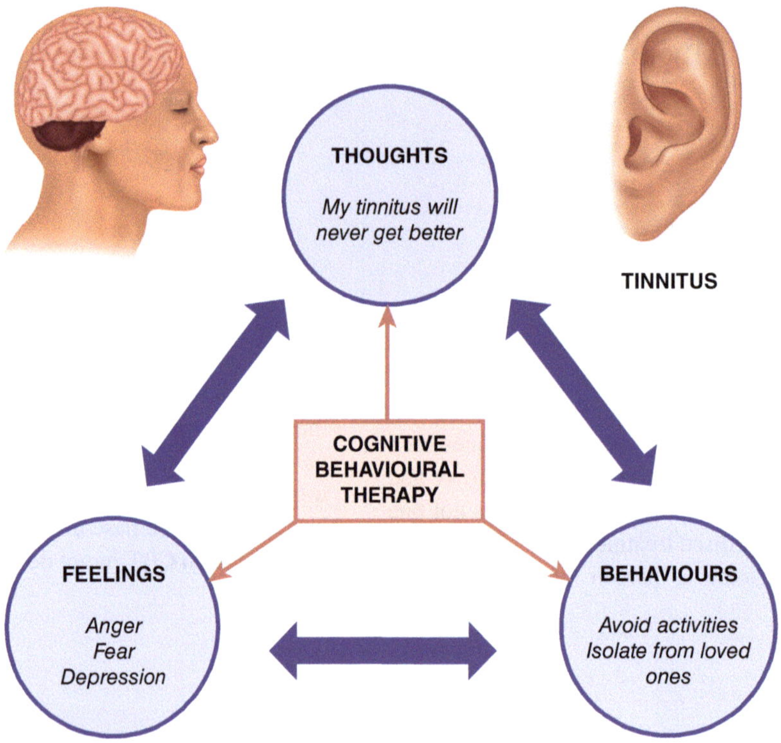

Rationale for Using CBT to Alleviate Distress and Disability

To understand why CBT is used for tinnitus, we will provide an overview of four psychological models used to explain why distress and disability can result from tinnitus. Psychological models of tinnitus are appealing because the level of tinnitus-related distress correlates weakly with psychoacoustic measures of tinnitus loudness [1, 2] and moderately with self-reported tinnitus loudness [3, 4]. Psychological models of tinnitus also have appeal in their own right through their ability to provide a better understanding of the development and maintenance of disabling tinnitus. Additionally, they can be used to generate possible solutions to reversing its disabling effects. The models described here are the: *habituation* model [5]; the *neurophysiological* model [6, 7]; a *cognitive behavioural (CB) model* of tinnitus [8]; and, the *fear avoidance (FA)* model [9, 10]. Table 44.1 summarises each of the models' core assumptions, predictions, and comment on the level of empirical support.

The Habituation Model of Disabling Tinnitus

Habituation is a process whereby reaction(s) to a stimulus decrease in response to repeated presentations of the same stimulus [19]. It is considered to be context- and individual-specific, influenced by and susceptible to indirect learning and motivational factors [20]. The principle of habituation was first applied to tinnitus in 1984 by Hallam and colleagues to explain reductions in tinnitus-related distress over time. It has some intuitive appeal as, for most people, it appears that sustained perception of tinnitus leads to them learning that it is a stimulus not worthy of attentional resources, thereby becoming a nonaversive stimulus [5]. Tinnitus-related distress according to this model occurs when there is a "failure" to habituate and attention or some other response continues to be directed to tinnitus.

Operant conditioning, a form of associative learning where the frequency of a behaviour is increased through rewards (i.e. positive or negative reinforcement) or an unwanted behaviour decreased through positive or negative

Table 44.1 Overview of psychological models of disabling tinnitus

Model	Fundamental assumptions	Core predictions	Empirical support
Habituation model [5]	That tinnitus is stable, consistent or constant enough to enable learning processes to account for a decrease in response to tinnitus, i.e. habituation	If failures in habituation occur when attentional processes malfunction, most often in situations of heightened physiological arousal, then relaxation and other stress reduction techniques should be used as a treatment to facilitate the reappraisal of the meaning of the tinnitus and habituation	Limited empirical support exists for the habituation model [11]
Neurophysiological model [6, 12]	The perception of tinnitus is paired, through classical conditioning, with an aversive emotional reaction; conscious negative evaluation of tinnitus is not required for this process. The model also assumes that animal models of tinnitus are valid and applicable to humans	If classical conditioning accounts for the association between tinnitus and an aversive emotional experience, then presenting the conditioned stimulus without the unconditioned stimulus (i.e. extinction) would result in decreased tinnitus distress. Jastreboff proposed that through counselling and sound therapy, the learned association between tinnitus and an aversive emotional response is broken and habituation is made possible	The empirical basis for the model is based on animal models of tinnitus and assumed to be applicable to humans. Mixed evidence of effectiveness of tinnitus retraining therapy (the indicated therapeutic treatment according to Jastreboff) is available [13, 14] (see Chap. 47)
Cognitive Behavioural model [8]	Negative automatic evaluation of tinnitus is primarily responsible for the/a dysfunctional emotional and behavioural response to tinnitus	If negative automatic thoughts about and appraisals of one's ability to cope with tinnitus are fundamentally responsible for disabling tinnitus, then cognitive and behavioural treatments should focus on this to achieve therapeutic benefits	McKenna et al. [8] cite numerous studies that provide evidence for components of the model (.g. the role of selective attention in distorting the perception of tinnitus) although the studies themselves were not designed to test the model itself. Low to moderate quality evidence exists for the effectiveness of CBT to reduce tinnitus-related distress and interference which indirectly supports this model [15]. Handscomb et al. [16] used path analysis to assess how well different configurations of this model fit, concluding different configurations, e.g. a beliefs driven model, a loudness-driven model, may be more appropriate to different groups of people with tinnitus
Fear avoidance model of tinnitus [9, 10]	Catastrophic interpretations of auditory stimuli and associative learning are responsible for a cascade of emotional and behavioural reactions to tinnitus. It is also assumed that fear is the dominant (or at least primary) emotional response to tinnitus	If classical and operant mechanisms initiate and maintain disabling tinnitus, and fear is the primary emotional response, then exposure therapy leading to extinction will be an effective treatment. Further, if catastrophic (mis)interpretations of tinnitus precipitate a cycle of negative emotional and behavioural responses then interpreting it as a neutral (even positive) stimulus leads to a functional response to tinnitus	Some evidence for the role of cognitive and emotional processes within the fear avoidance model of tinnitus exists [10, 17, 18]. Low to moderate quality evidence exists for the effectiveness of CBT to reduce tinnitus-related distress and interference that indirectly supports this model [15]

punishment [21], was later included into the habituation model (referred to as "operant" factors). Operant factors were added to the model to account for learning and emergence of avoidant behaviours [22]. For example, negative reinforcement (where an aversive stimulus is removed) is thought to explain an increase in or maintenance of avoidance behaviours.

There are, however, limitations of the habituation model as it is applied to tinnitus. The model inherently assumes that the characteristics of tinnitus (e.g. pitch, loudness, frequency, and context in which it is experienced) are stable for most people. However, this assumption seems problematic as the dynamic characteristics of tinnitus are well known [23]. Furthermore, any changes in which or how tinnitus is experienced could reasonably be considered as a "new" presentation of the stimulus and thus require attentional resource allocation. A further issue relates to the bidirectional arrow between "tinnitus sensation" and "disability due to tinnitus" which implies that hearing tinnitus itself is enough to cause disability. Given the presence of cognitive factors in the habituation model, it seems inherently inconsistent to propose that perception, without some form of evaluation or belief about the tinnitus, leads to disability. Further to these limitations, there is scant empirical evidence in support of the habituation model overall [11].

A Neurophysiological Model of Tinnitus (See Also Chap. 20)

Jastreboff expanded the work of Hallam in a neurophysiological model focussing on tinnitus generation and perception rather than tinnitus-related disability. This model proposed that the association between tinnitus and an aversive emotional state emerges through classical conditioning mechanisms [6, 12]. According to Jastreboff, successful habituation to tinnitus is expedited through counselling the patient that there is nothing to worry about or fear and using sound therapy to partially mask tinnitus and make it more constant//stable and not worthy of conscious attention. This combined treatment approach was named Tinnitus Retraining Therapy; TRT; see Chap. 47) [24, 25].

Several theoretical and empirical limitations exist in relation to the neurophysiological model. First, the model does not clearly specify the unconditioned stimulus, conditioned stimulus, conditioned, and unconditioned responses [11]. Assuming tinnitus has become the conditioned stimulus and an aversive emotional arousal is the conditioned response, the use of a masking device appears contrary to current understandings of extinguishing learned responses, i.e. through exposure therapy [26]. That is, the use of a masking device can be conceptualised as an avoidance and/or safety behaviour that is usually considered counterproductive in the therapeutic context. It has been demonstrated in tinnitus patients that avoidance behaviours mediate the relationship between anxiety sensitivity and tinnitus distress [27]. Similarly, Hesser et al. [28] found that efforts to control the salience of tinnitus using sounds is associated with increased levels of disability. Furthermore, within anxiety research safety behaviours and avoidance have also been shown to preserve threat expectancies [29, 30].

A Cognitive-Behavioural Model of Tinnitus (See Also Chap. 21)

The cognitive-behavioural (CB) model of tinnitus distress proposed by McKenna et al. [8] emphasises the key role of cognition and the subsequent effects that specific thoughts about tinnitus have on attentional processes and, to a lesser degree, on the behavioural response to tinnitus sounds. McKenna's approach is based on the dual appraisal model [31], which differentiates between primary and secondary appraisals. The primary appraisal of tinnitus concerns the causal attributions ("what is it and where does it come from?"), whereas the secondary appraisal concerns the beliefs about the possibilities to reduce it ("what can I do about it?"). For example, a person might initially think of the tinnitus as a symptom of brain damage, and then, potentially, think that neurosurgery is the only solution available. Once the fight or flight response is activated, the model predicts that increasing physiological arousal leads to further monitoring and selectively attending to tinnitus. Beliefs about tinnitus and the capacity to cope with it underpin automatic negative thoughts and motivate the use of safety behaviours that might be used to better endure the tinnitus. The CB model's main strengths lie in its empirical foundation, compatibility with cognitive models of insomnia and chronic pain, and its compatibility with CBT. Importantly also, it can be used to generate testable hypotheses.

The CB model has limitations. First, it does not consider motivational, social, environmental, or personal resilience factors that might moderate distress. Second, the evidence for some components of the model is limited. This is particularly relevant to tinnitus-related safety behaviours where research on this topic is in its infancy. Third, a qualitative evaluation of the model found that tinnitus patients did not identify with or recognise all parts of the model [32]. Furthermore, path analyses of the model using questionnaire data for each variable suggested several configurations of the model were a good fit to the data, one conclusion being that different configurations might be more applicable than others to different individuals [32].

Fear Avoidance Model of Tinnitus

Chronic pain and chronic tinnitus appear to share numerous conceptual similarities, including the perception of a sensation whose source is neither identifiable nor indicative of (further) physical harm [33–35] (for similarities between tinnitus and pain see also Chap. 8). Within the field of chronic pain research, the fear avoidance (FA) model [36–38] has been highly influential in providing a basis for understanding why some people might experience dysfunctional responses to chronic pain, and what therapeutic strategies might be effective. Given the commonalities between chronic pain and tinnitus, tinnitus researchers have adopted the FA model [9, 10] and begun applying it as a basis for treatments to manage tinnitus.

The FA model of tinnitus proposes that regardless of the cause of the tinnitus, once it is detected, negative cognitive appraisals (e.g. catastrophic misinterpretations) and aversive emotional reactions (e.g. fear) elicit or can lead to behavioural safety responses. These behavioural responses (e.g. avoidance) might be relieving in the short term but paradoxically can lead to severe impairment in the longer-term. Conversely, neutral or positive evaluation of the tinnitus does not lead to any fear or interference in daily activities.

The FA model of tinnitus distress shares features with both the neurophysiological and the CB model but differs from both in its serial nature and in providing a clear point at which a person perceiving tinnitus might move towards a neutral or negative response. A particular strength of the FA model is that it draws on classical and operant conditioning, which can be used to inform predictions about the acquisition, generalisation [i.e. the spread of the effects of conditioning (either classical or operant) to stimuli different from the stimulus present during original conditioning [39]], and extinction of conditioned responses. While there is a large body of empirical support for the FA model of chronic pain [38, 40], the evidence for the FA model of tinnitus is limited [10, 17].

The FA model of tinnitus has been criticised. Wideman et al. [41] have questioned the assumption of the FA model of chronic pain that the fear of pain (and by extension, fear of tinnitus) is analogous to a phobia and thus exposure the most empirically supported treatment. By extension there is an inherent assumption that fear is the only or dominant emotional response in disabling tinnitus. Further, Wideman, Sullivan [42] have argued that an accumulation of risk factors such as higher pain catastrophising, fear of movement, and depression, is a better predictor of disability than the individual factors included in the FA model. It remains to be seen whether this also applies in the context of tinnitus. If however the FA model of tinnitus and underlying assumptions that fear of tinnitus is analogous to a phobia are valid, then by extension, there exists an absence of evidence regarding the role that generalisation of tinnitus-related fear might play in maintaining or exacerbating disability. Lastly, the FA model of tinnitus does not take in to consideration personal motivational factors or the social context in which patients exist. [Note that the FA model of chronic pain does [43], but the FA model of tinnitus and evidence base for it, lags behind.]

Summary

These four models of tinnitus differ and overlap in varying degrees from each other but all identify mechanisms, predominantly of a cognitive or behavioural nature that might account for disabling tinnitus, at least in subgroups of people with tinnitus. Further, the models provide the underpinning and rationale for a range of psychological interventions. If as the models propose, cognitive appraisals are prominent in the causing or precipitating distress and disability, then it follows that interventions targeting these appraisals could be an effective point at which to intervene. Consequently, from the models, it appears that the main goals of an intervention should be to reduce autonomic arousal associated with tinnitus, challenge or modify the negative or catastrophic cognitive appraisals of the tinnitus which led to fear and other strong emotional responses and redress the behavioural responses that lead to maintenance of distress and disability.

CBT for Tinnitus

The development of behavioural, cognitive, and cognitive behavioural therapies (combined) for tinnitus has largely been derived from the principles and interventions of CBT used for treating depression and other psychological disorders. This is possible because the behavioural and cognitive models of depression and other psychopathology, respectively, are generalisable across emotional, behavioural, or psychosocial outcomes. The core idea underlying CBT is that it is our interpretation or thoughts about experiences, sensations, and events that initiate a cascade of emotional and behavioural responses. Further, it is inherently assumed that these thoughts and evaluative processes can be modified; principally through interpreting information and experiences from a new perspective and based on personal empiricism. That is, patients working together with a clinician (most often a psychologist) select from numerous behavioural and cognitive interventions to test and re-examine assumptions and interpretations of experiences (including memories) that are maintaining emotional distress (etc).

Behavioural interventions such as exposure therapy are based on principles of classical and operant conditioning. They create opportunities for patients to develop/learn new associations between tinnitus and a productive response to it. Additionally, they often generate or provoke the thoughts, memories, or evaluative processes that led to and maintain distress or disability, that can in turn become the basis of or complement cognitive interventions. Cognitive interventions focus on the relationship between thoughts and emotions and were first developed in the 1950s by psychologists such as Albert Ellis and Aaron Beck. They are used to challenge and modify irrational beliefs held about a person's world, and/or the negatively biased assumptions and methods of interpreting experience, so-called cognitive distortions. *Filtering* is just one example and is a process whereby an individual filters out positive events/interpretations/experience/memories, etc. and instead dwells on the negatives. More recently, so-called *third-wave CBT* interventions such as mindfulness based cognitive therapy (see Chap. 45) and acceptance and commitment therapy have been applied to tinnitus. They focus more on the observation of thoughts and experiences and consciously choosing a productive response to thoughts, experiences, or sensations, rather than trying to change the negatively biased information processing style. A comparative study by Brown et al. [44] of the characteristics of CBT and third-wave therapies noted this divergence in the techniques used in these therapies but no major differences in the background or attitude between traditional CBT and its contemporaries. Moreover, third-wave therapies emphasise clarification of the patient's values and a more contextual approach to behaviour change, not unlike in existential therapy and interpersonal approaches, respectively [45].

CBT uses both behavioural and cognitive interventions over the course of therapy. It is usually time limited (typically between 6 and 20 sessions), although the frequency of sessions (e.g. daily, weekly, and fortnightly) and length of sessions can vary. Content is generally structured, and patients are encouraged to engage in activities outside the sessions to reinforce what they have learned during the session and to stimulate new experiences that can form content in future sessions. Modes of delivering CBT include group sessions, one-to-one, face-to-face, telephone, via Apps, or via the internet with or without remote support from someone (for E-health-based approaches see also Chap. 57). Other variables include who delivers the CBT (e.g. psychotherapist, psychologist, audiologist, social worker, nurse, and computer program) and the setting (e.g. hospital, health centre, private clinic, and at home).

The following section provides a description and examples of the treatment components that are used within CBT for tinnitus.

Cognitive Restructuring or Reframing

Cognitive restructuring or reframing involves structured, goal-directed, and collaborative strategies to explore, evaluate, and substitute maladaptive thoughts, appraisals, and beliefs that maintain psychological disturbance [46]. In the case of tinnitus, there may be a tendency to allocate attention to anticipating negative consequences and catastrophising, and thoughts such as, for example, "I can't cope with this." "I'm never going to be OK again." The patient and therapist can work together to examine these fearful thoughts as a hypothesis, searching for discrepant evidence to disconfirm these maladaptive thoughts. Ultimately, these thoughts are replaced with more functional ones, supporting new, more functional behaviour. Cognitive restructuring of thoughts and beliefs associated with tinnitus is considered a necessary feature of therapy [47], and the use of cognitive restructuring is reported consistently in the CBT for tinnitus literature.

Guided Discovery

Guided discovery is an overarching strategy in CBT. Typically, the therapist acquaints themselves with the patient viewpoint and then uses questions and prompts designed to challenge beliefs and facilitate an experimental frame of mind to broaden thinking [48]. For example, the patient is asked to give evidence that supports their viewpoint, and evidence that does not. In this process the patient learns to view things from new perspectives and choose a more helpful path. Guided Discovery through Socratic Dialogue is a particular example following an inductive process that bypasses deductions based on the patient's negative beliefs. It usually involves a series of questions that progress from analytic questions (to elicit and unpack problems), through evaluative questions (exploring meaning and potentially "re-packing" problems in a new way), and finally to summaries and synthesising questions (to collate what has emerged so that patients can be prompted to make new conclusions [48].

Perhaps because it is an overarching meaning there is limited evaluation or even reference to the term Guided Discovery in the tinnitus literature. Aazh et al. [49] mention the importance of Guided Discovery through careful questioning in describing their audiologist-delivered CBT for tinnitus. Olsson [50] also mentions use of discovery as a technique to help tinnitus patients to identify the relationship between irrational beliefs and their consequences. However, it was described as the ideal approach but that teaching the patient may be a necessary alternative, perhaps due to the patient's engagement level of ability to participate, and/or the competence level of the delivering clinician. Guided Discovery is reportedly the most difficult CBT competency to master [51].

Exposure Therapy

When people are fearful of something, they tend to avoid the feared objects, activities or situations. This might be helpful in the short-term but not necessarily so in the long-term. Exposure therapy is used to help break patterns of avoidance and fear. It involves exposure of the patient to the feared object, activity, thought, memory or situation in the absence of the feared outcome to ultimately reduce anxiety and help the patients cope [26, 52]. Exposure to a feared stimulus can be done in varying increments of difficulty, in vivo, through guided imagery, or using virtual reality.

Use of exposure therapy is reported widely within the CBT for tinnitus literature as a technique to reduce tinnitus-related anxiety and avoidance [45]. For example, Hubbard [53] describes using exposure therapy to gradually reverse avoidance, reintroduce the patient to sound, to silence, and to the activities they may have formerly believed to be [impaired] by tinnitus. Lindberg et al. [54] described their technique as involving exposure to tinnitus provoking environmental noise, directing attention to the tinnitus sound, and then asking the patient to relax quickly and turn their attention to environmental noise. This technique was trained under increasingly trying acoustic conditions to achieve a generalised coping strategy.

Journaling and Thought Records

Journaling and thought records are writing exercises used in CBT and many other psychological treatment approaches to help the patient deepen self-reflection and facilitate the therapeutic change process. They can also help the patient keep an account of new thoughts and behaviours they put into practice between therapy sessions and provide a record of their progress. Journaling is an outlet that provides a valuable means of self-exploration for patients. Daily journal writing is widely advocated as providing a meditative period of self-reflection and examination of one's own mental and emotional processes. This opens the patient up to personal inspection of their actions, values, and beliefs [55].

Within the literature on CBT for tinnitus, diaries are reported within protocols as quantitative daily measures of tinnitus variables such as subjective loudness, discomfort, sleep disturbance, interference with activity, control of tinnitus, hours per day of ignored, often only measured on a visual analogue scale rather than qualitative reflection [45]. An example of journaling appears in Aazh et al. [56] who used a Diary of Thoughts and Feelings (DTF) as a structured method for the patient to make notes about their tinnitus-related problems and any associated thoughts and emotions The DTF was completed by patients between sessions, and then during sessions the audiologist used Socratic questioning to encourage the patient to think through the thoughts they had recorded, replacing unrealistic or unhelpful thoughts with an alternative statements (for App-based diaries see also Chap. 7.15).

Activity Scheduling and Behavioural Activation

Activity scheduling is a technique used within CBT to help patients engage in behaviours they have withdrawn from or avoid because of depression, anxiety, or other health problem such as tinnitus. This CBT technique generally involves working with a patient to identify a rewarding infrequent behaviour and scheduling time to increase the frequency of that behaviour. Pleasant activity scheduling is recognised as an evidence-based treatment that is effective in reducing a variety of mental health symptoms. It is perhaps most widely used and evidenced in the treatment for depression to re-introduce rewarding behaviours and positive social interaction into a patient's routine [57]. Activity scheduling can help establish good habits and provide ample opportunity to put what has been learned in treatment into practice.

Avoidance behaviours are common in those who have tinnitus, and many patients report effects of having tinnitus on their social, work and individual activities [58]. Activity scheduling and behavioural activation therefore have clear applications for tinnitus. Some explicit examples in the tinnitus literature include Sweetow [59] who required patients to maintain a detailed log of activity schedule to discuss in therapy each week, to combat negative behaviour. Kaldo-Sandstrom et al. [60] describe a specific treatment component to increase the patients' level of physical activity, to enhance well-being and better manage stress and tinnitus. Tyler et al. have developed a treatment strategy which is primarily based on motivating tinnitus patients to engage in activities (see also Chap. 49)

Behavioural Experiments

Behavioural experiments are typically used for disorders that involve catastrophic thinking. The experiments are planned activities to gather information with which to test the accuracy of a patient's beliefs about themselves, about others, and about the world, or to test more adaptive beliefs [61]. So, for example, before undertaking a task that makes the patient anxious, they are asked to predict what will happen, and later discuss the actual outcome compared to the predicted (catastrophic) outcome. There is also a strong theoretical basis that behavioural experiments promote greater cognitive, affective, and behavioural change than purely cognitive techniques.

The use of behavioural experiments within CBT for tinnitus do appear occasionally in the literature. Aazh et al. [49] listed the technique as being included in their audiologist-delivered CBT. Sweetow [59] provided a little more detail of its use and a process, whereby the patient identifies a behaviour they would like to modify, the therapy groups consider whether this behaviour can be modified, and thereafter [behavioural] experiments recorded in the form of a diary as part of homework assignments.

Relaxation and Stress Reduction Techniques

Relaxation and stress reduction techniques are commonly used within CBT to help patients regulate their physiological stress reactions [62]. Common techniques include guided imagery, breathing exercises, progressive muscle relaxation, and mindfulness exercises. These techniques help patients recognise bodily signs of stress and relax to alleviate stress. They also help patients become more thoughtful and intentional in how they respond to stress, which can support their use of other skills learned in CBT [63]. Stress is synonymous with tinnitus although the direction of relationship is not consistent; stress causes or exacerbates tinnitus, tinnitus causes or exacerbates stress, and for some patients, stress provides a distraction from tinnitus [64]. Regardless, relaxation techniques appear widely in the tinnitus literature [45, 65].

Role-Playing

Role-play has many applications within CBT. It is used to help patients discover automatic thoughts, practise new responses, or modify core beliefs. It is also a useful tool for improving communication skills and developing skills such as assertiveness [65]. Playing out possible scenarios can lessen fear and generate familiarity and confidence in certain situations. Role-playing does not feature heavily in the tinnitus literature. In the cognitive treatment described by Jakes et al. [66], patients practiced challenging their cognitions in the sessions primarily by using role-reversal. Role-playing has also got an important place in clinician training to use CBT techniques for tinnitus [67].

Successive Approximation

Successive approximation, or "shaping", is a CBT technique for patients who have difficulty completing a task, either because they are not familiar with the task or because they are overwhelmed by it. So, for example, if the patient was alcohol dependent the overwhelming task might be to abstain from alcohol. The technique would involve supporting the patient to master steps to completing a similar but easier task (reduced daily intake, abstinence for 1 day) [68]. In successive approximation, each step taken is recognised and rewarded to build confidence. Having experienced and rehearsed one behaviour the previously overwhelming task becomes more manageable. Successive approximation does not explicitly appear in the tinnitus literature although some techniques involving exposure therapy could be considered here also.

Empirical Evidence for the Effects of CBT for Tinnitus

CBT for tinnitus is widely regarded as the intervention with the largest and strongest body of research evidence supporting its efficacy in alleviating tinnitus distress and disability rather than for it changing any sound characteristic of the tinnitus. This view reflects consistent results from systematic reviews, meta-analyses, and randomised controlled trials. Further evidence supporting the use of CBT comes from observational studies of CBT delivered in routine care although process evaluations, and qualitative data supporting the implementation of CBT are rare.

Before giving an overview of the evidence base for CBT for tinnitus, it is important to consider against what or how CBT is being judged efficacious and effective. Studies examining the efficacy and effectiveness of CBT typically use a measures of tinnitus distress or disability (e.g. [69]) as the primary outcome measure. Tinnitus distress or disability is usually assessed by self-report questionnaires such the Tinnitus Handicap Inventory [70], Tinnitus Questionnaire [71, 72], or the Tinnitus Functional Inventory [73]. However, the construct of tinnitus-related distress or disability is not usually defined in studies but is used as an umbrella term for aversive or unpleasant emotional responses to tinnitus. It is also important to note that tinnitus-related distress is distinct from depression or anxiety which is also often measured in tinnitus studies using questionnaires such as the Hospital Anxiety and Depression Scale [74] or Beck Depression Inventory [75].

Systematic Reviews of CBT for Tinnitus

Systematic reviews and meta-analyses provide a useful overview: for consumers of research (i.e. patients, policy makers, researchers, insurance companies, and service providers); of the research questions that have been asked, the quality of evidence on a given topic; and the confidence one can be that the results reflect the "true" (albeit impossibly unknown) result or effect of a treatment.

At least 11 systematic reviews of CBT for tinnitus have been completed since the first by Andersson, Lyttkens [76], which despite differences in methods and inclusions, are largely consistent in their conclusions about the evidence for CBT for tinnitus. Table 44.2 provides an example of some of the similarities and differences between four recent systematic reviews regarding their scope, methodologies, and conclusions. The main conclusions relate to the: efficacy of CBT and duration of effects; effect of CBT on tinnitus characteristics, anxiety, and depression; quality of evidence and risk of biases.

Table 44.2 Characteristics and main conclusions from recent systematic reviews and meta-analyses of CBT for tinnitus

Study	Design and focus of the review	Included study designs and total number of included studies size	Comparators	Primary outcome and time points	Analysis	Risk of bias and tool used to measure quality of the evidence	Author's conclusions
Beukes et al. [77]	Systematic review and meta-analysis of internet-based CBT interventions for hearing loss, tinnitus, and vestibular disorders	RCTs $N = 9$ (targeting tinnitus)	1. Inactive controls (n = 7) 2. Active controls (n = 5)	Impact of tinnitus on quality of life at end of treatment or post-intervention follow-up	Random effects pair wise comparison	Cochrane risk of bias 2; GRADE	This review indicates the potential of internet interventions for tinnitus to provide evidence-based accessible care. There is a need for additional high-quality evidence before conclusive results can be established regarding the effects of audio vestibular internet interventions
Rademaker et al. [78]	Systematic review of mindfulness based interventions (MBIs)	RCTs, retrospective and prospective cohort studies, case series ($n \geq 5$) $N = 7$	1. Any other therapy (n = 2) 2. Waitlist control (n = 2)	Impact of tinnitus on quality of life	Narrative synthesis	Cochrane risk of bias tool; MINORS	A decrease of tinnitus distress scores in MBIs can be observed directly post-therapy based on moderate- to high-quality studies. This was found regardless of the heterogeneity of patients, study design, type of MBI, and outcome assessment
Fuller et al. [15]	Systematic review and meta-analysis of behavioural, cognitive, cognitive behavioural interventions including mindfulness and acceptance and commitment therapy	RCTs $N = 28$	1. Waitlist control (n = 14) 2. Audiological treatment (n = 3) 3. TRT (n = 1) 4. Any other active control (n = 16)	Impact of tinnitus on quality of life at end of treatment, 6- and 12-months	Random effects and fixed effect (when possible) pair wise comparison	Cochrane risk of bias 2; GRADE	CBT may be effective in reducing impact of tinnitus on quality of life. An absence of evidence at 6- and 12-months follow-up prevents conclusions being made about the duration of effects
Landry et al. [79]	Systematic review and meta-analysis of behavioural, cognitive, cognitive behavioural interventions including mindfulness and acceptance and commitment therapy	RCTs $N = 19$	1. Waitlist control (n = 12) 2. Cognitive and/or behavioural therapies compared to one another and waitlist control (n = 19)	Impact of tinnitus on quality of life. Unclear which time point was used in the analysis	Random effects, pair wise comparison; Network meta-analysis	Cochrane risk of bias 2; GRADE	CBT is an effective therapy for tinnitus. While guided self-administered forms of CBT had largest effect sizes

Note. GRADE grading of recommendations assessment, development and evaluation, *MINORS* methodological index for non-randomised studies

Efficacy and Duration of Effects of CBT for Tinnitus on Tinnitus-Related Distress and Disability

Reviews have consistently reported small to medium effect sizes of CBT on the impact of tinnitus on quality of life as measured by tinnitus questionnaires. The size of the effect when CBT is compared with a waitlist control group is often medium and exceeding criteria for minimally important clinical differences. When CBT is compared to an active treatment, the size of the effect in favour of CBT are often small, but still close to minimally important clinical differences [15]. Overall, CBT appears to be superior to no treatment and probably better than other available interventions.

This is all very promising, but does it matter if CBT is delivered in a group rather than individually? Or does CBT have to be delivered face to face rather than via the internet with remote support from someone? And what does the evidence say about the type of CBT? That is, is any one of behavioural, cognitive, cognitive *and* behavioural therapy, mindfulness or acceptance and commitment therapy superior to the others?

From the perspective of policymakers and healthcare funders, results are largely encouraging. Although there is limited evidence for the superiority of one form of CBT over another, all forms of CBT appear effective. Furthermore, results show that there is no meaningful difference between improvements made by patients receiving CBT via the internet with additional communication from a clinician compared to in-person therapy. Similarly, results suggest that benefits of group-based CBT interventions are equivalent to CBT delivered to individuals. It is important to note though that these comments are based on analyses of data at a group level and not from studies where determining the best mode of delivery has been the aim of the study. Unquestionably, some people will not benefit from CBT, and nor will everyone benefit to the same degree regardless of how CBT is delivered. Moreover, it should also be considered that people participating in clinical trials of CBT for tinnitus may not be representative of all tinnitus patients.

An additional consideration is that while these results are very encouraging, they are limited by the absence of follow-up data beyond 6–12-months. This is despite authors stressing, from the earliest systematic reviews and meta-analyses on this topic, the importance of and need for more, and longer term follow-up data to be collected and reported (e.g. [76]). The follow-up data that is available, largely at less than 6-months, suggest that the benefits of CBT are at least maintained up to this time point.

Effect of CBT for Tinnitus on Tinnitus-Related Characteristics, Anxiety, Depression, and Quality of Life

Many reviews of CBT for tinnitus have considered outcomes such as perceived loudness, measures of symptoms of anxiety and depression, typically as secondary outcomes, with consistent findings. First, CBT is considered not to have a direct impact on the tinnitus percept. That is, it does not directly affect the perceived loudness a person experiences. Meta-analyses have also indicated that the effects of CBT for tinnitus on anxiety and depression are small at best. Given that, CBT for tinnitus is derived from the core principles of CBT that are largely generalisable, this is simultaneously surprising and disappointing. That said, it probably reflects the specific and unique features of the respective conditions and CBT interventions.

Quality of Evidence and Risk of Biases

Recent systematic reviews and meta-analyses have consistently used two measures to assess biases that might affect the results of RCTs and rate the overall quality of the body of evidence, respectively (Table 44.2). First, the Cochrane Risk of Bias 2 tool [80] assesses: random sequence generation (selection bias); allocation concealment (selection bias); blinding of participants and personnel (performance bias); blinding of outcome assessment (detection bias); incomplete outcome data (attrition bias); selective reporting (reporting bias); and, other biases. Each element is judged as having a *low*, *uncertain*, or *high* risk of bias. For example, an RCT might be judged as having a low risk of bias associated with random sequence generation if the investigators in the study used an internet-based randomisation system such as www.randomization.com to allocate participants to groups. Second, the Grading of Recommendations Assessment, Development and Evaluation (GRADE; [81]) tool is used to rate the overall level of confidence in the evidence that CBT has on a given outcome. Working from a starting point of *high certainty* (i.e. that true effect of the results is close to the estimate of effect reported), reviewers potentially downgrade the certainty or level of confidence in the findings according to a range of criteria to a minimum of *very low certainty* (i.e. having very little confidence in the effect estimates). Reasons that a study might be downgraded include but are not limited to risk of bias, inconsistency, or imprecision of the results (associated with small sample sizes). Although these tools provide guidelines, judgments are still subjective, and differences arise between reviews by different authors. For example, Fuller et al. [15] rate 7 of the RCTs of CBT for tinnitus as being at *uncertain* or *high* risk of "other" biases, whereas Landry et al. [79] rates all their included trials as representing a *high* risk of bias.

Randomised Controlled Trials of CBT for Tinnitus

We now move from systematic reviews of CBT for tinnitus, to describe two examples of RCTs: Cima et al. [82] and Beukes et al. [83]. These two trials were chosen to illustrate some of similarities and differences that can exist between CBT treatments and how they are implemented.

Case Study 1: Specialised Treatment Based on Cognitive Behaviour Therapy Versus Usual Care for Tinnitus: A Randomised Controlled Trial [82]

Published in 2012 in The Lancet, the RCT by Cima and colleagues not only reinvigorated research into CBT for tinnitus but also grabbed the attention of audiologists and medical professionals in a way that previous studies had failed to do. As highlighted in the editorial associated with the article, this RCT not only challenged a view that nothing can be done to help people suffering from tinnitus, but it also demonstrated how psychological interventions could be tested according to the highest methodological standards [84]. What did the trial do exactly?

The aim of the trial was to test how well specialised CBT for tinnitus delivered in a stepped-care manner compared to standard audiological treatment as delivered in the Netherlands. Following recruitment, a research assistant independent from the study team, using computer generated sequences for randomisation, allocated participants to receive either specialised CBT (n = 245) or "treatment as usual" (n = 247). Participants had an average age of 54 years and were mostly male (308 males, 184 females). Seventy percent had experienced tinnitus for more than 1 year. Treatment comprised two steps. Step 1, conducted within a 3-month period, involved all participants undergoing an audiological assessment, attending a 2-hour group education session, and having a psychological assessment. Audiological care (i.e. the control condition) in Step 1 included: audiological diagnostics; assessment and explanation from a clinical physicist in audiology about of the results from the assessment as well as information about hearing loss and tinnitus; prescription of a hearing aid if indicated; and referral to a social worker when required.

Step 2. This consisted of three different 12-week group treatment options with levels of care dependent on tinnitus severity and hearing loss. Session content included psychoeducation; cognitive restructuring; exposure to tinnitus; mindfulness-based exercises; stress relief and attention redirecting techniques by means of movement therapy; and applied relaxation. If indicated from the psychological assessment, an individual course of treatment was available. In the control condition, Step 2 involved an intake conducted by a social worker (60 min), a general inventory of tinnitus complaints and use of hearing aids or maskers and up to a maximum of nine follow-up contacts of 60 min each. Follow-up social work contacts could be counselling sessions, telephone contacts, and appointments with third parties or home visits.

The primary outcome measures were health-related quality of life, tinnitus severity, and disability at pre, post, and 4 months after treatment. On all outcomes, the group who received CBT improved more than the group who received audiological care; effect sizes were small to medium [82]. In addition, a treatment fidelity check and cost-effectiveness study were completed. The treatment fidelity check revealed a high level of protocol adherence with only a small number of forbidden treatment elements being observed within the intervention as it was delivered. The cost-effectiveness study established that specialised CBT for tinnitus was cost effective compared to the audiological treatment [85]. Risk of bias in this trial was low or uncertain on most domains of bias [15], which means that whilst we can have some confidence in the estimate of effect, it was difficult to assess some potential limitations or problems.

Case Study 2: Audiologist-Guided Internet-Based Cognitive Behaviour Therapy for Adults with Tinnitus in the United Kingdom: A Randomised Controlled Trial [83]

Expanding access to evidence-based interventions is an ongoing challenge for policy makers and service providers. Inherent with this challenge are the issues of providing a service that can be accessed by many people and having a qualified workforce available to deliver the treatment. One approach to address these issues has been to examine whether CBT for tinnitus can be delivered effectively via the internet. This is not a new idea; internet interventions for tinnitus have been tested since 2004 [86]. However, examining whether health professionals other than psychologists can deliver effective CBT is a relatively new topic of research. This is an important consideration in expanding access to treatment as the numbers of psychologists providing CBT for tinnitus is small. With these issues in mind, Beukes and colleagues [83] recently examined whether patients benefited from a CBT for tinnitus intervention delivered via the internet with "minimal" support from an experienced audiologist.

Beukes and colleagues recruited 146 participants (63 females, 83 males) from advertisements and information available online, newspapers, magazines, support groups, and healthcare professionals (e.g. general practitioners and audiologists) in the UK. Participants were on average 57 years of age and had experienced tinnitus for over 11 years. An independent researcher used a computer-generated sequence for participant allocation to either the intervention or the control group. The design of the study meant that the research team was not blinded to group allocation. The intervention that participants received was CBT for tinnitus, delivered via the internet, over an 8-week period. The content of the intervention was based on self-help material developed by Andersson and Kaldo [86] and included a set of core and optional modules. The 16 core modules included applied relaxation, thought analysis, cognitive restructuring, imagery, and exposure techniques. Five optional modules were available to add an element of tailoring, and these focused on topics such as sleep, concentration, and sound sensitivity. A registered audiologist (without formal CBT training) would during phone calls to participants: introduce weekly modules, provide feedback, answer queries, provide guidance, support, and encourage engagement. A clinical psychologist supervised the audiologist throughout the intervention. Participants not allocated to the intervention condition joined a waiting list to access the treatment and thus acted as the control group.

Tinnitus distress was specified as the primary outcome of interest and measured at pre, post, and 2 months after the completion of treatment. Secondary outcomes included insomnia, anxiety, depression, and quality of life. The results showed that after completing the intervention, participants had a greater reduction in tinnitus distress compared to the control condition (medium effect size). When this was examined more closely, analyses revealed that 51% of people who received CBT improved by a clinically meaningful amount, compared to 5% of the control group. Participants' superior level of improvement was also reflected across the secondary outcome measures. The benefits of the intervention were maintained at 2-months follow-up. Risk of bias in this trial varied from low on four domains, to high on three domains of bias [15], which indicated some methodological limitations that may affect confidence in the effects reported.

Reflections on the Case Studies

Despite their methodological differences, both RCTs indicate that CBT for tinnitus can make a meaningful difference to patients' lives. Both trials examined the issue of expanding access to treatment but tested different means of doing so. That is, Cima and colleagues stratified treatment according to need with those with greatest need receiving longer and more intensive treatment. Beukes and colleagues on the other hand explored this challenge by testing a model of service delivery via the internet that avoids the need for patients to travel. Results from both studies favoured CBT over the comparison condition and in doing so demonstrated the promise for these models of service delivery.

Which intervention should be more widely adopted you might ask? It is not possible to answer this question from the evidence presented so far. Additional sources of information are required to inform such recommendations. It is important to understand, for example, how well an intervention works in everyday clinical practice, as well as understanding how acceptable it is to the clinicians required to provide it and the patients who engage in it. In the following section, we examine evidence that addresses these questions.

CBT for Tinnitus in Everyday Clinical Practice

Effectiveness or pragmatic trials are conducted to ask whether an intervention works as a treatment in the messy and (experimentally) uncontrolled world of everyday clinical practice. Effectiveness trials also collect information on what people who receive and provide treatment think of it. In conjunction with results from systematic reviews and RCTs, this information is critical for informing decisions on whether to fund new treatments on a wide scale, and/or on how interventions that have proven efficacious in RCTs might be improved or made more appealing to clinicians and patients. If, for example, a new format of CBT for tinnitus is efficacious in an RCT, but is extremely unpopular with patients and clinicians, then it would be unlikely to make a difference on a wide scale if funded and delivered on a national level.

Effectiveness

Compared with the number of published RCTs, effectiveness studies are relatively few, possibly reflecting that services providing CBT for tinnitus are relatively rare. However, the effectiveness studies that have been published (Table 44.3) demonstrate that patients completing a variety of types of CBT for tinnitus, delivered in differing formats in routine practice, benefit substantially. Furthermore, there is some evidence that when interventions are adapted or tailored to local contexts and resources, they can continue to be beneficial for patients [91]. The studies in Table 44.3 reveal that what is considered "routine" or "everyday" clinical practice varies between studies. For example, in one study "routine practice" consists of audiologist-delivered CBT, while in another it constitutes a therapist guided internet-based CBT intervention. Thus, as with RCTs of CBT, it is important to consider in effectiveness studies what elements of CBT are actually included in a given intervention as well as the mode(s) of delivery (to name a few characteristics) before directly comparing the results. Similarly, long-term outcome data on the effectiveness of interventions are lacking. This is a concern because it would yield information on trajectory of recovery and rates of relapse.

Overall, this gap in knowledge about the long-term efficacy and effectiveness of CBT for tinnitus could be addressed by ensuring that funding for longer term follow-up periods is included in grant applications and that participants' response burden at follow-up time points is minimised. Incentives for participants to complete the long-term follow-up measures regardless of whether they have improved or not might also be required to minimise response bias in the datasets, i.e. e.g., it might be that participants who fare well in the long-term are more likely to respond than those who do not.

Facilitators and Barriers to Implementation of CBT for Tinnitus

Little research has been conducted that specifically examines facilitators and barriers to implementation of interventions for disabling tinnitus in practice. A notable exception though comes from the US where researchers have systematically developed and tested a stepped care model of interventions for American military personnel and veterans suffering from tinnitus; that is, progressive tinnitus management (PTM). While the treatment does not constitute CBT, the later steps offer individualised services of which CBT is included. Two studies on the implementation of PTM have found that it varied substantially across locations. The reasons for the devia-

Table 44.3 Examples of evaluations of CBT for tinnitus in routine care

Study	Country	Design	Participants	Treatment	Outcome measures and time points	Authors' conclusion
Aazh, Moore [87]	United Kingdom	Retrospective, observational	$N = 68$; mean age 52.5 years; 57% female; 72% had no detectable hearing loss	Audiological assessment session (90 min) and individual, face-to-face, audiologists-delivered CBT sessions lasting 60 min, once per week for 6 weeks	THI, VAS for tinnitus annoyance, impact, loudness, HQ, ISI, Pre and post treatment	Audiologist-delivered CBT led to significant improvements in self-report measures of tinnitus-related handicap, hyperacusis, and insomnia
Kaldo et al. [88]	Sweden	Prospective, observational	$N = 374$; mean age 47.4 (full ICBT) and 47.1 (low-intensity CBT); 36% (full ICBT) and 33% (low-intensity CBT) females; tinnitus duration 8.4 years (full ICBT), 6.8 years (low-intensity CBT); no hearing loss 32% both groups	Nonrandomised allocation of participants to one of two treatments depending on assessed need. *Therapist guided internet-based CBT* treatment of 6 modules completed over 6–9 weeks *Low-intensity CBT* constituted reading the same material as provided in the therapist-guided treatment but without the need to complete the homework exercises or have contact with a therapist	TRQ*, HADS, ISI, sound sensitivity. Pre, post and 3-months after treatment	ICBT can be used in a regular clinical setting to reduce tinnitus distress… for help-seeking patients with lower distress, a low-intensity version of ICBT can be used
Kaldo-Sandstrom et al. [60]	Sweden	Prospective, observational	$N = 77$; mean age 46.1 years; 48% female; duration of tinnitus suffering 7 years	Internet-based CBT self-help program that included 6 modules to be completed in a 6–10 week period. Therapists provided feedback on homework assignments via email; 1–3 "booster" sessions could be provided by therapists upon request	TRQ, HADS, ISI Pre, post, and 3-months after treatment	Internet-based cognitive–behavioral therapy holds some promise as a treatment modality for tinnitus
McKenna et al. [89]	United Kingdom	Prospective observational	$N = 182$; mean age 59 years; 57% female; all participants had tinnitus for a minimum of 3 months	Group mindfulness- based cognitive therapy (MBCT) over 8 weeks delivered by clinical psychologists. The course followed the standard 8-week course developed by Segal et al. [90] for depression, but adapted for tinnitus	TQ*, CORE*, MAAS, TAQ at pre, post, and 6 weeks after treatment	MBCT was associated with significant and reliable improvements in patients with chronic, distressing tinnitus. Changes were associated with increases in tinnitus acceptance and dispositional mindfulness

Note: * indicates specified primary outcome measure; *CORE* clinical outcomes in routine evaluation-outcome measure, *FTQ* fear of tinnitus questionnaire, *HADS* hospital anxiety and depression scale, *HQ* hyperacusis questionnaire, *HUI* health utilities index-III, *ISI* insomnia severity index, *MAAS* mindful attention awareness scale, *TAQ* tinnitus acceptance questionnaire, *TCS* tinnitus catastrophising scale, *TDI* tinnitus disability index, *THI* tinnitus handicap inventory, *TQ* tinnitus questionnaire, *TRQ* tinnitus reaction questionnaire

tion from the intended model of delivery were a product of numerous factors but included limited resources and staff capacity, low prioritisation of the service, and a lack of skilled staff [92, 93]. Although several proposals were made by the authors of these studies for ways to overcome these barriers, there is an absence of evidence when it comes to evidence-based interventions for facilitating the successful implementation of CBT for tinnitus services within or instead of pre-existing services.

Treatment Acceptability of CBT for Tinnitus

Research on the acceptability of CBT for tinnitus interventions comes from studies conducted in preparation for [94] and evaluation of [95, 96] RCTs and service evaluations [49, 56]. Quantitative and qualitative evidence from these studies indicates that acceptability is high regarding the content of CBT for tinnitus interventions, whether CBT is delivered via internet or face-to-face, and for audiologists to deliver

CBT. Within the context of effectiveness studies, clinicians have not been surveyed as to how acceptable they find CBT to deliver.

Who Benefits from CBT?

Currently, it is not possible to predict at an individual level precisely who will benefit from CBT for tinnitus; nor is it possible to predict by how much if at all. However, based on the findings from the samples included in RCTs and effectiveness studies, we can say that CBT for tinnitus (on average) benefits:

- Adults typically aged between 40 and 70 years with or without hearing loss, but without severe comorbid psychological conditions. Potential study participants with severe depression (for example) but seeking help for tinnitus have usually been excluded from tinnitus trials to date. Similarly, people under 18 years have also been excluded from most studies. Given this, it is not possible to comment on what effect CBT for tinnitus has for these groups of patients.
- People who have had tinnitus and/or suffered from tinnitus for at least 3 months. It is worth noting that some studies have not distinguished between or specified the period that someone has had tinnitus compared with the period that they have suffered from it.
- People seeking help to alleviate the impact that tinnitus has on quality of life and daily activities. This seems self-evident but serves as a reminder that most people with tinnitus do not seek help for it and many studies do not specify a minimum level of distress or disability for participation. Studies that do not specify a minimum severity instead typically require people to be primarily seeking help for their tinnitus (or tinnitus-related complaints).

It is important to recognise that most research into tinnitus and CBT has been conducted in Europe, Sweden, the UK, and the US. Contributions to the evidence base though are being made in countries including South Korea, Australia, China, Israel, Turkey, and Iran. Incorporating results from these countries into future evidence syntheses will help determine the extent to which the conclusions about the efficacy and effectiveness of CBT can be generalised.

Lastly, it is also fair to acknowledge and reiterate that CBT might not be effective (or even the preferred course of treatment) for everyone. Minority groups (e.g. immigrants, people with impaired communication or intellectual abilities) have traditionally been underrepresented in RCTs and thus it is unknown how efficacious or effective CBT is within these subgroups. This too should be kept in mind when considering whom CBT is likely to benefit.

Key points regarding the evidence base for CBT for tinnitus

- Systematic reviews, meta-analyses, and RCTs consistently demonstrate that CBT for tinnitus (in all its forms) is an efficacious intervention for alleviating distress and disability associated with tinnitus
- Effectiveness or pragmatic trials of CBT for tinnitus are relatively rare, but consistently show that it can be successfully delivered in routine clinical practice
- Evidence regarding the long-term efficacy of CBT for tinnitus is lacking
- CBT for tinnitus, while not for everyone, is largely considered to be an acceptable intervention from a patient perspective

Key topics for future research on CBT for tinnitus

- What is the optimal protocol of CBT for tinnitus?
- Which forms of CBT works best for whom?
- What is the longer term effectiveness of CBT for tinnitus (6–12 months and beyond) and what factors contribute to benefits being maintained?
- What is the clinical and cost-effectiveness of CBT for adults with tinnitus delivered by appropriately trained healthcare professionals other than psychologists (for example, audiologists)?
- Which patients can be adequately treated with online-based approaches and which require face-to-face treatment?
- What is the clinical and cost-effectiveness of CBT for children and young people who have tinnitus-related distress?
- What is the clinical and cost-effectiveness of CBT for specific populations such as people who are d/deaf or who have a severe-to-profound hearing loss and tinnitus-related distress?
- Which outcome measures are most specific and sensitive to the effects of CBT for tinnitus?
- What adverse effects are associated with CBT for tinnitus?

References

1. Andersson G. Tinnitus loudness matchings in relation to annoyance and grading of severity. Auris Nasus Larynx. 2003;30(2):129–33.
2. Kuk FK, Tyler RS, Russell D, Jordan H. The psychometric properties of a tinnitus handicap questionnaire. Ear Hear. 1990;11(6):434–45.
3. Wallhäusser-Franke E, Brade J, Balkenhol T, D'Amelio R, Seegmüller A, Delb W. Tinnitus: distinguishing between subjectively perceived loudness and tinnitus-related distress. PLoS One. 2012;7(4):e34583. https://doi.org/10.1371/journal.pone.0034583.
4. Hiller W, Goebel G. Factors influencing tinnitus loudness and annoyance. Arch Otolaryngol Head Neck Surg. 2006;132(12):1323–30. https://doi.org/10.1001/archotol.132.12.1323.
5. Hallam RS, Rachman S, Hinchcliffe R. Psychological aspects of tinnitus. Contributions to medical psychology. Oxford: Pergamon Press; 1984. p. 31–53.
6. Jastreboff PJ. Phantom auditory perception (tinnitus): mechanisms of generation and perception. Neurosci Res. 1990;8(4):221–54. https://doi.org/10.1016/0168-0102(90)90031-9.
7. Jastreboff PJ, Hazell JW, Graham RL. Neurophysiological model of tinnitus: dependence of the minimal masking level on treatment outcome. Hear Res. 1994;80(2):216–32.
8. McKenna L, Handscomb L, Hoare DJ, Hall DA. A scientific cognitive-behavioral model of tinnitus: novel conceptualizations of tinnitus distress. Front Neurol. 2014;5:196. https://doi.org/10.3389/fneur.2014.00196.

9. Cima RFF, Crombez G, Vlaeyen JW. Catastrophizing and fear of tinnitus predict quality of life in patients with chronic tinnitus. Ear Hear. 2011;32(5):634–41. https://doi.org/10.1097/AUD.0b013e31821106dd.
10. Kleinstäuber M, Jasper K, Schweda I, Hiller W, Andersson G, Weise C. The role of fear-avoidance cognitions and behaviors in patients with chronic tinnitus. Cogn Behav Ther. 2013;42(2):84–99. https://doi.org/10.1080/16506073.2012.717301.
11. Baguley D, Andersson G, McFerran D, McKenna L, Baguley D, Andersson G, et al. Psychological models of tinnitus. Tinnitus: a multidisciplinary approach. Chichester: Wiley; 2013. p. 102–9.
12. Jastreboff PJ, Brennan JF, Coleman JK, Sasaki CT. Phantom auditory sensation in rats: an animal model for tinnitus. Behav Neurosci. 1988;102(6):811–22.
13. Phillips JS, McFerran D. Tinnitus retraining therapy (TRT) for tinnitus. Cochrane Database Syst Rev. 2010;2010(3):CD007330. https://doi.org/10.1002/14651858.CD007330.pub2.
14. Bauer CA, Berry JL, Brozoski TJ. The effect of tinnitus retraining therapy on chronic tinnitus: a controlled trial. Laryngoscope Investig Otolaryngol. 2017;2(4):166–77. https://doi.org/10.1002/lio2.76.
15. Fuller TE, Cima RFF, Langguth B, Mazurek B, Vlaeyen JW, Hoare DJ. Cognitive behavioural therapy for tinnitus. Cochrane Database Syst Rev. 2020;1:Cd012614. https://doi.org/10.1002/14651858.CD012614.pub2.
16. Handscomb L, Shorter GW, Hoare DJ, Hall DA. Evaluation of a cognitive behavioral model of tinnitus distress: a cross-sectional study using structural equation modeling. Ear Hear. 2020;41(4):1028–39. https://doi.org/10.1097/aud.0000000000000826.
17. Cima RFF, van Breukelen G, Vlaeyen JWS. Tinnitus-related fear: mediating the effects of a cognitive behavioural specialised tinnitus treatment. Hear Res. 2018;358:86. https://doi.org/10.1016/j.heares.2017.10.003.
18. Blaesing L, Kroener-Herwig B. Self-reported and behavioral sound avoidance in tinnitus and hyperacusis subjects, and association with anxiety ratings. Int J Audiol. 2012;51(8):611–7. https://doi.org/10.3109/14992027.2012.664290.
19. Bouton ME. Learning and behavior: a contemporary synthesis. 2nd ed. Sunderland: Sinauer Associates, Inc.; 2016.
20. De Paepe AL, Williams ACC, Crombez G. Habituation to pain: a motivational-ethological perspective. Pain. 2019;160:1693. https://doi.org/10.1097/j.pain.0000000000001533.
21. Skinner BF. The behavior of organisms. New York: Appleton-Century-Crofts; 1938.
22. Kroner-Herwig B, Frenzel A, Fritsche G, Schilkowsky G, Esser G. The management of chronic tinnitus: comparison of an outpatient cognitive-behavioral group training to minimal-contact interventions. J Psychosom Res. 2003;54(4):381–9. https://doi.org/10.1016/s0022-3999(02)00400-2.
23. Cederroth CR, Gallus S, Hall DA, Kleinjung T, Langguth B, Maruotti A, et al. Editorial: towards an understanding of tinnitus heterogeneity. Front Aging Neurosci. 2019;11:53. https://doi.org/10.3389/fnagi.2019.00053.
24. Jastreboff PJ, Hazell JW. A neurophysiological approach to tinnitus: clinical implications. Br J Audiol. 1993;27(1):7–17. https://doi.org/10.3109/03005369309077884.
25. Jastreboff PJ, Hazell JWP. Tinnitus retraining therapy: implementing the neurophysiological model. Cambridge: Cambridge University Press; 2004.
26. Craske MG, Hermans D, Vervliet B. State-of-the-art and future directions for extinction as a translational model for fear and anxiety. Philos Trans R Soc Lond Ser B Biol Sci. 2018;373(1742):20170025. https://doi.org/10.1098/rstb.2017.0025.
27. Hesser H, Andersson G. The role of anxiety sensitivity and behavioral avoidance in tinnitus disability. Int J Audiol. 2009;48(5):295–9.
28. Hesser H, Pereswetoff-Morath CE, Andersson G. Consequences of controlling background sounds: the effect of experiential avoidance on tinnitus interference. Rehabil Psychol. 2009;54(4):381–9. https://doi.org/10.1037/a0017565.
29. Lovibond PF, Mitchell CJ, Minard E, Brady A, Menzies RG. Safety behaviours preserve threat beliefs: protection from extinction of human fear conditioning by an avoidance response. Behav Res Ther. 2009;47(8):716–20. https://doi.org/10.1016/j.brat.2009.04.013.
30. van Uijen SL, Dalmaijer ES, van den Hout MA, Engelhard IM. Do safety behaviors preserve threat expectancy? J Exp Psychopathol. 2018;9(4):2043808718804430. https://doi.org/10.1177/2043808718804430.
31. Lazarus RS. Progress on a cognitive-motivational-relational theory of emotion. Am Psychol. 1991;46(8):819–34. https://doi.org/10.1037//0003-066x.46.8.819.
32. Handscomb L. A systematic evaluation of the cognitive behavioural model of tinnitus distress. Nottingham: University of Nottingham; 2018.
33. Møller AR. Similarities between chronic pain and tinnitus. Am J Otol. 1997;18(5):577–85.
34. Møller AR. Similarities between severe tinnitus and chronic pain. J Am Acad Audiol. 2000;11(3):115–24.
35. De Ridder D, Elgoyhen AB, Romo R, Langguth B. Phantom percepts: tinnitus and pain as persisting aversive memory networks. Proc Natl Acad Sci U S A. 2011;108(20):8075–80. https://doi.org/10.1073/pnas.1018466108.
36. Lethem J, Slade PD, Troup JD, Bentley G. Outline of a fear-avoidance model of exaggerated pain perception-I. Behav Res Ther. 1983;21(4):401–8. https://doi.org/10.1016/0005-7967(83)90009-8.
37. Vlaeyen JWS, Linton SJ. Fear-avoidance and its consequences in chronic musculoskeletal pain: a state of the art. Pain. 2000;85(3):317–32. https://doi.org/10.1016/S0304-3959(99)00242-0.
38. Vlaeyen JWS, Linton SJ. Fear-avoidance model of chronic musculoskeletal pain: 12 years on. Pain. 2012;153(6):1144–7. https://doi.org/10.1016/j.pain.2011.12.009.
39. American Psychological Association: APA Dictionary of psychology. 2020. https://dictionary.apa.org/stimulus-generalization. Accessed 22 June 2020.
40. Markfelder T, Pauli P. Fear of pain and pain intensity: meta-analysis and systematic review. Psychol Bull. 2020;146(5):411–50. https://doi.org/10.1037/bul0000228.
41. Wideman TH, Asmundson GG, Smeets RJ, Zautra AJ, Simmonds MJ, Sullivan MJ, et al. Rethinking the fear avoidance model: toward a multidimensional framework of pain-related disability. Pain. 2013;154(11):2262–5. https://doi.org/10.1016/j.pain.2013.06.005.
42. Wideman TH, Sullivan MJL. Development of a cumulative psychosocial factor index for problematic recovery following work-related musculoskeletal injuries. Phys Ther. 2012;92(1):58–68. https://doi.org/10.2522/ptj.20110071.
43. Claes N, Karos K, Meulders A, Crombez G, Vlaeyen JWS. Competing goals attenuate avoidance behavior in the context of pain. J Pain. 2014;15(11):1120–9. https://doi.org/10.1016/j.jpain.2014.08.003.
44. Brown LA, Gaudiano BA, Miller IW. Investigating the similarities and differences between practitioners of second- and third-wave cognitive-behavioral therapies. Behav Modif. 2011;35(2):187–200. https://doi.org/10.1177/0145445510393730.
45. Thompson DM, Hall DA, Walker DM, Hoare DJ. Psychological therapy for people with tinnitus: a scoping review of treatment components. Ear Hear. 2017;38(2):149–58. https://doi.org/10.1097/aud.0000000000000363.
46. Clark DA. Cognitive restructuring. In: Hofmann SG, Dozois DJA, Rief W, Smits JAJ, editors. The Wiley handbook of cognitive behavioral therapy. Wiley; 2013. p. 1–22.

47. Andersson G, Vretblad P, Larsen HC, Lyttkens L. Longitudinal follow-up of tinnitus complaints. Arch Otolaryngol Head Neck Surg. 2001;127(2):175–9. https://doi.org/10.1001/archotol.127.2.175.
48. Wills F. CBT skills. In: Dryden W, Branch R, editors. The CBT handbook. London: Sage Publishing; 2012.
49. Aazh H, Moore BC, Lammaing K, Cropley M. Tinnitus and hyperacusis therapy in a UK National Health Service audiology department: patients' evaluations of the effectiveness of treatments. Int J Audiol. 2016;55(9):514–22. https://doi.org/10.1080/14992027.2016.1178400.
50. Olsson RJ. A practical guide to managing the tinnitus patient. (Unpublished doctoral dissertation). USA: Central Michigan University; 2001.
51. Waltman S, Hall BC, McFarr LM, Beck AT, Creed TA. In-session stuck points and pitfalls of community clinicians learning CBT: qualitative investigation. Cogn Behav Pract. 2017;24(2):256–67. https://doi.org/10.1016/j.cbpra.2016.04.002.
52. Craske MG, Treanor M, Conway CC, Zbozinek T, Vervliet B. Maximizing exposure therapy: an inhibitory learning approach. Behav Res Ther 2014;58(0):10–23. https://doi.org/10.1016/j.brat.2014.04.006.
53. Hubbard B. Cognitive behavioural therapy for tinnitus. Tinnitus Today. 2014;39.
54. Lindberg P, Scott B, Melin L, Lyttkens L. The psychological treatment of tinnitus: an experimental evaluation. Behav Res Ther. 1989;27(6):593–603. https://doi.org/10.1016/0005-7967(89)90143-5.
55. Lent J. Journaling enters the 21st century: the use of therapeutic blogs in counseling. J Creat Ment Health. 2009;4(1):67–73. https://doi.org/10.1080/15401380802705391.
56. Aazh H, Bryant C, Moore BCJ. Patients' perspectives about the acceptability and effectiveness of audiologist-delivered cognitive behavioral therapy for tinnitus and/or hyperacusis rehabilitation. Am J Audiol. 2019;28(4):973–85. https://doi.org/10.1044/2019_AJA-19-0045.
57. Orgeta V, Brede J, Livingston G. Behavioural activation for depression in older people: systematic review and meta-analysis. Br J Psychiatry J Ment Sci. 2017;211(5):274–9. https://doi.org/10.1192/bjp.bp.117.205021.
58. Hall DA, Fackrell K, Li AB, Thavayogan R, Smith S, Kennedy V, et al. A narrative synthesis of research evidence for tinnitus-related complaints as reported by patients and their significant others. Health Qual Life Outcomes. 2018;16(1):61. https://doi.org/10.1186/s12955-018-0888-9.
59. Sweetow RW. Cognitive aspects of tinnitus patient management. Ear Hear. 1986;7(6):390–6. https://doi.org/10.1097/00003446-198612000-00008.
60. Kaldo-Sandstrom V, Larsen HC, Andersson G. Internet-based cognitive-behavioral self-help treatment of tinnitus: clinical effectiveness and predictors of outcome. Am J Audiol. 2004;13(2):185–92.
61. Bennett-Levy J, Butler G, Fennell M, Hackmann A, Mueller M, Westbrook D, et al. Oxford guide to behavioural experiments in cognitive therapy. New York, NY: Oxford University Press; 2015.
62. Benhamou K, Piedra A. CBT-informed interventions for essential workers during the COVID-19 pandemic. J Contemp Psychother. 2020;50:275–83. https://doi.org/10.1007/s10879-020-09467-3.
63. Dugas MJ, Brillon P, Savard P, Turcotte J, Gaudet A, Ladouceur R, et al. A randomized clinical trial of cognitive-behavioral therapy and applied relaxation for adults with generalized anxiety disorder. Behav Ther. 2010;41(1):46–58. https://doi.org/10.1016/j.beth.2008.12.004.
64. Elarbed A, Fackrell K, Baguley DM, Hoare DJ. Tinnitus and stress in adults: a scoping review. Int J Audiol. 2020;60:171–82. https://doi.org/10.1080/14992027.2020.1827306.
65. Beck JS. Cognitive behavior therapy: basics and beyond. 3rd ed. New York, NY: The Guilford Press; 2020.
66. Jakes SC, Hallam RS, McKenna L, Hinchcliffe R. Group cognitive therapy for medical patients - an application to tinnitus. Cogn Ther Res. 1992;16(1):67–82. https://doi.org/10.1007/BF01172957.
67. Taylor JA, Thompson DM, Hall DA, Walker DM, McMurran M, Casey A, et al. The TinMan study: feasibility trial of a psychologically informed, audiologist-delivered, manualised intervention for tinnitus. Int J Audiol. 2020;59(12):905–14. https://doi.org/10.1080/14992027.2020.1788730.
68. Papas RK, Gakinya BN, Mwaniki MM, Lee H, Keter AK, Martino S, et al. A randomized clinical trial of a group cognitive-behavioral therapy to reduce alcohol use among human immunodeficiency virus-infected outpatients in western Kenya. Addiction. 2021;116(2):305–18. https://doi.org/10.1111/add.15112.
69. Hesser H, Weise C, Westin VZ, Andersson G. A systematic review and meta-analysis of randomized controlled trials of cognitive-behavioral therapy for tinnitus distress. Clin Psychol Rev. 2011;31(4):545–53. https://doi.org/10.1016/j.cpr.2010.12.006.
70. Newman CW, Jacobson GP, Spitzer JB. Development of the tinnitus handicap inventory. Arch Otolaryngol Head Neck Surg. 1996;122(2):143–8. https://doi.org/10.1001/archotol.1996.01890140029007.
71. Hallam RS. Manual of the tinnitus questionnaire (revised 2008). London: Polpresa Press; 2008.
72. Hallam RS, Jakes SC, Hinchcliffe R. Cognitive variables in tinnitus annoyance. Br J Clin Psychol. 1988;27:213–22. https://doi.org/10.1111/j.2044-8260.1988.tb00778.x.
73. Meikle MB, Henry JA, Griest SE, Stewart BJ, Abrams HB, McArdle R, et al. The tinnitus functional index: development of a new clinical measure for chronic, intrusive tinnitus. Ear Hear. 2012;33(2):153–76. https://doi.org/10.1097/AUD.0b013e31822f67c0.
74. Zigmond AS, Snaith RP. The hospital anxiety and depression scale. Acta Psychiatr Scand. 1983;67(6):361–70.
75. Beck AT, Epstein N, Brown G, Steer RA. An inventory for measuring clinical anxiety: psychometric properties. J Consult Clin Psychol. 1988;56(6):893–7.
76. Andersson G, Lyttkens L. A meta-analytic review of psychological treatments for tinnitus. Br J Audiol. 1999;33(4):201–10.
77. Beukes EW, Manchaiah V, Allen PM, Baguley DM, Andersson G. Internet-Based interventions for adults with hearing loss, tinnitus, and vestibular disorders: a systematic review and meta-analysis. Trends Hear. 2019;23:2331216519851749. https://doi.org/10.1177/2331216519851749. PMID: 31328660; PMCID: PMC6647231.
78. Rademaker MM, Stegeman I, Ho-Kang-You KE, Stokroos RJ, Smit AL. The effect of mindfulness-based interventions on tinnitus distress. A Systematic Review. Front Neurol. 2019;10:1135. https://doi.org/10.3389/fneur.2019.01135. PMID: 31736854; PMCID: PMC6838968.
79. Landry EC, Sandoval XCR, Simeone CN, Tidball G, Lea J, Westerberg BD. Systematic review and network meta-analysis of cognitive and/or behavioral therapies (CBT) for tinnitus. Otol Neurotol. 2020;41(2):153–66. https://doi.org/10.1097/MAO.0000000000002472. PMID: 31743297.
80. Sterne JAC, Savović J, Page MJ, Elbers RG, Blencowe NS, Boutron I, et al. RoB 2: a revised tool for assessing risk of bias in randomised trials. BMJ. 2019;366:l4898. https://doi.org/10.1136/bmj.l4898.
81. Schünemann HJ, Brożek J, Guyatt GH, Oxman A, editors. GRADE handbook for grading quality of evidence and strength of recommendations. guidelinedevelopment.org/handbook: The GRADE Working Group; 2013.
82. Cima RFF, Maes IH, Joore MA, Scheyen DJ, El Refaie A, Baguley DM, et al. Specialised treatment based on cognitive behaviour therapy versus usual care for tinnitus: a randomised controlled

trial. Lancet. 2012;379(9830):1951–9. https://doi.org/10.1016/s0140-6736(12)60469-3.
83. Beukes EW, Baguley DM, Allen PM, Manchaiah V, Andersson G. Audiologist-guided internet-based cognitive behavior therapy for adults with tinnitus in the United Kingdom: a randomized controlled trial. Ear Hear. 2018;39(3):423–33. https://doi.org/10.1097/aud.0000000000000505.
84. Langguth B. Tinnitus: the end of therapeutic nihilism. Lancet. 2012;379(9830):1926–8. https://doi.org/10.1016/S0140-6736(12)60561-3.
85. Maes IH, Cima RFF, Anteunis LJ, Scheijen DJ, Baguley DM, El Refaie A, et al. Cost-effectiveness of specialized treatment based on cognitive behavioral therapy versus usual care for tinnitus. Otol Neurotol. 2014;35(5):787–95. https://doi.org/10.1097/mao.0000000000000331.
86. Andersson G, Kaldo V. Internet-based cognitive behavioral therapy for tinnitus. J Clin Psychol. 2004;60(2):171–8. https://doi.org/10.1002/jclp.10243.
87. Aazh H, Moore BCJ. Effectiveness of audiologist-delivered cognitive behavioral therapy for tinnitus and hyperacusis rehabilitation: outcomes for patients treated in routine practice. Am J Audiol. 2018;27(4):547–58. https://doi.org/10.1044/2018_aja-17-0096.
88. Kaldo V, Haak T, Buhrman M, Alfonsson S, Larsen HC, Andersson G. Internet-based cognitive behaviour therapy for tinnitus patients delivered in a regular clinical setting: outcome and analysis of treatment dropout. Cogn Behav Ther. 2013;42(2):146–58. https://doi.org/10.1080/16506073.2013.769622.
89. McKenna L, Marks EM, Vogt F. Mindfulness-based cognitive therapy for chronic tinnitus: evaluation of benefits in a large sample of patients attending a tinnitus clinic. Ear Hear. 2018;39(2):359–66. https://doi.org/10.1097/aud.0000000000000491.
90. Segal ZV, Williams JM, Teasdale JD. Mindfulness-based cognitive therapy for depression. 2nd ed. New York: Guildford Press; 2012.
91. Beck JE, Zaugg TL, Egge JL, Lima EN, Thielman EJ. Progressive tinnitus management at two Veterans Affairs Medical Centers: clinical implementation with modified protocols. Am J Audiol. 2019;28(1s):162–73. https://doi.org/10.1044/2018_aja-ttr17-18-0040.
92. Tuepker A, Elnitsky C, Newell S, Zaugg T, Henry JA. A qualitative study of implementation and adaptations to progressive tinnitus management (PTM) delivery. PLoS One. 2018;13(5):e0196105. https://doi.org/10.1371/journal.pone.0196105.
93. Zaugg TL, Thielman EJ, Carlson KF, Tuepker A, Elnitsky C, Drummond KL, et al. Factors affecting the implementation of evidence-based progressive tinnitus management in Department of Veterans Affairs Medical Centers. PLoS One. 2020;15(12):e0242007. https://doi.org/10.1371/journal.pone.0242007.
94. Beukes EW, Vlaescu G, Manchaiah V, Baguley DM, Allen PM, Kaldo V, et al. Development and technical functionality of an internet-based intervention for tinnitus in the UK. Internet Interv. 2016;6:6–15. https://doi.org/10.1016/j.invent.2016.08.002.
95. Nyenhuis N, Zastrutzki S, Jäger B, Kröner-Herwig B. An internet-based cognitive-behavioural training for acute tinnitus: secondary analysis of acceptance in terms of satisfaction, trial attrition and non-usage attrition. Cogn Behav Ther. 2012;42(2):139–45. https://doi.org/10.1080/16506073.2012.724081.
96. Beukes EW, Manchaiah V, Baguley DM, Allen PM, Andersson G. Process evaluation of internet-based cognitive behavioural therapy for adults with tinnitus in the context of a randomised control trial. Int J Audiol. 2017;57:98. https://doi.org/10.1080/14992027.2017.1384858.

Mindfulness and Tinnitus

45

Laurence McKenna and Florian Vogt

Abstract

The evidence supporting the use of mindfulness in tinnitus management is discussed. Overall, the evidence is encouraging, suggesting that there are benefits in terms of reduced tinnitus distress post intervention and at follow-up including the likelihood of continued benefit several years post intervention. More mixed results were found for the impact of mindfulness on psychological wellbeing and on perceived tinnitus loudness. There is, however, a need for an expanded database and further rigorous trials. A widely accepted definition of mindfulness (viz., what comes from paying attention, on purpose, in the present moment, non-judgementally) is explored. There are several likely processes implied in this definition including exposure, acceptance, the reduction of ironical or paradoxical information processing, cognitive change, including meta-cognitive awareness, compassion, regulation of the self, together with body awareness and changes in self-perspective. The possible roles of such processes in helping reduce tinnitus distress are discussed. Mindfulness is recognised as being diametrically opposite from tinnitus management approaches involving masking, partially masking, substituting an alternative signal for tinnitus or distracting from tinnitus. It is also distinct from relaxation programmes. The use of mindfulness in tinnitus management remains in its infancy and a systematic approach to its development is this context is required.

Highlights

- This chapter outlines the introduction of mindfulness-based programmes into the western medicine.
- The evidence supporting it use in tinnitus management is reviewed.
- This evidence is still limited as relatively few studies have been completed; nonetheless, that evidence suggests that the use of mindfulness has a beneficial effect in reducing tinnitus related distress and that this approach merits further exploration.
- The nature of mindfulness is discussed through an exploration of a commonly accepted working definition.
- Consideration is given to the process through which it might influence the experience of tinnitus.

The psychiatrist, neuroscientist and Oxford literary scholar, Iain McGilchrist argues that the kind of attention we bring to the world alters the nature of the world we experience: 'Attention changes what kind of a thing comes into being for us: in that way it changes the world' ([1], p. 28). Attention is also seen as having a pivotal role in the way that cognitive-behavioural therapy (CBT) conceptualises tinnitus distress [2], and CBT has reliably shown to be effective in the treatment of tinnitus distress (NICE). Mindfulness approaches, including Mindfulness Based Cognitive Therapy, are about paying attention and McGilchrist's words seem directly relevant to this process and its application to managing tinnitus. According to a UK Government Advisory Group more than 500 peer-reviewed scientific journal papers were being published on mindfulness every year at that time; this figure is likely to be higher now [3]. This chapter aims to offer a sample of the evidence and some basic reflections on the processes likely to be involved in the application of mindfulness to tinnitus.

L. McKenna (✉) · F. Vogt
Royal National ENT and Eastman Dental Hospital, University College Hospitals, London, UK
e-mail: laurence.mckenna@nhs.net

W. Schlee et al. (eds.), *Textbook of Tinnitus*, https://doi.org/10.1007/978-3-031-35647-6_45

Mindfulness in Health Care and Tinnitus Management

Mindfulness-based approaches were introduced to mainstream western medicine by Jon Kabat-Zinn of the University of Massachusetts Medical School. He put mindfulness into a scientific context, separating it from its Buddhist associations and in the mid-1980s developed a programme of meditation and yoga for people with chronic pain. This programme was known as mindfulness based stress reduction (MBSR) [4, 5]. The key finding of the programme was that people were able to tolerate pain better, even if the pain was unchanged. It is usually taught to groups of about twelve people over eight weekly sessions. The classes educate people about links between the body, the mind and stress. Groups then practice a series of meditation exercises that highlight these links and support people in exploring different ways of responding to stress. Today, MBSR continues to be used in a wide range of health care settings, and it is now also found in education and employment settings and is even included in the training of some military units [6].

Psychologists went on to combine the structure and process of the MBSR programme with aspects of Cognitive Behaviour Therapy (CBT) to form mindfulness based cognitive therapy (MBCT). Originally, MBCT was developed as a treatment approach for people experiencing recurrent depression [7, 8]. It now forms part of the recommended guidelines from the UK National Institute for Health and Care Excellence's (NICE) guidelines for the treatment of depression [9]. MBCT has also been found to be an effective treatment for anxiety and stress [10]. There are now many studies indicating that mindfulness is also a helpful approach in the care of people with a range of physical conditions [11, 12], including pain, diabetes and cancer [13, 14]. Comparisons with other interventions suggest that mindfulness based programmes produce better outcomes than psycho-education and support groups and comparable outcomes to CBT and maintenance antidepressant medication [15, 16].

Mindfulness first appeared in the tinnitus literature in 2008 [17]. Since then, there has been a growing interest in its use of this approach in tinnitus management [18] and it is now integral to the care of tinnitus patients in a small number of specialist centres. This growth is taking place in the context of a still emerging evidence base and with some misconceptions about the actual nature of the approach and so merits careful consideration.

The Evidence for Mindfulness

A search of the literature reveals that at the time of writing there are nine studies examining the impact of a mindfulness-based intervention in adults. We considered randomized controlled trials (RCTs), and observational studies, such as case series. The evidence is encouraging but limited, as the total number of participants referred to in the published literature is less than 300. All nine included at least a baseline to post intervention comparison, and six of these also included a baseline-to follow-up comparison. Five out of the eight studies included a control group, four of which allocated group membership at random. Three of the four RCTs used relaxation therapy as the comparison group, the other used a waiting list control group. There was substantial heterogeneity in the content of the mindfulness-based programme used, in terms of duration, frequency and content as well as study design, such as, sample size, length of follow-up and type of measures used. For example, one study used 1-h sessions of conventional CBT and education for 25 tinnitus patients [17], with mindfulness meditation introduced in the third session, while another used eight 2-h sessions and 39 patients [19]. Several different measures were used to assess tinnitus distress, psychological distress and loudness. Among others, measures of tinnitus distress included the tinnitus questionnaire (TQ), the Tinnitus Functional Index (TFI) and the Tinnitus Handicap Index (THI), all of which have been reviewed elsewhere [20]. Two reviews have considered the effect of mindfulness in the context of tinnitus, both of which suggested that mindfulness has a role in the management of tinnitus [21, 22]. The evidence will now be considered in more detail and include all recent studies.

Impact on Tinnitus Distress

The evidence suggests that mindfulness-based interventions result in lower tinnitus distress post intervention compared to baseline. Eight studies looked at the effect of mindfulness post-intervention, and seven found that compared to baseline, those who received mindfulness saw their distress decrease [17, 19, 23–27]. The one study that did not detect a significant difference post intervention had only eight participants and therefore was at risk of a Type 1 error [28]. Still, the study detected a medium to large effect on distress, despite this not being significant. Two studies also compared mindfulness interventions to a waitlist control group [17, 25]. One of these was an RCT and found that those in the mindfulness group had lower levels of tinnitus distress at the end of the intervention (i.e. 9 weeks after baseline) [25]. The other study that included a waitlist control group tested if tinnitus distress reduced only in the control group [17], which it did not; the study did not formerly compare the mindfulness group to the control group. It also allocated participants consecutively and not randomly. Two RCTs evaluated the impact of mindfulness post intervention by comparing it to relaxation therapy. One study found that mindfulness was significantly more effective at reducing tinnitus distress [23]. The other study [19] found that both mindfulness and relaxation training significantly reduced tinnitus distress; no significant difference was observed between the treatments at the post-intervention point (but see longer term outcome below).

The evidence also favours an assessment that mindfulness reduces distress about tinnitus over the longer term. All six studies that examined tinnitus distress at a follow-up stage found that, on average, those who completed mindfulness had reduced distress compared to their baseline score [19, 24–27, 29]. One RCT found that compared to a waitlist control group, there was no difference at follow-up (i.e. 24 weeks after baseline) [25]. Both RCTs that compared mindfulness to relaxation therapy found that mindfulness was associated with greater reduction in tinnitus distress at follow-up [19, 29].

Typically, patients are not interested in statistical significance but whether improvement is going to be noticeable for them and whether they can expect to live a 'normal' life. Some studies reported findings in terms of the proportion of participants who responded, experienced reliable change, clinically significant change and recovery [30]. A reliable change means that the change is unlikely to be due to inaccuracies in its measurement. Clinically significant change is when the dysfunction is greatly reduced. Two studies reported on reliable change [19, 26]. In one study, post-treatment, reliable change (≥11 change on TQ) in tinnitus distress was observed in 59% of participants in the mindfulness group, which climbed to 62% at the 6-month follow-up [19]. In another study, post-treatment, reliable change (≥11 change on TQ) in tinnitus distress was observed in 50% of participants who had undertaken mindfulness training, and in 52.8% at the 6-week follow-up [26]. Clinically significant change was also investigated by two studies [24, 27]. In one, 60% showed a clinically significant decline in distress (≥13 change on TFI) pre- to post-intervention, and 58% from pre-intervention to follow-up after 16 weeks [24]. The second study used two measures of tinnitus distress, finding that 62% (≥13 change on TFI) and 77% (≥7 change on THI) achieved clinically significant change at the 4-week follow-up [27]. A further study defined a responder as >5 change on TQ and found that 88% of participants fit this criterion at post mindfulness intervention, and 69% did so after 24 weeks [25]; among the waitlist control group 47% were classified as responders post intervention and 59%, were so classified at follow-up. Of the studies that reported findings with some definition of improvers, at least 50% saw meaningful change at least up to 6 months. We found only one study that also looked at such change in a waitlist control group, this group also saw considerable reduction in dysfunction, but not as high as those who underwent the mindfulness intervention.

Impact on Psychological Distress

Alongside tinnitus distress, all the reviewed studies also studied psychological distress more broadly. Some studies included separate measures of anxiety and depression, and others included composite measures of psychological distress, which combine both constructs, for example the Clinical Outcomes in Routine Evaluation (CORE) [31]. The evidence suggests that the impact of mindfulness on psychological distress in tinnitus patients is not as favourable as that on tinnitus distress. Five out of eight studies that examined psychological distress post-intervention found that mindfulness significantly reduced it [19, 23, 25–27]; three did not [17, 28, 29]. A contributing factor may have been that all three that did not detect a significant difference had a small sample size; each had fewer than 16 people in their intervention group. One of these was an RCT, and it found that those in the mindfulness group had lower levels of psychological distress at the end of the intervention than those in the waitlist control group but the difference did not reach significance [25]. None of the three RCTs that used relaxation as a control group detected a significant difference between the intervention in terms of psychological distress post intervention [19, 23, 29]. A meta-analysis combined two of the datasets [19, 29] and made comparisons post-intervention. This analysis observed a trend favouring mindfulness over relaxation and at follow-up in terms of impact on psychological state, but this trend did not reach significance [21].

The long-term impact on psychological distress of mindfulness was studied by five studies, three of which detected a significant impact [19, 25, 26], while the remaining two did not [25, 29]. The RCT showed that mindfulness continued to have a superior reduction in psychological distress compared to the waitlist control (i.e. 24 weeks after baseline) [25]. Neither of the two studies that examined psychological distress at follow-up in comparison to relaxation detected a significant difference [19, 29].

Two studies reported in terms of meaningful change of mindfulness on psychological distress. Post-treatment, 42% [26] and 49% [19] of participants in a mindfulness intervention showed reliable change (>5 change on CORE), and recovery for 29% (reliable change and no longer in dysfunctional range) [26]. At 6-week follow-up, 37% [26] and at 6-month follow-up 49% [19] of the participants showed reliable change (>5 change on CORE) and recovery for 22% (reliable change and no longer in dysfunctional range) [26].

Impact on Loudness

Three studies looked at the impact of mindfulness on tinnitus loudness. Two studies observed a reduction in reported tinnitus loudness among the mindfulness group to post-intervention [19, 23], and one study found no difference [25]. At follow-up, one study continued to detect a significant reduction in loudness [19] while another did not [25]. The three studies that used relaxation in the control group found no difference between mindfulness and relaxation in their impact on loudness, neither at post intervention or at follow-up [19, 23, 25].

Remarks on Evidence

Overall, there is reasonable evidence to suggest that mindfulness is effective at reducing tinnitus distress. The evidence is weaker for psychological distress, and there is extremely limited evidence of any impact on tinnitus loudness although the latter is unlikely to be a therapeutic goal for mindfulness. The few direct comparisons that were made between mindfulness, a waitlist control group or relaxation, suggest that mindfulness may be more effective.

While many studies continue to identify benefits over the long term, the longest any effect was studied was 6 months, although one study reported on a sub-sample after 12 month [24]. Another study reported on feedback collected from people who had participated in mindfulness-based cognitive therapy for tinnitus between one to over five years previously [32]. Eighty-four percent of those who provided feedback (response rate of 58%) reported an immediate reduction in tinnitus distress following the course and 32% described increasing benefits in terms of tinnitus distress and wellbeing in the years following the course. Only a minority (3–6%) reported that they no longer noticed benefits from the treatment. These finding are consistent with the suggestion that mindfulness-based cognitive therapy has lasting benefits.

An Operational Definition of Mindfulness and Its Possible Mechanisms

With the evidence supporting the use of mindfulness-based interventions in patients with tinnitus, we will now consider how mindfulness may exert its effect in people with tinnitus. There is already a challenge in trying to define mindfulness, which has been likened to 'trying to pin jelly to the wall' ([33], p. 17). This maybe because it is a subtle blend of psychology and philosophy, particularly Buddhist philosophy. Nonetheless, in a health care setting mindfulness is neither religious nor esoteric in its nature; we will focus on the psychology. Given the difficulty in defining mindfulness there is unsurprisingly also some debate about the mechanisms of action involved in it. Various theories have suggested common mechanisms of mindfulness that underlie positive changes associated with mindfulness-based programmes [34]. Several factors have been suggested across the models, including exposure, acceptance, cognitive change, compassion, regulation of the self, of attention or of emotions together with body awareness and changes in self-perspective. The evidence concerning possible neuropsychological pathways, however, is still weak [35]. Instead, we will consider the possible mechanism by considering mindfulness itself, and what better place to start than by considering how it has been defined. Kabat-Zinn offers a definition of mindfulness that allows the process to be operationalized in a practical way ([36], p. 4). He suggests that mindfulness is what comes from:

> *paying attention, on purpose, in the present moment and without judgment.*

These few words refer to several processes each of which is challenging in it's own way. It is helpful to explore this definition and in so doing consider some of the possible mechanisms involved, as well as the possible relevance to tinnitus.

Paying Attention

It is argued that most people do not ordinarily engage in the process of paying careful attention [36]. Rather, for most people 'a fog of preoccupation and preconceptions habitually clouds the present moment much of the time' ([33], p. 21). The suggestion is that people operate on 'Autopilot'. This refers to a state in which a person caries out tasks without conscious intention or awareness of present moment sensory perception. The Autopilot is routinely employed not only in completing physical tasks but also in habitual thinking and problem solving. People process information quickly by fitting it into existing 'themes' and have many well-rehearsed 'behavioural scripts'. This reduces the effort involved in navigating the many demands of everyday life. While habitual problem-solving skills can be helpful it also reduces a person's conscious choices about how to respond to experiences. A Nobel prize was awarded to the research outlining the interplay between habitual processing and their impact on our decision making [37].

The mindfulness concept connects to this lack of careful attention and the automatic processes that are employed in managing the demands of life by suggesting two broad modes of mind: a Doing mode and a Being mode [8]. The Doing mode is engaged when a person is involved in practical tasks and problem solving. It registers discrepancies between an idea of how things are and an idea of how the person wants them to be. It is a goal-oriented approach aimed at reducing the gap between a desired state and how the person is experiencing things in the present. If practical actions can reduce the circumstances provoking an unpleasant emotional state, then they should be enacted. The automatically triggered and well-rehearsed goal-oriented strategies of the Doing mode, however, can be unhelpful if the standard methods of managing unpleasant states, viz. escape or avoidance, are not available. Then their continued implementation is likely to maintain or worsen the distress. For example, in the absence of a means of removing tinnitus, attempts to avoid or escape it are likely to be unhelpful. Not only is the energy spent on trying to treat tinnitus unlikely to be rewarded, leading to disappointment, it likely increases the focus on the tinnitus.

It is likely that attempts to avoid thinking about tinnitus lead to paradoxical or ironical information processing. The nature of ironical processing was highlighted by Fyodor Dostoevskyin in 1863 in his account of his travels in Western Europe: *'Try to pose for yourself this task: not to think of a polar bear, and you will see that the cursed thing will come to mind every minute'* [38]. This point was demonstrated experimentally in a classic study that observed that when subjects were instructed to not think of a white bear they continued to do so anyway [39]. When these subjects were subsequently instructed to deliberately think of a white bear they did so even more often than a different group of participants who had been told from the beginning to think of white bears. The results suggested that attempting to suppress the thought caused it to 'rebound' even more prominently into the participants' minds later. The suggestion is that paradoxical or ironic information processing makes it hard to reduce unwanted thoughts. This ironic process can be made worse by stress [40]. A person's efforts to not think about tinnitus, particularly if the experience of tinnitus is very stressful, may therefore lead to frustration and even greater awareness of the symptom. Clinical experience suggests that there is substance to the assumptions made here but experimental demonstrations have so far not been consistent [41].

This attempted avoidance of the undesirable stimulus is generally recognised formally as avoidance behaviour, a process that is seen as maintaining tinnitus related distress [42]. In addition to the ironical processing mentioned above, a CBT conceptualisation suggests that avoidance behaviour can have additional undesirable consequences of preventing negative beliefs about the feared object from being updated, i.e. it stops the person from finding out whether or not their negative thought is accurate [2]. In the context of tinnitus, patients commonly report fears that they will not be able to take their attention away from the tinnitus or that it might make tinnitus worse if they actively paid attention to it. Avoidance maintains such beliefs and the behaviour that it motivates can be exhausting. Ultimately, the apparent helplessness that characterise the Doing mode's avoidance attempts can lead to self-criticism, anxiety and anxiety about anxiety itself (e.g., 'why can't I get rid of this noise' or 'I will no longer be able to deal with the stress'). If the Doing mode offers few natural solutions, perhaps the Being mode offers an alternative.

The Being mode is about paying attention to one's experience in the present moment, putting on hold the tendency to problem solve. It places its emphasis on experiencing the world by focusing on the physical senses—seeing, hearing, smelling, feeling and tasting. The Being mode offers a sense of connection with internal experience and with the world and permits an awareness of the multidimensional complexity of experiences. This emphasis on experience can reduce the multiple ways in which the mind simplifies experiences by quickly and automatically categorizing stimuli and can reduce avoidance when (if the stimuli is categorized as unpleasant) or approach (if the stimuli is categorized as pleasurable). A classic introduction to mindfulness involves paying careful attention to a single raisin, including its many wrinkles, shadows and reflections, its stickiness between fingers, its pneumatic squeeziness, the squelching sound it makes when squeezed and smelling its sweet odour. Commonly, people are surprised about the intense taste of the raisin when they are ultimately asked to eat it. Without instruction to pay mindful attention, most people who categorize raisins as pleasurable, would automatically swallow the raisin, missing most of its qualities. The generalisation that the raisin exercise demonstrates is the highly nuanced nature of all experience, both pleasant and unpleasant experiences. There is no suggestion that one mode is more or less correct or helpful. Each is regarded as valuable in its own right. Each, however, represents a different paradigm that allows only certain types of questions and experiences. Given the dominance of the Doing mode in the everyday lives of most people the intention of mindfulness is to increase the person's awareness of the Being or experiential mode in order to provide a more inclusive experience.

In the context of tinnitus, the Being mode seems to pose a particular challenge with its intended activation of the sensory experiences. Certainly, the object for which people are seeking help is not regarded pleasantly, like a raisin usually is. In the initial stages of mindfulness training people commonly ask the questions: 'Will paying attention to (unpleasant) tinnitus lead to greater awareness of it?' The answer maybe yes, at least in the short term. There may, however, be a misconception here that mindfulness-based interventions are based around paying attention exclusively to tinnitus. Instead, the emphasis is on paying attention to *all* sensory experiences, including a soundscape rather than just one particular sound. This greater connection with experience may offer a mixture of pleasure and pain. It does create the opportunity for a more accurate perspective on 'what is', rather than a selective attention on the tinnitus that is consistent with a solution-focused attempt to remove awareness of it. Of course, mindfulness-based programmes will also include awareness of the tinnitus itself. By paying attention to unpleasant stimuli and resisting the automatic avoidance processes, features of the stimuli may become apparent that are neither pleasant nor unpleasant. This can trigger a more intricate categorization of a previously unapproachable stimuli. Paying attention to tinnitus may help to create a more nuanced experience and allow the identification of specific aspects of the tinnitus that are more manageable and some that are less manageable.

Attention On Purpose

The next clause in Kabat Zinn's definition suggests that paying attention is done *deliberately*. This point is also made by Feldman et al. [43] (p. 14) 'Mindfulness is seen as an intentional process; attention and awareness are deployed deliberately. ... Attention can be intentionally placed in different sense modalities. Including a hearing, seeing, body fencing, tasting and smelling. Each sense can come to be the primary focus for our attention. ... Attention can also be placed in the realm of thoughts, images and moods' . Mindfulness exercises encourage not only the deliberate but the willing deployment of attention. While it might be supposed that most tinnitus patients do pay attention to their tinnitus it can also be supposed that most do not do so willingly, hence the ironic processing. A patient who is aware of her tinnitus despite her best efforts to avoid it is likely to feel frustrated, distressed and lacking in control. Mindfulness suggests that allowing oneself to be aware of an experience such as tinnitus can provide a very different experience. Mindfulness is described as an Acceptance-based therapy. The meaning of the word Acceptance is different in this context from its everyday use. It does not mean the same as accepting a gift or being resigned or defeated in a struggle. Rather, it means allowing one's physical, cognitive or emotional experiences to be present without seeking to change those experiences. In the context of tinnitus it means allowing tinnitus to be present and observing it without trying to change it, escape it or struggling against it in any other way. Less struggle means less suffering and less emotional exhaustion. Acceptance has been described as the opposite of avoidance and suppression. The process of acceptance is likely to be regarded as counter intuitive by people who believe that exercising control is crucial to their wellbeing. In a clinical context, however, 'accepting' or 'allowing' simply represents stepping back from a futile attempt to control unpleasant experiences that cannot be controlled through avoidance. This is likely to be a more helpful, less distressing way of responding to experiences, including tinnitus. The alternative perspective that the process of acceptance offers is that greater control is achieved by allowing experiences to be present rather than by unsuccessful attempts to remove them. The paradoxical information processing is removed, and the reduced avoidance and greater exposure create an opportunity to test the accuracy of negative thoughts. It has been demonstrated that tinnitus acceptance mediates between initial tinnitus distress and later depression, quality of life and distress [44]. These points provide a distinction between the unhelpful selective attention to tinnitus referred to in the CBT model of tinnitus [2] and the attention that mindfulness exercises invite. The selective attention referred to by McKenna et al. [2] is largely involuntary, tunnel vision, fuelled by a negative appraisal of tinnitus while the mindfulness process invites voluntary awareness that is more inclusive and within the context of a different appraisal process (see below).

This point is further developed through a consideration of the practicality of paying attention during meditation. When a person seeks to pay attention in the way described it is almost inevitable that their mind will wander. When practicing of mindfulness exercises, the person is encouraged to recognise mind wandering; when the person becomes aware that attention has moved away from the object of meditation (e.g. the breath, a particular body part, etc.) then they are encouraged to return their focus to the object. This process is likely to happen repeatedly during meditation, and it is suggested that this back-and-forth movement of attention develops cognitive flexibility or self-regulation of attention [8, 45]. Several functional and structural MRI studies on mindfulness training have investigated neuroplasticity in brain regions supporting attention regulation [46]. Reduced control of the ability to switch attention is a factor in maintaining awareness of and the severity of tinnitus [47].

Present Moment Attention

The next part of Kabat Zinn's definition refers to a timescale: 'in the present moment'. The philosophy and practice of mindfulness relies heavily on this concept of 'the present' and on the simple truth: you are alive in only one moment—this one! (setting aside the realm of quantum physics). Assuming you are reading this at some point during the daytime then the moment when you got out of bed this morning is passed; it no longer exists. The time when you will go to bed tonight does not yet exist. Literally, the only moment that does exist is this one. This appeals to the (reasonable) supposition that people spend much of the time thinking about the future or the past. The future and the past can be very distant or very proximal to the person's current position; considering getting to the end of this paragraph is as much a focus on the future as contemplating one's distant retirement.

A focus on past and (possible) future *events* is particularly relevant in context of heightened emotional states such as anxiety where the focus of thinking is future based; something *shall* (future tense) go wrong, something bad *shall* happen. This future focus is characteristic of the catastrophic thinking associated with greater tinnitus distress [48–50]. By focusing on the present, the person is therefore giving less weight to negative thoughts that concern the past and the future. This may include fewer thoughts and a reduced sense of loss of having experiences spoiled by the tinnitus. It might also lessen negative thoughts about the ability to cope with tinnitus. A focus on the future or the past removes attention from the present. As the present moment is the only one that exists it is also the only one that a person needs to cope with and the only one that it is possible to cope with. The process of 'present moment existence' focuses the requirements on the person to cope with this moment rather than the next 5 min/hours/days/years. The thought 'I have to cope with this tinnitus for the rest of my life' has a different emotional feel from 'I have to cope with this tinnitus for the next 10 seconds'. Another assumption underpinning mindfulness is that life is lived in a state of flux. All experiences are impermanent. Most people will recognize the flux in terms of good and bad days or weeks. This variability can also be observed at a micro-level as taking place moment by moment. The assumption is that flux exists as much in people's physical, emotional and cognitive experiences as it does in the weather. If tinnitus seems unbearable now, perhaps the next moment will be different. Mindfulness exercises therefore invite the person to look at their experience right now, and only right now. This focus on the present may encourage people to 'smell the roses' or 'smell the coffee' and being aware of the moment can offer an opportunity to engage with life in richer way. Present moment awareness provides a focus for the self-regulation of attention that is posited as a key mechanism in mindfulness [8, 45].

Non-judgemental Attention

The final part of Kabat Zinn's definition suggests that the person pays attention, on purpose, in the present moment, *non-judgementally*. It is a common-place recognition that people make judgements about their experiences all the time. At a fundamental level, this judgement is about whether the experience is pleasant, unpleasant or neutral. This may translate in terms of an appraisal about whether the experience will help us or hurt us or any of a myriad of other thoughts. Negative cognitions are common among tinnitus sufferers and associated with anxiety, depression and tinnitus severity [49]. This is a clear recognition of the importance of the cognitive component of CBT [51]. Unsurprisingly, the CBT model of tinnitus distress [2] attributes a primary role to cognition (negative automatic thinking) in the creation of tinnitus distress and suggests that the ensuing processes influence the way in which a person perceives tinnitus. In this sense, it is in keeping with McGilchrist's assertion that 'Attention changes what kind of a thing comes into being for us' ([1], p. 28). McKenna et al. [2] posit that these *overly* negative thoughts provoke stress arousal and, through that, a process of selective attention that may distort the perception of tinnitus. A number of vicious cycles of involving thinking, arousal attention, distorted perception and behavioural avoidance follow from this. Mindfulness practices create the possibility of breaking these vicious cycles in a several ways. One way is that the process of deliberately directing awareness to specific body parts, or to the breath facilitates a disengagement from the judgemental analytic Doing mode of mind. The alternative foci occupy attention that would otherwise be used to ruminate or think negatively about tinnitus. This point is also relevant when tinnitus is deliberately made the focus of attention in the present moment. By attending to the direct physical representation of the tinnitus, e.g., its frequency, rhythm, intensity and its position in a wider soundscape the opportunity to disengage from the Doing mode of mind is created, and it is possible to distinguish tinnitus *per se* from thinking about tinnitus.

Mindfulness exercises, however, do encourage the recognition of thought processes. Each time the person's attention wanders from the breath, or other focus, the person is encouraged to acknowledge the content of the thought process that has captured the attention before returning awareness to the breath or other focus. This turns off the Automatic Pilot information processing. By repeatedly doing this, the person becomes more aware of the existence and emotional influence of the thought process and comes to recognize repeating themes or narratives within their cognitive set. This improved cognitive and meta-cognitive awareness can provide the person with greater agency over the influence of their thought processes. The mindfulness process, however, suggests a different way of responding to thoughts from the mainstream CBT approach. The mindful approach suggests that thoughts are viewed as transient mental events and not as representations of reality. It is evident, for example, that a person can think of an imaginary piece of chocolate and understand that this thought is not the same thing as an actual piece of chocolate. This is equally true of less tangible things such as anxiety or happiness. Furthermore, the transient, changing, nature of experiences, including thoughts, is appealed to in this context. The changing nature of thoughts is evidenced by processes such as cognitive distortion in clinical settings [51], the use of heuristics [37] and priming or 'nudging' [52] in everyday settings. Such process leads one person to interpret an event in different ways at different times and different people to interpret the same event in different ways at the same time. These processes challenge the commonly held assumption that there is a fusion between thoughts and reality. The mindful approach therefore invites the person to 'de-centre' from their thoughts by regarding them as ephemeral mental events and simply to observe the shifting nature of them without having to react (Doing mode) to them in any other way. This can allow individuals to establish a different relationship with thoughts and other experiences [45]. The intention is not to remove negative thinking but rather that the new, different, relationship may diminish the potency and destructive nature of negative thoughts. Through this the experience of tinnitus may become less aversive. The process involves bringing attention to the physicality of the event being observed rather than to the narrative about the event. This supports a focus on the actuality of the present moment rather than on the discrepancy between it and some other state. In this way, a moment of very intrusive tinnitus is no longer experienced as a *life ruined*, but rather as just *a moment of intrusive tinnitus*.

Mindfulness requires that 'paying attention, on purpose, in the present moment, non-judgmentally' is done with an attitude of compassion. The Mindfulness paradigm offers a clear recognition that experiences of emotional disturbance and of physical illness are distressing. Alongside this the concept of a 'healthy and happy normality' is challenged. The prevalence and incidence of physical and emotional disorders are highlighted and the ubiquitous nature of suffering is recognised [8]. There is also a clear acknowledgment that mindfulness exercises may be challenging. Through this recognition people's experiences and their struggles in coping are normalised; negative judgements that lead to anxiety about being anxious or depression about being depressed may be contained. Mindfulness programmes therefore explicitly encourage participants to adopt an attitude of kindness and compassion towards themselves and their experiences. In referring to compassion [53] state that '*it is the* acknowledgment that not all pain can be "fixed" or "'solved" but all suffering is made more approachable in a landscape of compassion' (p. 144). They go on to define compassion as 'an orientation of mind that recognises pain and the universality of pain in human experience and the capacity to meet that pain with kindness, empathy, equanimity and patience' (p.145). A psychological perspective on compassion is offered by Gilbert [54]. He explains the concept in terms of an evolved psychological capacity that is part of human beings' care giving and attachment systems that allow young and vulnerable individuals to be supported. In addition to its possible evolutionary roots compassion is seen as a quality that can be cultivated. In this way, mindfulness programmes have some commonality with Compassion Focused Therapy [55]. This compassionate attitude is seen as a crucial component of mindfulness training; without it the focus of attention on difficult experiences might indeed be counter-productive [2].

An interpretative phenomenological analysis (IPA) carried out with tinnitus patients who had completed a course in Mindfulness Based Cognitive Therapy [56] identified four superordinate themes associated with therapeutic outcome: two describing *what* changed: 'Relating to Tinnitus in a New Way' and 'Holistic Benefits' and two describing *how* this was cultivated: 'Connection, Kindness and Compassion' and factors that 'support engagement and change'. Every participant reported a transformation in their relationship with tinnitus. The shift from 'being at war with it' to 'allowing it' was the core process and outcome shared across the group. The more specific processes of behavioural exposure, self-regulation of attention and meta-cognitive awareness underpinned these changes. The analysis also suggested that attitudes of gentleness, kindness and permissiveness, potentially enabling acceptance of tinnitus, rather than just tolerance of it. These processes reported by people with tinnitus practicing mindfulness are the same as those that are proposed as the active ingredients in mindfulness-based therapy more generally [34].

Risks

It is reasonable to suppose that any therapy that is powerful enough to have significant benefit might also be powerful enough to do harm. A review of the sparse literature concludes that while mindfulness may involve practices that are difficult and distressing the rate of adverse effects and serious adverse effects is like that seen in other psychological therapies [57]. While Baer et al. [57] call for greater conceptual clarity in the mindfulness literature it would seem that there is no reason to be more concerned about the risks of mindfulness programmes than about other psychological interventions.

Summary and Conclusion

Being mindful means intentionally turning off the Autopilot through which we operate for much of the time. Judgements and the pursuit of goals are suspended for a time; the focus becomes the present moment *as it is* rather than as the person wishes it to be. Participants practice developing mindful awareness towards all experience, including tinnitus and practice allowing experiences to be present rather than avoiding them. Mindfulness is therefore diametrically opposite from those approaches to tinnitus management that involve masking, partially masking, substituting an alternative signal for tinnitus or distracting the person from it. It is also distinct from relaxation programmes. Many tinnitus patients assume that learning to meditate will be relaxing or even serene. Any given mindfulness meditation, which may involve quietly sitting still, may not be inherently relaxing and may be even less so when tinnitus is added to the experience. The experience is challenging rather than serene. Further, relaxation strategies involve exercises intended to change a person's physical and mental state; mindfulness supports the establishment of gentle toleration of the existing state. It is interesting to note that relaxation training has been used as a control condition in several of the studies examining the efficacy of mindfulness in tinnitus management. Unlike in CBT, the mindfulness practice does not involve challenging thoughts explicitly. Instead, participants simply observe physical and mental experiences and learn for themselves how the different ways of responding impact on their wellbeing. This experience provides the person with information about the ephemeral nature of their experiences, including their thoughts, emotions and their physical state including the impact of their tinnitus. The psychological processes that underpin this are exposure, compassion, the development of attention and attention control and cognitive and metacognitive awareness. The intention is not the removal of tinnitus but the development of a different, less threatening relationship with it.

The reduction in tinnitus distress, observed in the, albeit small, literature supports the implementation of mindfulness programmes in the management of distressing tinnitus. The challenges inherent in it mean that it is unlikely to be suitable for all tinnitus patients but it certainly merits inclusion in the tinnitus 'toolbox'. Further research is of course needed. In the absence of a clear regulatory process around mindfulness, it will be helpful if research and clinical practice do adhere to a clear protocol. The one offered by Segal et al. [8] has an evidence base supporting its use in clinical settings. The evidence to date derives from targeted interventions carried out by clinicians trained in mindfulness and familiar with tinnitus. There is no data about whether tinnitus patients benefit from joining generic mindfulness programmes.

The use of mindfulness represents a radically different approach from traditional tinnitus management methods. In keeping with McGilchrist's arguments, paying attention in a mindful way may 'change the kind of thing' that tinnitus is for us and create an opportunity for an easier relationship with it. Its implementation within tinnitus clinics requires resources in terms of time, clinic space and trained clinicians. Ultimately, these costs are justified by a reduction in the revolving door of help seeking that is often observed in tinnitus services [58].

References

1. McGilchrist I. The master and his emissary: the divided brain and the making of the Western World (Reprint edition). New Haven: Yale University Press; 2009.
2. McKenna L, Handscomb L, Hoare DJ, Hall DA. A scientific cognitive-behavioral model of tinnitus: novel conceptualizations of tinnitus distress. Front Neurol. 2014;5:196. https://doi.org/10.3389/fneur.2014.00196.
3. Mindfulness All-Party Parliamentary Group. 2015. Mindful Nation UK. The Mindfulness Initiative. https://www.themindfulnessinitiative.org/mindful-nation-report.
4. Kabat-Zinn J. An outpatient program in behavioral medicine for chronic pain patients based on the practice of mindfulness meditation: theoretical considerations and preliminary results. Gen Hosp Psychiatry. 1982;4(1):33–47. https://doi.org/10.1016/0163-8343(82)90026-3.
5. Kabat-Zinn J, Lipworth L, Burney R. The clinical use of mindfulness meditation for the self-regulation of chronic pain. J Behav Med. 1985;8(2):163–90. https://doi.org/10.1007/BF00845519.
6. Zanesco AP, Denkova E, Rogers SL, MacNulty WK, Jha AP. Mindfulness training as cognitive training in high-demand cohorts: an initial study in elite military servicemembers. Prog Brain Res. 2019;244:323–54. https://doi.org/10.1016/bs.pbr.2018.10.001.
7. Kuyken W, Byford S, Taylor RS, Watkins E, Holden E, White K, Barrett B, Byng R, Evans A, Mullan E, Teasdale JD. Mindfulness-based cognitive therapy to prevent relapse in recurrent depression. J Consult Clin Psychol. 2008;76(6):966–78. https://doi.org/10.1037/a0013786.
8. Segal ZV, Williams JMG, Teasdale JD. Mindfulness-based cognitive therapy for depression: a new approach to preventing relapse. 2nd ed. Taylor & Francis Ltd.; 2012.
9. NICE. Depression: the treatment and management of depression in adults (clinical guideline no. CG90). 2009. National Institute for Health and Clinical Excellence. http://www.nice.org.uk/CG90.
10. Nyklíček I, Mommersteeg PMC, Van Beugen S, Ramakers C, Van Boxtel GJ. Mindfulness-based stress reduction and physiological activity during acute stress: a randomized controlled trial. Health Psychol. 2013;32(10):1110–3. https://doi.org/10.1037/a0032200.
11. Bohlmeijer E, Prenger R, Taal E, Cuijpers P. The effects of mindfulness-based stress reduction therapy on mental health of adults with a chronic medical disease: a meta-analysis. J Psychosom Res. 2010;68(6):539–44. https://doi.org/10.1016/j.jpsychores.2009.10.005.
12. Khoury B, Lecomte T, Fortin G, Masse M, Therien P, Bouchard V, Chapleau M-A, Paquin K, Hofmann SG. Mindfulness-based therapy: a comprehensive meta-analysis. Clin Psychol Rev. 2013;33(6):763–71. https://doi.org/10.1016/j.cpr.2013.05.005.
13. Gardner-Nix J, Backman S, Barbati J, Grummitt J. Evaluating distance education of a mindfulness-based meditation programme for chronic pain management. J Telemed Telecare. 2008;14(2):88–92. https://doi.org/10.1258/jtt.2007.070811.
14. Ludwig DS, Kabat-Zinn J. Mindfulness in medicine. JAMA. 2008;300(11):1350–2. https://doi.org/10.1001/jama.300.11.1350.
15. Goldberg SB, Tucker RP, Greene PA, Davidson RJ, Wampold BE, Kearney DJ, Simpson TL. Mindfulness-based interventions for psychiatric disorders: a systematic review and meta-analysis. Clin Psychol Rev. 2018;59:52–60. https://doi.org/10.1016/j.cpr.2017.10.011.
16. Kuyken W, Warren FC, Taylor RS, Whalley B, Crane C, Bondolfi G, Hayes R, Huijbers M, Ma H, Schweizer S, Segal Z, Speckens A, Teasdale JD, Van Heeringen K, Williams M, Byford S, Byng R, Dalgleish T. Efficacy of mindfulness-based cognitive therapy in

prevention of depressive relapse: an individual patient data meta-analysis from randomized trials. JAMA Psychiat. 2016;73(6):565–74. https://doi.org/10.1001/jamapsychiatry.2016.0076.
17. Sadlier M, Stephens SDG, Kennedy V. Tinnitus rehabilitation: a mindfulness meditation cognitive behavioural therapy approach. J Laryngol Otol. 2008;122(1):31–7. https://doi.org/10.1017/S0022215107007438.
18. Hoare DJ, Broomhead E, Stockdale D, Kennedy V. Equity and person-centeredness in provision of tinnitus services in UK National Health Service audiology departments. Eur J Pers Cent Healthc. 2015;3(3):318–26. https://doi.org/10.5750/ejpch.v3i3.984.
19. McKenna L, Marks EM, Hallsworth CA, Schaette R. Mindfulness-based cognitive therapy as a treatment for chronic tinnitus: a randomized controlled trial. Psychother Psychosom. 2017;86(6):351–61. https://doi.org/10.1159/000478267.
20. Cima RFF, Mazurek B, Haider H, Kikidis D, Lapira A, Noreña A, Hoare DJ. A multidisciplinary European guideline for tinnitus: diagnostics, assessment, and treatment. HNO. 2019;67(Suppl 1):10–42. https://doi.org/10.1007/s00106-019-0633-7.
21. NICE. Tinnitus: assessment and management (clinical guideline no. 155). 2020. National Institute for Health and Clinical Excellence. https://www.nice.org.uk/guidance/ng155.
22. Rademaker MM, Stegeman I, Ho-Kang-You KE, Stokroos RJ, Smit AL. The effect of mindfulness-based interventions on tinnitus distress. A systematic review. Front Neurol. 2019;10:1135. https://doi.org/10.3389/fneur.2019.01135.
23. Arif M, Sadlier M, Rajenderkumar D, James J, Tahir T. A randomised controlled study of mindfulness meditation versus relaxation therapy in the management of tinnitus. J Laryngol Otol. 2017;131(6):501–7. https://doi.org/10.1017/S002221511700069X.
24. Husain FT, Zimmerman B, Tai Y, Finnegan MK, Kay E, Khan F, Menard C, Gobin RL. Assessing mindfulness-based cognitive therapy intervention for tinnitus using behavioural measures and structural MRI: a pilot study. Int J Audiol. 2019;58(12):889–901. https://doi.org/10.1080/14992027.2019.1629655.
25. Kreuzer PM, Goetz M, Holl M, Schecklmann M, Landgrebe M, Staudinger S, Langguth B. Mindfulness-and body-psychotherapy-based group treatment of chronic tinnitus: a randomized controlled pilot study. BMC Complement Altern Med. 2012;12:235. https://doi.org/10.1186/1472-6882-12-235.
26. McKenna L, Marks EM, Vogt F. Mindfulness-based cognitive therapy for chronic tinnitus: evaluation of benefits in a large sample of patients attending a tinnitus clinic. Ear Hear. 2018;39(2):359–66. https://doi.org/10.1097/AUD.0000000000000491.
27. Roland LT, Lenze EJ, Hardin FM, Kallogjeri D, Nicklaus J, Wineland AM, Fendell G, Peelle JE, Piccirillo JF. Effects of mindfulness based stress reduction therapy on subjective bother and neural connectivity in chronic tinnitus. Otolaryngol Head Neck Surg. 2015;152(5):919–26. https://doi.org/10.1177/0194599815571556.
28. Gans JJ, Cole MA, Greenberg B. Sustained benefit of mindfulness-based tinnitus stress reduction (MBTSR) in adults with chronic tinnitus: a pilot study. Mindfulness. 2015;6(5):1232–4. https://doi.org/10.1007/s12671-015-0403-x.
29. Philippot P, Nef F, Clauw L, de Romrée M, Segal Z. A randomized controlled trial of mindfulness-based cognitive therapy for treating tinnitus. Clin Psychol Psychother. 2012;19(5):411–9. https://doi.org/10.1002/cpp.756.
30. Evans C, Margison F, Barkham M. The contribution of reliable and clinically significant change methods to evidence-based mental health. Evid Based Ment Health. 1998;1(3):70–2. https://doi.org/10.1136/ebmh.1.3.70.
31. Evans C, Connell J, Barkham M, Margison F, McGrath G, Mellor-Clark J, Audin K. Towards a standardised brief outcome measure: psychometric properties and utility of the CORE–OM. Br J Psychiatry. 2002;180(1):51–60. https://doi.org/10.1192/bjp.180.1.51.
32. Marks E, McKenna L, Vogt F. Mindfulness based cognitive therapy for tinnitus: evaluation of long-term outcomes. Clin Psychol Forum. 2020a;334:45–50.
33. Crane R. Mindfulness-based cognitive therapy: distinctive features. 1st ed. Routledge; 2008.
34. Shapiro SL, Carlson LE, Astin JA, Freedman B. Mechanisms of mindfulness. J Clin Psychol. 2006;62(3):373–86.
35. Lao S-A, Kissane D, Meadows G. Cognitive effects of MBSR/MBCT: a systematic review of neuropsychological outcomes. Conscious Cogn. 2016;45:109–23. https://doi.org/10.1016/j.concog.2016.08.017.
36. Kabat-Zinn J. Wherever you go, there you are: mindfulness meditation in everyday life. 1st ed. Hyperion; 1994.
37. Kahneman D. Thinking, fast and slow (01 edition). Penguin; 2012.
38. Dostoevsky F. Winter notes on summer impressions: New Translation: Fyodor Dostoevsky (K. Zinovieff, Trans.; 1st edition). Alma Books Ltd.; 2016.
39. Wegner DM, Schneider DJ, Carter SR, White TL. Paradoxical effects of thought suppression. J Pers Soc Psychol. 1987;53(1):5–13. https://doi.org/10.1037//0022-3514.53.1.5.
40. Wegner DM. White bears and other unwanted thoughts: suppression, obsession, and the psychology of mental control (Reprint edition). New York: The Guilford Press; 1994.
41. Andersson G, Jüris L, Classon E, Fredrikson M, Furmark T. Consequences of suppressing thoughts about tinnitus and the effects of cognitive distraction on brain activity in tinnitus patients. Audiol Neurootol. 2006;11(5):301–9. https://doi.org/10.1159/000094460.
42. Cima RFF, Andersson G, Schmidt CJ, Henry JA. Cognitive-behavioral treatments for tinnitus: a review of the literature. J Am Acad Audiol. 2014;25(1):29–61. https://doi.org/10.3766/jaaa.25.1.4.
43. Feldman C, Kuyken W, Segal ZV. Mindfulness: ancient wisdom meets modern psychology. 1st ed. New York, NY: Guilford Publications; 2019.
44. Westin V, Hayes SC, Andersson G. Is it the sound or your relationship to it? The role of acceptance in predicting tinnitus impact. Behav Res Ther. 2008;46(12):1259–65. https://doi.org/10.1016/j.brat.2008.08.008.
45. Bishop SR, Lau M, Shapiro S, Carlson L, Anderson ND, Carmody J, Segal ZV, Abbey S, Speca M, Velting D, Devins G. Mindfulness: a proposed operational definition. Clin Psychol Sci Pract. 2004;11(3):230–41. https://doi.org/10.1093/clipsy.bph077.
46. Tang Y-Y, Hölzel BK, Posner MI. The neuroscience of mindfulness meditation. Nat Rev Neurosci. 2015;16(4):213–25. https://doi.org/10.1038/nrn3916.
47. Trevis KJ, McLachlan NM, Wilson SJ. Cognitive mechanisms in chronic tinnitus: psychological markers of a failure to switch attention. Front Psychol. 2016;7:1262. https://doi.org/10.3389/fpsyg.2016.01262.
48. Baguley D, Andersson G, McFerran D, McKenna L. Tinnitus: a multidisciplinary approach. 2nd ed. Wiley-Blackwell; 2013. https://doi.org/10.1002/9781118783009.
49. Cima RFF, Crombez G, Vlaeyen JWS. Catastrophizing and fear of tinnitus predict quality of life in patients with chronic tinnitus. Ear Hear. 2011;32(5):634–41. https://doi.org/10.1097/AUD.0b013e31821106dd.
50. Weise C, Hesser H, Andersson G, Nyenhuis N, Zastrutzki S, Kröner-Herwig B, Jäger B. The role of catastrophizing in recent onset tinnitus: its nature and association with tinnitus distress and medical utilization. Int J Audiol. 2013;52(3):177–88. https://doi.org/10.3109/14992027.2012.752111.
51. Beck AT. Depression: causes and treatment. University of Pennsylvania Press; 1967.
52. Thaler RH, Sunstein CR. Nudge: improving decisions about health, wealth, and happiness. New York: Penguin Books; 2009. https://

www.amazon.de/Nudge-Improving-Decisions-Health-Happiness/dp/014311526X

53. Feldman, C. & Kuyken, W. (2013) Compassion in the landscape of suffering. In Mindfulness: Diverse perspectives on its meaning, origin and applications, ed. M Williams & J Kabat-Zinn, Oxon: Routledge.
54. Gilbert P. The compassionate mind. London: Robinson; 2010.
55. Gilbert P, Choden. Mindful compassion: how the science of compassion can help You understand your emotions, live in the present, and connect deeply with others. New Harbinger Publications; 2003.
56. Marks E, Smith P, McKenna L. I wasn't at war with the noise: how mindfulness based cognitive therapy changes patients' experiences of tinnitus. Front Psychol. 2020b;11:483. https://doi.org/10.3389/fpsyg.2020.00483.
57. Baer R, Crane C, Miller E, Kuyken W. Doing no harm in mindfulness-based programs: conceptual issues and empirical findings. Clin Psychol Rev. 2019;71:101–14. https://doi.org/10.1016/j.cpr.2019.01.001.
58. McFerran D, Hoare DJ, Carr S, Ray J, Stockdale D. Tinnitus services in the United Kingdom: a survey of patient experiences. BMC Health Serv Res. 2018;18(1):110. https://doi.org/10.1186/s12913-018-2914-3.

46 Auditory Treatments of Tinnitus

Magdalena Sereda and Derek J. Hoare

Abstract

Auditory stimulation is one of the most widely used management options for tinnitus and a part of many tinnitus management programmes. Auditory treatments for tinnitus can amplify, modulate, or convert sound to compensate for hearing impairment, or produce sound to achieve a therapeutic effect. While many treatments aim to make tinnitus less audible, auditory stimulation can also provide distraction from tinnitus, promote relaxation, promote habituation, and reverse maladaptive tinnitus-related changes in brain activity. There is limited evidence from controlled trials for the effectiveness of auditory treatments and the decision to offer such treatment is usually based on the clinical experience and patient preferences. This chapter provides an overview of the role and mechanisms of action of the available auditory stimulation options, including hearing aids, sound generators, combination hearing aids, acoustic CR® neuromodulation, modified music, and cochlear implants. A summary of clinical guideline recommendations and a review of the empirical evidence for the use of auditory treatments for tinnitus is provided, together with recommendations for further research and clinical practice.

M. Sereda (✉) · D. J. Hoare
NIHR Nottingham Biomedical Research Centre, Nottingham, UK

Hearing Sciences, Mental Health and Clinical Neurosciences, School of Medicine, University of Nottingham, Nottingham, UK
e-mail: Magdalena.Sereda@nottingham.ac.uk; Derek.Hoare@nottingham.ac.uk

W. Schlee et al. (eds.), *Textbook of Tinnitus*, https://doi.org/10.1007/978-3-031-35647-6_46

Graphical Abstract

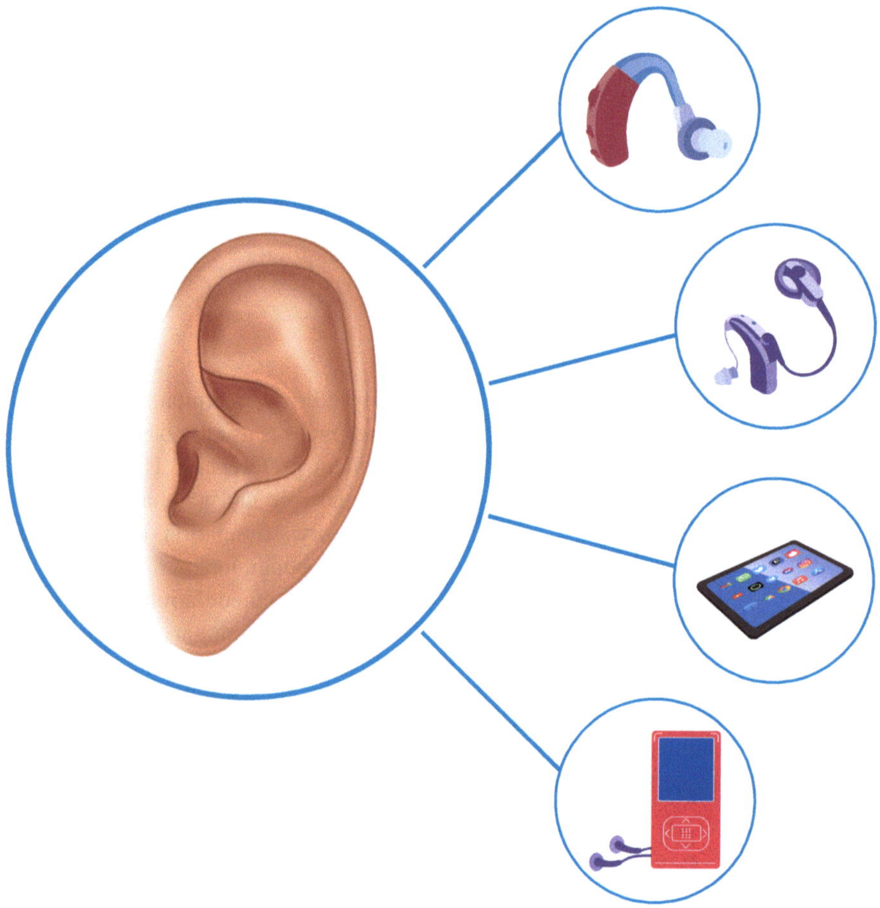

Highlights

- There are many different tinnitus treatment using auditory stimulation, offering options for personal preference and personalisation.
- Putative mechanisms of auditory treatment include reducing the tinnitus intrusiveness by masking it and promoting relaxation.
- Auditory treatments may also affect change in auditory neurophysiology, particularly with long term use.
- Evidence from controlled trials is limited but in general support the usefulness and acceptability of auditory treatments for many people with tinnitus.

Role of Auditory Stimulation in the Treatment of Tinnitus

Auditory stimulation might be the oldest treatment approach proposed for tinnitus and resulted from the observations that people with tinnitus often report that they are more aware of their tinnitus in quiet, and that environmental sounds are making their tinnitus less audible and provide relief from tinnitus. In general, auditory treatments for tinnitus either amplify, modulate, or convert the sound to compensate for hearing loss (hearing aids or cochlear implants) or produce sound (environmental sound enrichment or sound generators) with the view of producing a therapeutic effect [1]. Combinations of these approaches have also been introduced in the form of combination devices (hearing aids with built in sound generator) or through wireless streaming of sound from external sound players via hearing aids [2]. Auditory stimulation is among the most widely used tinnitus management options and is a component of many tinnitus management programmes such as tinnitus retraining therapy (TRT, see Chap. 47), Tinnitus Activities Treatment (TAT, see Chap. 49), Progressive Tinnitus Management (PTM), and Neuromonics© treatment.

Auditory stimulation has been used in clinical practice for over 70 years. Hearing aids have been proposed for the management of tinnitus since 1940s [3] and sound generators (ear-level devices that produce sounds for therapeutic use) were first introduced in 1976 [4]. Historical approaches to auditory stimulation aimed to provide tinnitus relief by partially or fully 'masking' the tinnitus percept. Vernon [4, 5] proposed a 'masking' method, where tinnitus was made inaudible or 'masked' by a more acceptable sound (in this case white noise), therefore providing a distraction and relief from tinnitus. Later, together with the introduction of combination hearing aids, the concept of partial masking was introduced as an acceptable outcome of tinnitus therapy [6]. Partial masking meant that the tinnitus was still audible but less so. In the 1990s, Jastreboff introduced a neurophysiological model of tinnitus (see Chap. 20), which proposed that to promote 'habituation' to tinnitus, auditory stimulation (broadband noise) should be used at or below the "mixing" or "blending point" (where the sound/noise starts to reduce how much tinnitus is heard but does not completely mask it) [7]. To accommodate those approaches the term "sound generator" was introduced to describe devices that are used for partial masking or sound enrichment as opposed to "maskers" used to achieve total masking of tinnitus.

Current views on auditory stimulation for tinnitus acknowledge that making tinnitus less audible is only one of the many goals and that tinnitus relief can be achieved through multiple different mechanisms, even without achieving complete or even partial masking of tinnitus [8]. Those include providing distraction from tinnitus, promoting relaxation and providing relief from stress or tension caused by tinnitus, providing "sound enrichment", and reducing contrast between environment and tinnitus which may promote habituation [1]. Moreover, several audiometric treatment approaches assume that acoustic stimulation can trigger neuroplastic changes in the brain and reverse tinnitus-related maladaptive changes. Those treatments use specific sound algorithms or modified sounds (e.g. notched music, patterned tones), which they postulate target abnormal tinnitus-related activity in the brain [9, 10].

Historically, broadband noise and specifically white noise, was the sound of choice for tinnitus masking or tinnitus habituation [4, 5, 7]. While broadband noises such as white (equal power across the frequency spectrum, resembles waterfall), pink (similar to white but with reduced high frequencies, resembles steady rainfall or wind), or brown (high frequencies reduced more than pink noise, resembles the roar of the river current or strong wind) noise are still standard options on most auditory treatment devices for tinnitus, manufacturers also offer options for filtering and modulating the noise, and options such as noise shaped to the patient's individual audiogram, noise centred either at or away from the tinnitus frequency, nature sounds, or specific sound algorithms aimed at neuromodulation. Moreover, the introduction of wireless streaming meant unlimited sound options for tinnitus treatment, including music, environmental sounds, or even individually modified sounds [2]. Availability of different sound options means that treatments can be highly personalised, depending on the aim of the treatment and individual patient preferences. For example, Henry et al. [11] proposed categories of sound options differentiating (a) soothing sounds (to produce a sense of relief from tinnitus-associated stress), (b) background sounds (passively diverting attention from tinnitus by reducing contrast between environment and tinnitus), and (c) interesting sounds (actively diverting attention away from tinnitus).

Clinical guidelines for tinnitus list several options for auditory stimulation that are used in clinical practice, including use of environmental enrichment devices (e.g., CD recordings, table-top sound generators, smartphones, and tablets with mobile applications offering different sound options), hearing aids, behind-the-ear and in-the-ear sound generators, combination hearing aids that offer patients with both tinnitus and hearing loss a single device for both, and cochlear implants for patients with severe to profound hearing loss. They also listed different approaches using sound as a main component of treatment or in combination with other approaches such as relaxation or psychological counselling [12, 13]. For example, acoustic CR® neuromodulation uses patterned stimuli that are individualised to each person by selecting pure tones at specific intervals above and below around the frequency most closely matched to the patient's dominant tinnitus pitch [14]. This treatment targets pathological neural synchronous activity thought to be associated with tinnitus. Neuromonics© treatment uses a combination of counselling, and music and broadband noise adjusted to each person's hearing loss, to provide stimulation within the deprived region and to promote relaxation [15, 16]. Notched music stimulation uses music with a one octave wide notch around the tinnitus frequency with the view of suppressing tinnitus-related cortical activity within the notch [9, 17]. Customised, spectrally altered music stimulation aims to compensate for the reduced sensory inputs due to hearing loss and reverse tinnitus-related changes in the brain [18]. The TRT approach comprises directive counselling and sound therapy administered according to a specific protocol [19]. See also Chap. 47 for a comprehensive overview. The protocol for the therapy was developed by Jastreboff based on his Neurophysiological Model [20] with an aim to promote habituation to tinnitus over several months. Depending on patients' hearing loss, hearing aids, behind-the-ear sound generators, or combination hearing aids delivering broadband noise can be used [21]. Since then, various modifications of TRT that are typically less intensive have also been used [19]. The PTM protocol introduces acoustic stimulation (soothing, background, and interesting sounds) for those patients for whom education and counselling were not sufficient. The use of therapeutic sound within PTM is flexible to meet individual needs and preferences [11].

Despite listing multiple approaches, clinical practice guidelines for tinnitus do not offer specific recommendations regarding the use of auditory stimulation for the management of tinnitus. This reflects the limited number of controlled clinical trials of their effectiveness as tinnitus treatments. There is a considerable variability in the recommendations and availability of different auditory treatment options in different countries. A systematic review of clinical guidelines for tinnitus identified five national clinical guidelines (Denmark, Germany, The Netherlands, Sweden, and US) and concluded that the greatest variation between guidelines occurred in recommendations for use of sound, and therapies such as TRT, which involves sound [22]. The Dutch, Swedish, and US guidelines all recommend use of TRT, however specify different criteria for eligibility for the therapy. The Dutch guideline states that TRT can only be recommended for those with very mild tinnitus. The Swedish guideline recommends sound stimulation as part of the TRT for people with no hearing loss. And the US guideline states that clinicians may recommend sound therapies such as TRT or tinnitus masking to patients with persistent, bothersome tinnitus, stating that patient preferences should play a significant role when deciding which option should be chosen [22]. Neither the subsequent European tinnitus guideline [12] nor the National Institute for Health and Care Excellence (NICE) guideline for tinnitus assessment and management [23] make recommendations regarding use of auditory treatments for tinnitus due to the limited research evidence.

Effectiveness of hearing aids in ameliorating hearing function is well established [24]. As such, clinical practice guidelines for tinnitus generally recognise the need to address hearing loss and hearing difficulties in patients with tinnitus. The use of hearing aids is consistently recommended for those who have clinically meaningful hearing loss and tinnitus [12, 22]. However, guidelines lack recommendations regarding specific fitting parameters that might be beneficial for tinnitus, or characteristics of the patients that might benefit from different available options (e.g. hearing aids vs combination hearing aids). They also lack specific recommendations when to provide hearing aids to primarily address the complaint of tinnitus. This can be the case, for example, where there is no hearing handicap or only a mild hearing loss. NICE guidelines make different recommendations depending on whether individuals have both tinnitus and communication difficulties [23]. For people with tinnitus, hearing loss, and communication difficulties, NICE guideline recommend fitting hearing aids; however, for people with tinnitus and hearing loss who do not have communication difficulties hearing aids were presented as an option to offer according to individual clinical judgements. These guidelines do no detail which circumstances should be taken into consideration within clinical judgements, or for which individuals within that group hearing aids might be considered a good option. Fitting of hearing aids for tinnitus in the absence of hearing loss was not recommended [23]. A more detailed guidance document specific to combination hearing aids was produced by the British Society of Audiology [25] providing instruction on the topics of candidacy, expectation setting, and fitting procedures that can support informed shared decision-making with respect to this class of device.

Cochlear implantation has become a standard option for people with severe-to-profound bilateral hearing loss who receive little or no benefit from hearing aids [26]. However, using cochlear implants to primarily suppress tinnitus has not been accepted worldwide and most tinnitus management guidelines recommend cochlear implantation only for patients meeting the hearing loss criteria for candidacy [12, 13, 23]. The current German tinnitus guideline recommends the use of CIs for unilaterally or bilaterally deafened patients with tinnitus, stating that CI fitting can provide good tinnitus suppression [27].

So, how widely are these treatment options used? An evaluation of clinical practices across Europe, involving clinical experts, researchers, and policy makers highlighted differences in the availability of auditory treatments between countries and regions [28]. Sound-based therapy (including hearing aids) was the most commonly available treatment in the northern and southern regions of Europe with almost 70% of departments offering those options. In contrast only 26% of departments in eastern Europe offered this treatment option. The use of TRT (including its modified versions) also differed between southern, eastern, and northern Europe, with 31, 16, and <1% of departments, respectively, offering it.

Mechanisms of Auditory Treatments for Tinnitus

The use of sound stimuli in the treatment of tinnitus may be beneficial by multiple mechanisms. Individual mechanisms include changes in neurophysiology, that is, altering tinnitus-related brain activity. Neurophysiological effects may involve a change, reduction, or reversal of tinnitus-related neuronal activity in the central auditory system. Such activity, and often associated with hearing loss, includes increased central gain, reorganisation, or 'retuning' of neurons within the auditory cortex (leading to over-representation of certain frequencies), or a loss of lateral inhibition within the auditory system leading to aberrant activity, and pathological neural synchrony (see Chaps. 17, 18, 20) [29, 30]. Altering or reducing tinnitus-related brain activity should change the sound qualities of tinnitus, which in turn may alter how an individual reacts to it, and how intrusive it is on their daily lives.

Treatments involving sound stimuli may additionally or alternatively have a primary effect of changing reaction to tinnitus, i.e., how much a person attends to or is aware of their tinnitus, or how stressed or disrupted they are by it. Whilst some auditory stimulation treatments are explicit about their hypothesised mechanism, most are not, and likely all treatments involving auditory stimulation will be beneficial, or not, because of various factors. So, before we review the evidence of benefits derived from clinical trials, let us consider how some common treatments may be exerting their effects.

Hearing aids amplify external sound. They primarily function to support communication, [24] and this alone can improve quality of life, cognitive performance, and general well-being for individuals with hearing loss. Hearing aids improve speech perception, which can be depleted in tinnitus, independent of comorbid hearing loss [31]. Hearing aids may additionally act as tinnitus maskers, reducing awareness of tinnitus and thereby reducing stress [32]. There is also some tinnitus-specific evidence for improvements in cognitive performance attributed to hearing aid use [33]. Hearing aids may also act directly against tinnitus generation by reducing drivers of central gain adaptation or inhibition. For example, central gain is a process whereby cochlear injury results in reduced activity in the cochlear nerve but increased neural activity at virtually all levels of the central auditory system [34]. This imbalance is hypothesised to result in tinnitus. The use of amplified environmental sound, however, increases or 'restores' a level of peripheral neural activity, redressing this imbalance and restoring normal levels of gain within the auditory system.

Sound generators are devices, which deliver one or more sound options, typically broadband (white) noise or narrowband sounds at a low, comfortable level. Intuitively, these have a controllable masking effect and are often described as offering relief or distraction from tinnitus, and an opportunity for the user to develop coping, or 'habituate' to tinnitus [35]. They may also have a neurophysiological effect in diminishing or reversing enhanced central gain. Indeed, there is substantial evidence in the animal literature to suggest long-term use of low-level noise can lead to changes such as substantial hypoactivity in regions of the auditory system with specificity corresponding to the stimulus; there are also however observations of hyperactivity or tonotopic enhancement as a primary result of long-term low-level noise exposure, so the picture is not clear (for a review see [36]). Nonetheless, sound generators are an important treatment option with strong evidence of an effect on coping; in a large qualitative study, Munir and Pryce [37] found that sound generators helped create a sense of escapism and control over tinnitus, and that even going through the necessary process to obtain their devices created a sense of validation for the person and their tinnitus, restoring a sense of self.

Combination hearing aids combine the functions of hearing aids and sound generators so can be used to mask, distract, relax or sooth and reduce tinnitus distress, and may promote neurophysiological change over long-term use [2]. One caveat with combination hearing aids is the potential trade-off between maximising for effects on tinnitus versus maximising for hearing abilities [25].

Cochlear implants, unlike hearing aids, bypass the normal acoustic hearing process, and replace it with electrical signals that directly stimulate the auditory nerve. They are primarily indicated to help provide a sense of sound to a person who is profoundly deaf or severely hard-of-hearing, and binaural hearing to those with a unilateral deafness [38, 39]. For most people, they do so successfully. For example, a scoping review of cochlear implant studies found an improvement in word perception ability from an average of just 8% before implantation to 54% after implantation [40]. As with hearing aids, this improved function can lead to general improvements in quality of life and consequently may reduce tinnitus distress. More specifically for tinnitus, however, cochlear implants are of interest as both a primary treatment of tinnitus, and in terms of understanding mechanisms, a treatment that can suppress tinnitus in many recipients but also induce tinnitus in those who did not have it prior to implantation [41]. Since 2008 there has been an interest in applications of CIs primarily for tinnitus [42]. However, the exact mechanisms that provide tinnitus suppression are not yet clear [43]. For many CI users, tinnitus returns shortly after the device is taken off, e.g. before going to bed. Then tinnitus abates again when the CI is put on in the morning. Studies in tinnitus have observed different effects in implant recipients concluding a multimodal mechanism of tinnitus suppression. Mallen and colleagues [44] found that 65% of implant recipients reported improvement in tinnitus at the time of cochlear implant activation, but that 93% reported improvements after 2 months. This might suggest masking effects in the immediate improvers and neuroplastic changes due to ongoing electrical stimulation leading to later improvements; Mallen and colleagues hypothesised the latter may be a direct inhibitory effect at the auditory cortex or inferior colliculus.

Acoustic coordinated Reset (CR®) neuromodulation involves a patterned sound stimulation using pure tones at frequencies above and below the frequency closest matched to the pitch of tinnitus. This makes it only suitable to those who have tonal tinnitus and who can reliably pitch match. It was one of the first treatment to use auditory stimulation to target a specific putative mechanism of tinnitus, i.e., to reverse pathological neural synchrony within the auditory system [45]. This approach involves a spatiotemporal stimulus pattern whereby sub-populations of neurons within a population showing abnormal synchrony are stimulated to fire out of sync, ultimately inducing sustained, long-lasting desynchronisation. For tinnitus, this approach is still under scrutiny with recent work from the developers to devise more 'perceptually-relevant' tones than those used previously which account for the consequences of additional variables such as hearing thresholds on tone selection [46].

Modified music involves either inserting a notch or otherwise customising it to alter its stimulation properties. Notched music requires a broadband music which is filtered to remove a narrow band of sound, e.g., between 1 and

1.6 kHz. Listening to such spectrally "notched" music was found to reduce cortical activity corresponding to the notch centre frequency, so in this example, 1.3 kHz, possibly through lateral inhibition. For tinnitus, this would mean creating a notch centred on the dominant tinnitus pitch, such that the music, having no energy in the tinnitus region, would only promote lateral inhibition of cortical regions corresponding to tinnitus generation [9, 47]. In addition to changes in the auditory system, there is also evidence this approach influences attention control, with demonstrated increases in responsiveness of the posterior cingulate cortex to cognitive tasks [48].

Another approach to modifying music for tinnitus involves customising it to the tinnitus or hearing loss of an individual. Mahboubi and colleagues [49] describe their customised masking strategy as specifically designed to deliver targeted sound energy, using the individuals pitch-matched frequency, intra-aural and inter-frequency attenuation characteristics to create sound stimuli composed of a series of narrow-band noise peaks that provide partial masking; in terms of mechanism, they describe auditory stimulation treatment as a distraction tool and providing a soothing sensation through masking.

Empirical Evidence for the Use of Auditory Treatments for Tinnitus

A 2018 Cochrane review summarised the evidence for effectiveness of three auditory treatments (hearing aids, sound generators, and combination hearing aids) used in clinical practice [1]. The review included eight studies (with a total of 590 participants), of which seven investigated the effects of hearing aids, four investigated combination hearing aids, and three investigated sound generators. The review found no randomised controlled trials (RCTs) comparing any of those treatments to a typical control group (waiting list control, placebo, or education/information only with no device). Data comparing these devices with each other were also limited. There were also methodological shortcomings in the included studies such as limited detail on methods for randomisation, little or no use of blinding, and no reports whether there were adverse effects. Authors concluded there might be little or no difference in the effects on tinnitus symptom severity of combination devices, hearing aids, or sound generators [1]. A review by Hesse [50] which included less stringent evidence such as non-randomised trials and cohort studies surmised the evidence was inconclusive and often contradictory.

Auditory stimulation is often used in combination with other treatment approaches in which cases it can be difficult to distinguish the specific effects of the auditory stimulation on tinnitus. One such study by McKinney and colleagues [51] compared the effectiveness of counselling alone to counselling in combination with the use of maskers, hearing aids, or combination hearing aids, in the context of TRT. Authors concluded that counselling is the main active component leading to improvements in tinnitus; the additional use of any of the devices provided only minimal additional benefit.

Hearing Aids

Whilst hearing aids are demonstrated to improve listening ability, hearing specific and general health-related quality of life [24], their effects on the tinnitus percept or tinnitus symptom severity are less well evidenced. Indeed, there is no high-level evidence that hearing aids are an effective treatment for tinnitus [1]. When compared to other treatment options such as sound generators or combination hearing aids, there was no evidence for superiority or inferiority of hearing aids over the other options [1].

There is no clear consensus which patients might benefit from amplification for their tinnitus. A service evaluation of UK clinical practice and a Delphi review on hearing aid provision concluded that clinicians are more likely to prescribe hearing aids if patients with hearing loss also have tinnitus, and that they would offer hearing aids for milder hearing loss if the patient also had tinnitus [52, 53]. Clinicians would also offer hearing aids if there was a complaint of tinnitus without reported hearing difficulties [53]. Beck [54] proposed that hearing aids can lead to significant improvements in tinnitus in people with very mild to moderate sensorineural hearing losses. Those patients might not typically look for or be prescribed a hearing aid. However, Henry et al. [55] postulated that a crucial step in tinnitus therapy is to determine if patient needs intervention for their tinnitus, hearing loss, or both. They proposed different approaches depending on whether patients report distress mainly due to tinnitus or hearing loss; only patients that showed hearing-related problems would be offered amplification.

There are many options available for hearing aid fitting. However, it is not clear which would be optimal for tinnitus. In general, there is an agreement that open-fit hearing aids should be fitted whenever possible for patients who have tinnitus. This avoids occlusion and makes use of the residual hearing, allowing natural environmental sounds to enter the ear [56, 57].

One question is whether patients with tinnitus should be offered one or two hearing aids. A UK clinical consensus study showed that clinicians agree that bilateral hearing aids should always be fitted for someone who has bothersome tinnitus, even if the patient has unilateral or asymmetric hearing loss [53]. Del Bo and Ambrosetti [56] also suggested that the best results for tinnitus are achieved with bilateral fittings. However, several studies report that a reduction in tinnitus symptom severity (regardless of tinnitus laterality) can be achieved with either unilateral or bilateral fitting [58–60]. Trotter and Donaldson [60] described a 25-year experience of using hearing aids for tinnitus therapy and did not find a difference in tinnitus improvement between unilaterally and bilaterally fitted patients. Other authors suggested that laterality of fitting should depend on the laterality of hearing loss and tinnitus. While in the case of a unilateral hearing loss and tinnitus fitting the impaired ear is sufficient, bilateral complaints require bilateral fitting [61, 62]. However, the main goal of the above-mentioned studies was to assess the efficacy of hearing aid fitting for tinnitus and not the laterality of fitting per se, and there are no studies that offer high quality evidence for the superiority or equivalence of unilateral and bilateral fitting.

Another question of interest regards the relationship between the amplification bandwidth and tinnitus pitch. Some authors consider amplification is only effective where the tinnitus pitch falls within the amplified frequency range, typically up to 6 kHz [63–65]. Moffat and colleagues [63] offered patients either conventional amplification or high-bandwidth amplification (with less gain at frequencies below 1 kHz and more gain at frequencies above 1 kHz). While the tinnitus percept was not affected in the group receiving high-bandwidth amplification, there was a significant reduction of low-frequency components of the tinnitus spectrum in the group receiving conventional amplification. In a pilot study by Schaette and colleagues [64], effects of conventional hearing aids on tinnitus symptom severity and loudness were compared in patients whose tinnitus pitch fell below or above 6 kHz (the typical upper limit of most hearing aids). Reduction of both tinnitus symptom severity and self-reported tinnitus loudness was observed in participants whose tinnitus pitch was below 6 kHz, but not in those participants whose tinnitus pitch was above 6 kHz. McNeil and colleagues [65] equally concluded that tinnitus masking was more likely to be achieved when tinnitus pitch falls into the frequency range of the hearing aids. In their study, participants who achieved masking with hearing aids reported a greater reduction in tinnitus symptom severity. In a further trial by Yakunina and colleagues [33], the effects of different types of amplification on tinnitus in participants with high frequency hearing loss were compared. Participants were randomly assigned to receive either hearing aids with wide dynamic range compression (WDRC), hearing aids with frequency translation, or hearing aids with linear frequency transposition. After 3 months, authors reported an improvement in tinnitus symptom severity in all three groups regardless of the amplification strategy used. Similarly, a crossover trial by Hodgson and colleagues [66] compared WDRC and frequency compression in participants who had high-frequency sensorineural hearing loss, concluding that while amplification with frequency compression was effective in reducing tinnitus symptom severity in some, it was not superior to WDRC, which should therefore remain the default hearing aid processing strategy for tinnitus.

Whilst there is limited high-level evidence for the benefit or superiority of hearing aids specifically for tinnitus, they clearly have an important role in improving speech perception and reducing hearing loss-related impairments in quality of life. Whether directly or indirectly they may also have a role in reducing the percept or symptom severity of tinnitus, and there is clinical consensus on their potential as a treatment for tinnitus. Patient choice and preference will also be an important determinant in adherence to this treatment option.

Cochlear Implants

Cochlear implants are offered to people with severe to profound hearing loss and deafness to improve hearing [67]. Several systematic reviews of the effects of cochlear implantation on tinnitus have been conducted. Ramakers and colleagues [68] presented an overview of the effects of cochlear implantation on tinnitus patients with bilateral sensorineural hearing loss. They concluded a lack of high-level evidence for effects of cochlear implantation on tinnitus. The 10 included studies reported reductions in tinnitus symptom severity after unilateral cochlear implantation. However, an increased burden of existing tinnitus and the induction of tinnitus were also reported. Total suppression of tinnitus was found in 30–37% of patients, a decrease in 29–72% of patients, no change in 0–30% of patients and a worsening in 0–25% of patients across the included studies.

A systematic review by Peter and colleagues [69] considered the effects of cochlear implantation on tinnitus in patients with single-sided deafness. No RCTs were identified and only cohort studies were included. In general, a reduction in tinnitus symptom severity was observed after cochlear implantation. Across the 13 included studies, 34% of patients showed complete suppression of tinnitus, 54% showed an improvement, 7% showed no change and 5% showed an increase in tinnitus symptom severity. None of the patients reported induction of tinnitus after implantation.

It is not clear which factors influence the outcomes of cochlear implantation for tinnitus, and studies often report inconsistent or contradictory results. Factors such as the level of pre-operative tinnitus handicap, pre-operative hearing loss, pre-operative stress levels, age at implantation, duration of hearing loss, additional hearing loss post-operation, and phoneme scores after implantation have been proposed to predict or correlate with positive or negative outcome for tinnitus [70–76]. A study by Kloostra and colleagues [77] aimed to create prognostic models, using binary logistic regression analyses to predict positive or negative changes in tinnitus after cochlear implantation. Authors reported that it was not possible to create a significant model to predict a positive effect of cochlear implantation on tinnitus, while lower preoperative tinnitus symptom severity and preoperative hearing handicap were predictive factors associated with worsening of tinnitus after implantation.

Cochlear implant programming is usually optimised for speech discrimination; however, those parameters might not necessarily be optimal for tinnitus suppression [78]. A review of optimal programming parameters for tinnitus suppression by Perreau and colleagues [79] concluded that there is no clear evidence for specific parameters yielding better results for tinnitus suppression in all patients. Authors suggested that adjusting cochlear implants to specifically suppress tinnitus is complex and that optimal parameters are likely to be different for different patients. Across reviewed studies parameters that led to tinnitus suppression varied greatly. Low and high-rate stimulation, different electrode numbers, and low T-levels were helpful in suppressing tinnitus. Authors concluded that more studies with greater numbers of participants are needed.

An additional study from van Zon and colleagues [80] compared the effects of unilateral versus simultaneous bilateral implantation on tinnitus symptom severity. There was no significant difference between the unilateral and bilateral groups, with 80% of patients overall demonstrating a reduction in tinnitus symptom severity after implantation. Secondary analyses as part of a multi-center RCT compared simultaneous and sequential bilateral cochlear implantation for tinnitus [68]. The median difference scores of tinnitus symptom severity were equal in both groups. Five participants developed tinnitus within 1 year of implantation, all in the simultaneous group. In the sequential group, four patients achieved a total suppression of tinnitus with the second implant compared to none in the unilateral implantation group.

CIs can be life changing in restoring hearing abilities, and there is positive evidence and increasing recommendation for use to treat tinnitus. CIs of course carry risks of surgery and so as with any treatment, informed decision making is crucial. The encouraging results of CI care in tinnitus suppression have led to scientific research on broader applications of this technique [81]. One aspect of the research is the focus on fully implanted systems, another aspect is the question whether there is a place for a "tinnitus implant" in the sense of a system that can also be used by people with better hearing. The ideas here are new positioning of specific electrodes or even an implant without insertion (at the round window) [82, 83].

Sound Generating Devices

A Cochrane review by Sereda and colleagues [1] concluded little evidence for effectiveness of sound generators. Recommendations regarding the choice and level of sound that should be used for tinnitus treatment varied greatly across the literature. Some programmes such as Tinnitus Masking allow use of any type of sound if it provides maximum masking benefit [84]. The choice of sound in such case depends strongly on patients' feedback and preferences. TRT recommends the use of broadband noise adjusted to mixing or blending point to allow for habituation [85].

A few mixed methods studies have explored preferences and perceived benefits of sound generating device use from the patient perspective. Handscomb [86] explored preferences for different sounds produced by the bedside sound generator *Naturecare*™. Participants were asked about how these sounds assisted with sleep, and why they preferred certain sounds over others. Semi-structured interviews revealed that the main reason for choosing a particular sound was because it had a pleasant emotional effect, rather than for its sound quality or perceived effect on tinnitus. The most frequently preferred sounds were nature sounds ('brook' and 'birds') with 'white noise' being the least popular. When selected as a favourite, participants tended to use that one sound only rather than alternate to other sounds. This study found a significant improvement in self-reported sleep quality as a result of using these devices.

Sound generating devices are also used widely in the self-management of tinnitus, such as the use of mobile applications (apps). A web-based survey showed that sound was the main component of mobile apps chosen by people for management of their tinnitus [87]. Mobile apps not only offer a wide selection of sounds but also offer multiple options for personalisation, such as adjusting sound balance, variance, speed, intensity, pitch, and frequency shaping. Some apps allow the user to record and play their preferred sounds or to create personalised soundscapes by mixing and adjusting multiple sounds and adding random sound effects. Authors recommended that further research should consider the place for apps in tinnitus management (stand-alone self-management intervention versus part of management by a hearing professional). As a relatively low risk treatment option, patients should be supported to make informed decision about the judicious use (avoiding safety behaviour) of sound generators in tinnitus management.

Combination Hearing Aids

The Cochrane review of sound therapy for tinnitus [1] included three RCTs of combination devices that measured improvements in tinnitus symptom severity using a validated questionnaire [88–90]. All trials compared combination hearing aids with hearing aids providing amplification only. The review concluded that there was no evidence of superiority of combination devices over hearing aids and that the use of either type of device was associated with a clinically significant reduction in tinnitus symptom severity. No RCTs comparing combination hearing aids to no intervention, placebo, or waiting list control were identified. A scoping review by Tutaj et al. [2] identified 34 studies involving combination hearing aids for tinnitus. Most records supported the use of combination hearing aids in tinnitus therapy, reporting improvements in tinnitus symptom severity, regardless of the sound used, device and sound settings, or management program followed. The review usefully highlighted variabilities in recommendations on combination hearing aids, and variables that may be important to consider in trials and in clinical practice. For example, several records were found stipulating that tinnitus should be clinically significant, bothersome, or even debilitating to warrant fitting combination hearing aids (e.g., [91, 92]). Other studies specified that tinnitus should be a primary complaint (e.g., [93]). Several authors postulated that amplification should always be trialled first and only when it proves not to adequately reduce tinnitus symptom severity, should combination aids be offered (e.g., [94]). Additional criteria mentioned in the literature that should be taken into consideration when offering combination hearing aids included patients' motivation to comply with the intervention, minimum masking levels that would indicate that the level of sound delivered through devices would be sufficient to mask tinnitus, and difficulty sleeping [2].

Combination hearing aids with wireless streaming may also be beneficial for tinnitus [2]. Barozzi and colleagues [95] compared the efficacy of nature sounds wirelessly streamed to participants' hearing aids and a conventional broadband noise available on combination aids. The study concluded that both options were effective in improving patients' coping with tinnitus. Searchfield and colleagues [96] compared customised spatial (3D) masking, which allowed presentation of masking sound at the same location in auditory space as patient's tinnitus with conventional bilateral masking, finding participants preferred 3D masking to conventional masking for tinnitus relief.

Combination hearing aids are used as a part of many different management programs including TRT, Tinnitus Masking (TM), Zen Therapy, PTM, and others [2]. Wherever combination hearing aids are used, optimal settings to address both problems with hearing loss and tinnitus will need to be carefully balanced, and for success, meet the preferences and be acceptable to the patient.

Acoustic Coordinated Reset (CR®) Neuromodulation

A systematic review of Acoustic CR® Neuromodulation by Wegger and colleagues [10] included eight publications with a total of 329 patients. Based on the available evidence authors concluded that the treatment was safe but that the evidence for effectiveness was insufficient to warrant clinical implementation. The review also questioned the postulated mechanism of action. In a further controlled trial Hall and colleagues [97] compared acoustic CR neuromodulation to a well-matched control condition (patterned sound stimulation delivered using the same device but predicted not to affect neuromodulation). They found no significant difference between groups on any self-report measures, or on oscillatory activity as measured using electroencephalography [97, 98]. Finally, a non-inferiority trial conducted by Theodoroff and colleagues compared 24-week of the treatment (now named Desyncra™) to a brief course of Cognitive Behaviour Therapy (CBT), concluding it was not inferior in terms of changes in tinnitus symptom severity [99]. The clinical picture is unchanged by these additional trials insofar as acoustic CR neuromodulation involves significant device use over time with no evidence of superiority over other sound- or CBT-based treatments.

Notched Music Stimulation

Two clinical trials investigated the effects of notched music stimulation on tinnitus [9, 17]. Okamoto et al. [9] compared the effects of the 12-month stimulation with target notch music (frequency band of one octave width centred at the individual tinnitus frequency removed from the music energy spectrum) with a placebo notch music (moving filter of one octave width not including the tinnitus frequency). Filtering was applied to the favourite music provided by participants. The study found a reduction in self-reported tinnitus loudness in those who received target notch stimulation (n = 8) but not those in the placebo group (n = 8). There was also reduced evoked activity in auditory cortex areas corresponding to the tinnitus frequency, as measured with magnetoencephalography, in the treatment group compared to placebo [9]. In a similar trial by Stein et al. [17] loudness of tinnitus was significantly reduced in the treatment group in comparison to placebo at 1-month follow-up after 3 months of treatment. Notable in this trial however was no between group difference on their primary outcome measures, which were all measures of tinnitus symptom severity. Further large-scale trials would be needed to progress this treatment to clinical use.

Customised Music Stimulation

An RCT by Li et al. [18] investigated the effects of classical music customised to individual's audiogram and tinnitus characteristics using a computational model and compared it with the effects of unaltered music. Authors postulated that the model could predict changes in neural connectivity and activity that may underlie the tinnitus development and the stimulation with customised music aims to reverse those changes. The study found a significant reduction in tinnitus symptom severity in the treatment group as measured with one of their tinnitus questionnaires (Tinnitus Handicap Inventory) but not the other (Tinnitus Functional Index) at 3, 6 and 12 months from baseline. Clinical utility of this approach is therefore far from clear.

Tinnitus Masking Therapy

The main goal of the tinnitus masking therapy is to provide immediate relief from tinnitus using ear-level devices and whichever sound provides maximum tinnitus masking. The choice of sound therefore depends on its effectiveness and acceptability for the patient. The level of noise for tinnitus masking should not be louder than necessary and should be tolerable by the patient [100, 101]. In many studies, investigating the effectiveness of tinnitus masking the choices (noise generators, hearing aids, combination hearing aids, and one or two devices) was driven by maximum tinnitus relief after trialling all available options [101–104] with devices used 'as needed' throughout the day and adjustments by the patient to their preferred level of noise. Due to the flexibility of candidacy, fitting parameters, settings on masking devices, differences in protocols and outcome measures, and studies of effectiveness of this therapy are often not comparable. Only some studies have used placebo controls. A lack of high-level evidence for the effectiveness of tinnitus masking therapy was concluded in the Cochrane review of sound therapy [1].

Tinnitus masking has also been compared to masking in combination with education or counselling. Henry and colleagues [101] compared partial masking therapy and TRT (partial masking plus education). Both approaches led to improvements in tinnitus symptom severity. However, TRT was more effective for patients with more severe tinnitus. While improvements in tinnitus with masking alone occurred quicker, within the first 3 months, TRT achieved greater benefit in the longer term (6 and 12 months). An RCT by Tyler and colleagues [105] compared counselling with complete tinnitus masking using bilateral noise generators, counselling with bilateral noise generators set to a mixing point, counselling only, and finding no difference in tinnitus symptom severity between groups after treatment. Only a minority of patients in each group showed a meaningful improvement (4/11, 6/19 and 3/18, respectively). A study by von Wedel and colleagues [106] found that patients who reported partial masking when using their devices (hearing aids or sound generators) showed greater reductions in tinnitus symptom severity than those patients reporting complete masking.

Masking as a technique has a place in many tinnitus treatments. It is important that patients are informed and make judicious use of this technique in the longer term (e.g. as part of their relapse prevention plan) rather than develop dependence on it for everyday functioning.

Conclusions

Auditory treatments for tinnitus make intuitive sense. Sound stimuli can be emotive, relaxing, distracting, they can mask other sounds, are infinitely varied, and malleable to individual tastes and preferences. Despite a lack of large controlled clinical trials, auditory treatments (hearing aids and CIs) and general advice about the use of environment sound for tinnitus are common in many clinical settings. In the absence of empirical evidence that they work, the strongest evidence to drive decisions whether to opt for auditory treatments is clinical experience and patient preferences through informed shared decision-making [107]. These can be guided by decision aids and clinical guidance where available [25, 108]. It may be that we never see a significant number of RCTs testing specific devices for auditory treatment, and perhaps that is not the best way forward in any case. Technology is ever changing, and so major investment to trial a new device that is quickly superseded by a next generation of that device would be suboptimal. Nevertheless, continued and more concerted work in this field is important, particularly to understand the neurobiological basis of benefit from auditory treatments (e.g. CIs), to more consistently and accurately measure outcomes that are most important to key stakeholders, [109] and to amass data that will inform subtyping (who benefits from what and why). Ultimately, this will turn auditory treatments such as hearing aids, CIs, and other emerging treatments options that can be personalised with more predictable outcomes for an individual patient.

References

1. Sereda M, Xia J, El Refaie A, Hall DA, Hoare DJ. Sound therapy (using amplification devices and/or sound generators) for tinnitus. Cochrane Database Syst Rev. 2018;12(12):CD013094.
2. Tutaj L, Hoare DJ, Sereda M. Combined amplification and sound generation for tinnitus: a scoping review. Ear Hear. 2018;39(3):412–22.
3. Saltzman M, Ersner MS. A hearing aid for the relief of tinnitus aurium. Laryngoscope. 1947;57(5):358–66.
4. Vernon J. The use of masking for relief of tinnitus. In: Silverstein H, Norrell H, editors. Neurological surgery of the ear, vol. II. Birmingham: Aesculapius Publishing Co; 1976. p. 104–18.
5. Vernon J. Attemps to relieve tinnitus. J Am Audiol Soc. 1977;2(4):124–31.
6. Vernon JA. Current use of masking for the relief of tinnitus. In: Kitahara M, editor. Tinnitus: pathophysiology and management. Tokyo: Igaku-Shoin; 1988. p. 96–106.
7. Jastreboff PJ, Jastreboff MM. Tinnitus retraining therapy (TRT) as a method for treatment of tinnitus and hyperacusis patients. J Am Acad Audiol. 2000;11(3):162–77.
8. Hoare DJ, Searchfield GD, El Refaie A, Henry JA. Sound therapy for tinnitus management: practicable options. J Am Acad Audiol. 2014;25(1):62–75.
9. Okamoto H, Stracke H, Stoll W, Pantev C. Listening to tailor-made notched music reduces tinnitus loudness and tinnitus-related auditory cortex activity. Proc Natl Acad Sci U S A. 2010;107(3):1207–10.
10. Wegger M, Ovesen T, Larsen DG. Acoustic coordinated reset neuromodulation: a systematic review of a novel therapy for tinnitus. Front Neurol. 2017;8:36.
11. Henry JA, Zaugg TL, Myers PJ, Schechter MA. Using therapeutic sound with progressive audiologic tinnitus management. Trends Amplif. 2008;12(3):188–209.
12. Cima RFF, Mazurek B, Haider H, Kikidis D, Lapira A, Noreña A, Hoare DJ. A multidisciplinary European guideline for tinnitus: diagnostics, assessment, and treatment. HNO. 2019;67(Suppl 1):10–42.
13. Tunkel DE, Bauer CA, Sun GH, Rosenfeld RM, Chandrasekhar SS, Cunningham ER Jr, et al. Clinical practice guideline: tinnitus. Otolaryngol Head Neck Surg. 2014;151(2 Suppl):S1–S40.
14. Hauptmann C, Tass PA. Therapeutic rewiring by means of desynchronizing brain stimulation. Biosystems. 2007;89(1-3):173–81.
15. Davis PB, Paki B, Hanley PJ. Neuromonics tinnitus treatment: third clinical trial. Ear Hear. 2007;28(2):242–59.
16. Davis PB, Wilde RA, Steed LG, Hanley PJ. Treatment of tinnitus with a customized acoustic neural stimulus: a controlled clinical study. Ear Nose Throat J. 2008;87(6):330–9.
17. Stein A, Wunderlich R, Lau P, Engell A, Wollbrink A, Shaykevich A, Kuhn JT, Holling H, Rudack C, Pantev C. Clinical trial on tonal tinnitus with tailor-made notched music training. BMC Neurol. 2016, Mar 17;16:38.
18. Li SA, Bao L, Chrostowski M. Investigating the effects of a personalized, spectrally altered music-based sound therapy on treating tinnitus: a blinded, randomized controlled trial. Audiol Neurootol. 2016;21(5):296–304.
19. Phillips JS, McFerran D. Tinnitus retraining therapy (TRT) for tinnitus. Cochrane Database Syst Rev. 2010;2010(3):CD007330.
20. Jastreboff PJ. Phantom auditory perception (tinnitus): mechanisms of generation and perception. Neurosci Res. 1990;8(4):221–54.
21. Jastreboff PJ, Hazell JWP. Tinnitus retraining therapy: implementing the neurophysiological model. New York: Cambridge University Press; 2004.
22. Fuller TE, Haider HF, Kikidis D, Lapira A, Mazurek B, Norena A, et al. Different teams, same conclusions? A systematic review of existing clinical guidelines for the assessment and treatment of tinnitus in adults. Front Psychol. 2017;8:206.
23. National Institute for Health and Care Excellence. Tinnitus: assessment and management. NICE guideline [NG155]. [Internet]. 2020 [cited 2021 Jan 29]. https://www.nice.org.uk/guidance/ng155.
24. Ferguson MA, Kitterick PT, Chong LY, Edmondson-Jones M, Barker F, Hoare DJ. Hearing aids for mild to moderate hearing loss in adults. Cochrane Database Syst Rev. 2017;9(9):CD012023.
25. British Society of Audiology. Practice guidance: fitting of combination hearing aids for subjects with tinnitus. [Internet] 2020 [cited 2021 Jan 29. https://www.thebsa.org.uk/wp-content/uploads/2020/03/OD104-88-BSA-Combination-aids-practice-guidance.pdf.
26. Buchman CA, Gifford RH, Haynes DS, Lenarz T, O'Donoghue G, Adunka O, Biever A, Briggs RJ, Carlson ML, Dai P, Driscoll CL. Unilateral cochlear implants for severe, profound, or moderate sloping to profound bilateral sensorineural hearing loss: a systematic review and consensus statements. JAMA Otolaryngol Head Neck Surg. 2020;146(10):942–53.
27. The Association of the Scientific Medical Societies. 2021. German S3 Guideline 017/064: Chronic Tinnitus [AWMF-Register Nr. 017/064 Klasse: S3 Chronischer Tinnitus]. https://www.awmf.org/uploads/tx_szleitlinien/017-0641_S3_Chronischer_Tinnitus_2021-09_1.pdf.
28. Cima RFF, Kikidis D, Mazurek B, Haider H, Cederroth CR, Noreña A, et al. Tinnitus healthcare: a survey revealing extensive variation in opinion and practices across Europe. BMJ Open. 2020;10(1):e029346.
29. Shore SE, Wu C. Mechanisms of noise-induced tinnitus: insights from cellular studies. Neuron. 2019;103(1):8–20.
30. Pienkowski M. Rationale and efficacy of sound therapies for tinnitus and hyperacusis. Neuroscience. 2019;407:120–34.
31. Jagoda L, Giroud N, Neff P, Kegel A, Kleinjung T, Meyer M. Speech perception in tinnitus is related to individual distress level-a neurophysiological study. Hear Res. 2018;367:48–58.
32. Shekhawat GS, Searchfield GD, Stinear CM. Role of hearing aids in tinnitus intervention: a scoping review. J Am Acad Audiol. 2013;24(8):747–62.
33. Yakunina N, Lee WH, Ryu YJ, Nam EC. Tinnitus suppression effect of hearing aids in patients with high-frequency hearing loss: a randomized double-blind controlled trial. Otol Neurotol. 2019;40(7):865–71.
34. Noreña AJ. An integrative model of tinnitus based on a central gain controlling neural sensitivity. Neurosci Biobehav Rev. 2011;35(5):1089–109.
35. Mondelli MF, Cabreira AF, de Matos IL, Ferreira MC, Rocha AV. Sound generator: analysis of the effectiveness of noise in the habituation of tinnitus. Int Arch Otorhinolaryngol. 2020;25:e205.
36. Sheppard A, Stocking C, Ralli M, Salvi R. A review of auditory gain, low-level noise and sound therapy for tinnitus and hyperacusis. Int J Audiol. 2020;59(1):5–15.
37. Munir S, Pryce H. How can sound generating devices support coping with tinnitus? Int J Audiol. 2020;60:312–8.
38. Levy DA, Lee JA, Nguyen SA, McRackan TR, Meyer TA, Lambert PR. Cochlear implantation for treatment of tinnitus in single-sided deafness: a systematic review and meta-analysis. Otol Neurotol. 2020;41(8):e1004–12.
39. Sharma SD, Cushing SL, Papsin BC, Gordon KA. Hearing and speech benefits of cochlear implantation in children: a review of the literature. Int J Pediatr Otorhinolaryngol. 2020;133:109984.
40. Boisvert I, Reis M, Au A, Cowan R, Dowell RC. Cochlear implantation outcomes in adults: a scoping review. PLoS One. 2020;15(5):e0232421.

41. van Heteren JA, Arts RA, Killian MJ, Assouly KK, van de Wauw C, Stokroos RJ, Smit AL, George EL. Sound therapy for cochlear implant users with tinnitus. Int J Audiol. 2021;60:374–84.
42. Van de Heyning P, Vermeire K, Diebl M, Nopp P, Anderson I, De Ridder D. Incapacitating unilateral tinnitus in single-sided deafness treated by cochlear implantation. Ann Otol Rhinol Laryngol. 2008;117(9):645–52.
43. Knipper M, van Dijk P, Schulze H, Mazurek B, Krauss P, Scheper V, Warnecke A, Schlee W, Schwabe K, Singer W, Braun C, Delano PH, Fallgatter AJ, Ehlis AC, Searchfield GD, Munk MHJ, Baguley DM, Rüttiger L. The neural bases of tinnitus: lessons from deafness and Cochlear implants. J Neurosci. 2020;40(38):7190–202.
44. Mallen JR, Chiu J, Marquis H, Ottochian A, Perez E, Kuo CL, Otto S, Ryan T, Roberts DS. Quantifying tinnitus suppression in cochlear implantation using tinnitus interval-limited tracking. Laryngoscope. 2020;130(8):2047–52.
45. Tass PA, Adamchic I, Freund HJ, von Stackelberg T, Hauptmann C. Counteracting tinnitus by acoustic coordinated reset neuromodulation. Restor Neurol Neurosci. 2012;30(2):137–59.
46. Tass PA, Silchenko AN, Popelka GR. Acoustic coordinated reset therapy for tinnitus with perceptually relevant frequency spacing and levels. Sci Rep. 2019;9(1):1–6.
47. Pantev C, Wollbrink A, Roberts LE, Engelien A, Lütkenhöner B. Short-term plasticity of the human auditory cortex. Brain Res. 1999;842(1):192–9.
48. Pape J, Paraskevopoulos E, Bruchmann M, Wollbrink A, Rudack C, Pantev C. Playing and listening to tailor-made notched music: cortical plasticity induced by unimodal and multimodal training in tinnitus patients. Neural Plast. 2014;2014:516163.
49. Mahboubi H, Haidar YM, Kiumehr S, Ziai K, Djalilian HR. Customized versus noncustomized sound therapy for treatment of tinnitus: a randomized crossover clinical trial. Ann Otol Rhinol Laryngol. 2017;126(10):681–7.
50. Hesse G. Evidence and evidence gaps in tinnitus therapy. GMS Curr Top Otorhinolaryngol Head Neck Surg. 2016;15:Doc04.
51. McKinney C, Hazell J, Graham R. An evaluation of the TRT method. In: Hazell J, editor. Proceedings of the 6th international tinnitus seminar. Cambridge: THC; 1999. p. 99–105.
52. Hoare DJ, Gander PE, Collins L, Smith S, Hall DA. Management of tinnitus in English NHS audiology departments: an evaluation of current practice. J Eval Clin Pract. 2012 Apr;18(2):326–34.
53. Sereda M, Hoare DJ, Nicholson R, Smith S, Hall DA. Consensus on hearing aid candidature and fitting for mild hearing loss, with and without tinnitus: Delphi review. Ear Hear. 2015;36(4):417.
54. Beck DL. Hearing aid amplification and tinnitus: 2011 overview. Hear J. 2011;64(6):12–4.
55. Henry JA, Zaugg TL, Myers PJ, et al. The role of audiologic evaluation in progressive audiologic tinnitus management. Trends Amplif. 2008;12:170–87.
56. Del Bo L, Ambrosetti U. Hearing aids for the treatment of tinnitus. Prog Brain Res. 2007;166:341–5.
57. Forti S, Crocetti A, Scotti A, Costanzo S, Pignataro L, Ambrosetti U, Del Bo L. Tinnitus sound therapy with open ear canal hearing aids. Acta Otorhinolaryngol Belg. 2010;6(3):195.
58. Brooks DN, Bulmer D. Survey of binaural hearing aid users. Ear Hear. 1981;2(5):220–4.
59. Bentler RA, Tyler RS. Tinnitus management. ASHA. 1987;29(5):27–32.
60. Trotter MI, Donaldson I. Hearing aids and tinnitus therapy: a 25-year experience. J Laryngol Otol. 2008;122(10):1052–6.
61. Melin L, Scott B, Lindberg P, Lyttkens L. Hearing aids and tinnitus--an experimental group study. Br J Audiol. 1987;21(2):91–7.
62. Zagólski O. Management of tinnitus in patients with presbycusis. Int Tinnitus J. 2006;12(2):175–8.
63. Moffat G, Adjout K, Gallego S, Thai-Van H, Collet L, Norena AJ. Effects of hearing aid fitting on the perceptual characteristics of tinnitus. Hear Res. 2009;254(1–2):82–91.
64. Schaette R, König O, Hornig D, Gross M, Kempter R. Acoustic stimulation treatments against tinnitus could be most effective when tinnitus pitch is within the stimulated frequency range. Hear Res. 2010;269(1–2):95–101.
65. McNeill C, Távora-Vieira D, Alnafjan F, Searchfield GD, Welch D. Tinnitus pitch, masking, and the effectiveness of hearing aids for tinnitus therapy. Int J Audiol. 2012;51(12):914–9.
66. Hodgson SA, Herdering R, Singh Shekhawat G, Searchfield GD. A crossover trial comparing wide dynamic range compression and frequency compression in hearing aids for tinnitus therapy. Disabil Rehabil Assist Technol. 2017;12(1):97–103.
67. Zenner HP, Delb W, Kröner-Herwig B, Jäger B, Peroz I, Hesse G, Mazurek B, Goebel G, Gerloff C, Trollmann R, Biesinger E. A multidisciplinary systematic review of the treatment for chronic idiopathic tinnitus. Eur Arch Otorhinolaryngol. 2017;274(5):2079–91.
68. Ramakers GGJ, Kraaijenga VJC, Smulders YE, van Zon A, Stegeman I, Stokroos RJ, Free RH, Frijns JHM, Huinck WJ, Van Zanten GA, Grolman W. Tinnitus after simultaneous and sequential bilateral cochlear implantation. Front Surg. 2017;4:65.
69. Peter N, Liyanage N, Pfiffner F, Huber A, Kleinjung T. The influence of cochlear implantation on tinnitus in patients with single-sided deafness: a systematic review. Otolaryngol Head Neck Surg. 2019;161(4):576–88.
70. Olze H, Szczepek AJ, Haupt H, et al. Cochlear implantation has a positive influence on quality of life, tinnitus, and psychological comorbidity. Laryngoscope. 2011;10:2220–7.
71. Souliere CR Jr, Kileny PR, Zwolan TA, Kemink JL. Tinnitus suppression following cochlear implantation. A multifactorial investigation. Arch Otolaryngol Head Neck Surg. 1992;12:1291–7.
72. Pan T, Tyler RS, Ji H, Coelho C, Gehringer AK, Gogel SA. Changes in the tinnitus handicap questionnaire after cochlear implantation. Am J Audiol. 2009;2:144–51.
73. Olze H, Szczepek AJ, Haupt H, Zirke N, Graebel S, Mazurek B. The impact of cochlear implantation on tinnitus, stress and quality of life in postlingually deafened patients. Audiol Neurootol. 2011;1:2–11.
74. Amoodi HA, Mick PT, Shipp DB, Friesen LM, Nedzelski JM, Chen JM, Lin VY. The effects of unilateral cochlear implantation on the tinnitus handicap inventory and the influence on quality of life. Laryngoscope. 2011;121(7):1536–40.
75. Kompis M, Pelizzone M, Dillier N, Allum J, Demin N, Senn P. Tinnitus before and 6 months after cochlear implantation. Audiol Neurootol. 2012;3:161–8.
76. Dixon PR, Crowson M, Shipp D, Smilsky K, Lin VY, Le T, Chen JM. Predicting reduced tinnitus burden after cochlear implantation in adults. Otol Neurotol. 2020;41(2):196–201.
77. Kloostra FJJ, Arnold R, Hofman R, Burgerhof JGM, van Dijk P. Models to predict positive and negative effects of cochlear implantation on tinnitus. Laryngoscope Investig Otolaryngol. 2018;4(1):138–42.
78. Andersson G, Baguley DM, McKenna L, McFerran D. Tinnitus: a multidisciplinary approach. London: Whurr; 2005.
79. Perreau A, Tyler R, Mancini PC. Programming a cochlear implant for tinnitus suppression. J Am Acad Audiol. 2020;31(4):302–8.
80. van Zon A, Smulders YE, Ramakers GG, Stegeman I, Smit AL, Van Zanten GA, Stokroos RJ, Hendrice N, Free RH, Maat B, Frijns JH, Mylanus EA, Huinck WJ, Topsakal V, Tange RA, Grolman W. Effect of unilateral and simultaneous bilateral cochlear implantation on tinnitus: a prospective study. Laryngoscope. 2016;126(4):956–61.

81. Mitchell-Innes A, Saeed SR, Irving R. The future of cochlear implant design. Adv Otorhinolaryngol. 2018;81:105–13.
82. Wenzel GI, Sarnes P, Warnecke A, Stöver T, Jäger B, Lesinski-Schiedat A, Lenarz T. Non-penetrating round window electrode stimulation for tinnitus therapy followed by cochlear implantation. Eur Arch Otorhinolaryngol. 2015;272(11):3283–93.
83. Chen M, Min S, Zhang C, Hu X, Li S. Using extracochlear multichannel electrical stimulation to relieve tinnitus and reverse tinnitus-related auditory-somatosensory plasticity in the cochlear nucleus. Neuromodulation. 2021;25:1338. https://doi.org/10.1111/ner.13506.
84. Henry JA, Jastreboff MM, Jastreboff PJ, Schechter MA, Fausti SA. Assessment of patients for treatment with tinnitus retraining therapy. J Am Acad Audiol. 2002;13(10):523–44.
85. Jastreboff PJ, Jastreboff MM. Tinnitus retraining therapy: a different view on tinnitus. ORL. 2006;68(1):23–30.
86. Handscomb L. Use of bedside sound generators by patients with tinnitus-related sleeping difficulty: which sounds are preferred and why? Acta Otolaryngol Suppl. 2006;556:59–63.
87. Sereda M, Smith S, Newton K, Stockdale D. Mobile apps for management of tinnitus: users' survey, quality assessment, and content analysis. JMIR Mhealth Uhealth. 2019;7(1):e10353.
88. dos Santos G, Bento R, de Medeiros I, et al. The influence of sound generator associated with conventional amplification for tinnitus control: randomized blind clinical trial. Trends Hear. 2014;18:1–9.
89. Henry JA, Frederick M, Sell S, Griest S, Abrams H. Validation of a novel combination hearing aid and tinnitus therapy device. Ear Hear. 2015;36(1):42–52.
90. Henry JA, McMillan G, Dann S, Bennett K, Griest S, Theodoroff S, Silverman SP, Whichard S, Saunders G. Tinnitus management: randomized controlled trial comparing extended-wear hearing aids, conventional hearing aids, and combination instruments. J Am Acad Audiol. 2017;28(6):546–61.
91. Hicks M, Abrams H, Henry J, Frederick M, Sell S, Griest S. Clinical validation of a novel combination hearing aid and tinnitus therapy device. Proceedings of the 8th International TRI Tinnitus Conference. Tinnitus Research Initiative, Auckland, New Zealand. 2014 Mar 10–13. p. 237–238.
92. Johansen JD, Skellgaard PH, Caporali S. Effect of counseling, amplification and fractal tones in tinnitus management. J Commun Disord Deaf Stud Hear Aids. 2014;2:124.
93. Sweetow RW, Sabes JH. Effects of acoustical stimuli delivered through hearing aids on tinnitus. J Am Acad Audiol. 2010;21(7):461–73.
94. Piskosz M. The role of wireless streaming in tinnitus management. Hear Rev. 2012:12–5.
95. Barozzi S, Del Bo L, Crocetti A, Dyrlund O, Passoni S, Zolin A, Panicucci E, Mancuso A, Kaur M, Searchfield GD. A comparison of nature and technical sounds for tinnitus therapy. Acta Acust United Ac. 2016;102(3):540–6.
96. Searchfield GD, Kobayashi K, Hodgson SA, Hodgson C, Tevoitdale H, Irving S. Spatial masking: development and testing of a new tinnitus assistive technology. Assist Technol. 2016;28(2):115–25.
97. Hall DA, Pierzycki RH, Thomas H, Greenberg D, Sereda M, Hoare DJ. Systematic evaluation of the T30 neurostimulator treatment for tinnitus: a double-blind randomised placebo-controlled trial with open-label extension. Brain Sci. 2022;12(3):317.
98. Pierzycki RH, McNamara AJ, Hoare DJ, Hall DA. Whole scalp resting state EEG of oscillatory brain activity shows no parametric relationship with psychoacoustic and psychosocial assessment of tinnitus: a repeated measures study. Hear Res. 2016;331:101–8.
99. Theodoroff SM, McMillan GP, Schmidt CJ, Dann SM, Hauptmann C, Goodworth MC, Leibowitz RQ, Random C, Henry JA. Randomised controlled trial of interventions for bothersome tinnitus: DesyncraTM versus cognitive behavioural therapy. Int J Audiol. 2021;61:1035–44.
100. Henry JA, Schechter MA, Zaugg TL, Griest S, Jastreboff PJ, Vernon JA, Kaelin C, Meikle MB, Lyons KS, Stewart BJ. Outcomes of clinical trial: tinnitus masking versus tinnitus retraining therapy. J Am Acad Audiol. 2006;17(2):104–32.
101. Henry JA, Schechter MA, Zaugg TL, Griest S, Jastreboff PJ, Vernon JA, Kaelin C, Meikle MB, Lyons KS, Stewart BJ. Clinical trial to compare tinnitus masking and tinnitus retraining therapy. Acta Otolaryngol. 2006;126(sup556):64–9.
102. Vernon JA, Meikle MB. Tinnitus masking. In: Tyler R, editor. Tinnitus Handbook. San Diego: Singular; 2000. p. 313–56.
103. Henry JA, Schechter MA, Nagler SM, Fausti SA. Comparison of tinnitus masking and tinnitus retraining therapy. J Am Acad Audiol. 2002;13(10):559–81.
104. Schechter MA, Henry JA. Assessment and treatment of tinnitus patients using a "masking approach". J Am Acad Audiol. 2002;13(10):545–58.
105. Tyler RS, Noble W, Coelho CB, Ji H. Tinnitus retraining therapy: mixing point and total masking are equally effective. Ear Hear. 2012;33(5):588–94.
106. Von Wedel H, Von Wedel UC, Streppel M, Walger M. Effectiveness of partial and complete instrumental masking in chronic tinnitus. Studies with reference to retraining therapy. HNO. 1997;45(9):690–4.
107. Pryce H, Hall A, Marks E, Culhane BA, Swift S, Straus J, Shaw RL. Shared decision-making in tinnitus care–an exploration of clinical encounters. Br J Health Psychol. 2018;23(3):630–45.
108. Pryce H, Durand MA, Hall A, Shaw R, Culhane BA, Swift S, Straus J, Marks E, Ward M, Chilvers K. The development of a decision aid for tinnitus. Int J Audiol. 2018;57(9):714–9.
109. Hall DA, Smith H, Hibbert A, Colley V, Haider HF, Horobin A, Londero A, Mazurek B, Thacker B, Fackrell K. Core outcome measures in tinnitus (COMiT) initiative. The COMiT'ID study: developing core outcome domains sets for clinical trials of sound-, psychology-, and pharmacology-based interventions for chronic subjective tinnitus in adults. Trends Hear. 2018;22:2331216518814384.

47 Tinnitus Retraining Therapy

Pawel J. Jastreboff and Margaret M. Jastreboff

Abstract

Tinnitus retraining therapy (TRT) is a clinical implementation of the neurophysiological model of tinnitus. The primary goal of TRT is the habituation of reactions evoked by bothersome tinnitus without attempting to remove tinnitus. Habituation is initiated, and further facilitated, using the method of modified passive extinction of conditioned reflexes and involves: (1) teaching/counseling aimed at reclassification of bothersome tinnitus signal (i.e., tinnitus-related neuronal activity) to the category of neutral stimuli and (2) sound therapy, which decreases the strength of the tinnitus signal by providing an enhanced sound background. Once a sufficient level of habituation of reactions is achieved, then habituation of perception occurs automatically.

If present, the decreased sound tolerance is treated concurrently with tinnitus using specific protocols. Many centers reported an over 80% success rate of TRT in the treatment of tinnitus. Specific long-term studies, evaluating the stability of results after stopping of treatment, confirmed the persistence of positive effects with a tendency to further improvement.

P. J. Jastreboff (✉)
Department Otolaryngology, Emory University School of Medicine, Atlanta, GA, USA

JHDF, Inc., Guilford, CT, USA

M. M. Jastreboff
JHDF, Inc., Guilford, CT, USA

W. Schlee et al. (eds.), *Textbook of Tinnitus*, https://doi.org/10.1007/978-3-031-35647-6_47

Graphical Abstract

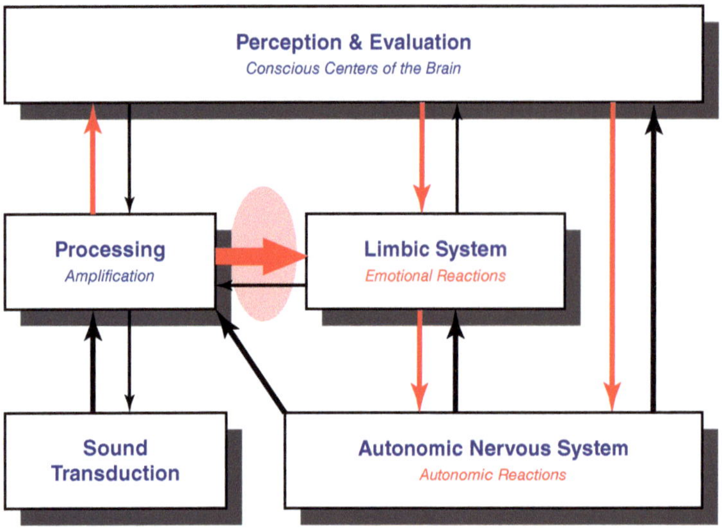

Subconscious functional connections between the auditory and the limbic and autonomic nervous systems are governed by conditioned reflexes and they are responsible for negative reactions of patients with tinnitus.

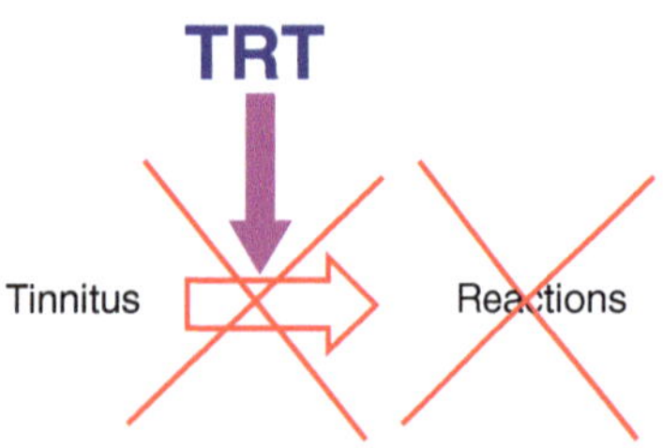

TRT aims at blocking the spread of tinnitus signal from the auditory to other centers in the brain involved in negative reactions. Consequently, in TRT etiology of tinnitus is irrelevant.

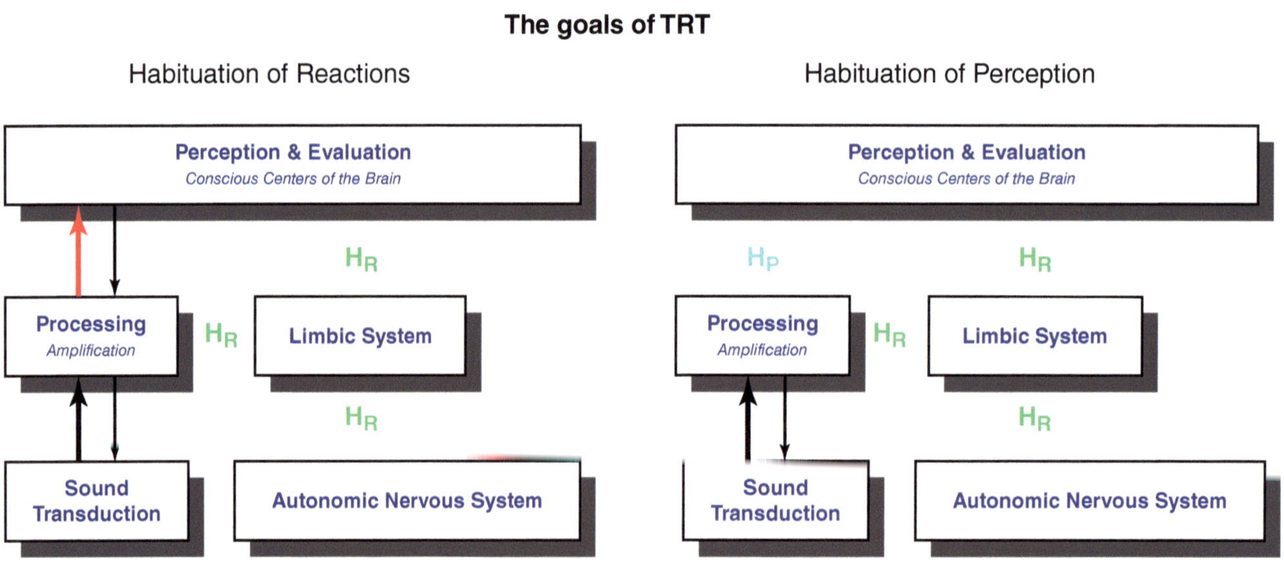

Abbreviations

DPOAE	Distortion Product Otoacoustic Emission
DST	Decreased Sound Tolerance
HA	Hearing Aid
IHC	Inner Hair Cells
LDLs	Loudness Discomfort Levels
MML	Minimal Masking Level
OHC	Outer Hair Cells
TRT	Tinnitus Retraining Therapy

Highlights

1. Tinnitus retraining therapy (TRT) is based on the neurophysiological model of tinnitus.
2. The primary goal of TRT is the habituation of reactions evoked by bothersome tinnitus without attempting to remove or weaken the tinnitus signal.
3. Habituation is initiated and further facilitated using the method of modified passive extinction of the conditioned reflexes and involves:
   (a) Teaching/counseling aimed at reclassification of the signal of bothersome tinnitus to the category of neutral stimuli.
   (b) Sound therapy, which decreases the strength of the tinnitus signal by increasing the level of background neuronal activity in the auditory system, is achieved by providing an enhanced sound background.
4. Once a sufficient level of habituation of reactions is achieved, then habituation of perception takes place automatically.
5. If present, the decreased sound tolerance must be treated first, concurrently with tinnitus.
6. Different protocols need to be used for hyperacusis than for misophonia.
7. Classification of patients into one of 5 categories determines treatment protocol. It is determined by the following factors:
   (a) Impact of tinnitus on patients' lives and/or duration of clinically significant tinnitus.
   (b) The presence of hyperacusis.
   (c) The presence of significant hearing loss.
   (d) Prolonged exacerbation of tinnitus/hyperacusis by sound.
8. Misophonia is treated independently with the use of specific protocols, concurrently with tinnitus, hyperacusis, and hearing loss.
9. Results from many centers have confirmed the effectiveness of TRT for tinnitus treatment, reporting a success rate of more than 80%.
10. Specific studies performed to assess the stability of improvement 18 months and 4 years after stopping the treatment revealed that improvement continued and a trend toward increased improvement was evident.

Outline of Main Concepts of the Neurophysiological Model of Tinnitus Utilized in TRT

Tinnitus retraining therapy (TRT) is a treatment based on the neurophysiological model of tinnitus (see Chap. 20). The model points out the difference between people experiencing tinnitus and those who suffer from it. The experience of tinnitus is frequent and commonly ignored, but unfortunately, the life of some people is negatively affected by it [1]. Tinnitus evokes annoyance, anxiety, and panic and affects concentration, sleep, and ability to enjoy life activities. People with "clinically significant tinnitus" are bothered by it to such an extent that they seek a treatment in an attempt to remove it. It is postulated that in clinically significant tinnitus the neuronal activity, which is perceived as tinnitus (i.e., tinnitus signal), spreads from the auditory pathways to non-auditory parts of the brain, particularly (while not exclusively) to emotional (limbic system) and autonomic nervous systems [2] (see Chap. 20). These two systems are essential and are responsible for negative reactions evoked by tinnitus with the overstimulation of the sympathetic part of the autonomic nervous system playing a crucial role. Other systems in the brain such as the prefrontal cortex, thalamus, reticular formation, and cerebellum are involved as well [3–5].

All systems involved in clinically significant tinnitus may act within the norms, but newly developed inappropriate functional connections are responsible for the presence of negative behavioral reactions. Consequently, utilizing brain plasticity, TRT is aimed at retraining of these abnormal functional connections without trying to modify the tinnitus signal itself, removing or attenuating it, or changing the function of systems involved in tinnitus-evoked reactions. The main goal of TRT is to eliminate reactions induced by tinnitus by preventing the spread of tinnitus signal to other systems in the brain – to achieve habituation of tinnitus-evoked reactions. Habituation of tinnitus perception develops subsequently, and it is inevitable. Brain plasticity is essential and indispensable in developing the habituation of tinnitus.

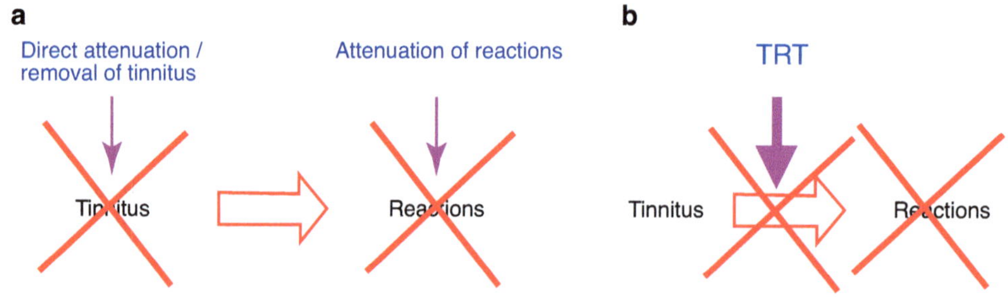

Fig. 47.1 General approaches utilized in tinnitus treatment. (**a**) Aimed at attenuation/removal of tinnitus signal (e.g., medications aimed at the cochlea, electrical stimulation of cochlea or various brain areas, acoustic masking, or aimed at decreasing negative reactions) (e.g., psychotropic medications, improving coping with tinnitus, or other psychological methods); (**b**) TRT approach aimed at blocking connections of the auditory system with parts of the brain involved in negative reactions to tinnitus—habituation of tinnitus. Once these connections are blocked by definition there are no reactions

These principles of the neurophysiological model of tinnitus and TRT are illustrated in Fig. 47.1b and contrasted with other approaches Fig. 47.1a.

Tinnitus retraining therapy (TRT) is a treatment based on the neurophysiological model of tinnitus, which postulated that in the clinically significant tinnitus the neuronal activity, which is perceived as tinnitus (i.e., tinnitus signal) spreads from the auditory pathways to non-auditory parts of the brain, particularly (while not exclusively) to emotional (limbic system) and autonomic nervous systems.

The main goal of TRT is to eliminate reactions induced by tinnitus by preventing the spread of tinnitus signal to other systems in the brain—to achieve habituation of tinnitus evoked reactions. Then a person still perceiving tinnitus, but is not bothered by it anymore. Habituation of tinnitus perception develops subsequently, and it is inevitable. Brain plasticity is essential and indispensable in developing the habituation of tinnitus.

The concept of habituation has been known for a long time and started to be extensively studied from the end of the nineteenth-century [6]. In general terms, habituation describes "becoming accustomed, used to something," enabling us to selectively ignore irrelevant stimuli. Note, that this process has to occur at a subconscious level, and it is impossible to achieve habituation by conscious effort.

It is possible to distinguish between two main categories of negative responses evoked by tinnitus: (1) physiological (e.g., problems with anxiety, depression, sleep, increased stress level) and (2) behavioral responses/consequences (e.g., attention and concentration problems, decreased joy of life, trouble with social interactions, work, family problems) [1].

The successful outcome of TRT leaves a person still perceiving tinnitus, but not being bothered by it anymore, thus achieving habituation of tinnitus-evoked reactions. Notably, once a sufficient level of habituation of reactions is achieved, habituation of perception automatically follows and a person is gradually aware of tinnitus for smaller proportions of time as the brain automatically habituates and disregards all stimuli that are not important [1, 7]. An individual with tinnitus changes from being a tinnitus sufferer to a person who just experiences tinnitus and is not bothered by it. It is important to note that this treatment will not work when attempts are made to induce habituation of perception first before achieving habituation of reactions [1, 8] (see Fig. 47.2).

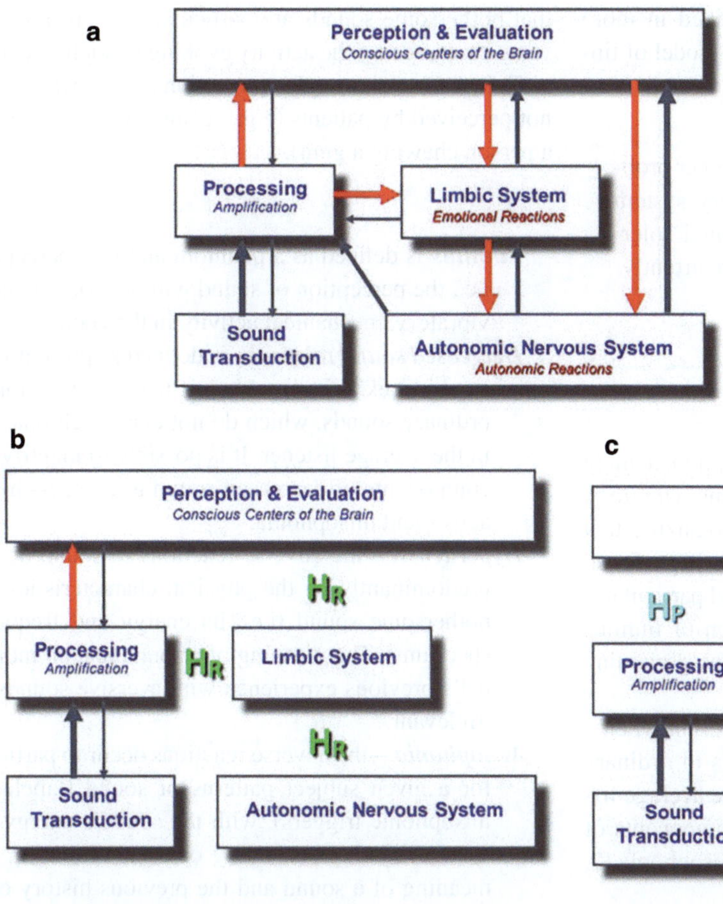

Fig. 47.2 The figure presents a simplified diagram of the block diagram of the model presented in accompanied Chap. 20 as shown to the patients. (**a**) Interconnections between the auditory and the limbic and autonomic nervous systems in patients suffering from tinnitus. (**b**) Primary goal of TRT, i.e., habituation of reactions (removing tinnitus-induced negative reactions by preventing the spread of tinnitus signal to other parts of the brain). The subject still perceives tinnitus, but she/he is not bothered by it. (**c**) Habituation of reactions and perception of tinnitus

Clinical Goals of Tinnitus Retraining Therapy

TRT is a habituation-based treatment that utilizes counseling to decrease the strength of tinnitus-evoked reactions and sound to decrease the strength of the tinnitus signal. The primary goal of TRT is to achieve habituation of tinnitus-evoked negative reactions and remove the effect of tinnitus on patients' lives. As pointed out above, once habituation of reactions has been achieved at least partially, habituation of perception develops automatically without the need for any additional action. At the end of a successful treatment, people are not bothered by tinnitus (or bothered very little), even when perceiving it, and tinnitus has no impact on their lives. Additionally, their awareness of tinnitus typically drops to 10–20% of their waking time.

As postulated by the neurophysiological model, tinnitus should not be treated disregarding other problems and dysfunctions involving the auditory system (including hearing loss and decreased sound tolerance). These problems should be treated concurrently as they are interacting with each other and treating only one in isolation with the other problems will be much less successful.

The idea of TRT, first introduced over 30 years ago, is based on a particular view on tinnitus and its treatment. Therefore, definitions of tinnitus and decreased sound tolerance (hyperacusis and misophonia), as referred to in this chapter, will be briefly presented here (described in more detail in the chapter on the neurophysiological model of tinnitus [7] (see Chap. 20).

Tinnitus should not be treated disregarding other problems and dysfunction involving the auditory system (including hearing loss and decreased sound tolerance). These problems should be treated concurrently.

Definitions

Tinnitus is defined as a phantom auditory perception, namely the perception of sound without corresponding vibratory, mechanical activity in the cochlea [1, 9]. Recognizing that tinnitus is a phantom auditory perception has a profound impact on the approach to tinnitus treatment and particularly at sound therapy as it specifies that interaction of tinnitus with external sounds is not following the rules governing interactions of external sounds [7].

Decreased sound tolerance is defined as present when a subject exhibits any kind of negative reactions to ordinary sounds, which do not elicit such reactions in the average listener [10–12]. It is possible to identify two components of decreased sound tolerance—hyperacusis and misophonia [2, 13, 14].

A characteristic property of ***hyperacusis*** is that the reactions to sound depend predominantly on the physical characteristics of a bothersome sound, such as its energy and frequency spectrum. The meaning of a sound and an individual's previous experience with aversive sounds are irrelevant [1, 13, 14]. It has been proposed that the neural mechanisms of hyperacusis involve abnormally high amplification within the auditory system, with activation of other centers in the brain responsible for negative reactions (i.e., the limbic and autonomic nervous systems) occurring only as a secondary consequence [14].

A characteristic feature of ***misophonia*** is that the adverse reactions occur to particular for a given subject patterns of sound (labeled as misophonic triggers), with the sound's energy and spectrum being secondary or even irrelevant. The meaning of a sound and the previous history of an individual relevant to this sound are crucial. Frequently described misophonic triggers include, e.g., boiling water, sound of a refrigerator, crumpling or wrinkling paper, hum of a computer, laughter, nail clipping breathing, sounds of eating, swallowing, chewing, flushing toilet, dog walking on a hardwood floor. Note, that there is nothing particular or specific about the misophonic triggers themselves, and any sound can become a bothersome misophonic trigger. "Specific/particular" is directed to the relation of "a sound" to "a patient," i.e., that bothersome sounds are particular to a given patient. In some cases, seeing the activity evoking misophonic trigger is sufficient to evoke negative reactions, even when sound is not perceived by patients (e.g., seeing a lawn mower, seeing a person chewing a gum).

Tinnitus is defined as a phantom auditory perception, i.e., the perception of sound without corresponding vibratory, mechanical activity in the cochlea.

Decreased sound tolerance is defined as present when a subject exhibits any kind of negative reactions to ordinary sounds, which do not elicit such reactions in the average listener. It is possible to identify two components of decreased sound tolerance—hyperacusis and misophonia.

Hyperacusis—the adverse reactions to sound depend predominantly on the physical characteristics of a bothersome sound (i.e., its energy and frequency spectrum). The meaning of a sound and an individual's previous experience with aversive sounds are irrelevant.

Misophonia—the adverse reactions occur to particular for a given subject patterns of sound (labeled as misophonic triggers), with the sound's energy and spectrum being secondary or even irrelevant. The meaning of a sound and the previous history of an individual relevant to this sound are crucial.

Postulated mechanisms of hyperacusis and misophonia differs significantly. The mechanisms of hyperacusis reflects abnormally strong reactivity of the subconscious part of the auditory pathways to sound, which in turn yields the activation of the limbic and autonomic nervous systems (Fig. 4a in [7]). The mechanism of misophonia involves the development of conditioned reflexes linking specific patterns of a sound with a negative reinforcement ([14] Fig. 4b in [7]) In people with misophonia, the auditory system itself functions normally; however, selective connections from the auditory system to the limbic and autonomic nervous systems for certain sound patterns are abnormally created or intensified.

Methods of Collecting Information Needed for Diagnosis

Structured Interviews and Questionnaires

Before starting the treatment, proper identification of patients' problems and comprehensive diagnosis are crucial. While following the main ideas of the neurophysiological model of tinnitus, the specific implementation of TRT for tinnitus, hyperacusis, and misophonia is not the same. Patients' detailed initial interview is crucial and audiological evaluation alone is not sufficient for proper diagnosis.

To efficiently collect information about patients' complaints the use of structured interviews and forms for facilitating the interview is suggested [15–17]. The examples of such forms for initial and follow-up visits are attached in Appendix A. The structured interview form consists of a series of questions and scales, which allow to assess the specifics and severity of existing problems as well as to follow their changes during subsequent follow-up contacts.

While the information provided by the interview gives good insight into many aspects of tinnitus and decreased sound tolerance (DST) and allows to predict the extent of problems with a high level of accuracy, it is used only as a secondary measure and it is necessary to use generally accepted, validated questionnaires as a primary measure of severity and treatment outcome [18–21]. The changes of the scores over time offer an accepted and internationally comparable way to monitor the treatment progress and outcome. There are many questionnaires available for tinnitus. Unfortunately, at the moment, no questionnaires are allowing to distinguish hyperacusis from misophonia.

> While the information provided by the interview gives good insight into many aspects of tinnitus and DST and allows to predict the extent of problems with a high level of accuracy, it is used only as a secondary measure and it is necessary to use generally accepted, validated questionnaires as a primary measure of severity and treatment outcome.

Questions asked to differentiate between hyperacusis and misophonia focus on finding out whether there are inconsistencies between the extent of negative reactions and acoustical characteristics of sounds. In the case of hyperacusis, the reactions depend on sound intensity with a tendency to stronger reactions to sounds with a higher proportion of high-frequency components (e.g., clicking dishes, knife hitting china). In the case of misophonia, as described earlier, the reactions depend on other factors and patients can listen to some loud sound without a problem while other, softer sounds are bothersome (e.g., boiling water, sound of a refrigerator, crumpling or wrinkling paper, hum of a computer, laughter, nail clipping, breathing, sounds of eating, swallowing, chewing, flushing toilet, and dog walking on a hardwood floor). Questions aimed at finding out whether reactions to a sound depend on the situation and who is generating it are important as well. It is one of the factors differentiating misophonia from hyperacusis.

Audiological Evaluation

Many tinnitus patients have DST that is negatively affecting their lives and requires intervention. Additionally, approximately 80% of tinnitus patients have hearing loss as well. The main role of audiological evaluation is to assess to which extent hearing loss is hindering perception of the environmental sounds, creates problems with communication, and affects everyday life while coexisting with tinnitus. Determination of sound tolerance is crucial as well. It has an impact on the overall diagnosis of coexisting problems, counseling, and determining a choice of sound therapy. In this respect, normal values of loudness discomfort levels (LDLs) allow for eliminating the presence of hyperacusis.

> Recommended audiological evaluation includes (1) pure-tone audiometry (up to at least 12 kHz); (2) evaluation of speech discrimination in quiet; (3) determination of pure-tone Loudness Discomfort Levels (LDLs); (4) determination of speech discomfort level (UCL); (5) high-frequency resolution distortion product otoacoustic emission (DPOAE); (6) psychoacoustical evaluation of tinnitus (pitch and loudness match and minimum masking levels—MMLs).

Audiogram and speech discrimination scores delineate the patient's hearing ability. Expanded frequency range including ultrahigh frequencies is particularly helpful in young patients and in patients with misophonia as misophonic patients are more sensitive to the presence of distortions, which predominantly are present in higher frequencies. Furthermore, comparing hearing tested up to at least 12 kHz (where typically some hearing loss is present), with LDLs helps in differentiation between hyperacusis and misophonia. Evaluation of speech discrimination in quiet provides guidance when amplification (e.g., hearing aids) is needed in patients with tinnitus and hearing loss.

LDLs are crucial to exclude the presence of hyperacusis and are helpful in assessing the presence and extent of misophonia. Note, that testing of acoustic reflexes and reflex decay is not recommended as a part of routine evaluation. Since a large proportion of patients with tinnitus have decreased sound tolerance as well, the exposure to loud sounds (necessary for testing acoustic reflexes) may cause worsening of their symptoms (particularly misophonia) and make subsequent interaction with patients more difficult.

Patients without DST have an average value of LDLs of about 100 dB HL. Comparison of the shape of audiogram and shape of LDLs is helpful in differentiation of hyperacusis from misophonia, and this is one of the reasons why it is recommended to measure LDLs for all frequencies measured in the audiogram (see Fig. 47.3). In the case of pure hyper-

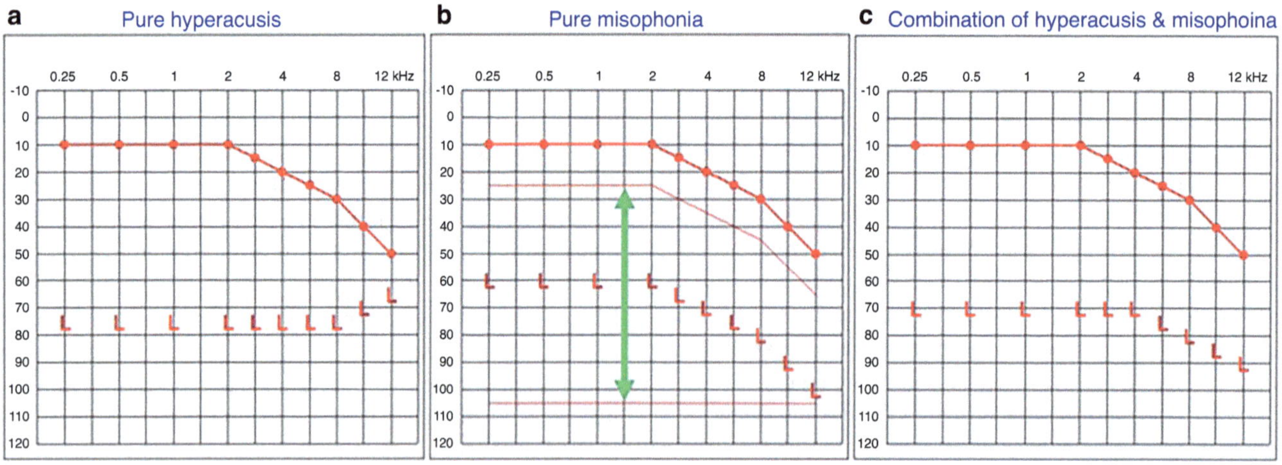

Fig. 47.3 Comparison of shapes of audiograms and LDLs typically observed in the clinic. (**a**) Pure hyperacusis (note flat LDLs independent of audiogram with a tendency to lower values for higher frequencies); (**b**) pure misophonia (note comparable shapes of audiogram and LDLs which is observed not only for shown typical high-frequency hearing loss but is observed for all configurations of hearing loss); (**c**) mixture of hyperacusis and misophonia (note stable LDLs until HL become stronger)

acusis, the values of LDLs are decreased, but the values are constant, since in hyperacusis reaction depends on the total energy carried by a sound, which is not dependent on the hearing threshold but depends on physical properties of a sound. There is a tendency of LDLs being even worse at higher frequencies [1, 13].

In case of misophonia, due to recruitment induced by the presence of hearing loss, patients will have a tendency to perceive sounds as having similar loudness, which are at the same distance from the hearing threshold (Sensation Level). Consequently, many individuals with misophonia react to sounds perceived as "louder than" a certain level, yielding LDLs values following the shape of the audiogram. This promotes recommendation for testing hearing and LDLs to at least 12 kHz as majority of people have some hearing loss for this frequency.

> LDLs are crucial to exclude the presence of hyperacusis and are helpful in assessing the presence and extent of misophonia. Comparison of the shape of audiogram and shape of LDLs is helpful in differentiation hyperacusis from misophonia.

Results of DPOAEs are extremely helpful during counseling, especially in patients with tinnitus and normal hearing, when discussing discordant dysfunction theory is particularly useful [1, 9] (presented later in the chapter).

Evaluation of psychoacoustical properties of tinnitus (pitch and loudness match and MMLs is done for counseling purposes only.

Diagnosis

The following information is used for diagnosis, identification of patient categories, and consequently, recommended treatment specifications: (1) impact of tinnitus on patients' lives and/or the duration of clinically significant tinnitus; (2) the presence and significance of hearing loss; (3) hyperacusis; and (4) prolonged exacerbation of tinnitus/hyperacusis by sound. Note, that the presence of misophonia is not affecting categorization.

Impact of Tinnitus on Patients' Lives and/or Duration of Clinically Significant Tinnitus

The severity of tinnitus varies significantly between patients, and tinnitus variably affects patients' lives. The severity of tinnitus reflects the strength of neuronal connections involved in the processing of tinnitus signal. In the case of low severity tinnitus, the connections are likely to be weaker. In recently developed clinically significant tinnitus (just during the past last few weeks) even when patients report severe tinnitus, the connections are still relatively weak due to lack of sufficient time needed to establish strong neuronal connections. Note, that the duration of the symptoms to be taken into account relates to *clinically significant tinnitus* and not the duration of the tinnitus perception or duration of non-bothersome tinnitus. Tinnitus may be present and perceived for many years, without bothering a person, before becoming a problem.

The Presence and Significance of Hearing Loss

As mentioned before, as much as 80% of individuals with tinnitus have some degree of hearing loss (typically less than 60 dB HL in the frequency range up to 8 kHz), which may have an impact on their everyday life. The same degree of hearing loss can be of large significance to one person (e.g., professions requiring communication in noise or musicians) while having no significance to another person (e.g., farmers or computer programmers working from home). Hearing loss may induce a "strain to hear" effect in everyday life, which increases stress levels and frequently results in worsening of tinnitus as well.

Hearing loss decreases stimulation of the auditory pathways by environmental sounds and as such has a tendency to increase the strength of the tinnitus signal. Note that hearing loss commonly affects the higher frequencies range. At the same time, there is less sound energy in an environment in this frequency range. Due to the tonotopic organization of all parts of the auditory pathways, including the auditory cortex, the high-frequency areas of the brain are understimulated mimicking a situation similar to Heller and Bergman's experiment when keeping subjects in a low level of sound environment, which was sufficient to induce tinnitus [22].

Hyperacusis

> There is a need to differentiate between hyperacusis and misophonia as their treatments are distinctively different. A detailed interview typically provides enough information to differentiate these problems. A positive diagnosis of hyperacusis requires that the average value of LDLs is less than 90 dB. However, low values of LDLs do not prove the presence of hyperacusis, as a low value of LDLs may be due to misophonia. The behavioral reactions evoked by hyperacusis and misophonia are very similar, frequently identical, thus they cannot be used for differentiation either.

The presence of hyperacusis requires specific counseling and creates some limitations during the use of sound therapy, as compared with tinnitus sound therapy. Additionally, there is a need to differentiate between hyperacusis and misophonia as their treatments are distinctively different. On the behavioral level problems reported by hyperacusis and misophonic patient are very similar causing that the distinction between hyperacusis and misophonia is complex. A detailed interview, together with a comparison of the shape of a person's audiogram and that of the LDLs, typically provides enough information to differentiate these problems [13, 14]. A positive diagnosis of hyperacusis requires that the average value of LDLs is less than 90 dB (typically in the 70–80 dB HL range). However, low values of LDLs do not prove the presence of hyperacusis, as a low value of LDLs may be due to misophonia as well. The behavioral reactions evoked by hyperacusis and misophonia are very similar, frequently identical, thus they cannot be used exclusively for differentiation either. A detailed interview with attention to specific sounds evoking negative reactions (misophonic triggers) and other sounds is crucial. During the interview, the focus is on detecting whether the characteristic features of misophonia are present (such as the independence of reaction from acoustical/physical characterization of the bothersome sounds, the ability to tolerate some sounds with *energy* larger than bothersome sounds, the dependence of reactions on a place, situation or who is making/producing sound [7, 14]. If the patient's problems include tinnitus, hyperacusis, and hearing loss, the first phase of treatment always focuses on treating the hyperacusis.

Prolonged Exacerbation of Tinnitus/Hyperacusis by Sound

> Short-lasting worsening is common and irrelevant for the treatment.

Many patients report that their tinnitus and/or DST becomes worse for some time (ranging from minutes to hours) after exposure to sound (loud, moderate, or even soft). This short-lasting worsening is common and irrelevant for the treatment. Some patients, however, report that this effect persists to the next day, even after a "good night's sleep," or sometimes lasts even for several days. This prolonged worsening may be due to (1) "kindling" or "wind-up" phenomena [1, 17], (2) or due to strong misophonia. "Kindling" is a term from the field of epilepsy that describes the phenomenon when a weak stimulus that initially does not evoke a seizure evokes epileptic seizures after being presented repeatedly over a period of time. The "wind-up" phenomenon is a term from the field of chronic pain. It describes the situation when the second presentation of a painful stimuli causes a stronger reaction than the first one. Another situation is when a stimulus is presented for a limited time (e.g., a few minutes) it is not painful, but when the duration is longer, it becomes painful. This is similar to what happens when a sound, which initially is without any effect, causes a worsening of tinnitus or hyperacusis after it has been presented for a longer period. Worsening of tinnitus or hyperacusis can be observed in some medical conditions, which affect functions of the brain in a significant manner, e.g., brain injury (after a car accident), blast injury (e.g., during military operations), brain surgery, and some hormonal changes (e.g., menopause). It is worth checking for the presence of undiagnosed and untreated Lyme disease as it has been reported that hyperacusis was present in 48% of Lyme disease cases [23]. Since untreated Lyme disease can cause significant brain impairment, it is not surprising that some patients report the presence of this effect similar to patients with brain injury.

In cases with long-term worsening the presence of undiagnosed and untreated Lyme Disease should be done as it has been reported that hyperacusis was present in 48% of Lyme Disease cases.

In the past, it was not recognized that the presence of misophonia may result in the perception of prolonged worsening of tinnitus and/or hyperacusis after sound exposure. People with tinnitus sometimes become afraid of sound (phonophobia). They are afraid that exposure to sound may cause their tinnitus to become permanently worse. Consequently, they start avoiding sounds (or start using ear protection) causing enhancement of tinnitus, which results in a prolonged worsening of the problem. Clinical observations showed that most patients with prolonged worsening had misophonia and only a small proportion of patients experienced a relevant medical problem. Nevertheless, when prolonged worsening of tinnitus and/or hyperacusis after sound exposure is reported by a patient, potential medical reasons should be considered.

Most patients with prolonged worsening had misophonia and only a small proportion of patients experience a relevant medical problem.

Recognizing the four factors discussed above [1, 8, 24] five main categories of patients were identified, and a specific variant of TRT treatment associated with each one of the categories has been proposed (see Table 47.1). These categories provide general treatment directions. It is important to recognize that there is a continuum of patients' problems and treatment. Notice, presence of misophonia is not affecting categorization, and misophonia is treated independently.

Table 47.1 Concise description of patients' categorization and main features of elements of TRT used. Abbreviations: *T.* tinnitus, *H.* hyperacusis, *HL* hearing loss, *SG* sound generators, *HA* hearing aids, *Combi* combination instruments

Cat	Problem	Counseling	Sound therapy
0	T (and/or H) is of low severity or developed very recently. Normal hearing	Abbreviated, focused on understanding habituation, reassurance	"Avoid silence." SG not suggested
1	T is significant, established problem. No H or HL	Extensive, related to T	"Avoiding silence" SG used as much as possible during waking time with the sound set close but below level evoking annoyance. Stable sound level during the block of time of their use
2	T and HL are both problems	Extensive, with stress on issues related to consequences of HL	"Avoid silence" Combi with SG part set as for Cat 1. HAs used to counteract the effects of sound introduced from SGs and to enhance the frequency range and amount of enriched sound background
3	H is the dominant problem, T and/or HL may or maybe not present	Focused on mechanisms of H. T and/or HL, if present, are briefly discussed during first session and addressed in more detail later in the treatment	"Avoid silence" SGs (or SG part of Combi) used as in Cat 1 but with the recommendation of increasing their level before entering the environment with expected bothersome sound. Even more stress on sound use 24/7 than in Cat 1
4	T and/or H are problems that worsen for a prolonged period of time after sound exposure	Highly individual, with exploring medical issues which may be involved	"Avoid silence" Highly individual with stress on avoiding sound level which may trigger worsening

Misophonia is treated independently with specific counseling and sound therapy from the very beginning of the treatment. It is not affecting categorization and described above recommendations related to a specific category

Category 0

Patients in Category 0 experience tinnitus or hyperacusis with a low degree of severity, or a problem developed relatively recently. They experience normal hearing. They need abbreviated counseling, with information focused on reclassification of tinnitus into a category of neutral stimuli. The problem should not be discussed as worse than currently reported, and patients should be advised about the enrichment of background sound. Hyperacusis patients need counseling regarding ear overprotection, avoiding silence, and benefits of the use of environmental sounds.

While an initial visit is typically sufficient to achieve a noticeable improvement in these patients, short follow-up visits or telephone/video contacts after the initial visit are recommended.

Category 1

Patients in Category 1 have significant tinnitus, no hyperacusis. They do not have hearing loss significantly affecting their life, or experience sound-induced prolonged worsening of tinnitus. The treatment involves intensive counseling focused on the patient's tinnitus. If present, misophonia is addressed as well. Patients are advised to avoid silence, and more extensive sound therapy including the use of ear-level instruments is strongly suggested (see more about sound therapy and instruments later in this chapter). Follow-up visits, supplemented with telephone or Internet contacts, are more frequent (at 1, 2, 3 months) at the beginning of the treatment, than after 3 months. This is continued in 6 month intervals for up to 9–18 months, which is usually the duration of the treatment.

Category 2

Patients classified as Category 2 differ from Category 1 by the presence of significant hearing loss. Extensive counseling similar as in Category 1 is advised, but stress is put on issues focusing on the aspects of hearing loss that impact tinnitus, as well as the hearing loss itself. Similarly, as in Category 1, follow-up visits with particular attention to the use of sound enrichment are recommended.

Category 3

Patients in Category 3 may suffer from tinnitus and may have misophonia as well, but they have significant hyperacusis. In the first stage of the therapy, stress is put on the treatment of hyperacusis while other coexisting hearing problems are concurrently addressed. Consequently, the counseling session focuses on central mechanisms controlling amplification within the auditory pathways. Discussion of sound therapy aimed at desensitization is crucial. At the beginning of treatment, contacts with these patients are frequent and LDLs measurements are repeated. In most patients with the proper treatment, their problem with hyperacusis is resolved in half a year. At this point, other problems reported by patients are directly addressed.

Category 4

Patients in Category 4 may have tinnitus and/or hyperacusis, and they experience a prolonged exacerbation of their worst problem (typically, hyperacusis). This worsening may last at least "after a good night's sleep," and is not resulting from effects of misophonia, which is treated independently.

The treatment of patients experiencing a long-lasting worsening of hyperacusis or tinnitus who do not have relevant medically treatable problems is challenging. It requires extensive counseling and many adjustments in sound therapy tailored to the needs of the individual patient. The patient's understanding of physiological mechanisms which are utilized in TRT is particularly important.

- Category 0—tinnitus or hyperacusis with a low degree of severity, or a problem developed relatively recently.
- Category 1—significant tinnitus, no hyperacusis. They do not have hearing loss significantly affecting their life, or experience sound-induced prolonged worsening of tinnitus.
- Category 2—differ from Category 1 by the presence of significant hearing loss.
- Category 3—significant hyperacusis; may suffer from tinnitus and may have misophonia as well.
- Category 4—prolonged exacerbation of their worst problem (typically, hyperacusis); may have tinnitus and/or hyperacusis.

Treatment

Combined information from initial interview and audiological evaluation allows for diagnosis of existing hearing disorders, for determination of their relative impact on the patient's life and adjusting both counseling and sound therapy to the needs of the individual patient. The goal of TRT is

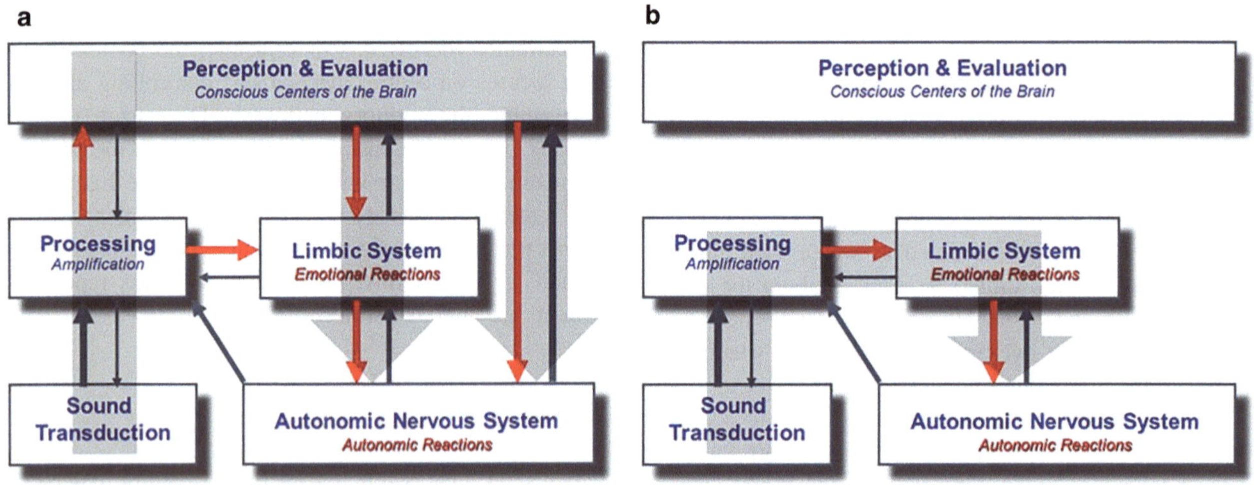

Fig. 47.4 Two loops transmitting tinnitus signal to the autonomic nervous system—(**a**) high loop, (involving cognition, verbalizations, and conscious analysis) and (**b**) low loop, connecting the auditory system with the limbic and autonomic nervous systems at a subconscious level

to neutralize neural functional confections, which are responsible for the overstimulation of the limbic and sympathetic part of the autonomic nervous systems by the tinnitus signal. Overexcitation of these systems is responsible for behavioral and physiological negative tinnitus-evoked reactions. In this process, brain plasticity plays a crucial role.

Discussion of clinical goals of TRT is an important part of counseling. Two loops linking tinnitus signal in the auditory system with systems involved in reactions to tinnitus can be recognized – the "low" subconscious loop and "high" loop which involves higher, cognitive areas and functions in the brain (Fig. 47.4a, b). These loops and their role have been extensively discussed, including a description in the chapter on the neurophysiological model of tinnitus (see Chap. 20) [1, 7]. Analysis of the contribution of various attributes of tinnitus in patients revealed that the low, subconscious loop (Fig. 47.4b) plays a dominant role in chronic, clinically significant tinnitus [25]. Consequently, it is postulated that clinical efforts in tinnitus treatment should focus on extinction (removal) of this subconscious loop.

Two loops exist linking tinnitus signal in the auditory system with systems involved in reactions to tinnitus—the "low" subconscious loop and "high" loop which involves higher, cognitive areas, and functions in the brain (Fig. 47.4).

The low, subconscious loop plays a dominant role in chronic, clinically significant tinnitus.

Consequently, clinical efforts in tinnitus treatment should focus on extinction (removal) of this subconscious loop.

The extent of excitation of the autonomic nervous system represents a sum of activity carried by the conscious path (high loop) and the subconscious path (low loop). There is no method allowing to directly modify the function of the low loop; but the high loop, which involves cognition, perception, and analysis, can be modified by appropriate counseling. Clinical data indicate that subconscious connections play a dominant role in chronic tinnitus [7, 25]. Therefore, when performing TRT, the focus is on restoring ("retraining") the functional connections which create this low loop.

Retraining of Conditioned Reflexes

From the time of Pavlov, it is well known that a conditioned reflex (created by simultaneous exposure of a subject to a sensory stimulus and a reinforcement), undergoes extinction if reinforcement is removed (e.g., in the classical example of the Pavlovian dog, the bell keeps ringing but the food is no longer given). This process is known as passive extinction of conditioned reflexes, or habituation of reaction [1, 26]. Unfortunately, while effective, this technique cannot be applied in its original form to tinnitus (or misophonia) because negative reinforcement is provided by reactions of the limbic and autonomic nervous systems and cannot be removed. Consequently, the reflexes are self-reinforcing. This observation explains why spontaneous habituation of established, clinically significant tinnitus is not observed. A comparable situation exists for misophonia, with the difference being that the neuronal activity evoking negative reactions from the limbic and autonomic nervous systems is induced by external sounds (misophonic triggers) rather than by internally generated neuronal activity within the auditory system, as is the case with tinnitus.

The process of passive extinction of conditioned reflexes is known as well as habituation of reaction.
The modified version of passive extinction of conditioned reflexes, using a simultaneous decrease of the sensory signal and decrease of reinforcement is used in TRT.

To solve the problem of retraining self-reinforced conditioned reflexes, the modified version of passive extinction of conditioned reflexes was introduced. This version uses a simultaneous decrease of the sensory signal and decrease of reinforcement [1]. In the case of the Pavlovian dog, it would correspond to making the ringing of the bell softer and giving less food, which is not as tasty. Note that to create a conditioned reflex it is necessary to present a conditioned stimulus (e.g., sound) and a reinforcement (e.g., electrical shock) at the same time or close in time. The same principle applies when an attempt is made to modify the established reflex—modification of the strength of sensory stimulus, and strength of reinforcement should be present at the same time. Therefore, it is important that decrease of both the strength of tinnitus signal and the negative reactions evoked by tinnitus occurs concurrently, and patients' counseling visit is close in time with the starting of the sound therapy, which is introduced to decrease the strength of the tinnitus signal.

It is impossible to modify the activity of the subconscious low loop directly [1], but it is possible to attenuate and finally remove the contribution of cognitive components (the high loop—Fig. 47.4a). As both, the high and low loops contribute to the final activation of the limbic and autonomic nervous systems, the decrease of activation of these systems can be achieved by removing, or at least decreasing, the transmission and processing of tinnitus signals in the high loop, thus removing its contribution. This process is effective, but it requires more time than classical passive extinction when reinforcement is totally removed. These interventions must be carried on for some time to obtain good results.

Decreasing the contribution of the upper loop can be accomplished by (1) reclassifying tinnitus to the category of neutral stimuli, (2) showing its benign character, (3) providing an explanation about its origin and mechanisms, and (4) pointing out that the patients reacts properly but to a wrong stimulus. It is important to answer patients' questions as well. It is possible to eliminate transmission of the tinnitus signal in the high loop in a relatively short time. Unfortunately, even complete interruption of tinnitus signal processing and transmission in the high loop is not sufficient to eliminate negative reactions evoked by the tinnitus because the low, subconscious loop remains active and unchanged, providing overstimulation of the limbic and autonomic nervous systems by the tinnitus signal.

Decreasing the contribution of the upper loop can be accomplished by

1. Reclassifying tinnitus to the category of neutral stimuli.
2. Showing its benign character.
3. Providing an explanation about its origin and mechanisms.
4. Pointing out that the patients reacts properly but to a wrong stimulus.

Another, more general mechanism of attenuation of the effects of the high loop in tinnitus is based on the fact that people react stronger to unknown dangers than to even significant but known dangers. Therefore, once patients are able to understand and predict the behavior of their tinnitus (e.g., typical increase of the tinnitus when in quiet places or in a stressful situation) and their own increased reactions to tinnitus, they may still be annoyed and bothered by tinnitus, but gradually to a smaller extent. The decrease of the strength of the tinnitus signal is achieved by sound therapy (described subsequently)

With time, the negative reactions to tinnitus or misophonia will undergo gradual extinction. On average, patients show clear improvement after just 1–3 months of TRT treatment. The total treatment typically takes 9–18 months as seen in the literature describing results from various centers and is reported to be successful in about 80% of patients [27–45].

Unfortunately, while searching for information and answers, many patients acquire a lot of misconceptions and worry about their tinnitus. This frequently causes an initially not bothersome problem to become much worse and more threatening. Patients believe that tinnitus is a significant health issue. This became a strong obstacle in the habituation-based treatment as it is particularly difficult to habituate stimuli, which have strong negative connotations. Therefore, the intensive teaching about tinnitus origin, its mechanism, and benign nature of its perception, demystification of tinnitus, is crucial to remove the negative impact of cognitive processes, which prevent achieving extinction of subconscious conditioned reflexes, dominant for inducing negative reactions to tinnitus.

Proper counseling can relatively easily modify the functional connections from the cognitive areas down to the limbic and autonomic nervous systems and other parts of the brain, but only indirectly affects the subconscious connections between the auditory system and the limbic and autonomic nervous systems. In conclusion, counseling alone is helpful by consistently decreasing the negative impact of conscious thinking on the limbic and autonomic nervous systems, but there is a need to utilize other methods specific to retrain the conditioned reflexes.

Specific General Aspects of Counseling for Tinnitus Patients with Hearing Loss

Tinnitus and hearing loss coexist very frequently. Typically, patients blame tinnitus for problems that are known to result from hearing loss. Many patients believe that tinnitus causes or is closely related to hearing loss and with progressing hearing loss tinnitus is going to become worse. Some patients believe that tinnitus masks speech, causing problems with understanding. All these (incorrect) beliefs are discussed during counseling sessions.

Some tinnitus patients have normal or almost normal hearing and often intensively search for the cause of their tinnitus. In this situation the discussion of the concept of Discordant Dysfunction Theory, supported by the results of DPOAE, is particularly useful. This theory has risen from the clinical and research observations that tinnitus emerges when outer hair cells (OHC) are affected, while inner hair cells (IHC) are in better functional condition [1, 9]. A classic example of that is aspirin. A high dose of aspirin (above 7 g) evokes tinnitus in 100% of people. The effect is fully reversible, and tinnitus disappears 24–48 h after stopping aspirin administration. Research has shown that such a dose of aspirin causes OHC to lose their normal internal turgor. While they survive, they are unable to transfer their vibration to structures of the organ of Corti. They become dysfunctional. At the same time, aspirin is not affecting the functionality of IHC. Another good example is tinnitus induced by cisplatin, but then tinnitus is permanent due to OHC being destroyed by this medication.

The IHC and OHC are innervated by two different types of fibers in the auditory nerve—Type I for IHC and Type II for OHC. Discordant Dysfunction Theory postulates that the tinnitus related neuronal activity (i.e., tinnitus signal) is generated in the dorsal cochlear nucleus, as a result of discordant information coming from IHC and OHC (Type I and Type II auditory nerve fibers respectively) [9, 46]. Each part of the cochlear basilar membrane where the OHC are dysfunctional or damaged, while IHC are still functioning reasonably well, acts as a source of a tinnitus signal. The strength of the signal depends on the difference in functional properties between OHC and IHC that are localized on a particular part of the basilar membrane. If there is only one area with a discordant dysfunction of OHC and IHC, the subject will perceive tonal tinnitus. However, in typical cases of complex tinnitus perception, the final tinnitus is composed of signals created by many local sources. Tinnitus signal is further enhanced in the subconscious part of the auditory pathways; and finally perceived at the cortical level [1, 9]. The Discordant Dysfunction Theory has been supported by an animal experiment which showed relation of neuronal hyperactivity in dorsal cochlear nucleus to the extent of OHC damage, Interestingly, as predicted by discordant dysfunction theory the hyperactivity decreased when IHC were damaged as well [47].

Discordant Dysfunction Theory can explain several observations inexplicable by other theories:

1. noise exposure as the main factor associated with inducing tinnitus perception,
2. salicylate (aspirin), quinine, cisplatin as the most powerful drugs to induce tinnitus,
3. tinnitus in patients with normal hearing,
4. absence of tinnitus in total deafness,
5. pitch of tinnitus associated with the bottom of the audiogram slope.

In this respect, high-frequency resolution DPOAE (8–10 points per octave) is very useful as it allows documentation of the presence of minor irregularities in OHC functionality. This observation is extremely helpful in counseling all patients with tinnitus, and particularly with tinnitus and normal hearing. Discordant Dysfunction Theory, supported by results of DPOAE, allows to show patients that indeed there is something incorrect with their hearing, but this is irrelevant from the point of view of their ability to hear, and that tinnitus does not indicate medical problems.

General Aspects of Counseling for Patients with Decreased Sound Tolerance (DST)

In patients with hyperacusis, counseling is shorter than in patients with tinnitus and focuses on presumed neural mechanisms of hyperacusis, i.e., abnormally high amplification within the subconscious part of the auditory pathways. The activation of other centers of the brain responsible for patients' negative reactions to sound occur only as a secondary consequence [14]. During counseling, this concept is presented to patients, and the focus is put on the role of sound therapy. Pure hyperacusis is relatively rare and hyperacusis commonly coexists with misophonia. In cases of strong hyperacusis, misophonia is created automatically as negative reactions evoked by hyperacusis serve as a negative reinforcement and create conditioned reflexes which become the basis for misophonia [48]. Moreover, when hyperacusis coexisting with misophonia is successfully treated, then the misophonic component increases, and at behavioral level, only a small or negligible change may be observed. These issues need to be carefully discussed with the patient as it does not necessarily indicate unsuccessful treatment of hyperacusis.

Pure hyperacusis is relatively rare and hyperacusis commonly coexists with misophonia.
When hyperacusis coexisting with misophonia is successfully treated, then the misophonic component increases, and at behavioral level, only a small or negligible change may be observed.

In patients with misophonia, the counseling focuses on the demystification of mechanisms of misophonia, with stress on answering questions such as why it is impossible to ignore reactions to misophonic triggers, why misophonia has developed, and explaining in detail the protocols to be used for removing these reactions. In addition to part of the counseling that follows, the path of reasoning as for tinnitus, the approach based on active extinction of conditioned reflexes and complex conditioned stimuli is explained. Mechanisms underlying the sound protocols for misophonia are discussed in detail as well and described later in this chapter. All patients, those with tinnitus, hyperacusis, and misophonia are consulted on the use of sound therapy with great detail.

Sound Therapy

General Principles

Sound therapy utilizes the principle, which governs all sensory perception and processing the neuronal signal in the brain, namely that the assessment of the strength of the neuronal signal within the brain depends on the difference/contrast between a signal and background neuronal activity, which is a sum of spontaneous activity and activity evoked by environmental sounds. Therefore, it is possible to decrease the strength of the tinnitus signal (i.e., neuronal activity perceived as tinnitus), or the strength of neuronal activity evoked by bothersome sounds (in case of hyperacusis and misophonia) by increasing the background neuronal activity. This can be achieved by increasing background sound levels in the patients' environment (Fig. 47.5).

Since it is possible to induce tinnitus in the majority of subjects without preexisting tinnitus by keeping them for minutes in an environment with a very low level of sound [22, 49] and pre-existing tinnitus is enhanced in the environment with a low level of sound, all patients are recommended to "Avoid Silence" since silence enhances the perception of tinnitus and perception of bothersome sounds.

A type of used sound and its level should not evoke annoyance or any kind of negative reaction. It should neither be too soft nor too loud. The specific principles governing the type and level of sound are presented in detail later in this chapter.

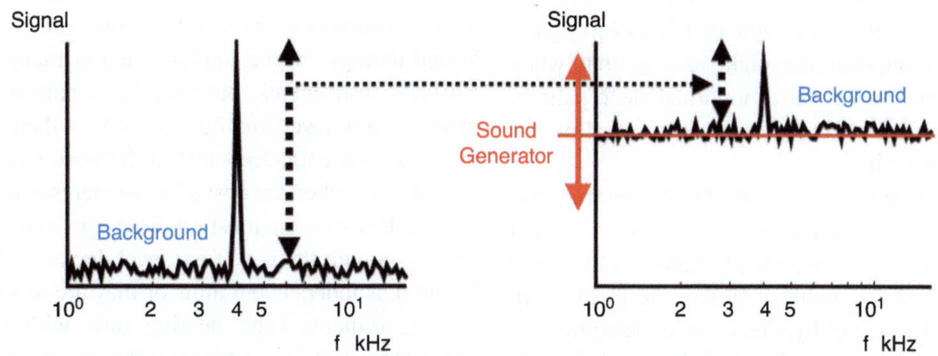

Fig. 47.5 Illustration of the contrast principle determining the strength of the sensory signal and all signals in the brain. Increasing background neuronal activity (e.g., by increasing the level of background sound) yields a decrease of the strength of tinnitus signal or of activity evoked by the misophonic trigger. Sound generators provide an easy way of adjusting the background level of the sound (red double arrow)

In principle, many different methods may be used to decrease the tinnitus signal (e.g., by using some drugs, electrical stimulation, transcranial magnetic stimulation, and sound), but in practice, the use of sound is simple. It can be easily implemented, controlled, and adapted to the needs of an individual patient. It is recommended to use sound enrichment, as much as possible, preferably all the time (24/7) and to use more than one type of sound source. As humans have a high level of acceptance of sounds of nature, these sounds are best to use to enrich sound background. Sounds should be stable, neutral, and not bringing attention to it (e.g., the sound of gently flowing water, stream, or steady rain, rather than the sound of waves, which changes in time).

> As humans have a high level of acceptance of sounds of nature, these sounds are best to use to enrich sound background.

Sound Therapy and Sleep

Moreover, the majority of tinnitus patients report problems with sleep because of tinnitus (falling asleep and sleeping continuously throughout the night). There is a common misconception that tinnitus is awakening them during the night. In reality, patients are sleeping in approximately 90-min cycles (like everyone else), go through normal phases of sleep, and sleep very shallowly, or wake up for short periods every 90 min. If at the time of awakening there is no environmental sound and tinnitus is the dominant perceived sound, it appears to be strong, increases arousal, evokes anxiety, and consequently makes it more difficult to fall asleep again. Providing sound throughout the night assures that when patients are awakened as a result of a normal sleep pattern, the external sound weakens tinnitus sufficiently to allow for easier falling asleep again.

Since the auditory pathways up to the level of inferior colliculi are fully functional during sleep, the use of sound throughout the night is recommended. Additionally, these subconscious levels of the auditory system are involved in abnormal gain (in the case of hyperacusis), in detecting tinnitus signal and activity evoked by misophonic triggers. If patients are not using sound during the night, they might partially lose improvement achieved during the day.

> Providing sound throughout the night assures that when patients are awakened as a result of a normal sleep pattern, the external sound weakens tinnitus sufficiently to allow for easier falling asleep again.

Instrumentation

The easy and inexpensive way to enrich background sound is to use table-top sound delivering devices, smartphones, computers, or iPads, downloads from the internet, specific smartphone apps, TV, radio, playing music, and other general methods of sound enrichment. However, attention needs to be paid to the quality of sound. Sounds delivered directly from smartphones or computers are to be avoided due to their higher level of distortion and bias toward higher frequencies. Therefore, playing sound directly from smartphones or computers is not recommended, and patients are advised to use external good-quality speakers or headphones. With the popularity of Bluetooth technology, this is easy to implement.

Ear level sound generating devices have a specific advantage unique to them because the sound does not change when patients are moving around or moving their head. Moreover, sounds received in the left and right ear are not correlated. This situation is identical to tinnitus where the perception is not correlated between ears and does not change when the subject is moving around or moving their head. At the same time, patients have full control over the sound from these devices, the sound is neutral, and as such, easy to habituate. The brain learns to habituate the sound from devices (with unique characteristics shared with tinnitus), and it makes habitation of tinnitus easier. Note, that sound from the internet (or apps) provided via earbuds does not have the property of lack of correlation between ears, while it shares the property of not changing with head movements, so it offers only a partial benefit of sound generators.

All patients with tinnitus and DST are advised to keep their environment enriched by sound and to avoid silence. Sound therapy can be implemented in many cases without ear-level instruments, particularly in patients with normal hearing, low-level tinnitus severity, when any ear-level instruments are unacceptable in the work environment (e.g., military), or when the cost of instruments is prohibitive for a patient. But still, the most efficient way to implement sound therapy is with the use of ear-level devices. They are manufactured as independent units or they are a part of combination instruments (i.e., hearing aids with built-in sound generator parts). It is important that the patient understands that "It is the sound and not any particular device, which is important" when they are using TRT.

Main Rule of Sound Therapy in TRT

The main rule to consider to successfully implement sound therapy is "Never use the sound as a part of sound therapy which evokes annoyance, discomfort or problems for any reason." The use of a sound that would elicit any negative reactions would further negatively activate the limbic and autonomic nervous system, worsening the situations and making habituation more difficult to achieve.

Specific Recommendations for Sound Therapy

When using ear-level devices, patients should have full control over the adjustment of sound level independently in each of the two devices. Adjusting the spectrum of sound to the patient's audiogram or using one of the sounds with spectra as offered by manufacturers of instruments is not recommended.

Patients should have a good understanding of how to choose the sound level. Tinnitus patients are asked to use sound on the same comfortable level through a block of time of their use ("Set the level of sound in the morning, considering the use of sound throughout the whole day"). Patients are discouraged from making changes to the sound level during the one block of time of their use (except when the sound becomes annoying). Patients set the sound level again if they discontinue their use because of any reason during the day and restart their use. Ear-level devices should be fitted in both ears to preserve the symmetry of sound stimulation.

Some patients use the "Step Method," increasing the sound level above the threshold of hearing by one "Just Noticeable Difference" at the time (it corresponds for low-level sound to about 1.5–2.0 dB per step). The goal is to be at least 6 dB above the threshold of hearing (6 dB SL) reflecting an attempt to be above the range of stochastic resonance (discussed below). After making 4 steps, patients are advised to go as high as they can to reach annoyance level and then decrease sound level by 1–2 steps. Currently, the majority of patients are using smartphones to remotely control their devices. The change of intensity corresponding to one step of change on the smartphone depends on manufacturers and the specific of programing of the device, but typically it is 2 dB. Therefore, 3 steps above the threshold of hearing are sufficient to reach the minimal recommended sound level of 6 dB SL. In the case of the Tranquil II sound generators (SoftTouch Labs), which are popular in the USA, each push of the toggle switch produces a 1 dB increase or decrease of sound level, so it is easy to determine reaching the level of at least 6 dB SL simply by counting the number of pushes.

In clinical practice, the suppression of tinnitus perception ("masking") is very infrequent. Short periods of masking (i.e., minutes, single hours) are irrelevant. However, if it happens, the recommendation is to go up to the point when external sound and tinnitus start to mix, blend with each other (mixing point), and use sound at this level, if the sound does not induce annoyance.

The Issue of the "Mixing Point"

It is important to clarify the concept of setting the sound generators level at the "mixing point" – a concept promoted during the 1990s. The theoretical basis for this recommendation was based on the analysis of factors involved in decreasing the strength of a sound.

An additional important factor to consider relates to the fact that since the goal is to retrain the brain's reactions to perceived sound of tinnitus, the spectrum of this sound should not be substantially modified. In the process of decreasing the strength of complex sound by another external sound (e.g., by a broad-band noise), it is necessary to consider the change of the composition and spectrum of the masked signal by broadband noise. In such a situation, it is important to reasonably preserve the composition of the original sound because otherwise retraining will occur not for the original, but for the modified pattern, and consequently will be less effective. Therefore, from a theoretical point of view, the optimal point would be the beginning of partial suppression of the first sound, where its spectral composition would remain nearly the same. In the case of tinnitus, the intensity of an external sound would correspond to the situation when this sound starts blending, mixing with tinnitus – thus labeled "blending, mixing point." Consequently, at the beginning of the 1990s, patients were instructed to try to reach this point but not to go above it.

While optimal in theory, this approach was not working in clinical practice. When we initiated doing real ear measurements (REM) on all patients during the fitting appointment and during follow-up visits, it turned out that the level at which patients were starting to be annoyed by sound from sound generators was lower than mixing point [50]. Therefore, setting of sound generators at mixing point is counterproductive, because, while at "mixing point," the decrease of the strength of tinnitus signal is largest without modification of the spectrum, but if this level induces negative activation of limbic system, it consequently hinders the process of habituation. From this time, the recommendation of the sound level to be used has changed from "mixing point" to a level which does not induce annoyance.

Stochastic Resonance

Adding a low level of noise to the signal results in decreasing the threshold of detection of periodic signal and increases its strength (then labeled as suprathreshold stochastic resonance). This phenomenon is known as a stochastic resonance and is an inherent property of all nonlinear systems [51, 52]. Indeed, the impact of stochastic resonance on tinnitus has been shown during the evaluation of the impact of added white noise (range of −9 dB SL to 9 dB SL) at tinnitus loudness match; and revealed that tinnitus loudness match increased by 11% as compared with the situation without white noise concurrently present. For white noise intensity range from −6 dB SL to 3 dB SL, the increase was highly statistically significant. Even for a noise level of 6 dB SL some increase was observed (3%) [53, 54].

While the increase of loudness match was highly statistically significant, it is not clear whether it has clinical significance. The interesting insight is provided by results of Katherine McKinney [28], who evaluated the effectiveness of TRT using one group of participants without sound, other groups with a variety of sound levels, and no treatment in the waiting group. While treatment with or without sound showed improvement in all groups as compared with the waiting list group, the worst improvement was observed in the group with sound generators set at the threshold of hearing. As the goal of sound therapy in TRT is to decrease the tinnitus signal, setting the sound level higher than 6 dB SL is recommended to avoid the effects of stochastic resonance [1, 53, 54].

As the too low level of sound is not recommended, the increase of the level of sound and reaching total suppression of tinnitus perception ("masking") is contraindicated as well. The brain cannot be retrained for the signal that the brain cannot detect any more. It is possible to speculate that even if awareness of tinnitus is suppressed by sound the brain is still able to *detect* the tinnitus signal. Such a scenario is unlikely and there is no data supporting it.

If the goal of the treatment is simply to eliminate the signal, total suppression (masking) may be a solution. It has been shown, however, that total suppression of tinnitus can be achieved only for a short time. If an attempt is made to keep tinnitus masked for 30 min, it may be necessary to increase the level of broadband noise by as much as 45 dB, which makes the method impossible to implement in practice [55], so, it does not have a clinical applicability.

Combining limitations imposed on sound use, i.e., stochastic resonance, annoyance level, mixing point, and masking can be presented in graphic form (see Fig. 47.6).

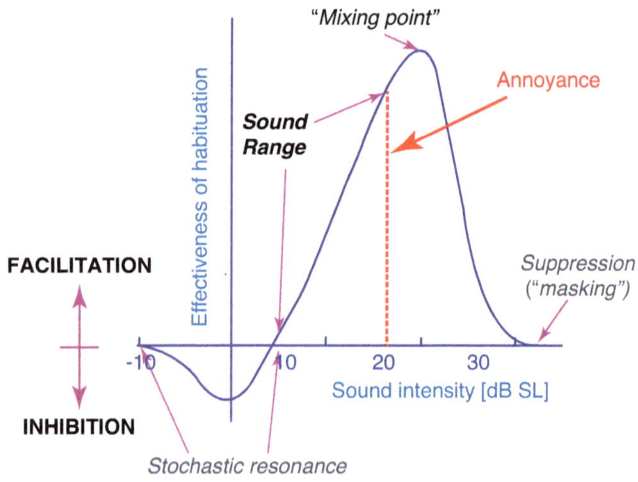

Fig. 47.6 Dependence of habituation from sound level

Sound Therapy when Significant Hearing Loss Is Present in Tinnitus and/or Hyperacusis Patients

Hearing aids/combination instruments are implemented to extend stimulation of the auditory system but only secondarily to alleviate "strain-to-hear," as instruments are used primarily for the treatment of tinnitus and DST, and communication is a secondary benefit. Amplification can work only when there is sound to be amplified and therefore understanding of enrichment of environmental sound by patients is crucial. Consequently, it is recommended to block in hearing aids all features related to "noise reduction," except preserving some directionality. As the aim is to retrain the brain, hearing aids should be worn during all waking hours and not only when needed for improving communication.

Since decreasing the "strain-to-hear" is one of the goals, the evaluation of speech discrimination in noise (QuickSIN performed in free field with and without instrumentation) is highly recommended to assess to which extent instruments are helping. An attempt is made to restore the symmetry of auditory pathways stimulation, and therefore, bilateral devices are always recommended.

Tinnitus and DST patients are typically more sensitive to the quality of sound than those without these problems, therefore attention is paid to keeping a low level of distortion of amplified sound, with a tendency to use minimal amplitude compression and not using frequency compression, if not necessary. In all patients, and particularly with DST, initial amplification of hearing aids or hearing aids part of combination instruments is set below "target" recommended by manufacturers, and patients are given large control over the volume (gain of amplification) [56].

For unilateral losses, an approach based on multisensory integration is recommended, i.e., the use of CROS (contralateral routing of signals) or BiCROS (bilateral CROS) systems, which transform the signal from the deaf (or heavily affected) side to the other ear. The use of special exercises with the use of sound and visual guides is recommended to train the auditory system in the interpretation of binaural signals provided through one ear only, and the training facilitates recalibration of the auditory space localization. It is speculated that due to this multisensory (auditory combined with visual integration) neuronal activity in the ipsilateral to deaf ear pathways is enhanced, weakening tinnitus signal.

Sound generators or combination instruments are not used. Our clinical results fully support the effectiveness of this approach [57].

Proper diagnosis and treatment of DST and its components are crucial for the successful outcome of tinnitus treatment. Hyperacusis is relatively easy to treat with the desensitization protocol [14], and typically hyperacusis can be attenuated or eliminated within a few months of the treatment.

The use of sound generators is very helpful. They are set at close to the level which would evoke annoyance, but still at a comfortable level. Patients are advised to increase their sound level when they are or plan to be in the surrounding with an uncomfortable level of sound. Patients are advised to gradually stop using ear protection (if they use it) in situations when the average person is not using it. Ear-level sound generators are particularly helpful for hyperacusis, more than for tinnitus and misophonia. With proper use of sound generators, hyperacusis patients improve fast, up to the point of achieving a cure and being able to tolerate sounds as people around them.

Misophonia

Misophonic patients are bothered by specific patterns of sound (misophonic triggers), and their lives are negatively affected by these sounds. Similar to tinnitus, their problems develop as a consequence of an enhancement of functional connections between auditory, limbic, and autonomic nervous systems; and the negative responses to bothersome sounds had to be neutralized to decrease conditioned reflex-based responses. The range of bothersome sounds gradually expand to include other previously not bothersome sounds due to generalization of stimuli (i.e., sounds similar to initially evoking reactions start to be bothersome as well) and explains typical observation that untreated misophonia is gradually worsening with time.

Sound therapy is important in misophonia treatment, as for tinnitus and hyperacusis, but it follows specific rules, which are only partially overlapping with sound therapy recommended for tinnitus or hyperacusis. The recommendation of avoiding silence and enhancing the background sound level is the common element. Similar to sound therapy in hyperacusis, misophonic patients are advised to increase the background sound before and when entering an environment in which patients are expecting to experience problems as well. This approach decreases the strength of neuronal activity evoked by misophonia triggers. The use of sound generators is not crucial to achieve a successful outcome of the treatment, as bothersome sounds are not constantly present, but the majority of patients benefit significantly from their use as sound generators are giving patients an opportunity to adjust the extent of protection from bothersome sounds.

> Sound therapy is important in misophonia treatment, as for tinnitus and hyperacusis, but it follows specific rules which are only partially overlapping with sound therapy recommended for tinnitus or hyperacusis.

However, the above-described approaches are not sufficient to positively resolve the problem of misophonia. The main goal of sound therapy in misophonia treatment is to create an association of sounds with a pleasant situation, and as mentioned previously, all four protocols for misophonia have this element. Music plays a significant role in sound therapy for misophonia [14]. Music has a strong impact on emotions and may affect human behavior even when people are not aware of its presence. The majority of patients are able to identify some type of music they like, and therefore, music is typically used in exercise protocols for misophonia to evoke positive emotional reactions associated with sound. Furthermore, music has shown to be able to reduce stress, anxiety, improve the quality of sleep, mood, and mental alertness, which helps many patients on the behavioral level.

> Music plays a significant role in sound therapy for misophonia.

Complex Conditioned Stimuli

By utilizing the concept of complex conditioned stimuli, it is possible to recondition and remove reactions to specific misophonic triggers. When a conditioned reflex is purposefully created in animals or humans, the sensory stimulus is kept simple and clearly different from other sensory stimuli present at the moment to achieve conditioning at this specific stimulus. In misophonia, this is a typical situation, with cognition contributing to focusing on a specific aspect, e.g., eating, speech, with the inability to control the situation further linking a situation with negative reactions. A complex conditioned stimulus describes a situation in which the conditioned stimulus consists of several components that are treated by the brain as one pattern. Notably, the reaction to the complex conditioned stimulus can be totally different from responses to its individual components. For example, it is possible to train animals to have negative reactions to tone alone and to noise alone and positive reactions when both tone and noise are presented at the same time. A complex stimulus may have components belonging to different modalities, e.g., acoustic, smell, surrounding. An interesting clinical example has been described regarding the reactions of patient to tinnitus alone and tinnitus perceived when patient was going to sleep [9].

This concept is utilized in the treatment of misophonia, in the protocol (4), when the complex stimulus is purposefully created by combining a misophonic trigger with other stimuli, which already have a positive connotation (e.g., favorite music, favorite food, smell, and relaxing situation) aiming at having an outcome that the reactions to this new, complex stimulus are less bothersome, preferably neutral, or even slightly positive. Patients' contribution is crucial in creating a proper composition of the misophonic trigger and positive stimuli. Therefore, they need to understand the principles and the goal of this approach. Next, the positive stimuli gradually decreased, slowly changing the composition of this complex stimulus over weeks (e.g., gradually decreasing the level of favorite music played during a meal).

Protocols Used for Misophonia Treatment

Four main classes of protocols are used for misophonia treatment. All protocols aim to create a positive association with sound but differ regarding the extent of control the patient has over the sound environment and protocol (4) is based on using the concept of complex conditioned stimuli.

Protocol (1) gives full control to a patient over the selection of sound, its level, and duration. The focus is on selecting the sound, which is most favorable to listen to in a given moment. Another feature is that the patient needs to listen to sound attentively. As such, it can be used even when significant hyperacusis coexists and can be implemented from the very beginning of the treatment.

Protocol (2) gives the patient full control over the type of sound, but only indirect control over the sound level (e.g., listening to a favorite movie at home). This control is given to someone close to a patient who is instructed to set the volume of the sound at the level she/he thinks the patient would accept. After the listening session, the patient provides feedback regarding whether the sound level was too high, too low, or just fine. This exercise is repeated the next day, aiming at a comfortable level.

Protocol (3) allows the patient for selection of sound type, but the sound level is outside of the patient's control (e.g., going to a movie theater to see a favorite movie or to a mall). This protocol can be used only when significant hyperacusis is absent, or hyperacusis has been already eliminated. Therefore, the introduction of this protocol is typically delayed until significant hyperacusis (if present) is successfully treated.

Protocol (4) utilizes the concept of complex conditioned stimuli and combines the exposure to sounds evoking negative reactions simultaneously with the exposure to highly positive sound. Furthermore, positive stimulation from other sensory modalities is used. With time, the extent of positive stimulation is gradually decreased.

> Four main classes of protocols are used for misophonia treatment:
>
> Protocol (1) gives full control to a patient over the selection of sound, its level, and duration. Stress is on selecting the sound which is most favorable to listen to in a given moment.
>
> Protocol (2) gives the patient full control over the type of sound, but only indirect control over the sound level.
>
> Protocol (3) allows the patient for selection of sound type, but the sound level is outside of the patient's control. This protocol can be used only when significant hyperacusis is absent, or hyperacusis has been already eliminated.
>
> Protocol (4) utilizes the concept of complex conditioned stimuli and combines the exposure to misophonic trigger simultaneously with the exposure to highly positive sound, together with positive stimulation from other sensory modalities.

The duration of misophonia treatment varies substantially, but generally, it is similar to the duration of tinnitus treatment. It is not surprising, as tinnitus and misophonia share the same systems in the brain, and the difference being that internally generated tinnitus signal is replaced by neuronal activity evoked by misophonic triggers. The success rate is very high (83%), and in many cases, it is possible to achieve a cure (i.e., ex-patients do not have any problem with sounds that previously were acting as misophonic triggers) [14]. Moreover, the successful treatment restores habituation of external environmental sounds and somatosounds about which misophonic patients are frequently aware.

Notably, TRT is very effective for the treatment of both hyperacusis and misophonia. Total elimination of hyperacusis and misophonia (a cure) is possible in many patients. Another positive aspect is that after successful treatment of misophonia, the tensor tympani syndrome, which frequently accompanies misophonia, disappears as well, and that tinnitus, if still bothersome, typically also improves [14].

Results of TRT

TRT is not attempting to modify the tinnitus signal, but to prevent the spread of this signal outside of the auditory system to other systems of the brain. Therefore, the etiology of tinnitus is irrelevant, and TRT can be successfully used for any type of tinnitus, e.g., bilateral, unilateral, continuous, or intermittent, as well as for somatosounds (described by others as objective tinnitus, see Chap. 40). The results from our patients showed significant improvement in over 80% of the patients after 12 months from the beginning of treatment, disregarding the etiology of tinnitus [1, 28, 58]. Furthermore, results from consecutive over 300 patients showed statistically significant improvement after 3 months of TRT treatment, with further improvement when the treatment was continued [12, 59].

The treatment typically takes 9–18 months, after which there is no need for patients to do anything special or use sound generators. To prevent relapse, the minimal duration of the treatment is set at 9 months, and we observe relapse extremely infrequently. The treatment of hyperacusis usually takes about 6 months.

The results of open studies and clinical trials reported from various centers using TRT consistently showed significant improvement in over 80% of the patients [29–31, 44, 45, 60–66].

Of interest is a report presenting results of a randomized, clinical trial, which showed that TRT is particularly effective for patients with severe symptoms typically reported to be difficult to treat using other approaches, while being highly effective for patients with all levels of tinnitus severity [67]. Interestingly, there was no indication of the improvement reaching a plateau after the 18 months of treatment, suggesting the possibility for achieving even better results with the further continuation of the treatment.

Long-Term Evaluation of TRT

Specific investigations performed 18 months and 4 years after finalizing the treatment showed that not only patients kept their high level of improvement of tinnitus (as evaluated by Tinnitus Handicap Inventory) but also other parameters related to tinnitus severity, assessed by visual-analog scales kept improving, despite not following any treatment [29, 30]. Results showed that a high level of statistically significant improvement, reported immediately following the treatment, and persisted for the 18 months after TRT completion [30]. Moreover, the proportion of patients reporting the disappearance of their tinnitus-evoked difficulties, while attempting to relax and concentrate and reporting problems with sleep, social interaction, and work, increased continuously after treatment completion. The study performed with 4 years follow-up [29] showed very similar results. These observations have been predicted by the model, as achieved habituation should result in decreased activity in functional connections between systems in the brain involved in tinnitus and then, due to Hebb principle [68] (i.e., unused connections become weaker and frequently used become stronger), these connections become even weaker providing further betterment of patients' condition.

Specific studies assessing long-term effect of TRT revealed that a high level of statistically significant improvement reported immediately following the treatment persisted for the 18 and 48 months after TRT completion.

Conclusions

Tinnitus retraining therapy (TRT) is a habituation-based treatment based on the neurophysiological model of tinnitus [1, 8, 9] (see Chap. 20 and Fig. 47.2), which stresses the necessity of including a network of interaction between many different systems in the brain involved in tinnitus, hyperacusis, and misophonia. The model and TRT stresses the importance of the strength of functional connections between brain centers involved in evoking negative reactions (mainly but not exclusively, the limbic and autonomic nervous systems), the role of the subconscious brain, conditioned reflexes, and brain plasticity are crucial.

TRT utilizes counseling to reclassify tinnitus to the category of neutral stimuli and sound therapy, to decrease tinnitus related neuronal activity and to promote habituation of tinnitus induced reactions. This is followed automatically by habituation of tinnitus perception. After successful treatment, patients may still perceive tinnitus, but they are not bothered by it. TRT offers effective treatment for hyperacusis and misophonia as well.

- Tinnitus retraining therapy (TRT) is a habituation-based treatment based on the neurophysiological model of tinnitus
- The crucial characteristic features of the model and TRT are
  1. Stresses on the importance of the strength of functional connections between brain centers involved in evoking negative reactions rather than functional properties of these centers themselves
  2. Dominant involvement of the limbic and autonomic nervous systems
  3. Dominant role of the subconscious brain and subconscious conditioned reflexes
  4. Crucial role of brain plasticity.

Changes in Implementation of TRT over 30 Years of Its Use

While the basic principles of the neurophysiological model of tinnitus utilized in TRT remained unchanged, the implementation of TRT underwent many modifications since its first use in 1988.

In counseling, main changes are

1. Emphasis on conditional reflexes
2. Emphasis on the subconscious processing of information
3. Specific description of using a modified version of passive extinction of conditioned reflexes
4. Introduction of the concept of misophonia.

In sound therapy:

1. Stress on avoiding sounds used as a part of sound therapy that evoke annoyance, discomfort, or problems because of any reason
2. Abandoning the need for reaching a "mixing point"
3. Stress on avoiding too low level of sound which could evoke stochastic resonance
4. Different instruction for sound use in patients with hyperacusis
5. Omitting gradual increase of sound level and gradual increase of time of using instruments,
6. Introduction of specific protocols for misophonia,
7. Higher stress on hearing rehabilitation, hearing aids/combination instruments recommended to a larger proportion of patients, and
8. Stress on expanded high frequency of amplification.

These modifications in counseling and sound therapy resulted in a significant reduction of the time needed to achieve statistically significant improvement in the patients' problems, from 1 year to 3 months. During this time, not all patients notice significant changes at the behavioral level, but in the end, most patients finish the treatment successfully within 18 months if they do not have additional medical issues.

Results from many tinnitus treatment centers show that TRT causes noticeable improvements or treatment outcomes in and above 80% of patients with any type of tinnitus. A search in Medline for "Tinnitus Retraining Therapy" showed over 180 papers, majority of which report positive results of TRT. Notably, refined counseling and sound therapy increased the effectiveness of TRT in the treatment of DST, so that it now becomes possible to achieve complete elimination (cure) of DST in most patients.

Forms for Structured Initial and Follow-Up Interviews

Form 1: Tinnitus/Hyperacusis Initial Interview Form

FU JHDF **FOLLOW-UP TINNITUS / DST INTERVIEW FORM**

Clinic ID: Diagnosis
Name: Instr
Current Date: Initial

TINNITUS

Days worse than average Y / N Frequency
Ear overprotection Y / N % of time, in quiet Y / N
Any other T treatments
Why is T a problem
Activities affected by tinnitus. Change
Sleep 0 1 2 3 4 N/A
Falling asleep Y / N Wakes up Y / N Hours
Restaurants 0 1 2 3 4 N/A *Work* 0 1 2 3 4 N/A
Concentration 0 1 2 3 4 N/A *Social* 0 1 2 3 4 N/A
FAM 0 1 2 3 4 N/A *QRA* 0 1 2 3 4 N/A
Other 0 1 2 3 4 N/A
% of time when (1st) Aware (1st) Annoyed

Has it changed
0 1 2 3 4 5 6 7 8 9 10 *Loudness of tinnitus*
0 1 2 3 4 5 6 7 8 9 10 *Annoyance*
0 1 2 3 4 5 6 7 8 9 10 *Effect on Life*

SOUND TOLERANCE

DST Y / N Change Physical discomfort Y / N Change Description
Description of troublesome sounds

Miso prot used 1 2 3 4. Description of used positive sounds
Reactions to bothersome sounds

Ear [over]protection Y / N % of time In quiet Y / N
Changes of DST: None / Better/ Worse
Why is DST a problem
Activities prevented or affected by DST. Change
Restaurants 0 1 2 3 4 N/A *Work* 0 1 2 3 4 N/A
Loud events 0 1 2 3 4 N/A *Social* 0 1 2 3 4 N/A
Housekeeping 0 1 2 3 4 N/A *Childcare* 0 1 2 3 4 N/A
Kitchen sounds 0 1 2 3 4 N/A *Shopping* 0 1 2 3 4 N/A
Movie theater 0 1 2 3 4 N/A *Church* 0 1 2 3 4 N/A
High pitch snds 0 1 2 3 4 N/A *Other* 0 1 2 3 4 N/A

0 1 2 3 4 5 6 7 8 9 10 *Loudness of sounds*
0 1 2 3 4 5 6 7 8 9 10 *Annoyance*
0 1 2 3 4 5 6 7 8 9 10 *Effect on Life*

HL

Hearing problem Y / N

Ranking problems
0 1 2 3 4 5 6 7 8 9 10 **T**
0 1 2 3 4 5 6 7 8 9 10 **DST**
0 1 2 3 4 5 6 7 8 9 10 **HL**

How would you feel if you had to give back your instruments
Main problem discussed

Are you glad that you started this program Y / N / NS

MM & PJ Jastreboff, 2020

Legend:

T - tinnitus **HL** - hearing loss **TTS** - Tensor Tympani Syndrome
DST - decreased sound tolerance **H** - hyperacusis **M** - misophonia
Ear [over]protection - Ear **[over]**protection - asking patient about ear protection allows you to judge if they over protect or extensively use ear protection "just in case."
FAM - family oriented activities and interactions
QRA - quiet recreational activities, e.g., reading a book, working on tablet, meditating. - Is your **T** interfering with QRA
Loud events - e.g., concerts, sport events, sport activities
Scales: 0 to 4 (0 - no problem, 4 - you cannot do it or doing with big effort, "N/A" not applicable)
0 to 10 (0 - no problem, 10 - as big problems as you can imagine)
Change: since the beginning of the treatment, "Better / Worse / None" or "Weaker / Stronger / None"

T

Is your **T** preventing or affecting any activities in your life
On scale 0 to 4 how much is your T affecting **given activity**
% of time when: **Aware** - What % of time were you aware of your T over last month?
Annoyed - What % of the time over last months T bothered you?
Loudness - On scale 0 to 10, How strong or loud was your T on average over last month?
Annoyance - On scale 0 to 10, How much was T annoying you on average over last month?
Effect on life - On scale 0 to 10, How much was T affecting your life on average over last month?
Any other T specific treatments - Have you tried or are you currently using any treatments for your T.

DST

Sound tolerance - Is your tolerance to sounds the same as people around you?
Loudness - On scale 0 to 10 estimate minimal loudness of sounds which are bothersome (0 - very quiet, 10 - very loud
Annoyance - On scale 0 to 10, How much was DST annoying you on average over last month?
Effect on life - On scale 0 to 10, How much was DST affecting your life on average over last month?

HL

Hearing - Do you think you have a hearing problem?
Ear sensations - fullness, blockage, pulsation, itching, sound distortion, pain

Ranking - On scale 0 to 10 estimate importance of each problems separately

MM & PJ Jastreboff, 2020 Follow-up_112120.wpd

Form 2: Tinnitus/Hyperacusis Follow-Up Interview Form

I

JHDF **INITIAL TINNITUS / DST INTERVIEW FORM**

Clinic ID: Diagnosis
Name: Instr
Date:

TINNITUS

Description of T sound(s)
R / L / Both / Head = > Intermittent / *Constant* *Volume fluctuations* Y / N
Onset *Gradual / Sudden* When
Days worse than average Y / N Frequency
Ear [over]protection Y / N % of time, in quiet Y / N
Why is T a problem
Activities affected by tinnitus:
Sleep 0 1 2 3 4 N/A
Falling asleep Y / N Wakes up Y / N Hours
Restaurants 0 1 2 3 4 N/A *Work* 0 1 2 3 4 N/A
Concentration 0 1 2 3 4 N/A *Social* 0 1 2 3 4 N/A
FAM 0 1 2 3 4 N/A *QRA* 0 1 2 3 4 N/A
Other 0 1 2 3 4 N/A
% of time when Aware Annoyed

0 1 2 3 4 5 6 7 8 9 10 *Loudness of tinnitus*
0 1 2 3 4 5 6 7 8 9 10 *Annoyance*
0 1 2 3 4 5 6 7 8 9 10 *Effect on Life*
Past & current treatments for tinnitus
T instr used / tried Y / N

SOUND TOLERANCE

DST Y / N First noticed Physical discomfort Y / N Description
Description of troublesome sounds
Are you bothered by: all loud sounds Y / N e.g.,
specific sounds Y / N e.g.,
only in specific situations Y / N e.g.,
only produced by specific person(s) Y / N e.g.,
Reactions to bothersome sounds
Favorite sounds

Ear [over]protection Y / N % of time In quiet Y / N
Changes of DST with time: None / Better/ Worse
Why is DST a problem
Activities prevented or affected by DST:
Restaurants 0 1 2 3 4 N/A *Work* 0 1 2 3 4 N/A
Loud events 0 1 2 3 4 N/A *Social* 0 1 2 3 4 N/A
Housekeeping 0 1 2 3 4 N/A *Childcare* 0 1 2 3 4 N/A
Kitchen sounds 0 1 2 3 4 N/A *Shopping* 0 1 2 3 4 N/A
Movie theater 0 1 2 3 4 N/A *Church* 0 1 2 3 4 N/A
High pitch snds 0 1 2 3 4 N/A *Other* 0 1 2 3 4 N/A

0 1 2 3 4 5 6 7 8 9 10 *Loudness of sounds*
0 1 2 3 4 5 6 7 8 9 10 *Annoyance*
0 1 2 3 4 5 6 7 8 9 10 *Effect on Life*
Past & current treatments for DST

HL

Hearing problem Y / N Ranking problems 0 1 2 3 4 5 6 7 8 9 10 **T**
Hearing Aid(s) Y / N Type 0 1 2 3 4 5 6 7 8 9 10 **DST**
Other sensations in the ear 0 1 2 3 4 5 6 7 8 9 10 **HL**

Examples:

MM & PJ Jastreboff, 2020

Legend:

T - tinnitus **HL** - hearing loss **TTS** - Tensor Tympani Syndrome
DST - decreased sound tolerance **H** - hyperacusis **M** - misophonia
Ear [**over**]protection - asking patient about ear protection allows you to judge if they over protect or extensively use ear protection "just in case."
FAM - family oriented activities and interactions
QRA - quiet recreational activities, e.g., reading a book, working on tablet, meditating. - Is your **T** interfering with QRA
Loud events - e.g., concerts, sport events, sport activities
Scales: 0 to 4 (0 - no problem, 4 - you cannot do it or doing with big effort, "N/A" not applicable)
0 to 10 (0 - no problem, 10 - as big problems as you can imagine)

T

Is your **T** preventing or affecting any activities in your life
On scale 0 to 4 how much is your T affecting **given activity**
% of time when: **Aware** - What % of time were you aware of your T over last month?
Annoyed - What % of the time over last months T bothered you?
Loudness - On scale 0 to 10, How strong or loud was your T on average over last month?
Annoyance - On scale 0 to 10, How much was T annoying you on average over last month?
Effect on life - On scale 0 to 10, How much was T affecting your life on average over last month?
Any other T specific treatments - Have you tried or are you currently using any treatments for your T.

DST

Sound tolerance - Is your tolerance to sounds the same as people around you?
Loudness - On scale 0 to 10 estimate minimal loudness sounds which are bothersome (0 - very quiet, 10 - very loud
Annoyance - On scale 0 to 10, How much was DST annoying you on average over last month?
Effect on life - On scale 0 to 10, How much was DST affecting your life on average over last month?

HL

Hearing - Do you think you have a hearing problem?
Ear sensations - fullness, blockage, pulsation, itching, sound distortion, pain

Ranking - On scale 0 to 10 estimate importance of each problems separately

References

1. Jastreboff PJ, Hazell JWP. Tinnitus retraining therapy: implementing the neurophysicological model. Cambridge: Cambridge University Press; 2004. p. xiii, 276p.
2. Jastreboff PJ, Jastreboff MM. Decreased sound tolerance: hyperacusis, misophonia, diplacousis, and polyacousis. Handb Clin Neurol. 2015;129:375–87.
3. Bauer CA, Kurt W, Sybert LT, Brozoski TJ. The cerebellum as a novel tinnitus generator. Hear Res. 2013;295:130–9.
4. Mennink LM, van Dijk JMC, van Dijk P. The cerebellar (Para)flocculus: a review on its auditory function and a possible role in tinnitus. Hear Res. 2020;398:108081.
5. Lanting CP, de Kleine E, van Dijk P. Neural activity underlying tinnitus generation: results from PET and fMRI. Hear Res. 2009;255(1–2):1–13.
6. Jennings HS. The interpretation of the behavior of the lower organisms. Science. 1908;27(696):698–710.
7. Jastreboff PJ, Jastreboff MM. The neurophysiological model of tinnitus and decreased sound tolerance. In: Moller A, editor. Textbook of tinnitus. 2nd ed. Springer; 2022.
8. Jastreboff PJ. Tinnitus habituation therapy (THT) and tinnitus retraining therapy (TRT). In: Tyler R, editor. Tinnitus handbook. San Diego: Singular, Thomson Learning; 2000. p. 357–76.
9. Jastreboff PJ. Phantom auditory perception (tinnitus): mechanisms of generation and perception. Neurosci Res. 1990;8:221–54.
10. Jastreboff PJ, Jastreboff MM. Tinnitus and decreased sound tolerance: theory and treatment. In: Huges G, Pensak M, editors. Clinical otology. 3rd ed. New York: Thieme Medical Publishers, Inc.; 2007.
11. Jastreboff PJ, Jastreboff MM. Decreased sound tolerance. In: Snow JB, editor. Tinnitus: theory and management. Hamilton, London: BC Decker; 2004. p. 8–15.
12. Jastreboff P, Jastreboff M. Tinnitus and decreased sound tolerance. In: Wackym P, Snow J, editors. Ballenger's otorhinolaryngology head and neck surgery. 18th ed. Shelton, CT: People's Medical Publishing House; 2018. p. 391–404.
13. Jastreboff MM, Jastreboff PJ. Decreased sound tolerance and tinnitus retraining therapy (TRT). Aust N Z J Audiol. 2002;21(2):74–81.
14. Jastreboff P, Jastreboff M. Treatment for decreased sound tolerance (Hyperacusis and Misophonia). Semin Hear. 2014;35:105–20.
15. Henry JA, Jastreboff MM, Jastreboff PJ, Schechter MA, Fausti SA. Guide to conducting tinnitus retraining therapy initial and follow-up interviews. J Rehabil Res Dev. 2003;40(2):157–77.
16. Jastreboff MM, Jastreboff PJ. Questionnaires for assessment of the patients and treatment outcome. In: Hazell JWP, editor. Proceedings of the sixth international tinnitus seminar, 1999, Cambridge, UK. London: THC; 1999. p. 487–90.
17. Jastreboff PJ. Tinnitus retraining therapy. In: Moller A, Kleinjung T, Langguth B, De Ridder D, editors. Texbook of tinnitus. New York: Springer; 2010. p. 575–96.
18. Newman CW, Sandridge SA, Jacobson GP. Psychometric adequacy of the tinnitus handicap inventory (THI) for evaluating treatment outcome. J Am Acad Audiol. 1998;9(2):153–60.
19. Newman CW, Wharton JA, Jacobson GP. Retest stability of the tinnitus handicap questionnaire. Ann Otol Rhinol Laryngol. 1995;104:718–23.
20. Henry JA, Griest S, Thielman E, McMillan G, Kaelin C, Carlson KF. Tinnitus functional index: development, validation, outcomes research, and clinical application. Hear Res. 2016;334:58–64.
21. Meikle MB, Henry JA, Griest SE, Stewart BJ, Abrams HB, McArdle R, et al. The tinnitus functional index: development of a new clinical measure for chronic, intrusive tinnitus. Ear Hear. 2012;33(2):153–76.
22. Heller MF, Bergman M. Tinnitus in normally hearing persons. Ann Otol. 1953;62:73–93.
23. Nields JA, Fallon BA, Jastreboff PJ. Carbamazepine in the treatment of Lyme disease-induced hyperacusi. J Neuropsychiatry Clin Neurosci. 1999;11(1):97–9.
24. Jastreboff PJ. Categories of the patients and the treatment outcome. In: Hazell JWP, editor. Proceedings of the sixth international tinnitus seminar, 1999, Cambridge, UK. London: THC; 1999. p. 394–8.
25. Jastreboff PJ. The role of subconscious pathways in tinnitus and decreased sound tolerance. 9th international tinnitus seminar, Goeteborg, Sweden; 2008.
26. Konorski J. Integrative activity of the brain. Chicago: University of Chicago Press; 1967. p. 1967.
27. Henry JA, Schechter MA, Zaugg TL, Griest S, Jastreboff PJ, Vernon JA, et al. Outcomes of clinical trial: tinnitus masking versus tinnitus retraining therapy. J Am Acad Audiol. 2006;17(2):104–32.
28. McKinney CJ, Hazell JWP, Graham RL. An evaluation of the TRT method. In: Hazell JWP, editor. Proceedings of the sixth international tinnitus seminar, 1999, Cambridge, UK. London: THC; 1999. p. 99–105.
29. Lux-Wellenhof G, Hellweg FC. Longterm follow up study of TRT in Frankfurt. In: Patuzzi R, editor. Proceedings of the seventh international tinnitus seminar. Perth: The University of Western Australia; 2002. p. 277–9.
30. Forti S, Costanzo S, Crocetti A, Pignataro L, Del BL, Ambrosetti U. Are results of tinnitus retraining therapy maintained over time? 18-month follow-up after completion of therapy. Audiol Neurootol. 2009;14(5):286–9.
31. Molini E, Faralli M, Calenti C, Ricci G, Longari F, Frenguelli A. Personal experience with tinnitus retraining therapy. Eur Arch Otorhinolaryngol. 2009;267(1):51–6.
32. Lee K, Makino K, Yamahara K. Evaluation of tinnitus retraining therapy for patients with normal audiograms versus patients with hearing loss. Auris Nasus Larynx. 2018;45(2):215–21.
33. Nemade SV, Shinde KJ. Clinical efficacy of tinnitus retraining therapy based on tinnitus questionnaire score and visual analogue scale score in patients with subjective tinnitus. Turk Arch Otorhinolaryngol. 2019;57(1):34–8.
34. Barozzi S, Ambrosetti U, Callaway SL, Behrens T, Passoni S, Bo LD. Effects of tinnitus retraining therapy with different colours of sound. Int Tinnitus J. 2017;21(2):139–43.
35. Park JM, Kim WJ, Ha JB, Han JJ, Park SY, Park SN. Effect of sound generator on tinnitus and hyperacusis. Acta Otolaryngol. 2018;138(2):135–9.
36. Bauer CA, Berry JL, Brozoski TJ. The effect of tinnitus retraining therapy on chronic tinnitus: a controlled trial. Laryngoscope Investig Otolaryngol. 2017;2(4):166–77.
37. Lee SY, Rhee J, Shim YJ, Kim Y, Koo JW, De Ridder D, et al. Changes in the resting-state cortical oscillatory activity 6 months after modified tinnitus retraining therapy. Front Neurosci. 2019;13:1123.
38. Bauer CA, Berry J, Brozoski TJ. Clinical trials supported by the tinnitus research consortium: lessons learned, the Southern Illinois University experience. Hear Res. 2016;334:65–71.
39. Ostermann K, Lurquin P, Horoi M, Cotton P, Hervé V, Thill MP. Somatic tinnitus prevalence and treatment with tinnitus retraining therapy. B-ENT. 2016;12(1):59–65.
40. Han JJ, Lee JH, Oh SH, Chang SO, Suh MW. Assessing the effects of tinnitus retraining therapy in patients lost to follow-up: a telephone survey. Otol Neurotol. 2015;36(4):581–7.
41. Han M, Yang X, Lv J. Efficacy of tinnitus retraining therapy in the treatment of tinnitus: a meta-analysis and systematic review. Am J Otolaryngol. 2021;42(6):103151.
42. Seydel C, Haupt H, Szczepek AJ, Hartmann A, Rose M, Mazurek B. Three years later: report on the state of well-being of patients with chronic tinnitus who underwent modified tinnitus retraining therapy. Audiol Neurootol. 2015;20(1):26–38.

43. Thong JF, Ibrahim JB, Wong MC, Chan YM. Habituation following tinnitus retraining therapy in tinnitus sufferers. Ann Acad Med Singap. 2013;42(12):681–6.
44. Hatanaka A, Ariizumi Y, Kitamura K. Pros and cons of tinnitus retraining therapy. Acta Otolaryngol. 2008;128(4):365–8.
45. Madeira G, Montmirail C, Decat M, Gersdorff M. TRT: results after one year treatment. Rev Laryngol Otol Rhinol (Bord). 2007;128(3):145–8.
46. Jastreboff PJ. Tinnitus as a phantom perception: theories and clinical implications. In: Vernon J, Moller AR, editors. Mechanisms of tinnitus. Boston: Allyn & Bacon; 1995. p. 73–94.
47. Kaltenbach JA, Rachel JD, Mathog TA, Zhang J, Falzarano PR, Lewandowski M. Cisplatin-induced hyperactivity in the dorsal cochlear nucleus and its relation to outer hair cell loss: relevance to tinnitus. J Neurophysiol. 2002;88(2):699–714.
48. Jastreboff MM, Jastreboff PJ. Misophonia enforced by strong hyperacusis. 12th International Tinnitus Research Initiative Conference & 3rd Cross-Strait Tinnitus Seminar May 17–19, 2019. Taipei, Taiwan; 2019.
49. Tucker DA, Phillips SL, Ruth RA, Clayton WA, Royster E, Todd AD. The effect of silence on tinnitus perception. Otolaryngol Head Neck Surg. 2005;132(1):20–4.
50. Jastreboff PJ, Jastreboff MM, Payne L. Real ear measurements in tinnitus retraining therapy. 7th international tinnitus seminar, Freemantle, Australia; 2002.
51. Gammaitoni L, Hänggi P, Jung P, Marchesoni F. Stochastic resonance. Rev Mod Phys. 1998;70(1):223–87.
52. Lindner JF, Bennett M, Wiesenfeld K. Stochastic resonance in the mechanoelectrical transduction of hair cells. Phys Rev E Stat Nonlinear Soft Matter Phys. 2005;72(5 Pt 1):051911.
53. Jastreboff PJ, Payne L, Jastreboff MM. Effects of stochastic resonance on tinnitus loudness match. 7th international tinnitus seminar, Fremantle, Western Australia; 2002.
54. Jastreboff PJ, Jastreboff MM. Potential impact of stochastic resonance on tinnitus and its treatment. Assoc Res Otolaryngol. 2000;5542.
55. Penner MJ, Brauth S, Hood L. The temporal course of the masking of tinnitus as a basis for inferring its origin. J Speech Hear Res. 1981;24:257–61.
56. Jastreboff PJ, Jastreboff MM. In: Derebery J, Luxford W, editors. The role of hearing aids in tinnitus management. Hearing Aid Book: Plural Publishing; 2009. p. 119–31.
57. Jastreboff PJ. Tinnitus retraining therapy. In: Snow JB, editor. Tinnitus: theory and management. Hamilton: BC Decker; 2004. p. 295–309.
58. Jastreboff PJ, Jastreboff MM. Tinnitus retraining therapy (TRT) as a method for treatment of tinnitus and hyperacusis patients. J Am Acad Audiol. 2000;11(3):156–61.
59. Jastreboff PJ. Tinnitus retraining therapy. Prog Brain Res. 2007;166:415–23.
60. Sheldrake JB, Hazell JWP, Graham RL. Results of tinnitus retraining therapy. In: Hazell JWP, editor. Proceedings of the sixth international tinnitus seminar, 1999, Cambridge, UK. London: THC; 1999. p. 292–6.
61. Bartnik G, Fabijanska A, Rogowski M. Effects of tinnitus retraining therapy (TRT) for patients with tinnitus and subjective hearing loss versus tinnitus only. Scand Audiol Suppl. 2001;52:206–8.
62. Heitzmann T, Rubio L, Cardenas MR, Zofio E. The importance of continuity in TRT patients: results at 18 months. In: Hazell JWP, editor. Proceedings of the sixth international tinnitus seminar, 1999, Cambridge, UK. London: THC; 1999. p. 509–11.
63. Mazurek B, Fischer F, Haupt H, Georgiewa P, Reisshauer A, Klapp BF. A modified version of tinnitus retraining therapy: observing long-term outcome and predictors. Audiol Neurootol. 2006;11(5):276–86.
64. Seydel C, Haupt H, Szczepek AJ, Klapp BF, Mazurek B. Long-term improvement in tinnitus after modified tinnitus retraining therapy enhanced by a variety of psychological approaches. Audiol Neurootol. 2010;15(2):69–80.
65. Herraiz C, Hernandez FJ, Plaza G, De los SG. Long-term clinical trial of tinnitus retraining therapy. Otolaryngol Head Neck Surg. 2005;133(5):774–9.
66. Baracca GN, Forti S, Crocetti A, Fagnani E, Scotti A, Del BL, et al. Results of TRT after eighteen months: our experience. Int J Audiol. 2007;46(5):217–22.
67. Henry JA, Schechter MA, Zaugg TL, Griest S, Jastreboff PJ, Vernon JA, et al. Clinical trial to compare tinnitus masking and tinnitus retraining therapy. Acta Otolaryngol Suppl. 2006;556:64–9.
68. Hebb DO. The organization of behavior; a neuropsychological theory. New York: Wiley; 1949. p. xix, 335 p.

Tinnitus Pharmacotherapy

48

Ana Belén Elgoyhen and Berthold Langguth

Abstract

Tinnitus is a common symptom for which, in most cases, there is no proved and reliable causal treatment. Thus, it is still a clinically unmet need. The proposed interventions for the management of tinnitus are diverse and most patients would welcome a compound that finally abolishes their phantom sound. The observation that tinnitus can be transiently suppressed by lidocaine indicates that the symptom is susceptible to pharmacotherapy.

In this chapter, we review clinical studies investigating pharmacological compounds for the treatment of tinnitus. A wide variety of different drugs have been investigated. However, at present, there is no approved drug to treat tinnitus. Evidence-based pharmacological approaches are limited to the treatment of comorbidities such as depression, anxiety, or insomnia.

Finally, we discuss challenges in tinnitus drug discovery and potential strategies to overcome them.

A. B. Elgoyhen (✉)
Instituto de Investigaciones en Ingeniería Genética y Biología Molecular "Dr. Héctor N. Torres," Consejo Nacional de Investigaciones Científicas y Técnicas, Buenos Aires, Argentina
e-mail: elgoyhen@dna.uba.ar

B. Langguth
Department of Psychiatry and Psychotherapy, Universität Regensburg Bezirksklinikum, Regensburg, Germany
e-mail: berthold.Langguth@medbo.de

W. Schlee et al. (eds.), *Textbook of Tinnitus*, https://doi.org/10.1007/978-3-031-35647-6_48

Graphical Abstract

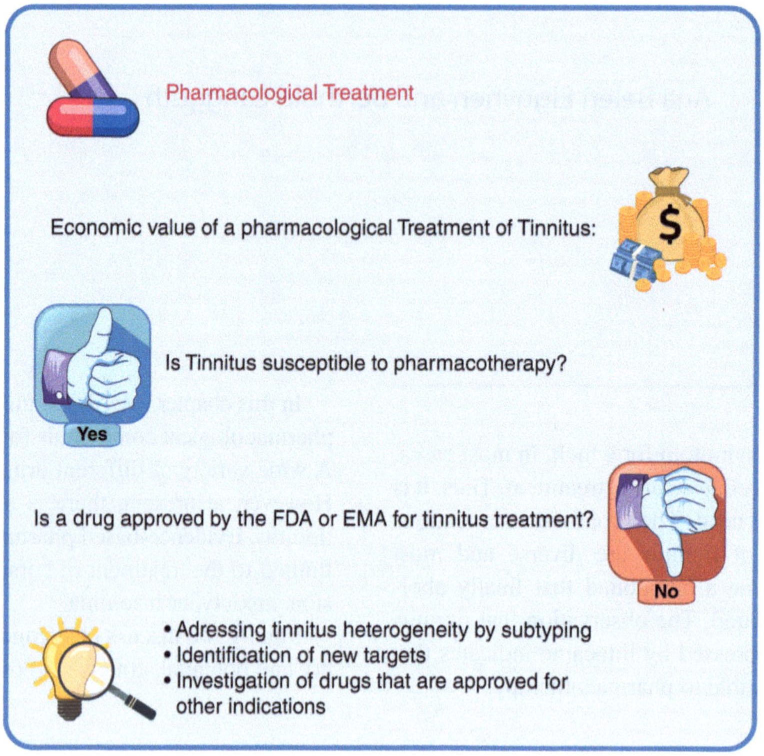

Highlights

- Tinnitus is a common symptom for which, in most cases, there is no proved and reliable causal treatment. Thus, it is still a clinically unmet need.
- The proposed interventions for the management of tinnitus are diverse and most patients would welcome a compound that finally abolishes their phantom sound.
- The observation that tinnitus can be transiently suppressed by the use of lidocaine indicates that the symptom is susceptible to pharmacotherapy.
- At present, there is no approved drug to treat tinnitus. Nevertheless, in clinical practice, drugs are frequently used off-label to relieve the perception of the phantom sound or its associated symptoms (e.g. insomnia, depression, anxiety).
- Since tinnitus is a very heterogeneous disorder, even if a specific drug has failed to demonstrate efficacy in controlled clinical trials in a large sample, it might have beneficial effects in a subgroup of tinnitus patients. Thus, subtyping tinnitus patients is crucial for the search of a tinnitus pharmacotherapy.
- Even a drug that produces a small, but significant effect would have an enormous therapeutic impact for patients.

Introduction

The treatments used for the management of tinnitus patients are diverse and mainly depend upon the specialty of the treating physician. These include counseling and cognitive behavioral therapies, neurobiofeedback, different forms of sound therapies, hearing aids or cochlear implants that attempt to increase input to the auditory system, various forms of brain stimulation (implanted electrodes or transcranial magnetic stimulation), and pharmacotherapy [1–9]. However, meta-analyses of hearing aids [10], sound maskers [11], the use of pharmacotherapeutics like antidepressants

[12], anticonvulsants [13] and cognitive enhancers [14], neuromodulation [15], oxygen therapy [16] and cognitive behavioral therapy [17], have shown no effect on tinnitus loudness. Nevertheless, cognitive behavioral therapy has a beneficial effect on the quality of life of tinnitus patients [17], indicating that some treatments do benefit patients suffering from tinnitus and that further search for better treatments is urgently needed.

At present there is not a single Food and Drug Administration (FDA) nor European Medicines Agency (EMA) approved drug on the market. However, already in 2005 it was reported that over four million prescriptions are written each year for tinnitus relief in Europe and the US [18], but these are all off-label from a wide variety of therapeutic drugs. Although in some cases, these drugs target the tinnitus-associated distress symptoms, they are ineffective in relieving tinnitus perception. Thus, there is still a significant unmet clinical need for a safe and effective drug-targeting tinnitus relief. Even a drug that produces a small but significant effect would have a huge therapeutic impact.

The fact that a transient dose-dependent reduction of tinnitus in up to 70% of patients after intravenous infusion of the voltage-gated sodium channel blocker lidocaine is observed [19–25], is a proof-of-principle for tinnitus pharmacotherapy. Growing evidence indicates that tinnitus pathophysiology involves changes in neuronal activity not only in different parts of the auditory pathway, including the dorsal cochlear nucleus, inferior colliculus, thalamus, and/or auditory, but in non-auditory areas as well [26–28]. Since neuronal excitability can be modulated by different neurotransmitters, neuromodulators, and voltage-gated channel acting compounds [29–33], compounds other than lidocaine should result effective in relieving tinnitus. Due to its poor bioavailability after oral intake, its short-lasting effect, and considerable side effects [34–36], the use of lidocaine in tinnitus pharmacotherapy is limited. Several other oral antiarrhythmic drugs like tocainide, flecainide, and mexiletine have been studied for tinnitus. None of these compounds have been demonstrated to be particularly useful. Almost all of them exhibit severe side effects and are now in disuse [37–39], urging the need to search for the discovery of novel drugs that target tinnitus.

Pharmacological Treatment of Acute Tinnitus

Acute tinnitus is generally defined as tinnitus with a duration of less than 3 months. Neuronal mechanisms and networks underlying acute versus chronic tinnitus differ, thus requiring different treatment approaches. Acute tinnitus frequently resolves spontaneously, therefore therapeutic strategies for short-term tinnitus should aim to provide an environment that facilitates tinnitus recovery. In some cases, acute tinnitus is associated to sudden hearing loss, characterized by the abrupt loss of hearing, typically unilateral, with severities that range from mild to profound. No specific sound frequency region in the cochlea appears to be preferentially affected and spontaneous recovery is seen in up to 65% of patients. In most cases, the exact etiology of sudden hearing loss remains unknown and could involve vascular, inflammatory, and infectious factors. Subjects with good recovery usually resolve in 2 weeks of the onset of hearing loss. Several treatments have been used including systemic or intratympanic steroids [40, 41], vasodilators [42], antiviral agents [43, 44], and hyperbaric oxygen [16]. Although some studies report positive results in a subset of patients, none have proven effective in well-controlled studies [16, 44]. Although oral and intratympanic steroids are widely used, neither a systematic review [45] nor a placebo-controlled study demonstrates a beneficial effect of this group of drugs in acute unilateral tinnitus [46].

Of special interest is hearing loss and tinnitus resulting from the exposure to overly loud sounds. Single, repeated, or continuous exposure to high levels of noise can cause noise-induced hearing loss and tinnitus. Noise at levels of 85 dBA and higher is considered to produce mechanical and metabolic damage of the cochlea and can generate excitotoxic effects on the sensory nerve terminals [47, 48]. Moreover, the exposure to leisure noise among the young (like attending rock concerts or discos or the use of MP3 players) is expected to have a substantial, deleterious impact on hearing loss and tinnitus incidence in older generations in the near future [18, 49, 50]. Hearing loss is a major public health problem, given that its impact on human communication and quality of life is devastating. It affects about 10% of the world's population and approximately one-third of persons over 65 years. Unless action is taken, it is likely that the number of people with disabling hearing loss will grow over the coming years. Projections show that the number could rise over 15% by 2050 (https://www.who.int/news-room/fact-sheets/detail/deafness-and-hearing-loss).

Population-based observational studies have shown that hearing impairment is strongly related to accelerated cognitive decline and dementia risk in older adults [51–53]. Indeed, hearing loss is now known to be the largest modifiable risk factor for developing dementia, exceeding that of smoking, high blood pressure, lack of exercise, and social isolation [54]. Hearing impairment is typically permanent and results from a variety of causes, including genetic predisposition, loud sounds, aging, antibiotics, chemotherapeutic agents, and infections. What is common to these various causes is that they damage or destroy sensory cells, auditory neurons, and other specialized cells in the inner ear [55]. Mammalian supporting cells in the organ of Corti do not proliferate to replace lost hair cells [56]. Therefore, loss of cochlear hair cells is irreversible, leading to permanent damage. Neuronal loss, whether accompanying or independent of hair cell loss, is an important factor contributing to the degree of sensory impairment in cases of inner ear pathology. It should be noted that a new pathology known as "hidden hearing loss" has been described. It is a cochlear synaptopathy produced by exposure to noise levels that cause only transient auditory threshold elevations, it affects many people, it evades detection by a regular audiogram and is believed to contribute to hearing disorders like tinnitus [57].

Preclinical studies in animals show that growth factors and drugs directed against apoptosis, excitotoxicity, and oxidative stress can provide protection from hearing loss and tinnitus if applied during exposure [58]. Otoprotectants have been used clinically with variable results in order to prevent noise-induced hearing loss and associated tinnitus. This include oral Mg granulate and the glutathione prodrug N-acetylcysteine. Sound Pharmaceuticals is developing SPI-1005 (ebselen), an antioxidant and small molecule mimic and inducer of glutathione peroxidase (https://soundpharma.com/technology/#tech-oto) [59]. In a single center, randomized, double-blind, placebo-controlled phase 2 trial, 400 mg of oral ebselen of twice for 4 days, beginning 2 days before a calibrated sound challenge was safe and effective in preventing noise-induced temporary threshold shifts [60]. On the other hand, Auris Medical performed a Phase II trial to test AM-101 (esketamine hydrochloride), a NMDA antagonist for the treatment of tinnitus derived from excitotoxicity in the cochlea due to noise trauma [61, 62]. In a double-blind, randomized, placebo-controlled phase II trial including 248 subjects with persistent tinnitus no longer than 3 months after acute noise trauma, otitis media, or sudden deafness received three intratympanic injections of AM-101 (810 µg/mL) for 3 consecutive days. The study showed statistically significant reduction in tinnitus loudness, sleep impact, and tinnitus impairment in patients suffering from acute tinnitus with established cochlear origin. Based on these results, AM-101 was investigated in a phase III program (https://aurismedical.com/product-candidates/am-101), which, however, was not able to demonstrate efficacy of the compound (https://clinicaltrials.gov/ct2/show/results/NCT01803646).

It has long been known that the activation of the medial olivocochlear system prevents damage produced to the cochlea by the exposure to loud sounds [63, 64]. Efferent cholinergic neurotransmission to hair cells is served by α9α10 acetylcholine nicotinic receptors nAChRs [65–71]. The use of genetically modified mice has shown that hidden hearing loss in animals is inversely correlated to the cholinergic efferent activity [72]. Thus, it is enhanced in an α9 gene (CHRNA9) *knockout* mouse model and reduced in a CHRNA9 *knockin* model that harbors a gain of function mutation in the second transmembrane domain (TM2) of the α9 subunit (L9′T). Therefore, it has been proposed to develop compounds that target α9α10 nAChRs in order to prevent noise-induced hearing loss and associated tinnitus [73]. However, this is not a trivial endeavor. Being α9α10 a very peculiar member of the nAChR family [74, 75], it is not activated by the majority of known cholinergic agonists [76–80]. Therefore, alternative strategies to increase receptor activity are needed. Drugs that mimic the kinetic effects rendered by the α9 point mutation of the CHRNA9 *knockin* appear as attractive molecules to use as pharamcotherapeutic approaches to prevent hearing loss. In this regard, in recent years, new compounds known as positive allosteric modulators (PAMs) of neuronal nAChRs have emerged and have similar effects as those induced by the L9′T mutation. These compounds reinforce the endogenous cholinergic neurotransmission without directly stimulating the target receptors [81]. Allosteric modulation, whether positive or negative, has become a very attractive area for the development of modulators for a variety of receptor classes as they, potentially, can add significant advantages over the orthosteric ligands, since they circumvent receptor desensitization. PAMs have a long and successful clinical track record, exemplified by the benzodiazepine family of drugs (e.g., diazepam), which function as allosteric modulators of $GABA_A$ receptors [82]. However, this approach is completely novel in the case of nAChRs. PAMs targeting α7 and α4β2 nAChRs are now being investigated in preclinical settings for central nervous system (CNS) disorders like Alzheimer disease and schizophrenia [83].

In summary, although there is consensus that acute tinnitus deserves specific attention and that there might be a short therapeutic window for specific pharmacologic interventions, there are no treatments available which have shown repeated efficacy in controlled trials. This probably derives from the etiologic heterogeneity of acute hearing loss and the high rate of spontaneous recovery. Further clinical trials to validate treatments for acute tinnitus and development of better strategies are urgently needed.

Pharmacological Treatment of Chronic Tinnitus

As mentioned before, there are no pharmacological treatments approved for the management of chronic tinnitus. However, a large variety of drugs developed for other indications are used off-label in the treatment of chronic tinnitus, mainly based upon the specialty of the prescribing physician and the comorbidities associated with the phantom sound. For a comprehensive description of compounds used off-label in tinnitus, see the Table 48.1 in [84] and previous reviews [1, 2, 84, 85].

Antidepressants are commonly used for the management of chronic tinnitus [37–39] due to the well-described comor-

Table 48.1 Pharmaceutical treatment effects on chronic tinnitus (from [84])

Drugs	Authors	Subjects	Placebo controlled	Dosage	Results
Na-channel blocker					
Lidocaine	Israel et al. (1982)	26	Randomized placebo controlled	1–2 mg per kg of body weight intravenously for 3–4 min	Complete or partial tinnitus suppression in 19 out of 26 patients treated with lidocaine i.v.; no effect of saline i.v.
Antidepressants					
Amitryptilin	Bayar et al. (2001)	37	Randomized placebo controlled	50–100 mg daily for 6 weeks	Decreased tinnitus intensity and subjective relief as compared to placebo
Nortriptyline	Sullivan et al. (1993)	92	Randomized placebo controlled	50–150 mg/mL for 6 weeks	Depression and tinnitus loudness decreased as compared to placebo
Paroxetine	Robinson et al. (2005)	115	Randomized placebo controlled	Maximum of 50 mg per day for 100 days	No significant difference
Sertraline	Zoger et al. (2006)	76	Randomized placebo controlled	25–50 mg daily for 16 weeks	Improved loudness and severity as compared to placebo
Trimipramine	Mihail et al. (1988)	19	Placebo controlled cross-over		No significant difference
Anticonvulsants					
Carbamazepine	Donalson I (1981)	62	Randomized placebo controlled	100 mg	No significant difference
	Hulshoff and Vermeij (1985)		Randomized placebo controlled		No significant difference
Gabapentin	Bauer et al. (2006)	39	Randomized placebo controlled	Maximum 2400 mg/day for 20 weeks	Decrease in annoyance
	Witsell et al. (2006)	76	Randomized placebo controlled	1800 mg/day for 5 weeks	No significant difference
	Dehkordi et al. (2011)	80	Randomized placebo controlled		No significant difference
	Piccirillo et al. (2007)	135	Randomized placebo controlled	900–3600 mg/day for 8 weeks	No significant difference
Lamotrigine	Simpson et al. (1999)	31	Randomized placebo controlled	25–100 mg daily for 8 weeks	No significant difference
Benzodiazepines/GABAergic drugs					
Alprazolam	Johnson et al. (1993)	36	Randomized placebo controlled	0.25 or 0.5 mg for 1 week, increased to maximum of 1.0 mg for some for 56 days	Reduction in loudness as compared to placebo
	Jalali et al. (2009)	36	Randomized placebo controlled	0.5 mg 1–3 times per day for 8 weeks	No significant difference
Baclofen	Westerberg et al. (1996)	30	Randomized placebo controlled	Maximum 60 mg/day for 3 weeks	No significant difference
Clonazepam	Bah mad et al. (2006)	30	Randomized placebo controlled		Reduction of tinnitus annoyance and intensity (measured with a VAS scale) as compared to placebo
	Han et al. (2012)	38	Open-label comparison to Ginkgo biloba	0.5 mg Clonazepam; 4.0 mg GB increased from 1 to 4 doses per day for 5 weeks	Clonazepam more effective than GB; tinnitus annoyance, duration, and loudness decreased

(continued)

Table 48.1 (continued)

Drugs	Authors	Subjects	Placebo controlled	Dosage	Results
Diazepam	Kay et al. (1981)	21	Placebo controlled cross-over		No significant difference
Glutamatergic drugs					
Acamprosate	Azevedo et al. (2007)	50	Randomized placebo controlled	333 mg 3× daily for 3 months	Improvement over placebo
	Sharma et al. (2012)	40	Randomized placebo controlled	333 mg TDS 3× daily for 45 days	Significant improvement over placebo
Memantine	Figueiredo et al. (2008)	43	Placebo controlled cross-over	5–10 mg 1–2 times per day for 90 days	No significant difference
Neremexane	Suckfull et al. (2011)	320	Randomized placebo controlled	25–75 mg daily for 16 weeks	Decreased annoyance and impact on life at higher dosage
Others					
Atorvastatin	Olzowy et al. (2007)	50 patients with age between 60 and 75	Randomized placebo controlled	40 mg/day for 13 months	Trend toward relief from tinnitus without reaching statistical significance
Betahistine	Sonmez et al. (2013)	68	Randomized placebo controlled	48 mg per day for 3 months	Slight improvement in loudness and on THI
Cilostazol	Lim et al. (2016)	50	Randomized placebo controlled	200 mg Colistazol/day for 4 weeks	Statistically significant difference between cilostazol and placebo in the VAS score but not in the Tinnitus Handicap Inventory
Cyclandelate	Hester et al. (1998)	59	Randomized placebo controlled	Cyclandelate for 3 months	No significant difference
Deanxit	Menus et al. (2011)	28	Placebo-controlled cross-over	1 mg per day for 3 weeks add-on to clonazepam	3/28 report tinnitus improvement
Gingko Biloba	Hilton et al. (2013)	1543	Cochrane Meta-analysis	Ginkgo for the treatment of tinnitus	No evidence for efficacy
Melatonin	Rosenberg et al. (1998)	30	Placebo-controlled cross-over	3 mg melatonine for 30 days	No significant difference for the whole group, tendency to a beneficial effect in patients with tinnitus and insomnia
	Hurtuk et al. (2011)	61	Placebo-controlled cross-over	3 mg melatonine for 30 days	statistically significant decrease in tinnitus intensity and improved sleep quality
MIsoprostol	Yilmaz et al. (2004)	40	Randomized placebo controlled	Treatment at increasing dosage for 4 months	Statistically significant difference between misoprostol and placebo in tinnitus loudness, but not in subjective tinnitus scoring
Odansetron	Taslimi et al. (2013)	60	Randomized placebo controlled	16 mg Odansetron/day for 4 weeks	Statistically significant difference between odansetron and placebo in the Tinnitus Severity Index score but not in the VAS score and the Tinnitus Handicap Inventory
Oxytocin	Azevedo et al. (2017)	16	Placebo-controlled cross-over	Single dose of 16 IU oxytocin	Statistically significant difference between oxytocin and placebo in the CGI score but not in the VAS score
Piribedil	De Azevedo et al. (2009)	56	Randomized placebo controlled	50 mg daily	No difference from placebo

Table 48.1 (continued)

Drugs	Authors	Subjects	Placebo controlled	Dosage	Results
Pramipexole	Sziklai et al. (2011)	40	Randomized placebo controlled	maximum dosage: 0.7 mg 3×/day for 4 weeks	35% of pramipexole group improved in tinnitus annoyance
Vardenafil	Mazurek et al. 2009	42	Randomized placebo controlled	20mg Vardenafil/day for 12 weeks	No significant difference
Vitamin B12	Berkiten et al. (2013)	83 patients with Vit B12 deficiency	Randomized placebo controlled	1 g/mL injected daily for 5 days, then once a month for 12 months	No significant change
	Singh et al. (2016)	40	Randomized placebo controlled	2500 mcg Vitamin B12 weekly for a period of 6 weeks	Significant improvement in patients with Vitamin B12 deficiency
Zinc	Person et al. (2016)	209	Cochrane meta-analysis	Zinc supplementation	No significant effect

bidity between depressive disorders and tinnitus [86, 87]. Based upon the proposed commonalities between the pathophysiology underlying tinnitus and chronic pain [88], and the beneficial effects of tricyclic antidepressants in chronic pain syndromes [89], amitriptyline, trimipramine and nortriptyline have been analyzed in tinnitus patients. In a small scale, single-blind placebo-washout study involving patients with severe tinnitus and major depression, nortriptyline significantly reduced depression and tinnitus loudness (10 dB reduction) [90]. This was followed up by a double blind placebo-controlled study involving subjects with severe tinnitus and severe depression or depressive symptom. Nortriptyline significantly reduced depression scores, tinnitus disability scores, and tinnitus loudness compared to placebo [91]. There was a significant correlation between the reduction in tinnitus disability scores and depression scores, suggesting that nortriptyline is effective in reducing tinnitus loudness and severity in severely depressed tinnitus patients, but has less benefit in non-depressed individuals [92]. One study has compared amitriptyline with placebo and found that after 6 weeks of 100 mg amitriptyline there is a significant reduction of tinnitus complains and tinnitus loudness compared to the placebo group [93]. On the other hand, no difference was found between trimipramine and placebo in a small double-blind placebo crossover study [94].

Selective serotonin reuptake inhibitors (SSRI) such as paroxetine or sertraline have been tested. In a randomized double-blind placebo-controlled study of patients without severe hearing loss, but with depression, anxiety, and a high risk for developing severe tinnitus, sertraline was significantly more effective than placebo in reducing tinnitus loudness and tinnitus severity [95]. On the contrary, paroxetine showed no effect in controlled studies [96]. In a further trial, paroxetine was investigated in combination with the neurokinin-1 receptor antagonist vestipitant with no beneficial effects on tinnitus [97]. The serotonin reuptake enhancer tianeptine has shown beneficial effects on depressive symptoms and tinnitus handicap in an open-label study in patients with both tinnitus and depression [98]. It should be noticed that a meta-analysis that included all randomized-controlled clinical studies of antidepressant drugs versus placebo in patients with tinnitus, concluded that there is yet insufficient evidence to say that antidepressant drug therapy improves tinnitus [12]. Moreover, they found that except the trial using SSRI, none of the other included trials met the highest quality standard, due to use of inadequate outcome measures, large drop-out rates or failure to separate the effects on tinnitus from the effects on symptoms of anxiety and depression. The meta-analysis suggests that the use of SSRI merits further investigation.

Benzodiazepines are widely prescribed in tinnitus patients. This is based upon the proposal that tinnitus results from an imbalance between excitatory and inhibitory neurotransmission, favoring excitation [99, 100] and that benzodiazepines are positive allosteric modulators of gamma amino butyric type A ($GABA_A$) receptors, the major inhibitory neurotransmitter in the CNS [101]. Moreover, it derives from the fact that severe tinnitus is very often accompanied by anxiety and insomnia, thus requiring intervention for these comorbidities. Alprazolam has been prescribed as an anxiolytic and antidepressant. In a double-blind placebo control study, 12 weeks of alprazolam administration at an individually adjusted dosage reduced tinnitus loudness in 76% of subjects, whereas only 5% showed a reduction in tinnitus loudness in the control group [102]. An additional trial also studied the effects of alprazolam on tinnitus relief, with no beneficial effects [103]. A double-blind triple cross-over trial involving 21 tinnitus patients, indicated that diazepam had no effect on tinnitus loudness [104]. In a retrospective study of medical records from over 3000 patients taking clonazepam (0.5–1 mg/day, 60–180 days) for vestibular or cochleovestibular disorders, 32% reported an improvement in their tinnitus [105]. A randomized, single-blind clinical trial involving 10 patients per group, showed that clonazepam significantly reduced tinnitus loudness and annoyance relative to the control group [106]. The effect of clonazepam (0.5–2 mg/day) compared to *Ginkgo biloba* (40–160 mg/day) was further analyzed in an open-label, randomized, crossover study, during a three weeks' treatment with increasing dosages. Significant improvement in tinnitus loudness, annoyance, and Tinnitus Handicap Inventory score was observed only with clonazepam [107]. Although these studies suggest that benzodiazepines might have some beneficial effect, additional larger and well-controlled trials are needed in order to evaluate the efficacy of benzodiazepines on tinnitus. Moreover, caution should be taken since protracted tinnitus has been reported after discontinuation of benzodiazepines [108]. In addition, drug dependence should be considered when prescribing benzodiazepines.

Anticonvulsants are increasingly used in the treatment of several non-epileptic conditions, including various psychiatric disorders and pain syndromes [109] and tinnitus. Based on the increased neuronal excitability, anticonvulsants should exert beneficial effects on tinnitus treatment due to their effects on voltage-gated sodium and calcium channels, and on synaptic transmission—mainly mediated by $GABA_A$ receptors [110]. For example, carbamazepine binds to voltage-gated sodium channels and stabilizes the sodium inactivation state, thereby reducing neural firing [111, 112]. Based on the similarities between carbamazepine and lidocaine in their mechanism of action, three studies investigated the effect of carbamazepine in tinnitus patients who previously had responded to intravenous lidocaine [113–115] with some positive results. However, placebo-controlled studies have not demonstrated benefits [116–118]. A significant benefit from carbamazepine has been reported for a rare group of patients who have intermittent tinnitus that sounds like a typewriter, popcorn, or ear clicking, and which is caused by a neurovascular conflict [119, 120]. On the other hand, the results with gabapentin, which acts on voltage-gated calcium channels and is used for the treatment of seizures, neuropathic pain, and migraine, are contradictory. One controlled trial has shown a significant improvement in tinnitus annoyance and loudness for a subgroup of participants with tinnitus related to acoustic trauma [121]. An additional study reported a significant improvement in tinnitus annoyance when compared to placebo [122]. However, further controlled trials did not show any beneficial effect of gabapentine on tinnitus annoyance or loudness [123, 124]. Thus, although the effects of gabapentin are limited, it might benefit a subpopulation of patients in which tinnitus is associated with acoustic trauma [125]. Lamotrigine, a blocker of voltage-sensitive sodium channels, failed to demonstrate a beneficial effect in a small trial [126]. Modulators of voltage-gated potassium channels have been recently analyzed. Thus, retigabine and other KCNQ2/3-specific channel activators, have been shown to prevent the development of tinnitus in animal models [127, 128]. Anecdotal reports collected from patients suggest that retigabine may also reduce tinnitus severity in humans [129]. Autifony Therapeutics registered a trial for AUT00063, a modulator of voltage-gated potassium channels (Kv3.1), but results are not yet published (ClinicalTrials.gov ID NCT02315508), and the compound is not in their pipeline as described in their webpage (https://autifony.com/pipeline/hearing-disorders/). A Cochrane meta-analysis concluded that studies of anticonvulsants for tinnitus show small effects of doubtful clinical significance [13].

Glutamate receptor antagonists have been used in tinnitus sufferers in order to reduce the increased neuronal excitation observed [100, 130]. The putative nonselective NMDA receptor antagonist acomprosate has been tried in a double-blind study [131]. Patients received placebo or acamprosate (333 mg, 3 times per day) and rated the loudness and annoyance of their tinnitus before and at monthly intervals of treatment. Acamprosate had a significant effect at 90 days. Approximately 87% of the subjects in the acamprosate group showed some improvement, including 3 subjects in which tinnitus disappeared, compared to 44% in the placebo group. An additional trial with acamprosate showed beneficial effects [132]. A randomized double-blind crossover study using the Tinnitus Handicap Inventory to assess efficacy, 90-day treatment with the non-selective NMDA antagonist memantine should no efficacy [133]. The memantine analogue neramexane, which blocks both NMDA [134] and α9α10 nAChRs [135], was tested in a phase II study [136] with some positive results which could not be confirmed in phase III and the drug has not been approved. A recent trial has shown that the AMPA antagonist selurampanel (BGG492) reduces tinnitus loudness after a single does and tinnitus handicap after 2 weeks' treatment (ClinicalTrials.gov ID NCT01302873).

Dopaminergic pathways in limbic and prefrontal areas may be involved in mediating emotional aspects of tinnitus [27, 28, 137, 138]. Thus, both dopaminergic and antidopaminergic drugs have been proposed for treating tinnitus. Sulpiride significantly reduced subjective ratings of tinnitus and tinnitus visual analogue scores in one double-blind, placebo-controlled study, and the effect was more pronounced when sulpiride was combined with either hydroxyzine (an antihistamine and anxiolytic) or melatonin [139]. The dopamine agonist piribedil was tested in a double-blind placebo-controlled cross-over study with negative results. However, a post hoc analysis suggested that a subgroup of patients with specific findings in the electrocochleography may benefit from piribedil [140]. Although these results are preliminary and need further studies, they are encouraging and indicate that the dopaminergic pathway might be a promising target for tinnitus relief. The D2/D3 receptor agonist pramipexol reduced the THI score and tinnitus loudness significantly in a placebo-controlled trial [141].

A wide variety of other compounds with different underlying mechanisms of action have been used in tinnitus therapy with varying results and need further testing. These include cyclobenzaprine [142], atorvastatin [143], cyclandelate [144, 145], furosemide [146–148], Ginkgo biloba [149–153], melatonin [139, 154, 155], misoprostol [156–158], nimodipine [159, 160], vardenafil [161], oxytocin [162], naltrexone [163], ondansetron [164], cannabinoids [165, 166], vitamin B12 [167], and zinc [168–173].

Challenges in Tinnitus Drug Discovery

Serendipity has played a major role in the initial discovery of CNS-acting drugs, even though a detailed understanding of the pathophysiology and etiology of CNS disorders remains elusive. This is true, for example, for the first psychotropic drugs. Thus, clozapine was developed as a chlorpromazine analogue, whose antipsychotic actions were discovered serendipitously when used as a preanesthetic agent in psychiatric patients [174] and led to modern pharmacological treatment of psychiatric diseases. In the case of modern antipsychotics (with the exceptions of aripiprazole and the substituted benzamides), the design strategy has been to create clozapine-like compounds, devoid of its more serious side effects [175, 176]. A similar scenario can be described for drugs used for anxiety, depression, and epilepsy. Thus, the gold standard of drug discovery as from the 1960s has been the design of more selective drugs with ideally one specific target, with the aim of reducing side effects [175–178]. However, serendipity has not favored tinnitus, and no compounds that alleviate phantom sounds have been discovered by chance, with the exception of the use of lidocaine. This discovery should be followed up in order to understand the mechanisms underlying tinnitus alleviation. For example, brain imaging studies have shown changes in activity in several CNS regions after lidocaine infusion [179–181]. This should be matched to the dynamic multiple parallel overlapping brain networks known to be involved in tinnitus pathophysiology [26, 27, 100, 182, 183], in order to gain further understanding of the tinnitus relieving effect.

Another challenge for the search of tinnitus pharmacotherapeutics is the design of adequate animal models that can faithfully recapitulate the pathology, in order to be used in preclinical studies. The basic dilemma faced by the animal researcher who wants to study tinnitus is the generation and further assessment of the phantom sound [184, 185]. One additional important challenge is imposed by the fact that, in humans, tinnitus is accompanied by insomnia, distress, anxiety, depression and this is probably not recapitulated in the animal models. However, even in diseases for which there exists a more comprehensive mechanistic understanding, there are still significant disparities between the animal models used in discovery validation and the human diseases being targeted for treatment [186]. Thus, if we look at animal models that were developed for complex CNS disorders such as depression or schizophrenia, they have proven useful, even if they can serve only as models of disease mechanisms but not of the disease itself. However, as with other CNS pathologies, caution is needed in the direct translation of tinnitus animal research to humans, especially research into novel treatments, since treatments that showed benefit in preclinical tinnitus trials, failed to show positive effects in humans [13, 187, 188].

An additional challenge for drug discovery is that tinnitus is a symptom that might encompass a wide variety of patients with different underlying pathophysiologies. Thus, subtyping tinnitus patients is an added complexity that should be undertaken in order to pave the way for drug discovery [189–194]. In addition, the subjective nature of the disease makes tinnitus assessment difficult. Moreover, being a CNS disorder, tinnitus pharmacotherapy will not follow the "one gene, one drug, one disease" paradigm best known as the Paul Ehrlich's "magic bullet" concept of chemotherapy [195]. A better fit might be the strategies of "magic shotguns," "promiscuous," or "dirty drugs" that target "disease-causing networks" as described for brain acting drugs [176, 178, 196, 197]. For example, the pleiotropic actions of clozapine are probably responsible for its exceptionally beneficial actions in schizophrenia and related disorders and many newer generation anti-psychotics might have failed in the clinics because of higher target specificity [176]. Likewise, the "dual- and triple-action" antidepressants, which inhibit the reuptake of both 5-HT and other biogenic amines (for example, dopamine and noradrenaline), have been shown to be more effective than 'single-action' antidepressants [176, 198]. However, the finding of the right combination of drugs to deliver a tinnitus "magic shotgun/s" is not trivial. A recent review of network physiology and pharmacology concepts proposes some avenues [199].

A recent work has used a novel network pharmacological approach in order to identify proteins that may be relevant for tinnitus generation, which may also represent potential targets for pharmacological treatments [200]. They integrated available drug side effect information with knowledge concerning the drugs' mechanisms of action to build a drug-target tinnitus network. A network of 1313 drug–target pairs, based on 275 compounds that elicit tinnitus as side effect and their targets reported in databases, was constructed, and a quantitative score was applied to identify emergent targets that were more common than expected at random. In order to control for potential nonspecific effects, these analyses were complemented with similar analyses for hearing impairment and hyperacusis. The analysis confirmed targets known to be involved in tinnitus generation, such as cyclooxygenase inhibitors and serotonin receptors, and also identified novel emergent protein targets such as the angiotensin converting enzyme (ACE). The role of ACE in tinnitus generation is worth investigating.

Conclusions

Despite the significant unmet clinical need for a safe and effective drug targeting tinnitus relief, there is currently not a single approved drug on the market. A wide variety of drugs, with a plethora of therapeutic uses, have been used off-label with some effect in a subset of patients. Although the available treatments for the management of the tinnitus patient are diverse, most patients and clinicians would welcome a drug or a combination of drugs that can suppress or significantly reduce tinnitus once and for all. Thus, there is a pressing need to develop a drug targeting tinnitus relief. Although the tinnitus and hearing loss market are huge, big pharma companies still see it as a risky endeavor. Therefore, the tinnitus field is still dependent upon governmental and philanthropic research funding to move forward. These will eventually provide advances in the understanding of tinnitus pathophysiology and heterogeneity, as well as a methodological improvement of clinical research that might attract more biotech and large pharmaceutical companies to enter the hearing and tinnitus field.

References

1. Elgoyhen AB, Langguth B. Pharmacological approaches to the treatment of tinnitus. Drug Discov Today. 2010;15(7-8):300–5.
2. Langguth B, Elgoyhen A. Emerging pharmacotherapy of tinnitus. Expert Opin Emerg Drugs. 2011;16:603–6.
3. Langguth B, Hajak G, Kleinjung T, Pridmore S, Sand P, Eichhammer P. Repetitive transcranial magnetic stimulation and chronic tinnitus. Acta Otolaryngol Suppl. 2006;(556):102–105
4. Jastreboff PJ, Jastreboff MM. Tinnitus retraining therapy: a different view on tinnitus. ORL J Otorhinolaryngol Relat Spec. 2006;68(1):23–9; discussion 9-30.
5. Güntensperger D, Thüring C, Meyer M, Neff P, Kleinjung T. Neurofeedback for tinnitus treatment - review and current concepts. Front Aging Neurosci. 2017;9:386.
6. Lefaucheur JP, André-Obadia N, Antal A, Ayache SS, Baeken C, Benninger DH, et al. Evidence-based guidelines on the therapeutic use of repetitive transcranial magnetic stimulation (rTMS). Clin Neurophysiol. 2014;125(11):2150–206.
7. Peter N, Liyanage N, Pfiffner F, Huber A, Kleinjung T. The influence of cochlear implantation on tinnitus in patients with single-sided deafness: a systematic review. Otolaryngol Head Neck Surg. 2019;161(4):576–88.
8. McKenna L, Vogt F, Marks E. Current validated medical treatments for tinnitus: cognitive behavioral therapy. Otolaryngol Clin North Am. 2020;53(4):605–15.
9. National Guideline Centre (UK). Evidence review for sound therapy and amplification devices: tinnitus: assessment and management: evidence review M. London: National Institute for Health and Care Excellence (UK); 2020.
10. Hoare DJ, Edmondson-Jones M, Sereda M, Akeroyd MA, Hall D. Amplification with hearing aids for patients with tinnitus and co-existing hearing loss. Cochrane Database Syst Rev. 2014;(1):Cd010151.
11. Hobson J, Chisholm E, El Refaie A. Sound therapy (masking) in the management of tinnitus in adults. Cochrane Database Syst Rev. 2012;11(11):Cd006371.
12. Baldo P, Doree C, Molin P, McFerran D, Cecco S. Antidepressants for patients with tinnitus. Cochrane Database Syst Rev. 2012;2012(9):Cd003853.
13. Hoekstra CE, Rynja SP, van Zanten GA, Rovers MM. Anticonvulsants for tinnitus. Cochrane Database Syst Rev. 2011;(7):CD007960.
14. Hilton MP, Zimmermann EF, Hunt WT. Ginkgo biloba for tinnitus. Cochrane Database Syst Rev. 2013;(3):Cd003852.
15. Meng Z, Liu S, Zheng Y, Phillips JS. Repetitive transcranial magnetic stimulation for tinnitus. Cochrane Database Syst Rev. 2011;(10):Cd007946.
16. Bennett MH, Kertesz T, Perleth M, Yeung P, Lehm JP. Hyperbaric oxygen for idiopathic sudden sensorineural hearing loss and tinnitus. Cochrane Database Syst Rev. 2012;10:Cd004739.
17. Hesser H, Weise C, Westin VZ, Andersson G. A systematic review and meta-analysis of randomized controlled trials of cognitive-behavioral therapy for tinnitus distress. Clin Psychol Rev. 2011;31(4):545–53.
18. Vio MM, Holme RH. Hearing loss and tinnitus: 250 million people and a US$10 billion potential market. Drug Discov Today. 2005;10(19):1263–5.
19. Duckert LG, Rees TS. Treatment of tinnitus with intravenous lidocaine: a double-blind randomized trial. Otolaryngol Head Neck Surg. 1983;91(5):550–5.
20. Israel JM, Connelly JS, McTigue ST, Brummett RE, Brown J. Lidocaine in the treatment of tinnitus aurium. A double-blind study. Arch Otolaryngol. 1982;108(8):471–3.
21. Kalcioglu MT, Bayindir T, Erdem T, Ozturan O. Objective evaluation of the effects of intravenous lidocaine on tinnitus. Hear Res. 2005;199(1-2):81–8.
22. Lenarz T. Treatment of tinnitus with lidocaine and tocainide. Scand Audiol Suppl. 1986;26:49–51.
23. Melding PS, Goodey RJ, Thorne PR. The use of intravenous lignocaine in the diagnosis and treatment of tinnitus. J Laryngol Otol. 1978;92(2):115–21.
24. Merchant SN, Merchant N. Intravenous lignocaine in tinnitus. J Postgrad Med. 1985;31(2):80–2.
25. Trellakis S, Lautermann J, Lehnerdt G. Lidocaine: neurobiological targets and effects on the auditory system. Prog Brain Res. 2007;166:303–22.
26. Elgoyhen AB, Langguth B, De Ridder D, Vanneste S. Tinnitus: perspectives from human neuroimaging. Nat Rev Neurosci. 2015;16(10):632–42.
27. De Ridder D, Elgoyhen AB, Romo R, Langguth B. Phantom percepts: Tinnitus and pain as persisting aversive memory networks. Proc Natl Acad Sci U S A. 2011;108:8075–80.
28. De Ridder D, Vanneste S, Weisz N, Londero A, Schlee W, Elgoyhen AB, et al. An integrative model of auditory phantom perception: tinnitus as a unified percept of interacting separable subnetworks. Neurosci Biobehav Rev. 2014;44:16–32.
29. Lambert RC, Bessaih T, Leresche N. Modulation of neuronal T-type calcium channels. CNS Neurol Disord Drug Targets. 2006;5(6):611–27.
30. Surmeier DJ, Ding J, Day M, Wang Z, Shen W. D1 and D2 dopamine-receptor modulation of striatal glutamatergic signaling in striatal medium spiny neurons. Trends Neurosci. 2007;30(5):228–35.

31. Wonnacott S, Barik J, Dickinson J, Jones IW. Nicotinic receptors modulate transmitter cross talk in the CNS: nicotinic modulation of transmitters. J Mol Neurosci. 2006;30(1-2):137–40.
32. Slassi A, Isaac M, Edwards L, Minidis A, Wensbo D, Mattsson J, et al. Recent advances in non-competitive mGlu5 receptor antagonists and their potential therapeutic applications. Curr Top Med Chem. 2005;5(9):897–911.
33. Blank T, Nijholt I, Kye MJ, Spiess J. Small conductance Ca2+-activated K+ channels as targets of CNS drug development. Curr Drug Targets CNS Neurol Disord. 2004;3(3):161–7.
34. Gil-Gouveia R, Goadsby PJ. Neuropsychiatric side-effects of lidocaine: examples from the treatment of headache and a review. Cephalalgia. 2009;29(5):496–508.
35. ALQuadeib BT, Eltahir EK, Alagili MF. The oral administration of lidocaine HCl biodegradable microspheres: formulation and optimization. Int J Nanomed. 2020;15:857–69.
36. Tucker GT, Mather LE. Clinical pharmacokinetics of local anaesthetics. Clin Pharmacokinet. 1979;4(4):241–78.
37. Patterson MB, Balough BJ. Review of pharmacological therapy for tinnitus. Int Tinnitus J. 2006;12(2):149–59.
38. Darlington CL, Smith PF. Drug treatments for tinnitus. Prog Brain Res. 2007;166:249–62.
39. Dobie RA. A review of randomized clinical trials in tinnitus. Laryngoscope. 1999;109(8):1202–11.
40. Slattery WH, Fisher LM, Iqbal Z, Friedman RA, Liu N. Intratympanic steroid injection for treatment of idiopathic sudden hearing loss. Otolaryngol Head Neck Surg. 2005;133(2):251–9.
41. Slattery WH, Fisher LM, Iqbal Z, Liu N. Oral steroid regimens for idiopathic sudden sensorineural hearing loss. Otolaryngol Head Neck Surg. 2005;132(1):5–10.
42. Narozny W, Kuczkowski J, Kot J, Stankiewicz C, Sicko Z, Mikaszewski B. Prognostic factors in sudden sensorineural hearing loss: our experience and a review of the literature. Ann Otol Rhinol Laryngol. 2006;115(7):553–8.
43. Stokroos RJ, Albers FW, Tenvergert EM. Antiviral treatment of idiopathic sudden sensorineural hearing loss: a prospective, randomized, double-blind clinical trial. Acta Otolaryngol. 1998;118(4):488–95.
44. Westerlaken BO, Stokroos RJ, Dhooge IJ, Wit HP, Albers FW. Treatment of idiopathic sudden sensorineural hearing loss with antiviral therapy: a prospective, randomized, double-blind clinical trial. Ann Otol Rhinol Laryngol. 2003;112(11):993–1000.
45. Lavigne P, Lavigne F, Saliba I. Intratympanic corticosteroids injections: a systematic review of literature. Eur Arch Otorhinolaryngol. 2016;273(9):2271–8.
46. Lee HJ, Kim MB, Yoo SY, Park SN, Nam EC, Moon IS, et al. Clinical effect of intratympanic dexamethasone injection in acute unilateral tinnitus: a prospective, placebo-controlled, multicenter study. Laryngoscope. 2018;128(1):184–8.
47. Lim DJ. Effects of noise and ototoxic drugs at the cellular level in the cochlea: a review. Am J Otolaryngol. 1986;7(2):73–99.
48. Puel JL, Ruel J, Gervais d'Aldin C, Pujol R. Excitotoxicity and repair of cochlear synapses after noise-trauma induced hearing loss. Neuroreport. 1998;9(9):2109–14.
49. Biassoni EC, Serra MR, Richtert U, Joekes S, Yacci MR, Carignani JA, et al. Recreational noise exposure and its effects on the hearing of adolescents. Part II: development of hearing disorders. Int J Audiol. 2005;44(2):74–85.
50. Holley MC. Keynote review: The auditory system, hearing loss and potential targets for drug development. Drug Discov Today. 2005;10(19):1269–82.
51. Deal JA, Goman AM, Albert MS, Arnold ML, Burgard S, Chisolm T, et al. Hearing treatment for reducing cognitive decline: design and methods of the aging and cognitive health evaluation in elders randomized controlled trial. Alzheimers Dement (N Y). 2018;4:499–507.
52. Loughrey DG, Kelly ME, Kelley GA, Brennan S, Lawlor BA. Association of age-related hearing loss with cognitive function, cognitive impairment, and dementia: a systematic review and meta-analysis. JAMA Otolaryngol Head Neck Surg. 2018;144(2):115–26.
53. Livingston G, Sommerlad A, Orgeta V, Costafreda SG, Huntley J, Ames D, et al. Dementia prevention, intervention, and care. Lancet. 2017;390(10113):2673–734.
54. Wilson BS, Tucci DL, Merson MH, O'Donoghue GM. Global hearing health care: new findings and perspectives. Lancet. 2017;390(10111):2503–15.
55. Liberman MC. Noise-induced and age-related hearing loss: new perspectives and potential therapies. F1000Res. 2017;6:927.
56. Brigande JV, Heller S. Quo vadis, hair cell regeneration? Nat Neurosci. 2009;12(6):679–85.
57. Kujawa SG, Liberman MC. Adding insult to injury: cochlear nerve degeneration after "temporary" noise-induced hearing loss. J Neurosci. 2009;29(45):14077–85.
58. Lynch ED, Kil J. Compounds for the prevention and treatment of noise-induced hearing loss. Drug Discov Today. 2005;10(19):1291–8.
59. Kil J, Pierce C, Tran H, Gu R, Lynch ED. Ebselen treatment reduces noise induced hearing loss via the mimicry and induction of glutathione peroxidase. Hear Res. 2007;226(1-2):44–51.
60. Kil J, Lobarinas E, Spankovich C, Griffiths SK, Antonelli PJ, Lynch ED, et al. Safety and efficacy of ebselen for the prevention of noise-induced hearing loss: a randomized, double-blind, placebo-controlled, phase 2 trial. Lancet. 2017;390(10098):969–79.
61. Muehlmeier G, Biesinger E, Maier H. Safety of intratympanic injection of AM-101 in patients with acute inner ear tinnitus. Audiol Neurootol. 2011;16(6):388–97.
62. Staecker H, Morelock M, Kramer T, Chrbolka P, Ahn JH, Meyer T. Safety of repeated-dose intratympanic injections with AM-101 in acute inner ear tinnitus. Otolaryngol Head Neck Surg. 2017;157(3):478–87.
63. Reiter ER, Liberman MC. Efferent-mediated protection from acoustic overexposure: relation to slow effects of olivocochlear stimulation. J Neurophysiol. 1995;73(2):506–14.
64. Maison SF, Liberman MC. Predicting vulnerability to acoustic injury with a noninvasive assay of olivocochlear reflex strength. J Neurosci. 2000;20(12):4701–7.
65. Elgoyhen AB, Johnson DS, Boulter J, Vetter DE, Heinemann S. a9: an acetylcholine receptor with novel pharmacological properties expressed in rat cochlear hair cells. Cell. 1994;79:705–15.
66. Elgoyhen AB, Vetter D, Katz E, Rothlin C, Heinemann S, Boulter J. Alpha 10: a determinant of nicotinic cholinergic receptor function in mammalian vestibular and cochlear mechanosensory hair cells. Proc Natl Acad Sci U S A. 2001;98:3501–6.
67. Ballestero J, de San Z, Martin J, Goutman J, Elgoyhen AB, Fuchs PA, Katz E. Short-term synaptic plasticity regulates the level of olivocochlear inhibition to auditory hair cells. J Neurosci. 2011;31(41):14763–74.
68. Gomez-Casati ME, Wedemeyer C, Taranda J, Lipovsek M, Dalamon V, Elgoyhen AB, et al. Electrical properties and functional expression of ionic channels in cochlear inner hair cells of mice lacking the alpha10 nicotinic cholinergic receptor subunit. J Assoc Res Otolaryngol. 2009;10(2):221–32.
69. Goutman JD, Elgoyhen AB, Gomez-Casati ME. Cochlear hair cells: the sound-sensing machines. FEBS Lett. 2015;589(22):3354–61.
70. Vetter D, Lieberman M, Mann J, Barhanin J, Boulter J, Brown M, et al. Role of a9 nicotinic ACh receptor subunits in the development and function of cochlear efferent innervation. Neuron. 1999;23:93–103.

71. Vetter DE, Katz E, Maison SF, Taranda J, Turcan S, Ballestero J, et al. The alpha10 nicotinic acetylcholine receptor subunit is required for normal synaptic function and integrity of the olivocochlear system. Proc Natl Acad Sci U S A. 2007;104(51):20594–9.
72. Boero LE, Castagna VC, Di Guilmi MN, Goutman JD, Elgoyhen AB, Gomez-Casati ME. Enhancement of the medial olivocochlear system prevents hidden hearing loss. J Neurosci. 2018;38(34):7440–51.
73. Elgoyhen AB, Katz E, Fuchs PA. The nicotinic receptor of cochlear hair cells: a possible pharmacotherapeutic target? Biochem Pharmacol. 2009;78(7):712–9.
74. Marcovich I, Moglie MJ, Carpaneto Freixas AE, Trigila AP, Franchini LF, Plazas PV, et al. Distinct evolutionary trajectories of neuronal and hair cell nicotinic acetylcholine receptors. Mol Biol Evol. 2020;37(4):1070–89.
75. Franchini LF, Elgoyhen AB. Adaptive evolution in mammalian proteins involved in cochlear outer hair cell electromotility. Mol Phylogenet Evol. 2006;41(3):622–35.
76. Verbitsky M, Rothlin C, Katz E, Elgoyhen AB. Mixed nicotinic-muscarinic properties of the a9 nicotinic cholinergic receptor. Neuropharmacology. 2000;39:2515–24.
77. Rothlin C, Verbitsky M, Katz E, Elgoyhen A. The α9 nicotinic acetylcholine receptor shares pharmacological properties with type A γ-aminobutyric acid, glycine and type 3 serotonin receptors. Molec Pharmacol. 1999;55:248–54.
78. Rothlin CV, Katz E, Verbitsky M, Vetter D, Heinemann S, Elgoyhen AB. Block of the a9 nicotinic receptor by ototoxic aminoglycosides. Neuropharmacology. 2000;39:2525–32.
79. Rothlin CV, Lioudyno MI, Silbering AF, Plazas PV, Casati ME, Katz E, et al. Direct interaction of serotonin type 3 receptor ligands with recombinant and native alpha 9 alpha 10-containing nicotinic cholinergic receptors. Mol Pharmacol. 2003;63(5):1067–74.
80. Elgoyhen AB, Wedemeyer C, Di Guilmi MN. Efferent innervation to the cochlea. In: Kandler K, editor. The Oxford handbook of the auditory brainstem. New York: Oxford University Press; 2019. p. 59–93.
81. Albuquerque EX, Santos MD, Alkondon M, Pereira EF, Maelicke A. Modulation of nicotinic receptor activity in the central nervous system: a novel approach to the treatment of Alzheimer disease. Alzheimer Dis Assoc Disord. 2001;15(Suppl 1):S19–25.
82. Olsen JA, Balle T, Gajhede M, Ahring PK, Kastrup JS. Molecular recognition of the neurotransmitter acetylcholine by an acetylcholine binding protein reveals determinants of binding to nicotinic acetylcholine receptors. PLoS One. 2014;9(3):e91232.
83. Bertrand D, Gopalakrishnan M. Allosteric modulation of nicotinic acetylcholine receptors. Biochem Pharmacol. 2007;74(8):1155–63.
84. Langguth B, Elgoyhen AB, Cederroth CR. Therapeutic approaches to the treatment of tinnitus. Annu Rev Pharmacol Toxicol. 2019;59:291–313.
85. Langguth B, Salvi R, Elgoyhen AB. Emerging pharmacotherapy of tinnitus. Expert Opin Emerg Drugs. 2009;14(4):687–702.
86. Langguth B, Kleinjung T, Fischer B, Hajak G, Eichhammer P, Sand PG. Tinnitus severity, depression, and the big five personality traits. Prog Brain Res. 2007;166:221–5.
87. Langguth B, Landgrebe M, Kleinjung T, Sand GP, Hajak G. Tinnitus and depression. World J Biol Psychiatry. 2011;12(7):489–500.
88. Moller AR. Tinnitus and pain. Prog Brain Res. 2007;166:47–53.
89. Mico JA, Ardid D, Berrocoso E, Eschalier A. Antidepressants and pain. Trends Pharmacol Sci. 2006;27(7):348–54.
90. Sullivan MD, Dobie RA, Sakai CS, Katon WJ. Treatment of depressed tinnitus patients with nortriptyline. Ann Otol Rhinol Laryngol. 1989;98(11):867–72.
91. Sullivan M, Katon W, Russo J, Dobie R, Sakai C. A randomized trial of nortriptyline for severe chronic tinnitus. Effects on depression, disability, and tinnitus symptoms. Arch Intern Med. 1993;153(19):2251–9.
92. Katon W, Sullivan M, Russo J, Dobie R, Sakai C. Depressive symptoms and measures of disability: a prospective study. J Affect Disord. 1993;27(4):245–54.
93. Bayar N, Boke B, Turan E, Belgin E. Efficacy of amitriptyline in the treatment of subjective tinnitus. J Otolaryngol. 2001;30(5):300–3.
94. Mihail RC, Crowley JM, Walden BE, Fishburne J, Reinwall JE, Zajtchuk JT. The tricyclic trimipramine in the treatment of subjective tinnitus. Ann Otol Rhinol Laryngol. 1988;97(2 Pt 1):120–3.
95. Zoger S, Svedlund J, Holgers KM. The effects of sertraline on severe tinnitus suffering--a randomized, double-blind, placebo-controlled study. J Clin Psychopharmacol. 2006;26(1):32–9.
96. Robinson S. Antidepressants for treatment of tinnitus. Prog Brain Res. 2007;166:263–71.
97. Roberts C, Inamdar A, Koch A, Kitchiner P, Dewit O, Merlo-Pich E, et al. A randomized, controlled study comparing the effects of vestipitant or vestipitant and paroxetine combination in subjects with tinnitus. Otol Neurotol. 2011;32(5):721–7.
98. Hwang SM, Lim SH, Oh DJ, Kim SK, Jung HH, Im GJ. Effect of tianeptine on depressed tinnitus patients. J Audiol Otol. 2016;20(2):90–6.
99. Eggermont JJ. Tinnitus: neurobiological substrates. Drug Discov Today. 2005;10(19):1283–90.
100. Eggermont JJ, Roberts LE. The neuroscience of tinnitus. Trends Neurosci. 2004;27(11):676–82.
101. Olsen RW. GABA(A) receptor: positive and negative allosteric modulators. Neuropharmacology. 2018;136(Pt A):10–22.
102. Johnson RM, Brummett R, Schleuning A. Use of alprazolam for relief of tinnitus. A double-blind study. Arch Otolaryngol Head Neck Surg. 1993;119(8):842–5.
103. Jalali MM, Kousha A, Naghavi SE, Soleimani R, Banan R. The effects of alprazolam on tinnitus: a cross-over randomized clinical trial. Med Sci Monit. 2009;15(11):Pi55–60.
104. Kay NJ. Oral chemotherapy in tinnitus. Br J Audiol. 1981;15(2):123–4.
105. Gananca MM, Caovilla HH, Gananca FF, Gananca CF, Munhoz MS, da Silva ML, et al. Clonazepam in the pharmacological treatment of vertigo and tinnitus. Int Tinnitus J. 2002;8(1):50–3.
106. Bahmad FM Jr, Venosa AR, Oliveira CA. Benzodiazepines and GABAergics in treating severe disabling tinnitus of predominantly cochlear origin. Int Tinnitus J. 2006;12(2):140–4.
107. Han SS, Nam EC, Won JY, Lee KU, Chun W, Choi HK, et al. Clonazepam quiets tinnitus: a randomized crossover study with Ginkgo biloba. J Neurol Neurosurg Psychiatry. 2012;83(8):821–7.
108. Busto U, Fornazzari L, Naranjo CA. Protracted tinnitus after discontinuation of long-term therapeutic use of benzodiazepines. J Clin Psychopharmacol. 1988;8(5):359–62.
109. Ettinger AB, Argoff CE. Use of antiepileptic drugs for nonepileptic conditions: psychiatric disorders and chronic pain. Neurotherapeutics. 2007;4(1):75–83.
110. Neligan A, Shorvon SD. The history of status epilepticus and its treatment. Epilepsia. 2009;50(Suppl 3):56–68.
111. Catterall WA. Molecular properties of brain sodium channels: an important target for anticonvulsant drugs. Adv Neurol. 1999;79:441–56.
112. Willow M, Gonoi T, Catterall WA. Voltage clamp analysis of the inhibitory actions of diphenylhydantoin and carbamazepine on voltage-sensitive sodium channels in neuroblastoma cells. Mol Pharmacol. 1985;27(5):549–58.
113. Melding PS, Goodey RJ. The treatment of tinnitus with oral anticonvulsants. J Laryngol Otol. 1979;93(2):111–22.
114. Sanchez TG, Balbani AP, Bittar RS, Bento RF, Câmara J. Lidocaine test in patients with tinnitus: rationale of accomplishment and relation to the treatment with carbamazepine. Auris Nasus Larynx. 1999;26(4):411–7.

115. Shea JJ, Harell M. Management of tinnitus aurium with lidocaine and carbamazepine. Laryngoscope. 1978;88(9 Pt 1):1477–84.
116. Donaldson I. Tegretol: a double blind trial in tinnitus. J Laryngol Otol. 1981;95(9):947–51.
117. Hulshof JH, Vermeij P. The value of carbamazepine in the treatment of tinnitus. ORL J Otorhinolaryngol Relat Spec. 1985;47(5):262–6.
118. Marks NJ, Onisiphorou C, Trounce JR. The effect of single doses of amylobarbitone sodium and carbamazepine in tinnitus. J Laryngol Otol. 1981;95(9):941–5.
119. Levine RA. Typewriter tinnitus: a carbamazepine-responsive syndrome related to auditory nerve vascular compression. ORL J Otorhinolaryngol Relat Spec. 2006;68(1):43–6; discussion 6-7.
120. Mardini MK. Ear-clicking "tinnitus" responding to carbamazepine. N Engl J Med. 1987;317(24):1542.
121. Bauer CA, Brozoski TJ. Effect of gabapentin on the sensation and impact of tinnitus. Laryngoscope. 2006;116(5):675–81.
122. Witsell DL, Hannley MT, Stinnet S, Tucci DL. Treatment of tinnitus with gabapentin: a pilot study. Otol Neurotol. 2007;28(1):11–5.
123. Bakhshaee M, Ghasemi M, Azarpazhooh M, Khadivi E, Rezaei S, Shakeri M, et al. Gabapentin effectiveness on the sensation of subjective idiopathic tinnitus: a pilot study. Eur Arch Otorhinolaryngol. 2008;265(5):525–30.
124. Piccirillo JF, Finnell J, Vlahiotis A, Chole RA, Spitznagel E Jr. Relief of idiopathic subjective tinnitus: is gabapentin effective? Arch Otolaryngol Head Neck Surg. 2007;133(4):390–7.
125. Bauer CA, Brozoski TJ. Gabapentin. Prog Brain Res. 2007;166:287–301.
126. Simpson JJ, Gilbert AM, Weiner GM, Davies WE. The assessment of lamotrigine, an antiepileptic drug, in the treatment of tinnitus. Am J Otol. 1999;20(5):627–31.
127. Kalappa BI, Soh H, Duignan KM, Furuya T, Edwards S, Tzingounis AV, et al. Potent KCNQ2/3-specific channel activator suppresses in vivo epileptic activity and prevents the development of tinnitus. J Neurosci. 2015;35(23):8829–42.
128. Kumar M, Reed N, Liu R, Aizenman E, Wipf P, Tzounopoulos T. Synthesis and evaluation of potent KCNQ2/3-specific channel activators. Mol Pharmacol. 2016;89(6):667–77.
129. Langguth B, Elgoyhen AB, Schlee W. Potassium channels as promising new targets for pharmacologic treatment of tinnitus: Can Internet-based 'crowd sensing' initiated by patients speed up the transition from bench to bedside? Expert Opin Ther Targets. 2016;20(3):251–4.
130. Eggermont JJ. Pathophysiology of tinnitus. Prog Brain Res. 2007;166:19–35.
131. Azevedo AA, Figueiredo RR. Treatment of tinnitus with acamprosate. Prog Brain Res. 2007;166:273–7.
132. Sharma DK, Kaur S, Singh J, Kaur I. Role of acamprosate in sensorineural tinnitus. Indian J Pharmacol. 2012;44(1):93–6.
133. Figueiredo RR, Langguth B, Mello de Oliveira P, Aparecida de Azevedo A. Tinnitus treatment with memantine. Otolaryngol Head Neck Surg. 2008;138(4):492–6.
134. Danysz W, Parsons CG, Jirgensons A, Kauss V, Tillner J. Amino-alkyl-cyclohexanes as a novel class of uncompetitive NMDA receptor antagonists. Curr Pharm Des. 2002;8(10):835–43.
135. Plazas PV, Savino J, Kracun S, Gomez-Casati ME, Katz E, Parsons CG, et al. Inhibition of the alpha9alpha10 nicotinic cholinergic receptor by neramexane, an open channel blocker of N-methyl-D-aspartate receptors. Eur J Pharmacol. 2007;566(1-3):11–9.
136. Suckfüll M, Althaus M, Ellers-Lenz B, Gebauer A, Görtelmeyer R, Jastreboff PJ, et al. A randomized, double-blind, placebo-controlled clinical trial to evaluate the efficacy and safety of neramexane in patients with moderate to severe subjective tinnitus. BMC Ear Nose Throat Disord. 2011;11:1.
137. Lockwood AH, Salvi RJ, Coad ML, Towsley ML, Wack DS, Murphy BW. The functional neuroanatomy of tinnitus: evidence for limbic system links and neural plasticity. Neurology. 1998;50(1):114–20.
138. Jastreboff PJ, Hazell JW. A neurophysiological approach to tinnitus: clinical implications. Br J Audiol. 1993;27(1):7–17.
139. Lopez-Gonzalez MA, Moliner-Peiro F, Alfaro-Garcia J, Esteban-Ortega F. Sulpiride plus hydroxyzine decrease tinnitus perception. Auris Nasus Larynx. 2007;34(1):23–7.
140. Azevedo A, Langguth B, de Oliveira P, Figueiredo R. Tinnitus treatment with piribedil guided by electrocochleography and acoustic otoemisions. Otol Neurotol. 2009;30(5):676–80.
141. Sziklai I, Szilvássy J, Szilvássy Z. Tinnitus control by dopamine agonist pramipexole in presbycusis patients: a randomized, placebo-controlled, double-blind study. Laryngoscope. 2011;121(4):888–93.
142. Coelho C, Figueiredo R, Frank E, Burger J, Schecklmann M, Landgrebe M, et al. Reduction of tinnitus severity by the centrally acting muscle relaxant cyclobenzaprine: an open-label pilot study. Audiol Neurootol. 2012;17(3):179–88.
143. Olzowy B, Canis M, Hempel JM, Mazurek B, Suckfull M. Effect of atorvastatin on progression of sensorineural hearing loss and tinnitus in the elderly: results of a prospective, randomized, double-blind clinical trial. Otol Neurotol. 2007;28(4):455–8.
144. Memin Y. Perceived efficacy of cyclandelate in the treatment of cochleovestibular and retinal disturbances related to cerebrovascular insufficiency. A study in general practice comprising 2772 patients. Drugs. 1987;33(Suppl 2):120–4.
145. Hester TO, Theilman G, Green W, Jones RO. Cyclandelate in the management of tinnitus: a randomized, placebo-controlled study. Otolaryngol Head Neck Surg. 1998;118(3 Pt 1):329–32.
146. Risey JA, Guth PS, Amedee RG. Furosemide distinguishes central and peripheral tinnitus. Int Tinnitus J. 1995;1(2):99–103.
147. Futaki T, Kitahara M, Morimoto M. A comparison of the furosemide and glycerol tests for Meniere's disease. With special reference to the bilateral lesion. Acta Otolaryngol. 1977;83(3-4):272–8.
148. Kuchar DL, O'Rourke MF. High dose furosemide in refractory cardiac failure. Eur Heart J. 1985;6(11):954–8.
149. Mahadevan S, Park Y. Multifaceted therapeutic benefits of Ginkgo biloba L.: chemistry, efficacy, safety, and uses. J Food Sci. 2008;73(1):R14–9.
150. Holstein N. Ginkgo extract helps patients suffering from tinnitus. Review of the literature shows: tinnitus decreases. MMW Fortschr Med. 2000;142(47):46.
151. Morgenstern C, Biermann E. The efficacy of Ginkgo special extract EGb 761 in patients with tinnitus. Int J Clin Pharmacol Ther. 2002;40(5):188–97.
152. Drew S, Davies E. Effectiveness of Ginkgo biloba in treating tinnitus: double blind, placebo controlled trial. BMJ. 2001;322(7278):73.
153. Rejali D, Sivakumar A, Balaji N. Ginkgo biloba does not benefit patients with tinnitus: a randomized placebo-controlled double-blind trial and meta-analysis of randomized trials. Clin Otolaryngol Allied Sci. 2004;29(3):226–31.
154. Megwalu UC, Finnell JE, Piccirillo JF. The effects of melatonin on tinnitus and sleep. Otolaryngol Head Neck Surg. 2006;134(2):210–3.
155. Rosenberg SI, Silverstein H, Rowan PT, Olds MJ. Effect of melatonin on tinnitus. The Laryngoscope. 1998;108(3):305–10.
156. Briner W, House J, O'Leary M. Synthetic prostaglandin E1 misoprostol as a treatment for tinnitus. Arch Otolaryngol Head Neck Surg. 1993;119(6):652–4.
157. Yilmaz I, Akkuzu B, Cakmak O, Ozluoglu LN. Misoprostol in the treatment of tinnitus: a double-blind study. Otolaryngol Head Neck Surg. 2004;130(5):604–10.
158. Akkuzu B, Yilmaz I, Cakmak O, Ozluoglu LN. Efficacy of misoprostol in the treatment of tinnitus in patients with diabetes and/or hypertension. Auris Nasus Larynx. 2004;31(3):226–32.

159. Theopold HM. Nimodipine (Bay e 9736) a new therapy concept in diseases of the inner ear? Laryngol Rhinol Otol (Stuttg). 1985;64(12):609–13.
160. Davies E, Knox E, Donaldson I. The usefulness of nimodipine, an L-calcium channel antagonist, in the treatment of tinnitus. Br J Audiol. 1994;28(3):125–9.
161. Mazurek B, Haupt H, Szczepek AJ, Sandmann J, Gross J, Klapp BF, et al. Evaluation of vardenafil for the treatment of subjective tinnitus: a controlled pilot study. J Negat Results Biomed. 2009;8:3.
162. Azevedo AA, Figueiredo RR, Elgoyhen AB, Langguth B, Penido NO, Schlee W. Tinnitus treatment with oxytocin: a pilot study. Front Neurol. 2017;8:494.
163. Vanneste S, Azevedo A, De Ridder D. The effect of naltrexone on the perception and distress in tinnitus: an open-label pilot study. Int J Clin Pharmacol Ther. 2013;51(1):5–11.
164. Taslimi S, Vahidi H, Pourvaziri A, Modabbernia A, Fallah AY, Yazdani N, et al. Ondansetron in patients with tinnitus: randomized double-blind placebo-controlled study. Eur Arch Otorhinolaryngol. 2013;270(5):1635–41.
165. Narwani V, Bourdillon A, Nalamada K, Manes RP, Hildrew DM. Does cannabis alleviate tinnitus? A review of the current literature. Laryngoscope Investig Otolaryngol. 2020;5(6):1147–55.
166. Perin P, Mabou Tagne A, Enrico P, Marino F, Cosentino M, Pizzala R, et al. Cannabinoids, inner ear, hearing, and tinnitus: a neuroimmunological perspective. Front Neurol. 2020;11:505995.
167. Singh C, Kawatra R, Gupta J, Awasthi V, Dungana H. Therapeutic role of Vitamin B12 in patients of chronic tinnitus: A pilot study. Noise Health. 2016;18(81):93–7.
168. Shambaugh GE Jr. Zinc for tinnitus, imbalance, and hearing loss in the elderly. Am J Otol. 1986;7(6):476–7.
169. Coelho CB, Tyler R, Hansen M. Zinc as a possible treatment for tinnitus. Prog Brain Res. 2007;166:279–85.
170. Ochi K, Kinoshita H, Kenmochi M, Nishino H, Ohashi T. Zinc deficiency and tinnitus. Auris Nasus Larynx. 2003;30(Suppl):S25–8.
171. Yetiser S, Tosun F, Satar B, Arslanhan M, Akcam T, Ozkaptan Y. The role of zinc in management of tinnitus. Auris Nasus Larynx. 2002;29(4):329–33.
172. Paaske PB, Pedersen CB, Kjems G, Sam IL. Zinc in the management of tinnitus. Placebo-controlled trial. Ann Otol Rhinol Laryngol. 1991;100(8):647–9.
173. Arda HN, Tuncel U, Akdogan O, Ozluoglu LN. The role of zinc in the treatment of tinnitus. Otol Neurotol. 2003;24(1):86–9.
174. Delay J, Deniker P, Harl JM. Therapeutic method derived from hiberno-therapy in excitation and agitation states. Ann Med Psychol (Paris). 1952;110(2 2):267–73.
175. Conn PJ, Roth BL. Opportunities and challenges of psychiatric drug discovery: roles for scientists in academic, industry, and government settings. Neuropsychopharmacology. 2008;33(9):2048–60.
176. Roth BL, Sheffler DJ, Kroeze WK. Magic shotguns versus magic bullets: selectively non-selective drugs for mood disorders and schizophrenia. Nat Rev Drug Discov. 2004;3(4):353–9.
177. Hopkins AL. Network pharmacology. Nat Biotechnol. 2007;25(10):1110–1.
178. Hopkins AL. Network pharmacology: the next paradigm in drug discovery. Nat Chem Biol. 2008;4(11):682–90.
179. Andersson G, Lyttkens L, Hirvela C, Furmark T, Tillfors M, Fredrikson M. Regional cerebral blood flow during tinnitus: a PET case study with lidocaine and auditory stimulation. Acta Otolaryngol. 2000;120(8):967–72.
180. Mirz F, Pedersen B, Ishizu K, Johannsen P, Ovesen T, Stodkilde-Jorgensen H, et al. Positron emission tomography of cortical centers of tinnitus. Hear Res. 1999;134(1-2):133–44.
181. Reyes SA, Salvi RJ, Burkard RF, Coad ML, Wack DS, Galantowicz PJ, et al. Brain imaging of the effects of lidocaine on tinnitus. Hear Res. 2002;171(1-2):43–50.
182. Schlee W, Hartmann T, Langguth B, Weisz N. Abnormal resting-state cortical coupling in chronic tinnitus. BMC Neurosci. 2009;10:11.
183. Schlee W, Mueller N, Hartmann T, Keil J, Lorenz I, Weisz N. Mapping cortical hubs in tinnitus. BMC Biol. 2009;7:80.
184. Bauer CA. Animal models of tinnitus. Otolaryngol Clin North Am. 2003;36(2):267–85. vi
185. Turner JG. Behavioral measures of tinnitus in laboratory animals. Prog Brain Res. 2007;166:147–56.
186. Hurko O, Ryan JL. Translational research in central nervous system drug discovery. NeuroRx. 2005;2(4):671–82.
187. Zheng Y, Hooton K, Smith PF, Darlington CL. Carbamazepine reduces the behavioural manifestations of tinnitus following salicylate treatment in rats. Acta Otolaryngol. 2008;128(1):48–52.
188. Hilton MP, Zimmermann EF, Hunt WT. Ginkgo biloba for tinnitus. Cochrane Database Syst Rev. 2013;3:CD003852.
189. Genitsaridi E, Hoare DJ, Kypraios T, Hall DA. A review and a framework of variables for defining and characterizing tinnitus subphenotypes. Brain Sci. 2020;10(12):938.
190. Landgrebe M, Zeman F, Koller M, Eberl Y, Mohr M, Reiter J, et al. The Tinnitus Research Initiative (TRI) database: a new approach for delineation of tinnitus subtypes and generation of predictors for treatment outcome. BMC Med Inform Decis Mak. 2010;10:42.
191. Michiels S, Harrison S, Vesala M, Schlee W. The presence of physical symptoms in patients with tinnitus: international web-based survey. Interact J Med Res. 2019;8(3):e14519.
192. Schecklmann M, Landgrebe M, Langguth B. Phenotypic characteristics of hyperacusis in tinnitus. PLoS One. 2014;9(1):e86944.
193. Schecklmann M, Lehner A, Poeppl TB, Kreuzer PM, Hajak G, Landgrebe M, et al. Cluster analysis for identifying sub-types of tinnitus: a positron emission tomography and voxel-based morphometry study. Brain Res. 2012;1485:3–9.
194. Vielsmeier V, Strutz J, Kleinjung T, Schecklmann M, Kreuzer PM, Landgrebe M, et al. Temporomandibular joint disorder complaints in tinnitus: further hints for a putative tinnitus subtype. PLoS One. 2012;7(6):e38887.
195. Kaufmann SH. Paul Ehrlich: founder of chemotherapy. Nat Rev Drug Discov. 2008;7(5):373.
196. Sams-Dodd F. Target-based drug discovery: is something wrong? Drug Discov Today. 2005;10(2):139–47.
197. Csermely P, Agoston V, Pongor S. The efficiency of multi-target drugs: the network approach might help drug design. Trends Pharmacol Sci. 2005;26(4):178–82.
198. Millan MJ. Multi-target strategies for the improved treatment of depressive states: Conceptual foundations and neuronal substrates, drug discovery and therapeutic application. Pharmacol Ther. 2006;110(2):135–370.
199. Elgoyhen AB, Langguth B, Vanneste S, De Ridder D. Tinnitus: network pathophysiology-network pharmacology. Front Syst Neurosci. 2012;6:1.
200. Elgoyhen AB, Langguth B, Nowak W, Schecklmann M, De Ridder D, Vanneste S. Identifying tinnitus-related genes based on a side-effect network analysis. CPT Pharmacometrics Syst Pharmacol. 2014;3(1):e97.

Tinnitus Activities Treatment

49

Ann E. Perreau and Richard S. Tyler

Abstract

Tinnitus activities treatment (TAT) is a holistic approach to tinnitus management that includes listening to the patient, understanding the patient's needs, and providing comprehensive counseling to address their concerns. We use three principles including picture-based counseling on tinnitus and related problems, coping strategies and homework to practice activities learned in the session, and sound therapy using partial masking. TAT was developed in the 1980s by Dr. Richard Tyler at the University of Iowa and since has been implemented worldwide by many audiologists and clinicians. The content for TAT includes four areas that are largely impacted by tinnitus: thoughts and emotions, hearing and communication, sleep, and concentration. The picture-based materials provide helpful illustrations of difficult concepts on tinnitus and the hearing mechanism, though the presentation can be modified to include relevant information for the patient. Before providing therapy using TAT, we suggest administering the Tinnitus Primary Functions Questionnaire that evaluates tinnitus in these four areas. The outcomes from the questionnaire can be used to determine the sessions that are relevant for the patient and to document treatment effectiveness as therapy progresses. TAT uses a collaborative approach that nurtures patient expectations and provides a sense of hope.

A. E. Perreau (✉)
Department of Communication Sciences and Disorders, Augustana College, Rock Island, IL, USA

Department of Otolaryngology—Head and Neck Surgery, University of Iowa, Iowa City, IA, USA
e-mail: annperreau@augustana.edu

R. S. Tyler
Department of Otolaryngology—Head and Neck Surgery, University of Iowa, Iowa City, IA, USA

Department of Communication Sciences and Disorders, University of Iowa, Iowa City, IA, USA
e-mail: rich-tyler@uiowa.edu

W. Schlee et al. (eds.), *Textbook of Tinnitus*, https://doi.org/10.1007/978-3-031-35647-6_49

Graphical Abstract

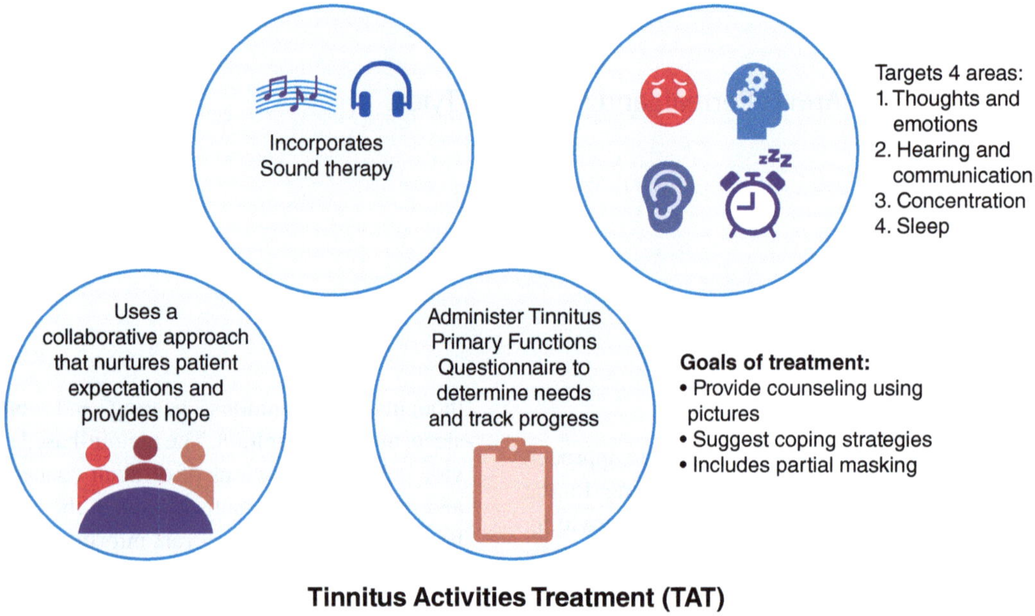

Abbreviations

COSIT	Client oriented scale of improvement for tinnitus
TAT	Tinnitus activities treatment
THQ	Tinnitus handicap questionnaire
TPFQ	Tinnitus primary functions questionnaire

Highlights

- Tinnitus activities treatment (TAT) aims to address the needs of tinnitus patients through three primary goals: (a) to provide informational counseling on tinnitus and related problems, (b) to suggest coping strategies, and (c) to recommend partial masking.
- TAT uses picture-based counseling to explain concepts that can be easily adapted to each patient and transferred across clinicians. Images were updated in 2019.
- TAT includes four broad topic areas of thoughts and emotions, hearing and communication, sleep, and concentration along with an introduction session, homework, and practice activities.
- We suggest using the Tinnitus Primary Functions Questionnaire to determine the sessions that are relevant for the patient and to document treatment effectiveness.
- We focus on a collaborative and holistic approach to helping patients manage their tinnitus. We emphasize nurturing patient expectations and providing hope.

History and Overview of Treatment

Tinnitus activities treatment (TAT), a counseling (see Chap. 43), and sound therapy (see Chap. 46) program for patients with tinnitus, began in the 1980s at the University of Iowa. We established this program to address the needs of patients with bothersome tinnitus that were not being met by audiologists, hearing healthcare professionals, and ENT physicians at that time. In the development of TAT, we relied on the guidance and expertise of previous researchers and audiologists [1–4].

TAT aims to address the needs of tinnitus patients through three primary goals: (a) to provide informational counseling on tinnitus and related problems, (b) to suggest coping strategies, and (c) to recommend partial masking [5–8]. Informational counseling is often a required component in initial sessions with tinnitus patients, as we educate patients on the causes and mechanisms of tinnitus. The famous quote by Francis Bacon that "knowledge is power" applies here, as educating patients about tinnitus is often the first step to managing their reactions to it. Coping strategies are incorporated throughout the therapy to allow patients to identify and explore their thoughts and reactions to their tinnitus (both positive and negative) and, with the help of the clinician, implement useful strategies to address these concerns. Cognitive behavioral therapy (CBT) (see Chap. 44) was included following the recommendations of Henry and Wilson [3]. Lastly, partial masking using a low-level background sound is recommended because it can provide adequate relief from tinnitus [5, 9, 10], yet not potentially worsen the tinnitus or interfere with speech perception as is often experienced with total masking. We recognize that not all patients will benefit from sound therapy and that sound therapy should not be used at all times given the listening demands of the situation, especially as it relates to patients with hearing loss.

A unique feature of TAT is that it uses picture-based counseling [11] using images and charts to explain complicated concepts. Picture-based counseling has several advantages in that the sessions proceed in an orderly fashion without overlooking important concepts, it is easy for patients to understand challenging concepts (i.e., increased neural activity as a mechanism for tinnitus), and sessions can be easily adapted or transferred across clinicians. TAT materials were updated in 2019 with new images and notes for the clinician and are available to clinicians from the University of Iowa at no cost (https://medicine.uiowa.edu/oto/research/tinnitus-and-hyperacusis).

The Essential Role of the Clinician

In TAT, we focus on a collaborative and holistic approach to helping the patient manage their tinnitus. Using a person-centered approach to care ensures that the patient is an integral part of the therapy process, rather than the clinician assuming the needs of the patient and providing directive counseling to address a perceived need. We recommend that clinicians nurture patient expectations and provide hope, and to that effort, have suggested the following characteristics of a competent and caring clinician [12]:

- Connect personally with the patient.
- Understand where the patient is in process of managing their tinnitus.
- Understand the patient's needs and desires.
- Provide a clear therapy plan.
- Show the patient that you care.
- Be a good 'listener'.

Considering the patient's difficulties holistically rather than solely focusing on their tinnitus is an important aspect of TAT. For example, in an early study [6] of 70 tinnitus patients, we identified and classified the problems related to tinnitus into four broad categories: (a) Thoughts and Emotions (e.g., causes distress, anxiety, and/or depression), (b) Hearing Difficulties (e.g., causes communication difficulties to hear over the tinnitus), (c) Sleep, and (d) Concentration. Related to the International Classification of Functioning, Disability and Health or ICF [13–15], patients who suffer from hearing loss and/or tinnitus may experience participation restrictions, such as not being able to engage in social activities, do their job, or volunteer in their local community. Experiencing such restrictions can further exacerbate the tinnitus, as the patient becomes more focused on their tinnitus and less engaged in other activities. Therefore, we have developed a management plan that addresses the issues reported by tinnitus patients using the four categories as the framework. TAT should be delivered across multiple sessions, typically in 1–1.5 h sessions at 1–2 week intervals. Completing TAT over several weeks ensures adequate information is covered on each topic without being excessive and allows patients to practice activities in their daily life between sessions. There is considerable flexibility in TAT because the clinician can cover any or all of the modules of TAT. Sessions can be adapted to the needs and interests of the patient. Consistent with the goals of TAT, all sessions provide informational counseling, suggest coping strategies, and recommend sound therapy (when appropriate).

Questionnaires for Planning Tinnitus Therapy and Documenting Outcomes

To determine which TAT sessions to include and to document patient outcomes from the therapy, we recommend administering several questionnaires to your tinnitus patient (see also Chap. 27). First, we administer the 12-item Tinnitus Primary Functions Questionnaire (TPFQ) [16] to measure the patient's reactions to their tinnitus and specifically, the impact of tinnitus on primary or everyday activities. The four subscales of the TPFQ (thoughts and emotions, hearing, sleep, and concentration) are consistent with the TAT sessions that are used to devise an individual treatment plan including, which areas may need to be addressed in the counseling sessions. The questionnaire takes less than 5 min to complete, and a simple average of the three items in each subscale makes for easy interpretation of the patient's responses. There are a variety of questionnaires available for measuring patients' reactions to tinnitus, including the Tinnitus Questionnaire (TQ; [17]), the Tinnitus Handicap Inventory (THI, [18]), and the Tinnitus Functional Index (TFI; [19]). Regardless of the questionnaire used, it is important that the clinician select a validated, reliable, and sensitive tool for assessing reactions to tinnitus [20] and administer this before and after therapy to document changes. Our preference is for use of the TPFQ for its ease of use and focus on how tinnitus impacts daily activities. In addition to the TPFQ, we also create patient-centered goals for the therapy sessions and recommend the open-ended Client-Oriented Scale of Improvement for Tinnitus (COSIT) [21, 22] to determine up to five specific problems caused by the tinnitus. The COSIT is a great tool for goal setting and establishing treatment effectiveness, as clinicians can identify three to five goals with the patient and then measure the patient's progress with therapy overtime.

Beginning TAT: The Introduction Session

We begin the first counseling session with a tinnitus patient by providing a brief, 15-min overview of TAT. After this introduction, clinicians will have a clear understanding of the patient's needs and concerns and can determine with the patient's input the approximate number and types of counseling sessions that are warranted. Relevant topics for the introduction session include:

- Why is the patient here? What does he/she/they expect from therapy? Is the patient alone, or does he/she/they have support?
- What do they think caused their tinnitus?
- When tinnitus began, what was your life like?
- How has tinnitus influenced your life?
- How do you think we can help?

We start by asking these straightforward questions about the patient's expectations, anticipated outcomes, and level of support because we cannot assume that we know what is best for the patient. Asking these probing questions will provide helpful information for the counseling sessions and nurture the patient's expectations that there is support from you—the clinician—and reason for hope. We ask about what caused their tinnitus as this quickly informs the clinician of how the patient views their tinnitus and what education is needed to help further the patient's understanding. Questions about their lifestyle more generally (e.g., were you sick, stressed, or having problems at work/home?) can influence the direction of counseling whereas questions about the impact of tinnitus on one's life (e.g., how has tinnitus affected you?) often lead to a conversation about the difficulties they have faced since tinnitus began. Clinicians may want to have patients list the difficulties that they have experienced and then discuss them in depth.

During the initial session, we emphasize that it is THEIR counseling session and likewise customize the counseling to each patient. TAT should include only relevant sessions for the patient that may be based on the results from the TPFQ (i.e., which areas are significantly impacted by the tinnitus?) and the patient's input about the direction of therapy. The picture-based counseling materials should be discussed by the patient and clinician, and we include activities throughout TAT to better understand the patient's problems, interests, and motivations. We have developed homework and practice activities to keep patients engaged in the therapy process and allow the patients to practice the strategies introduced in each session. Clinicians should be familiar with all of the TAT modules because some techniques discussed in one module (e.g., muscle relaxation and visual imagery training in the sleep module) might be helpful in another module (e.g., for concentration). Despite the approach taken by the clinician, we suggest that there is no right or wrong way to therapy as long as the patient and clinician are engaged and progress is being made. Clinicians should recognize the individual differences among tinnitus patients and tailor their approach accordingly.

At the conclusion of the initial TAT session, we answer any remaining questions with the patient and provide support and hope. We often set goals for the counseling sessions using the COSIT, if not already administered, and teach the patient a mantra, such as "I am ok" or "This is ok." Developing a positive message will help patients to counternegative thoughts about their tinnitus and begin the necessary coping process.

Components of TAT

As we begin TAT, we focus on the four broad topic areas of thoughts and emotions, hearing and communication, sleep, and concentration, knowing that these areas are associated with functional impairments such as social and work problems for many tinnitus patients [6]. Educating patients on the physiological mechanisms of tinnitus is a first step as it often alleviates the fears and the unknowns related to having tinnitus. As shown in Fig. 49.1, we explain that tinnitus is the result of increased spontaneous neural activity or excessive input to the brain (see Part III). We provide a brief background to describe the role of the auditory nerve in coding sound and how hearing loss causes a reduction in spontaneous neural activity. This explanation is often met with a sense of relief as patients begin to understand that there is a physiological reason for tinnitus rather than tinnitus signaling mental illness or inherently leading to senility. These explanations can set up discussions with the patient about the biggest problem that has resulted from their tinnitus, which can be further addressed in each of the four TAT sessions.

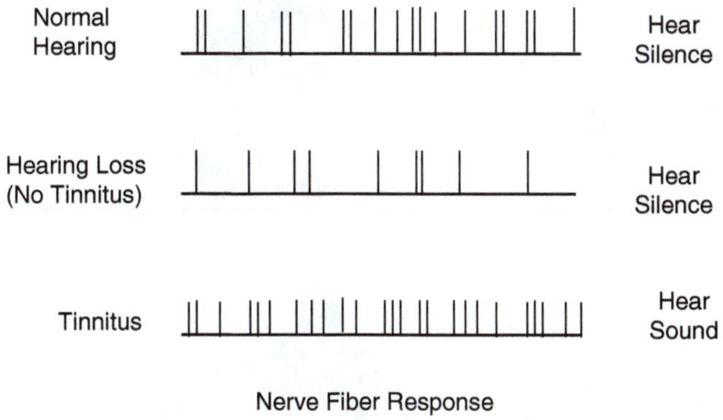

Fig. 49.1 Sound coded by nerve impulses (vertical lines) and transmitted to the brain. Tinnitus is often attributed to an increase in spontaneous activity of the auditory nerve

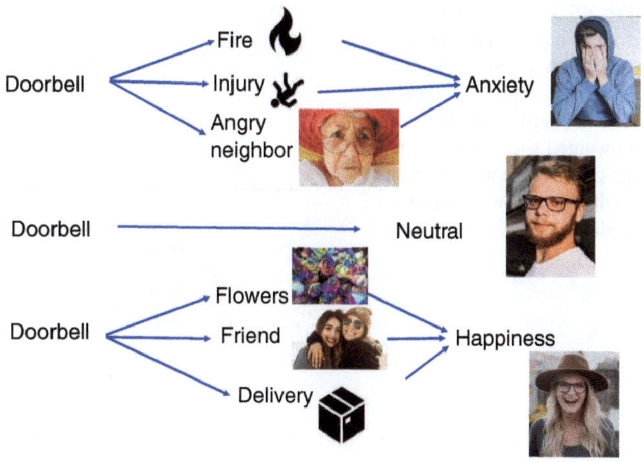

Fig. 49.2 The brain can learn different responses to the same sound (e.g., doorbell). Tinnitus often causes negative thoughts and emotional reactions, but more neutral or positive thoughts can be produced depending on the context and interpretation of the tinnitus

Thoughts and Emotions

We focus on three aspects in this session, including

- How tinnitus captures our conscious attention.
- How our thoughts about tinnitus dictate our emotions.
- How we can change our reactions to tinnitus.

To help determine that tinnitus is not important and can be ignored, we distinguish two types of attention, conscious attention (or the level of awareness when we think about and analyze various stimuli) and subconscious attention (or the level of awareness when we monitor information, but do not consciously analyze it). We review the various types of stimuli that compete for our attention, including tactile, visual, olfactory, gustatory, and finally, auditory (e.g., tinnitus!). Through this discussion of conscious attention and competing stimuli, we can make the connection that people simultaneously monitor these stimuli all the time as suggested by Hallam [2]. Further, important stimuli that are unusual, important, scary, or unexpected will capture our conscious attention. Tinnitus is often defined by all of these aspects, and therefore, is deemed important and monitored at a conscious level. This discussion provides an opportunity to discuss how patients can divert their attention away from the tinnitus if it is decided that tinnitus is no longer important. However, doing so requires that there be no medical concerns for having tinnitus (i.e., an ENT examination reveals no tumor or other immediate concerns). With time, most patients are able to learn how to divert their attention away from the tinnitus typically in at least 18 months [2], though we acknowledge this process varies significantly from patient to patient.

To understand the connection between our thoughts and emotions, we explain that thoughts generally fall into three categories: positive, negative, and neutral that will give rise to the three related categories of emotions (i.e., positive, negative, and neutral). We explore the patient's thoughts about their tinnitus, identifying unhealthy or negative thoughts about tinnitus, and working to restructure these thoughts to be neutral or even positive. At this point, educating the tinnitus patient that they (and their brain!) can learn a response to a particular sound (e.g., a doorbell) and later learn a different response to the same sound is appropriate. Figure 49.2 provides an example slide from TAT that illustrates how the brain automatically attaches an emotional reaction to the sound, which varies from negative, neutral, and positive depending on the consequence. We use this visual aid to help understand how tinnitus might produce an entirely different emotional reaction depending on our thoughts about tinnitus.

In changing our reactions to tinnitus, we emphasize four main actions:

- Demote the importance of tinnitus.
- Unlearn negative thoughts about tinnitus.
- Refocus on other activities.
- Reduce the contrast between tinnitus and background sounds.

To demote or change the importance of tinnitus, reviewing the facts about tinnitus is an effective strategy, such as stating that tinnitus is the result of increased spontaneous neural activity and that the prevalence of tinnitus is relatively high (i.e., 30 million persons living in the United States and 27% of elderly individuals) [23]. We reiterate that tinnitus and one's reaction to it are different and one coping method is to decrease or demote its importance. Practice activities such as focusing on tinnitus and then on something else (e.g., listening to music, reading a book) are often used to demonstrate how to divert away from tinnitus. This message pro-

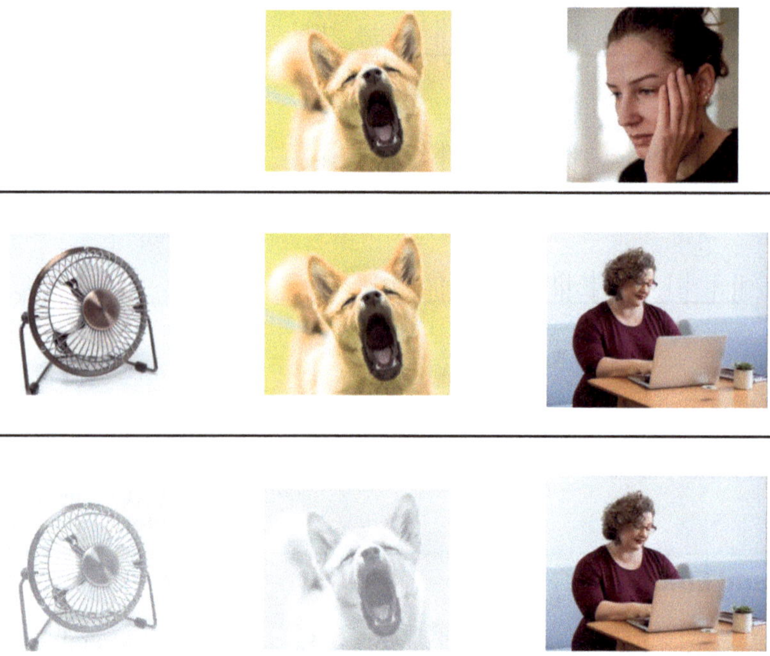

Fig. 49.3 Background sounds can partially mask unwanted sounds (e.g., dog barking to represent tinnitus). The background and unwanted sound will often be less noticeable and reactions to the tinnitus will improve with time

vides hope as patients realize that overtime they may be less bothered by tinnitus if less attention is paid to it. Unlearning negative thoughts about tinnitus (e.g., I hate this noise! I can't live like this with this noise in my head!) takes considerable effort given the heighted emotional reactions that many patients have and the resulting depression, anxiety, and distress that are correlated with tinnitus [24, 25]. We recommend use of a tinnitus diary to assist patients in changing how they react emotionally to tinnitus and learning positive self-talk. Diaries often include patients logging their negative thoughts and worries about tinnitus, checking to see if these thoughts actually happen, and listing alternate ways of thinking about tinnitus (neutral or positive). We recommend that diaries should be kept for only 2 weeks, as consistent use of a diary will often bring one's attention to their tinnitus, rather than the intended purpose to identify and restructure negative thoughts about tinnitus. For patients who need additional counseling and/or medications to manage mental distress, we readily refer to and work collaboratively with trained mental health professionals.

We also explore with the patient other activities such as engaging in hobbies, exercise, and social activities that bring intrinsic value and will help to focus away from their tinnitus. The use of the tinnitus diary can be used to identify how activities affect the tinnitus and select those activities that are enjoyable and will refocus their attention in a helpful way. Sound therapy is an important consideration at the beginning of tinnitus counseling because the use of background sound often makes tinnitus less noticeable, for most patients. Not all patients will have explored sound therapy adequately on their own. Therefore, we explain the mechanism for sound therapy and how it makes tinnitus more difficult to detect (i.e., interferes with the brain's neural input). We use visual aids to explain these concepts, such as shown in Fig. 49.3, which displays how a background sound can decrease the neural prominence of tinnitus and eventually, reduce negative emotional reactions to the tinnitus. Many patients are concerned that adding a second sound will only exacerbate their tinnitus that is why appropriate counseling on sound therapy is so critical for its success. We use the tinnitus diary to assist patients in conducting a "Sound Search" that documents the sounds they listen to (e.g., static sounds like white noise, environmental sounds like rain or ocean waves, and music) and their effect on the tinnitus. Many tinnitus patients benefit from sound therapy [26–28] that can be added to their environment with little expense and in a variety of formats (Apps, stand-alone sound generators, CDs, personal recorded sounds, etc.).

Hearing

Recognizing the importance of communication in our everyday lives and the significant number of patients with tinnitus and hearing loss, the goals of this session are to educate patients about their hearing and reduce communication and hearing difficulties. We explain the patient's audiogram thoroughly and in detail so that they understand if they have hearing loss and if so, the severity and type of loss. We review causes of hearing loss including the most prevalent causes of noise and age and compare this to the patient's own cause of hearing loss and tinnitus, if known. Using helpful visual aids like diagrams of the ear and the everyday sound audiogram explain how the auditory system works to code sounds and how hearing loss affects communication. We use the audiogram to distinguish low- and high-frequency sounds and their importance for speech perception and relate this to the patient's hearing abilities and the communication difficulties resulting from hearing loss. Patients will often attribute their communication difficulties to the tinnitus even in cases of significant hearing loss. Thus, education is needed to better understand the hearing mechanism and the influence of tinnitus on communication, such as masking some speech sounds. Certainly, tinnitus can mask some sounds [29, 30] and can be confused with external sounds that have a similar pitch percept. We emphasize that tinnitus does not cause hearing loss, though can make it harder to hear sounds or distract from listening.

The influence of background noise is also significant for patients with tinnitus and hearing loss, which should be addressed by discussing how to improve the signal-to-noise ratio (e.g., eliminating distracting noise sources and increasing the distance from a noise source such as a noisy kitchen at a restaurant). Additional factors that influence communication are discussed including the ability to see the talker, the familiarity with the talker, the familiarity with the discussion topic, and the overall stress level of the patient during communication. We suggest (and demonstrate) the advantages of asking the talker to slow down and speak clearly.

It should be clearly mentioned that a first step in managing hearing loss is through amplification [31] via hearing aids, cochlear implants, hearing assistive technology, or other hearing devices (e.g., Personal Sound Amplification Products) as appropriate (see Chap. 46). The benefits of amplification are discussed including better audibility for sounds and speech, improved hearing in noise and localization of sounds in our environment, and less effortful listening. Advantages of proper and well-fit amplification are compared to the limitations, such as amplification of unwanted sounds, unnatural sound quality, and inconvenience of wearing devices. With proper counseling, we help patients navigate these issues and concerns, and we also offer hearing aid trials to patients so they can experience the benefits of amplification firsthand. Many hearing aid manufacturers today offer multiple options for tinnitus relief that include sound therapy using static and modulated sounds, music, notch therapy, and mixing sounds, along with smartphone Apps to further adjust tinnitus therapy sounds.

Beyond reducing background noise and using amplification (in cases of hearing loss) to improve communication, we also suggest that patients use speech reading, adopt repair strategies, and implement an effective communication style. Our tips for improved communication include:

- Position and eye contact.
  - Always face the talker. Look at the mouth and eyes for nonverbal cues.
  - Sit close to the talker, but within a safe distance.
  - Do not have a conversation walking side by side with someone.
- Lighting and visibility.
  - Communicate in good lighting, making sure your face is well lit.
  - Use a clear mask or face shield to maximize visual cues (during pandemic times).
- Clear speech.
  - Speak slowly and clearly and pause occasionally. Do not shout or over-articulate.
  - Rephrase your questions or comments rather than repeating the same words.
  - Use gestures and hand signs like "thumbs" up.
- Background noise.
  - Close a door or window to reduce background noise.
  - Turn off all other noise sources.
- Technology.
  - Rely on written communication (email, text) whenever possible.
  - Use captioning for TV watching and viewing videos and lectures.
  - Try smartphone apps to transcribe live speech. Check out Google Live Transcribe (Android only), Ava, Otter, and Live Caption.

We also encourage patients to adopt an assertive communication style (e.g., interacts appropriately, guides communication partner) rather than a passive (e.g., withdraws from conversations or pretends to understand) or aggressive communication style (e.g., dominates conversation, is unwilling to take responsibility for breakdowns). Therefore, a discussion of effective communication and repair strategies along with activities to track their communication style and use of communication strategies for later reflection will benefit many patients.

Sleep

Sleep disturbances are commonly reported by tinnitus patients [6, 32, 33], typically causing difficulties in falling asleep or falling back asleep once awake at night. Fatigue is often a consequence of poor sleep that exacerbates the severity of the tinnitus and one's emotional reactions to it. Fortunately, there are many medications to help manage sleep problems (e.g., melatonin, over-the-counter sleep aids, and prescription medications), and we refer patients to physicians to manage chronic insomnia (see Chaps. 42 and 48). Additionally, counseling about sleep and improving sleep hygiene is an important component and is often well received by tinnitus patients with sleep problems. We review normal sleep patterns, including the four sleep stages, and expectations for good sleep that averages about 6.5–9 h, depending on the individual. Some patients will expect the same amount and same type of deep sleep they had when younger, not realizing that the duration and number of awakenings increase as we age. Using a sleep chart to describe the sleep stages and average hours of sleep can be particularly useful in setting realistic expectations. We discuss the factors that affect the quality and amount of sleep, including stress and emotions (depression and anxiety), environmental considerations (noise, lighting, and temperature), work schedules and learned sleeplessness patterns, among others. To reduce stress and prepare for sleep, patients are encouraged to create a curfew, about 1.5 h before bed at which time they should avoid stress, exercise, eating, alcohol, caffeine, etc. Before the curfew, patients can write down their concerns and worries so they are less focused on these concerns and better able to relax. We encourage patients to engage in regular exercise at least 3–4 h before bedtime that sufficiently exhausts the body and mind. When there is a bad night of sleep (that impacts all people from time to time), patients should be encouraged to lead as normal a day as possible, avoiding the lack of sleep that was experienced. Sleep is best when we make the least amount of effort.

Other suggestions to better prepare for sleep include the following:

- Eliminating or reducing any distractions and nonsleep related items, including a TV, computer, laptop, food/drink, etc.
- Adding comfortable mattresses, pillows, and blankets to make the bedroom cozy.
- Darkening the bedroom to avoid being awaken by light.
- Setting the room temperature cool at 58–68 °F (14–20 °C).
- Listening to low-level background sound.

There are a number of options for adding background sound to the bedroom, which will help many patients who report increased tinnitus in quiet situations. For example, there are many Apps or sound generators for sleep that are used by individuals with insomnia, not just the tinnitus patient. Apps and sound generators have the ability to combine and select a variety of sounds and also options for setting a sleep timer that will gradually reduce the volume of the sound rather than turning off abruptly. Other patients will take a more traditional approach such as a fan, but the level of sound is not controlled as with an App or Sound Pillow. To ascertain the benefit of using background sound, and learning more about the patient's sleep patterns, patients can create a sleep diary similar to a tinnitus diary. The sleep diary should be specific to address the patient's concerns and may include the average hours of sleep, the impact of better sleep hygiene including use of a curfew or rearranging the bedroom, and the use and effect of background sound in the bedroom.

Preparing for sleep using relaxation exercises, such as progressive muscle relaxation, guided imagery, and body scanning, are great techniques to facilitate good sleep. We have implemented progressive muscle relaxation in TAT adopted by Henry & Wilson [34] that teaches patients to systematically tense and relax groups of muscles [35]. Progressive muscle relaxation includes deliberately applying tension to certain muscles (i.e., arms, legs, and feet) and then relaxing the muscle and focusing on the release after tension is stopped. Guided or visual imagery, as shown in Fig. 49.4, is a mindfulness activity that uses all five senses to recreate an experience that patients find relaxing. We use pictures and sound via an App to create that experience, starting with the visualization of a beach, birds flying overhead, and blue water, and then guiding the patient through the smells of the air and saltwater, the sounds of the ocean waves and birds squawking, and then feel of the sand and taste of the ocean. This example is easily relatable for most patients, though it should be tailored to meet the needs of the individual patient if there is a favorite relaxation scene (e.g., forest, mountains) preferred by the patient. Other relaxation techniques include body scanning or mindfulness meditation by doing a quick replay of the day right before bedtime [36]. These relaxation techniques are demonstrated during the clinical session so that patients can choose a technique that suits them. We encourage daily practice to help manage negative reactions to their tinnitus (e.g., increased stress or anxiety) and prepare for sleep. We also recommend Apps for meditation and mindfulness such as *Resound Relief, Tinnitus Calmer, Relax Melodies, Headspace, and Zenways* that were found to be acceptable and of sufficient quality when studied in 120 tinnitus patients [37].

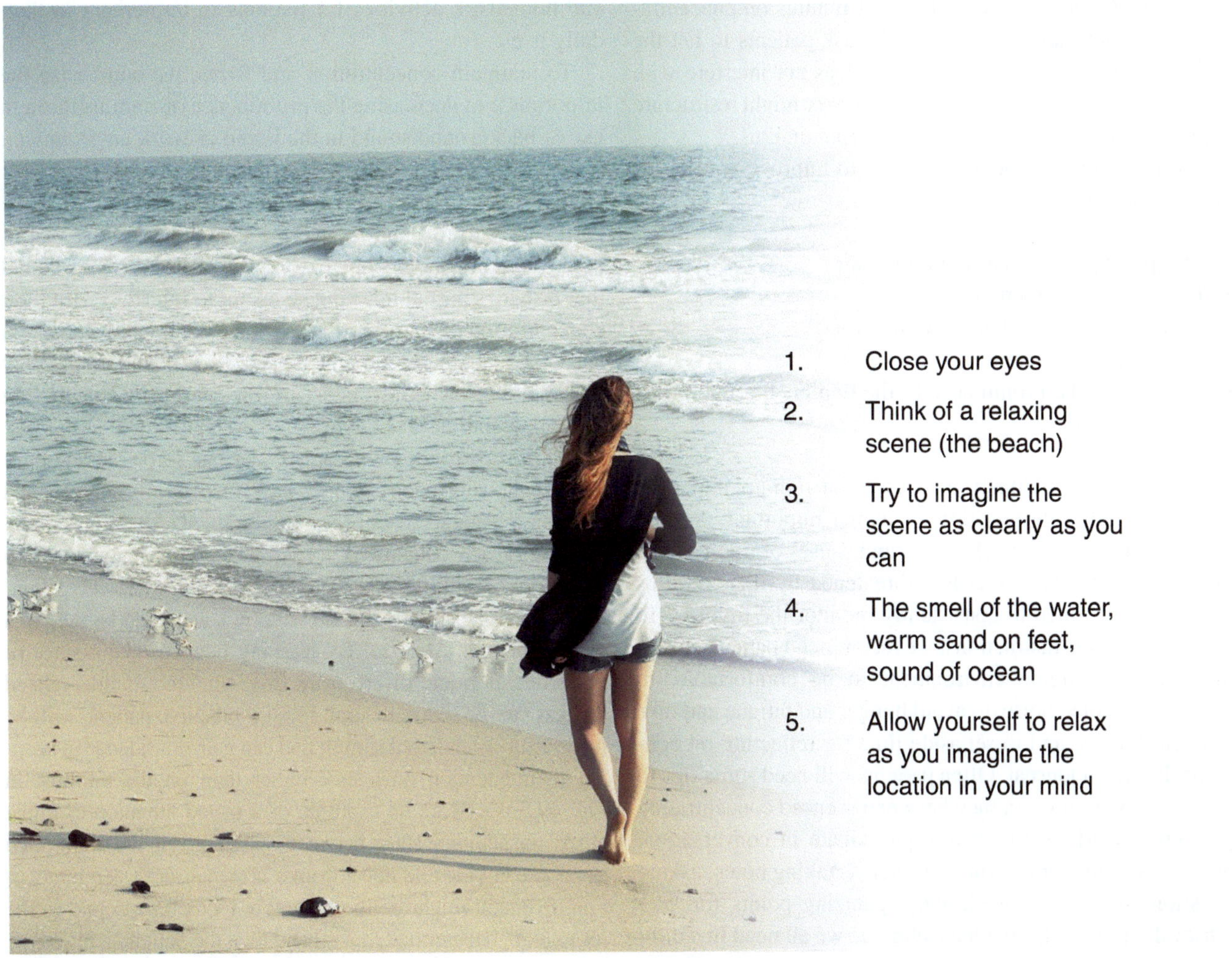
1. Close your eyes
2. Think of a relaxing scene (the beach)
3. Try to imagine the scene as clearly as you can
4. The smell of the water, warm sand on feet, sound of ocean
5. Allow yourself to relax as you imagine the location in your mind

Fig. 49.4 A guided imagery example for use during counseling and promoting relaxation. Patients should imagine a favorite scene that elicits all five senses

Concentration

Tinnitus patients often remark that the tinnitus interferes with their ability to focus and concentrate on certain tasks. Recognizing these difficulties, we have developed the concentration session to do the following: describe how tinnitus affects concentration including the influence of task complexity, review strategies to improve concentration such as adjusting work habits, and learn how to take volitional control of attention through attention control exercises.

To understand how tinnitus affects concentration, we review the importance of concentration to complete tasks and remember information. An inability to concentrate, as described by many tinnitus patients, will cause frustration and increase stress that can further worsen their tinnitus. There are multiple factors that would result in an inability to concentrate, including excessive background noise, auditory or visual distractions (TV, radio), poor lighting, having a challenging physical state such as hunger, fatigue, and poor health, and finally, being in a negative emotional state such as anxiety, depression, or fear. We acknowledge that all people can be distracted by stimuli, especially those that are annoying, fearful, competing with other things, loud, etc., as would be experienced with tinnitus. To engage patients during this session, we ask that they rate their ability to concentrate on a given task and reflect on the concentration problems that they experience in everyday life.

Tinnitus can affect individuals with tinnitus in various ways, and not all patients will be distracted by it. However, we know that if attention is focused on tinnitus, focusing on other tasks or problems will be hindered because we consciously respond to only one stimulus at a given time. Examining the specific effects of tinnitus on concentration often begins by observing the influence of task complexity. For some patients, working on a simple tasks like reading or responding to email are not stimulating enough and tinnitus might be very distracting. Comparatively, complex tasks like composing a music piece or crafting a new quilt will be more demanding cognitively. When conscious attention is focused away from tinnitus, patients will often find that their tinnitus will be less noticeable. Of course, these effects of tinnitus on concentration vary from patient to patient. We ask patients to list the situations or tasks where the tinnitus does not interfere with concentration and use this to frame how they might restructure their day to minimize the distractions from tinnitus.

We recommend several strategies to improve concentration, including

- Interpreting tinnitus as not important.
- Eliminating distractions.
- Staying focused and attentive on tasks.
- Adjusting work habits.
- Decreasing the prominence of the tinnitus through background sound.

As reviewed previously, a necessary step in not attending to tinnitus is to interpret tinnitus as not important. A good understanding of the mechanisms and causes of tinnitus will often help patients to feel less threatened by their tinnitus and be less inclined to consistently monitor the tinnitus. To eliminate outside distractions, we recommend patients adjust their work or home environment to be comfortable, to remove unwanted noise, to avoid hunger and fatigue and take frequent breaks, and to set aside time for reflecting on concerns through a journal. Often patients will need some tips to help stay focused when they have experienced concentration problems. Working to actively participate in conversation, problem solving, or meetings, as well as taking notes, asking questions to stay engaged, and organizing points for later retrieval will be helpful. One technique we all need in a digital age is to adjust work habits by working in short time spans of 20–40 min with a break. Working at a realistic pace is critical to avoid fatigue and maintain adequate concentration. Complex tasks require advanced task management skills such as reducing the project into smaller tasks, working on priorities, and stopping for reflection and modification. In our sessions, we provide handouts of these strategies and homework activities for patients to implement in their daily lives.

To maintain concentration and focus, we emphasize the importance of decreasing the prominence of tinnitus through use of background sound in the home or work environment. For patients who have difficulty concentrating, especially for simple tasks, playing background sounds or music may be particularly useful and reduce the distracting nature of tinnitus. Patients should opt for low-level background sound that provides partial masking so as not to interfere with their concentration on a given task. We have completed studies on use of sound therapy using Apps [38–40] and found that many patients benefit from use of low-level sounds including for concentration [41].

Taking control of attention is under one's voluntary control and attention diversion exercises have successfully been applied to tinnitus patients to improve attention [3]. Attention control exercises teach patients to consciously switch their attention from one stimulus (e.g., visual object in room) to another stimulus (e.g., visual stimuli outside window), as would be seen in a visual attention exercise. By learning how to take control of one's attention and divert away from tinnitus, tinnitus-related distress can be reduced. With regular practice, patients will be more aware of external stimuli and can gain confidence in keeping their attention on a task rather than on the tinnitus. In Fig. 49.5, we share an example of a sound attention example where the attention shifts between two sounds in the room, such as people talking and noise from a heater. A next step in attention diversion might be to alternately focus on a sound in the room (e.g., background music) and then the patient's tinnitus or between a sound in the room and reading. Switching back and forth between external stimuli (e.g., sounds, reading) and their tinnitus improves voluntary control of one's attention and provides a level of confidence that concentration can be maintained with practice. Regular practice of these exercises is encouraged and outcomes are reviewed with patients as they return for future sessions.

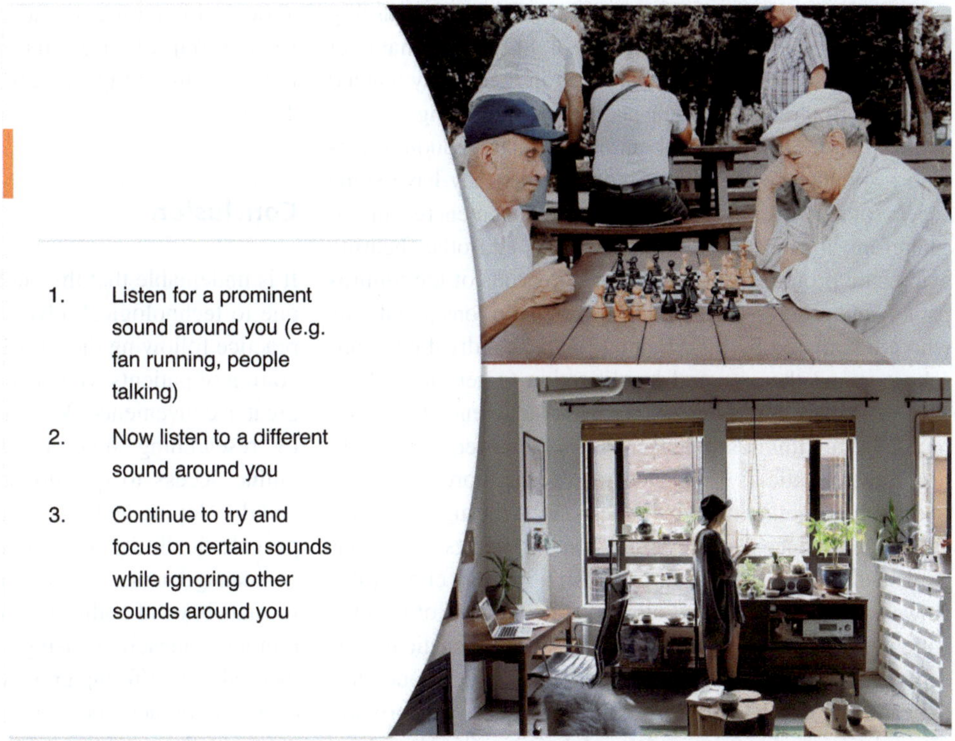

Fig. 49.5 An attention diversion example that uses sound around the listener (e.g., people talking, background fan or heater noise) and compares this to another sound in the room

Evidence for TAT

To document treatment effectiveness with TAT, we have presented and published case studies of tinnitus patients [42, 43] and also conducted a clinical trial at the University of Iowa with 184 tinnitus patients with and without hearing aids [44]. Participants were assigned to one of three groups: counseling, counseling plus total masking, and counseling plus partial masking. Outcomes were compared pre- and post-treatment using the Tinnitus Handicap Questionnaire (THQ) [45]. Results revealed that, for the participants without hearing aids, 48/59 (81%) of participants reported a reduction in THQ scores, which was significant in 24/59 or 41% of these participants when a criterion of 20% reduction was applied. For the participants with tinnitus using hearing aids, THQ post-treatment scores improved in 34 of 43 (79%) participants. Using the 20% reduction as significant, there were 14 of 43 (33%) participants who reported a significant reduction in THQ scores. Group differences between the pre- and post-treatment THQ scores were compared and no significant group effect was observed. Similar results were obtained with the TPFQ. Many, but not all, received significant benefit in each of the four areas affected by tinnitus. Overall, the study found that TAT was effective for some tinnitus patients with and without sound therapy. However, not all patients benefitted from counseling and sound therapy from TAT, which is consistent with our experience in clinical practice and also applies to other therapy approaches for tinnitus. Reasons for why some tinnitus patients benefit from counseling and sound therapy, and others do not deserve more attention and research. In part, we believe that many tinnitus patients get involved in research studies because they are seeking the 'cure'.

Ways to Start TAT in Your Practice

TAT is a long-standing tinnitus management program, backed by years of clinical expertise at the University of Iowa and implemented at other tinnitus clinics around the world. We offer training on TAT to clinicians and hearing healthcare professionals at the University of Iowa's annual conference on the Management of the Tinnitus and Hyperacusis Patient. TAT materials, including the Introduction session and four individual sessions, are available free from the University of Iowa on our website (https://medicine.uiowa.edu/oto/research/tinnitus-and-hyperacusis). We also have created practice and homework activities for each session as described here and developed a TAT summary session that provides a general overview of counseling and sound therapy. For additional descriptions of TAT, please see *Tinnitus Treatment: Clinical Protocols* [12] and the *Katz Handbook of Clinical Audiology* [46].

Tinnitus patients often have difficulty finding help from medical professionals to address their tinnitus-related distress, including receiving basic information and learning how to cope with tinnitus. Husain et al. [47] found that over 60% of 230 tinnitus patients surveyed in their study wanted more information from their audiologist regarding tinnitus management. Conversely, about 67% of the 68 audiologists who responded to the survey reported that they have some access (or less) to appropriate tinnitus management resources. Therefore, it is critical that audiologists and other hearing healthcare professionals respond to the needs of the tinnitus patient and provide multiple management options to patients who are bothered by their tinnitus, such as individual counseling, sound therapy, and amplification (when needed) as offered in TAT. Specialized training or adherence to certain protocols for tinnitus management is not a requirement to help tinnitus patients. Clinicians who desire more training in tinnitus management can gain these skills through the Iowa annual conference or other professional meetings, or see our published papers on how to establish a tinnitus clinic [48]. However, we advocate that clinicians taking care of tinnitus patients have the expertise needed to address medical concerns raised by tinnitus patients (i.e., knowledge about anatomy and physiology of the ear and brain) and already provide counseling to address a variety of hearing disorders (i.e., hearing loss) that uniquely prepares them to respond to the needs of tinnitus patients [48].

In addition to individual counseling for tinnitus, clinicians may also want to consider offering group educational sessions [49]. Group sessions are effective because helpful information about tinnitus can be shared with a larger group of individuals in a single session, realistic expectations for managing tinnitus can be set in a clear manner, and people with tinnitus and their partners are able to share their questions and concerns with others to validate their experience. Patients with bothersome tinnitus often want to know that they are not alone, which can be addressed in a group setting. We facilitate the discussion during group educational sessions to ensure that we cover relevant topics and manage time well, however, also allow for adequate discussion time amongst participants in the group session as their questions and concerns arise.

Many tinnitus patients also report hyperacusis (see Chaps. 3 and 41) and additional counseling should be provided to help them manage their hyperacusis symptoms. In our clinics, we offer Hyperacusis Activities Treatment [46], a holistic approach to hyperacusis management that includes counseling and sound therapy. Counseling for hyperacusis can include providing helpful education about hyperacusis, exploring one's emotional reactions to sound, and reviewing helpful management strategies in a collaborative, supportive manner. Many patients respond well to the use of mindfulness exercises, which should be used daily to lessen stress and anxiety about bothersome sounds. A recent publication from a focus group of 11 adults with hyperacusis outlined steps in providing group education using Hyperacusis Activities Treatment [50].

Conclusion

It is undeniable that the landscape of healthcare is changing due to technological advancements, the emergence of telepractice following the COVID-19 pandemic, and a new generation of patients who desire digital access to healthcare for greater convenience. We have responded to these demands by researching smartphone Apps for tinnitus, providing online access to questionnaires and counseling materials, and developing and researching online tinnitus therapies. To provide flexibility for patients and expand services in tinnitus management, clinicians may want to consider a variety of formats beyond traditional one-on-one counseling, including remote counseling using synchronous or asynchronous methods and offering group educational sessions. Regardless of the approach, person-centered care that addresses the needs of the patient is critical to delivering beneficial and effective intervention. TAT focuses on the four areas impacted by the tinnitus (i.e., thoughts and emotions, hearing, sleep, and concentration) using an outcome-based approach by documenting treatment effectiveness via the TPFQ. The collaborative nature of TAT counseling, along with easy-to-use visual aids, provides the audiologist with helpful materials to establish a successful practice in counseling the tinnitus patient.

References

1. Coles RRA. Tinnitus and its management. In: Stephens D, Kerr AG, editors. Scott-Brown's otolaryngology, vol. 2, Chapter 10. Guildford: Butterworth; 1987. p. 368–414.
2. Hallam RS. Tinnitus: living with the ringing in your ears. New York, NY: Harper Collins Publishing; 1989.
3. Henry JL, Wilson PH. The psychological management of chronic tinnitus: a cognitive-behavioral approach. Boston, MA: Allyn & Bacon Publishers; 2001.
4. Sweetow RW. Cognitive-behavioral modification in tinnitus management. Hear Instru. 1984;35:14–52.
5. Tyler RS, Babin RW. Tinnitus. In: Cummings CW, Fredrickson JM, Harker L, Krause CJ, Schuller DE, editors. Otolaryngol Head Neck Surg, vol. 4. St. Louis, MO: Mosby; 1986. p. 3201–17.
6. Tyler RS, Baker LJ. Difficulties experienced by tinnitus sufferers. J Speech Hear Disord. 1983;48:150–4.
7. Tyler RS, Stouffer JL, Schum R. Audiological rehabilitation of the tinnitus client. J Acad Rehabil Audiol. 1989;22:30–42.
8. Stouffer JL, Tyler RS, Kileny P, Dalzell L. Tinnitus as a function of duration and etiology: counseling implications. Am J Otol. 1991;12:188–94.
9. Bentler RA, Tyler RS. Tinnitus management. ASHA. 1987;29(5):27–32.

10. Tyler RS, Bentler RA. Tinnitus maskers and hearing aids for tinnitus. Semin Hear. 1987;8(1):49–61.
11. Tyler RS, Bergan C. Tinnitus retraining therapy: a modified approach. Hear J. 2001;54(11):36–42.
12. Perreau A, Tyler R, Mancini P, Witt S. Tinnitus activities treatment. In: Tyler RS, Perreau A, editors. Tinnitus treatment: clinical protocols (2nd ed). Thieme; 2022. p. 42–70.
13. World Health Organization. International Classification of Functioning (ICF), Disability and Health. Geneva, Switzerland. 2001.
14. Hickson L, Scarinci N. Older adults with acquired hearing impairment: applying the ICF in rehabilitation. Semin Speech Lang. 2007;28(4):283–90.
15. Newman C, Sandridge S, Jacobsen GP. Assessing outcomes of tinnitus intervention. J Am Acad Audiol. 2014;25:76–105.
16. Tyler RS, Perreau AE, Ji H, Witt S, Noble W, Coelho C. The development and validation of the tinnitus primary functions questionnaire. Am J Audiol. 2014;23(3):260–72.
17. Hallam RS, Jakes SC. Cognitive variables in tinnitus annoyance. Br J Clin Psychol. 1988;27(3):213–22.
18. Newman CW, Jacobson GP, Spitzer JB. Development of the tinnitus handicap inventory. Arch Otolaryngol Head Neck Surg. 1996;122(2):143–8.
19. Meikle MB, Henry JA, Griest SE, Stewart BJ, Abrams HB, McArdle R, et al. The tinnitus functional index: development of a new clinical measure for chronic, intrusive tinnitus. Ear Hear. 2012;33(2):153–76.
20. Tyler RS. Tinnitus disability and handicap questionnaires. Semin Hear. 1993;14(4):377–84.
21. Dillon H, et al. Client oriented scale of improvement (COSI) and its relationship to several other measures of benefit and satisfaction provided by hearing aids. J Am Acad Audiol. 1997;8:27–43.
22. Searchfield GD. A client-oriented scale of improvement in tinnitus for therapy goal planning and assessing outcomes. J Am Acad Audiol. 2019;30(4):327–37.
23. Kochkin S, Tyler R, Born J. MarkeTrak VIII: the prevalence of tinnitus in the United States and the self-reported efficacy of various treatment. Hear Rev. 2011;18(12):10–26.
24. Andersson G, Baguley DM, McKenna L, McFerran DJ. Tinnitus: a multidisciplinary approach. London: Whurr; 2005.
25. Dobie RA. Depression and tinnitus. Otolaryngol Clin N Am. 2003;36:383–8.
26. Hazell JWP, Wood SM, Cooper H, Stephens SDG, Corcoran AL, Coles RRR, et al. A clinical study of tinnitus maskers. Br J Audiol. 1985;19:65–116.
27. Henry J, McMillan G, Dann S, Bennett K, Griest S, Theodoroff S, et al. Tinnitus management: randomized controlled trial comparing extended-wear hearing aids, conventional hearing aids, and combination instruments. J Am Acad Audiol. 2017;28:546–61.
28. Hobson J, Chisholm E, El Refaie A. Sound therapy (masking) in the management of tinnitus in adults. Cochrane Database Syst Rev. 2010;12(11):CD006371.
29. Melin L, Scott B, Lindberg P, Lyttkens L. Hearing aids and tinnitus—an experimental group study. Br J Audiol. 1987;21(2): 91–7.
30. Surr R, Montgomery A, Mueller H. Effect of amplification on tinnitus among new hearing aid users. Ear Hear. 1985;6:71–5.
31. Searchfield GD. Hearing aids and tinnitus. In: Tyler RS, editor. Tinnitus treatment: clinical protocols. New York, NY: Thieme; 2006. p. 161–75.
32. McKenna L. Tinnitus and insomnia. In: Tyler RS, editor. Tinnitus handbook. San Diego, CA: Singular; 2000. p. 59–84.
33. McKenna L, Daniel HC. Tinnitus-related insomnia treatment. In: Tyler RS, editor. Tinnitus treatment: clinical protocols. New York, NY: Thieme; 2006. p. 81–95.
34. Henry JL, Wilson PH. Tinnitus: a self-management guide for the ringing in your ears. Boston, MA: Allyn & Bacon Publishers; 2002.
35. Davison GC, Neale JM. Abnormal psychology. 3rd ed. New York: Wiley; 1982.
36. Calistoga Press. Mindfulness made simple. New York: Fall River Press; 2014.
37. Sereda M, Smith S, Newton K, Stockdale D. Mobile apps for management of tinnitus: users' survey, quality assessment, and content analysis. JMIR Mhealth Uhealth. 2019;7(1):e10353.
38. Tyler RS, Keiner AJ, Walker K, Deshpande AK, Witt S, Killian M, et al. A series of case studies of tinnitus suppression with mixed background stimuli in a cochlear implant. Am J Audiol. 2015;22:398–410.
39. Tyler R, Owen R, Bridges J, Gander P, Mancini PC, Perreau A. Tinnitus suppression in cochlear implant patients using a sound therapy app. Am J Audiol. 2018;27:316–23.
40. Perreau A, Tyler RS, Frank V, Watts A, Mancini P. Use of a smartphone app for cochlear implant patients with tinnitus. Am J Audiol. 2021;30;676–87.
41. Tyler R, Perreau A, Powers T, Watts A, Owen R, Ji H, et al. Tinnitus sound therapy trial shows effectiveness for those with tinnitus. J Am Acad Audiol. 2020;31:6–16.
42. Perreau A, Tyler R. Tinnitus and hyperacusis activities treatment: counseling for adults and children. Paper presented at the Illinois Academy of Audiology Annual Convention. Normal, IL. Jan 2020.
43. Perreau A, Tyler R. Tinnitus treatment following acoustic neuroma and Meniere's disease: a single case study. Tinnitus and sound sensitivity casebook. New York, NY: Thieme; 2022.
44. Tyler RS, Stocking C, Ji H, Witt S, Mancini PC. Tinnitus activities treatment with total and partial masking. J Am Acad Audiol. 2021;32:501–9.
45. Kuk FK, Tyler RW, Russell D, Jordan H. The psychometric properties of a tinnitus handicap questionnaire. Ear Hear. 1990;11:434–45.
46. Tyler RS, Noble W, Coelho C, Roncanci ER, Jun HJ. In: Katz J, Chasin M, English K, Hood LJ, Tillery KL, editors. Handbook of clinical audiology. 7th ed. New York: Wolters Kluwer; 2015. p. 647–58.
47. Husain FT, Gander PE, Jansen JN, Shen S. Expectations for tinnitus treatment and outcomes: a survey study of audiologists and patients. J Am Acad Audiol. 2018;29(4):313–36.
48. Tyler RS, Haskill GB, Gogel SA, Gehringer AK. Establishing a tinnitus clinic in your practice. Am J Audiol. 2008;17:25–37.
49. Mancini P, Witt S, Perreau A, Tyler R. Establishing a tinnitus and hyperacusis clinic in your practice. In: Tyler RS, Perreau A, editors. Tinnitus treatment: clinical protocols (2nd ed). Thieme; 2022, 206–18.
50. Perreau AE, Tyler RS, Mancini PC, Witt S, Elgandy MS. Establishing a group educational session for hyperacusis patients. Am J Audiol. 2019;28(2):245–50.

Neural Therapy, Botulinum Toxin

50

Eberhard Biesinger, Jose Miguel Lainez, Marlene M. Speth, and Veronika Vielsmeier

Abstract

Local anaesthesia of peripheral structures and nerves with lidocaine or related drugs can reduce central tinnitus-related activity. The physiology underlaying this phenomenon is the fact that the somatosensory systems and the trigeminal nerves can have a significant impact to the central auditory systems. Inhibition of pathologic afferencies from these structures to the brain is the intention of the described therapeutic procedures. Trigger points in muscles and tendons in head and neck area and the shoulder girdle are examined by specific active and passive tests in a silent chamber and then treated with needle injection of local anaesthesia.

The trigeminal nerve plays another role. Well described by S. Shore, this nerve system has enormous influence on the dorsal cochlear nucleus. The deafferentation here can be accomplished by administering the local anesthetic to the otic ganglion. The proper application is done intraorally, which is in contrast to mostly described procedures in the literature.

The application of Botulinum toxin is helpful for the palatal myoclonus, when muscles are contracting irregularly. The toxin acts here by blocking the neuromuscular action. Another effect is an antinoceptive one which might also be helpful for inhibitation of central trigeminovascular neurons. The application is done around the ear and to cervical muscles.

E. Biesinger
Private Practice, Centre of Otorhinolaryngology, Lindenberg, Germany
e-mail: eberhard@biesinger.email

J. M. Lainez
Department of Neurology, University Clinic Hospital, Catholic University of Valencia, Valencia, Spain
e-mail: miguel.lainez@sen.es

M. M. Speth
Department of Otorhinolaryngology - Head and Neck Surgery, Kantonsspital Aarau, Aarau, Switzerland

V. Vielsmeier (✉)
Department of Otorhinolaryngology, University of Regensburg, Regensburg, Germany
e-mail: veronika.vielsmeier@ukr.de

Highlights

Local anaesthesia to peripheral structures is effective in treating somatosensory tinnitus. Diagnostic tools are the passive and active examinations of head and neck in a silent chamber. Application of local anesthetic to the otic ganglion is a specific therapy for tinnitus and pain caused by the trigeminal nerve system. Botulinum toxin is the only possible therapy for the palatal myoclonus and potentially also for special forms of somatosensory tinnitus.

Introduction

Neural therapy goes back to the German doctor G. Spiess [1], who in 1902 published for the first time about the healing properties of local anaesthetics. Later, it was Huneke [2] who introduced the term neural therapy and examined the topic scientifically. The principle of neural therapy involves the application of local anaesthetics to peripheral nerves and to trigger points of the musculoskeletal system. The mechanism of action of neural therapy is the inhibition of action potentials at peripheral nerves by the blockage of sodium channels. As non-physiologic information from the periphery can thereby get eliminated, a reorganisation of central neurons and reduction of pathologic neuronal activity (here so-called tinnitus related activity) can take place. This fundamental value of neural therapy has been examined for acute and chronic pain and can have therapeutic potential in the same way for acute and chronic tinnitus.

W. Schlee et al. (eds.), *Textbook of Tinnitus*, https://doi.org/10.1007/978-3-031-35647-6_50

Substances

All neural therapeutics go back to cocaine, which has been isolated from cocoa leaves in 1855 by Gaedeke (chemical substance: Benzoylecgoninmethylesther) [3]. Most known today are the synthetically produced drugs procaine and lidocaine. Due to their chemical composition they both differ profoundly: procaine is composed of an ester bond, whereas lidocaine is made up of an amide bond. Hence, there is a different distribution of each of the substances in tissue. Procaine spreads very little in tissue and therefore has to be applied very precisely. On the contrary, lidocaine spreads very well in tissue, which is why it is the preferred substance in clinical practice. Furthermore, when applied locally, allergic reactions to lidocaine are rare and mostly only additives are responsible (for example, methylparaben) for allergic reactions. Today, the medical substances used differ in their effect duration, i.e. procaine lasts up to 0.5 h whereas bupivacaine last between 2 and 8 h [4]. All local anaesthetics function little or not at all in inflamed tissue.

Lidocaine 1% without adrenaline is recommended for the measures shown here. The therapist applying the drugs is responsible for the consideration of potential risks and contraindications for each individual patient.

The Clinical Importance of Neural Therapy for Tinnitus

The neural mechanisms underlying these phenomena were first described by Shore et al. in 2007 [5]. As explained in Chap. X sensations from the head, face and neck can influence the activity in the central auditory pathway [5]. Projections from the somatosensory system to the inferior colliculus and to the cochlear nucleus were detected [5, 6].

This involvement of somatosensory structures offers additional treatment options for tinnitus, but the involvement varies in tinnitus patients. Thus, it is expected that treatment options targeting the somatosensory system will be particularly effective in groups of patients where the somatosensory system is critically involved in the individual pathophysiology.

In this context, neural therapy is understood as a complementary therapy for the treatment of somatosensory tinnitus (SST) (see Chap. X). Mostly, it is seen as a part or as an addition to further measures including manual therapy, osteopathy and trigger point treatment [7], as well as to drugs like muscle relaxants and antiphlogistics.

Furthermore, somatic tinnitus is clinically observed by modulation of pitch. By muscle contraction and pressure applied to the head, neck and limbs a different pitch of tinnitus can be seen. This is the case for up to 60% of all tinnitus patients [8].

A review showed that treatment of the cervical spine has positive effects on patients with subjective tinnitus [9]. This could also be in patients with comorbid temporomandibular joint disorders [10, 11] or in patients whose musculoskeletal system seems influences the individual tinnitus [12, 13]. This group of patients can often modulate their tinnitus by jaw movements (43%), head movements (39%), using muscle pressure (13%), eye movements and by applying a global muscular effort (9%) [14].

However, the identification of somatic tinnitus can be complex in some cases. The modulation of tinnitus regarding volume and frequency can only be perceived in quiet environment. This is why the patient should be examined in a totally silent environment. In accordance to Travell [7], myofascial trigger points when stimulated, can modulate the volume and frequency of tinnitus. They can be identified in the clinical examination. Those trigger points may also have distant effects equivalent to the so-called referred pain. Such trigger points are then also useful for neural therapy.

In the following, we explain two examples for clinical practice:

1. Applying pressure to the muscular insertion point of the M. levator scapulae (Fig. 50.1) often leads to a modulation of tinnitus. This muscle typically inserts at the facet

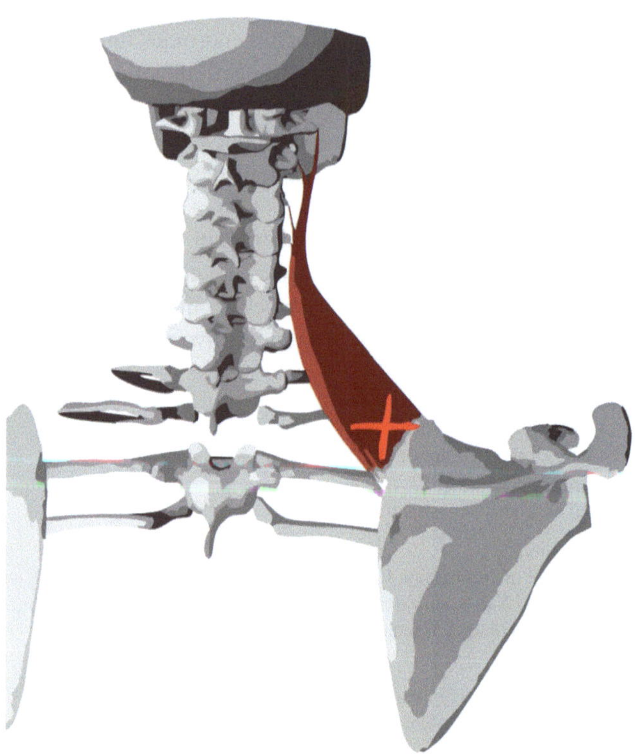

Fig. 50.1 The insertion point of the levator scapulae as an often diagnosed trigger point

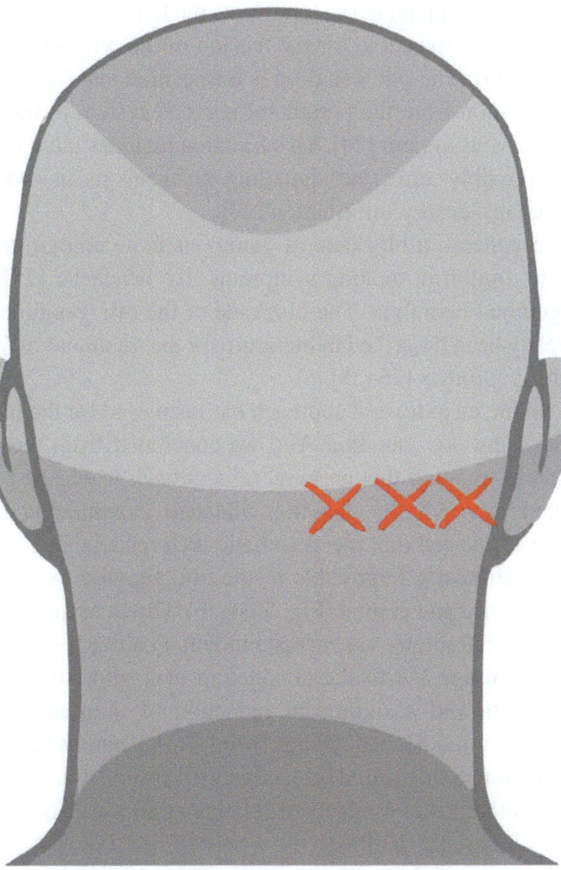

Fig. 50.2 Neural therapeutic points at the suboccipital muscles

joints C2 to C3 and thereby has great biodynamic effects to the upper cervical spine. Neural therapy consists of injecting approximately 0.5 ml lidocaine to the insertion points of the muscle at the medial part of the scapula.

2. Often, myogelosis and trigger points can be found at the insertion points of the suboccipital muscles (splenius capitis muscle, semispinalis capitis muscle). Lidocaine (approximately 0.3 ml) can then be specifically targeted and applied to those structures (Fig. 50.2). Caveat: suboccipital muscles show a high density of vestibular afferences. As side effect of neural therapy dizziness can result. Therefore, it is recommended not to apply more than 2 ml of lidocaine in total.

It can be preceded accordingly at other structures, which lead to a modulation of tinnitus once stimulated.

Treatment Aspects

Cervical Spine

The neuronal interconnection of the afferences of the upper cervical spine to the central neurons of the dorsal cochlear nucleus were first described by Bankoul, Neuhuber and Pfaller in 1990 and 1988, respectively [15, 16]. The neuroanatomic interconnections were made visible by using horseradish peroxidase. Those afferences are collected from the periphery by the cervical root C2 and are then interconnected by monosynaptic connections and lead to the centre. Shore et al specify this anatomic connection and describe the meaning of somatic inputs to the dorsal cochlear nucleus [5, 17] (Chap. X).

The convergence of neuronal impulses to the radix C2 is essential for neural therapy: by injecting lidocaine to the supply area of this radix, pathologic afferences can be inhibited and thus, a central tinnitus related activity can be inhibited indirectly. In daily clinical practice, the application of lidocaine to this area can be carried out safely (Fig. 50.3). One has to only be cautious not to inject too deeply into the facet joints and therefore not directly to the radix.

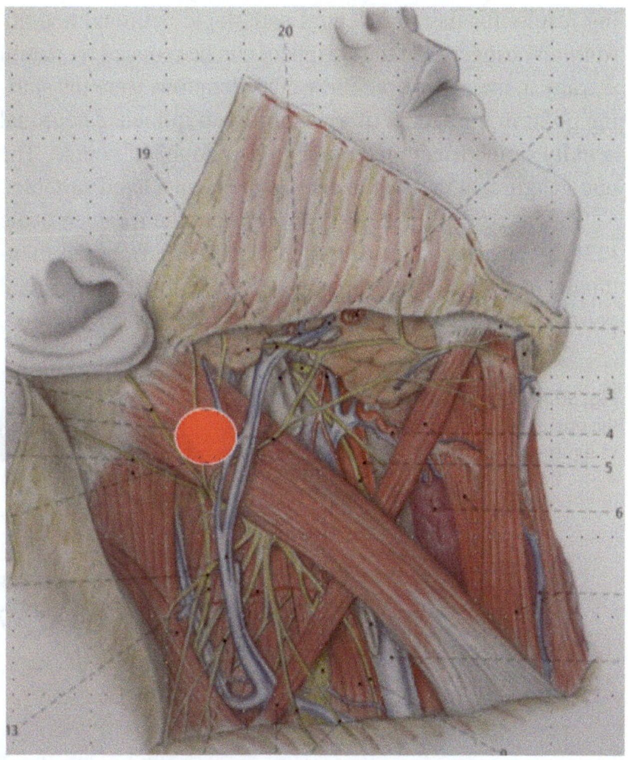

Fig. 50.3 Access to the afferences to radix C2 (mod. from Sobotta, Atlas der Anatomie, Elsevier)

More invasive methods for this deafferentation are described by Gritsenko [18] and Klessinger [19], who successfully carry out the ablation of C2/3 using radiofrequency after bupivacaine application that is the direct deafferentation to the radix.

The superior cervical sympathetic ganglion has a similar meaning as a link for sympathetic afferences to the central hearing system [20]. However, local anaesthesia of this ganglion can be accompanied by severe side effects and is therefore not recommended in classic neural therapy.

Otic Ganglion, Trigeminal Structures and Muscles of the Temporomandibular Joint

Shore and colleagues have described the significance and linkage of the trigeminal centres to the dorsal cochlear nucleus in a large number of important publications. They have described how somatic tinnitus, triggered by the trigeminal nerve, can potentially develop (see Chap. X) [5]. Neuroanatomic connections from the trigeminal nerve to the cochlea and to central nuclei have been examined using horseradish peroxidase [21]. As a consequence, the following results for therapy: central pathologic neuronal activity (tinnitus) triggered in the periphery can be reduced by neural therapy to the periphery. These considerations were the starting point in the search of a possibility to influence neuronal activity of the trigeminal nerve in its peripheral course. The otic ganglion at the scull base was then considered suitable.

The otic ganglion is located inferior to the foramen ovale [22]. It consists of a sensory part originating from the mandibular nerve, a parasympathetic part from the superficial petrosal nerve and a sympathetic part [22, 23]. In addition, the tensor tympani nerve innervates the tensor tympani muscle and is responsible for the tension of the tympanic membrane [23]. The otic ganglion is a transition site for sensory information from the peripheral nervous system to the central nervous system [24]. This function includes intercellular and possibly autocrine signalling mechanisms in order to modulate sensory information [24].

In general, a blockade of ganglions is a common therapeutic option in treating symptoms like headache [25] and trigeminal neuralgia. The blockade of the otic ganglion has already been described in literature for the treatment of facial pain syndromes [26–28].

So far, an extra oral approach has been used for the blockade of the otic ganglion. Yet, we concluded from the anatomical situation that an intraoral approach would be better suited to reach the ganglion: detailed examination on a cadaver showed that the zygomatic arch renders an external approach nearly impossible as the otic ganglion is situated more dorsal and cranial (Fig. 50.4a, b). Direct access is only possible intraorally via the open mouth. Positive results from clinical usage led to the conduction of a pilot study [29], which showed a significant reduction of tinnitus distress (Mini Tinnitus Questionnaire (Mini-TQ), Tinnitus severity) and loudness (measured subjectively) over time. Interestingly though the positive effects of this injection are also observable for chronic tinnitus.

Because of these positive results, the application of this method can only be recommended. It is especially suitable for single sided tinnitus and for tinnitus which can be modulated by movement and which is caused by pathologies of the temporomandibular joint. However, in those cases, further functional therapies are necessary to eliminate the underlying causes affecting the temporomandibular joint.

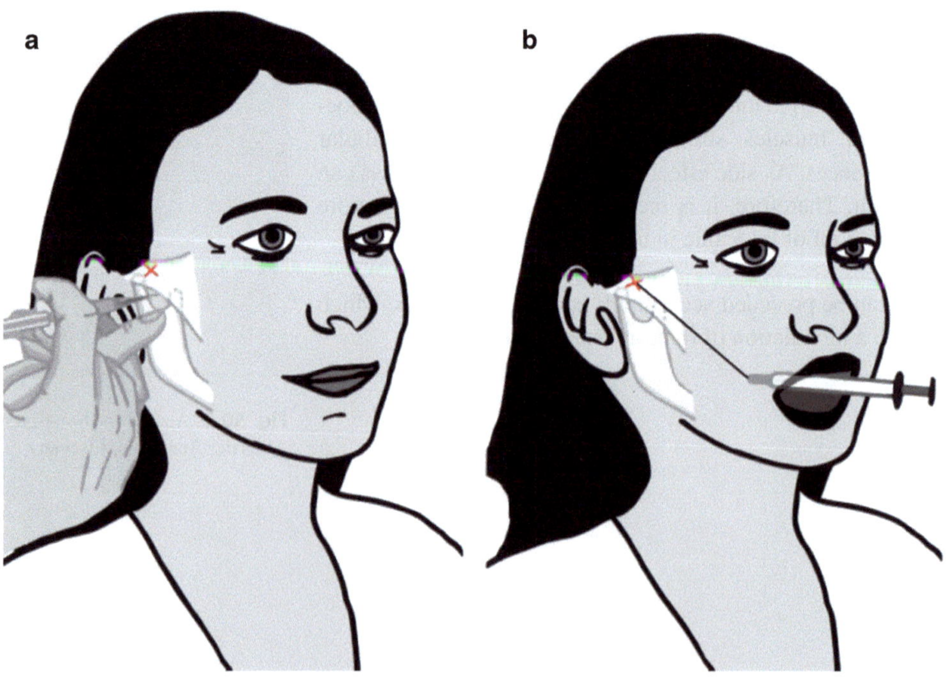

Fig. 50.4 (**a**, **b**) Location of the otic ganglion (red cross) in figure a, intraoral access in figure b

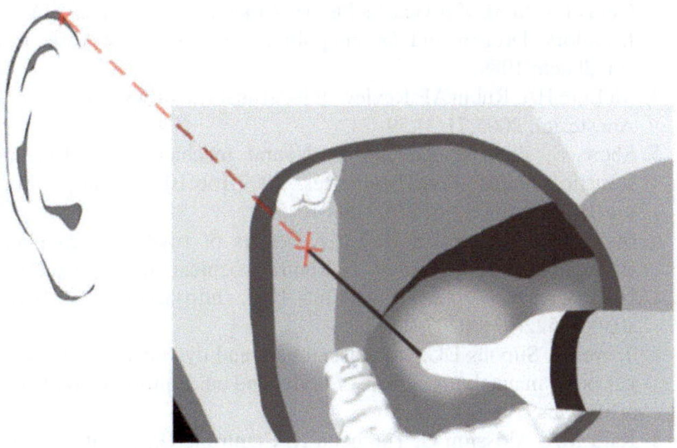

Fig. 50.5 Correct application of the local anaesthetics to the otic ganglion

Method: the mouth of the patient is opened and after disinfection of the mucous membrane approximately 0.5 ml lidocaine is applied using an about 45° to the top angled needle. The tip of the needle is aimed at the upper edge of the outer ear (Fig. 50.5). The needle is advanced until connection is made to the scull base. The injection is made after aspiration.

Potential side effects: in over 3000 documented applications, there has not yet been reported a single case resulting in chronic side effects. Due to the injection of the anaesthetic to the muscles of the temporomandibular joint, 70% of patients have reported a slight irritation and mild pain in this area. These symptoms can last up to 3 h and can be reduced with an antiphlogistic during this time. For a short and limited amount of time (maximum 15–20 min), the following can occur (<1%): Facial palsy, ocular motility disorder, dysgeusia. A pleasant feeling of warmth is often observed in the treated ear for about 20 min.

The attending physician is responsible to inform the patient about the procedure of the injection and its potential side effects.

Special Characteristics: Botulinum Toxin

General Considerations

This specific therapy is only used for the rarely occurring palatal myoclonus. Those patients show rhythmic involuntary contractions of the palatal muscles, which then produce a pulsatile type of tinnitus. Reasons for this phenomenon can be found centrally in the brainstem, but also psychological reasons have been described [30]. A central origin, for example, a stroke in the area of the basal ganglia should always be excluded.

A therapy with Botulinum toxin is therefore always only symptomatic, and the neurotoxin is carefully injected into the affected palatal muscles. Only few researchers have dealt with this phenomenon yet and give concrete instructions [31–33]. In the past, it has been tried to inject Botulinum toxin close to the ear in order to reduce tinnitus, but no reports about the effectiveness of this application have yet been found in literature.

Aspects of Treatment

OnabotulinumtoxinA (OBTA) is a focally administered neurotoxin, which inhibits the release of acetylcholine at the neuromuscular junction and is used therapeutically in disorders characterized by muscular hyperactivity like dystonia. Due to this effect, OBTA is useful in the treatment of tinnitus due to essential palatal tremor [34].

Preclinical in vitro and in vivo evidence demonstrates that OBTA also inhibits the release of nociceptive mediators such as glutamate, substance P and calcitonin gene-related peptide (CGRP) from nociceptive fibres, suggesting that BoNT-A may have a direct antinociceptive action different to its neuromuscular action, through its effects in the autonomic nervous system [35]. Moreover, through a peripheral mechanism, OBTA has also been shown to inhibit central sensitization of central trigeminovascular neurons, which is felt to be integral in the development, progression and chronification of migraine.

OBTA may inhibit the release of CGRP and other neuropeptides from the nociceptive C-fibres. This would not only prevent the C-fibre nociceptor from becoming sensitized but would also prevent the activation of nearby A-delta fibres by CGRP released from the C-fibre nerve terminals [36]. Thus, the afferent flow into the trigeminocervical complex (TCC) would be greatly reduced. These are the mechanisms by which OBTA is effective and widely used in the treatment of chronic migraine [37].

For these reasons, it is easy to think that a reduction in flow into the TCC could produce an improvement in patients with somatic tinnitus [38].

Stidham et al. [39] published a prospective double-blinded study with BoNT-A in thirty patients with tinnitus. Twenty-six patients completed both injections and were included in the analysis—the first arm with BoNT-A at the first injection and placebo with saline injection 4 months later, the second arm with saline injection at the first time and BoNT-A 4 months later—to evaluate tinnitus and hearing with subjective questionnaires like Tinnitus Handicap Inventory (THI), full audiograms with pure tone average- 2 (PTA-2) and speech discrimination scores (SDS), recorded for each prior to the first and second injection. Following BoNT-A injection in subjective tinnitus, 7 patients improved, 3 worsened and 16 showed no change, whereas following placebo, 2 patients improved, 7 worsened and 17 showed no change. Comparison of the treatment and placebo groups was statistically significant ($p < 0.05$) when including better, worse and same effects.

A significant decrease in THI scores between pre-treatment and 4 months post BoNT-A injection ($p = 0.04$) was recorded. Thus, this study found a significant difference in patients' subjective results and THI scores following BoNT-A injection compared to placebo, suggesting the possible benefit of BoNT-A in tinnitus management. The technique used to inject BoNT-A or placebo was into three sites around the ear; 1 cm above the superior aspect of the auricle, 1 cm behind the auricle at 2 o'clock position and 1 cm behind the auricle at 5 o'clock position [39]. This study has shown a possible potential of a benefit of BoNT-A in tinnitus treatment, even with small doses, and opens a new way of investigation with promising future results; perhaps if we could extend the area of injection to modulate the inputs from occipito-cervical and temporal homolateral muscles and use several doses of BoNT-A, we could obtain better control of somatic tinnitus.

Besides this study, there are only some references to small open studies. There it is shown that OBTA can significantly improve somatic tinnitus in a significant percentage of patients and the area of injection is extended to cervical muscles [40].

Due to the pathophysiology of tinnitus, there are different sensory inputs, which are modulated by autonomic pathways when they converge in the DNA—from the face, the external and middle ears, glossopharyngeal and vagus nerves and the neck.

Similar to the treatment of chronic migraine, management of peripheral inputs from cervical, temporal, frontal and periauricular contracted muscles could be possible using OBTA injections, in order to achieve less impulses from peripheral areas which might modify tinnitus perception.

Larger studies with a higher number of patients with somatic tinnitus would be needed to confirm the potential of this approach in the management of patients with tinnitus.

Conclusion

Local anaesthesia to trigger points in the head and neck area and the shoulder girdle, found by proper examination in a silent chamber are relevant tools for the effective therapy of somatosensory tinnitus. An outstanding role plays the anaesthesia of the otic ganglion especially in patients with unilateral tinnitus and when involvement of the trigeminal nerve system is evident. Botulinum toxin is the specific drug for the treatment of palate myoclonus.

References

1. Spiess G. Die Heilwirkung der Anaesthesie. Med Welt Zbl Inn Med. 1902;23:222–3.
2. Huneke F. Unbekannte Fernwirkungen in der Lokalanästhesie. Fortschritte der Medizin. Z des praktischen Arztes. 1934;52:213–23.
3. Gunkelmann M. Zur Geschichte des Kokains. In: Scheerer S, Vogt I, editors. Drogen und Drogenpolitik, vol. 359. New York: Ein Handbuch; 1989.
4. McLure HA, Rubin AP. Review of local anaesthetic agents. Minerva Anestesiol. 2005;71(3):59–74.
5. Shore S, Zhou J, Koehler S. Neural mechanisms underlying somatic tinnitus. Prog Brain Res. 2007;166:107–23. https://doi.org/10.1016/S0079-6123(07)66010-5.
6. Shore SE, El Kashlan H, Lu J. Effects of trigeminal ganglion stimulation on unit activity of ventral cochlear nucleus neurons. Neuroscience. 2003;119(4):1085–101. https://doi.org/10.1016/s0306-4522(03)00207-0.
7. Travell J, Simons DG. Myofascial pain and dysfunction. The trigger point manual, upper half of body. 2nd ed. Baltimore: Williams & Wilkins; 1999.
8. Ralli MA, Altissimi G, Turchetta R, Cianfrone G. Somatic modulation of tinnitus: a review and some open questions. Otolaryngol Open J. 2016;2:111–4. https://doi.org/10.17140/OTLOJ-2-125.
9. Michiels S, Naessens S, Van de Heyning P, Braem M, Visscher CM, Gilles A, De Hertogh W. The effect of physical therapy treatment in patients with subjective tinnitus: a systematic review. Front Neurosci. 2016;10:545. https://doi.org/10.3389/fnins.2016.00545.
10. Vielsmeier V, Strutz J, Kleinjung T, Schecklmann M, Kreuzer PM, Landgrebe M, Langguth B. Temporomandibular joint disorder complaints in tinnitus: further hints for a putative tinnitus subtype. PLoS One. 2012;7(6):e38887. https://doi.org/10.1371/journal.pone.0038887.
11. Edvall NK, Gunan E, Genitsaridi E, Lazar A, Mehraei G, Billing M, Tullberg M, Bulla J, Whitton J, Canlon B, Hall DA, Cederroth CR. Impact of temporomandibular joint complaints on tinnitus-related distress. Front Neurosci. 2019;13:879. https://doi.org/10.3389/fnins.2019.00879.
12. Haider HF, Hoare DJ, Costa RFP, Potgieter I, Kikidis D, Lapira A, Nikitas C, Caria H, Cunha NT, Paco JC. Pathophysiology, diagnosis and treatment of somatosensory tinnitus: a scoping review. Front Neurosci. 2017;11:207. https://doi.org/10.3389/fnins.2017.00207.
13. Rocha CB, Sanchez TG. Efficacy of myofascial trigger point deactivation for tinnitus control. Braz J Otorhinolaryngol. 2012;78(6):21–6. https://doi.org/10.5935/1808-8694.20120028.
14. Kapoula Z, Yang Q, Le TT, Vernet M, Berbey N, Orssaud C, Londero A, Bonfils P. Medio-lateral postural instability in subjects with tinnitus. Front Neurol. 2011;2:35. https://doi.org/10.3389/fneur.2011.00035.
15. Bankoul S, Neuhuber WL. A cervical primary afferent input to vestibular nuclei as demonstrated by retrograde transport of wheat germ agglutinin-horseradish peroxidase in the rat. Exp Brain Res. 1990;79(2):405–11. https://doi.org/10.1007/BF00608252.
16. Pfaller K, Arvidsson J. Central distribution of trigeminal and upper cervical primary afferents in the rat studied by anterograde transport of horseradish peroxidase conjugated to wheat germ agglutinin. J Comp Neurol. 1988;268(1):91–108. https://doi.org/10.1002/cne.902680110.
17. Shore SE, Zhou J. Somatosensory influence on the cochlear nucleus and beyond. Hear Res. 2006;216-217:90–9. https://doi.org/10.1016/j.heares.2006.01.006.
18. Gritsenko K, Caldwell W, Shaparin N, Vydyanathan A, Kosharskyy B. Resolution of long standing tinnitus following radiofrequency ablation of C2-C3 medial branches--a case report. Pain Physician. 2014;17(1):E95–8.
19. Klessinger S. Cervical medial branch blocks for the diagnosis of somatosensory tinnitus. A pilot study. J Otolaryngol Adv. 2016;30:14.
20. Koning HM, Dyrbye BA, van Hemert FJ. Percutaneous radiofrequency lesion of the superior cervical sympathetic ganglion in patients with tinnitus. Pain Pract. 2016;16(8):994–1000. https://doi.org/10.1111/papr.12348.

21. Vass Z, Shore SE, Nuttall AL, Jancso G, Brechtelsbauer PB, Miller JM. Trigeminal ganglion innervation of the cochlea--a retrograde transport study. Neuroscience. 1997;79(2):605–15. https://doi.org/10.1016/s0306-4522(96)00641-0.
22. Goldstein B. Anatomy of the peripheral nervous system. Phys Med Rehabil Clin N Am. 2001;12(2):207–36.
23. Barop H. Lehrbuch und Atlas Neuraltherapie. Stuttgart: Haug; 2014.
24. Messlinger K, Russo AF. Current understanding of trigeminal ganglion structure and function in headache. Cephalalgia. 2019;39(13):1661–74. https://doi.org/10.1177/0333102418786261.
25. Iwanaga J, Wilson C, Simonds E, Vetter M, Schmidt C, Yilmaz E, Choi PJ, Oskouian RJ, Tubbs RS. Clinical anatomy of blockade of the pterygopalatine ganglion: literature review and pictorial tour using cadaveric images. Kurume Med J. 2018;65(1):1–5. https://doi.org/10.2739/kurumemedj.MS651001.
26. Jankovic D. Regionalblockaden & Infiltrationstherapie: Lehrbuch und Atlas; 2008.
27. Weinschenk S. Handbuch Neuraltherapie: Diagnostik und Therapie mit Lokalanästhetika. Thieme Verlag; 2019.
28. Maier C. Ganglionäre lokale Opioidanalgesie. Thieme Verlag; 1996.
29. Vielsmeier V, Schlee W, Langguth B, Kreuzer PM, Hintschich C, Strohmeyer L, Simoes J, Biesinger E. Lidocaine injections to the otic ganglion for the treatment of tinnitus—a pilot study. Prog Brain Res. 2020;260:355. https://doi.org/10.1016/bs.pbr.2020.08.006.
30. Zadikoff C, Lang AE, Klein C. The 'essentials' of essential palatal tremor: a reappraisal of the nosology. Brain. 2006;129(Pt 4):832–40. https://doi.org/10.1093/brain/awh684.
31. Anis MM, Pollak N. Treatment of palatal myoclonus with botulinum toxin injection. Case Rep Otolaryngol. 2013;2013:231505. https://doi.org/10.1155/2013/231505.
32. Selvadurai C, Schaefer SM. Focal unilateral palatal myoclonus causing objective clicking tinnitus without uvula elevation diagnosed by concurrent auscultation. J Mov Disord. 2020;13(3):223–4. https://doi.org/10.14802/jmd.20010.
33. Sinclair CF, Gurey LE, Blitzer A. Palatal myoclonus: algorithm for management with botulinum toxin based on clinical disease characteristics. Laryngoscope. 2014;124(5):1164–9. https://doi.org/10.1002/lary.23485.
34. Slengerik-Hansen J, Ovesen T. Botulinum toxin treatment of objective tinnitus because of essential palatal tremor: a systematic review. Otol Neurotol. 2016;37(7):820–8. https://doi.org/10.1097/MAO.0000000000001090.
35. Aoki KR. Evidence for antinociceptive activity of botulinum toxin type A in pain management. Headache. 2003;43(Suppl 1):S9–15. https://doi.org/10.1046/j.1526-4610.43.7s.3.x.
36. Pellesi L, Do TP, Ashina H, Ashina M, Burstein R. Dual therapy with anti-CGRP monoclonal antibodies and botulinum toxin for migraine prevention: is there a rationale? Headache. 2020;60(6):1056–65. https://doi.org/10.1111/head.13843.
37. Becker WJ. Botulinum toxin in the treatment of headache. Toxins (Basel). 2020;12(12):803. https://doi.org/10.3390/toxins12120803.
38. Lainez MJ, Piera A. Botulinum toxin for the treatment of somatic tinnitus. Prog Brain Res. 2007;166:335–8. https://doi.org/10.1016/S0079-6123(07)66031-2.
39. Stidham KR, Solomon PH, Roberson JB. Evaluation of botulinum toxin A in treatment of tinnitus. Otolaryngol Head Neck Surg. 2005;132(6):883–9. https://doi.org/10.1016/j.otohns.2005.02.015.
40. Minguez A. Piera A. Toxina Botulínica en pacientes con acúfenos somáticos Paper presented at the LXIX Reunión Anual de la Sociedad Española de Neurología, Valencia, 2017.

Neurofeedback

51

Patrick Neff and Martin Meyer

Abstract

Neurofeedback (NFB) for tinnitus is currently under research in several independent labs. In recent times, NFB established itself as a clinical intervention option for a variety of chronic brain diseases, while its efficacy and exact mechanisms of action are still under scrutiny.

In this chapter, we present and review the current state of research of NFB in the context of tinnitus, discuss results, identify open issues, new methodological avenues, and finally conclude with recommendations for NFB research and application.

The majority of studies identified employ EEG NFB based on an early finding of diminished auditory alpha band power in individuals with tinnitus. These studies iterated on either better localization of the aberrant tinnitus neural activity, individualization of NFB protocols, or mobile application. A single study diverged from this pattern by targeting a different putative neural correlate of tinnitus. FMRI NFB approaches are still under development, with merely two low-evidence pilot studies published to this day.

In future, NFB research in tinnitus would profit from better-controlled reproducible studies, further individualization of protocols and consideration of tinnitus heterogeneity, application of novel technology and methods, and multicenter transdisciplinary research efforts.

P. Neff (✉)
Neuro-X Institute, École Polytechnique Fédérale de Lausanne (EPFL), Geneva, Switzerland

Department of Radiology and Medical Informatics, University of Geneva, Geneva, Switzerland

Center for Cognitive Neuroscience (CCNS) and Department of Psychology, University of Salzburg, Salzburg, Austria

Department of Psychiatry and Psychotherapy, University of Regensburg, Regensburg, Germany

Department of Otorhinolaryngology - Head and Neck Surgery, University Hospital of Zurich, University of Zurich, Zurich, Switzerland
e-mail: Patrick.neff@uzh.ch

M. Meyer
University Research Priority Program "Dynamics of Healthy Aging", University of Zurich, Zurich, Switzerland

Department of Comparative Language Science, University of Zurich, Zurich, Switzerland

Center for the Interdisciplinary Study of Language Evolution (ISLE), University of Zurich, Zurich, Switzerland

Cognitive Psychology Unit, Alpen-Adria University Klagenfurt, Klagenfurt am Wörthersee, Austria
e-mail: Martin.meyer@uzh.ch

W. Schlee et al. (eds.), *Textbook of Tinnitus*, https://doi.org/10.1007/978-3-031-35647-6_51

Graphical Abstract

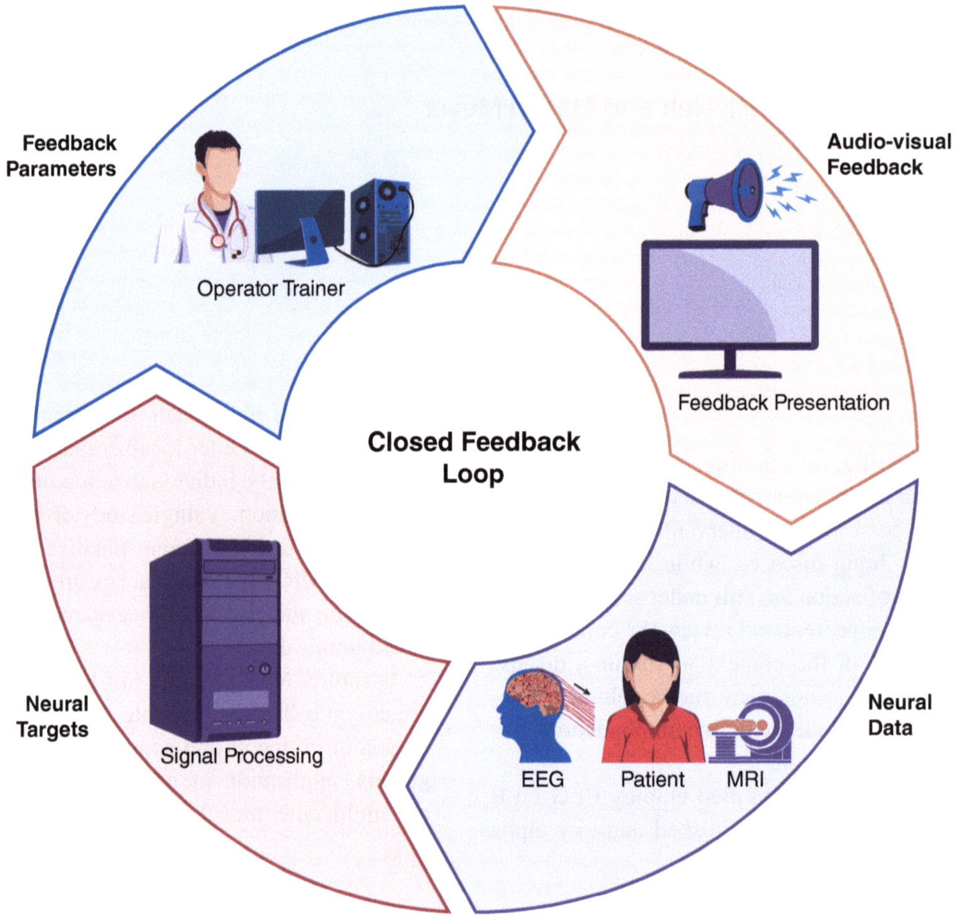

Highlights

- The first study of EEG neurofeedback for tinnitus treatment was conducted 20 years ago.
- We here present an updated assessment of neurofeedback in tinnitus.
- A surge of studies, including fMRI studies, can be observed in recent years.
- Most studies do not adhere to high standard principles of neurofeedback and clinical research.
- Advantages and limitations of current methods and protocols are discussed.
- Further studies are needed to corroborate current promising results and optimize protocols for tinnitus treatment.
- An outlook on emerging topics and technologies in general and tinnitus neurofeedback is provided.

Background and Aim

In the absence of a general-purpose cure [1], neurofeedback (NFB) is one of the tinnitus treatment options currently under research in several labs [2]. In contrast to neuromodulatory approaches (also presented in this textbook #REF), NFB is neither an invasive nor a passive intervention as it mainly builds on the self-regulatory learning mechanisms of the brain [3]. Under this open self-regulatory framework, different modes of learning are implied beyond the classical theories of operant or instrumental conditioning [4].

NFB is not an entirely new approach but had entered the scene in the 1960s [3]. However, the first theoretical models about the malleability of (human) brain functions by means of operant conditioning approaches were discussed starting even in the 1930s [5, 6]. First exploratory studies that aimed at modulating brain activity in animals (cats) were performed in the 1960s [7]. The approach preceding present NFB was better known as *biofeedback* which was based on heartbeat or respiratory patterns as the physiological variable to be modulated. The label *Neuro*feedback implies that neural signals rather than visceral activity are modulated. Quite frequently, one reads also the notion of "EEG-based" NFB because electrophysiological signals generated by ensembles of several ten or hundred thousands of neurons in cortical and subcortical patches of the human brain are recorded from a set of surface electrodes that are systematically distributed across the scalp while a participant receives a visual, auditory, or sensorimotor feedback that is linked to the real time measured brain activity. The overarching purpose of EEG NFB is the establishment of a self-regulatory loop that is meant to help altering an unwanted symptom or to reinforce a wanted behavior based on the principle of operant conditioning or other modes of learning [4, 8]. Although the neurofeedback approach demonstrated amazing success in its application, the method could not establish itself as an intervention for a long time and almost fell into oblivion. This was due to the fact that, apart from the subjective self-report of the treated patients, there was no objective evidence of its effectiveness. The suspicion that EEG NFB is largely based on the placebo effect diminished its popularity, at least in the scientific community. Only recently has the method experienced a renaissance, as advances in the field of EEG analysis have provided the means to demonstrate objective effect in changes in electrophysiological activity as a function of effective NFB treatment.

Typically, NFB systems are dovetailed with a device for electrophysiological (EEG) recordings which typically collects neural resting state activity and present it, or derivatives thereof, as target variable for the modification of behavior. Self-regulation is enabled by a closed-loop therapeutic setting where individuals actively modulate their neural activity which is mostly presented through an audiovisual feedback [8]. NFB seems to be a promising treatment option for many chronic CNS diseases and a surge in basic as well as clinical research can be noticed in the last decade [3]. Yet, given the inherent complexity and the infinite parameter space of the method as well as the large spectrum of the targeted diseases, there are still many issues and open questions which have to be addressed with scientific scrutiny. On top of that, this is also pertinent to tinnitus as a targeted disease, which per se is a complex and subjective condition with a large inherent heterogeneity [9–11]. Notably, the first studies in humans that were based on EEG NFB and were meant as an intervention training in attention deficit hyperactivity disorder were published soon in the 1970s, while NFB protocols aiming at alleviating tinnitus symptoms were first performed in the y2ks [12, 13]. Currently, the NFB method still lacks a solid and replicable demonstration of neural and/or behavioral mechanisms of action, which sparked a controversial debate about possible (neuro-)placebo effect of NFB in the absence of *true* brain training [14–16]. It may thus come as no surprise that NFB with its inherent complexity of multiple interacting systems and parameters faces many scientific challenges. In consequence, NFB research is highly demanding with respect to human, infrastructure, time, and monetary resources which may hinder rapid progress in the classical academic environment. Furthermore, it has to be considered that not all treated persons' response to the NFB intervention in the same effective way. The reason for the existence of responders and non-responders is still widely unknown [17]. Nevertheless, NFB seems to be an effective clinical intervention even in the absence of putative neurobehavioral effects [15] and some research also demonstrated that training of neural activity related to certain disorders can indeed reverse maladaptive neural signatures while improving the disorder's symptoms. While the discussion about efficacy and possible mechanisms of action of NFB is still ongoing, it can be also pointed out that fundamental issues of brain–behavior relation and causation permeate all fields of cognitive neuroscience [18].

In the following sections, we present and review the current state of research of NFB in tinnitus, discuss results, identify open issues and new methodological avenues, and finally conclude with recommendations for NFB research and application in tinnitus.

EEG Neurofeedback for Tinnitus Treatment

In what follows we summarize published studies that applied NFB protocols of different kinds to fathom the possibilities associated with this approach as a counteracting intervention for chronic subjective tinnitus. All NFB studies based on EEG and fMRI that are described below are additionally alphabetically listed in Table 51.1.

Early Attempts

First unspecific attempts in treating tinnitus with NFB were based on general assumptions of beneficial aspects of relaxation and applied simple electrode montages targeting global EEG states. [12] conducted the first study with the aim to increase α activity over right parietal electrodes and concomitantly decrease β activity over the same location. Results of this initial study were reported as highly promising in that all of the 40 participants indicated some form of self-reported tinnitus relief, also persisting during the 6 month follow-up period. Furthermore, authors could show changes in the trained EEG frequency bands in the desired direction (i.e., increase in average α power, decrease in β power). In a follow-up study by an independent group [13], the training of α and β band was split in the active study group, whereas a

Table 51.1 Neurofeedback studies in tinnitus. (Adapted from [2]). Novel EEG studies are highlighted with bold face. TI = tinnitus. TC = tinnitus controls (i.e., sham feedback, or waiting list). HC = healthy controls. NFB = neurofeedback. FDT = frequency discrimination task. rTMS = repetitive transcranial magnetic stimulation. IAF = individual alpha frequency. AC = auditory cortex. LG = lingual gyrus. BOLD = blood oxygenation level dependent

EEG							
Authors	*Participants/ groups*	*Training sessions*	*Neural training targets*	*Electrodes/ Location*	*Behavioral results*	*Neural results*	*Study control*
Abtahi et al. (2021)	TI = 30	20	α ↑ ↓ (ratio) δ	F3, F4, Fc1, Fc2	Distress ↓	–	–
Crocetti et al. (2011)	TI = 15	12	α ↑ ↓ (ratio) δ	F3, F4, Fc1, Fc2	Distress ↓ loudness ↓	α/δ -ratio ↑	–
Dohrmann et al. (2007a, b)	TI = 21, TC = 27 (FDT)	10	α ↑ ↓ (ratio, δ n = 11), α ↑ (n = 5), δ ↓ (n = 5)	F3, F4, Fc1, Fc2	Distress ↓ loudness ↓	α ↑ and δ ↓, correlation with decrease in loudness	Active control
Gosepath et al. (2001)	TI = 40, HC = 15	15	α ↓ ↑β	P4	Distress ↓	α ↑β ↓	–
Güntensperger et al. (2019)	TI = 24	15	α ↑ ↓ (ratio, IAF) δ	F3, F4, Fc1, Fc2	Distress ↓ loudness ↓	α/δ-ratio ↑, correlation of IAF with decrease in distress	–
Güntensperger et al. (2020)	TI = 24, TC = 24 (NFB)	15	α ↑ ↓ (ratio, IAF) δ	F3, F4, Fc1, Fc2 / bilateral AC	Distress ↓ loudness ↓	α/δ-ratio ↑	Active control
Guillard et al. (2020)	TI = 33	10	α ↑ ↓ (ratio) δ	F3, F4, Fc1, Fc2	Distress ↓ loudness ↓	α ↑ (within and not between sessions)	–
Hartmann et al. (2013)	TI = 8, TC = 9 (rTMS)	10	α ↑	Bilateral AC	Distress ↓	α ↑	Active control
Jensen et al. (2020) (in prep.)	TI = 40, TC = 80 (1 sham, 1 diary)	10	α ↑ ↓ (ratio) δ	F3, F4, Fc1, Fc2	Distress ↓ (preliminary)	–	Sham, diary
Schenk et al. (2005)	TI = 40	12	α ↓ (n = 4), α ↑ ↑β (n = 23), β ↓ (n = 13)	P4, C3	Distress ↓	α ↑	–
Vanneste et al. (2016)	TI = 23, TC = 35 (1 sham, 1 waiting list)	15	α ↓γ ↓ ↑β	PCC / LG	Distress ↓	Changes in connectivity	Sham, waiting list
fMRI							
Authors	*Participants/ groups*	*Training sessions*	*Neural training targets*	*Location*	*Behavioral results*	*Neural results*	*Study control*
Haller et al. (2010)	TI = 6	4	BOLD signal ↓	Bilateral AC	–	BOLD signal ↓	–
Emmert et al. (2017)	TI = 14 (2 groups)	9	BOLD signal ↓	Bilateral AC	–	BOLD signal ↓	–

small group ($n = 4$) trained the two frequency bands simultaneously. Again, all participants, irrespective of the NFB protocol, apparently profited from the intervention. To this day, this specific protocol has never been reused and no replication or extension studies exists. Notably, the control group without tinnitus was not able to train any of the frequency bands while, on the other hand, tinnitus patients were successful in both neural training and alleviating their tinnitus symptoms. This could possibly be an example of NFB-unspecific placebo effects like demand characteristics in clinical studies (i.e., fulfillment of expectations of study), interaction with a practitioner or generally a health professional, overestimation of technology also driven by its price, among others [3]. Eventually, this research avenue may also have been discarded due to the lack of solid theoretical background of the NFB protocol with regards to tinnitus specificity.

Neural Signature of Chronic Tinnitus to Inform EEG Neurofeedback Studies

As a next step, following early work on M/EEG resting-state neural correlates of tinnitus in the human brain [19, 20], α and δ oscillations in the auditory cortex have afterward become primary neural targets for NFB training [21–27]. These original findings about a chronic maladaptive signature related to tinnitus were substantiated in theory and with data from general considerations about deafferentation and potential thalamo-cortical dysrhythmia [28, 29]. In contrast to the previous studies targeting tinnitus-unspecific activity [12, 13], the current neural targets were based on putatively tinnitus specific neural alterations. Other neuromodulatory approaches for tinnitus treatment were also based on these principles (e.g., in α band power neuromodulation, TMS [30], tACS [31], acoustic stimulation [32, 33], see chapter #REF for more information). In NFB research and application, this specific concept of NFB is coined frequency band training [34]. In this spirit, tinnitus can be seen as an acquired *oscillopathy* (i.e., in α, δ, and γ bands) and a respective normalization of aberrant band power through NFB training a method to counteract tinnitus symptoms, namely distress and intensity. The observed decrease in α band power over temporal auditory regions was mainly interpreted as a failure of the tinnitus brain to suppress peripheral auditory input or generally a lack of inhibition [20, 35]. Event-related α decrease has been theorized as a gating mechanism of perception [36] and is key in event-related (de)synchronization of neural signals [37]. Γ oscillations are suggested as neural correlates of conscious perception or memory binding processes of the brain [38, 39] and are often at interplay with lower carrier frequencies like α or θ throughout several brain networks. In tinnitus, following original reasonings of the Weisz group [20, 40], correlational studies of tinnitus loudness or distress [41–44], as well as more recent data by Sedley and colleagues [38, 39, 45], have demonstrated changes in γ activity in relation to tinnitus. It was mostly theorized that γ oscillations were related to the actual auditory sensation of tinnitus while, in the light of predictive brain theories, it was also speculated that γ could actually reflect inhibitory or prediction-updating efforts of the brain [38, 39, 46, 47]. Δ activity is generally associated with sleep or drowsy states and is attributed with general deafferentation of peripheral input which is also applicable for the majority of tinnitus models, where peripheral hearing loss leads to deafferentation cascade along the auditory pathway up to the primary auditory cortex [28]. In tinnitus research, increased δ band power has been identified as a neural correlate of the phantom sound in original work of the Weisz group [19, 40] as a possible consequence of deafferentation. Further studies corroborated these findings of increased δ band power in relation to tinnitus [41, 48].

To this day, these neural correlates in the form of band power changes are still disputed with some evidence pointing to an absence thereof [49, 50] and a lack of replication with different methods, especially source localization using LORETA methods (e.g., [51]). For more details, the reader is referred to the M/EEG chapter of this book (#REF) and to the Supplemental Materials of two recent publications [2, 52].

EEG Neurofeedback Targeting Auditory α and δ Band Power

Given the data and theoretical considerations of these early findings of altered band power, [21] performed a NFB study with the aim of counteracting the maladaptive band power changes in α and δ bands. In 10 sessions of 30 min participants either trained (1) α and δ ratio, (2) α upregulation, or (3) δ downregulation at frontocentral electrodes F3, F4, FC1, and FC2, putatively covering auditory cortex activity, whereas an independent control group performed an auditory frequency discrimination task [53]. Results were indicative of reduced tinnitus distress, intensity, and α and δ ratio after the training period, but not in the follow-up period. In addition, tinnitus intensity changes were negatively correlated to α and δ ratio changes in support of the hypothesized relation between behavior and brain activity. There was no change of tinnitus parameters in the group performing the auditory frequency discrimination task and the α and δ ratio changes were most predictive of treatment success.

An independent research group aimed at replicating this protocol in a population of 15 tinnitus sufferers in the absence of a control group or condition [22]. The behavioral results of the original study could be replicated, namely a reduction of tinnitus distress and intensity after the training period but not in the follow-up, whereas α and δ ratio merely showed a trend and its changes were negatively correlated with THI score changes and not with tinnitus intensity.

[23] further iterated on the NFB protocol in focusing on α power exclusively and applying a tomographic approach by confining the trained region to bilateral temporal auditory areas. Similar to the original study of the group [21], NFB was compared to a standard treatment approach in the form of rhythmic transcranial magnetic stimulation (rTMS) including a sham condition (1000 1 Hz pulses in 10 sessions). Again, results indicated superior performance of the NFB protocol in contrast to rTMS and sham in both behavioral tinnitus questionnaire data as well as in the targeted α band and temporal auditory cortex location. Moreover, authors could demonstrate an (uncorrected) increase in connectivity in and near the regions of α power changes.

In a further replication attempt and iteration on protocol parameters, [24] individualized the neural target in the frequency domain by training the individual α frequency [54] and feedbacking α and δ power separately (i.e., rewarding α increases and δ power decreases, respectively). In contrast to previous studies [22, 23] and similar to the original study [21] 26 individuals were enrolled for the study, while a control condition or group was not included. Furthermore, the amount of training sessions was increased to 15 and a large comprehensive set of descriptive as well as outcome variables were assessed better describe the study population, outcomes, and allow for subgroup analyses. In line with previous findings, decreases in tinnitus questionnaire scores and intensity were found, which partly also persisted through the follow-up period up to 6 months after treatment end. Neural data partly corroborated the behavioral findings, especially in the case of α-δ ratio analyses on all electrodes when tinnitus was attended in the outcome resting state EEG recordings (cf. [55]). Following up this study and explicitly addressing low spatial specificity of the surface electrode-based approaches of former studies except [23, 25] performed a study applying sLORETA-based NFB over bilateral auditory cortex targeting identical frequency bands as in the former study [24]. Forty-eight participants were enrolled and randomly allocated to either the sLORETA or surface electrode-based condition and trained in 15 sessions. Interestingly, no differences was found between the groups with regard to symptom reduction and neurophysiological changes outcomes except a reduction in tinnitus loudness after the training for the sLORETA group. THI scores and neurophysiological α-δ ratio changes remained stable over the course of the 3-months follow-up period. The authors concluded that, given the current data and knowledge, there seems to be no significant added value of source-localized approaches for NFB training in tinnitus, at least as long as auditory cortical regions are the distinct target of the feedback.

[27] ported the established α δ ratio surface electrode-based NFB protocol to the mobile use case of home training in a single arm, non-controlled clinical pilot study. Thirty-three participants were enrolled and (merely) α band power was trained in 10 sessions à 50 min at the common FC1, FC2, F3, and F4 electrode locations. Authors report a 23% decrease in THI scores after training and a 31% reduction in the follow-up as well as reductions of loudness and intrusion measured by means of a visual analog scale (VAS) at the same time points. On the neurophysiological level, α band power increases could be observed within but not between sessions. Overall, this study indicated the potential of home application of the NFB protocol while again positive behavioral effects of the established protocol could be reported.

Finally, a recent publication [56] further adds to the body of putatively positive evidence of the protocol by demonstrating THI and VAS (severity) decreases in a prospective clinical trial with no control group or condition. Tinnitus patients underwent 20 NFB training sessions with the established α δ protocol. Tinnitus scores were lower after the training and continued to decrease in the 1, 3, and 5 month follow-up assessments. Follow-up data including neuroscientific outcomes are therefore advisable to further validate the current findings.

Besides these 7 original studies building on the protocol of [21], one other group [26] has been currently conducting a randomized controlled trials with 3 study arms including sham treatment and a diary control group. This ongoing study is the first study in EEG NFB applying the α δ on frontocentral electrodes for tinnitus treatment which actually employs a well-controlled design. The study is still running and expected to be finished by the end of 2021 resulting in a predicted outcome (i.e., NFB better than control conditions) (personal communication).

Differential EEG Neurofeedback Protocol

[57] investigated a differential approach using source-localized sLORETA NFB on the posterior cingulate cortex (PCC), which was found to be an integral hub in tinnitus [58]. This novel protocol aimed at an upregulation of α band power while downregulating β and γ power. Fifty-eight tinnitus patients were enrolled in total and allocated to a verum group receiving the PCC training (n = 23), a sham group with the same protocol but targeting the lingual gyrus which is not implied in tinnitus (n = 17), and a waiting list control group (n = 18). Behavior results were indicative of a decrease in tinnitus distress in the verum condition which was not found for the two control conditions. No effects were found for tinnitus loudness or the trained power bands in the PCC. An ancillary sLORETA connectivity analysis unveiled various changes including cross frequency coupling of the PCC as a function of treatment outcome. This study was the first one in tinnitus NFB to produce hypothesized effects with the application of a genuine NFB sham control condition and even an untreated waiting list to counteract possible placebo effects. Yet, no link could be established between trained neural targets and behavioral effects. Furthermore, no follow-up assessments were performed to further observe the trajectory of the tinnitus distress reduction.

We refrain from discussing case studies [59, 60] in this chapter due to their low value compared to the line of research including clinical trials presented here.

Discussion of EEG Neurofeedback Protocols

Taken together, the bulk of the aforementioned studies iterating on the original protocol from [21] yielded convening results which certainly speak in favor of the NFB approach. The various neural target strategies with regard to frequency bands (upregulation of α power, upregulation of α-δ ratio, concomitant downregulation of higher frequency band power like β or γ) did not produce significantly different outcomes with respect to behavioral outcomes. Looking at neural outcomes and their relation to behavioral outcomes, results are heterogeneous that may come as no surprise given the current state of evidence in NFB research in general [61]. Merely the original study of Dohrmann and colleagues [21] could demonstrate effects for all planned outcomes.

Technical details of signal processing including frequency band filtering and feedback generation including success/failure thresholds are rather individual throughout the studies, also depending on applied systems and refinement. Furthermore, the targeted frequency bands α, δ, and γ present specific challenges with regard to neural signal processing which can critically influence neural targeting of NFB and in consequence study outcomes. α band activity is generally sufficiently accessible with common electrophysiological methods and has distinct roles in audition [35]. Yet, the signal in this frequency band may be contaminated by strong competing posterior sources from the visual cortex and/or neighboring source of the sensorimotor cortex (i.e., activity in the SMR band). Two approaches have been suggested recently which counteract this shortcoming and enable accurate targeting of the specific auditory α activity [62, 63]. Applying these methods or other approaches like auditory localizer methods should thus become mandatory for targeting auditory α in tinnitus NFB. Γ band activity is challenging due to its low amplitudes compared to lower frequency bands which makes it highly susceptible to noise e.g. stemming from muscle activity and/or suboptimal montage of electrodes. Generally, this frequency band is filtered out starting at its lower bound for any M/EEG analysis with a lowpass filter with a cutoff frequency around 30 Hz. It therefore may come as no surprise, that only the study of [57] targeted γ activity in their NFB protocol. Finally, activity in the δ band, contrary to higher frequencies, is driven by high amplitude (changes) which could also originate from various physiological and non-physiological sources. As the susceptibility to artifacts is especially high in real-time data acquisition and analysis pipelines like NFB, where no (offline) preprocessing is performed, these inherent issues of the targeted frequency bands are even more exacerbated. In any case, future studies would profit from an extensive and transparent description of the signal pipeline ever so critical for the highly complex science of NFB [61]. This is also true for training style (i.e., intermittent vs. continuous), instructions, and possible transfer strategies [4]. Beyond reporting, careful consideration of these aspects following state of the art guidelines should be integral to any current study of tinnitus NFB. Training session duration, amount of training sessions, and training intervals also deferred between studies while most of variability here is certainly explainable by either study type (pilot study vs. clinical trial) or available resources. It is though conceivable that more training sessions would certainly increase the observed effects if participants are responsive to the NFB treatment. Finally, participant selection [10] and general heterogeneity within the tinnitus population [9] can be identified as another source of variability influencing the outcomes.

Applying novel techniques like tomographic approaches targeting distinct local brain regions have not yet demonstrated a clear supremacy towards protocols that utilized a more global feedback via widely distributed electrodes [25]. However, it is worth mentioning that the present evidence on the efficacy of tomographic approaches is parsimonious, and it cannot be excluded that protocols that are meant to modulate brain activity in extra-auditory areas, namely the anterior cingulate or the insula, will provide more compelling results (see our current ongoing study, https://clinicaltrials.gov/ct2/show/NCT03895047). This has practical implications in that materials (e.g., number of electrodes) and efforts (i.e., electrode montage and system handling in general) are minimal even allowing for mobile or home use scenarios [27]. Notably, a source-localized NFB protocol with 19 [57] or 32 electrodes [25] takes considerable time to set up which may not be suitable for daily clinical routine anyways.

fMRI Approaches

Real-time (rt)-fMRI NFB is a more recent subform of NFB which has been surging since 2010, with very few studies before that [64]. While EEG NFB targets direct neural activity or instantaneous derivatives thereof with good temporal resolution, rt-fMRI NFB tracks blood oxygenation level dependent (BOLD) signals in the brain, which is a putative vascular coupling to actual neural activity with both a time lag and low temporal resolution but high spatial resolution.

In a preliminary study, [65] pioneered a NFB paradigm where BOLD activity in bilateral auditory cortex was targeted applying an auditory localizer task. Participants ($n = 6$) were trained to lower the BOLD levels in the target region while being presented with an activation bar displaying the BOLD activity directly. Five participants learned to successfully downregulate their BOLD activity and 2 participants furthermore reported a reduction of their tinnitus.

In a follow-up pilot study, [66] compared two NFB strategies, namely continuous vs. intermittent feedback, in a group of 14 participants with tinnitus. Seven participants were allocated to the continuous feedback condition and 7 participants to the intermittent condition, respectively. The study protocol succeeded at temporary deactivation of auditory cortex, especially with continuous feedback, while a behavioral effect measured by the TFI [67] could not be reported for either of the conditions.

Besides these two pilot studies with an actual tinnitus population, another group developed an fMRI NFB protocol to volitionally downregulate auditory cortex activation with the goal of tinnitus treatment [68, 69]. The experiments were conducted on a healthy population and sham-controlled ($n = 27$, and $n = 41$, respectively). In both studies, auditory cortex activity could be successfully downregulated over time and vs. sham. Furthermore, the downregulation could be correlated with a behavioral sense of control over the feedback [69].

Taken together, tinnitus fMRI tinnitus NFB is still in its infancy with ongoing iterations on protocols, while no sufficiently powered clinical trial has been performed so far. Yet, considerable efforts are spent in order to establish fMRI NFB for tinnitus treatment [64, 70, 71]. Currently, the research group of Van De Ville in Geneva is conducting a clinical trial where the fMRI NFB protocol of auditory cortex downregulation is compared to standard cognitive behavioral psychotherapy for tinnitus relief https://www.kofam.ch/en/snctp-portal/search/122590/study/38838. Furthermore, this ongoing trial also includes an arm with EEG NFB building following the line of research starting with thus training α and δ ratio using a custom-built system. Results will both inform current knowledge about feasibility of fMRI NFB in tinnitus but also be able to provide a head-to-head comparison of the two neuroscientific approaches.

At this point, differences between the methods should be discussed—not only with respect to their scientific details but also in assessing clinical practicability. First, fMRI NFB allows for more precise localization of neural targets but lacks temporal resolution compared to electrophysiological methods. Localization naturally improves neural target specificity where MRI can provide millimeter precision in contrast to centimeter precision in the case of source-localized EEG NFB protocols (e.g., with sLORETA [25, 57]). Timing is critical when temporal contingency between the neural activity to be trained and the presented feedback needs to be optimized. Here, electrophysiological methods can produce round times (i.e., time needed from neural signal recording to e.g. feedback presentation on a computer screen) in the millisecond domain, whereas an fMRI feedback loop takes several seconds. Second, settings of fMRI and EEG NFB differ considerably in that EEG allows for naturalistic, comfortable clinical environments, whereas MRI NFB is currently bound to scanning facilities where the participants are forced to lie quiet on the scanner bed, are not allowed to move, and usually are presented feedback stimuli with low-quality media (e.g., mirrored screens, headphones presenting sound with scanner noise attenuation in the absence of active noise cancelling). Furthermore, scanner noise is a considerable issue, especially in the case of tinnitus and related hyperacusis [72]. While this may be considered acceptable and ethical in basic research, this can be very burdensome when multiple training sessions have to be performed and certain instructions or mental strategies require auditory attention. EEG NFB currently putatively provides a more naturalistic and engaging environment, which may also enable better engagement and learning by the participants. Head-to-head comparisons of the two approaches on a tinnitus population, possibly even in a within-person design, may help to elucidate such differences. Third, MRI infrastructure is in need of considerable material, human, and monetary resources in order to maintain its operation. Moreover, MRI devices are usually deployed and reserved for clinical and basic research purposes in single sessions. Inherently, MRI technology is not mobile at all in contrast to emerging ubiquitous electrophysiological mobile solutions [27].

Taken together, both methods currently provide insightful results in tinnitus NFB basic research with their respective inherent limitations, whereas EEG can certainly be considered the method with more translational value in respect to clinical routine. In addition, NFB research is generally in need of substantial resources and very time consuming in the form of well-controlled longitudinal studies. In times of disruptive events like the ongoing pandemic such resourceful and effortful research may be severely hampered, which can be seen in all currently ongoing studies in Zurich, Geneva, and Marburg [26]. PhD candidates and further personnel may also be completely absorbed by study management, training, and technical challenges instead of focusing on scientific output. Unfortunately, funding agencies may not be completely aware of all the resources and efforts needed for high-standard NFB research and thus the acquisition of sufficient funding may pose considerable challenges. It may therefore come as no surprise that gold-standard study control is still largely absent from longitudinal trials and sample sizes are still very low on average [73]. Raising and promoting awareness for the specific needs of high-quality NFB research is therefore essential to further the field. Related to that, no multicenter studies or comparable initiatives are on the horizon in tinnitus NFB research to this day.

General Discussion

NFB, among others, is a tinnitus treatment option which is currently under investigation in many labs while the first studies date back to as early as 2001 [12]. This ongoing interest is partly due to recent technological advances and availability of systems but also due to a general re-invoked interest in the method. While this is certainly true for EEG NFB, fMRI NFB, with a surge of publications since 2010, may have partly contributed to this *renaissance* of NFB especially with its inherently better localization of neural targets compared to electrophysiology. While NFB conveys clinical promises for many chronic, maladaptive diseases, its general and specific efficacy is still under scrutiny [3].

In the case of tinnitus, current guidelines do not (yet) list NFB as a feasible treatment option [74], which may reflect the inconclusive results especially in the absence of a solid line of research with well-controlled randomized clinical trials. We thus surmise that it is critical to adhere to high scientific standards and focus on publishing randomized clinical trials especially with the established and effective protocol of α upregulation (with an optional δ downregulation) over auditory temporal cortex [21–27]. [26] is the first group that adheres to such standards in application of this specific NFB protocol with promising but yet unpublished results (personal communication). Besides that [57] presented data of a well-controlled study on their genuine NFB protocol including sham and waiting list control while follow-up measurements to probe long-lasting treatment effects were missing. Furthermore, no follow-up study or modified version has been performed on this protocol to this day.

The CRED-nf guidelines [61] devised by international leading experts in NFB research and practice is a valid reference to plan and conduct future studies in tinnitus NFB. Besides general considerations of concurrent open and reproducible science, authors specifically recommend methodological best practices pertinent to NFB.

A key issue is the use of adequate control conditions [3, 75], which has to be carefully considered with respect to targeted conditions and neural assemblies. Several strategies exist here from presenting neural data and related feedback stimuli of a different participant, presentation of generic signals or feedbacks, inversion of feedback, or presentation of feedback generated from different neural sources. These strategies differ in various aspects but most importantly in the sense of control over the feedback, which is low in the case of generic feedback or feedback from other individuals. On the other hand, the other two strategies provide a high sense of control while introducing further issues. Inverted feedback is most probably not suited for tinnitus NFB because it may increase symptoms in an undesirable manner. Feedback from independent neural sources may thus be optimal for tinnitus and probably most NFB experiments, whereas the choice of such brain loci in the widespread tinnitus networks of the brain may constitute a challenge in itself. The choice of the lingual gyrus [57] is certainly reasonable, yet, some evidence exists showing that this region might be involved in tinnitus pathology [76–78].

A further central issue is applied (learning) strategies, sense of control and motivation, and possible transfer runs after actual training sessions. It is advocated to properly define and track these aspects during the NFB training sessions which allows for critical correlations of neural and behavioral training effects as well as overall improvement or individualization of NFB protocols. Standardized psychometric tools are currently missing here, but the application of such assessment tools is encouraged. In tinnitus NFB research, which mostly predates current methodological considerations, these data traces are largely absent. Related to that, careful consideration of intra- and inter-session training outcomes on the neural level is deemed crucial to increase validity of results of NFB studies. In contrast to outcome measures at the end of treatments very common in clinical trials, this strategy allows for tracking training trajectories in more detail and finally link them to the overall neural and behavioral outcomes. Again, this concept has not been applied to tinnitus NFB research with the exception of a recent study with mobile devices [27]. Tracking these neural changes is deemed critical to properly track absolute changes in band power and adapt thresholds of the feedback reward. The application of (relative) dynamic thresholds of feedback generation is also widespread and does not per se hamper tracking of absolute neural intra- and inter-session changes.

Finally, related to both the specific NFB protocol and its targets as well as to applied strategies, the mode of learning during NFB is a critical factor which has to be considered [4, 79]. In general, but also in tinnitus, NFB learning is loosely attributed to operant conditioning, where the feedback serves as the reward structure, or even completely ignored. While the neural and behavioral outcomes are usually clearly defined aiming at reverting maladaptive plasticity of the targeted pathology, the exact mechanisms of reaching these goals are often undefined or underinvestigated. On the neural level, neuroplastic changes related to NFB are coarsely theorized to be either of Hebbian, homeostatic, or (in consequence) structural nature [80]. Behaviorally, besides operant or instrumental learning, where desired brain activity is simply reinforced by rewarding feedback outcomes, several other modes of learning are currently discussed [4]: The dual process theory tries to integrate feedforward and feedback learning processes to describe the individual's attempts to find strategies to control the feedback voluntarily. If a successful strategy is found NFB may even become automatic and thus non-cognitive. Alternatively, a dual process learning mode can also be acquired without actual effective cognitive strategies. In any case, this mode of learning can be experimentally controlled by respective measures of providing or assessing mental strategies of NFB control. The awareness theory simply proposes that the organism or brain may become aware about its own physiology (i.e., brain activity) and therefore actively engages in its self-regulation. Looking at the global network level of the brain, the global workspace theory of NFB surmises that control over neural activity is acquired by the wide distribution of the feedback signal throughout the brain which thus becomes conscious and controllable [80]. Similar to the dual process theory, it has been shown that conscious learning or strategies may not be necessary for successful NFB learning. Finally, skill learning, which plays a critical role in brain-computer, or more generally brain-machine interfacing [81, 82], has also been proposed as a mode of NFB learning. It is characterized by the typical asymptotic temporal trajectory of learning where rapid skill acquisition is followed by a slower skill consolidation. Critically, this mode of NFB learning has been substantiated by a recent meta-analysis where global, thus mostly unspecific, activation of several regions and networks key to awareness, learning, movement, self-regulation, and executive control have been identified [83]. The skill learning theory of NFB constitutes itself as a conscious pro-active strategy in contrast to the other theories presented here. Furthermore, the identified unspecific and learning-related brain regions and networks are considered very useful to tune NFB protocols to the specific need of neural targets in many pathologies. In tinnitus, there might be a considerable overlap of regions in limbic, medial or subcortical brain regions with such NFB-global or unspecific activations. These overlaps may not be detrimental in the case of the omnipresent auditory temporal EEG NFB protocols [21], with the exception of motor activity from neighboring motor cortex or NFB-related activity of underlying insular structures [83], but certainly informative for source-localized NFB [57] and possible fMRI approaches beyond auditory cortex. Returning to modes of learning, tinnitus NFB research has largely ignored this aspect until recently when transfer runs (i.e., mentalization strategies to reinstate modes of learning during real NFB) were integrated to the protocol [26] or several strategies were presented as options to the participants during training sessions [27]. In the latter case, suggested strategies reach from unspecific relaxation instructions (e.g., "Try to relax and meditate"), to auditory distractor instructions (e.g., "Play a music you like in your head"), and tinnitus-specific instructions (e.g., "Try to move the sound of tinnitus between your ears"). These strategies were tracked in and between sessions and the best strategies were selected and applied in the second half of the training sessions. These attempts of integrating (individual) strategies are laudable, yet in need of more refinement for application in tinnitus NFB.

The fundamental discussion about active engagement to the tinnitus percept or even suffering in NFB vs. distraction strategies may be of central interest here. Active engagement and reduction of tinnitus in the sense of instrumental conditioning or skill learning may prove as a feasible strategy. This is further backed by the assumptions of the process-based NFB framework of [84], where highly contingent, sensory-rich NFB environments and strategies (e.g., to abolish a drinking habit while avoiding a liquor store in a virtual reality environment) are theorized to be especially efficient NFB approaches. Notably at this point, virtual environments have been proposed for tinnitus treatment but not linked to NFB yet [85–87]. On the other hand, a passive strategy solely relying on self-regulatory processes of the NFB loop akin to the awareness theory or dual process learning may prove as the more productive choice of tinnitus NFB strategies. In any case, a study design specifically tailored to investigate differences between active and passive strategies could produce the needed insights. Ultimately, as with the identification of individual neural targets, the choice and actual form of strategies might be ideally chosen individually including respective pre-training sessions to consolidate strategies. Overall, in comparison to other *neuromodulatory* approaches, NFB can be categorized as an active learning neuromodulatory intervention, whereas transcranial electric, magnetic, and bimodal stimulations are clearly passive versions of neuromodulation. This difference may be critical when it comes mechanisms of action, trainability, and sustainability of neural changes and their putative behavioral correlates. NFB may be advantageous here as induced changes are learned via self-regulation and in consequence self-efficacy or control with respect to the tinnitus sensation and burden can be experienced. At this point, this reasoning is speculative as both comparative studies are missing and evidence for either of the neuromodulatory concepts is inconclusive (for reviews see [2, 88, 89]).

To close, while neural targets and psychology of participants are understood rather well, we identify a research gap when it comes to esthetics of (mostly audiovisual) feedback stimuli and possibly the entire NFB setting. Here, it is generally assumed that simple visualizations like moving bars are sufficient to produce long-time motivation and engagement of the participants which is especially questionable in times of ubiquitous digital game esthetics and the concept of *gamification*. Furthermore, different age cohorts have different needs in that elderly individuals may neither be prone to digital hi-resolution aesthetics nor gamification, whereas younger individuals may be quickly unsatisfied given their exposition to these technologies in daily life. Nonetheless, technological advances are much needed with respect to feedback (design) esthetics, modalities, and ideally be accompanied by concurrent perceptual and learning psychology. Again, creating a sensory-rich, engaging, and motivating NFB environment might be beneficial for treatment success and specificity in the spirit of the process-based NFB framework [84].

Outlook and Conclusion

Beyond adhering to current standards of solid reproducible research and state of the art NFB experimental designs, iteration on technological advances (e.g., in localization [62, 63] or mobile systems [27]) and individualization of protocols (e.g., [17, 90]) may pave the way toward more effective protocols of tinnitus NFB. It is well known that not all individuals respond to NFB in general and that the neural heterogeneity with respect to tinnitus is large within the population and thus protocols may need to be individually tuned. Notably, no study in tinnitus NFB aimed at identifying individual neural targets and a subsequent training or modulation thereof besides two studies targeting individual α frequency peaks [2, 24]. Therefore, the research avenue of individual tinnitus NFB protocols may prove as especially innovative, which may be even enhanced by the addition of fitting individual mental and learning strategies. Neural targets are currently limited to frequency band power in tinnitus EEG NFB and BOLD signal in the case of fMRI NFB. This bias is also reflected in the traditional general literature of NFB. Novel targets, especially connectivity of ongoing brain activity [91], or to a lesser extent training on evoked responses [92], training of machine-learning features [93], or (non-linear) measures of signal complexity or information content like entropy [94–96] may also establish themselves as NFB protocols to be investigated in tinnitus given a partly vast bulk of basic literature (e.g., [97, 98] for connectivity, [99] for evoked responses, [47, 63] for machine-learning features, [100] for entropy). In the spirit of current research on bimodal treatment options of tinnitus [101], also discussed in a chapter of this book #REF, bimodal treatment combining NFB with auditory, magnetic, or electrical stimulation can also be envisioned.

NFB is an emerging tinnitus treatment option that is currently investigated in several labs. After 20 years of research, conclusive evidence from well-controlled clinical trials is still missing. The majority of studies apply EEG training mainly α upregulation of auditory sources on a minimal set of electrodes. Recent attempts with source-localized protocols have not been able to demonstrate superiority compared to the established electrode protocol. As in tinnitus treatment research in general, progress may be seriously hampered by the lack of reliable causal (neural) models. Related to that, research into individualized protocols has just been started and may prove as a promising novel research avenue. Currently, EEG NFB seems preferable compared to fMRI approaches due to some methodological aspects but ultimately with respect to their clinical practicability. Head-to-head comparisons and possibly studies simultaneously applying both methods may help to elucidate differences and complementary aspects. Mobile EEG devices and setups already have been shown to be feasible options, which may be especially useful in pandemic situations including social distancing but also reflects current trends of personalized mobile interventions. Novel neural targets derived from brain network measures, evoked responses, machine learning, and signal complexity theory may inform novel research avenues. To close, awareness for the complex and resource-consuming nature of NFB research has to be established to be able to satisfy current demands of high-quality, solid, and reproducible research. In that spirit, multicenter transdisciplinary collaborations and large-scale projects are encouraged.

Acknowledgments This research was supported by the Swiss National Fund "Postdoc Mobility" Grant P400PS_186670 and P5R5PS_203068 sponsoring PN.

References

1. McFerran DJ, Stockdale D, Holme R, Large CH, Baguley DM. Why is there no cure for tinnitus? Front Neurosci. 2019;13:802.
2. Güntensperger D, Thüring C, Meyer M, Neff P, Kleinjung T. Neurofeedback for tinnitus treatment - review and current concepts. Front Aging Neurosci. 2017;9:386.
3. Thibault RT, Lifshitz M, Raz A. The self-regulating brain and neurofeedback: experimental science and clinical promise. Cortex. 2016;74:247–61.
4. Sitaram R, Ros T, Stoeckel L, Haller S, Scharnowski F, Lewis-Peacock J, et al. Closed-loop brain training: the science of neurofeedback. Nat Rev Neurosci. 2017;18(2):86–100.
5. Loomis AL, Harvey EN, Hobart G. Electrical potentials of the human brain. J Exp Psychol. 1936;19(3):249.
6. Jasper H, Shagass C. Conditioning of the occipital alpha rhythm in man. J Exp Psychol. 1941;28(5):373.
7. Sterman MB, Wyrwicka W, Roth S. Electrophysiological correlates and neural substrates of alimentary behavior in the cat*. Ann N Y Acad Sci. 1969;157(2):723–39.
8. Papo D. Neurofeedback: principles, appraisal, and outstanding issues. Eur J Neurosci. 2019;49(11):1454–69.
9. Cederroth CR, Gallus S, Hall DA, Kleinjung T, Langguth B, Maruotti A, et al. Editorial: towards an understanding of tinnitus heterogeneity. Front Aging Neurosci. 2019;11:53.
10. Probst T, Pryss RC, Langguth B, Spiliopoulou M, Landgrebe M, Vesala M, et al. Outpatient tinnitus clinic, self-help web platform, or mobile application to recruit tinnitus study samples? Front Aging Neurosci. 2017;9:113.
11. Langguth B, Landgrebe M, Schlee W, Schecklmann M, Vielsmeier V, Steffens T, et al. Different patterns of hearing loss among tinnitus patients: a latent class analysis of a large sample. Front Neurol. 2017;8(10):46.
12. Gosepath K, Nafe B, Ziegler E, Mann WJ. Neurofeedback in der Therapie des Tinnitus. HNO. 2001;49(1):29–35.
13. Schenk S, Lamm K, Gündel H, Ladwig KH. Effects of neurofeedback-based EEG alpha and EEG beta training in patients with chronically decompensated tinnitus. HNO. 2005;53(1):29–38.
14. Schabus M, Griessenberger H, Gnjezda MT, Heib DPJ, Wislowska M, Hoedlmoser K. Better than sham? A double-blind placebo-controlled neurofeedback study in primary insomnia. Brain. 2017;140(4):1041–52.
15. Thibault RT, Lifshitz M, Raz A. Neurofeedback or neuroplacebo? Brain. 2017;140(4):862–4.
16. Thibault RT, Lifshitz M, Birbaumer N, Raz A. Neurofeedback, self-regulation, and brain imaging: clinical science and fad in the service of mental disorders. Psychother Psychosom. 2015;84(4):193–207.
17. Riha C, Güntensperger D, Kleinjung T, Meyer M. Accounting for heterogeneity: mixed-effects models in resting-state EEG data in a sample of tinnitus sufferers. Brain Topogr. 2020;33(4):413–24.
18. Krakauer JW, Ghazanfar AA, Gomez-Marin A, MacIver MA, Poeppel D. Neuroscience needs behavior: correcting a reductionist bias. Neuron. 2017;93(3):480–90.
19. Weisz N, Moratti S, Meinzer M, Dohrmann K, Elbert T. Tinnitus perception and distress is related to abnormal spontaneous brain activity as measured by magnetoencephalography. PLoS Med. 2005;2(6):e153.

20. Weisz N, Dohrmann K, Elbert T. The relevance of spontaneous activity for the coding of the tinnitus sensation. Prog Brain Res. 2007;166:61–70.
21. Dohrmann K, Elbert T, Schlee W, Weisz N. Tuning the tinnitus percept by modification of synchronous brain activity. Restor Neurol Neurosci. 2007;25(3–4):371–8.
22. Crocetti A, Forti S, Bo LD. Neurofeedback for subjective tinnitus patients. Auris Nasus Larynx. 2011;38(6):735–8.
23. Hartmann T, Lorenz I, Müller N, Langguth B, Weisz N. The effects of neurofeedback on oscillatory processes related to tinnitus. Brain Topogr. 2013;27(1):149–57.
24. Güntensperger D, Thüring C, Kleinjung T, Neff P, Meyer M. Investigating the efficacy of an individualized alpha/delta neurofeedback protocol in the treatment of chronic tinnitus. Neural Plast. 2019;2019(3–4):3540898–15.
25. Güntensperger D, Kleinjung T, Neff P, Thüring C, Meyer M. Combining neurofeedback with source estimation: evaluation of an sLORETA neurofeedback protocol for chronic tinnitus treatment. Restor Neurol Neurosci. 2020;38(4):283–99.
26. Jensen M, Hüttenrauch E, Schmidt J, Andersson G, Chavanon ML, Weise C. Neurofeedback for tinnitus: study protocol for a randomised controlled trial assessing the specificity of an alpha/delta neurofeedback training protocol in alleviating both sound perception and psychological distress in a cohort of chronic tinnitus sufferers. Trials. 2020;21(1):382–13.
27. Guillard R, Fraysse MJ, Simeon R, Cervoni T, Schmutz J, Piedfort B, et al. A portable neurofeedback device for treating chronic subjective tinnitus: feasibility and results of a pilot study. Prog Brain Res. 2021;260:167–85.
28. Ridder DD, Vanneste S, Langguth B, Llinás R. Thalamocortical dysrhythmia: a theoretical update in tinnitus. Front Neurol. 2015;6:124.
29. Llinás RR, Ribary U, Jeanmonod D, Kronberg E, Mitra PP. Thalamocortical dysrhythmia: a neurological and neuropsychiatric syndrome characterized by magnetoencephalography. Proc Natl Acad Sci U S A. 1999;96(26):15222–7.
30. Ridder DD, Loo E, Kelen KV, Menovsky T, Heyning P, Moller A. Theta, alpha and beta burst transcranial magnetic stimulation: brain modulation in tinnitus. Int J Med Sci. 2007;4(5):237.
31. Vanneste S, Walsh V, Heyning PV, Ridder DD. Comparing immediate transient tinnitus suppression using tACS and tDCS: a placebo-controlled study. Exp Brain Res. 2013;226(1):25–31.
32. Neff P, Michels J, Meyer M, Schecklmann M, Langguth B, Schlee W. 10 Hz amplitude modulated sounds induce short-term tinnitus suppression. Front Aging Neurosci. 2017;9:215–1.
33. Munro BA, Searchfield GD. The short-term effects of recorded ocean sound with and without alpha frequency binaural beats on tinnitus perception. Complement Ther Med. 2019;44:291–5.
34. Rogala J, Jurewicz K, Paluch K, Kublik E, Cetnarski R, Wróbel A. The do's and don'ts of neurofeedback training: a review of the controlled studies using healthy adults. Front Hum Neurosci. 2016;10(1005):301.
35. Weisz N, Hartmann T, Müller N, Lorenz I, Obleser J. Alpha rhythms in audition: cognitive and clinical perspectives. Front Psychol. 2011;2:73.
36. Jensen O, Mazaheri A. Shaping functional architecture by oscillatory alpha activity: gating by inhibition. Front Hum Neurosci. 2010;4:186.
37. Pfurtscheller G. Functional brain imaging based on ERD/ERS. Vis Res. 2001;41(10–11):1257–60.
38. Sedley W, Teki S, Kumar S, Barnes GR, Bamiou DE, Griffiths TD. Single-subject oscillatory γ responses in tinnitus. Brain. 2012;135(Pt 10):3089–100.
39. Sedley W, Cunningham MO. Do cortical gamma oscillations promote or suppress perception? An under-asked question with an over-assumed answer. Front Hum Neurosci. 2013;7:595.
40. Weisz N, Müller S, Schlee W, Dohrmann K, Hartmann T, Elbert T. The neural code of auditory phantom perception. J Neurosci Off J Soc Neurosci. 2007;27(6):1479–84.
41. Balkenhol T, Wallhäusser-Franke E, Delb W. Psychoacoustic tinnitus loudness and tinnitus-related distress show different associations with oscillatory brain activity. PLoS One. 2013;8(1):e53180.
42. van der Loo E, Gais S, Congedo M, Vanneste S, Plazier M, Menovsky T, et al. Tinnitus intensity dependent gamma oscillations of the contralateral auditory cortex. PLoS One. 2009;4(10):e7396.
43. van der Loo E, Congedo M, Vanneste S, Van De Heyning P, De Ridder D. Insular lateralization in tinnitus distress. Auton Neurosci. 2011;165(2):191–4.
44. Ridder DD, Congedo M, Vanneste S. The neural correlates of subjectively perceived and passively matched loudness perception in auditory phantom perception. Brain Behav. 2015;5(5):e00331.
45. Sedley W, Gander PE, Kumar S, Oya H, Kovach CK, Nourski KV, et al. Intracranial mapping of a cortical tinnitus system using residual inhibition. Curr Biol. 2015;25(9):1208–14.
46. Sedley W, Friston KJ, Gander PE, Kumar S, Griffiths TD. An integrative tinnitus model based on sensory precision. Trends Neurosci. 2016;39(12):799–812.
47. Partyka M, Demarchi G, Roesch S, Suess N, Sedley W, Schlee W, et al. Phantom auditory perception (tinnitus) is characterised by stronger anticipatory auditory predictions. bioRxiv. 2019;142:869842.
48. Moazami-Goudarzi M, Michels L, Weisz N, Jeanmonod D. Temporo-insular enhancement of EEG low and high frequencies in patients with chronic tinnitus. BMC Neurosci. 2010;11(1):40.
49. Zobay O, Palmer AR, Hall DA, Sereda M, Adjamian P. Source space estimation of oscillatory power and brain connectivity in tinnitus. PLoS One. 2015;10(3):e0120123.
50. Pierzycki RH, McNamara AJ, Hoare DJ, Hall DA. Whole scalp resting state EEG of oscillatory brain activity shows no parametric relationship with psychoacoustic and psychosocial assessment of tinnitus: a repeated measures study. Hear Res. 2016;331:101–8.
51. Vanneste S, Ridder DD, Baumert M. Brain areas controlling heart rate variability in tinnitus and tinnitus-related distress. PLoS One. 2013;8(3):e59728.
52. Elgoyhen AB, Langguth B, Ridder DD, Vanneste S. Tinnitus: perspectives from human neuroimaging. Nature reviews. Neuroscience. 2015;16(10):632–42.
53. Flor H, Hoffmann D, Struve M, Diesch E. Auditory discrimination training for the treatment of tinnitus. Appl Psychophysiol Biofeedback. 2004;29(2):113–20.
54. Haegens S, Cousijn H, Wallis G, Harrison PJ, Nobre AC. Inter- and intra- individual variability in alpha peak frequency. NeuroImage. 2014;92:46–55.
55. Neff P, Hemsley C, Kraxner F, Weidt S, Kleinjung T, Meyer M. Active listening to tinnitus and its relation to resting state EEG activity. Neurosci Lett. 2018;694:176–83.
56. Abtahi SH, Abtahi SM, Mirdamadi M, Nilforoush MH, Nazari SM, et al. The long- term effect of neurofeedback therapy as adjuvant therapy on the management of tinnitus: a prospective clinical trial. Caspian J Neurol Sci. 2021;7(1):17–21.
57. Vanneste S, Joos K, Ost J, Ridder DD. Influencing connectivity and cross-frequency coupling by real-time source localized neurofeedback of the posterior cingulate cortex reduces tinnitus related distress. Neurobiol Stress. 2016;8:211–24.
58. Ridder DD, Elgoyhen AB, Romo R, Langguth B. Phantom percepts: tinnitus and pain as persisting aversive memory networks. Proc Natl Acad Sci U S A. 2011;108(20):8075–80.

59. Milner R, Lewandowska M, Ganc M, Cieśla K, Niedziałek I, Skarżyński H. Slow cortical potential neurofeedback in chronic tinnitus therapy: a case report. Appl Psychophysiol Biofeedback. 2016;41(2):225–49.
60. Verment R. Tinnitus treatment with neurofeedback: a case study. Neurosci Lett. 2011;500:e5.
61. Ros T, Enriquez-Geppert S, Zotev V, Young KD, Wood G, Whitfield-Gabrieli S, et al. Consensus on the reporting and experimental design of clinical and cognitive-behavioural neurofeedback studies (CRED-nf checklist). Brain. 2020;143(6):1674–85.
62. Malekshahi A, Malekshahi R, Czornik M, Dax J, Wolpert S, Bauer H, et al. Real-time monitoring and regulating auditory cortex alpha activity in patients with chronic tinnitus. J Neural Eng. 2020;17(1):016032.
63. Liu Z, Yao L, Wang X, Monaghan JJM, Schaette R, He Z, et al. Generalizable sample-efficient Siamese autoencoder for tinnitus diagnosis in listeners with subjective tinnitus. IEEE Trans Neural Syst Rehabil Eng. 2021;29:1452–61.
64. Sulzer J, Haller S, Scharnowski F, Weiskopf N, Birbaumer N, Blefari ML, et al. Real-time fMRI neurofeedback: Progress and challenges. NeuroImage. 2013;76:386–99.
65. Haller S, Birbaumer N, Veit R. Real-time fMRI feedback training may improve chronic tinnitus. Eur Radiol. 2010;20(3):696–703.
66. Emmert K, Kopel R, Koush Y, Maire R, Senn P, Ville DVD, et al. Continuous vs. intermittent neurofeedback to regulate auditory cortex activity of tinnitus patients using real-time fMRI - a pilot study. Neuroimage Clin. 2017;14:97–104.
67. Meikle MB, Henry JA, Griest SE, Stewart BJ, Abrams HB, McArdle R, et al. The tinnitus functional index: development of a new clinical measure for chronic, intrusive tinnitus. Ear Hear. 2012;33(2):153–76.
68. Sherwood MS, Parker JG, Diller EE, Ganapathy S, Bennett K, Nelson JT. Volitional down-regulation of the primary auditory cortex via directed attention mediated by real-time fMRI neurofeedback. AIMS Neurosci. 2018;5(3):179–99.
69. Sherwood MS, Parker JG, Diller EE, Ganapathy S, Bennett KB, Esquivel CR, et al. Self-directed down-regulation of auditory cortex activity mediated by real-time fMRI neurofeedback augments attentional processes, resting cerebral perfusion, and auditory activation. NeuroImage. 2019;195:475–89.
70. Haller S, Kopel R, Jhooti P, Haas T, Scharnowski F, Lovblad KO, et al. Dynamic reconfiguration of human brain functional networks through neurofeedback. NeuroImage. 2013;81:243–52.
71. Weiskopf N. Real-time fMRI and its application to neurofeedback. NeuroImage. 2012;62(2):682–92.
72. Baguley DM. Hyperacusis. J R Soc Med. 2003;96(12):582–5.
73. Thibault RT, MacPherson A, Lifshitz M, Roth RR, Raz A. Neurofeedback with fMRI: a critical systematic review. NeuroImage. 2018;172:786–807.
74. Cima RFF, Mazurek B, Haider H, Kikidis D, Lapira A, Norena A, et al. A multidisciplinary European guideline for tinnitus: diagnostics, assessment, and treatment. HNO. 2019;10(4):391–33.
75. Sorger B, Scharnowski F, Linden DEJ, Hampson M, Young KD. Control freaks: towards optimal selection of control conditions for fMRI neurofeedback studies. NeuroImage. 2019;186:256–65.
76. Lehner A, Langguth B, Poeppl TB, Rupprecht R, Hajak G, Landgrebe M, et al. Structural brain changes following left temporal low-frequency rTMS in patients with subjective tinnitus. Neural Plast. 2014;2014:132058.
77. Han Q, Zhang Y, Liu D, Wang Y, Feng Y, Yin X, et al. Disrupted local neural activity and functional connectivity in subjective tinnitus patients: evidence from resting-state fMRI study. Neuroradiology. 2018;27(11):676–9.
78. Meyer M, Neff P, Liem F, Kleinjung T, Weidt S, Langguth B, et al. Differential tinnitus-related neuroplastic alterations of cortical thickness and surface area. Hear Res. 2016;342:1–12.
79. Franchi JAM, Jeunet C, Lotte F. Neurofeedback: a challenge for integrative clinical neurophysiological studies. Neurophysiol Clin. 2020;50(1):1–3.
80. Ros T, Baars BJ, Lanius RA, Vuilleumier P. Tuning pathological brain oscillations with neurofeedback: a systems neuroscience framework. Front Hum Neurosci. 2014;8:1008.
81. Koralek AC, Jin X II, JDL, Costa RM, Carmena JM. Corticostriatal plasticity is necessary for learning intentional neuroprosthetic skills. Nature. 2012;483(7389):331–5.
82. Birbaumer N, Ruiz S, Sitaram R. Learned regulation of brain metabolism. Trends Cogn Sci. 2013;17(6):295–302.
83. Emmert K, Kopel R, Sulzer J, Brühl AB, Berman BD, Linden DEJ, et al. Meta-analysis of real-time fMRI neurofeedback studies using individual participant data: how is brain regulation mediated? NeuroImage. 2016;124(Pt A):806–12.
84. Lubianiker N, Goldway N, Fruchtman-Steinbok T, Paret C, Keynan JN, Singer N, et al. Process-based framework for precise neuromodulation. Nat Hum Behav. 2019;3(5):436–45.
85. Malinvaud D, Londero A, Niarra R, Peignard P, Warusfel O, Viaud-Delmon I, et al. Auditory and visual 3D virtual reality therapy as a new treatment for chronic subjective tinnitus: results of a randomized controlled trial. Hear Res. 2016;333:127–35.
86. Searchfield GD, Sanders PJ, Doborjeh Z, Doborjeh M, Boldu R, Sun K, et al. A state-of-art review of digital technologies for the next generation of tinnitus therapeutics. Front Digital Health. 2021;3:724370.
87. Deshpande AK, Bhatt I, Rojanaworarit C. Virtual reality for tinnitus management: a randomized controlled trial. Int J Audiol. 2021;61(10):868–75.
88. Schoisswohl S, Agrawal K, Simoes J, Neff P, Schlee W, Langguth B, et al. RTMS parameters in tinnitus trials: a systematic review. Nat Publ Group. 2019;9(1):12190–11.
89. Peter N, Kleinjung T, Jeker R, Meyer M, Klaghofer R, Weidt S. Tinnitus functional index: validation of the German version for Switzerland. Health Qual Life Outcomes. 2017;15(1):94.
90. Riha C, Güntensperger D, Oschwald J, Kleinjung T, Meyer M. Application of latent growth curve modeling to predict individual trajectories during neurofeedback treatment for tinnitus. Prog Brain Res. 2021;263:109–36.
91. Koush Y, Rosa MJ, Robineau F, Heinen K, Rieger SW, Weiskopf N, et al. Connectivity-based neurofeedback: dynamic causal modeling for real-time fMRI. NeuroImage. 2013;81:422–30.
92. Rieger K, Rarra MH, Hernandez LD, Hubl D, Koenig T. Neurofeedback-based enhancement of single-trial auditory evoked potentials: treatment of auditory verbal hallucinations in schizophrenia. Clin EEG Neurosci. 2018;49(6):367–78.
93. Čukić M, López V, Pavón J. Classification of depression through resting-state electroencephalogram as a novel practice in psychiatry: review. J Med Internet Res. 2020;22(11):e19548.
94. Hsu WY. Assembling a multi-feature EEG classifier for left–right motor imagery data using wavelet-based fuzzy approximate entropy for improved accuracy. Int J Neural Syst. 2015;25(08):1550037.
95. Sho'ouri N, Firoozabadi M, Badie K. Neurofeedback training protocols based on selecting distinctive features and identifying appropriate channels to enhance performance in novice visual artists. Biomed Signal Process Control. 2019;49:308–21.
96. Sabeti M, Katebi S, Boostani R. Entropy and complexity measures for EEG signal classification of schizophrenic and control participants. Artif Intell Med. 2009;47(3):263–74.

97. Schlee W, Hartmann T, Langguth B, Weisz N. Abnormal resting-state cortical coupling in chronic tinnitus. BMC Neurosci. 2009;10(1):11.
98. Mohan A, Moreno N, Song JJ, De Ridder D, Vanneste S. Evidence for behaviorally segregated, spatiotemporally overlapping subnetworks in phantom sound perception. Brain Connect. 2017;7(3):197–210.
99. Azevedo AA, Figueiredo RR, Penido NO. Tinnitus and event related potentials: a systematic review. Braz J Otorhinolaryngol. 2020;86(1):119–26.
100. Sadeghijam M, Talebian S, Mohsen S, Akbari M, Pourbakht A. Shannon entropy measures for EEG signals in tinnitus. Neurosci Lett. 2021;762:136153.
101. Riffle TL, Martel DT, Jones GR, Shore SE. Bimodal auditory electrical stimulation for the treatment of tinnitus: preclinical and clinical studies. In: The behavioral neuroscience of tinnitus. Cham: Springer; 2020. p. 295–323.

Noninvasive Brain Stimulation

52

Sven Vanneste and Tobias Kleinjung

Abstract

The pathophysiological mechanisms that underlie the generation and maintenance of tinnitus are being unraveled progressively. Based on this knowledge, a large variety of different neuromodulatory interventions have been developed and are still being designed, adapting to the progressive mechanistic insights in the pathophysiology of tinnitus. Different forms of transcranial electrical and magnetic stimulation, applied over the frontal and temporal cortex, have been investigated in tinnitus patients. Next to direct stimulation targeting specific brain areas, also nerve stimulation has been investigated as a potential treatment for tinnitus. In this chapter, we discuss the therapeutic effect and mechanics of the noninvasive neuromodulation therapies for tinnitus, their risk profiles, and potential future directions and developments.

S. Vanneste (✉)
School of Psychology, Global Brain Health Institute and Trinity College Institute for Neuroscience, Trinity College Dublin, Dublin, Ireland
e-mail: sven.vanneste@tcd.ie; http://www.lab-clint.org

T. Kleinjung
Department of Otorhinolaryngology – Head and Neck Surgery, University Hospital of Zurich, Zürich, Switzerland

W. Schlee et al. (eds.), *Textbook of Tinnitus*, https://doi.org/10.1007/978-3-031-35647-6_52

Graphical Abstract

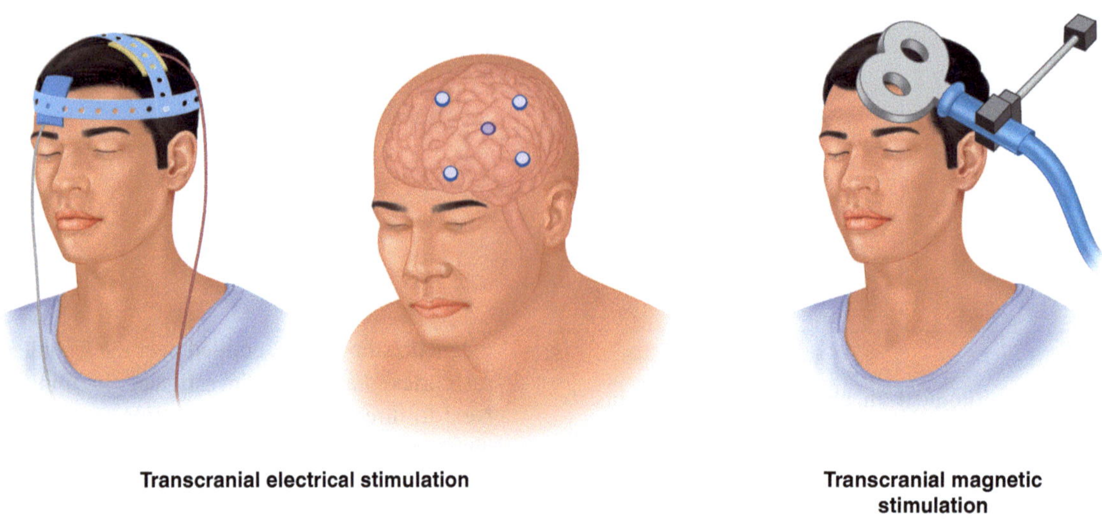

Highlights

- Based on the pathophysiological mechanisms that underlie the generation and maintenance of tinnitus, different noninvasive neuromodulation strategies for tinnitus suppression have been investigated.
- Different forms of transcranial electrical and magnetic stimulation have been applied over the temporal, frontal, and frontoparietal cortex.
- So far, there is no clear evidence for the recommendation of a specific noninvasive neuromodulatory approach in clinical routine practice.
- Systematic reviews reveal a potential effect of repetitive transcranial magnetic stimulation applied over the auditory cortex.
- Further research is needed for the translation of promising results into clinical practice.

Introduction

Despite major breakthroughs in pharmaceutical and nonpharmacological tinnitus management, these approaches are only effective in reducing the impact of tinnitus, rather than removing the tinnitus percept itself. There is increasing consensus among experts that tinnitus is a result of neuroplastic changes in auditory and nonauditory central nervous structures that occur because of peripheral deafferentation. This finding has opened the way for novel therapeutic procedures that attempt to influence the neuronal activity changes associated with tinnitus in a positive manner through stimulation. These techniques for tinnitus care include among others noninvasive neurostimulation technologies like transcranial electrical stimulation (tES) and transcranial magnetic stimulation (TMS). In recent years, they have gained popularity among researchers and physicians. The therapeutic effect and mechanisms of action associated with the noninvasive neuromodulation therapies for tinnitus, their risk profiles, and potential future directions and developments will be discussed in this chapter.

Transcranial Electrical Stimulation

Three different variants of tES are available, namely transcranial direct current stimulation, transcranial alternating current stimulation, and transcranial random noise stimulation. We also discuss transcutaneous electrical nerve stimulation as well as briefly examine vagus nerve stimulation and bimodal stimulation. In what follows, we will discuss these techniques one by one in relationship to the treatment and management of tinnitus symptoms.

Transcranial Direct Current (tDCS)

Regular tDCS

Regular tDCS uses one anode electrode and one cathode electrode on the scalp to target a specific brain area by producing a controlled electrical current from the anode to the cathode (see Figs. 52.1 and 52.2). Only 25 (to 50%) of the applied direct current reaches the brain due to the high electrical resistance of the skull, the rest being shunted through

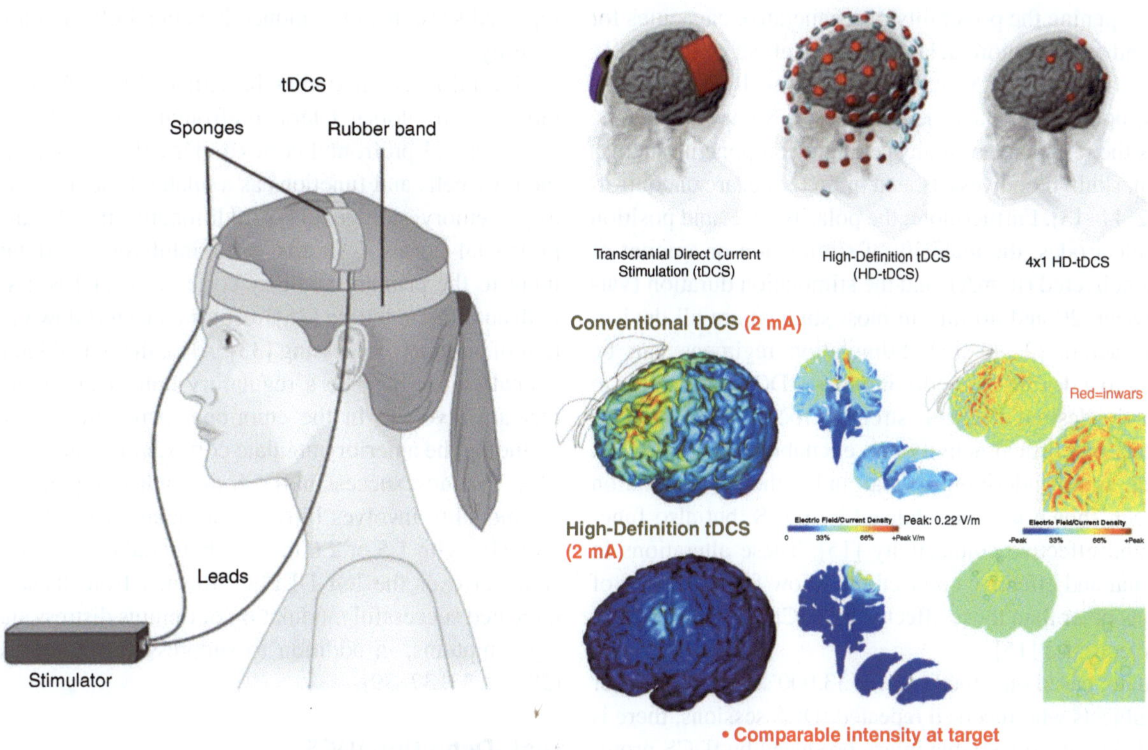

Fig. 52.1 Transcranial electrical stimulation setup for both regular and high definition and how deep the current goes

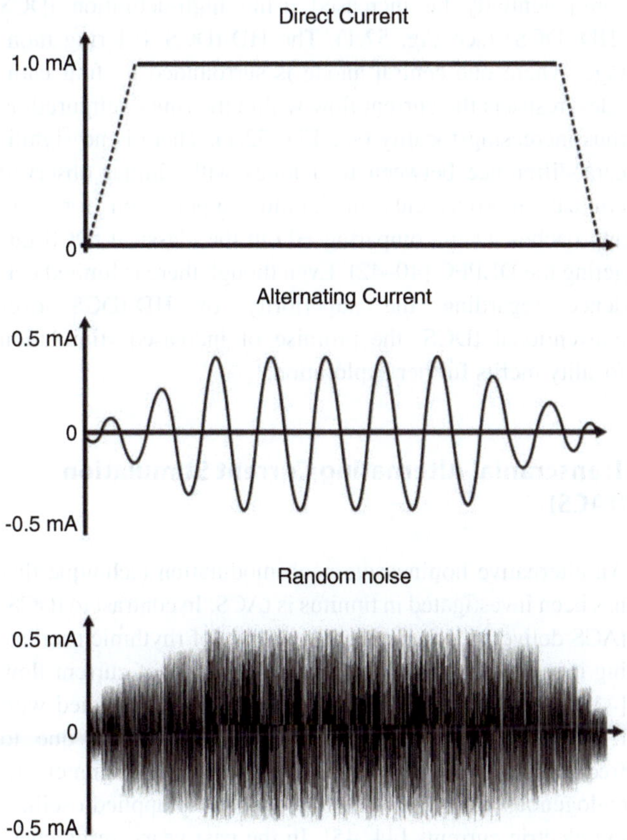

Fig. 52.2 Transcranial direct current stimulation (tDCS) delivers direct current, transcranial alternating current stimulation (tACS), and transcranial random noise stimulation (tRNS) deliver alternating current

the extracranial soft tissues, as demonstrated by calculations on realistic head models and validated both in animal and human experiments [1].

TDCS modulates cellular membrane potential and increase or suppress spontaneous neuronal activation [2, 3]. Anodal stimulation causes inward current flow, which causes depolarization of pyramidal cortical neurons and hyperpolarization of apical dendrites, whereas cathodal stimulation causes outward current flow, which causes somatic hyperpolarization of pyramidal cortical neurons and depolarization of apical dendrites [4, 5]. Under the anodal electrode, depolarization causes an increase in firing and excitability, whereas under the cathodal electrode, depolarization causes a decrease in firing and excitability [6]. However, the delayed clinical effect of tDCS on pyramidal and interneurons cell firing does not always result from an immediate effect [7]. Two additional pathways have been proposed to be influenced by tDCS, namely glial and stem cell regulation. TDCS seems to regulate microglia cells, a specific type of glial cells, under both the anode and cathode [8]. This may also delay the effect reported for tDCS as it is known that glial cells play a central role in synaptic formation, which takes time. Furthermore, tDCS may have a neuroimmunomodulatory effect by modulating the expression of immune-mediating genes via microglia and astrocytes [9, 10]. Apart from an immediate effect on neuronal cells, tDCS might also have a delayed effect via activating stem cells. TDCS seems to recruit proliferating neural stem cell under the cathode thereby opening the possibility of regenerative capacities for tDCS and an even more delayed clinical effect of tDCS [8].

The effects of tDCS are also influenced by a variety of factors, both patient- and device-related. Some parameters, such as the resistance of many cephalic components such as the skin, skull, blood vessels, and brain tissue, are uncontrollable [2, 11–13]. Furthermore, the polarity, size, and position of the electrodes, the intensity of stimulation or amount of current delivered (in mA), and the stimulation duration (varies between 20 and 40 min in most studies) are all device-related factors [2, 11–13]. Stimulation regimens can be adjusted to a degree by modifying these tDCS parameters to achieve the desired direction, strength, focality, and duration of effects on cortical activity and excitability [11, 14]. Not only the areas underlying anodal and cathodal stimulation have been shown to be modulated by tDCS, but also functional and effective connectivity [15]. These alterations in functional and effective connectivity allow for regulation of locations other than those affected by tDCS under the stimulation electrodes [15].

To date, based on a total of over 33,000 sessions and over 1000 subjects who received repeated tDCS sessions, there is no evidence for irreversible injury produced by tDCS protocols within a wide range of stimulation parameters (≤40 min, ≤4 mA) [16]. Another paper that summarizes the partially adverse effects of 567 tDCS sessions over different cortical areas revealed that tDCS is associated with relatively minor adverse effects in healthy humans and patients, according to the present safety guidelines [17].

TDCS delivers a low electrical current, commonly between 0.5 and 2 mA, to the cortex via positive (anodal) or negative (cathodal) scalp electrodes [18]. In subjects with tinnitus, anodal tDCS typically increases neural excitability through depolarization (i.e., increased brain activity), while cathodal tDCS achieves the opposite effect by inducing neural hyperpolarization (i.e., decreased brain activity). The effects of tDCS may last for an hour after a single treatment session and longer when stimulation duration is increased or provided over multiple session [6, 19].

Initial tinnitus-tDCS studies targeted the left-temporoparietal area and the auditory cortex (AC) with the goal of modulating primary auditory cortex, auditory association areas, and parts of the limbic system, specifically the amygdala and hippocampus [20–28]. Study findings were diverse. Some reports suggested that cathodal tDCS of the LTA with anodal tDCS over the contralateral supraorbital area had no effect [20, 21, 28], whereas others demonstrated suppression of tinnitus loudness [24, 25]. It is noteworthy that protocols for tDCS of the left-temporoparietal area and auditory cortex are heterogeneous, differing in stimulation parameters, polarity, and sham procedures. There is a likelihood that higher cathodal stimulation intensity (2 mA) of the left-temporoparietal area and auditory cortex, coupled with repeated sessions, may induce beneficial effects on tinnitus severity.

Several research studies investigated the effect of tDCS targeting the dorsal lateral prefrontal cortex [29–33]. The dorsal lateral prefrontal cortex reportedly contains auditory memory cells and functions as a bilateral facilitator of auditory memory storage [34]. Additionally, the dorsal lateral prefrontal cortex C exerts early inhibitory modulation of input to the primary auditory cortex [35] and is associated with auditory attention [36], resulting in a top-down modulation of auditory processing [33]. Also, the dorsal lateral prefrontal cortex may be a regulatory hub of brain structures that are involved in the emotional perception of tinnitus, including the anterior cingulate cortex, amygdala, and insula [37]. The most successful tDCS-dorsal lateral prefrontal cortex modality involves bifrontal stimulation for 20 minutes, typically with 1.5 or 2.0 mA, with anodal over the right and cathodal over the left DLPFC. Results from these studies indicated successful modulation of tinnitus distress and anxiety symptoms, in addition to suppressing tinnitus severity [29, 30, 33, 37–39].

High-Definition tDCS

One main limitation of tDCS is the use of saline-soaked sponges that stimulate a broad cortical region. The focality can potentially be increased using high-definition tDCS (HD-tDCS) (see Fig. 52.1). The HD-tDCS 4x1 ring montage, where one central anode is surrounded by four cathodes, restricts the current flow within the ring configuration, thus increasing focality (see Fig. 52.1). There is no significant difference between techniques with similar observed clinical improvements in tinnitus suppression for both approaches when comparing HD to the classical tDCS targeting the DLPFC [40–42]. Even though there is limited evidence regarding the superiority of HD-tDCS over conventional tDCS, the promise of increased stimulation focality merits further exploration.

Transcranial Alternating Current Stimulation (tACS)

An alternative noninvasive neuromodulation technique that has been investigated in tinnitus is tACS. In contrast to tDCS, tACS delivers a prespecified frequency of rhythmic oscillating current that is independent of direction of current flow [43] (see Fig. 52.2). The main mechanism associated with tACS is that it influences the neurophysiology due to frequency-specific entertainment, i.e., phase alignment of endogenous brain oscillations to externally applied oscillating electric currents [44, 45]. In the past years, researchers have utilized tACS to modulate the decreased alpha and increased gamma bands in the auditory cortex that has been stipulated to be associated with tinnitus percept [31, 45]. To date, there is a lack of evidence that tACS can deliver therapeutic outcomes in tinnitus. For example, when comparing tACS with tDCS in a sham-control designed study, results indicated that a single session of bifrontal tDCS, with anodal over the right DLPFC and cathodal over the left DLPFC, can reduce suppression of both annoyance and loudness, yet, alpha-frequency tACS of the DLPFC showed no significant effect [39]. Similar tACS-tinnitus studies have presented consistently negative results [31, 46], rendering a lack of merit in further pursuing trials examining the use of tACS in tinnitus management.

Transcranial Random Noise Stimulation (tRNS)

In contrast to tACS, the application of tRNS in tinnitus has generated more promising results. TRNS produces alternating current to the cortical region with a constantly changing frequency ranging from 0.1 to 600 Hz [47] (see Fig. 52.2). Currently, there are three postulated principles in regard to the mechanism of tRNS: (1) long-term potentiation [48], (2) repeated subthreshold stimulations that prevent the system from building up homeostasis and potentiating task-related neural activity [48], and (3) the occurrence of stochastic resonance where nonlinear neural signals are modulated by noise stimulation [49]. Research found that high-frequency tRNS increases excitability; however, the exact mechanism of action is unknown. It could possibly increase excitability by preventing system homeostasis through a stochastic resonance effect caused by repeated subthreshold stimulations [50, 51]. Desynchronization of (pathological) rhythms is another proposed mechanism of action, although none of the foregoing processes have been verified [52].

In a study comparing single sessions of tDCS, tACS or tRNS on the auditory cortex, tRNS induced a larger transient suppressive effect on tinnitus loudness and distress while tDCS and tACS generated small nonsignificant effects [31]. Also, there seems to be added beneficial value when prefrontal anodal tDCS is followed by auditory tRNS compared to absolute tDCS of the prefrontal cortex [53]. Although preliminary, findings from studies indicate that tRNS may be superior to tDCS and tACS in the management of tinnitus. Another avenue of tRNS research has focused on the effects of low-frequency tRNS and high-frequency tRNS. Preliminary results showed no differences in low-frequency tRNS and high-frequency tRNS, with both modalities eventuating in pronounced suppression of tinnitus loudness and distress [54, 55]. A feasibility multisite stimulation study reported that 2 weeks of daily low-frequency tRNS over the auditory cortex preceded by high-frequency tRNS over the dorsolateral prefrontal cortex had significant larger reduction in loudness and distress compared to auditory cortex low-frequency tRNS and sham [56]. Although promising, it is of note that tRNS studies are in the exploratory stage. At present, there is no clear mechanistic explanation for differences in low-frequency and high-frequency tRNS. In addition, to establishing the underlying mechanism, replication of the results for tRNS modalities in larger studies are needed to document their efficacy.

Transcutaneous Electrical Nerve Stimulation (TENS)

TENS is a safe, noninvasive neuromodulation method established in the field of chronic pain [57]. Research suggests that bothersome tinnitus may be successfully alleviated with application of TENS to a varied number of stimulation sites, with a wide range of modalities. Initially, studies showed that tinnitus suppression could be achieved through TENS of the median nerve [58]. Further studies reported reduction in tinnitus symptoms with application of TENS to the temporomandibular joint [59] and to the tragus of the ear [60].

In most studies, TENS was applied to the C2 dermatome around the ear. C2 stimulation reportedly increases activation of the dorsal cochlear nucleus (DCN) along the somatosensory pathway and, subsequently, enhances the inhibitory role of DCN on the central auditory nervous system. The result is suppression of tinnitus [61]. It has been reported that electrical stimulation of the C2 dermatome controls the inhibition and excitement of principal cells within the dorsal cochlear nucleus [61]. In one study, 240 patients received 10 minutes of 6 Hz followed by 10 minutes of 40 Hz stimulation and finally 10 minutes of sham [62]. Significant transient improvement of 42.9% was reported in 17.9% of patients [62].

When comparing the mechanisms of TENS, tDCS, and TMS, it has been suggested that TENS modulates the tinnitus brain circuit indirectly through the previously discussed somatosensory mechanisms. However, tDCS and TMS suppress tinnitus via a dual working method, one that involves a TENS-like somatosensory mechanism and a direct cortical modulating approach [32].

Transcutaneous Vagus Nerve Stimulation (tVNS)

TVNS exerts an effect on the vagus nerve through a nerve branch innervating the skin of the external auditory canal [63, 64]. Although still preliminary, studies have demonstrated that tVNS is feasible and safe in tinnitus patients [65]. The stimulation was well tolerated; however, there was no discernible reduction in tinnitus symptoms [65]. However, in treated patients, there was a trend toward a reduction in depression symptoms [65]. Another study adds to the evidence for tVNS-induced stress reduction [66]. The effect of tVNS on heart rate activity in 173 tinnitus patients was explored in this study, and it was discovered that tVNS can reduce sympathetic activation in tinnitus patients. TVNS was paired with auditory stimulation in two short pilot studies, and the results revealed potential efficacy on tinnitus [67, 68]. TVNS has been performed without auditory pairing and has shown some benefit [69] [69], raising doubts about the value of paired sound presentation. More studies are needed to confirm the efficacy of tVNS in the management of bothersome tinnitus. In the Chap. 54, more information can be found in regard to vagus stimulation.

Bimodal Stimulation

In recent years, various bi- or multimodal stimulation techniques for the treatment of tinnitus have been developed. Aside from vagal stimulation, transcranial electrical stimulation, and transcranial magnetic stimulation in combination with auditory stimulation, the combination of auditory stimulation and somatosensory stimulation has been studied. The trigeminal nerve or greater occipital nerve afferents were used to stimulate the somatosensory system. The combination of auditory and somatosensory manipulation is prompted by a growing awareness of the somatosensory system's importance in tinnitus pathogenesis [70] The interplay between somatosensory and auditory afferents on the level of the dorsal cochlear nucleus can explain the clinical phenomenon that many patients can regulate their tinnitus by moving their face or neck [71]. As a result of this understanding, two alternative approaches to simultaneous somatosensory and auditory stimulation were developed. An inhibitory impact on the level of the dorsal cochlear nucleus is one method for modulating activity in the central auditory pathway. Basic neurophysiological research in animals described stimulus timing-dependent plasticity in the dorsal cochlear nucleus; therefore, the somatosensory and auditory stimuli were provided at precise intervals [72]. These findings were put into practice in a clinical pilot study with 20 patients, in which noises were combined with transcutaneous electrical stimulation of the greater occipital nerve at the level of the neck for 28 days. The bimodal treatment decreased the loudness and intrusiveness of tinnitus, but the control condition (auditory stimulation alone) had no effect [72]. However, the effect was transient, particularly in terms of loudness perception, which did not extend beyond the 3-week bimodal stimulation period, and the reduction in distress lasted only 3 weeks.

Another approach aiming to modulate the trigeminal nerve in the combination of sound and electrical stimulation of the tongue tip. In an open-label pilot study that utilized a broad-band spectrum noise with temporal fluctuations paired with electrical stimulation of the tongue [73]. A significant reduction on the tinnitus handicap questionnaire and on minimal masking levels was revealed, in addition to a drop for tinnitus loudness. This study was followed by a large randomized and double-blind clinical study [74]. Participants were evaluated during the 12-week treatment period and for three follow-up visits for up to 12 months to assess long-term therapeutic effects after the end of treatment. Depending on the condition, 75–88% of these participants had a significant drop on tinnitus handicap inventory or tinnitus functional index scores. Bimodal neuromodulation with sound and tongue stimulation were able to achieve this improvement within 6–12 weeks of treatment that was generally maintained for 12 months after the end of treatment. More information about this approach can be found in the Chap. 54.

Transcranial Magnetic Stimulation

Transcranial magnetic stimulation (TMS) is a neurophysiological technique for stimulating neurons in the brain via brief magnetic pulses delivered by a coil placed on the scalp [75] (Fig. 52.3). This tool has a long established history of safety, tolerability, and efficacy [76]. In brief, the stimulator delivers a short lasting, high-intensity current pulse through an insulated stimulating coil. This induces a magnetic field perpendicular to the coil which penetrates the scalp and brain with little attenuation (see Fig. 52.4). The magnetic field reaches a maximum of approximately 1.5–2 Tesla (same size as that of an MRI scanner) in about 100 μs and then decays back to zero [77]. The magnetic coils that are used have different shapes. Round coils are relatively powerful. Figure-eight-shaped coils are more focal with a maximal current delivered at the intersection of the two round components [78] (see Fig. 52.4).

Because the magnetic field changes rapidly with time, it induces an electrical current in the brain under the coil which is similar in duration and amplitude to a conventional electrical stimulator used to activate peripheral nerves. Due to the strong decline of the magnetic field with increasing distance from the coil, the direct stimulation is limited to superficial cortical areas, but the stimulation effects can be propagated transsynaptically to functionally connected remote areas and thus indirectly affect large areas of the brain.

Whereas single magnetic pulses do not seem to have longer lasting effects on the brain, the application of multiple pulses (typically between 100 and 3,000), called repetitive TMS (rTMS), leads to effects on the brain that outlast the duration of the stimulation [79]. These effects

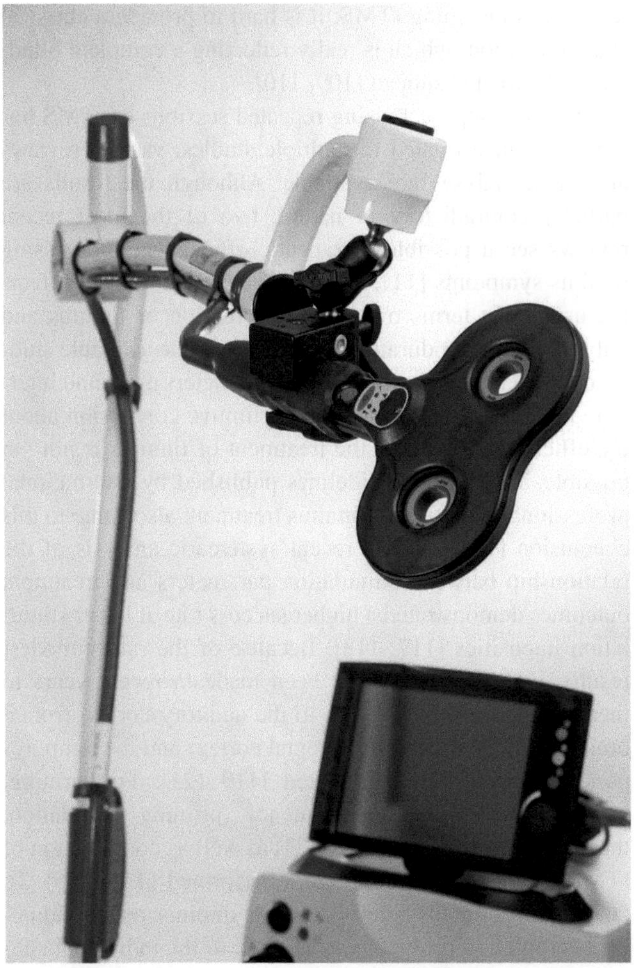

Fig. 52.3 Transcranial magnetic stimulation setup

resemble those seen in animal experiments where repeated stimulation of many pathways has been shown to produce changes in the effectiveness of synapses in the same circuits [80]. Low frequency (≤1 Hz) rTMS has been repeatedly shown to result in a decrease in cortical excitability [81], whereas high-frequency (5–20 Hz) rTMS results in an increase in excitability [82]. These changes include the phenomena of long-term potentiation (LTP) and long-term depression (LTD), which have been shown to be important in learning and memory [83]. Repetitive TMS can also be used to transiently disturb ongoing neural activity in the stimulated cortical area, thus creating a transient functional lesion. Such an approach can help to identify whether a given brain area is critically involved in a specific behavioral task.

Because of these unique and powerful features, rTMS has been widely used in various fields, including cognitive neuroscience and several clinical applications (for review, see [79, 84, 85]). Initially, TMS was mainly applied to study the function of the cerebral cortex for research and diagnostic issues. In the last two decades, it has increasingly become a routine tool for the treatment of certain diseases. Currently, the highest levels of evidence (A/B) exist for rTMS treatment in depression (dorsolateral prefrontal cortex), neuropathic pain (primary motor cortex), and promoting motor recovery at the postacute stage of stroke (primary motor cortex) [85]. However, despite its practical usefulness, the mechanisms of how rTMS stimulates neurons and interferes with neural functions are still incompletely understood.

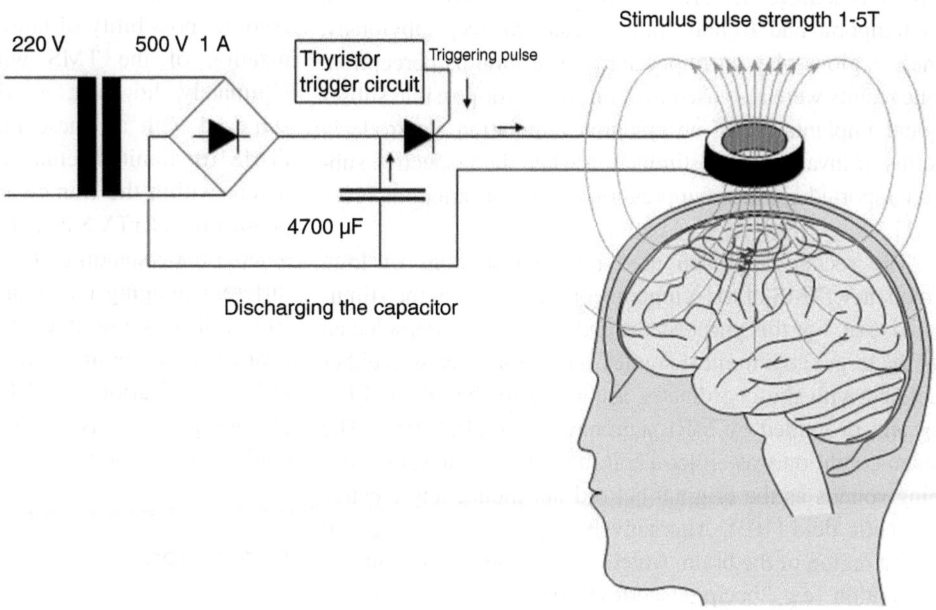

Fig. 52.4 Schematic overview of the magnetic field perpendicular to the coil which penetrates the scalp and brain with little attenuation

Rationale for the Application of TMS in Tinnitus

Tinnitus is often associated with a lesion in the peripheral auditory system. It often occurs together with presbycusis, Ménière's disease, noise trauma, sudden deafness, or drug-related ototoxicity [86–89]. However, these pathologies are not directly causing tinnitus. Rather, the neuroplastic changes which occur in the brain as reaction to sensory deafferentation represent the neural correlate of most forms of tinnitus [70, 90, 91].

Since rTMS has the ability to focally modulate cortical activity, it has been assumed that it can interfere with the abnormal neural activity in the auditory cortex associated with tinnitus and thereby influence the perception of tinnitus. If this is the case, repeated applications of rTMS might represent a potential treatment for some forms of tinnitus by producing shorter or longer lasting modulation of cortical activity. Additional support for this approach comes from clinical trials in which rTMS was used in an attempt to treat other pathological conditions with potential cortical hyperactivity, such as auditory hallucinations [92, 93], writers' cramp [94, 95], and obsessive compulsive disorders [96, 97].

rTMS for Tinnitus Diagnostics and Treatment

TMS has been used in two different ways in tinnitus research. One approach performed single sessions of rTMS to achieve temporary suppression of tinnitus perception by modulating activity in cortical areas in the sense of a "functional lesion." This was achieved in certain tinnitus sufferers by stimulation of temporal and frontal cortex areas [98, 99]. Obviously, these regions play an important role in tinnitus perception. The results were also used to define a site for possible subsequent implantation of an epidural stimulation electrode in terms of invasive neurostimulation when the respective subject reported tinnitus suppression during stimulation [100, 101].

The second approach used repeated sessions of low-frequency rTMS of the temporal cortex activity in the stimulated area. For this purpose, the auditory cortex was selected as the target area in most studies. The target area was either defined with the coordinates according to the 10–20 EEG system or guided by MRI-neuronavigation [102–105]. The sham condition was either a coil that emitted the same popping sounds as the original but did not induce any electromagnetic field [103]. Alternatively, a placement of the coil over a region of the brain, which are not relevant for tinnitus perception (e.g., occipital cortex) [106], the perpendicular placement of the coil [107] or the use of a system that delivers focal electrical activity to the scalp [108] can be considered. However, for most of noninvasive neurostimulation techniques including rTMS, it is hard to provide a classical sham condition, which is really reflecting a complete blinding of the treated subject [109, 110].

Since the approach using repeated sessions of rTMS has now been investigated in multiple studies, various reviews and meta-analyses are available. Although the results are partially contradictory in nature, two of the most recent reviews see a possible therapeutic efficacy in suppressing tinnitus symptoms [111, 112]. However, the clinical effects are usually in terms of partial suppression of tinnitus and only of temporary duration. Furthermore, the available studies differed in design, stimulation parameters used, and interindividual results [113]. Thus, a definitive conclusion about the efficacy of rTMS in the treatment of tinnitus is not yet possible. The various guidelines published by international professional societies on tinnitus treatment also came to this conclusion [114–116]. A recent systematic analysis of the relationship between stimulation parameters and treatment outcomes demonstrated a higher success rate at lower stimulation intensities [117, 118]. Because of the rather modest results, various efforts have been made in recent years to increase efficacy. In addition to the auditory cortex, frontal brain areas (dorsolateral prefrontal cortex) and the temporoparietal cortex were stimulated [119–121]. Furthermore, variations of stimulation frequency (priming stimulation, theta burst stimulation) [122, 123] as well as combination of rTMS with drug treatment were performed [124, 125]. To take into account the heterogeneity of tinnitus, an individualized stimulation protocol was tailored to the individual subjects in certain studies. After a trial phase with stimulation of different regions, the region that initially showed the greatest effect was stimulated for a longer period of time [126]. Another possibility of tailor-made protocols is the synchronization of the TMS with the individual EEG [127]. Ultimately, however, no decisive breakthrough could be achieved with all these modifications, so that the use of rTMS for tinnitus remains predominantly experimental in nature within the framework of studies. Besides the therapeutic effects, rTMS can also contribute important aspects to a better understanding of tinnitus pathogenesis. By means of different imaging techniques (PET, fMRI, structural MRI, EEG), it was possible to trace structural and functional changes in the brain of tinnitus patients after rTMS therapy [128–131]. Various model assumptions on tinnitus pathophysiology, such as the involvement of nonauditory areas, could be confirmed.

Conclusion

The last two decades' research in noninvasive neuromodulatory interventions for the treatment of tinnitus have significantly increased but have yet to result in regular clinical routine use. However, most recent meta-analyses suggest that a transition from experimental to clinical applications of noninvasive stimulation may be in view. Better insights in the pathophysiology of tinnitus and in the heterogeneous nature of tinnitus will provide novel approach that might be beneficial to apply new noninvasive neuromodulation approaches such as that better outcomes can be guaranteed.

References

1. Voroslakos M, Takeuchi Y, Brinyiczki K, Zombori T, Oliva A, Fernandez-Ruiz A, et al. Direct effects of transcranial electric stimulation on brain circuits in rats and humans. Nat Commun. 2018;9(1):483.
2. Moreno-Duarte I, Gebodh N, Schestatsky P, Guleyupoglu B, Reato D, Bikson M, et al. Transcranial electrical stimulation: transcranial direct current stimulation (tDCS), transcranial alternating current stimulation (tACS), transcranial pulsed current stimulation (tPCS), and transcranial random noise stimulation (tRNS). In: Kadosh RC, editor. Cognitive enhancement using non-invasive brain stimulation. London: Academia Press; 2014.
3. Nitsche MA, Cohen LG, Wassermann EM, Priori A, Lang N, Antal A, et al. Transcranial direct current stimulation: state of the art 2008. Brain Stimul. 2008;1(3):206–23.
4. Radman T, Ramos RL, Brumberg JC, Bikson M. Role of cortical cell type and morphology in subthreshold and suprathreshold uniform electric field stimulation in vitro. Brain Stimul. 2009;2(4):215–28, 28 e1-3.
5. Zaghi S, Acar M, Hultgren B, Boggio PS, Fregni F. Noninvasive brain stimulation with low-intensity electrical currents: putative mechanisms of action for direct and alternating current stimulation. Neuroscientist. 2010;16(3):285–307.
6. Nitsche MA, Paulus W. Sustained excitability elevations induced by transcranial DC motor cortex stimulation in humans. Neurology. 2001;57(10):1899–901.
7. Fujiyama H, Hyde J, Hinder MR, Kim SJ, McCormack GH, Vickers JC, et al. Delayed plastic responses to anodal tDCS in older adults. Front Aging Neurosci. 2014;6:115.
8. Rueger MA, Keuters MH, Walberer M, Braun R, Klein R, Sparing R, et al. Multi-session transcranial direct current stimulation (tDCS) elicits inflammatory and regenerative processes in the rat brain. PLoS One. 2012;7(8):e43776.
9. Goerigk S, Cretaz E, Sampaio-Junior B, Vieira ELM, Gattaz W, Klein I, et al. Effects of tDCS on neuroplasticity and inflammatory biomarkers in bipolar depression: results from a sham-controlled study. Prog Neuro-Psychopharmacol Biol Psychiatry. 2021;105:110119.
10. Rabenstein M, Unverricht-Yeboah M, Keuters MH, Pikhovych A, Hucklenbroich J, Vay SU, et al. Transcranial current stimulation alters the expression of immune-mediating genes. Front Cell Neurosci. 2019;13:461.
11. Brunoni AR, Nitsche MA, Bolognini N, Bikson M, Wagner T, Merabet L, et al. Clinical research with transcranial direct current stimulation (tDCS): challenges and future directions. Brain Stimul. 2012;5(3):175–95.
12. Medeiros LF, de Souza IC, Vidor LP, de Souza A, Deitos A, Volz MS, et al. Neurobiological effects of transcranial direct current stimulation: a review. Front Psych. 2012;3:110.
13. To WT, Hart J, De Ridder D, Vanneste S. Considering the influence of stimulation parameters on the effect of conventional and high-definition transcranial direct current stimulation. Expert Rev Med Devices. 2016;13(4):391–404.
14. Nitsche MA, Kuo M-F, Paulus W, Antal A. Transcranial direct current stimulation: protocols and physiological mechanisms of action in helena knotkova and dirk rasche, Textbook of Neuromodulation, Spirnger, New York, 2015:101–11.
15. To WT, De Ridder D, Hart J Jr, Vanneste S. Changing brain networks through non-invasive neuromodulation. Front Hum Neurosci. 2018;12:128.
16. Bikson M, Grossman P, Thomas C, Zannou AL, Jiang J, Adnan T, et al. Safety of transcranial direct current stimulation: evidence based update 2016. Brain Stimul. 2016;9(5):641–61.
17. Poreisz C, Boros K, Antal A, Paulus W. Safety aspects of transcranial direct current stimulation concerning healthy subjects and patients. Brain Res Bull. 2007;72(4–6):208–14.
18. Woods AJ, Antal A, Bikson M, Boggio PS, Brunoni AR, Celnik P, et al. A technical guide to tDCS, and related non-invasive brain stimulation tools. Clin Neurophysiol. 2016;127(2):1031–48.
19. Nitsche MA, Paulus W. Excitability changes induced in the human motor cortex by weak transcranial direct current stimulation. J Physiol. 2000;527(Pt 3):633.
20. Forogh B, Mirshaki Z, Raissi GR, Shirazi A, Mansoori K, Ahadi T. Repeated sessions of transcranial direct current stimulation for treatment of chronic subjective tinnitus: a pilot randomized controlled trial. Neurol Sci. 2016;37(2):253–9.
21. Garin P, Gilain C, Van Damme J-P, De Fays K, Jamart J, Ossemann M, et al. Short-and long-lasting tinnitus relief induced by transcranial direct current stimulation. J Neurol. 2011;258(11):1940–8.
22. Henin S, Fein D, Smouha E, Parra LC. The effects of compensatory auditory stimulation and high-definition transcranial direct current stimulation (HD-tDCS) on tinnitus perception–a randomized pilot study. PLoS One. 2016;11(11):e0166208.
23. Hyvärinen P, Mäkitie A, Aarnisalo AA. Self-administered domiciliary tDCS treatment for tinnitus: a double-blind sham-controlled study. PLoS One. 2016;11(4):e0154286.
24. Joos K, De Ridder D, Van de Heyning P, Vanneste S. Polarity specific suppression effects of transcranial direct current stimulation for tinnitus. Neural Plast. 2014;2014:1.
25. Minami SB, Oishi N, Watabe T, Uno K, Kaga K, Ogawa K. Auditory resting-state functional connectivity in tinnitus and modulation with transcranial direct current stimulation. Acta Otolaryngol. 2015;135(12):1286–92.
26. Pal N, Maire R, Stephan MA, Herrmann FR, Benninger DH. Transcranial direct current stimulation for the treatment of chronic tinnitus: a randomized controlled study. Brain Stimul. 2015;8(6):1101–7.
27. Shekhawat GS, Kobayashi K, Searchfield GD. Methodology for studying the transient effects of transcranial direct current stimulation combined with auditory residual inhibition on tinnitus. J Neurosci Methods. 2015;239:28–33.
28. Shekhawat GS, Stinear CM, Searchfield GD. Transcranial direct current stimulation intensity and duration effects on tinnitus suppression. Neurorehabil Neural Repair. 2013;27(2):164–72.
29. Faber M, Vanneste S, Fregni F, De Ridder D. Top down prefrontal affective modulation of tinnitus with multiple sessions of tDCS of dorsolateral prefrontal cortex. Brain Stimul. 2012;5(4):492–8.
30. Frank E, Schecklmann M, Landgrebe M, Burger J, Kreuzer P, Poeppl TB, et al. Treatment of chronic tinnitus with repeated sessions of prefrontal transcranial direct current stimulation: outcomes from an open-label pilot study. J Neurol. 2012;259(2):327–33.
31. Plazier M, Dekelver I, Vanneste S, Stassijns G, Menovsky T, Thimineur M, et al. Occipital nerve stimulation in fibromyalgia: a double-blind placebo-controlled pilot study with a six-month follow-up. Neuromodulation. 2013;17:256.
32. Vanneste S, Langguth B, De Ridder D. Do tDCS and TMS influence tinnitus transiently via a direct cortical and indirect somatosensory modulating effect? A combined TMS-tDCS and TENS study. Brain Stimul. 2011;4(4):242–52.

33. Vanneste S, Plazier M, Ost J, van der Loo E, Van de Heyning P, De Ridder D. Bilateral dorsolateral prefrontal cortex modulation for tinnitus by transcranial direct current stimulation: a preliminary clinical study. Exp Brain Res. 2010;202(4):779–85.
34. Bodner M, Kroger J, Fuster JM. Auditory memory cells in dorsolateral prefrontal cortex. Neuroreport: An international journal for the rapid communication of research. Neuroscience. 1996;7:1905.
35. Voisin J, Bidet-Caulet A, Bertrand O, Fonlupt P. Listening in silence activates auditory areas: a functional magnetic resonance imaging study. J Neurosci. 2006;26(1):273–8.
36. Mitchell TV, Morey RA, Inan S, Belger A. Functional magnetic resonance imaging measure of automatic and controlled auditory processing. Neuroreport. 2005;16(5):457.
37. Vanneste S, Plazier M, Van Der Loo E, Van de Heyning P, Congedo M, De Ridder D. The neural correlates of tinnitus-related distress. NeuroImage. 2010;52(2):470–80.
38. De Ridder D, Vanneste S, Kovacs S, Sunaert S, Menovsky T, van de Heyning P, et al. Transcranial magnetic stimulation and extradural electrodes implanted on secondary auditory cortex for tinnitus suppression. J Neurosurg. 2011;114(4):903–11.
39. Vanneste S, Walsh V, Van De Heyning P, De Ridder D. Comparing immediate transient tinnitus suppression using tACS and tDCS: a placebo-controlled study. Exp Brain Res. 2013;226(1):25–31.
40. Jacquemin L, Shekhawat GS, Van de Heyning P, Mertens G, Fransen E, Van Rompaey V, et al. Effects of electrical stimulation in tinnitus patients: conventional versus high-definition tDCS. Neurorehabil Neural Repair. 2018;32(8):714–23.
41. Shekhawat GS, Sundram F, Bikson M, Truong D, De Ridder D, Stinear CM, et al. Intensity, duration, and location of high-definition transcranial direct current stimulation for tinnitus relief. Neurorehabil Neural Repair. 2016;30(4):349–59.
42. Shekhawat GS, Vanneste S. High-definition transcranial direct current stimulation of the dorsolateral prefrontal cortex for tinnitus modulation: a preliminary trial. J Neural Transm. 2018;125(2):163–71.
43. Zaghi S, de Freitas RL, de Oliveira LM, El-Nazer R, Menning S, Tadini L, et al. Inhibition of motor cortex excitability with 15 Hz transcranial alternating current stimulation (tACS). Neurosci Lett. 2010;479(3):211–4.
44. Witkowski M, Garcia-Cossio E, Chander BS, Braun C, Birbaumer N, Robinson SE, et al. Mapping entrained brain oscillations during transcranial alternating current stimulation (tACS). NeuroImage. 2016;140:89–98.
45. Zaehle T, Rach S, Herrmann CS. Transcranial alternating current stimulation enhances individual alpha activity in human EEG. PLoS One. 2010;5(11):e13766.
46. Claes L, Stamberger H, Van de Heyning P, De Ridder D, Vanneste S. Auditory cortex tACS and tRNS for tinnitus: single versus multiple sessions. Neural Plast. 2014;2014:436713.
47. Terney D, Chaieb L, Moliadze V, Antal A, Paulus W. Increasing human brain excitability by transcranial high-frequency random noise stimulation. J Neurosci. 2008;28(52):14147–55.
48. Fertonani A, Pirulli C, Miniussi C. Random noise stimulation improves neuroplasticity in perceptual learning. J Neurosci. 2011;31(43):15416–23.
49. Moss F, Ward LM, Sannita WG. Stochastic resonance and sensory information processing: a tutorial and review of application. Clin Neurophysiol. 2004;115(2):267–81.
50. Fertonani A, Pirulli C, Miniussi C. Random noise stimulation improves neuroplasticity in perceptual learning. J Neurosci Off J Soc Neurosci. 2011;31(43):15416–23.
51. Terney D, Chaieb L, Moliadze V, Antal A, Paulus W. Increasing human brain excitability by transcranial high-frequency random noise stimulation. J Neurosci Off J Soc Neurosci. 2008;28(52):14147–55.
52. Paulus W. Transcranial electrical stimulation (tES - tDCS; tRNS, tACS) methods. Neuropsychol Rehabil. 2011;21(5):602–17.
53. To WT, Ost J, Hart J, De Ridder D, Vanneste S. The added value of auditory cortex transcranial random noise stimulation (tRNS) after bifrontal transcranial direct current stimulation (tDCS) for tinnitus. J Neural Transm. 2017;124(1):79–88.
54. Joos K, De Ridder D, Vanneste S. The differential effect of low-versus high-frequency random noise stimulation in the treatment of tinnitus. Exp Brain Res. 2015;233(5):1433–40.
55. Kreuzer PM, Poeppl TB, Rupprecht R, Vielsmeier V, Lehner A, Langguth B, et al. Daily high-frequency transcranial random noise stimulation of bilateral temporal cortex in chronic tinnitus–a pilot study. Sci Rep. 2019;9(1):1–6.
56. Mohsen S, Mahmoudian S, Talebian S, Pourbakht A. Prefrontal and auditory tRNS in sequence for treating chronic tinnitus: a modified multisite protocol. Brain Stimul. 2018;11(5):1177–9.
57. Nnoaham KE, Kumbang J. Transcutaneous electrical nerve stimulation (TENS) for chronic pain. Cochrane Database Syst Rev. 2008;3:CD003222.
58. Møller AR, Møller MB, Yokota M. Some forms of tinnitus may involve the extralemniscal auditory pathway. Laryngoscope. 1992;102(10):1165–71.
59. Herraiz C, Toledano A, Diges I. Trans-electrical nerve stimulation (TENS) for somatic tinnitus. Prog Brain Res. 2007;166:389–553.
60. Steenerson RL, Cronin GW. Tinnitus reduction using transcutaneous electrical stimulation. Otolaryngol Clin N Am. 2003;36(2):337.
61. Young ED, Nelken I, Conley RA. Somatosensory effects on neurons in dorsal cochlear nucleus. J Neurophysiol. 1995;73(2):743–65.
62. Vanneste S, Plazier M, Van de Heyning P, De Ridder D. Transcutaneous electrical nerve stimulation (TENS) of upper cervical nerve (C2) for the treatment of somatic tinnitus. Exp Brain Res. 2010;204(2):283–7.
63. Kreuzer PM, Landgrebe M, Husser O, Resch M, Schecklmann M, Geisreiter F, et al. Transcutaneous vagus nerve stimulation: retrospective assessment of cardiac safety in a pilot study. Front Psych. 2012;3:70.
64. Lehtimäki J, Hyvärinen P, Ylikoski M, Bergholm M, Mäkelä JP, Aarnisalo A, et al. Transcutaneous vagus nerve stimulation in tinnitus: a pilot study. Acta Otolaryngol. 2013;133(4):378–82.
65. Kreuzer PM, Landgrebe M, Resch M, Husser O, Schecklmann M, Geisreiter F, et al. Feasibility, safety and efficacy of transcutaneous vagus nerve stimulation in chronic tinnitus: an open pilot study. Brain Stimul. 2014;7(5):740–7.
66. Ylikoski J, Lehtimaki J, Pirvola U, Makitie A, Aarnisalo A, Hyvarinen P, et al. Non-invasive vagus nerve stimulation reduces sympathetic preponderance in patients with tinnitus. Acta Otolaryngol. 2017;137(4):426–31.
67. Lehtimaki J, Hyvarinen P, Ylikoski M, Bergholm M, Makela JP, Aarnisalo A, et al. Transcutaneous vagus nerve stimulation in tinnitus: a pilot study. Acta Otolaryngol. 2013;133(4):378–82.
68. Shim HJ, Kwak MY, An YH, Kim DH, Kim YJ, Kim HJ. Feasibility and safety of transcutaneous Vagus nerve stimulation paired with notched music therapy for the treatment of chronic tinnitus. J Audiol Otol. 2015;19(3):159–67.
69. Suk WC, Kim SJ, Chang DS, Lee HY. Characteristics of stimulus intensity in transcutaneousvagus nerve stimulation for chronic tinnitus. J Int Adv Otol. 2018;14(2):267–72.
70. Shore SE, Roberts LE, Langguth B. Maladaptive plasticity in tinnitus--triggers, mechanisms and treatment. Nat Rev Neurol. 2016;12(3):150–60.
71. Levine RA. Somatic (craniocervical) tinnitus and the dorsal cochlear nucleus hypothesis. Am J Otolaryngol. 1999;20(6):351–62.
72. Marks KL, Martel DT, Wu C, Basura GJ, Roberts LE, Schvartz-Leyzac KC, et al. Auditory-somatosensory bimodal stimulation

desynchronizes brain circuitry to reduce tinnitus in Guinea pigs and humans. Sci Transl Med. 2018;10(422):eaal3175.
73. Hamilton C, D'Arcy S, Pearlmutter BA, Crispino G, Lalor EC, Conlon BJ. An investigation of feasibility and safety of bi-modal stimulation for the treatment of tinnitus: An open-label pilot study. Neuromodulation. 2016;19(8):832–7.
74. Conlon B, Langguth B, Hamilton C, Hughes S, Meade E, Connor CO, et al. Bimodal neuromodulation combining sound and tongue stimulation reduces tinnitus symptoms in a large randomized clinical study. Sci Transl Med. 2020;12(564):eabb2830.
75. Barker AT, Jalinous R, Freeston IL. Non-invasive magnetic stimulation of human motor cortex. Lancet. 1985;1(8437):1106–7.
76. Barker AT, Shields K. Transcranial magnetic stimulation: basic principles and clinical applications in migraine. Headache. 2017;57(3):517–24.
77. Ridding MC, Rothwell JC. Is there a future for therapeutic use of transcranial magnetic stimulation? Nat Rev Neurosci. 2007;8(7):559–67.
78. Hallett M. Transcranial magnetic stimulation and the human brain. Nature. 2000;406(6792):147–50.
79. Lefaucheur JP. Transcranial magnetic stimulation. Handb Clin Neurol. 2019;160:559–80.
80. Post A, Keck ME. Transcranial magnetic stimulation as a therapeutic tool in psychiatry: what do we know about the neurobiological mechanisms? J Psychiatr Res. 2001;35(4):193–215.
81. Chen R, Classen J, Gerloff C, Celnik P, Wassermann EM, Hallett M, et al. Depression of motor cortex excitability by low-frequency transcranial magnetic stimulation. Neurology. 1997;48(5):1398–403.
82. Pascual-Leone A, Valls-Sole J, Wassermann EM, Hallett M. Responses to rapid-rate transcranial magnetic stimulation of the human motor cortex. Brain. 1994;117(Pt 4):847–58.
83. Wang H, Wang X, Scheich H. LTD and LTP induced by transcranial magnetic stimulation in auditory cortex. Neuroreport. 1996;7(2):521–5.
84. Burke MJ, Fried PJ, Pascual-Leone A. Transcranial magnetic stimulation: neurophysiological and clinical applications. Handb Clin Neurol. 2019;163:73–92.
85. Lefaucheur JP, Aleman A, Baeken C, Benninger DH, Brunelin J, Di Lazzaro V, et al. Evidence-based guidelines on the therapeutic use of repetitive transcranial magnetic stimulation (rTMS): An update (2014-2018). Clin Neurophysiol. 2020;131(2):474–528.
86. Dawes P, Newall J, Stockdale D, Baguley DM. Natural history of tinnitus in adults: a cross-sectional and longitudinal analysis. BMJ Open. 2020;10(12):e041290.
87. Langguth B, Kreuzer PM, Kleinjung T, De Ridder D. Tinnitus: causes and clinical management. Lancet Neurol. 2013;12(9):920–30.
88. Møller AR. Pathophysiology of tinnitus. In: Sismanis A, editor. Otolaryngologic clinics of North America. Amsterdam: W.B. Saunders; 2003. p. 249–66.
89. Møller AR. Tinnitus and pain. In: Langguth B, Hajak G, Kleinjung T, Cacace A, Møller AR, editors. Tinnitus: pathophysiology and treatment, progress in brain research. Amsterdam: Elsevier; 2007. p. 47–53.
90. Sedley W, Friston KJ, Gander PE, Kumar S, Griffiths TD. An integrative tinnitus model based on sensory precision. Trends Neurosci. 2016;39(12):799–812.
91. Vanneste S, Alsalman O, De Ridder D. Top-down and bottom-up regulated auditory phantom perception. J Neurosci. 2019;39(2):364–78.
92. Hoffman RE, Hawkins KA, Gueorguieva R, Boutros NN, Rachid F, Carroll K, et al. Transcranial magnetic stimulation of left temporoparietal cortex and medication-resistant auditory hallucinations. Arch Gen Psychiatry. 2003;60(1):49–56.
93. Marzouk T, Winkelbeiner S, Azizi H, Malhotra AK, Homan P. Transcranial magnetic stimulation for positive symptoms in schizophrenia: a systematic review. Neuropsychobiology. 2020;79(6):384–96.
94. Havrankova P, Jech R, Walker ND, Operto G, Tauchmanova J, Vymazal J, et al. Repetitive TMS of the somatosensory cortex improves writer's cramp and enhances cortical activity. Neuro Endocrinol Lett. 2010;31(1):73–86.
95. Siebner HR, Tormos JM, Ceballos-Baumann AO, Auer C, Catala MD, Conrad B, et al. Low-frequency repetitive transcranial magnetic stimulation of the motor cortex in writer's cramp. Neurology. 1999;52(3):529–37.
96. Mantovani A, Lisanby SH, Pieraccini F, Ulivelli M, Castrogiovanni P, Rossi S. Repetitive transcranial magnetic stimulation (rTMS) in the treatment of obsessive-compulsive disorder (OCD) and Tourette's syndrome (TS). Int J Neuropsychopharmacol. 2006;9(1):95–100.
97. Rapinesi C, Kotzalidis GD, Ferracuti S, Sani G, Girardi P, Del Casale A. Brain stimulation in obsessive-compulsive disorder (OCD): a systematic review. Curr Neuropharmacol. 2019;17(8):787–807.
98. De Ridder D, De Mulder G, Walsh V, Muggleton N, Sunaert S, Verlooy J, et al. Transcranial magnetic stimulation for tinnitus: a clinical and pathophysiological approach: influence of tinnitus duration on stimulation parameter choice and maximal tinnitus suppression. Otol Neurotol. 2005;147(5):495–501.
99. Plewnia C, Bartels M, Gerloff C. Transient suppression of tinnitus by transcranial magnetic stimulation. Ann Neurol. 2003;53(2):263–6.
100. De Ridder D, De Mulder G, Verstraeten E, Van der Kelen K, Sunaert S, Smits M, et al. Primary and secondary auditory cortex stimulation for intractable tinnitus. ORL J Otorhinolaryngol Relat Spec. 2006;68(1):48–54.
101. De Ridder D, De Mulder G, Walsh V, Muggleton N, Sunaert S, Møller A. Magnetic and electrical stimulation of the auditory cortex for intractable tinnitus. J Neurosurg. 2004;100(3):560–4.
102. Eichhammer P, Langguth B, Marienhagen J, Kleinjung T, Hajak G. Neuronavigated repetitive transcranial magnetic stimulation in patients with tinnitus: a short case series. Biol Psychiatry. 2003;54(8):862–5.
103. Folmer RL, Theodoroff SM, Casiana L, Shi Y, Griest S, Vachhani J. Repetitive transcranial magnetic stimulation treatment for chronic tinnitus: a randomized clinical trial. JAMA Otolaryngol Head Neck Surg. 2015;141(8):716–22.
104. Kleinjung T, Eichhammer P, Langguth B, Jacob P, Marienhagen J, Hajak G, et al. Long-term effects of repetitive transcranial magnetic stimulation (rTMS) in patients with chronic tinnitus. Otolaryngol Head Neck Surg. 2005;132(4):566–9.
105. Landgrebe M, Hajak G, Wolf S, Padberg F, Klupp P, Fallgatter AJ, et al. 1-Hz rTMS in the treatment of tinnitus: a sham-controlled, randomized multicenter trial. Brain Stimul. 2017;10(6):1112–20.
106. Khedr EM, Rothwell JC, Ahmed MA, El-Atar A. Effect of daily repetitive transcranial magnetic stimulation for treatment of tinnitus: comparison of different stimulus frequencies. J Neurol Neurosurg Psychiatry. 2008;79(2):212–5.
107. Vanneste S, De Ridder D. Differences between a single session and repeated sessions of 1 Hz TMS by double-cone coil prefrontal stimulation for the improvement of tinnitus. Brain Stimul. 2013;6(2):155–9.
108. Mennemeier M, Triggs W, Chelette K, Woods A, Kimbrell T, Dornhoffer J. Sham transcranial magnetic stimulation using electrical stimulation of the scalp. Brain Stimul. 2009;2(3):168–73.
109. Berlim MT, Broadbent HJ, Van den Eynde F. Blinding integrity in randomized sham-controlled trials of repetitive transcranial magnetic stimulation for major depression: a systematic review and meta-analysis. Int J Neuropsychopharmacol. 2013;16(5):1173–81.

110. Herwig U, Cardenas-Morales L, Connemann BJ, Kammer T, Schonfeldt-Lecuona C. Sham or real--post hoc estimation of stimulation condition in a randomized transcranial magnetic stimulation trial. Neurosci Lett. 2010;471(1):30–3.
111. Lefebvre-Demers M, Doyon N, Fecteau S. Non-invasive neuromodulation for tinnitus: a meta-analysis and modeling studies. Brain Stimul. 2021;14(1):113–28.
112. Liang Z, Yang H, Cheng G, Huang L, Zhang T, Jia H. Repetitive transcranial magnetic stimulation on chronic tinnitus: a systematic review and meta-analysis. BMC Psychiatry. 2020;20(1):547.
113. Dong C, Chen C, Wang T, Gao C, Wang Y, Guan X, et al. Low-frequency repetitive transcranial magnetic stimulation for the treatment of chronic tinnitus: a systematic review and meta-analysis of randomized controlled trials. Biomed Res Int. 2020;2020:3141278.
114. Cima RFF, Mazurek B, Haider H, Kikidis D, Lapira A, Norena A, et al. A multidisciplinary European guideline for tinnitus: diagnostics, assessment, and treatment. HNO. 2019;67(Suppl 1):10–42.
115. Ogawa K, Sato H, Takahashi M, Wada T, Naito Y, Kawase T, et al. Clinical practice guidelines for diagnosis and treatment of chronic tinnitus in Japan. Auris Nasus Larynx. 2020;47(1):1–6.
116. Tunkel DE, Bauer CA, Sun GH, Rosenfeld RM, Chandrasekhar SS, Cunningham ER Jr, et al. Clinical practice guideline: tinnitus. Otolaryngol Head Neck Surg. 2014;151(2 Suppl):S1–S40.
117. Langguth B. Non-invasive neuromodulation for tinnitus. J Audiol Otol. 2020;24(3):113–8.
118. Schoisswohl S, Agrawal K, Simoes J, Neff P, Schlee W, Langguth B, et al. RTMS parameters in tinnitus trials: a systematic review. Sci Rep. 2019;9(1):12190.
119. Kleinjung T, Eichhammer P, Landgrebe M, Sand P, Hajak G, Steffens T, et al. Combined temporal and prefrontal transcranial magnetic stimulation for tinnitus treatment: a pilot study. Otolaryngol Head Neck Surg. 2008;138(4):497–501.
120. Langguth B, Landgrebe M, Frank E, Schecklmann M, Sand PG, Vielsmeier V, et al. Efficacy of different protocols of transcranial magnetic stimulation for the treatment of tinnitus: pooled analysis of two randomized controlled studies. World J Biol Psychiatry. 2014;15(4):276–85.
121. Lehner A, Schecklmann M, Greenlee MW, Rupprecht R, Langguth B. Triple-site rTMS for the treatment of chronic tinnitus: a randomized controlled trial. Sci Rep. 2016;6:22302.
122. Langguth B, Kleinjung T, Frank E, Landgrebe M, Sand P, Dvorakova J, et al. High-frequency priming stimulation does not enhance the effect of low-frequency rTMS in the treatment of tinnitus. Exp Brain Res. 2008;184(4):587–91.
123. Schwippel T, Schroeder PA, Fallgatter AJ, Plewnia C. Clinical review: the therapeutic use of theta-burst stimulation in mental disorders and tinnitus. Prog Neuro-Psychopharmacol Biol Psychiatry. 2019;92:285–300.
124. Kleinjung T, Steffens T, Landgrebe M, Vielsmeier V, Frank E, Burger J, et al. Repetitive transcranial magnetic stimulation for tinnitus treatment: no enhancement by the dopamine and noradrenaline reuptake inhibitor bupropion. Brain Stimul. 2011;4(2):65–70.
125. Kleinjung T, Steffens T, Landgrebe M, Vielsmeier V, Frank E, Hajak G, et al. Levodopa does not enhance the effect of low-frequency repetitive transcranial magnetic stimulation in tinnitus treatment. Otolaryngol Head Neck Surg. 2009;140(1):92–5.
126. Kreuzer PM, Poeppl TB, Rupprecht R, Vielsmeier V, Lehner A, Langguth B, et al. Individualized repetitive transcranial magnetic stimulation treatment in chronic tinnitus? Front Neurol. 2017;8:126.
127. Schoisswohl S, Langguth B, Hebel T, Abdelnaim MA, Volberg G, Schecklmann M. Heading for personalized rTMS in tinnitus: reliability of individualized stimulation protocols in behavioral and electrophysiological responses. J Pers Med. 2021;11(6):536.
128. Carter G, Govindan RB, Brown G, Heimann C, Hayes H, Thostenson JC, et al. Change in EEG activity is associated with a decrease in tinnitus awareness after rTMS. Front Neurol Neurosci Res. 2021;2:100010.
129. James GA, Thostenson JD, Brown G, Carter G, Hayes H, Tripathi SP, et al. Neural activity during attentional conflict predicts reduction in tinnitus perception following rTMS. Brain Stimul. 2017;10(5):934–43.
130. Lehner A, Langguth B, Poeppl TB, Rupprecht R, Hajak G, Landgrebe M, et al. Structural brain changes following left temporal low-frequency rTMS in patients with subjective tinnitus. Neural Plast. 2014;2014:132058.
131. Mennemeier M, Chelette KC, Allen S, Bartel TB, Triggs W, Kimbrell T, et al. Variable changes in PET activity before and after rTMS treatment for tinnitus. Laryngoscope. 2011;121(4):815–22.

Invasive Brain Stimulation

53

Dirk De Ridder and Sven Vanneste

Abstract

There exist no FDA- or CE-approved pharmacological treatments for tinnitus. Based on network science, tinnitus is proposed to be an emergent property of dynamically changing interacting networks. It is related to a balance between three cardinal networks: the lateral "loudness" pathway, the medial "suffering" pathway, and the noise canceling pathway. Invasive and non-invasive neuromodulation are an option for tinnitus management. Invasive neuromodulation consists of implanting electrodes in or on the brain or nerves. Implants have been performed in all three cardinal pathways: auditory cortex (lateral pathway), dorsal anterior cingulate cortex and caudate (medial pathway), dorsolateral prefrontal cortex, parahippocampal area (noise canceling pathway), as well as in the thalamus and subthalamus. Despite the theoretical science network suggestions, no multitarget implants have been performed. Vagus nerve stimulation, with or without paired sound stimulation, has also been performed with some success. However, invasive neuromodulation requires further research before it can become a routine part of tinnitus management.

D. De Ridder (✉)
Section of Neurosurgery, Department of Surgical Sciences, University of Otago, Dunedin, New Zealand
e-mail: dirk.deridder@otago.ac.nz; http://www.brai3n.com

S. Vanneste
School of Psychology, Global Brain Health Institute and Trinity College of Dublin Institute for Neuroscience, Dublin, Ireland
e-mail: sven.vanneste@tcd.ie

W. Schlee et al. (eds.), *Textbook of Tinnitus*, https://doi.org/10.1007/978-3-031-35647-6_53

Graphical Abstract

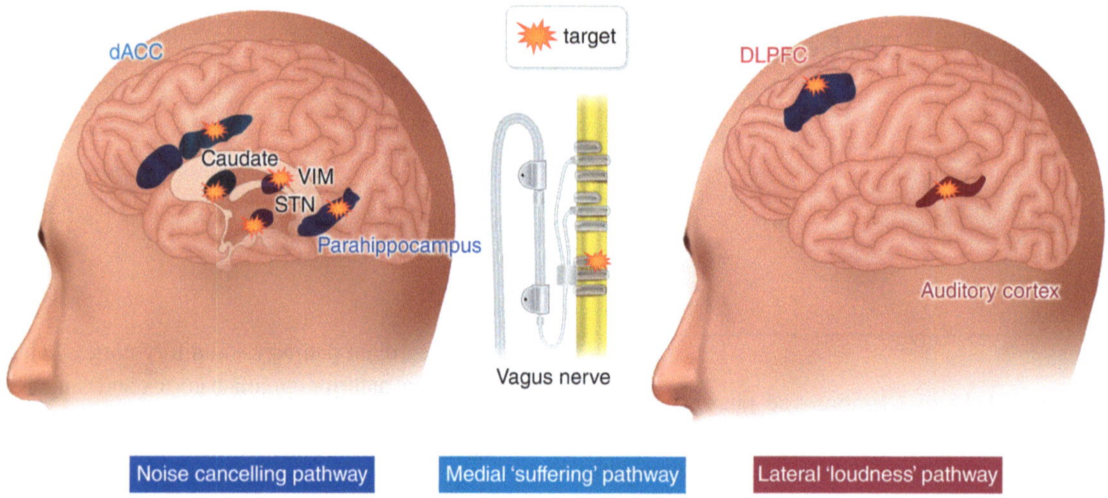

Highlights

- There exist no FDA- or CE-approved pharmacological treatments for tinnitus.
- Based on network science, tinnitus is proposed to be an emergent property of dynamically changing interacting networks.
- Tinnitus is related to an imbalance between three cardinal networks: the lateral "loudness" pathway, the medial "suffering" pathway, and the noise canceling pathway.
- Noninvasive and invasive neuromodulation are options for tinnitus management.
- Invasive neuromodulation consists of implanting electrodes in or on the brain or nerves.
- Implants have been performed in all three cardinal pathways: auditory cortex (lateral pathway), dorsal anterior cingulate cortex and caudate (medial pathway), dorsolateral prefrontal cortex, parahippocampal area (noise canceling pathway), as well as in the thalamus and subthalamus.
- No multitarget network implants have been performed.
- Vagus nerve stimulation, with or without paired sound stimulation, has also been performed with some success.
- Invasive neuromodulation requires further research before it can become a routine part of tinnitus management.

Introduction

Tinnitus is defined as the conscious awareness of a non-complex sound for which there is no identifiable corresponding external sound source [1], and can thus be regarded as a phantom sound [2]. Tinnitus occurs in about 15% of the population in the western world [3, 4], Asia [5–8], and Africa [9, 10]. Whereas most patients (80%) can learn to live with the phantom sound, quality of life is decreased in about 20% of the patients who cannot cope with the tinnitus [3, 11]. In these patients, tinnitus is frequently associated with suffering, which can be expressed as anxiety and depression, but also cognitive impairment, and sleep disturbances [12–14]. When tinnitus is associated with suffering, it is defined as tinnitus disorder [1].

Although many tinnitus treatments exist, both pharmacological and nonpharmacological, some of which are commercially available, evidence for a successful therapy that benefits everybody with tinnitus is lacking [15, 16], and thus almost all tinnitus treatments are off-label therapies. The lack of efficacious treatments for tinnitus likely originates from the heterogeneity of tinnitus and an incomplete understanding of the pathophysiology of the different forms of tinnitus [17].

Since 2011, the interest of big pharma for developing medications for psychiatric or neurological disorders has dramatically declined. Investments have decreased by 50% for brain-related disorders [18]. In contrast to heart medication, the chance of medication for brain disorders to reach the market is 50% smaller (6.2% vs 13.3%) [19]. Furthermore, it takes 30% longer to develop (19.3 vs 14.7 months) [19], and costs 30% more [19]. The main problem is that 80% of neuropharmacological products fail phase III trials [20], predominantly because they do not outperform placebo (46%) [20]. Thus, notwithstanding repurposing of existing medication [21], the likelihood of a pharmaceutical solution for tinnitus and tinnitus disorder is therefore limited [22]. Therefore, other treatment approaches are highly needed, one of which is brain stimulation, both non-invasive and invasive. In order to develop novel brain stimulation therapies, a better understanding of the brain mechanisms involved in the generation of tinnitus is mandatory. The evolution of the understanding of the pathophysiology of tinnitus goes hand in hand with the development of brain stimulation approaches and may benefit the rational development of novel technology for brain stimulation for tinnitus.

Advancing Insights in the Pathophysiology of Tinnitus

Since the Egyptian era, tinnitus has been considered a problem of the ear. This paradigm was changed in the 1990s when Jastreboff considered tinnitus to be triggered in the ear but related to maladaptive conditioning in the brain [2].

In 1999, Rodolfo Llinas published the first paper that specifically proposed a pathophysiological model implying the interaction between the auditory cortex and thalamus as the generator of tinnitus, called thalamocortical dysrhythmia [23]. Thalamocortical dysrhythmia is a pathophysiological model underlying multiple brain disorders such as tinnitus, depression, slow wave epilepsy, pain, and Parkinson's disease [23]. Intriguingly, based on Hippocrates, Celsus explained tinnitus as the result of a disbalance of the four humors, in the constellation of melancholia, too much black bile (=depression) and linked it to epilepsy [24], linking three of the thalamocortical dysrhythmias. Thalamocortical dysrhythmia is a deafferentation-based model and centers the treatment target on the auditory cortex. However, early research of TMS [24–27] and implants [24, 28–31] quickly revealed that not every person presenting with tinnitus could benefit from auditory cortex stimulation. Different explanations including the duration of the tinnitus [32, 33], the gender of the tinnitus patients [34], the amount of hearing loss [32], the tinnitus pitch [34], the perceived laterality, left or right side, of the tinnitus [34], laterality of the tinnitus generator in the brain [25, 35], and also TMS-related aspects such as the delivered dose [36] were investigated to explain the nonfulfillment of auditory cortex stimulation as a hypothesized universal approach to quiet tinnitus. Thus, a novel pathophysiological model was developed, in which the tinnitus percept was not phrenologically limited to the auditory cortex but considered the result of an emergent property of a tinnitus generating network [37, 38]. Translating theoretical concepts from network science [39] to brain stimulation, it was hypothesized that using more than one target could disrupt the tinnitus network more effectively than one single target. As the frontal cortex was already a somewhat successful target for transcranial direct current stimulation (tDCS) [40–45] and TMS [46–48], the first non-surgical multisite stimulations targeted the frontal and auditory cortex [49]. Later surgical attempts combined the auditory cortex and high cervical C2 area [50], using the same philosophy. Almost simultaneously to the network model, an alternative model was developed, in which tinnitus was the result of a deficient noise canceling mechanism [51, 52], analogous to pain [53, 54]. According to this model, the subgenual anterior cingulate cortex was the main hub in tinnitus generation, a difficult neuroanatomical target to reach with current brain stimulation technologies. Furthermore, other groups failed to replicate the imaging data on which the model was based. Other studies, using EEG rather than structural and functional MRI, suggested the main target for activating the deficient noise canceling mechanism was the pregenual to rostral anterior cingulate cortex, which is amenable to neurostimulation [55]. Indeed, bifrontal stimulation appears to activate the pregenual anterior cingulate cortex, as evidenced by EEG [44]. But this has not yet led to implants of the pregenual to rostral anterior cingulate cortex.

A further model was proposed that tinnitus could be the result of a Bayesian prediction error [56, 57]. According to this model, tinnitus can be understood as the result of a mismatch between the predicted sound percept and the actual neural input from the ear, which is reduced because of hearing loss. This has led to the description of the pathways in the brain associated with the tinnitus generating networks and the tinnitus inhibiting network (=noise canceling network) [58]. Potentially, combining activation of the noise canceling system and inhibiting the tinnitus generating network could be beneficial as a novel brain stimulation approach. These further elaborations of network stimulation approaches need to be seen in the larger concept of the brain as a complex adaptive system, and tinnitus as an emergent property of dynamically changing interacting brain networks (see Fig. 53.1).

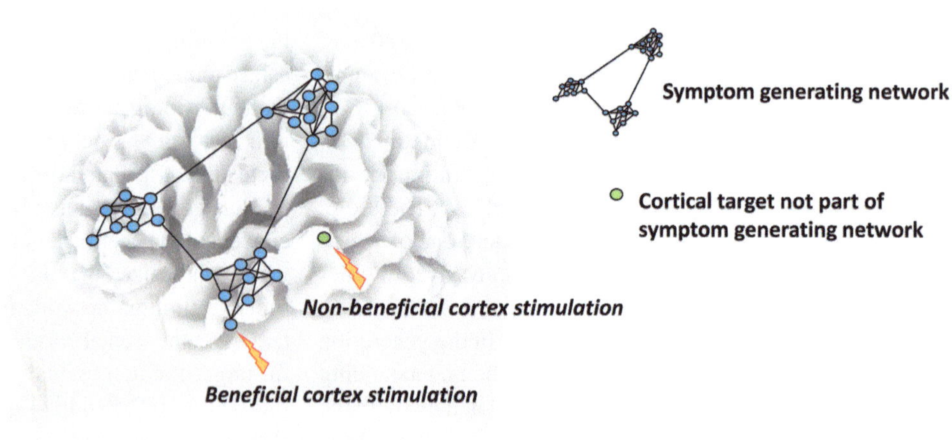

Fig. 53.1 Tinnitus is proposed to be an emergent property of a large tinnitus brain network, composed of different subnetworks, each characterizing a different aspect of the tinnitus percept. Neuromodulation has to reach the network directly or indirectly

A Theory of Symptom Generation in the Brain

The brain can be seen as a complex adaptive system [55, 59, 60], similar to the Internet, cities, the economy, the climate, social interactions, or an ant society [61]. In order to qualify as a complex adaptive system, a system has to fulfill two criteria [62]: (1) its structure is characterized by a small world topology and (2) the system has to embed noise [62]. These two criteria permit the system to be adaptive. Networks can be topologically organized in three ways [63]. At one extreme, the network can be topologically structured as a lattice (=regular) network [64]. In a lattice network, every stimulus will always result in exactly the same processing, which may be stable and efficient, but is not adaptive [65]. At the other extreme, a system can have a random topology, which is flexible, yet inefficient as every stimulus will evoke a random response. Therefore, an intermediate topology between lattice and random, called a small world (complex) topology, permits to incorporate the stability of a lattice and the flexibility of a random topology. Thus, small worlds permit flexible stability, i.e. adaptiveness to changing environments through variability. If combined with memory, such a small world topology can learn [66, 67]. The brain has a small world structure and thus fulfills the first criterion [66, 68–70]. The brain also embeds noise, both structurally and functionally [71, 72]. Thus, it fulfills the second criterion. The noise is structured, generally following a power law distribution [71]. Based on EEG [73–79] and fMRI [80], the underlying structure of the brain-derived activity is pink (1/f), yet in direct recordings from the brain's noise appears to be brown ($1/f^2$) [81]. This structured noise has an advantage that it has memory and can carry information, in contrast to white noise which is an unstructured completely random noise (=chaos) [82]. In summary, a small world system can learn, is flexible, while still maintaining stability. Implanting electrodes in an adaptive system such as the brain makes intuitive sense to change its network structure and thus its function. In a lattice or random topological system, stimulation would make little or no sense. Stimulating a random system would result in a different response for every stimulus; stimulation in a lattice system would result in always the same response, in other words very predictable, and not adaptive. The most essential characteristic of a complex adaptive system is emergence: the whole is more than the sum of its components and cannot be predicted from its constituent parts [22, 83]. The whole, i.e., the network, has new emerging properties that depend critically on the very specific connectivity between the parts. A collection of car parts is not a car. Only when all the constituent parts of a car are put together (i.e., connected) in a very specific way does a functional driving car emerge. But the analogy is limited: a car is complex but non-adaptive. A car does not reorganize itself, adapting to a changing environment, in contrast to a brain. This adaptive reorganization of the nervous system to a changing environment is called neuroplasticity. Emergentism in philosophy of mind explains consciousness as an emergent property of brain networks, and by extension, every thought, feeling, action is the consequence of specific connectivity patterns resulting from adaptive neuroplasticity. In keeping with this concept, every symptom or disease can be considered the emergent property of maladaptive plasticity resulting in pathology-related networks [84]. Implanting electrodes in the tinnitus generating network should change or use the brain's connectivity in order to create a change in the network configuration, reducing the tinnitus [22, 83].

From a clinical perspective, neuroplasticity can be visualized using structural and functional brain imaging as changes in structure, activity, and especially connectivity. Connectivity can be studied in different ways using structural, functional, and effective connectivity [66, 85]. Structural connectivity reflects anatomical connections in the brain [86], functional connectivity refers to co-activation patterns of different brain areas [87], and effective connectivity can be seen as directional functional connectivity, i.e., from which area in the brain to which other area does the information flow [87].

Neuromodulation as Targeted Neuroplasticity

Neuromodulation and neurostimulation or brain stimulation is being used interchangeably. Yet, neuromodulation is becoming the preferred term because it does not carry the connotation of activation, which seems to be inherently implied with neurostimulation [22]. Neuromodulation is more neutral, and basically states that the electrical stimulation influences brain activity and connectivity, without suggesting the influence is excitatory. If electrical stimulation is applied to a brain area with predominantly GABA receptors, the clinical effect can be inhibitory.

Neuromodulation can be operationally defined as the induction of neuroplastic changes via targeted application of electrical, magnetic, sound (including ultrasound), optical, or pharmacological stimuli [22].

Neuromodulation can be performed at any part of the nervous system or innervated organ with different stimulation devices [88]. This includes the peripheral nerve field, peripheral or autonomic nerves, the dorsal root ganglion (DRG), the spinal cord, the brainstem, or the brain. In brain stimulation, cortex stimulation is differentiated from deep brain stimulation, but the terminology is not always uniform [83]. For example, wire electrodes have been implanted in the anterior cingulate gyrus and this procedure was called deep brain stimulation (DBS) of the anterior cingulate [89], whereas paddle electrodes have been implanted onto the same target [90–92] and this qualifies as cortex stimulation. In the same vain, deep brain stimulation of the subgenual anterior cingulate cortex (Brodmann area 25) has been performed for major depressive disorder. In essence, deep brain stimulation is intracortical stimulation (with wire electrodes) of the subgenual anterior cingulate cortex, in which the electrodes are inserted inside the cortex, or more likely the underlying white matter tracts, rather than onto the cortex [93]. The same terminological confusion exists for tinnitus. Whereas in most studies the electrodes are implanted extradurally overlying the secondary auditory cortex or intradurally overlying the primary auditory cortex [24, 28–31, 94–97], in some patients, wire electrodes have been implanted inside the auditory cortex [98]. We define any form of stimulation that targets the cortex, whether intracortical or onto the cortex, as cortex stimulation, and define deep brain stimulation as brain stimulation that targets deep nuclei rather than cortical structures [22].

Mechanism of Action of Cortex Stimulation

Based on network science and within a monist emergentist framework, symptoms are considered emergent properties resulting from maladaptive network activity and connectivity, and not the result of phrenological hyper- or hypoactivity of one brain area [84, 99, 100]. When sound is presented to patients in vegetative state, who have no conscious awareness, their auditory cortex is functionally and metabolically activated, yet there is no conscious perception of the presented sound [101]. This suggests that activity restricted to the auditory cortex is insufficient for auditory conscious awareness. This is in keeping with the concept that visual cortex activation is insufficient for visual consciousness [102, 103]. Only if the activated auditory cortex is functionally connected to a consciousness enabling network do auditory stimuli reach consciousness, analogous to what has been shown for pain stimuli [104–106]. This is the basis of the global workspace model for consciousness [107, 108]. These consciousness enabling networks comprise the self-representational default mode network and the attentional frontoparietal network [109], also involved in goal oriented behavior [110, 111]. Based on this concept, it is expected that the auditory cortex must be functionally connected to the default mode network [112] and frontoparietal attention network to permit conscious awareness of an auditory stimulus [22]. If the auditory stimulus is generated in auditory memory, as suggested for tinnitus, then the parahippocampus has to be linked to the auditory cortex and default mode [112].

Functional connections between the target of stimulation and a wider network associated with the emergent property, i.e. tinnitus, are critical for the stimulation to be beneficial [91, 113, 114]. The presence of functional connectivity between the auditory cortex and the parahippocampus is critical for obtaining a beneficial result following auditory cortex stimulation via implanted electrodes [114]. The same holds for anterior cingulate implants for tinnitus [91]. When the implanted electrode contacts a network of hyperconnectivity, presumed to be part of the tinnitus network, the outcome is beneficial, when the electrode contacts an area of decreased functional connectivity, the stimulation is not beneficial [91]. The same concept has been proposed for non-invasive brain stimulation in multiple neurological and psychiatric disorders [113]. A lack of functional connectivity identified sites where stimulation was ineffective. These results suggest that the presence of resting-state functional connectivity to the stimulation target may be essential, both for optimizing treatment and identifying new stimulation targets [113].

In summary, if the target is part of a symptom generating network, the stimulation might be beneficial, whereas stimulation of a target that is not functionally connected to the symptom generating network might not be beneficial [83].

Brain Stimulation Techniques in the Treatment of Tinnitus

Brain stimulation can be performed in two ways, non-invasively and invasively, in other words with or without surgery involved. Non-invasive brain stimulation encompasses transcranial magnetic stimulation [115, 116] and transcranial electrical stimulation [117–119] and is detailed in another chapter of this book.

Invasive Auditory Cortex Stimulation

Auditory cortex stimulation via implanted electrodes [24] was developed 5 years before the network concept was proposed [37, 38], based on a phrenological pathophysiological model according to which the auditory cortex was the final common pathway in the generation of tinnitus. It was proposed that auditory cortex stimulation can alleviate tinnitus using a four-step rationale [120]:

1. Tinnitus is related to increased activity in the auditory cortex.
2. The anatomical location of the tinnitus generator in the auditory cortex can be determined by frequency-specific fMRI activation [94] (Fig. 53.2).
3. The abnormal neuronal activity of the auditory cortex can be modulated by neuronavigated TMS resulting in transient tinnitus reduction [24] (Fig. 53.3).
4. If TMS can transiently improve the tinnitus, electrical stimulation through an electrode implanted on the same area can provide permanent tinnitus suppression [24, 28, 30, 121] (Fig. 53.4).

Three different techniques have been developed: extradural auditory cortex stimulation (Fig. 53.4), intradural auditory cortex stimulation (Fig. 53.5), and intradural intracortical auditory cortex stimulation (Fig. 53.6).

A first case report detailing this approach was published [24] at the same time as the first case series of TMS for tinnitus [27]. Since then, no large randomized controlled trials have been performed, but multiple small and one larger case series of patients with auditory cortex electrodes have been published. One placebo-controlled study showed significant improvements in the Beck Depression Inventory and tinnitus questionnaires, although objective measures of tinnitus loudness remained fairly stable [96].

The largest study to date consists of 43 patients with severe or decompensated intractable tinnitus (grade 3 and 4 tinnitus based on the tinnitus questionnaire [122]) were implanted with an electrode overlying the secondary auditory cortex following transient tinnitus improvement with TMS [121]. Surgical eligibility was based on two positive TMS sessions with >20% tinnitus loudness reduction. Although all implanted patients responded to TMS, only one in three patients subsequently responded to the implant when tonic stimulation was applied [121]. There was a significant correlation between the loudness reduction during TMS and implantation, even though TMS could not predict who would and who would not respond to the implant [121]. This may be explained by a different mechanism of action of TMS and implanted electrodes [121].

In order to increase treatment success, burst stimulation was developed, based on the existence of burst TMS [34, 123–125], translated in an implantable version [95]. When switching from tonic stimulation to burst stimulation [95], half of the non-responding patients could be rescued, improv-

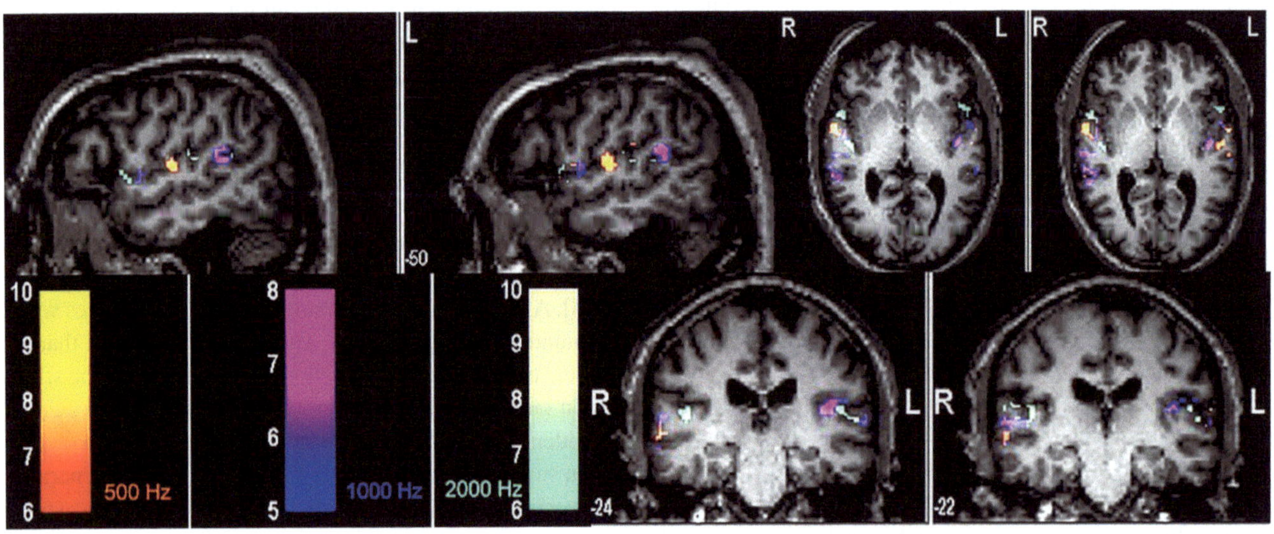

Fig. 53.2 The auditory cortex has a mirror tonotopic structure which can be visualized by fMRI

ing the total response rate from one in three to two in three patients. Burst stimulation was superior to tonic stimulation for suppressing noise-like tinnitus [121], analogous to what had been shown for burst TMS [34, 123]. In contrast to TMS, where the amount of improvement worsens with longer tinnitus duration, no such correlation was identified for electrical cortical stimulation in the same study population. This supported the concept that electrical cortical stimulation acts on tinnitus by a different mechanism than TMS.

The beneficial outcome also depended on the characteristics of the tinnitus. Pure tone tinnitus could be reduced more than narrow band noise or the combination of pure tone and narrow band noise, and unilateral tinnitus responded better than bilateral tinnitus [121].

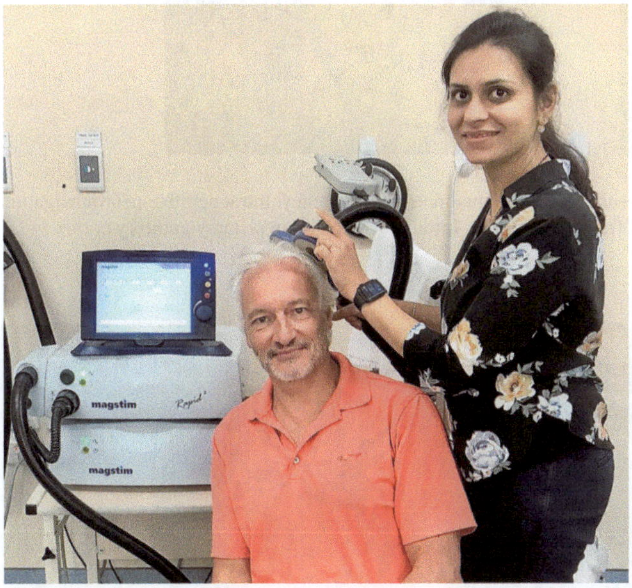

Fig. 53.3 Transcranial magnetic stimulation can transiently modulate the tinnitus network

Auditory cortex implants have been performed in a couple of neurosurgical centers. A French case report obtained 65% tinnitus loudness reduction in a woman using an fMRI-based extradural auditory cortex implant [97, 126]. This improvement persisted long term [97, 126]. A USA-based study of eight patients using a similar technique but different hardware found no persisting tinnitus loudness suppression [96]. Transient disappearance of tinnitus was observed in six of eight patients. However, tinnitus distress and depression scores decreased slowly over time, even without suppression of tinnitus intensity. An electrode with only two contacts was used, which limits the way the electrodes can be programmed. This habituation of the auditory cortex to electrical stimulation seems to be a feature that is noted in most patients, and can be overcome by recurrent programming, multitarget stimulation, and the development of novel noisy stimulation designs [121, 127].

In four patients, an intradural electrode was inserted in the Sylvian fissure, stimulating gray matter of the primary auditory cortex [24, 30]. In two of those patients, the purpose was to prevent habituation, as reprogramming was required every 2–3 days in order to maintain a beneficial effect. In both patients, the intradural positioning resulted in a stabilized improvement of their tinnitus.

Another approach has been proposed, inserting a wire electrode in the white matter beneath layer 6 of the primary auditory cortex, using magnetic source imaging for target localization. This has been performed successfully, resulting in tinnitus improvement [98]. Intriguingly, intracortical stimulation does not generate a sound percept associated with the delivered current in patients with tinnitus, in contrast to patients with epilepsy, in whom intracortical electrical stim-

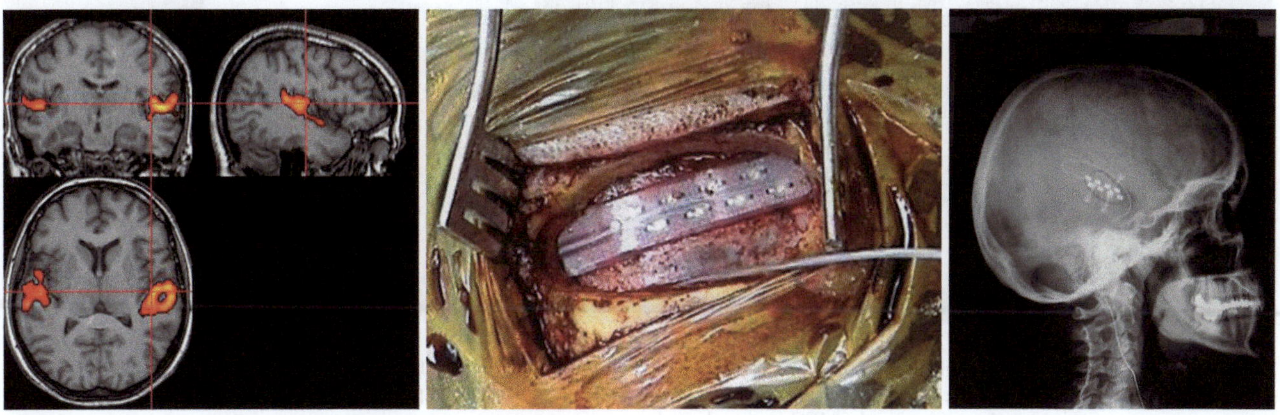

Fig. 53.4 Extradural auditory cortex implant. A fMRI is performed by presenting the tinnitus-matched frequency. Intraoperative picture of extradural paddle lead with eight electrodes, which is positioned using intraoperative neuronavigation. Postoperative X-ray demonstrating the implanted paddle lead

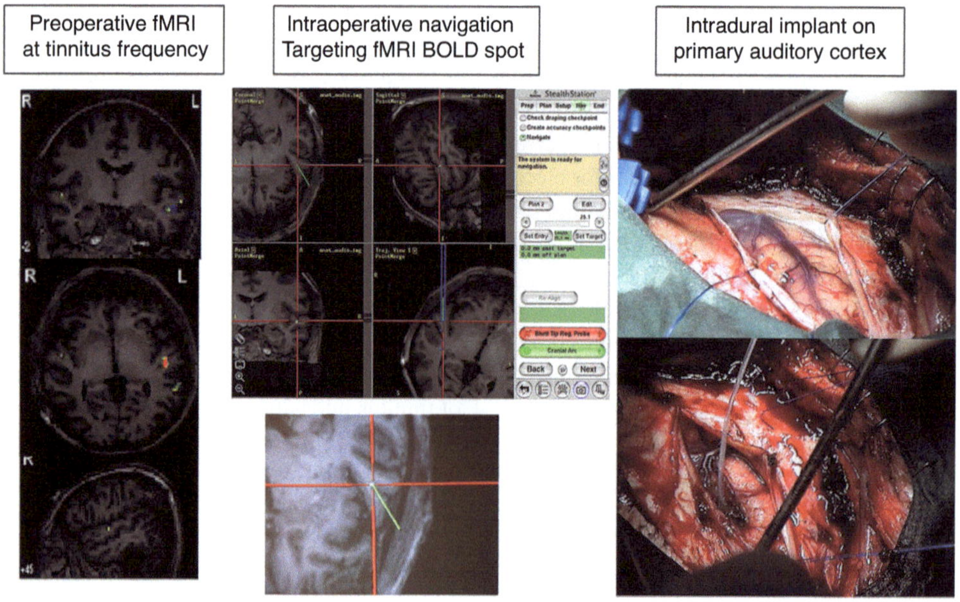

Fig. 53.5 Intradural auditory cortex implant. A fMRI is performed by presenting the tinnitus-matched frequency. Intraoperative neuronavigation demonstrating the BOLD spot, elicited by presenting the tinnitus-matched frequency (pitch). Intradural implant on primary auditory cortex

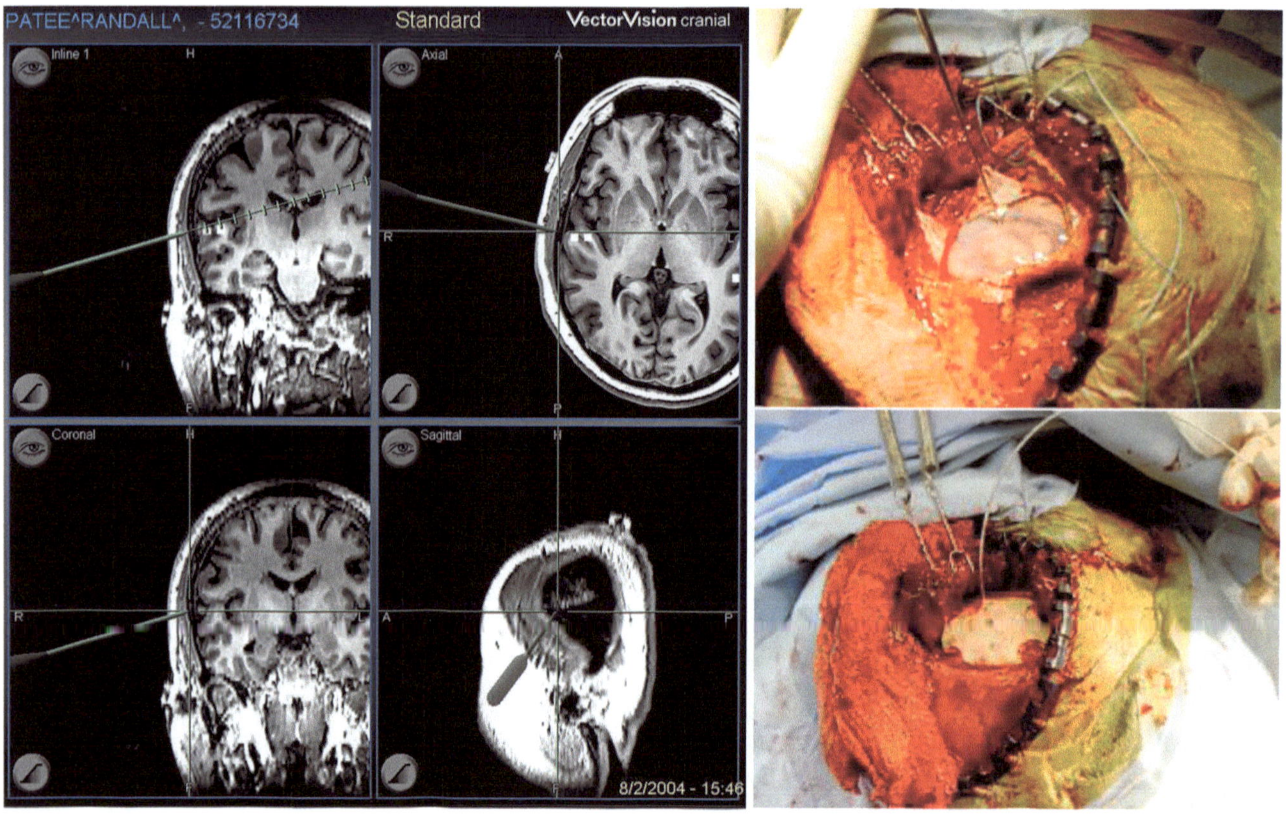

Fig. 53.6 Intradural intracortical implant. A magnetoencephalography is performed by presenting the tinnitus-matched frequency. Intraoperative neuronavigation demonstrating the MEG target, elicited by presenting the tinnitus-matched frequency (pitch). Intradural intracortical implant inside primary auditory cortex

ulation within Heschl's gyrus does generate sound perception, the loudness of which correlates with the delivered amplitude [128].

The success of the auditory cortex implants depends on its capacity to modulate activity in the parahippocampal area, known for its involvement in auditory memory [129]. Responders to the auditory cortex implant are characterized by high beta3 and gamma band activity in the parahippocampal area, even though the electrodes stimulate the auditory cortex. Only those patients who have functional connections between the area of the implant, i.e. the auditory cortex and the hyperactive parahippocampal area seem to benefit from the auditory cortex implant [114].

In agreement with the principles of network science [39], multisite stimulation may benefit tinnitus perception, analogous to what is noted in non-invasive neuromodulation [49, 130, 131]. In a patient who suffered from both pure tone and noise-like tinnitus, auditory cortex implantation resulted in a complete resolution of the pure tone component, without any beneficial effect on the noise-like component of the tinnitus, even after switching to burst stimulation [50]. After a successful trial with transcutaneous electrical nerve stimulation, capable of improving his noise-like tinnitus, a wire electrode was inserted subcutaneously in the C2 area for nerve field stimulation of the greater occipital nerve. With dual target stimulation, the pure tone tinnitus remains abolished after 5 years of stimulation and the noise-like tinnitus is reduced by 50%, from 8/10 to 4/10. This case report suggests that multisite stimulation might be better than single target implantation [50].

In some case reports, implants were also performed on other targets of the larger tinnitus generating network. Implants have been performed targeting the dorsolateral prefrontal cortex [47], anterior cingulate cortex [91], and parahippocampal area [120] following the same four-step approach. In the two rostral to dorsal anterior cingulate implants, one patient improved whereas another patient did not benefit from the implant. The responder was characterized by increased functional connectivity to a tinnitus distress network in contrast to the non-responder, who had decreased functional connectivity in comparison to healthy controls [91]. This suggests that analogous to non-invasive stimulation, brain stimulation via implanted electrodes requires functional connectivity to carry the delivered current throughout the symptom generating network [113].

Deep Brain Stimulation

Deep brain stimulation (DBS) has been performed as well targeting deeper brain structures involved in the tinnitus generating network. This was based on a serendipitous case report of a woman who became tinnitus-free following a stroke in the locus coerulous (LC) area of the caudate nucleus, while undergoing DBS for Parkinson's disease [132].

In a first study, tinnitus loudness reductions were found in three of seven patients when the DBS electrode was turned on, of which most clearly by ventral intermediate nucleus (VIM) stimulation, a typical target for tremor [133].

Based on the stroke of silence case report, tinnitus was prospectively evaluated in patients in whom DBS was performed to alleviate movement disorders, specifically evaluating the effect of caudate LC stimulation. In an observational study in six patients with comorbid tinnitus, in five participants where the DBS lead tip traversed area LC, tinnitus loudness in both ears was suppressed to a nadir of level 2 or lower on a 0–10 rating scale. In one subject where the DBS lead was outside area LC, tinnitus was not modulated [134, 135].

A large multicenter study evaluated the clinical impact of DBS on tinnitus in patients undergoing DBS for movement disorders [136]. The THI tinnitus questionnaire improved only after subthalamic nucleus stimulation, suggesting this target may be selected to treat tinnitus-related distress.

After encouraging results from these observational studies, a phase I study was performed targeting the caudate nucleus with a goal to treat severe intractable tinnitus. In this follow-up phase 1 trial, six patients were implanted in the caudate LC specifically for tinnitus suppression [137]. Based on minimal improvements required for clinical relevance, there were three responders determined by TFI ($\geq$ 13-point decrease) and four by THI ($\geq$20-point decrease) scores. One patient had a profound loudness suppression (7.8 points improvement on NRS). One patient was excluded due to suicidality, unrelated (stimulator off) to caudate stimulation. In the same patients, a study was performed to identify the caudate nucleus subdivisions that could be linked to tinnitus [138]. Acute tinnitus loudness reduction was observed at five caudate locations, four positioned at the body, and one at the head of the caudate nucleus in normalized Montreal Neurological Institute space. The remaining 15 electrical stimulation interrogations of the caudate head failed to reduce tinnitus loudness [138]. Compared to the caudate head, the body subdivision, which suppresses tinnitus better, has stronger functional connectivity to the auditory cortex on fMRI [138].

Vagus Nerve Stimulation (VNS)

Invasive vagus nerve stimulation has been performed for the treatment of tinnitus. Even though this is sensu stricto no brain stimulation the intriguing results warrant mentioning in this chapter.

The combination of vagal stimulation via implanted electrodes paired with simultaneous auditory stimuli has yielded highly impressive results in an animal model of tinnitus [139]. Based on the rationale that vagal stimulation renders the simultaneously presented sounds more salient, sounds were presented that exclude the tinnitus-matched frequencies. The sound-paired vagus stimulation almost completely reversed neurophysiological and behavioral signs of tinnitus, which was not the case with auditory stimulation alone [139]. In subsequent translational studies in humans, the efficacy of the invasive VNS paired to auditory stimuli was partially confirmed [140–142], albeit the clinical effects were clearly less pronounced than in animals. The relevance and necessity of pairing auditory stimuli to vagus nerve stimulation is yet unclear. A study in which vagus nerve stimulation was performed via implanted electrodes to treat epilepsy found equally good tinnitus attenuating results, without pairing the vagus stimulation to sounds [143].

Conclusion

In the last decades, neuroscientific research has contributed to an increasingly better understanding of the tinnitus generating network. The application of principles of network science has permitted to shift from a phrenological auditory cortex-centered approach to a network-based approach [22]. Cortex and deep brain stimulation with implanted electrodes have shown benefit, but the unsatisfactory results and insufficient data do not support their application for routine clinical use. Even though the theoretical framework of network stimulation is promising, invasive brain stimulation has not capitalized on it yet by performing multisite implants essential to disrupt the tinnitus generating network more effectively.

References

1. De Ridder D, et al. Tinnitus and tinnitus disorder: theoretical and operational definitions (an international multidisciplinary proposal). Prog Brain Res. 2021;260:1–25.
2. Jastreboff PJ. Phantom auditory perception (tinnitus): mechanisms of generation and perception. Neurosci Res. 1990;8(4):221–54.
3. Axelsson A, Ringdahl A. Tinnitus--a study of its prevalence and characteristics. Br J Audiol. 1989;23(1):53–62.
4. Heller AJ. Classification and epidemiology of tinnitus. Otolaryngol Clin N Am. 2003;36(2):239–48.
5. Xu X, et al. An epidemiologic study of tinnitus in a population in Jiangsu Province. China J Am Acad Audiol. 2011;22(9):578–85.
6. Manche SK, et al. Association of tinnitus and hearing loss in otological disorders: a decade-long epidemiological study in a south Indian population. Braz J Otorhinolaryngol. 2016;82(6):643–9.
7. Kim HJ, et al. Analysis of the prevalence and associated risk factors of tinnitus in adults. PLoS One. 2015;10(5):e0127578.
8. Park B, et al. Analysis of the prevalence of and risk factors for tinnitus in a young population. Otol Neurotol. 2014;35(7):1218–22.
9. Khedr EM, et al. Epidemiological study of chronic tinnitus in Assiut, Egypt. Neuroepidemiology. 2010;35(1):45–52.
10. Lasisi AO, Abiona T, Gureje O. Tinnitus in the elderly: profile, correlates, and impact in the Nigerian Study of Ageing. Otolaryngol Head Neck Surg. 2010;143(4):510–5.
11. Vanneste S, et al. Neuronal correlates of maladaptive coping: an EEG-study in tinnitus patients. PLoS One. 2014;9(2):e88253.
12. Bhatt JM, Bhattacharyya N, Lin HW. Relationships between tinnitus and the prevalence of anxiety and depression. Laryngoscope. 2017;127(2):466–9.
13. Vanneste S, et al. The neural correlates of cognitive dysfunction in phantom sounds. Brain Res. 2016;1642:170.
14. Wang Y, et al. The characteristics of cognitive impairment in subjective chronic tinnitus. Brain Behav. 2018;8(3):e00918.
15. Langguth B, et al. Tinnitus: causes and clinical management. Lancet Neurol. 2013;12(9):920–30.
16. Dobie RA. A review of randomized clinical trials in tinnitus. Laryngoscope. 1999;109(8):1202–11.
17. Elgoyhen AB, et al. Tinnitus: perspectives from human neuroimaging. Nat Rev Neurosci. 2015;16(10):632–42.
18. Yokley BH, Hartman M, Slusher BS. Role of academic drug discovery in the quest for new CNS therapeutics. ACS Chem Neurosci. 2017;8(3):429–31.
19. Gribkoff VK, Kaczmarek LK. The need for new approaches in CNS drug discovery: why drugs have failed, and what can be done to improve outcomes. Neuropharmacology. 2017;120:11–9.
20. Kesselheim AS, Hwang TJ, Franklin JM. Two decades of new drug development for central nervous system disorders. Nat Rev Drug Discov. 2015;14(12):815–6.
21. Pushpakom S, et al. Drug repurposing: progress, challenges and recommendations. Nat Rev Drug Discov. 2019;18(1):41–58.
22. De Ridder D, Adhia D, Langguth B. Tinnitus and Brain stimulation, vol. 51. Curr Top Behav Neurosci; 2021. p. 249–93.
23. Llinas RR, et al. Thalamocortical dysrhythmia: a neurological and neuropsychiatric syndrome characterized by magnetoencephalography. Proc Natl Acad Sci U S A. 1999;96(26):15222–7.
24. De Ridder D, et al. Magnetic and electrical stimulation of the auditory cortex for intractable tinnitus. Case report. J Neurosurg. 2004;100(3):560–4.
25. De Ridder D. Should rTMS for tinnitus be performed left-sided, ipsilaterally or contralaterally, and is it a treatment or merely investigational? Eur J Neurol. 2010;17(7):891–2.
26. Eichhammer P, et al. Neuronavigated repetitive transcranial magnetic stimulation in patients with tinnitus: a short case series. Biol Psychiatry. 2003;54(8):862–5.
27. Plewnia C, Bartels M, Gerloff C. Transient suppression of tinnitus by transcranial magnetic stimulation. Ann Neurol. 2003;53(2):263–6.
28. De Ridder D, et al. Electrical stimulation of auditory and somatosensory cortices for treatment of tinnitus and pain. Prog Brain Res. 2007;166:377–88.
29. De Ridder D, et al. Auditory cortex stimulation for tinnitus. Acta Neurochir Suppl. 2007;97(Pt 2):451–62.
30. De Ridder D, et al. Primary and secondary auditory cortex stimulation for intractable tinnitus. ORL J Otorhinolaryngol Relat Spec. 2006;68(1):48–54; discussion 54–5.
31. De Ridder D, Menovsky T, van de Heyning P. Auditory cortex stimulation for tinnitus suppression. Otol Neurotol. 2008;29(4):574–5; author reply 575.
32. Kleinjung T, et al. Which tinnitus patients benefit from transcranial magnetic stimulation? Otolaryngol Head Neck Surg. 2007;137(4):589–95.

33. De Ridder D, et al. Transcranial magnetic stimulation for tinnitus: influence of tinnitus duration on stimulation parameter choice and maximal tinnitus suppression. Otol Neurotol. 2005;26(4):616–9.
34. De Ridder D, et al. Theta, alpha and beta burst transcranial magnetic stimulation: brain modulation in tinnitus. Int J Med Sci. 2007;4(5):237–41.
35. Langguth B, et al. The impact of auditory cortex activity on characterizing and treating patients with chronic tinnitus--first results from a PET study. Acta Otolaryngol Suppl. 2006;556:84–8.
36. Plewnia C, et al. Dose-dependent attenuation of auditory phantom perception (tinnitus) by PET-guided repetitive transcranial magnetic stimulation. Hum Brain Mapp. 2007;28(3):238–46.
37. Schlee W, et al. Abnormal resting-state cortical coupling in chronic tinnitus. BMC Neurosci. 2009;10:11.
38. Schlee W, et al. Mapping cortical hubs in tinnitus. BMC Biol. 2009;7:80.
39. Albert R, Jeong H, Barabasi AL. Error and attack tolerance of complex networks. Nature. 2000;406(6794):378–82.
40. De Ridder D, Vanneste S. EEG driven tDCS versus bifrontal tDCS for tinnitus. Front Psych. 2012;3:84.
41. Frank E, et al. Treatment of chronic tinnitus with repeated sessions of prefrontal transcranial direct current stimulation: outcomes from an open-label pilot study. J Neurol. 2011;259:327.
42. Song JJ, et al. Transcranial direct current stimulation in tinnitus patients: a systemic review and meta-analysis. ScientificWorldJournal. 2012;2012:427941.
43. To WT, et al. The added value of auditory cortex transcranial random noise stimulation (tRNS) after bifrontal transcranial direct current stimulation (tDCS) for tinnitus. J Neural Transm (Vienna). 2017;124(1):79–88.
44. Vanneste S, De Ridder D. Bifrontal transcranial direct current stimulation modulates tinnitus intensity and tinnitus-distress-related brain activity. Eur J Neurosci. 2011;34(4):605–14.
45. Vanneste S, et al. Different resting state brain activity and functional connectivity in patients who respond and not respond to bifrontal tDCS for tinnitus suppression. Exp Brain Res. 2011;210(2):217–27.
46. De Ridder D, Song JJ, Vanneste S. Frontal cortex TMS for tinnitus. Brain Stimul. 2012;6(3):355–62.
47. De Ridder D, et al. Dorsolateral prefrontal cortex transcranial magnetic stimulation and electrode implant for intractable tinnitus. World Neurosurg. 2012;77(5–6):778–84.
48. Vanneste S, De Ridder D. The involvement of the left ventrolateral prefrontal cortex in tinnitus: a TMS study. Exp Brain Res. 2012;221(3):345–50.
49. Kreuzer PM, et al. Can temporal repetitive transcranial magnetic stimulation be enhanced by targeting affective components of tinnitus with frontal rTMS? A randomized controlled pilot trial. Front Syst Neurosci. 2011;5:88.
50. De Ridder D, Vanneste S. Multitarget surgical neuromodulation: combined C2 and auditory cortex implantation for tinnitus. Neurosci Lett. 2015;591:202–6.
51. Leaver AM, et al. Dysregulation of limbic and auditory networks in tinnitus. Neuron. 2011;69(1):33–43.
52. Rauschecker JP, Leaver AM, Muhlau M. Tuning out the noise: limbic-auditory interactions in tinnitus. Neuron. 2010;66(6):819–26.
53. Kong J, et al. Exploring the brain in pain: activations, deactivations and their relation. Pain. 2010;148(2):257–67.
54. Fields H. State-dependent opioid control of pain. Nat Rev Neurosci. 2004;5(7):565–75.
55. Freeman WJ, Kozma R, Werbos PJ. Biocomplexity: adaptive behavior in complex stochastic dynamical systems. Biosystems. 2001;59(2):109–23.
56. De Ridder D, Joos K, Vanneste S. The enigma of the tinnitus-free dream state in a Bayesian world. Neural Plast. 2014;2014:612147.
57. De Ridder D, Vanneste S, Freeman W. The Bayesian brain: phantom percepts resolve sensory uncertainty. Neurosci Biobehav Rev. 2014;44C:4–15.
58. De Ridder D, Vanneste S. The Bayesian brain in imbalance: medial, lateral and descending pathways in tinnitus and pain: a perspective. Prog Brain Res. 2021;262:309–34.
59. Sporns O, et al. Organization, development and function of complex brain networks. Trends Cogn Sci. 2004;8(9):418–25.
60. Morowitz H, Singer J, editors. The mind, the brain, and complex adaptive systems. Boulder, CO: Westview Press; 1994.
61. Holland J. Complexity. Very short introductions. Oxford: Oxford University Press; 2014.
62. Amaral LA, et al. Emergence of complex dynamics in a simple model of signaling networks. Proc Natl Acad Sci U S A. 2004;101(44):15551–5.
63. Bullmore E, Sporns O. The economy of brain network organization. Nat Rev Neurosci. 2012;13(5):336–49.
64. Watts DJ, Strogatz SH. Collective dynamics of 'small-world' networks. Nature. 1998;393(6684):440–2.
65. Catania KC. Tentacled snakes turn C-starts to their advantage and predict future prey behavior. Proc Natl Acad Sci U S A. 2009;106(27):11183–7.
66. Bassett DS, et al. Adaptive reconfiguration of fractal small-world human brain functional networks. Proc Natl Acad Sci U S A. 2006;103(51):19518–23.
67. Karuza EA, Thompson-Schill SL, Bassett DS. Local patterns to global architectures: influences of network topology on human learning. Trends Cogn Sci. 2016;20(8):629–40.
68. Achard S, et al. A resilient, low-frequency, small-world human brain functional network with highly connected association cortical hubs. J Neurosci. 2006;26(1):63–72.
69. Bullmore E, Sporns O. Complex brain networks: graph theoretical analysis of structural and functional systems. Nat Rev Neurosci. 2009;10(3):186–98.
70. Eguiluz VM, et al. Scale-free brain functional networks. Phys Rev Lett. 2005;94(1):018102.
71. Buzsaki G, Mizuseki K. The log-dynamic brain: how skewed distributions affect network operations. Nat Rev Neurosci. 2014;15(4):264–78.
72. He BJ. Scale-free brain activity: past, present, and future. Trends Cogn Sci. 2014;18:480.
73. To WT, et al. Thalamocortical dysrhythmia underpin the log-dynamics in phantom sounds. Prog Brain Res. 2021;262:511–26.
74. El Boustani S, et al. Network-state modulation of power-law frequency-scaling in visual cortical neurons. PLoS Comput Biol. 2009;5(9):e1000519.
75. Milstein J, et al. Neuronal shot noise and Brownian 1/f2 behavior in the local field potential. PLoS One. 2009;4(2):e4338.
76. He BJ, et al. The temporal structures and functional significance of scale-free brain activity. Neuron. 2010;66(3):353–69.
77. Dehghani N, et al. Comparative power spectral analysis of simultaneous elecroencephalographic and magnetoencephalographic recordings in humans suggests non-resistive extracellular media. J Comput Neurosci. 2010;29(3):405–21.
78. Radulescu A, Mujica-Parodi LR. Network connectivity modulates power spectrum scale invariance. NeuroImage. 2014;90:436–48.
79. He BJ. Scale-free properties of the functional magnetic resonance imaging signal during rest and task. J Neurosci. 2011;31(39):13786–95.
80. Akhrif A, et al. Fractal analysis of BOLD time series in a network associated with waiting impulsivity. Front Physiol. 2018;9:1378.
81. Freeman WJ, Zhai J. Simulated power spectral density (PSD) of background electrocorticogram (ECoG). Cogn Neurodyn. 2009;3(1):97–103.
82. Keshner MS. 1/f noise. Proc IEEE. 1982;70(3):212–8.
83. De Ridder D, Perera S, Vanneste S. State of the art: novel applications for cortical stimulation. Neuromodulation. 2017;20(3):206–14.

84. Fornito A, Bullmore ET. Connectomics: a new paradigm for understanding brain disease. Eur Neuropsychopharmacol. 2014;25:733.
85. Lewis CM, et al. Learning sculpts the spontaneous activity of the resting human brain. Proc Natl Acad Sci U S A. 2009;106(41):17558–63.
86. Hagmann P, et al. Mapping the structural core of human cerebral cortex. PLoS Biol. 2008;6(7):e159.
87. Friston KJ. Functional and effective connectivity: a review. Brain Connect. 2011;1(1):13–36.
88. Edwards CA, et al. Neurostimulation devices for the treatment of neurologic disorders. Mayo Clin Proc. 2017;92(9):1427–44.
89. Boccard SG, et al. Targeting the affective component of chronic pain: a case series of deep Brain stimulation of the anterior cingulate cortex. Neurosurgery. 2014;74:628.
90. De Ridder D, et al. Anterior cingulate implant for alcohol dependence. Neurosurgery. 2016;78:E883.
91. De Ridder D, Joos K, Vanneste S. Anterior cingulate implants for tinnitus: report of 2 cases. J Neurosurg. 2016;124(4):893–901.
92. Leong SL, et al. Anterior cingulate cortex implants for alcohol addiction: a feasibility study. Neurotherapeutics. 2020;17:1287.
93. Mayberg HS, et al. Deep brain stimulation for treatment-resistant depression. Neuron. 2005;45(5):651–60.
94. De Ridder D, et al. Theta-gamma dysrhythmia and auditory phantom perception. J Neurosurg. 2011;114(4):912–21.
95. De Ridder D, et al. Burst stimulation of the auditory cortex: a new form of neurostimulation for noise-like tinnitus suppression. J Neurosurg. 2010;112(6):1289–94.
96. Friedland DR, et al. Feasibility of auditory cortical stimulation for the treatment of tinnitus. Otol Neurotol. 2007;28(8): 1005–12.
97. Litre CF, et al. Surgical treatment by electrical stimulation of the auditory cortex for intractable tinnitus. Brain Stimul. 2009;2(3):132–7.
98. Seidman MD, et al. Direct electrical stimulation of Heschl's gyrus for tinnitus treatment. Laryngoscope. 2008;118(3):491–500.
99. Barabasi AL, Gulbahce N, Loscalzo J. Network medicine: a network-based approach to human disease. Nat Rev Genet. 2011;12(1):56–68.
100. Fornito A, Zalesky A, Breakspear M. The connectomics of brain disorders. Nat Rev Neurosci. 2015;16(3):159–72.
101. Boly M, et al. Cerebral processing of auditory and noxious stimuli in severely brain injured patients: differences between VS and MCS. Neuropsychol Rehabil. 2005;15(3–4):283–9.
102. Crick F, Koch C. Are we aware of neural activity in primary visual cortex? Nature. 1995;375(6527):121–3.
103. Melloni L, et al. Synchronization of neural activity across cortical areas correlates with conscious perception. J Neurosci. 2007;27(11):2858–65.
104. Demertzi A, Soddu A, Laureys S. Consciousness supporting networks. Curr Opin Neurobiol. 2012;23:239.
105. Laureys S, et al. Auditory processing in the vegetative state. Brain. 2000;123(Pt 8):1589–601.
106. Laureys S, et al. Cortical processing of noxious somatosensory stimuli in the persistent vegetative state. NeuroImage. 2002;17(2):732–41.
107. Baars BJ. Global workspace theory of consciousness: toward a cognitive neuroscience of human experience. Prog Brain Res. 2005;150:45–53.
108. Cho SB, Baars BJ, Newman J. A neural global workspace model for conscious attention. Neural Netw. 1997;10(7):1195–206.
109. Akeju O, et al. Disruption of thalamic functional connectivity is a neural correlate of dexmedetomidine-induced unconsciousness. elife. 2014;3:e04499.
110. Chand GB, Dhamala M. Interactions among the Brain default-mode, salience, and central-executive networks during perceptual decision-making of moving dots. Brain Connect. 2016;6(3):249–54.
111. Chen AC, et al. Causal interactions between fronto-parietal central executive and default-mode networks in humans. Proc Natl Acad Sci U S A. 2013;110(49):19944–9.
112. Song JJ, et al. The balance between Bayesian inference and default mode determines the generation of tinnitus from decreased auditory input: a volume entropy-based study. Hum Brain Mapp. 2021;42:4059.
113. Fox MD, et al. Resting-state networks link invasive and noninvasive brain stimulation across diverse psychiatric and neurological diseases. Proc Natl Acad Sci U S A. 2014;111(41):E4367–75.
114. De Ridder D, Vanneste S. Targeting the parahippocampal area by auditory cortex stimulation in tinnitus. Brain Stimul. 2014;7:709.
115. Barker AT. The history and basic principles of magnetic nerve stimulation. Electroencephalogr Clin Neurophysiol Suppl. 1999;51:3–21.
116. Barker AT, Jalinous R, Freeston IL. Non-invasive magnetic stimulation of human motor cortex. Lancet. 1985;1(8437):1106–7.
117. Moreno-Duarte I, et al. Transcranial Electrical Stimulation: Transcranial Direct Current Stimulation (tDCS), Transcranial Alternating Current Stimulation (tACS), Transcranial Pulsed Current Stimulation (tPCS), and Transcranial Random Noise Stimulation (tRNS). In: Kadosh RC, editor. The stimulated brain: cognitive enhancement using non-invasive brain stimulation. London: Academia Press; 2014.
118. Paulus W. Transcranial electrical stimulation (tES - tDCS; tRNS, tACS) methods. Neuropsychol Rehabil. 2011;21(5):602–17.
119. Vanneste S, Fregni F, De Ridder D. Head-to-head comparison of transcranial random noise stimulation, transcranial AC stimulation, and transcranial DC stimulation for tinnitus. Front Psych. 2013;4:158.
120. De Ridder D, et al. Surgical brain modulation for tinnitus: the past, present and future. J Neurosurg Sci. 2012;56(4):323–40.
121. De Ridder D, et al. Transcranial magnetic stimulation and extradural electrodes implanted on secondary auditory cortex for tinnitus suppression. J Neurosurg. 2011;114(4):903–11.
122. Goebel G, Hiller W. The tinnitus questionnaire. A standard instrument for grading the degree of tinnitus. Results of a multicenter study with the tinnitus questionnaire. HNO. 1994;42(3):166–72.
123. De Ridder D, et al. Do tonic and burst TMS modulate the lemniscal and extralemniscal system differentially? Int J Med Sci. 2007;4(5):242–6.
124. Meeus O, et al. Influence of tonic and burst transcranial magnetic stimulation characteristics on acute inhibition of subjective tinnitus. Otol Neurotol. 2009;30(6):697–703.
125. Vanneste S, et al. Burst transcranial magnetic stimulation: which tinnitus characteristics influence the amount of transient tinnitus suppression? Eur J Neurol. 2010;17(9):1141–7.
126. Litre CF, et al. Feasibility of auditory cortical stimulation for the treatment of tinnitus. Three case reports. Neurochirurgie. 2010;56(4):303–8.
127. De Ridder D, Vanneste S. Visions on the future of medical devices in spinal cord stimulation: what medical device is needed? Expert Rev Med Devices. 2016;13(3):233–42.
128. Donovan C, et al. Deep brain stimulation of Heschl gyrus: implantation technique, intraoperative localization, and effects of stimulation. Neurosurgery. 2015;77(6):940–7.
129. De Ridder D, et al. Amygdalohippocampal involvement in tinnitus and auditory memory. Acta Otolaryngol Suppl. 2006;556:50–3.
130. Burger J, et al. Transcranial magnetic stimulation for the treatment of tinnitus: 4-year follow-up in treatment responders--a retrospective analysis. Brain Stimul. 2011;4(4):222–7.
131. Lehner A, et al. Multisite rTMS for the treatment of chronic tinnitus: stimulation of the cortical tinnitus network--a pilot study. Brain Topogr. 2013;26(3):501–10.

132. Larson PS, Cheung SW. A stroke of silence: tinnitus suppression following placement of a deep brain stimulation electrode with infarction in area LC. J Neurosurg. 2013;118(1):192–4.
133. Shi Y, et al. Deep brain stimulation effects in patients with tinnitus. Otolaryngol Head Neck Surg. 2009;141(2): 285–7.
134. Cheung SW, Larson PS. Tinnitus modulation by deep brain stimulation in locus of caudate neurons (area LC). Neuroscience. 2010;169(4):1768–78.
135. Larson PS, Cheung SW. Deep brain stimulation in area LC controllably triggers auditory phantom percepts. Neurosurgery. 2011;70:398.
136. Smit JV, et al. The impact of deep brain stimulation on tinnitus. Surg Neurol Int. 2016;7(Suppl 35):S848–54.
137. Cheung SW, et al. Phase I trial of caudate deep brain stimulation for treatment-resistant tinnitus. J Neurosurg. 2019:1–10.
138. Perez PL, et al. Human caudate nucleus subdivisions in tinnitus modulation. J Neurosurg. 2019;132(3):705–11.
139. Engineer ND, et al. Reversing pathological neural activity using targeted plasticity. Nature. 2011;470(7332):101–4.
140. De Ridder D, et al. Placebo-controlled vagus nerve stimulation paired with tones in a patient with refractory tinnitus: a case report. Otol Neurotol. 2015;36(4):575–80.
141. De Ridder D, et al. Safety and efficacy of vagus nerve stimulation paired with tones for the treatment of tinnitus: a case series. Neuromodulation. 2014;17(2):170–9.
142. Tyler R, et al. Vagus nerve stimulation paired with tones for the treatment of tinnitus: a prospective randomized double-blind controlled pilot study in humans. Sci Rep. 2017;7(1):11960.
143. Wichova H, et al. Tinnitus perception in patients after vagal nerve stimulator implantation for epilepsy. Am J Otolaryngol. 2018;39(5):599–602.

Bimodal Stimulation for the Treatment of Tinnitus

54

Sven Vanneste and Berthold Langguth

Abstract

Sound stimulation combined with electrical vagus or trigeminal nerve stimulation has shown to modulate tinnitus-related brain plasticity. Sound stimulation paired with electrical nerve stimulation, also referred to as bimodal stimulation, has become an exciting new avenue for the treatment of tinnitus. This chapter discusses preclinical and clinical evidence for efficacy of bimodal stimulation treatments of tinnitus, the potential mechanisms of action involved, and the strengths and weakness of the different approaches.

S. Vanneste (✉)
School of Psychology, Global Brain Health Institute and Trinity College Institute for Neuroscience, Trinity College Dublin, Dublin, Ireland
e-mail: sven.vanneste@tcd.ie; http://www.lab-clint.org

B. Langguth
Klinik und Poliklinik für Psychiatrie, Psychosomatik und Psychotherapie, Universität Regensburg Bezirksklinikum, Regensburg, Germany
e-mail: berthold.langguth@medbo.de

W. Schlee et al. (eds.), *Textbook of Tinnitus*, https://doi.org/10.1007/978-3-031-35647-6_54

Graphical Abstract

paired vagus nerve stimulation

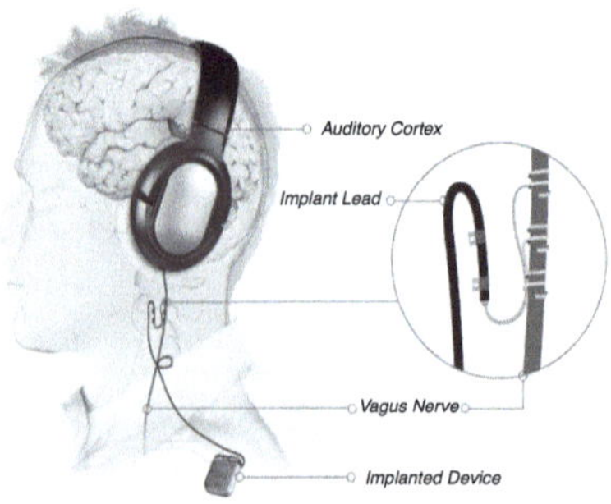

auditory somatosensory stimulation

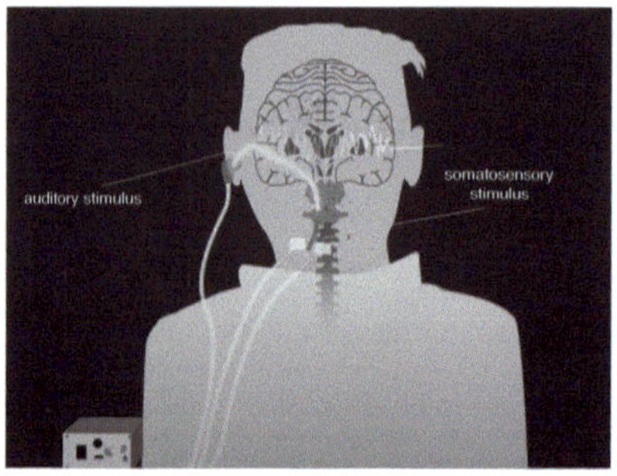

tongue stimulation combined with tone therapy

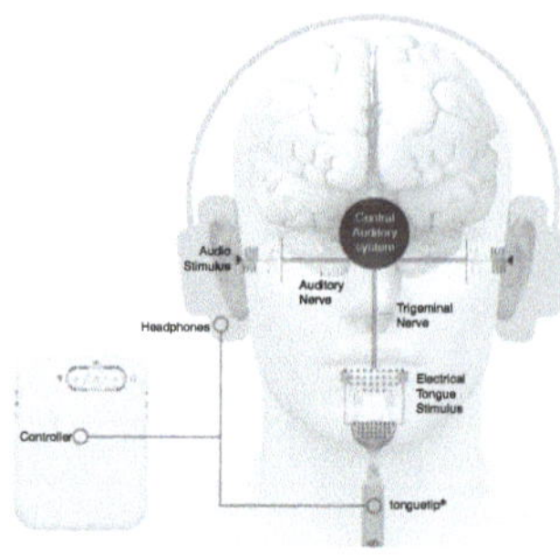

Highlights

- Animal research has demonstrated that bimodal stimulation consisting of sound combined with electrical vagus or trigeminal nerve stimulation can efficiently modulate neuronal plasticity in central auditory pathways.
- Pilot studies in humans have revealed very promising effects for different forms of bimodal auditory and electrical nerve stimulation.
- Further research is required to confirm these clinical findings, to identify the involved mechanisms in humans and to optimize stimulation parameters for patient subgroups.

Introduction

Several neural models of tinnitus propose that this phantom sound arises from aberrant cortical plasticity, which is in most cases due to a deafferentation of auditory input such as hearing loss or damage along the auditory pathway. It is assumed that the mechanism is similar to the emergence of phantom pain after limb amputation with somatosensory deafferentation [1, 2]. Research indicates that auditory deafferentation results in cortical changes including increases in neural synchrony, increases in spontaneous firing and excitability, expansion in receptor fields, and map reorganization in the auditory cortex [3]. Further research has shown that auditory deafferentation alters the excitatory and inhibitory balance on the thalamocortical level, which in turn generates the tinnitus percept [4–6]. Yet, another model suggests that the medial geniculate body is receiving tinnitus-related activity from the dorsal cochlear nucleus where changes have been seen in neural synchrony and spontaneous firing rates [7]. The more and more detailed knowledge about the pathophysiological mechanisms of tinnitus has led to the concept that modulation of the neuronal disbalance in auditory pathways might represent a promising treatment approach for tinnitus. Sound stimulation paired with electrical nerve stimulation, also referred to as bimodal stimulation, has been proposed as a technique to normalize tinnitus-related alterations of neuronal activity. In this chapter, we discuss the rationale for different bimodal stimulation approaches for the treatment of tinnitus. We will review preclinical and clinical findings, the strengths and weakness of the different approaches, and discuss future research avenues.

Inducing Map Plasticity Changes

Early investigations have shown that vagus nerve stimulation can enhance cortical plasticity [8]. By pairing vagus nerve stimulation with the presentation of tones, a reorganization of the tonotopic map in the primary auditory cortex could be induced [8]. Animals were repeatedly presented with a mid-frequency pure tone over the course of 20-day paired with vagus nerve stimulation. Repeated presentation of vagus nerve stimulation paired with the same number of tones increased the number of neurons that responded to the frequency near the paired tone. In a second batch with a high-frequency tone paired with vagus nerve stimulation, a similar map expansion was observed corresponding to the paired high-frequency tone, but not the mid-frequency area. This led to the idea that vagus nerve stimulation paired with tones can induce frequency-specific changes rather than a general-

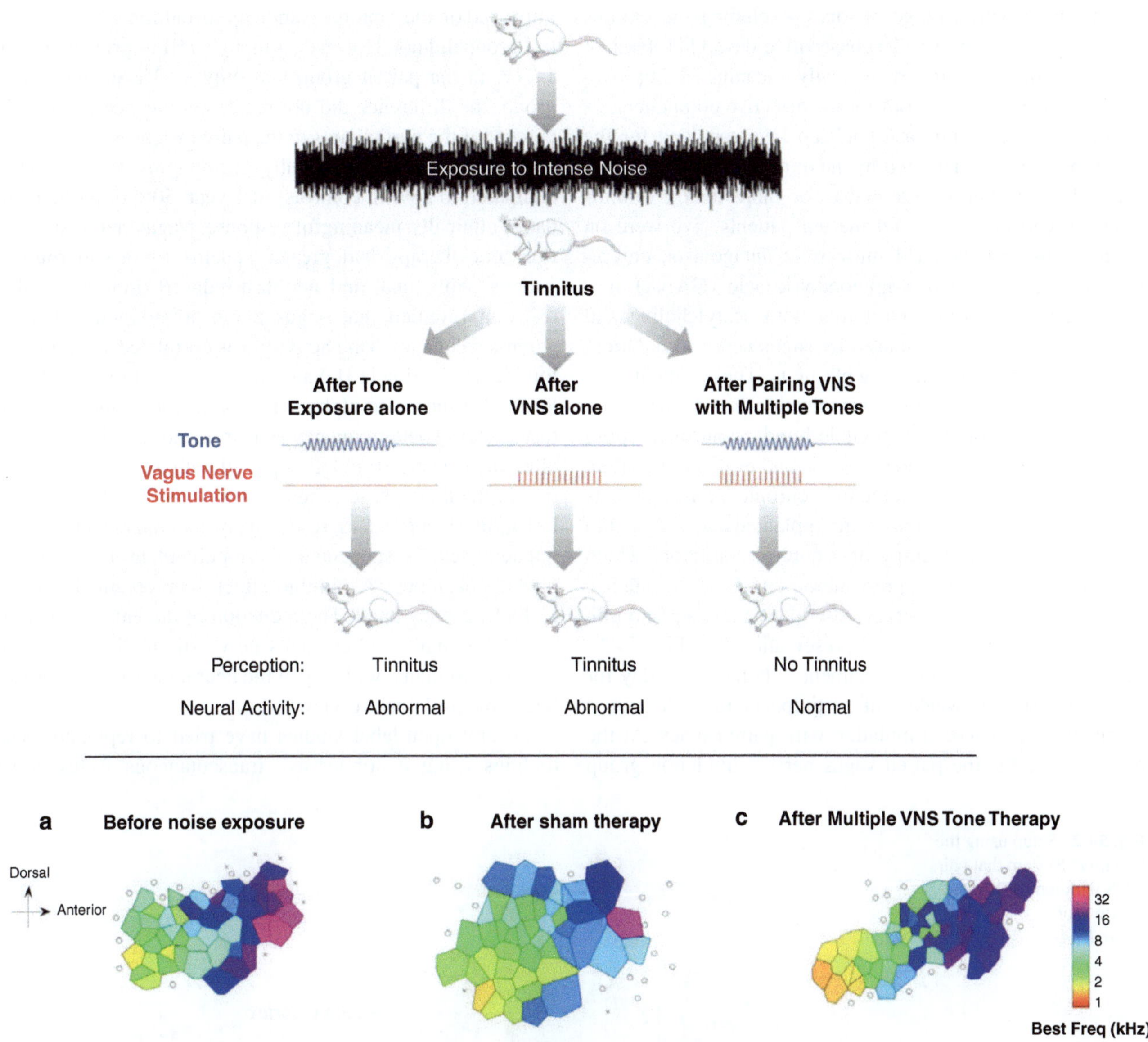

Fig. 54.1 Pairing vagus nerve stimulation (VNS) with tones reverses neural and behavioral correlates of tinnitus. Abnormal neural activity in noise exposed rats included reduced frequency selectivity, distorted frequency map organization, increased excitability, and greater neural synchronization. After exposure to intense noise, rats were treated with (1) tone exposure, (2) VNS, or (3) VNS paired with tones. Only the rats that received VNS paired with tones showed reversal of the abnormal neural activity and tinnitus. The color of each polygon indicates the characteristic frequency of each recording site. (Image courtesy of Engineer et al. [8])

ized modification in excitability in the primary auditory cortex.

Based on the assumption that a reorganization of the tonotopic map may cause tinnitus [9, 10], a reversal of these plasticity changes by vagus nerve stimulation paired with tones was tested as a treatment for tinnitus. In a seminal paper, Engineer et al. [8] evaluated the ability of vagus nerve stimulation-based targeted plasticity therapy to eliminate the tinnitus by reversing map plasticity in the auditory cortex. The rationale for the therapy was based on increasing the number of neurons tuned to frequencies other than the tinnitus frequency to reduce the overrepresented tinnitus frequency. Rats displaying a tinnitus percept centered on middle frequency tones were assigned to receive either vagus nerve stimulation tone therapy or sham therapy over the course of 4 weeks. The vagus nerve stimulation tone therapy consisted of vagus nerve stimulation with randomly interleaved tones that spanned the rat hearing range except for the tinnitus frequency. Intriguingly, within 2 weeks of vagus nerve tone therapy, the tinnitus percept was fully eliminated. A behavioral improvement was observed for up to 3 months after the end of the therapy, suggesting a permanent reversing of the tonotopic map (see Fig. 54.1).

Based on these preclinical findings, a first open-label trial was set up including 10 severe chronic tinnitus patients, where patients received invasive cervical vagus nerve stimulation paired with a range of tones, excluding the tinnitus frequency for 2.5 h over 20 consecutive days [11]. Four of the ten patients exhibited clinically meaningful improvements in their tinnitus, both for the affective component, as quantified by the Tinnitus Handicap Inventory and for the sound percept, as quantified by the minimum masking level. These improvements were stable for more than 2 months after the end of therapy. Of the ten patients, five were on medications that included muscarinic antagonists, norepinephrine agonists, and γ-aminobutyric acid (GABA) agonists, thereby possibly interfering with acetylcholine and norepinephrine release induced by vagus nerve stimulation, which is essential for inducing plasticity. These patients had no improvement in contrast to medication-free patients. In a prospective, randomized, double-blind, controlled pilot study, the aim was to further explore and evaluate the effect of paired vagus nerve stimulation in chronic tinnitus patients [12]. Thirty tinnitus patients were implanted and assigned to a vagus nerve tone therapy or a control condition, which included 10 min of tone presentation and 5 min of silence followed by 2 h of vagus nerve stimulation and again 5 min of silence and 10 min of tone presentation (see Fig. 54.2). Participants performed the treatment at home every day for 6 weeks. After 6 weeks, all participants in both groups received vagus nerve stimulation with paired tones. At the end of 6 weeks, the paired vagus nerve stimulation group improved on the Tinnitus Handicap Inventory, while the control group did not. However, although THI improvement was 17.7% in the paired group and only 10.3% in the control group, the difference did not reach significance level. Fifty percent of the participants in the paired vagus nerve stimulation group showed clinically meaningful improvements compared to 28% in controls. At 1 year, 50% of participants had a clinically meaningful response. Vagus nerve stimulation tone therapy had greater benefits for a subgroup of patients with tonal and nonblast-induced tinnitus. Further research revealed that vagus nerve stimulation paired of gamma frequency band activity was correlated with tinnitus loudness reduction [13]. Vagus nerve stimulation paired with tones also increased alpha synchronization in the left auditory cortex. Theta frequency synchronization did not change after vagus nerve stimulation paired with tones, but a reduction in the theta phase coherence was observed between the left auditory cortex and, respectively, the dorsal anterior cingulate cortex, the subgenual anterior cingulate cortex and the parahippocampus. A similar effect was obtained for the alpha frequency band. The reduction of the emotional component of tinnitus after vagus nerve stimulation treatment was not associated with any of the neural measures recorded. See Table 54.1 for overview.

Several open-label studies have tried to replicate these findings using a noninvasive transcutaneous vagus nerve

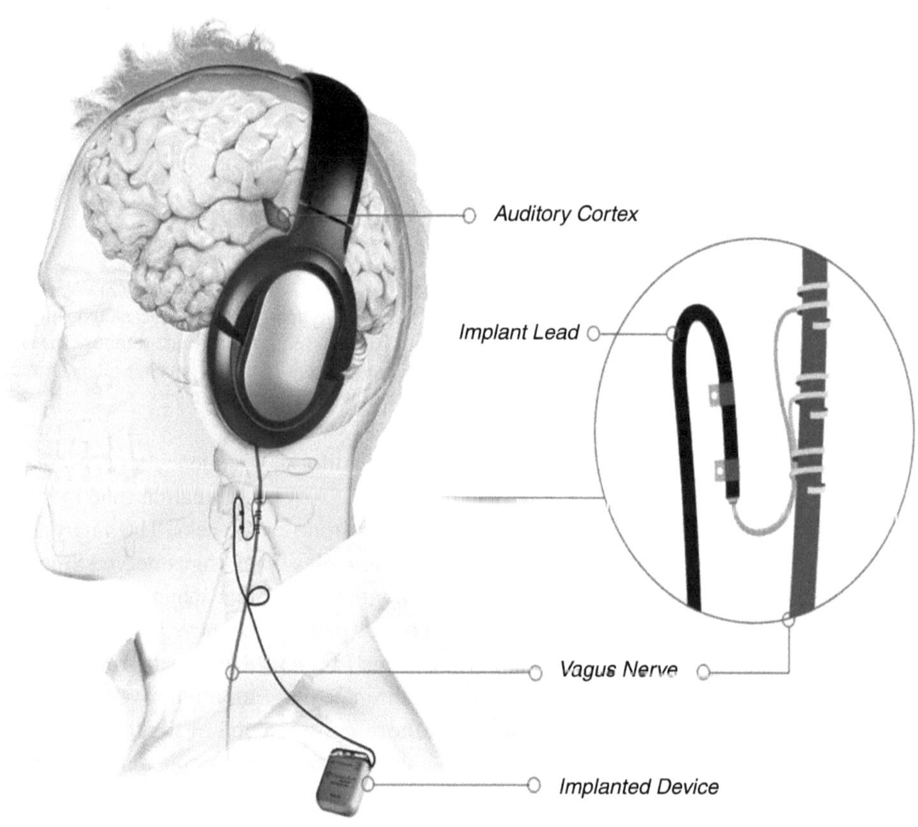

Fig. 54.2 Setup using the Serenity® System that pairs VNS with tones. (Image courtesy of *MicroTransponder, Inc.*)

Table 54.1 Human bimodal stimulation clinical studies: outcomes, parameters

	Bimodal stimulation tone therapy combined with		
	Vagus nerve	Somatosensory	Tongue
Study design	Double-blind sham-controlled delayed start	Double-blind sham-controlled cross-over	Double-blinded, exploratory parallel study
Device placement	Cuff electrode implanted at the cervical vagus nerve	Transcutaneous electrode on cheek or neck	Transcutaneous electrode on anterodorsal surface of the tongue
Participants	30 tinnitus patients	20 tinnitus patients	326 tinnitus patients
Treatment timeframe	6 weeks of paired or unpaired stimulation, followed by 6 weeks' paired stimulation	4 weeks of active or sham followed by 4 weeks of sham or active with a washout of 4 weeks followed after both conditions	12 weeks of treatment received 1 of the 3 active arms
Treatment usage	2.5 h a day	30 min a day	2 daily sessions of 30 min
Electrical stimuli	100 µs pulse width, 0.8 mA amplitude 30 Hz pulse rate, pulse train 0.5 s	Biphasic pulses, 100 µs duration, 2–5 mA amplitude	Arm 1, 2, 3: Biphasic anodic pulses between 5 and 210 µs duration, fixed amplitude
Auditory stimuli	Range of tones from 170 to 16,00 Hz excluding 1/2 octave around the tinnitus frequency. Tones presented at comfortable levels, 500-ms duration	Matched tinnitus spectrum presented at 40 dB SL, 10 ms duration with 1 ms linear rise and fall time	Arm 1 & 2: 500–8000 Hz tones, 15 ms, repetition 80 ms Arm 3: 100–550 Hz tones, repetition between 900 and 1100 ms
Pairing	Audio simultaneously with electrical stimulation	Audio is presented 5 ms prior to electrical stimulation	Arm 1: 80 ms between auditory and electrical stimulus Arm 2: 30–50-ms between auditory and electrical stimulus Arm 3: 900–1100-ms between auditory and electrical stimulus
Outcome measurement	THI, TFI, and MML	TFI, Tinn tester (tinnitus loudness matching)	THI and TFI
Results reported	Significant reduction in THI for paired group. 50% responder rate	Significant reduction in TFI and immediate effect on loudness. Responder rate = 50%	Significant reduction in THI and TFI; responder rate between 74% and 88.8%

stimulation approach paired with sound. Two studies utilized small electrodes placed on either the tragus or concha of the external ear to stimulate an afferent branch of the vagus nerve [14, 15]. In a first study, ten adults were tested using transcutaneous vagus nerve stimulation paired with classical music presented with a spectral notch corresponding to the participants tinnitus frequency [15]. Seven sessions over 10 days of 45–60 min resulted in a significant improvement on life impact questionnaires and a reduction in cortical N1m amplitude measured by magnetoencephalography. The other study tested 30 adults using transcutaneous vagus nerve stimulation paired with tailored notched music for 30 min for 10 sessions [14]. Results showed 50% of participants reported improvement measured on a global improvement questionnaire and a drop of 18% on tinnitus loudness, while scores on the tinnitus handicap inventory were unaffected. Transcutaneous vagus nerve stimulation alone (without paired tones) had no effect on tinnitus handicap [16].

Bimodal Auditory–Somatosensory Stimulation

A second bimodal stimulation approach aims to modulate a deep brain structure named the cochlear nucleus. The cochlear nucleus is an area that integrates auditory input from the cochlea and somatosensory input from the dorsal column and the trigeminal systems [17, 18]. This integration of auditory and somatosensory input involves spike-timing-dependent plasticity, so that the order and time interval between auditory and somatosensory stimuli determine whether increases or decreases in excitability will occur [19].

Several animal studies have shown that combining auditory–somatosensory bimodal stimulation elicits long-term potentiation or long-term depression depending on the order and the time interval between the auditory and somatosensory stimuli [7]. Based on these findings, a bimodal auditory and somatosensory stimulation paradigm was developed to treat tinnitus. Based on in vivo recordings in the dorsal cochlear nucleus of guinea pigs with behavioral signs of tinnitus, this tinnitus goes together with increased synchrony and spontaneous activity as well as a higher proportion of long-term potentiation [7]. Based on these findings, it was hypothesized that inducing long-term depression should induce a decrease in spontaneous firing and synchrony that would go together with a suppression of tinnitus. Transcutaneous electrical stimulation paired with tone presentation were randomly tested at six different conditions (somatosensory first followed by auditory stimulation or the other way around at intervals of 5, 10, and 20 ms each). The experiment revealed that auditory stimulation presented 5 ms before somatosensory stimulation produced the most pronounced long-term depression in dorsal cochlear nucleus cells. This protocol was then applied for 20 min per day in tinnitus animals on 25 consecutive days, resulting in a significant decrease in tinnitus that was paralleled by a reduction in spontaneous firing rate and synchrony.

Based on these findings, a pilot study was set up including 20 tinnitus patients that were able to modulate their tinnitus with a somatic maneuver. These patients were enrolled in a double-blind, sham-controlled, crossover study [7]. Participants received either bimodal auditory–somatosensory treatment or unimodal auditory treatment for 30 min per day for 28 consecutive days. After 4 weeks of washout, participants crossed over to the other treatment for 4 weeks. This was again followed by 4 weeks of wash-out. Participants were tested for changes in their tinnitus spectra using an interactive computer program and tinnitus life impact by using the tinnitus functional index. Participants that received the bimodal treatment showed a reduction of their tinnitus of −8 dB SPL over 4 weeks of treatment while unimodal treatment induced −3 dB SPL reduction. Two participants reported complete elimination of their tinnitus. For the tinnitus functional index, the bimodal group had a drop of 7.51 points, while unimodal stimulation induced a drop of approximately 3 points. Half of the participants had a minimal clinical important difference on the tinnitus functional index (at least 13 points drop). See Table 54.1 for overview. A recent study confirmed these findings, demonstrating that prolonged reduction in tinnitus symptoms can result from using an extended treatment duration of auditory-somatosensory stimulation.

Tongue Stimulation Combined With Tone Therapy

Based on previous research on the involvement of the somatosensory system in tinnitus, another approach of bimodal stimulation combines electrical tongue stimulation with tone therapy. In an open-label pilot study [20], 45 patients with chronic tinnitus used a broad-band spectrum noise with temporal fluctuations paired with electrical stimulation of the tongue for twice a day for 30 min for 10 weeks. This intervention led to a significant average reduction of 8.6 points on the tinnitus handicap questionnaire, and average reductions of 8.1 dB of minimal masking levels and 5.4 dB of tinnitus loudness match. In total, 45% of the participants had a minimal important difference (≥7 points) on the tinnitus handicap questionnaire, and 64% of the participants had a minimal important difference (≥5.3 points) for minimal masking levels. This pilot study was followed by a large randomized and double-blind clinical study enrolling 326 adult tinnitus subjects (see Fig. 54.3). Participants were randomized into three arms consisting of different parameter settings [21]. Participants were evaluated during the 12-week treatment period and for three follow-up visits for up to 12 months to assess long-term therapeutic effects after the end of treatment. Eighty-four percent of participants used the device at or above the minimum compliance level of 36 h over the 12-week treatment period, in which 75–88% of these treatment-compliant participants had tinnitus handicap inventory or tinnitus functional index scores that improved at the end of treatment. Overall, this corresponds to two-thirds of all enrolled participants showing improvements in tinnitus handicap inventory or tinnitus functional index scores, with an average change from baseline to the end of treatment of about 14 points in both questionnaires. These findings were quite encouraging considering that the extent of improvement observed in this study were comparable (TFI) or superior (THI) to what has been previously shown to be significant or clinically meaningful in well-designed clinical trials. Moreover, the improvement induced for 12-week treatment was generally maintained for 12 months after the end of treatment. This is remarkable, as such long-term improvement has not been demonstrated for any other treatment, not even for cognitive behavioral therapy [22]. Furthermore, different trends were observed in the extent of long-term effects that emerged between the three stimulation settings used in this study, in which the most synchronized setting between

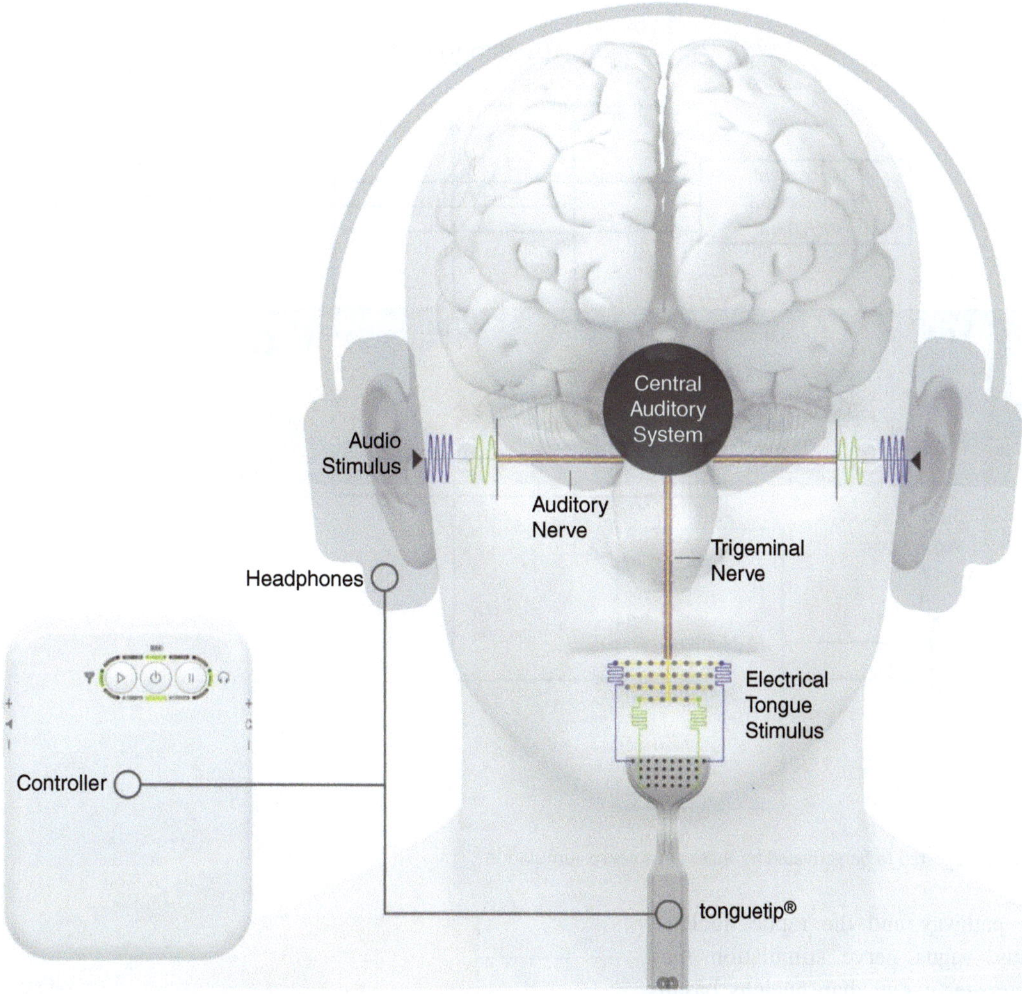

Fig. 54.3 Setup using the Lenire® System that pairs tongue stimulation with tones. The inset shows the electrode lead wrapped around the cervical vagus nerve. (Image courtesy of *Neuromod, Inc.*)

tongue and tone exhibited the best sustained effects [21]. See Table 54.1 for overview.

Mechanism of Action of Bimodal Stimulation

The methods of bimodal auditory electrical stimulation for the treatment of tinnitus are building on preclinical basic research. Interestingly, research on bimodal vagus nerve stimulation and the auditory–somatosensory approach suggest a different mechanism of action, while the tongue stimulation approach, although based on earlier research, does not have a direct translation from preclinical research.

About 80% of the afferent fibers of the human vagus nerve terminate on cells in the nucleus tractus solitarius [23]. These cells project to deep brain nuclei including the locus coeruleus, nucleus basalis, and the raphe nucleus that regulate the release of specific neuromodulators. Studies in rats have shown that electrical stimulation of the abdominal vagal afferents increases the activity of catecholamine neurons within the nucleus tractus solitaries, which in turn trigger the release of noradrenaline, acetylcholine, and serotonin in the cerebral cortex [24–28] (see Fig. 54.4). Other research indicated that noradrenaline, acetylcholine, and serotonin are key to regulate plasticity changes [24, 25]. Previous research already revealed that the deep brain stimulation of the nucleus basalis can facilitate powerful, specific, and long functional changes in the auditory cortex. Interestingly, stimulation of the vagus nerve can activate the same pathway but less invasively without deep brain stimulation [23, 29, 30]. Similar like nucleus basalis stimulation, vagus nerve stimulation drives cortex synchrony and excitability in the primary auditory system if paired with specific sounds [8]. However, whereas nucleus basalis stimulation mainly triggers the nucleus basalis-acetylcholine pathway, vagus nerve stimulation triggers in addition to this pathway also the locus

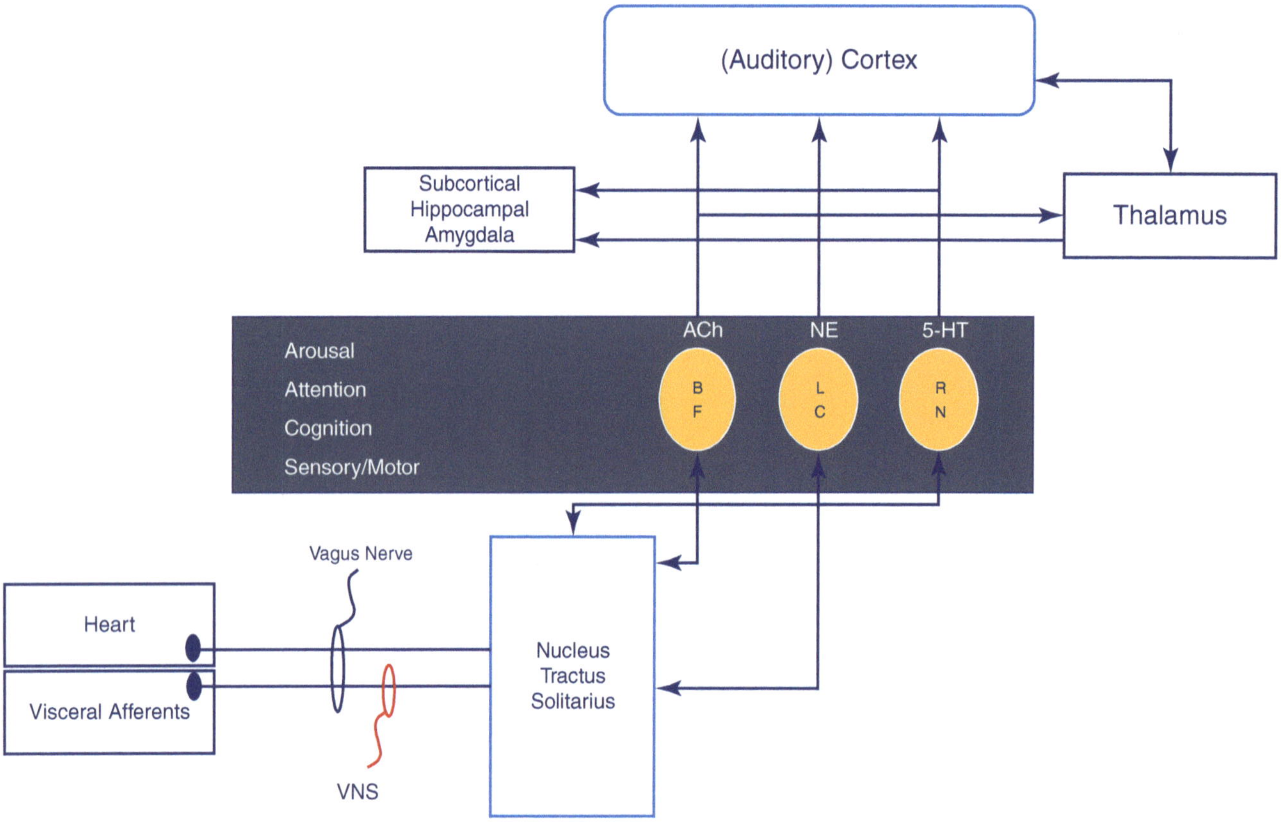

Fig. 54.4 The neural pathways suggested to be activated by that vagus nerve stimulation

coeruleus-noradrenaline pathway and the raphe nucleus-serotonin pathway. Thus, vagus nerve stimulation may enhance plasticity to a greater extent than nucleus basalis stimulation [24, 25]. In animals with tinnitus after noise trauma, vagus nerve stimulation paired with tones has shown to normalize alterations of the tonotopic map [8, 31]. Although earlier research suggests that alterations of the tonotopic map are associated with tinnitus [9, 10], more recent data suggest that this reorganization is due to hearing loss and does not represent a neuronal correlate of tinnitus [32].

A series of preclinical experiments preceded bimodal auditory–somatosensory stimulation [33]. In animals with tinnitus long-term potentiation, an increased spontaneous firing rate and synchrony have been demonstrated in the dorsal cochlear nucleus (see Fig. 54.5). A decrease in spontaneous firing rate and synchrony was achieved by presenting bimodal auditory–somatosensory stimulation [7]. Interestingly, vagus nerve stimulation also revealed changes in spontaneous firing rate and synchrony as well as changes in the inferior colliculus in addition to the auditory cortex [8]. This could suggest that bimodal auditory–somatosensory stimulation and vagus nerve stimulation share a similar mechanism of action. Moreover, it is also possible that similar to vagus nerve stimulation, auditory–somatosensory stimulation induces changes in the nucleus basalis-acetylcholine pathway, the locus coeruleus-noradrenaline pathway, as well as the raphe nucleus-serotonin pathway. Recent research revealed modulation of the locus coeruleus-

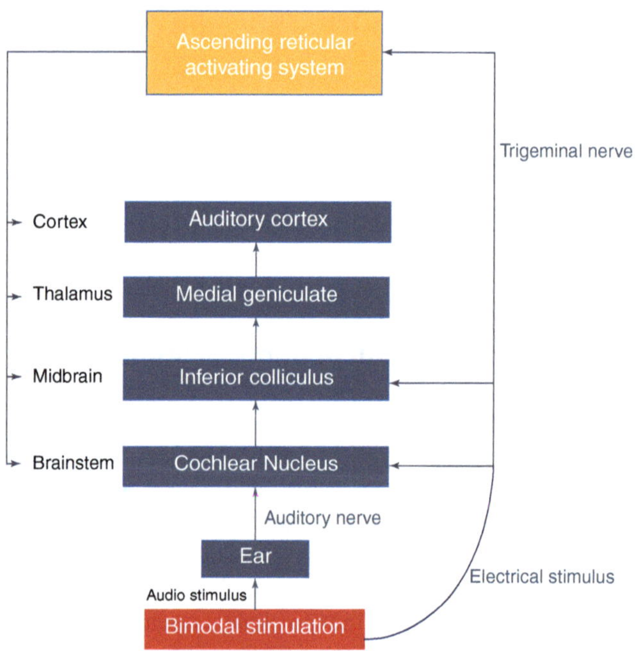

Fig. 54.5 The neural pathways suggested to be activated by that somatosensory stimulation

noradrenaline pathway by simulating the dorsal column pathway, i.e., the greater occipital nerve [34].

Electrical stimulation of the tongue presumably also modulates the trigeminal nerve, similar to the bimodal auditory–somatosensory stimulation approach [20]. Furthermore, animal studies have shown that sound paired with electrical stimulation of different body locations (or related nerves), such as the face, neck, ear, tongue, back, and limbs can all drive extensive neural plasticity across the auditory pathway, including the cochlear nucleus, inferior colliculus, and auditory cortex [7, 8, 35–39]. Further research is needed to explore to what extent these different approaches are unique from a mechanistic point of view and what they share.

In addition to the electrically stimulated structure, the used parameters (amplitude, pulses, the timeframe of treatment, the length of a daily session, specific auditory tones, pairing …) presumably play an important role. Moreover, variation of all these parameters may interact in a complex way. The identification of the optimal stimulus parameters for the individual patient remains a major challenge, especially when the heterogeneity of tinnitus is considered. Therefore, the success rate of a certain treatment may also depend on the characteristics of the treated patient sample.

Pairing and Habituation

Although basic research for both auditory–somatosensory stimulation and vagus nerve stimulation suggests that pairing seems to be essential and needs to be millisecond precise; it is not clear to what extent this applies in humans. The clinical trial on tongue stimulation revealed that synchronous (arm 1) and less synchronous (arms 2 and 3) bimodal stimulation had similar effects on tinnitus handicap inventory and tinnitus functional index [21] [40]. The clinical trial on vagus nerve stimulation revealed that vagus nerve stimulation unpaired with tone therapy did not significantly differ from paired stimulation, further questioning the relevance of millisecond pairing [12]. Moreover, in studies on vagus nerve stimulation paired with a motor task for the upper limb motor function after ischemic stroke, vagus nerve stimulation was effective even if the pairing was not millisecond precise [41].

These clinical results are in certain contrast with findings from animal research, where the comparison of different intervals (±5, ±10, and ±20 ms) of somatosensory and auditory stimulation revealed a clear relevance of the stimulation interval [7]. However, this finding still needs replication in humans.

Furthermore, recent research suggests that bimodal stimulation might have a habituation effect [40]. That is, in a large-scale clinical trial, bimodal sound and tongue stimulation drove significant treatment-related reductions in tinnitus symptom severity during the first 6 weeks, followed by a plateau during the second 6 weeks [21]. In a follow-up study, two different bimodal stimulation combinations (arm 1: 6 weeks of pure tone burst together with tongue stimulation, then switch to another 6 weeks of tongue stimulation immediately followed by pure tone burst; arm 2: 6 weeks of a brief tongue stimulation tone followed by a long pure tone burst with an interval of 700–800 ms in-between, then switched to another 6 weeks immediately followed by wideband noise) were compared. Significant improvements in tinnitus symptoms were observed in both arms within 6 weeks of initiating treatment. In arm 1, there was a mean reduction in tinnitus handicap inventory and tinnitus functional index score of 12.9 and 11.6 points, respectively, and in arm 2, there was a mean reduction of 11.5 and 11.7 points, respectively. There was no significant difference in outcomes between arm 1 and arm 2 for tinnitus handicap inventory or tinnitus functional index. Both arms exhibited significant reductions in tinnitus handicap inventory and tinnitus functional index scores, demonstrating that background noise is probably not necessary for patients to benefit from bimodal stimulation.

Outcome

All clinical studies used the tinnitus handicap inventory and/or tinnitus functional index as primary outcomes measure. This outcome measure reflects mainly changes in emotional state or distress, rather than the tinnitus loudness [42]. Both the clinical bimodal study on vagus nerve stimulation and auditory–somatosensory stimulation reported a proxy for tinnitus loudness using minimal masking levels or tinnitus spectra using an interactive computer program, respectively. In these measurements, short-term effects of the interventions have been shown [7, 12]. Future studies would ideally also incorporate physiological measures in addition to questionnaires and psychoacoustic measurements, in order to better understand how the various interventions exert their effects.

Conclusion

Bimodal stimulation represents an exciting new approach for the treatment of tinnitus. While the various approaches differ in many details, they have in common, that electrical nerve stimulation is combined with auditory presentation to induce neuronal plasticity in the central auditory pathways. It is important that rigorous, large-scale, double-blind, sham-controlled, and multicentric clinical trials will be performed to investigate the efficacy of the bimodal treatments. Tinnitus continues to prove to be a challenging area to research, especially in humans given the subjectivity and variability of the symptoms, as well as assessing the outcomes. Future research should investigate the effects of bimodal treatment for different tinnitus subtypes in order to enable a broader scope of treatment to be established and translational research to develop the best targets and approaches that could benefit the largest possible number of patients.

References

1. Eggermont JJ, Roberts LE. The neuroscience of tinnitus. Trends Neurosci. 2004;27(11):676–82. https://doi.org/10.1016/j.tins.2004.08.010.
2. Elgoyhen AB, Langguth B, De Ridder D, Vanneste S. Tinnitus: perspectives from human neuroimaging. Nat Rev Neurosci. 2015;16(10):632–42. https://doi.org/10.1038/nrn4003.
3. Shore SE, Roberts LE, Langguth B. Maladaptive plasticity in tinnitus--triggers, mechanisms and treatment. Nat Rev Neurol. 2016;12(3):150–60. https://doi.org/10.1038/nrneurol.2016.12.
4. De Ridder D, Vanneste S, Langguth B, Llinas R. Thalamocortical dysrhythmia: a theoretical update in tinnitus. Front Neurol. 2015;6:124. https://doi.org/10.3389/fneur.2015.00124.
5. Llinas R, Urbano FJ, Leznik E, Ramirez RR, van Marle HJ. Rhythmic and dysrhythmic thalamocortical dynamics: GABA systems and the edge effect. Trends Neurosci. 2005;28(6):325–33. https://doi.org/10.1016/j.tins.2005.04.006.
6. Llinas RR, Ribary U, Jeanmonod D, Kronberg E, Mitra PP. Thalamocortical dysrhythmia: a neurological and neuropsychiatric syndrome characterized by magnetoencephalography. Proc Natl Acad Sci U S A. 1999;96(26):15222–7.
7. Marks KL, Martel DT, Wu C, Basura GJ, Roberts LE, Schvartz-Leyzac KC, Shore SE. Auditory-somatosensory bimodal stimulation desynchronizes brain circuitry to reduce tinnitus in Guinea pigs and humans. Sci Transl Med. 2018;10(422):eaal3175. https://doi.org/10.1126/scitranslmed.aal3175.
8. Engineer ND, Riley JR, Seale JD, Vrana WA, Shetake JA, Sudanagunta SP, Kilgard MP. Reversing pathological neural activity using targeted plasticity. Nature. 2011;470(7332):101–4. https://doi.org/10.1038/nature09656.
9. Komiya H, Eggermont JJ. Spontaneous firing activity of cortical neurons in adult cats with reorganized tonotopic map following pure-tone trauma. Acta Otolaryngol. 2000;120(6):750–6. https://doi.org/10.1080/000164800750000298.
10. Muhlnickel W, Elbert T, Taub E, Flor H. Reorganization of auditory cortex in tinnitus. Proc Natl Acad Sci U S A. 1998;95(17):10340–3. https://doi.org/10.1073/pnas.95.17.10340.
11. De Ridder D, Kilgard M, Engineer N, Vanneste S. Placebo-controlled vagus nerve stimulation paired with tones in a patient with refractory tinnitus: a case report. Otol Neurotol. 2015;36(4):575–80. https://doi.org/10.1097/MAO.0000000000000704.
12. Tyler R, Cacace A, Stocking C, Tarver B, Engineer N, Martin J, et al. Vagus nerve stimulation paired with tones for the treatment of tinnitus: a prospective randomized double-blind controlled pilot study in humans. Sci Rep. 2017;7(1):11960. https://doi.org/10.1038/s41598-017-12178-w.
13. Vanneste S, Martin J, Rennaker RL 2nd, Kilgard MP. Pairing sound with vagus nerve stimulation modulates cortical synchrony and phase coherence in tinnitus: an exploratory retrospective study. Sci Rep. 2017;7(1):17345. https://doi.org/10.1038/s41598-017-17750-y.
14. Lehtimaki J, Hyvarinen P, Ylikoski M, Bergholm M, Makela JP, Aarnisalo A, et al. Transcutaneous vagus nerve stimulation in tinnitus: a pilot study. Acta Otolaryngol. 2013;133(4):378–82. https://doi.org/10.3109/00016489.2012.750736.
15. Shim HJ, Kwak MY, An YH, Kim DH, Kim YJ, Kim HJ. Feasibility and safety of transcutaneous Vagus nerve stimulation paired with notched music therapy for the treatment of chronic tinnitus. J Audiol Otol. 2015;19(3):159–67. https://doi.org/10.7874/jao.2015.19.3.159.
16. Kreuzer PM, Landgrebe M, Resch M, Husser O, Schecklmann M, Geisreiter F, et al. Feasibility, safety and efficacy of transcutaneous vagus nerve stimulation in chronic tinnitus: an open pilot study. Brain Stimul. 2014;7(5):740–7. https://doi.org/10.1016/j.brs.2014.05.003.
17. Shore SE, El Kashlan H, Lu J. Effects of trigeminal ganglion stimulation on unit activity of ventral cochlear nucleus neurons. Neuroscience. 2003;119(4):1085–101. https://doi.org/10.1016/s0306-4522(03)00207-0.
18. Zhou J, Shore S. Convergence of spinal trigeminal and cochlear nucleus projections in the inferior colliculus of the Guinea pig. J Comp Neurol. 2006;495(1):100–12. https://doi.org/10.1002/cne.20863.
19. Tzounopoulos T, Kim Y, Oertel D, Trussell LO. Cell-specific, spike timing-dependent plasticities in the dorsal cochlear nucleus. Nat Neurosci. 2004;7(7):719–25. https://doi.org/10.1038/nn1272.
20. Hamilton C, D'Arcy S, Pearlmutter BA, Crispino G, Lalor EC, Conlon BJ. An investigation of feasibility and safety of bi-modal stimulation for the treatment of tinnitus: an open-label pilot study. Neuromodulation. 2016;19(8):832–7. https://doi.org/10.1111/ner.12452.
21. Conlon B, Langguth B, Hamilton C, Hughes S, Meade E, Connor CO, Lim HH. Bimodal neuromodulation combining sound and tongue stimulation reduces tinnitus symptoms in a large randomized clinical study. Sci Transl Med. 2020;12(564):eabb2830. https://doi.org/10.1126/scitranslmed.abb2830.
22. Fuller T, Cima R, Langguth B, Mazurek B, Vlaeyen JW, Hoare DJ. Cognitive behavioural therapy for tinnitus. Cochrane Database Syst Rev. 2020;1:CD012614. https://doi.org/10.1002/14651858.CD012614.pub2.
23. Engineer ND, Moller AR, Kilgard MP. Directing neural plasticity to understand and treat tinnitus. Hear Res. 2013;295:58–66. https://doi.org/10.1016/j.heares.2012.10.001.
24. Hulsey DR, Hays SA, Khodaparast N, Ruiz A, Das P, Rennaker RL 2nd, Kilgard MP. Reorganization of motor cortex by Vagus nerve stimulation requires cholinergic innervation. Brain Stimul. 2016;9(2):174–81. https://doi.org/10.1016/j.brs.2015.12.007.
25. Hulsey DR, Shedd CM, Sarker SF, Kilgard MP, Hays SA. Norepinephrine and serotonin are required for vagus nerve stimulation directed cortical plasticity. Exp Neurol. 2019;320:112975. https://doi.org/10.1016/j.expneurol.2019.112975.
26. Manta S, Dong J, Debonnel G, Blier P. Enhancement of the function of rat serotonin and norepinephrine neurons by sustained vagus nerve stimulation. J Psychiatry Neurosci. 2009;34(4):272–80.
27. Sumal KK, Blessing WW, Joh TH, Reis DJ, Pickel VM. Synaptic interaction of vagal afferents and catecholaminergic neurons in the rat nucleus tractus solitarius. Brain Res. 1983;277(1):31–40. https://doi.org/10.1016/0006-8993(83)90904-6.
28. Van Bockstaele EJ, Peoples J, Telegan P. Efferent projections of the nucleus of the solitary tract to peri-locus coeruleus dendrites in rat brain: evidence for a monosynaptic pathway. J Comp Neurol. 1999;412(3):410–28. https://doi.org/10.1002/(sici)1096-9861(19990927)412:3<410::aid-cne3>3.0.co;2-f.
29. Kilgard MP, Merzenich MM. Cortical map reorganization enabled by nucleus basalis activity. Science. 1998;279(5357):1714–8.
30. Kilgard MP, Merzenich MM. Plasticity of temporal information processing in the primary auditory cortex. Nat Neurosci. 1998;1(8):727–31. https://doi.org/10.1038/3729.
31. Borland MS, Vrana WA, Moreno NA, Fogarty EA, Buell EP, Vanneste S, et al. Pairing vagus nerve stimulation with tones

drives plasticity across the auditory pathway. J Neurophysiol. 2019;122(2):659–71. https://doi.org/10.1152/jn.00832.2018.
32. Langers DR, de Kleine E, van Dijk P. Tinnitus does not require macroscopic tonotopic map reorganization. Front Syst Neurosci. 2012;6:2. https://doi.org/10.3389/fnsys.2012.00002.
33. Riffle TL, Martel DT, Jones GR, Shore SE. Bimodal auditory electrical stimulation for the treatment of tinnitus: preclinical and clinical studies. Curr Top Behav Neurosci. 2020; https://doi.org/10.1007/7854_2020_180.
34. Vanneste S, Mohan A, Yoo HB, Huang Y, Luckey AM, McLeod SL, et al. The peripheral effect of direct current stimulation on brain circuits involving memory. Sci Adv. 2020;6(45):eaax9538. https://doi.org/10.1126/sciadv.aax9538.
35. Basura GJ, Koehler SD, Shore SE. Multi-sensory integration in brainstem and auditory cortex. Brain Res. 2012;1485:95–107.
36. Gloeckner CD, Smith BT, Markovitz CD, Lim HH. A new concept for noninvasive tinnitus treatment utilizing multimodal pathways. Conf Proc IEEE Eng Med Biol Soc. 2013;2013:3122–5. https://doi.org/10.1109/EMBC.2013.6610202.
37. Koehler SD, Shore SE. Stimulus-timing dependent multisensory plasticity in the Guinea pig dorsal cochlear nucleus. PLoS One. 2013;8(3):e59828. https://doi.org/10.1371/journal.pone.0059828.
38. Koehler SD, Shore SE. Stimulus timing-dependent plasticity in dorsal cochlear nucleus is altered in tinnitus. J Neurosci. 2013;33(50):19647–56. https://doi.org/10.1523/JNEUROSCI.2788-13.2013.
39. Markovitz CD, Smith BT, Gloeckner CD, Lim HH. Investigating a new neuromodulation treatment for brain disorders using synchronized activation of multimodal pathways. Sci Rep. 2015;5:9462. https://doi.org/10.1038/srep09462.
40. Conlon B, Hamilton C, Meade E, Leong SL, O'Connor C, Langguth B, Vanneste S, Hall DA, Hughes A, Lim HH. Bimodal neuromodulation for tinnitus treatment: adjusting stimulus features over time achieves greater improvements in symptoms in a large randomized clinical study. Scientific Reports, 2022; 12:1–18.
41. Dawson J, Liu CY, Francisco GE, Cramer SC, Wolf SL, Dixit A, Alexander J, Ali R, Brown BL, Feng W, DeMark L, Hochberg LR, Kautz SA, Majid A, O'Dell MW, Pierce D, Prudente CN, Redgrave J, Turner DL, Engineer ND, Kimberley TJ. "Vagus nerve stimulation paired with rehabilitation for upper limb motor function after ischaemic stroke (VNS-REHAB): a randomised, blinded, pivotal, device trial." Lancet 397 (10284); 2021:1545–53.
42. Deklerck AN, Marechal C, Perez Fernandez AM, Keppler H, Van Roost D, Dhooge IJM. Invasive neuromodulation as a treatment for tinnitus: a systematic review. Neuromodulation. 2020;23(4):451–62. https://doi.org/10.1111/ner.13042.

Complementary and Alternative Therapies

55

Alain Londero and Deborah A. Hall

Abstract

In the absence of a validated therapy aimed at silencing their tinnitus, many patients turn to complementary alternative medicines (CAM) with the hope of finding a cure. A variety of therapies are proposed such as acupuncture and traditional Chinese medicine, herbal remedies, zinc and other oligo-elements, melatonin, homeopathy, and aromatherapy. A literature review demonstrates that there is poor scientific evidence supporting the use of any CAM in the field of tinnitus. The importance of the placebo effect and ethical issues linked to the use of CAM are discussed.

A. Londero (✉)
Service ORL et CCF Hôpital Européen Georges Pompidou, Assistance Publique—Hôpitaux de Paris. Faculté de Médecine Paris Descartes—Université de Paris, Paris, France

D. A. Hall
Hearing Sciences, Mental Health and Clinical Neurosciences, School of Medicine, University of Nottingham, Nottingham, UK

Department of Psychology, School of Social Sciences, Heriot-Watt University Malaysia, Putrajaya, Malaysia
e-mail: deborah.hall@hw.ac.uk

W. Schlee et al. (eds.), *Textbook of Tinnitus*, https://doi.org/10.1007/978-3-031-35647-6_55

Graphical Abstract

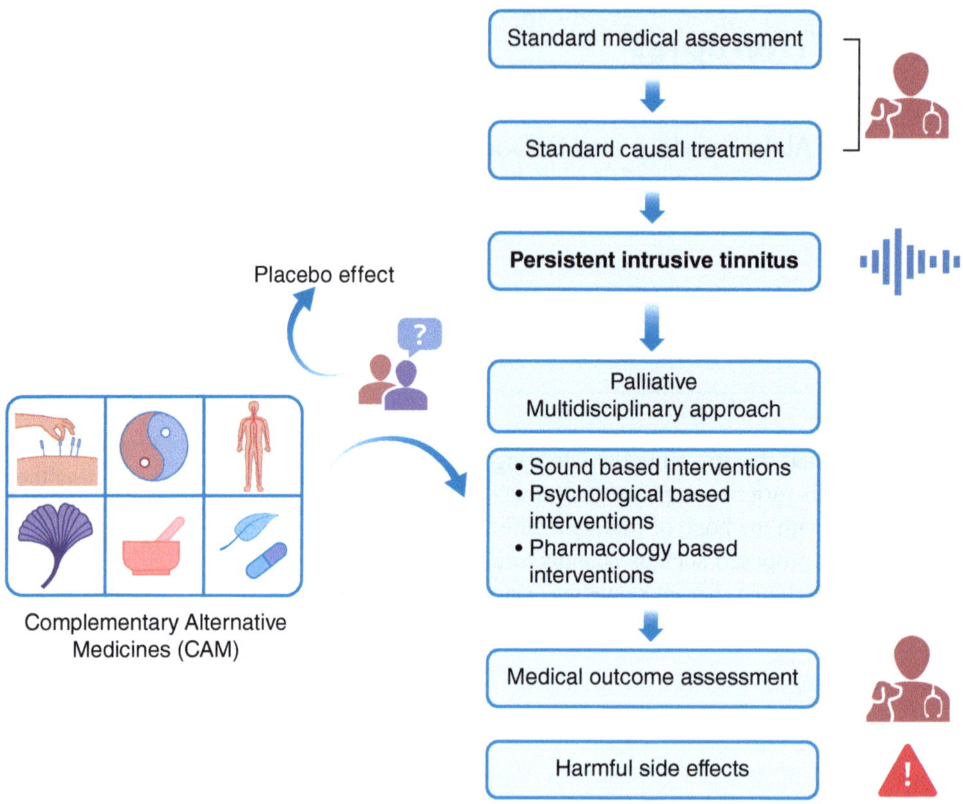

Highlights

- Many patients with subjective tinnitus turn to complementary and alternative therapies because of the lack of a cure and no standard treatment.
- There is little or no evidence suggesting that complementary and alternative approaches confer a specific therapeutic benefit for subjective tinnitus.
- For patients with mild-to-moderate depression, St John's Wort has similar efficacy and safety to selective serotonin reuptake inhibitors (antidepressants).
- For patients with anxiety, kava extract has similar efficacy to placebo.
- Complementary and alternative treatments do not mean absence of potential harmful side effects.
- In certain circumstances, the placebo effect could be a legitimate therapeutic option in subjective tinnitus management.
- If considered, alternative interventions should be integrated in a multidisciplinary approach under medical supervision.

Introduction

The majority of individuals with tinnitus know that, in most cases, there is no available medical or surgical intervention in the western medical practice to silence their auditory percept [1]. Conversely, it appears that many patients continue to look for a cure and thus turn to complementary and alternative approaches [2]. Complementary and alternative medicine (CAM) is the term for medical products and practices that are out of the medical mainstream. Complementary medicine refers to cases where these therapies are used along with traditional Western medicine, while alternative medicine refers to cases where these approaches are used instead of traditional Western medicine. The literature shows rather a lack of consistency in the definition of what treatments should be considered as complementary or alternative medicine. However, some of the most frequently used and well-known examples include oriental medicine such as acupuncture and herbal therapy, dietary supplements such as vitamins, chiropractic, aromatherapy, and homeopathy. For the purposes of this chapter, we do not consider cognitive behavioral therapy or mindfulness meditation as complementary or alternative treatments, in contrast to the review by Wolover et al. [3]. This is because they are now prescribed as conventional standalone treatments in a number of Western countries. A Swedish study in 1997 showed that almost 2/3 of patients (45 out of 69 consecutive patients) had already tried a complementary or alternative treatment before attending a specialized tinnitus clinic [4]. Of those 45, 19 had tried acupuncture, 13 had tried relaxation, and 13 had tried other treatments. The popularity of these treatments is also confirmed by a recent study that unveiled real-life patients' concerns about tinnitus by examining their social media conversations. Following previous works that analyzed text material freely available online using natural language processing techniques [5, 6], 130,000 posts from Reddit social media were studied using nonsupervised and automated text mining methods (cluster analysis and latent Derichlet allocation). Preliminary results of the cluster analysis revealed 16 clusters among which, two clusters relevant to complementary and alternative treatments emerged: "Hope for a cure," and "Use of dietary supplements" [7] (see Box 55.1).

Box 55.1
Illustrative text excerpts from the two clusters. Relevant words have been highlighted in bold.

Hope for a cure

- "i_ve had tinnitus for 4 months and reading stuff like this is some kind of a **relieve** i was **lucky** or w e you want to call it to live in an era of **technological breakthroughs** i **hope** someone finds a **cure** within my **lifetime**"
- "you just have to **realize** it_s a slight **handicap** and that if you want to keep your **sanity** we all just have to **learn to live with it** and **hope for a cure** sometime in the **future** they_re working on it"
- "i don_t **expect** a **cure** any time soon but i do **hope** they develop some kind of **effective treatment** within my **lifetime**".

Use of dietary supplements

- "i_ve been **vegan** this month as a challenge didn_t notice my t getting worse but could this be a side effect of lower **iron zinc** i take a **b12** supplement and **magnesium** nightly"
- "try **magnesium** almost everyone is deficient in it and it does have hand in spasms in the inner ear which can be linked to tinnitus in fact some people report after taking **vitamin d supplements** that pulsatile tinnitus develops"
- "so i haven_t spent much time on the road always aggravates it i_ve been taking **daily supplements** the usual **vitamins** and **magnesium** other than that i haven_t really been sleeping well not doing anything that differently that would be considered a **cure"**

In this chapter, we introduce some of the main concepts of the following CAM treatments: acupuncture, ginkgo biloba, and some other herbal remedies, zinc and other oligo-elements, melatonin, homeopathy, and aromatherapy. In keeping with a brief review, we limit our scope to reporting scientific findings from systematic reviews and meta-analyses that identify and pool together results from individual clinical trials. We consider the evidence for benefits (clinical effectiveness) and harms (adverse events), and comment on the overall strength and quality of the evidence. Our aim is to give the reader a broad appreciation of whether or not these different treatment approaches have clinical utility in alleviating the symptoms of subjective tinnitus.

Introduction to Traditional Chinese Medicine

Traditional Chinese Medicine (TCM) is a branch of oriental medicine originating and widely practiced in China. TCM is a form of holistic medicine which focuses on healing both physical and nonphysical aspects of health conditions. In contrast to Western medicine, TCM places less emphasis on anatomical structures and more on its unique system of nonphysical attributes collectively known as the three major functional entities. These are (1) the five fundamental substances (vital life force "qi," blood, body fluids, essence, and spirit); (2) a cycle of five zang organs, six fu organs, and their functions; and (3) the channels "meridians" through which qi flows. Ill health and disease are perceived as a disharmony (or imbalance) in the functions or interactions of these functional entities and/or of the interaction between the human body and the environment.

Taking this holistic approach, TCM does not conceive tinnitus as an auditory disorder. Instead, tinnitus is seen as the manifestation of a wider disorder affecting the major functional entities. A starting point for tinnitus is the kidneys, since TCM views the ears as the sensory organs related to the kidney, leading to disharmony between the kidney and the heart [8]. In this way, any ear problems, such as age-related hearing loss, tinnitus, and ear infections are signs that the kidney's energy may need extra support. There is some empirical evidence to support the association between age-related hearing loss and kidney deficiency. For example, Dong and colleagues [9] have shown that glutathione metabolism, amino acid metabolism, glucose metabolism, the *N*-methyl-d-aspartic acid (NMDA) receptor pathway, and the γ-aminobutyric acid (GABA) receptor pathway may be related to the pathogenesis of hearing loss. However, such evidence is not to say that tinnitus indicates damage to the patient's kidneys. Rather, the diagnosis means that the Chinese medical doctor will seek to influence the flow of blood and essential energies through the meridian circuit that is linked to the kidneys.

TCM doctors describe two types of tinnitus [10]. The first is a "deficiency type" and is attributed to a kidney-essence deficiency, as described above. The second is an "excess type" and is attributed to rising liver and gall-bladder fire. TCM theory connects this type of tinnitus to emotional strain, sometimes accompanied by headaches and dizziness. In summary, the deficiency type reflects a chronic shortage of essential energy while the excess type reflects a significant imbalance of energies in the patient's body. Each type of tinnitus requires a particular treatment approach.

Treatments often seek to exert influence via the meridians which operate as a highway throughout the entire body. Meridian points serve as the cornerstone for understanding how intervention might provide tinnitus relief. It is important to bear in mind that these meridians are nonphysical, and so there is no direct analogy within Western medicine since it focuses primarily on anatomy and physiology. However, similar to Western medicine, the goal for TCM is to address the root cause of the problem along with any other symptoms that may be present. Furthermore, the doctor's final decision about treatment is also influenced by other holistic factors such as the patient's general health status, their medical history, and any other comorbid symptoms are present. Prescribed interventions typically include acupuncture, diet, herbal therapy, meditation, physical exercise, and massage.

Acupuncture

Acupuncture involves the insertion of fine needles into the skin at certain points on the body to stimulate relevant acupoints. The overall aim is to clear any blockages along the meridians, thus restoring the flow of qi throughout the body [11]. Acupuncture is one of the more popular forms of complementary and alternative medicine, and it is a well-known treatment for tinnitus, in other countries as well as in China. In the case of the deficiency type of tinnitus, the specific purpose of acupuncture is to mobilize the whole body's essential energies and boost their circulation. While in the case of excess type, the specific purpose is to gather the body's energies, place them under control, and to re-establish a healthy balance in circulation.

While acupuncture has been the subject of numerous published studies, clinical trials, and systematic reviews, the conclusions are often mixed. Gilbey and colleagues (2013), [12] set out to review all those systematic reviews of acupuncture in an attempt to better answer the question "does acupuncture work and, if so, for what conditions?" Their search used the databases MEDLINE (via Ovid), Scopus and EbscoHost for the period 1991 to 2011, and search terms used were (systematic review) AND (acupuncture OR acupressure). Overall, 18 systematic reviews of acupuncture on humans were identified. These reviews considered acupuncture for a range of health conditions such as nausea/vomiting, headache, insomnia, chronic pain, arthritis, but only one considered tinnitus [13]. Overall, Gilbey et al. [12] erred on the side of caution by suggesting a need for more well-designed, large-scale clinical trials. However, they recommended focusing on acupuncture for chemotherapy-induced nausea and vomiting and for the pain of migraines, neck disorders, tension-type headaches, and peripheral joint arthritis since these were the indications showing the most promising results.

There have been several systematic reviews specifically of acupuncture for tinnitus [14, 15], but these reviews had a bias against articles published in Chinese. More recently, Liu et al. [16] conducted a focused systematic review and meta-analysis of randomized controlled trials (RCTs) using acupuncture to treat tinnitus. Their search used the following databases spanning the period 1966–2013: China Network Knowledge Infrastructure, Chinese Scientific Journal Database VIP, PubMed, EMBASE, and the Cochrane Library. Search terms used were (acupuncture) OR (acupressure) OR (acupoint) OR (electroacupuncture) AND (tinnitus). Overall, 18 RCTs were included in the systematic review (1086 participants), and 11 of those RCTs made it into the meta-analysis. Analysis of the pooled data suggested some advantage for acupuncture over conventional therapies (RR = 1.18, 95% CI = 1.02–1.37). No serious side effects were reported in any of the RCTs, and only some mild transient pain was reported in one RCT. Published in the same year, a focused systematic review of RCTs and quasi-RCTs using electroacupuncture to treat tinnitus (322 participants) came to similar conclusions about efficacy [17], and noted a lack of reporting adverse events. It is interesting to note that 10 out of the 18 studies were conducted in China and published in Chinese language, highlighting the importance of avoiding any Western-centric bias when reviewing the effectiveness of oriental medicine. The methodological flaws and high risk of bias, especially in the Chinese RCTs, prevent any firm conclusions that acupuncture is safe and effective in reducing tinnitus.

Ginkgo Biloba

Ginkgo biloba (Chinese Maidenhair) is a tree originating from China that is now common around the world as an ornamental tree. Its seeds have been used as snacks and medical materials in TCM, while over the last century, its leaf extracts have emerged as active ingredients to pharmaceutical products related to brain health in Western medicine. Ginkgo biloba is categorized as a "dietary supplement" in many tinnitus clinical guidelines (see section "Clinical Practice Guidelines and CAM"), but since it stems from TCM so we describe it here in this section of our chapter.

According to TCM, illness can enter the organs and channels of the body when the major functional entities are imbalanced. The five major flavors (bitter, sour, salty, pungent, and sweet) also indicate a food's therapeutic effect upon the body's systems because how a food tastes determines what organs and meridians it targets [18]. In this way, the botanical world provides a full palette of flavors for promoting harmony among the body's energies. Ginkgo leaves taste both bitter and sweet and so this herbal remedy has dual medicinal actions. Bitter flavors act first on the heart while sweet flavors act first on the spleen, extending to the lungs and stomach. TCM views the heart as the source of individual vitality, while the lungs are thought to be a key part of the production chain for qi and the body fluids that nourish the body.

In Western cultures, therapeutic benefit considers the physiological effects of the plant's active ingredients. For example, the leaf extract of ginkgo contains flavonoids, glycosides, and ginkgolides which improve blood flow through vasodilation and serve as an antioxidant [19]. Vascular problems and oxidative stress are two of the suggested causes for tinnitus. Vascular disease can cause problems in the blood supply to the labyrinthine artery and can thus induce hypoxia in the outer hair cells of the cochlea which in turn can lead to subjective tinnitus. Oxidative stress is caused by reactive molecules (free radicals) that form during the energy conversion of food to oxygen and can cause cochlear damage by attacking important cellular constituents such as lipids, proteins, and deoxyribonucleic acid (DNA) [20]. According to a Western medical model, the rationale for ginkgo biloba as a treatment for tinnitus is that adequate blood supply to the cochlea can stop this process of hypoxia and can counter oxidative stress by scavenging free radicals.

The Cochrane group has maintained an interest in the effects of ginkgo biloba for tinnitus. The first systematic review was published in 2004, and has been updated most recently in 2013 [21]. They searched the Cochrane Ear, Nose and Throat Disorders Group Trials Register; the Cochrane Central Register of Controlled Trials (CENTRAL); PubMed; EMBASE; Allied and complementary Medicine Database (AMED); Web of Science; BIOSIS Previews; Cambridge Scientific Abstracts; International Clinical Trials Registry Platform (ICTRP) as well as additional sources for published and unpublished trials over the period 1966–2013. Their search syntax looked for RCTs associated with (ginkgo biloba, and its name variants) AND (hearing disorders OR tinnitus). Four RCTs with a total of 1543 participants were included in the review. All four RCTs were rated as high-quality methodology and low risk of bias, since they were double-blind and placebo-controlled. The narrative synthesis led to the conclusion that there was no evidence for the therapeutic benefit of ginkgo biloba for tinnitus compared to placebo, although a meta-analysis could not be conducted because the studies reported different outcome measures. Some participants reported headaches and stomach upsets but these were just as common in the placebo group as in the treated group. These conclusions are based on articles published up to March 2012 and so it is perhaps unsurprising that Sereda and colleagues (2020) [22] made a call to prioritize an update on the Cochrane systematic review.

Dietary Supplements

The term dietary supplements is used to generalize nutritional and herbal substances promoted as remedies. Dietary supplements that come in the form of pills, capsules, powders, gel tabs, extracts, or liquids are added to the regular diet aiming at treating or preventing a variety of conditions including tinnitus [2, 23] and related symptoms such as anxiety or depression [24]. Some supplements are based on herbal ingredients (e.g., St John's Wort, kava), others are based on minerals (e.g., zinc, magnesium) or vitamins. Scientific evidence for the efficacy of these dietary supplements for subjective tinnitus is poor, yet they are commonly used by patients. In 2016, an Internet-based survey (1788 subjects from 53 countries) analyzed the benefit and harms of dietary supplements to treat tinnitus [25]. From this sample, 413 patients (23.1%) reported taking supplements, with a positive outcome in only 19% of them. There was no effect in 70.7% and even worsening in 10.3%. Some anecdotal side effects have been reported like bleeding, headache, or diarrhea (6.3%). One should stress that even if most of these dietary supplements and herbal medicines are freely available over the counter, that does not mean that they do not carry safety concerns. There can be negative side effects caused by herbs, plants, or by large doses of vitamin and mineral supplements [26]. Interactions with other prescribed drugs may also be a clinical issue [27].

St John's Wort for Symptoms of Depression

St John's Wort (SJW) or Hypericum perforatum is a flowering plant (Hypericaceae) that has been used for centuries in the traditional pharmacopeia. Although perhaps not prescribed for tinnitus per se, SJW may help relieve some of the common comorbidities of tinnitus, especially depressive feelings since it is commonly proposed as a natural antidepressant [28]. Studies have evaluated its effects compared to standard antidepressant drugs such as selective serotonin reuptake inhibitors (SSRI). For example, a systematic search of articles relevant to SJW and depression from 1960 to 2016 identified 27 clinical trials comparing the use of SJW and SSRI, with a total of 3808 participants with a mild-to-moderate depression [28]. Meta-analysis demonstrated a comparable benefit for SJW and standard SSRIs (RR = 0.98, 95% CI = 0.92–1.04) as measured using the Hamilton Rating Scale for Depression (HAM-D). In addition, SJW had a significantly smaller number of patients discontinuing treatment/dropping out due to adverse/side effects (OR = 0.59, 95% CI = 0.48–0.70). As observed in other reviews, the authors here also made the comment that studies from China had weaker methodological quality and also higher risk of bias. Although generally well tolerated in the short term, long-term intake of SJW may induce a variety of side effects: gastrointestinal (nausea, diarrhea, loss of appetite…), neurologic (fatigue, dizziness, headache ...), visual, dermatologic (sun sensitivity). It may also cause allergic reactions. Moreover, SJW has been shown to cause multiple drug interactions through induction of the cytochrome P450 enzymes CYP3A4 and CYP1A2. The increased metabolism leading to decreased plasma concentration of other drugs has a potential clinical effect, for example, in case of use of estrogen oral contraceptives. Then SJW can negatively interact with many prescribed drugs including the antipsychotics (e.g., risperidone), cyclosporine, digoxin, chemotherapies, or antiviral drugs. Conversely adding SJW to an antidepressant could provoke a serotonin syndrome [28].

Kava for Symptoms of Anxiety

Kava or Piper methysticum is a plant (Tracheophytes) whose root is consumed throughout the islands of the Pacific Ocean (Polynesia, Micronesia) for its sedating effects. To a lesser extent, kava extract is used in other countries as an herbal medicine. Although not prescribed for tinnitus per se, kava extract may help relieve feelings of generalized anxiety. A Cochrane systematic review identified publications up to 2005 describing double-blind, placebo-controlled randomized trials of kava extract for anxiety [29]. Twelve eligible RCTs reported data from 700 patients with anxiety, with seven trials providing data for meta-analysis based on the Hamilton Rating Scale for Anxiety (HAM-A). Findings showed a reduction of the HAM-A total score in patients receiving kava extract compared with patients receiving placebo (weighted mean difference = 3.9, 95% CI = 0.1–7.7). Four of seven RCTs in the meta-analysis had low risk of bias, while the remainder lacked either a description of randomization or double-blind procedures. In the review [29], six RCTs reported adverse effects experienced by patients receiving kava extract. Most frequent were stomach upsets, restlessness, drowsiness, tremor, headache, and tiredness. Four trials comprising 30% of patients in the reviewed trials report the absence of adverse events while taking kava extract. However, consumption of kava extracts produced with organic solvents, or excessive amounts of poor-quality kava products, may be linked to an increased risk of adverse health outcomes, including potential liver injury [30].

Zinc and Other Oligo-Elements

It has been observed that serum zinc levels decrease with age with a significant correlation between zinc levels and impairments in hearing thresholds, tinnitus severity, and tinnitus loudness [31]. Seemingly another study has shown that patients with tinnitus who had normal hearing had significantly lower serum zinc levels [32]. The same pattern of low serum magnesium levels in patients with tinnitus has been observed [33]. Since minerals have a role in cochlear physiology and in synaptic functioning within the central auditory system [34, 35], there is a plausible mechanism of action supporting the intake of minerals for auditory therapeutics. Some studies with a low quality of evidence have suggested that magnesium supplementation may improve hearing recovery in cases of idiopathic sudden hearing loss [36] or may have a beneficial effect on perception of tinnitus-related handicap [37].

In 2016, a Cochrane systematic review identified three RCTs comparing oral zinc supplementation with placebo with a total of 209 participants from a search of the ENT Trials Register, CENTRAL, PubMed, EMBASE, Cumulative Index to Nursing and Allied Health Literature (CINAHL), Web of Science, ClinicalTrials.gov, and ICTRP [22]. Overall, they reported no evidence that zinc supplementation improves subjective tinnitus over placebo. This conclusion was based on a narrative synthesis because different outcome measures precluded meta-analysis. We note that none of the included studies reported any significant adverse effects, and all studies were rated at a moderate to high risk of bias.

Melatonin

There is a large body of literature on the multiple effects of exogenous and endogenous melatonin on health (sleep disturbance, psychiatric, and neurologic conditions including tinnitus). Melatonin or *N*-acetyl-5-methoxy tryptamine is a hormone produced by the pineal gland and secreted into the blood. Melatonin controls circadian and circannual rhythms, and synchronizes the internal hormonal environment to the day–night cycle [38]. Melatonin is a natural compound available over the counter in many countries for the treatment of insomnia and depression. The security profile of melatonin is good despite the presence of mild side effects (dizziness, headache, nausea, and sleepiness) [39]. Melatonin displays a variety of biological effects (antioxidative, anti-inflammatory, antiapoptotic, antinociceptive, antihypertensive, cytoprotective, and neuroprotective) that have been suggested to be useful against cochlear damage induced by acoustic trauma and ototoxic agents [40]. Several clinical studies have reported the ability of melatonin to minimize the severity of tinnitus and to improve sleep disturbance linked to tinnitus [41]. Thus, melatonin has been proposed as a potential treatment option for the patient with tinnitus [42]. Nevertheless, a systematic review of trials published prior March 2014 and found through PubMed, MEDLINE, EMBASE, CENTRAL, and Google Scholar has highlighted the weakness of the evidence in this regard [43]. The authors' findings were inconclusive given the high risk of biases observed. Five clinical studies were included in this review. Three studies evaluated the effect of melatonin alone (n = 111 participants); one open-label single arm study and two double-blind, placebo-controlled randomized trials. Two further RCTs (n = 222 participants) evaluated the effects of melatonin co-administered with sulpiride (as an antidepressant and tranquilizer) or sulodexide (to improve blood flow in the microcirculation in the inner ear), compared to a placebo control group. No serious adverse events were reported, suggesting that melatonin was well tolerated. However, further details are not given in the review.

Homeopathy

According to its inventor, Samuel Hahnemann (1755–1843), homeopathy is based on a twofold counterintuitive postulate. First, the presupposition that the more a substance is diluted the more potent it becomes. And second, the so-called "like cures like" principle stating that a substance "which can produce a set of symptoms in a healthy individual, can treat a sick individual who is manifesting a similar set of symptoms." An initial homeopathy medical interview is aimed at making an in-depth assessment of the symptoms displayed by each individual patient for determining what homeopathic products have to be prescribed. From a practical point of view, the method for preparing a homeopathic remedy is a serial dilution (and shaking) of a given substance where the solvent (water, alcohol) is added to part of the previous mixture. The dilution is generally expressed according to the Hahnemann's "centesimal" or "C" scale, where the dilution is at a 100 factor at each stage. Meaning that for a C 6 dilution, the original substance is one part of one trillion. Unlikely after a C 12 dilution even a single molecule of the original substance is present in the solvent. But dilutions of C 15 up to C 200 are commonly used and thus considered as the most controversial and unconvincing aspect of homeopathy practice. This mainly is why the potential mechanisms of action of homeopathy and benefits have long been debated [44] and seldom used in the tinnitus field. Nevertheless, even if the reality of homeopathy effects is disputed, homeopathy is used by just over 2% of the US population, predominantly for respiratory, otorhinolaryngology, and musculoskeletal complaints [45]. In France, where homeopathy is still partially reimbursed by the social national health insurance, this figure is even higher with 10.6% of the general population regularly taking homeopathy remedies [46]. A review, in 2010, of all Cochrane reviews of RCTs prescribing homeopathy for any medical condition or disease (e.g., cancer, attention-deficit hyperactivity disorder, asthma, dementia, influenza, and induction of labor) failed to demonstrate any effects beyond placebo [47].

In the field of tinnitus, we found only one double-blind, placebo-controlled evaluation of a homeopathic preparation, although the sample was small (n = 28 participants) [48]. The remedy was taken in tablet form at a homeopathic D60 potency. Findings revealed that neither ratings of perceived tinnitus intensity nor intrusiveness were significantly different in the treated group compared to placebo. The conclusion for tinnitus therefore is consistent with that for other health conditions, namely homeopathy lacks any scientifically demonstrated therapeutic benefit.

Aromatherapy

Essential oils are concentrated liquids taken from trees (e.g., pine-tree), plants (e.g., lavender, cannabis), herbs (e.g., peppermint), and fruits (e.g., citruses) which are commonly used for their pleasant flavor and scent. They are available over the counter and in most countries their retailing is not regulated as for pharmaceutical drugs. Nevertheless, such aromatic plant extracts have been used for centuries for their supposed healing properties in a nonconventional practice called aromatherapy. Some claims have been made about usefulness of essential oils in health care for example as an adjunct to cancer care [49]. Seemingly, cannabidiol (CBD) oil, the nonintoxicating constituent of cannabis (marijuana) extract, has been the subject of scientific research in the field of anxiety [50] and epilepsy [50] with an approval of the US Food and Drug Agency (FDA) in this latter indication. Even if there is no approved essential oil for tinnitus relief, many extracts are proposed on commercial websites (e.g., basil, garlic, lavender, juniper, CBD…). As regards the CBD oil, there has been no controlled study in humans testing the effect of cannabinoids on tinnitus itself. And some animal data may even suggest a negative effect of CBD on central auditory processing and tinnitus [51]. Finally, one should note oil extract may induce allergic reactions, interact with other prescribed drugs, and display teratogenic properties and thus should not be administered during pregnancy or while nursing without medical advice. We were unable to find any published systematic review or meta-analysis of aromatherapy for tinnitus.

Clinical Practice Guidelines and CAM

In recent years, a number of guidelines have been published in various countries to provide clinicians managing patients with tinnitus with a set of evidence-based recommendations.

A systematic review of clinical guidelines for tinnitus identified four management guidelines from Germany, the Netherlands, Sweden, and the United States [52]. Table 55.1 summarizes recommendations made for various complementary and alternative therapies. The US guideline for bothersome tinnitus lasting at least 6 months [53] is perhaps the best known and is described in more detail here. This guideline was supported by the American Academy of Otolaryngology—Head and Neck Surgery Foundation. It was developed by a multidisciplinary panel including the disciplines otolaryngology, neurology, audiology, psychiatry, and family practice. The panel evaluated the evidence for dietary supplements and acupuncture, but they did not consider other forms of CAM [53].

Based on the evidence gathered, the panel recommended against dietary supplements including ginkgo biloba, melatonin, and zinc. On the one hand, they expressed low confidence in the potential for benefits due to methodological concerns, poor study quality, and limited ability to generalize the published results to patients with persistent, bothersome tinnitus. On the other hand, they expressed high confidence in the potential for harms related to these products, particularly in the elderly who may be taking other medications at the same time. The panel noted that dietary supplements do not require approval from any regulatory authorities and so there are no manufacturing controls on the content and dosage of the proposed active ingredients. This was another cause for concern, especially with respect to potential drug interactions.

Based on the evidence, the panel was unable to provide any specific recommendation for acupuncture. Similar to the conclusions for dietary supplements, they expressed low confidence in the potential for benefits due to the heterogeneity and methodological flaws in the clinical trials. Again they judged there to be high confidence in the potential for harms, although they did recognize that the likelihood of serious harm was rare. It is interesting to note that viewpoints were divided between making no recommendation and making a recommendation against the use of acupuncture, perhaps because the balance between benefits and harms is unclear from the literature.

Since the systematic review of clinical guidelines by Fuller [52], there have been several new guidelines and these have generally come to similar recommendations. For example, in 2019, a pan-European team of multidisciplinary experts published a general set of guidelines [54]. Consistent with the US guidelines [53], the panel made no recommendation in support of acupuncture and a recommendation against use of dietary supplements for tinnitus. In 2020, the National Institute for Health and Clinical Excellence (NICE) published a UK evidence-based guideline for managing tinnitus in primary, community, and secondary care settings [55]. However, CAM was outside the scope of the NICE guideline, and so the evidence was not evaluated.

Table 55.1 Tinnitus guideline recommendations regarding treatments for tinnitus. In the guidelines, "dietary supplements" refer to ginkgo biloba, zinc, and melatonin without distinguishing between them. N/A denotes that the topic was out of scope for the clinical practice guideline and so the evidence was not considered

	Acupuncture	Dietary supplements	Homeopathy	Aromatherapy
Europe	No recommendation	Recommended against	N/A	N/A
Germany	No evidence of effectiveness	Recommended against	N/A	N/A
Netherlands	Recommended against	Recommended against	N/A	N/A
Sweden	N/A	N/A	N/A	N/A
UK	N/A	N/A	N/A	N/A
USA	No recommendation	Recommended against	N/A	N/A

A Comment on the Placebo Effect

The placebo effect refers to any physiological and/or psychological changes that result from the meaning derived by an individual within some sort of healthcare setting, especially in situations when doctors and patients interact with each other. An example is when the doctor and the patient share a positive expectancy that the intervention will be effective. As we have seen in this chapter, placebo effects can be as large as treatment effects. Placebo effects can therefore be clinically meaningful, but they are seldom fully exploited in clinical practice perhaps because doctors worry that they would be deceiving patients in order to elicit placebo effects [56].

Keeping in mind the low level of evidence supporting their efficacy, the prescription of CAM in the field of tinnitus eventually poses a deontological problem regarding the morality of the doctor's action. Is it ethical to use the placebo effect in the clinical practice of tinnitus management? The answer to this question is not straightforward. Indeed, even in the research context where double-blind, placebo-controlled randomized trials are a gold standard, the use of placebo has been questioned and so even the absence of treatment of reference [57]. On the other hand, it has been demonstrated that the placebo can be an effective treatment of auditory conditions like Meniere's disease [58] or hearing loss [59] as well as for tinnitus [60]. Waiting for a treatment may also be beneficial [61], perhaps because it carries expectation about receiving a future therapeutic benefit.

An article in the *Journal of Medical Ethics* set out an argument that the placebo may even be morally imperative in select cases, especially when it can be an effective treatment and does not entail deception [62]. In this article, the authors published a set of guidelines to explain situations in which a placebo would be justified in clinical practice [62]. See Table 55.2.

Table 55.2 The following practical guidelines might help to consider cases where there is a legitimate use of the placebo in clinical practice. Taken from Lichtenberg et al. J Med Ethics 2004;30:pp.553. (Lichtenberg et al. J Med Ethics 2004;30:pp.553)

• The intentions of the physician must be benevolent: his/her only concern the well-being of the patient. No economical, professional, or emotional interest should interfere with his/her decision
• The placebo, when offered, must be given in the spirit of assuaging the patient's suffering, and not merely mollifying him, silencing him, or otherwise failing to address his distress.
• When proven ineffective the placebo should be immediately withdrawn. In these circumstances, not only is the placebo useless, but it also undermines the subsequent effectiveness of medication by undoing the patient's conditioned response and expectation of being helped
• The placebo cannot be given in place of another medication that the physician reasonably expects to be more effective. Administration of placebo should be considered when a patient is refractory to standard treatment, suffers from its side effects, or is in a situation where standard treatment does not exist
• The physician should not hesitate to respond honestly when asked about the nature and anticipated effects of the placebo treatment he is offering
• If the patient is helped by the placebo, discontinuing the placebo, in absence of a more effective treatment, would be unethical

Concluding Remarks: Is There a Role for Complementary and Alternative Therapies?

Scientific evidence supporting the use of alternative therapies in the field of tinnitus treatment remains poor according to the evidence-based medicine standards. Nonetheless, keeping in mind that there is no curative intervention aimed at making the tinnitus percept disappear, the use of nonharmful complementary therapies and their potential placebo effect may be worth consideration in tinnitus patients' multidisciplinary management. Conversely, one should discourage the use of such unconventional interventions without medical supervision because this could let the patients get lost in an irrational search for a miraculous cure made of false hopes and costly, nonvalidated and sometimes even detrimental alternative therapies.

References

1. McFerran DJ, Stockdale D, Holme R, Large CH, Baguley DM. Why is there no cure for tinnitus? Front Neurosci. 2019;13:802.
2. Luetzenberg FS, Babu S, Seidman MD. Alternative treatments of tinnitus: alternative medicine. Otolaryngol Clin N Am. 2020;53(4):637–50.
3. Wolever RQ, Price R, Hazelton AG, Dmitrieva NO, Bechard EM, Shaffer JK, et al. Complementary therapies for significant dysfunction from tinnitus: treatment review and potential for integrative medicine. Evid Based Complement Alternat Med. 2015;2015:1–8.
4. Andersson G. Prior treatments in a Group of Tinnitus Sufferers Seeking Treatment. Psychother Psychosom. 1997;66(2):107–10.
5. Manchaiah V, Ratinaud P, Andersson G. Representation of tinnitus in the US newspaper media and in Facebook pages: cross-sectional analysis of secondary data. Interact J Med Res. 2018;7(1):e9.
6. Palacios G, Noreña A, Londero A. Assessing the heterogeneity of complaints related to tinnitus and Hyperacusis from an unsupervised machine learning approach: an exploratory study. Audiol Neurootol. 2020;25(4):174–89.
7. Manchaiah V, Londero A, Deshpande AK, Revel M, Palacios G, Boyd RL, Ratinaud P. Online discussions about tinnitus: what can we learn from natural language processing of Reddit posts? Am J Audiol. 2022:1–10.
8. Dong J, Wang T, Zhao L, Chen X. Pattern of disharmony between the heart and kidney: theoretical basis, identification and treatment. J Tradit Chin Med Sci. 2017 Oct;4(4):317–21.
9. Dong Y, Ding Y, Liu P-Z, Song H-Y, Zhao Y-P, Li M, et al. Investigation of the material basis underlying the correlation between presbycusis and kidney deficiency in traditional Chinese medicine via GC/MS metabolomics. Evid Based Complement Alternat Med. 2013;2013:1–9.
10. HealthCMI Ltd. [Internet]. [cited 2022 April 4]. Available from: https://www.healthcmi.com/Acupuncture-Continuing-Education-News/1826-acupuncture-and-herbs-quiet-tinnitus.
11. Acumedic Ltd. [Internet]. [cited 2022 April 4]. Available from: https://clinic.acumedic.com/can-we-help/condition/tinnitus/.
12. Gilbey A, Ernst E, Tani K. A systematic review of reviews of systematic reviews of acupuncture: review. Focus Altern Complement Ther. 2013;18(1):8–18.
13. Linde K, Vickers A, Hondras M, ter Riet G, Thormählen J, Berman B, et al. Systematic reviews of complementary therapies - an annotated bibliography. Part 1: acupuncture. BMC Complement Altern Med. 2001;1:3. https://doi.org/10.1186/1472-6882-1-3.
14. Park J, White AR, Ernst E. Efficacy of acupuncture as a treatment for tinnitus: a systematic review. Arch Otolaryngol Head Neck Surg. 2000;126(4):489–92.
15. Kim J-I, Choi J-Y, Lee D-H, Choi T-Y, Lee MS, Ernst E. Acupuncture for the treatment of tinnitus: a systematic review of randomized clinical trials. BMC Complement Altern Med. 2012;12:97.
16. Liu F, Han X, Li Y, Yu S. Acupuncture in the treatment of tinnitus: a systematic review and meta-analysis. Eur Arch Otorhinolaryngol. 2016;273(2):285–94.
17. He M, Li X, Liu Y, Zhong J, Jiang L, Liu Y, et al. Electroacupuncture for tinnitus: a systematic review. Scherer RW, editor. PLOS One. 2016;11(3):e0150600.
18. Five Flavor Herbs Ltd. [Internet]. [cited 2022 April 4]. Available from: https://fiveflavorsherbs.com/blog/the-five-flavors-in-traditional-chinese-medicine/
19. von Boetticher A. Ginkgo biloba extract in the treatment of tinnitus: a systematic review. Neuropsychiatr Dis Treat. 2011;7:441.
20. Celik M, Koyuncu İ. A comprehensive study of oxidative stress in tinnitus patients. Indian J Otolaryngol Head Neck Surg. 2018;70(4):521–6.
21. Hilton MP, Zimmermann EF, Hunt WT. Ginkgo biloba for tinnitus. Cochrane Database Syst Rev. 2013;(3):CD003852.
22. Sereda M, McFerran D, Axon E, Baguley DM, Hall DA, Potgieter I, et al. A process for prioritising systematic reviews in tinnitus. Int J Audiol. 2020;59(8):640–6.
23. Laccourreye O, Werner A, Laccourreye L, Bonfils P. Benefits, pitfalls and risks of phytotherapy in clinical practice in otorhinolaryngology. Eur Ann Otorhinolaryngol Head Neck Dis. 2017;134(2):95–9.
24. Sarris J. Herbal medicines in the treatment of psychiatric disorders: 10-year updated review. Phytother Res. 2018;32(7):1147–62.
25. Coelho C, Tyler R, Ji H, Rojas-Roncancio E, Witt S, Tao P, et al. Survey on the effectiveness of dietary supplements to treat tinnitus. Am J Audiol. 2016;25(3):184–205.
26. Gryzlak BM, Wallace RB, Zimmerman MB, Nisly NL. National surveillance of herbal dietary supplement exposures: the poison control center experience. Pharmacoepidemiol Drug Saf. 2007;16(9):947–57.
27. Posadzki P, Watson L, Ernst E. Herb-drug interactions: an overview of systematic reviews. Br J Clin Pharmacol. 2013;75(3):603–18.
28. Ng QX, Venkatanarayanan N, Ho CYX. Clinical use of Hypericum perforatum (St John's wort) in depression: a meta-analysis. J Affect Disord. 2017;210:211–21.
29. Pittler MH, Ernst E. Kava extract for treating anxiety. Cochrane Database Syst Rev. 2003;(1):CD003383.
30. Licata A, Macaluso FS, Craxì A. Herbal hepatotoxicity: a hidden epidemic. Intern Emerg Med. 2013;8(1):13–22.
31. Berkiten G, Kumral TL, Yıldırım G, Salturk Z, Uyar Y, Atar Y. Effects of serum zinc level on tinnitus. Am J Otolaryngol. 2015;36(2):230–4.
32. Ochi K, Kinoshita H, Kenmochi M, Nishino H, Ohashi T. Zinc deficiency and tinnitus. Auris Nasus Larynx. 2003;30(Suppl):S25–8.
33. Uluyol S, Kılıçaslan S, Yağız Ö. Relationship between serum magnesium level and subjective tinnitus. Kulak Burun Bogaz Ihtis Derg. 2016 Aug;26(4):225–7.
34. Kalappa BI, Anderson CT, Goldberg JM, Lippard SJ, Tzounopoulos T. AMPA receptor inhibition by synaptically released zinc. Proc Natl Acad Sci U S A. 2015;112(51):15749–54.
35. Xiong M, Wang J, Yang C, Lai H. The cochlea magnesium content is negatively correlated with hearing loss induced by impulse noise. Am J Otolaryngol. 2013;34(3):209–15.
36. Gordin A, Goldenberg D, Golz A, Netzer A, Joachims HZ. Magnesium: a new therapy for idiopathic sudden sensorineural hearing loss. Otol Neurotol. 2002;23(4):447–51.
37. Cevette MJ, Barrs DM, Patel A, Conroy KP, Sydlowski S, Noble BN, et al. Phase 2 study examining magnesium-dependent tinnitus. Int Tinnitus J. 2011;16(2):168–73.
38. Posadzki PP, Bajpai R, Kyaw BM, Roberts NJ, Brzezinski A, Christopoulos GI, et al. Melatonin and health: an umbrella review of health outcomes and biological mechanisms of action. BMC Med. 2018;16(1):18.
39. Andersen LPH, Gögenur I, Rosenberg J, Reiter RJ. The safety of melatonin in humans. Clin Drug Investig. 2016;36(3):169–75.
40. Reiter RJ, Tan D-X, Korkmaz A, Fuentes-Broto L. Drug-mediated ototoxicity and tinnitus: alleviation with melatonin. J Physiol Pharmacol. 2011;62(2):151–7.

41. Megwalu UC, Finnell JE, Piccirillo JF. The effects of melatonin on tinnitus and sleep. Otolaryngol Head Neck Surg. 2006;134(2):210–3.
42. Hosseinzadeh A, Kamrava SK, Moore BCJ, Reiter RJ, Ghaznavi H, Kamali M, et al. Molecular aspects of melatonin treatment in tinnitus: a review. Curr Drug Targets. 2019;20(11):1112–28.
43. Miroddi M, Bruno R, Galletti F, Calapai F, Navarra M, Gangemi S, et al. Clinical pharmacology of melatonin in the treatment of tinnitus: a review. Eur J Clin Pharmacol. 2015;71(3):263–70.
44. Grimes DR. Proposed mechanisms for homeopathy are physically impossible: original article. Focus Altern Complement Ther. 2012;17(3):149–55.
45. Dossett ML, Yeh GY. Homeopathy use in the USA and implications for public health: a review. Homeopathy. 2018;107(1):3–9.
46. Piolot M, Fagot J-P, Rivière S, Fagot-Campagna A, Debeugny G, Couzigou P, et al. Homeopathy in France in 2011-2012 according to reimbursements in the French national health insurance database (SNIIRAM). Fam Pract. 2015;32(4):442–8.
47. Ernst E. Homeopathy: what does the 'best' evidence tell us? Med J Aust. 2010;192(8):458–60.
48. Simpson JJ, Donaldson I, Davies WE. Use of homeopathy in the treatment of tinnitus. Br J Audiol. 1998;32(4):227–33.
49. Reis D, Jones T. Aromatherapy: using essential oils as a supportive therapy. Clin J Oncol Nurs. 2017;21(1):16–9.
50. Blessing EM, Steenkamp MM, Manzanares J, Marmar CR. Cannabidiol as a potential treatment for anxiety disorders. Neurotherapeutics. 2015;12(4):825–36.
51. Zheng Y, Reid P, Smith PF. Cannabinoid CB1 receptor agonists do not decrease, but may increase acoustic trauma-induced tinnitus in rats. Front Neurol [Internet]. 2015 [cited 2020 Dec 27];6. Available from: https://www.ncbi.nlm.nih.gov/pmc/articles/PMC4364172/.
52. Fuller TE, Haider HF, Kikidis D, Lapira A, Mazurek B, Norena A, et al. Different teams, same conclusions? A systematic review of existing clinical guidelines for the assessment and treatment of tinnitus in adults. Front Psychol [Internet]. 2017 [cited 2018 Nov 21];8. Available from: https://www.ncbi.nlm.nih.gov/pmc/articles/PMC5319986/.
53. Tunkel DE, Bauer CA, Sun GH, Rosenfeld RM, Chandrasekhar SS, Cunningham ER, et al. Clinical practice guideline: tinnitus. Otolaryngol Head Neck Surg. 2014;151(2 Suppl):S1–40.
54. Cima RFF, Mazurek B, Haider H, Kikidis D, Lapira A, Noreña A, et al. A multidisciplinary European guideline for tinnitus: diagnostics, assessment, and treatment. HNO. 2019;67(1):10–42.
55. National Institute for health and Care Excellence (NICE). Tinnitus: assessment and management guideline [NG155]. [Internet]. Available from: https://www.nice.org.uk/guidance/ng155
56. Bishop FL, Coghlan B, Geraghty AW, Everitt H, Little P, Holmes MM, et al. What techniques might be used to harness placebo effects in non-malignant pain? A literature review and survey to develop a taxonomy. BMJ Open. 2017;7(6):e015516.
57. Millum J, Grady C. The ethics of placebo-controlled trials: methodological justifications. Contemp Clin Trials [Internet]. 2013 Nov [cited 2020 Dec 27];36(2). Available from: https://www.ncbi.nlm.nih.gov/pmc/articles/PMC3844122/.
58. Bretlau P, Thomsen J, Tos M, Johnsen NJ. Placebo effect in surgery for Meniere's disease: a three-year follow-up study of patients in a double blind placebo controlled study on endolymphatic sac shunt surgery. Am J Otol. 1984;5(6):558–61.
59. Dawes P, Hopkins R, Munro KJ. Placebo effects in hearing-aid trials are reliable. Int J Audiol. 2013;52(7):472–7.
60. Duckert LG, Rees TS. Placebo effect in tinnitus management. Otolaryngol Head Neck Surg. 1984;92(6):697–9.
61. Hesser H, Weise C, Rief W, Andersson G. The effect of waiting: a meta-analysis of wait-list control groups in trials for tinnitus distress. J Psychosom Res. 2011;70(4):378–84.
62. Lichtenberg P. The ethics of the placebo in clinical practice. J Med Ethics. 2004;30(6):551–4.

56 Public and Patient Involvement in Tinnitus Research

Patrick K. A. Neff, Maryam Shabbir, Hazel Goedhart, Markku Vesala, Georgina Burns-O'Connell, and Deborah A. Hall

Abstract

Public or patient involvement has only recently been established in tinnitus research. Citizen science (CS), community science, or participatory research are modes of scientific research which involve members of the general population with different levels of participation. CS covers a wide range of stakeholders, including patients, healthcare professionals, basic and clinical researchers, industry, governmental bodies, and funders. In this chapter, we aimed at systematically identifying current CS efforts and challenges in tinnitus research. To this day, CS in tinnitus has been almost exclusively performed in British academia. Beyond that, CS projects have often been initiated by charities or self-help organisations like the British Tinnitus Association (BTA) or Tinnitus Hub. Current challenges identified are the heterogeneity of tinnitus, misalignment between academic and patient interests, dissonance between stakeholders, and lack of academic incentives. We therefore recommend to better value the concept of CS, improve its evidence base and evaluation, further education and awareness, consider more diversity and inclusion, involve patients in all levels of research projects, and finally, encourage the use of new technologies including the internet and social media. Furthermore, transnational organisation and harmonisation could be achieved by raising awareness through scientific publishing, conference activities, and public dissemination.

P. K. A. Neff (✉)
Neuro-X Institute, École Polytechnique Fédérale de Lausanne (EPFL), Geneva, Switzerland

Department of Radiology and Medical Informatics, University of Geneva, Geneva, Switzerland

Department of Psychiatry and Psychotherapy, University of Regensburg, Regensburg, Germany

Centre for Cognitive Neuroscience and Department of Psychology, Paris-Lodron Universität Salzburg, Salzburg, Austria

Department of Otorhinolaryngology - Head and Neck Surgery, University Hospital of Zurich, University of Zurich, Zürich, Switzerland
e-mail: patrick.neff@uzh.ch

M. Shabbir
Hearing Sciences, Mental Health and Clinical Neurosciences, School of Medicine, University of Nottingham, Nottingham, UK
e-mail: maryam.shabbir@nottingham.ac.uk

H. Goedhart · M. Vesala
Tinnitus Hub, London, UK

Tinnitus Hub, Amsterdam, The Netherlands
e-mail: hazel@tinnitushub.com; markku@tinnitushub.com

G. Burns-O'Connell
British Tinnitus Association, Sheffield, UK
e-mail: info@tinnitus.org.uk

D. A. Hall
Hearing Sciences, Mental Health and Clinical Neurosciences, School of Medicine, University of Nottingham, Nottingham, UK

Department of Psychology, School of Social Sciences, Heriot-Watt University Malaysia, Putrajaya, Malaysia
e-mail: deborah.hall@hw.ac.uk

W. Schlee et al. (eds.), *Textbook of Tinnitus*, https://doi.org/10.1007/978-3-031-35647-6_56

Graphical Abstract

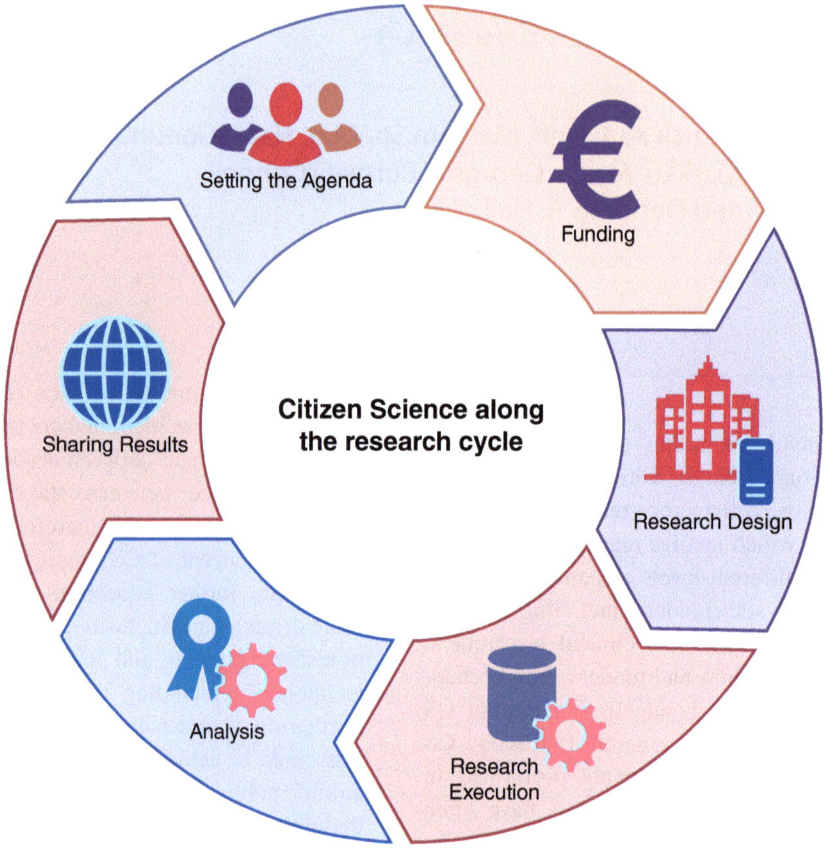

Highlights

- Individual champions and organisations in the UK and Europe are pioneering the involvement of the tinnitus community in research.
- Citizens with the lived experience of tinnitus have been involved in prioritising unanswered research questions about tinnitus, thus setting out an agenda for research.
- Good practice is illustrated through a case study by the COMiT initiative, involving the tinnitus community in the research team on an equal footing with professional experts.
- In the UK, general national practice standards have been developed for patient involvement in health research through active consultation with the public.
- We identify current limitations and challenges of patient involvement in tinnitus research.
- Our recommendations include valuing citizen science practices, better involvement of patients, and use of new technologies.

Defining Citizen Science and Levels of Involvement

Citizen science (CS) is a mode of scientific research which involves members of the general population with different levels of participation [1]. Historically, CS can be traced back to the nineteenth century where birdwatching by non-academic citizens informed and complemented "institutionalised" research [2, 3]. With large-scale digitalisation of all aspects of life towards the end of the twentieth century, CS started to establish itself as an emerging method for scientific knowledge gain. In a concerted international action, for example, citizens helped the Planetary Society and international space agencies decoding electromagnetic signals from space by contributing computing resources from their personal computers [4]. In recent times, CS has shifted away from data collection or resource-sharing between citizen partners to more inclusive and collaborative forms. Currently, participatory levels can be defined on a spectrum (from contractual to collaborative). The most collaborative being a collegial interaction between citizens and academic entities that co-create with equal responsibility [5]. In practice, participation often takes on very specific configurations driven by the needs of the individual project and working style of the lead researcher. For example, a biological field study observing water levels or animal behaviour does not directly affect citizen scientists and thus, their personal interest in proceedings or outcomes is relatively lower than if it were a chronic human disease.

CS seems to have established itself as an umbrella term encapsulating *community science* and *participatory research.* In medical research, it is commonly referred to as *patient and public involvement* (PPI) [6]. Other terminologies can be mostly considered as sub-forms of CS, fitting the different participatory levels described previously [1, 7, 8]. For example, *crowdsensing* or *participatory sensing* is a basic form where citizens simply provide data acting as "subjects" in scientific studies [9]. This form typically constitutes a participatory level that is somewhat passive. In current times, this especially holds true in real-life smartphone or sensor studies [10]. A related concept, *crowdsourcing*, refers to resource or work distribution among the stakeholders (i.e. all involved partners and interests) to reach a common goal as pioneered in, for example, the SETI@home project. The focus of crowdsourcing is set on shared resources while the actual research project is mostly planned and devised by the academic stakeholders. Finally, *patient involvement or participation* has recently emerged [6]. Patient involvement refers to the process of involving patients as collaborative partners in the research study team and this concept has naturally been expanded to medical research as an effective way to reduce the inherent power relation asymmetries between patients and physicians. However, for CS to be truly effective, clinical researchers need to be open-minded about modifying research questions or study designs based on patient input and willing to invest in developing a new skill set to support their CS work. If not, then there is a risk that the patient involvement endeavour might end up being detrimental to scientific progress, as well as personally dissatisfying. Stakeholder interests and related stakeholder dynamics are thus other important dimensions of any CS project [11]. Careful consideration and moderation is important particularly when the aim of CS is to achieve truly co-created science. This often means that the academic entities have to take on differential roles, namely primarily scientific expertise stakeholder, but also project management and critical moderation or facilitation of discussions and processes [3]. These multiple roles may pose conflicts of interests within the scientific stakeholder(s) and in consequence force scientific stakeholders to broaden their skill set accordingly. Alternatively, project management and moderation tasks might be delegated to an independent specialised entity (e.g. institutional centres or actions for CS, professional external moderators, or communication experts). In any case, early and exhaustive consideration of stakeholder interests, positions, and dynamics should be considered early on in any CS scenario to ensure productive proceedings and finally significant outcomes with the potential to surpass the knowledge gain of traditional institutionalised science [8, 12].

Taken together, CS is a scientific approach which is receiving increasingly more interest and uptake in various research fields while terminology, methodology, and implementation are still in development. This may come as no surprise given the inherent complexity and heterogeneity of CS configurations. However, the diversity may hamper convergence on general standards [7, 8]. Current CS projects have to therefore be carefully devised with stakeholder analyses, definition of roles and participation levels, and moderation as well as project management. Overall, some authors identify transformative potential in CS, both for science and society [13], which has been described as a transition between modes of knowledge gain [12]. This transition furthermore implies a putatively radical change in epistemic and ontological aspects of science itself [8].

In this chapter, we define CS projects as those taking a democratised approach using patient involvement methods in which citizens are considered to have epistemic privilege through their lived experience of tinnitus. As a consequence, we consider that CS maximally involves citizens in as many aspects of a research project as possible, from defining the research question to disseminating the study findings. In the following sections, we introduce current CS projects in tinnitus, discuss their weaknesses and potentials in the light of current good practices, and finally we suggest future directions for potentially transformative CS within the tinnitus field.

Citizen Science in Tinnitus Research

In 2018, a special session was dedicated to community science at the 11th Tinnitus Research Initiative (TRI) Meeting and TINNET conference in Regensburg, Germany. This session can be considered the first of its kind at a major tinnitus conference and was planned again as a symposium including a panel discussion with an extended set of stakeholders during the 13th TRI meeting in 2020. While these conference activities introduced the concepts and terminologies of CS to a broader academic community, CS research in tinnitus has typically been performed up until this point without specifically naming it CS [14–16]. Here, we therefore introduce some of the leading organisations and projects that are pioneering the involvement of the tinnitus community in research. This is by no means intended to be an exhaustive list, but provides illustrative examples of good practice.

British Tinnitus Association

Established in 1979, the British Tinnitus Association (BTA) describes itself as the only national UK charity dedicated to supporting people with tinnitus. Their work over the years has been influential, not only to patients, but also to researchers (Table 56.1). For researchers, the charity remains at the forefront of commissioning research into understanding

Table 56.1 List of completed and on-going BTA research since 2019

Date of research	Research topic	Level of involvement
Started 2021	Objective measures for tinnitus using Artificial Intelligence	Funder and contributor[a]
Started 2021	Identify tinnitus biomarkers	Funder and contributor[b]
2021	Externally Funded Project: The impact of tinnitus on musicians	BTA lead researcher and co-author[c]
Started 2020	Tinnitus and the arts	Contributor and helped with recruitment[d]
Started 2020	Hearing aids for tinnitus with hearing loss (HUSH) clinical trial	Contributor and will help with recruitment [15]
2020	A Delphi survey to determine a definition and description of hyperacusis by clinician consensus	BTA staff co-author [17]
2020	An evaluation of paediatric tinnitus services in UK National Health Service audiology departments	BTA staff co-author [18]
2020	A psychologically informed, audiologist-delivered, manualised intervention for tinnitus: Protocol for a randomised controlled feasibility trial (Tin Man study)	BTA staff co-author [19]
2020	NICE guidelines	BTA staff co-author [20]
2020	Changes in tinnitus experiences during the COVID-19 pandemic	BTA staff co-author [21]
2019	Eye movement desensitisation and reprocessing (EMDR) as a tinnitus treatment?	Funder [22]
2019	Using cortisol to measure the distress caused by tinnitus	Funder [23]
2019	Are children who have tinnitus more likely to be anxious?	Funder[e]
2019	Externally Funded Project: Establishing the impact of tinnitus on aged veterans in the UK	BTA lead researcher and co-author [24]

Funder: paid for research to be undertaken. Contributor: contributed ideas, undertook research methods. Lead researcher: BTA staff member undertaking project as lead research and conducting day-to-day running of project. Including leading on all stages of the research from proposal of idea to dissemination of findings. Helped with recruitment: BTA advertised the project to potential participants. Helped with recruitment/dissemination: BTA advertised the project to potential participants and helped to disseminate the findings and recommendations to the relevant people and organisations. BTA staff co-author: BTA member(s) of staff contributed to writing the journal article and/or report

[a] https://www.tinnitus.org.uk/Blog/were-investing-a-further-118k-for-research

[b] https://www.tinnitus.org.uk/Blog/large-research-grant-kcl

[c] https://www.tinnitus.org.uk/Pages/Category/musicians-with-tinnitus

[d] http://www.open.ac.uk/blogs/tinnitus/

[e] https://www.tinnitus.org.uk/anxiety-in-children-and-young-people-with-tinnitus-and-hyperacusis

mechanisms of tinnitus and identifying effective treatments. For people living with tinnitus, many of those affected are told by healthcare professionals to "learn to live with it" and "that nothing can be done". Through their helpline, network of support groups and face-to-face events, the BTA has helped hundreds of thousands of distressed people with tinnitus learn to successfully manage their symptoms and regain their quality of life.

Based on patient-based reports, the BTA has concluded that most people with tinnitus want their tinnitus loudness to be reduced and would prefer a pharmacological solution over other treatment options [25]. The BTA has therefore recently developed a "roadmap to a cure" in consultation with members of tinnitus patient support groups, members of the BTA and its Professional Advisers Committee and hearing healthcare professionals [25]. The map sets out three major research topics: (1) pre-discovery, (2) measurement of tinnitus, and (3) discovering a cure. Each topic is supported by a repository of evidence-based knowledge for the tinnitus community. It is designed to be free to access and easy to use, so that researchers can add to it over time. The BTA hopes that this roadmap can be used by charities, other patient groups, and individual tinnitus patients to demonstrate to politicians, research funders, the pharmaceutical industry, and healthcare organisations the size of the tinnitus problem and the need for a much enhanced research footprint.

Inequalities have been highlighted in other areas of chronic health conditions and provision [26] which demonstrate an urgency for tinnitus services to be inclusive of minority communities. The BTA is conducting research to explore equality, diversity, and inclusion within its own work. The aim of this work is to increase awareness of tinnitus and ultimately to offer help to a wider population. To do this, the first phase of the project is focussing on the inclusion of black, Asian and minority ethnic (BAME) citizens within the BTA's work. Focus groups and interviews with service users will be conducted to understand the lived experience of the potential barriers faced by BAME citizens when accessing the BTA services. To ensure the research is as inclusive as possible, BAME citizens with lived experience of tinnitus will be included throughout this work.

This project places CS prominently within the research design. Not only will BAME citizens with the lived experience of tinnitus contribute to the project design, but they will also conduct the focus groups and interviews. In this way, inclusion of those with lived experience of tinnitus ensures that the voice of those with epistemic privilege is prioritised.

James Lind Alliance

The James Lind Alliance (JLA) is a UK-based non-profit organisation whose very specific purpose is to give a voice to patients and clinicians to help shape future research agendas.

Table 56.2 Top ten research suggestions identified by the James Lind Alliance Tinnitus Priority Setting Partnership (taken from [27])

Research question related to an established uncertainty in the diagnosis, assessment, or treatment of tinnitus
What management strategies are more effective than a usual model of audiological care in improving outcomes for people with tinnitus?
Is CBT/psychological therapy, delivered by audiology professionals, effective for people with tinnitus? Here comparisons might be with usual audiological care or CBT delivered by a psychologist
What management strategies are more effective for improving tinnitus-related insomnia than a usual model of care?
Do any of the various available complementary therapies provide improved outcomes for people with tinnitus compared with a usual model of care?
What type of digital hearing aid or amplification strategy provides the most effective tinnitus relief?
What is the optimal set of guidelines for assessing children with tinnitus?
How can tinnitus be effectively managed in people who are deaf or have profound hearing loss?
Are there different types of tinnitus and can they be explained by different mechanisms in the ear or brain?
What is the link between tinnitus and hyperacusis (over-sensitivity to sounds)?
Which medications have proven to be effective in tinnitus management compared with placebo?

It was established in 2004 and has worked with patients experiencing a wide range of conditions and diseases from alcohol-related liver disease to womb cancer. In 2011, the British Tinnitus Association (BTA), in partnership with the National Institute for Health Research (NIHR) Nottingham Hearing Biomedical Research Unit, set up a tinnitus Priority Setting Partnership. Over a period of 11 months, this group engaged patients and clinicians to identify and prioritise uncertainties in the assessment, diagnosis, or treatment of tinnitus and the top ten is listed in Table 56.2 [28]. Working in consultation with the Professional Advisers' Committee of the BTA, the partnership also published ideas for future research projects to address each uncertainty (see [28]). These outcomes are being used to inform health research funders in the UK about what issues matter most to those people who live with the condition every day. For example, 5 years after the JLA project, the BTA reflected on the impact of the recommendations. It was positive to see that some funding had been awarded to support research projects that sought to answer some of the questions. The BTA itself has used the top ten list to commission several studies in neglected areas. For example, one commission awarded to another patient-centred charity, The Ear Foundation, gathered 1432 people's experiences with tinnitus and severe/profound hearing loss [29]. Those people with greater levels of hearing loss experienced the greatest impact of tinnitus, but they were more likely to be discharged from professional care or not given support at all. One recommendation was therefore for health professionals to take seriously the potential impact of tinnitus and include appropriate questions during clinic appointments especially for people who are deaf or have a severe hearing loss.

Table 56.3 Tinnitus Hub's citizen science projects

Date of research	Research topic	Level of involvement
Started 2020	Creating an inventory of tinnitus data in biobanks	Co-researcher
Started 2020	Monthly community voting on best tinnitus research paper	Initiator
2020	Collaboration with Dr. will Sedley on predictive brain processing research	Advisor
2020	NICE guidelines	Feedback provider
2019 and 2020	Somatic tinnitus	Data supplier and co-author
2019	Personalised tinnitus treatment	Data supplier and co-author
2019	Mapping white matter changes along the auditory pathway as a result of hearing loss	Funder (grantee selected through community vote)
2017	Analysis of treatment sentiment from discussions on the tinnitus talk forum	Co-author
2015	COMIT'iD	Contributor and co-author

Tinnitus Hub

The Tinnitus Hub is a not-for-profit patient organisation incorporated in the UK in 2015 and in the Netherlands in 2020. Tinnitus Hub is wholly managed by volunteers, all of whom have personal experience of the condition. The organisation is passionate about improving the lives of others with tinnitus, and above all seeks to promote the quest for a cure. Key activities include providing education and information, much of which is research oriented, for instance through the Tinnitus Talk Podcast, blogs, videos, and social media. Tinnitus Hub also provides a bridge function between patients and researchers (Table 56.3) by representing the "patient voice" in various EU-funded tinnitus research consortiums like TIN-ACT (Tinnitus Assessment Causes Treatments), ESIT (European School for Interdisciplinary Tinnitus Research, [27]), and UNITI (Unification of Treatments and Interventions for Tinnitus Patients, [30]).

Most importantly, Tinnitus Hub connects people from around the world virtually through the Tinnitus Talk forum, where people share experiences, advice, and information. This grassroots community informs Tinnitus Hub's strategy and priorities through a bottom-up process, and also lends itself particularly well to citizen science. An example of a bottom-up initiative that emerged from the Tinnitus Talk forum, as pertaining to research, is the creation of the Daniel Ballinger fund, which raised GBP 5000 in the name of a deceased forum member. PhD students were invited to apply for funding and then fund donors participated in a public and democratic voting process on which student should receive the grant. Another example of grassroots activity is the formation of a Tinnitus Talk working group to influence US government funding priorities of the National Institute on Deafness and Other Communication Disorders (NIDCD) in favour of cure-focussed tinnitus research.

Web-based platforms are growing in popularity within the tinnitus research community, and together with social media are replacing more traditional (and one-way) connection methods like newsletters and magazines. In particular, self-help discussion forums are starting to be used more widely for recruitment [31] and research data collection [32]. For researchers, the Tinnitus Talk forum is a specific example which offers a rapid and easy way to engage with a large number of people with tinnitus. Other advantages of such a forum are that it is more flexible and cost-effective than conventional paper-based or face-to-face methods. In partnership with various research teams, Tinnitus Hub has actively supported a number of citizen science activities through the Tinnitus Talk forum. This includes crowdsourcing of data in order to gather sample sizes that are typically not achievable through traditional academic methods. Tinnitus Hub conducted three surveys (2016–2020) with a response rate of 5000–8000 each. Sharing their data is a relatively simple way for Tinnitus Talk members to contribute to research causes, and most of them are happy to do so. The Tinnitus Talk forum has also been leveraged to recruit patients for clinical trials.

Tinnitus Hub's recent research activities are more explicitly designed to influence the course of research through agenda-setting. This includes a monthly poll on the Tinnitus Talk forum where people can vote on which research paper from the previous month they find most valuable. The outcomes of these polls will be shared with the research community to demonstrate what type or area of research is most valued by people with tinnitus. Furthermore, to foster co-creation, Tinnitus Hub has formed a Patient Expert Panel that works directly with researchers, preferably at the earlier stages of research, to help them shape and inform their research questions and methods.

An Illustrative Case Study Involving the Tinnitus Community in Research

In one recent example of citizen science, working with the NIHR Nottingham Biomedical Research Centre, the Tinnitus Hub team created a closed discussion group for invited participants [33, 34]. This project therefore was able to engage across geographical and time zone boundaries through a web-based platform. Participants who had previously taken part in a web-based survey (hosted using an academic software platform supported by the University of Liverpool) were invited to register for a follow-up web-based discussion forum. In this way, the project was a continuation of the Core Outcome Measures in Tinnitus (COMiT) initiative [35, 36]. The forum gave the research team a way to reach consensus on how to define and describe various tinnitus-related health concepts using plain language that could be understood by members of the public and professionals alike. This was achieved through a focus group-style semi-structured discussion and voting that was moderated by one of the research team. For the impact of tinnitus on concentration, the agreed description emphasised the importance of intentional control, highlighted the unavoidable prominence of tinnitus, and drew attention to the resulting cognitive effort and mental fatigue required when concentrating. Participants were 148 tinnitus experts including people living with tinnitus, healthcare professionals, clinical researchers, commercial representatives, and funders. Important to this study, none of the participants were required to identify what their expertise was and so everyone contributed their opinions on an equal footing. Another strength of this citizen science approach was that discussants were not just research participants; they also played an important role in shaping the research product. While the first benefit is perhaps easier to achieve using a web-based platform, the second benefit is certainly not restricted to an Internet approach. An unforeseen benefit from this work was that it identified recurring conversational themes relating to the lived experience of tinnitus that went beyond the original scope of the semi-structured discussion. For example, in the discussion forum, many of the participants referred to "tinnitus sufferers" and "suffering". Suffering emphasises intense distress. Usage of the word in academic literature is not widespread, perhaps because it is highly emotive language, but it was a very real experience for many with tinnitus.

The next stage of this COMiT project sought to identify how concentration could be adequately measured. The COMiT team's experience at this stage illustrates how CS may not be well suited in all circumstances. Considering measurement, a measure was deemed suitable if it assessed how well a person could control their attention and sustain focus on whatever it is they intended to focus upon, with ease and lack of effort. A systematic review first collated all of the potentially relevant instruments [37]. The investigators engaged members of the public to assess whether any of these instruments measured the given construct definition of concentration. Three professionals with expertise in cognitive psychology and three members of the public with tinnitus were invited to do the ratings using standardised psychometric criteria in a face-to-face meeting. The evaluation criteria assessed whether (1) the items were relevant for the construct of interest, (2) all key concepts were included, and (3) that the items and response options were understood as intended [38]. Since the ratings required an understanding of psychological and psychometric concepts, the investigators first provided a pre-meeting information pack to all participants with tinnitus for greater familiarisation. Immediately before the professional experts joined the meeting, members of the public participated in an orientation pre-meeting. During the meeting, a member of the research team served as a "buddy" to give them personalised support. Despite these preparations, the CS approach did create some challenges. Members of the public found it very hard to grasp some of the concepts and did not fully understand some of the rating tasks. The time was not used as effectively as hoped because the group discussion often veered off topic and lost focus. Feedback from the members of the public indicated that they had expected to discuss their own lived experience of tinnitus and found the rating tasks too demanding. This example is important to share as a lesson learned in making careful decisions about when and how to implement CS.

Citizen Science in Other Clinical Fields

Many people affected by health problems have already demonstrated a strong interest in and willingness to contribute to meaningful scientific research in health and medicine. The United States, Canada, European Union, and Australia have placed CS at the forefront of national science policy. For instance, in the United States, the Patient Centred Outcomes Research Institute (PCORI) encourages patients to submit research questions, provide input on funding applications, participate in events and become a public research ambassador. In addition, major international medical journals such as *Science*, *Nature*, and *Bioscience* regularly feature projects conducted by citizens. While numerous global communities, such as patientslikeme.com, also provide ways for individuals to share their real-world health experiences in order to help themselves and others, as well as to advance research in a wide range of clinical disciplines.

In this section, we provide an illustrative example of CS taken from the Core Outcome Measures in Effectiveness Trials (COMET) which is a clinical initiative funded by the Medical Research Council and the NIHR in the UK, and the European Commission. The overall aim of this initiative is to help researchers design clinical studies that provide the best evidence about what treatment works best for patients. At the moment, different clinical studies looking at treatments for the same condition often measure different outcomes, and this is very wasteful of limited resources. If all studies in a particular health condition used the same outcomes, they could all be compared and combined, making research much more efficient. To achieve this, COMET aims to encourage the development and uptake of an agreed standardised set of outcomes, known as a "Core Outcome Set" (COS), for a specific condition. A COS represents the minimum set of outcomes that should be measured and reported in all clinical trials for the condition of interest. To facilitate a meaningful role for citizens, COMET has a dedicated People and Patient Participation, Involvement and Engagement (PoPPIE) working group. The purpose of PoPPIE is to facilitate the involvement of citizens with the lived experience of the condition of interest. To support their work they have created resources including a plain language summary to explain some of the more difficult concepts used within the COMET network [39]. PoPPIE has also published research with suggestions on how to make COS development more meaningful and accessible for patients in order to ensure that they have a genuine say in the process [40].

The COMET approach has been applied to many different health conditions such as fibromyalgia, eczema, and various forms of cancer and pain. Common to all is the emphasis on the importance of patients, carers and healthcare professionals to ensure that the COS are relevant to all stakeholders. Over recent years, the patient voice has become more mainstream. For example, of those published COS studies involving public and patients, 64% (106/165) had a publication date in the last 5 years (2015–2019) [Susanna Dodd, personal communication]. The development of a COS for fibromyalgia provides a compelling example of the positive impact and new insights gained by involving the general public as key stakeholders in the research [41]. At an early stage of the research design, six focus groups were conducted across three clinical sites in the United States with 48 women living with fibromyalgia for at least 6 months. The purpose was to identify the greatest impacts of fibromyalgia on quality of life and functioning from a patient's perspective. Patients identified four symptom categories that had the greatest impact on their quality of life, notably physical factors such as sleep disturbance and fatigue, emotional/cognitive factors such as depression and anxiety, social factors such as disrupted relationships with family and friends and isolation, and activity-related factors such as avoidance of physical activity and inability to advance in career. These findings contributed important and novel insights since, up until then, clinical trials of interventions for fibromyalgia had rarely considered some of the symptoms identified by the focus groups as important to their everyday lives such as depressive and anxiety symptoms, and cognition. The authors therefore acknowledge the wider value of the CS approach as introducing the potential to redefine fibromyalgia in a way that has clinical relevance for patients and clinicians. Consistent with the narrow viewpoint held by professionals, diagnostic criteria for fibromyalgia at the time were characterised by pain and tenderness (e.g. American College of Rheumatology 1990, [42]), without recognition of the wider psychological and social factors reported by patients. It is interesting to note that the 2010 revised criteria considered fatigue, trouble thinking or remembering, waking up tired (unrefreshing sleep) and depression [43].

Limitations and Challenges

Professional research is governed by a range of legal standards which safeguard participants. This includes informed consent, an honest and transparent assessment of risks and benefits, and an equitable process to recruit and enrol participants. In CS, the underlying principles are the same. Nevertheless, new layers of ethical complexity are introduced when citizens themselves are driving the research or when they are taking on the role of research partners beyond providing data as subjects. For example, all three of the essential principles (respect for persons, beneficence, and justice) support expectations for collegial relationships, not clinician–patient or researcher–subject relationships. Developing and maintaining collegial relationships with a large pool of research partners incurs responsibilities for clearly communicating research progress and results, along with faithfully completing the planned work [44]. As you can imagine, this carries its own challenges. A potential solution lies in greater emphasis on training and support, not only for those citizens who get involved but also for those researchers to ensure they possess a minimum skill level and knowledge about public involvement [45].

Some researchers have acknowledged the tokenism that can exist and the narrowness of current patient and public involvement models, with few organisations explicitly mentioning empowerment or ensuring equality and diversity of representation so that citizens can genuinely influence the design, planning, and co-production of health and medical research [46].

The field of tinnitus is no different. Indeed, the involvement of citizens with tinnitus in research on tinnitus is still in its infancy. A poll on the Tinnitus Talk forum makes clear that the tinnitus patient community, overwhelmingly, would like to have more opportunities for involvement *earlier on in the research cycle*. Yet, the James Lind Alliance Priority Setting Partnership concluded in 2012 is perhaps the only formal example where tinnitus communities and patient organisations were directly involved in the identification of research priorities for new research projects (see section "James Lind Alliance"). More recently, patient organisations have been invited as partners to EU-funded tinnitus research consortia like ESIT, TIN-ACT, and UNITI, but only after the research agenda has been set. The role of patient organisations in these EU programmes has thus been limited mostly to communication of research outcomes. While this provides a good starting point for more meaningful participation in future, the status quo clearly leaves much to be desired and truly co-created research is still far off.

We take this opportunity to reflect on a number of challenges to overcome in order for the tinnitus community to achieve a truly democratised approach to CS.

The Heterogeneity of the Condition

Tinnitus is known to be highly heterogeneous, varying greatly in terms of type and intensity of sound perceived, the degree to which quality of life is affected, and the presence or absence of hearing loss and other comorbidities like hyperacusis and chronic pain. This makes it challenging for patient communities to speak with "one voice" or for researchers to know which patient representatives to approach. As a result, patient organisations may feel as though they have to "choose" which groups to represent. The interests of different groups can even be conflicting, particularly when it comes to (lobbying for) the allocation of sparse research. For instance, people who experience negative impact from both tinnitus *and* hyperacusis might be more likely to prioritise a research question about the links between tinnitus and hyperacusis (see Table 56.2), than people with tinnitus who do not experience hyperacusis. In this way, research topics that have a substantial impact on a small number of individuals might not make it onto the research agenda because they have only minority support.

Tinnitus Hub has formed a Patient Expert Panel to represent the voice of the tinnitus community towards the research community. In addition, Tinnitus Hub's leadership, who all suffer from tinnitus themselves, represents the patient community in various research forums and consortiums. One side effect of this approach is that the patient experts or representatives often become research experts over time and thus do not represent the average tinnitus patient per se. To counter this effect, Tinnitus Hub frequently calls on the wider tinnitus community through the Tinnitus Talk forum. The users of the forum tend to fall within the moderate to severe end of the tinnitus spectrum, and many also suffer from comorbidities like hyperacusis. Hence, the forum community is well suited when it comes to gathering input from this sub-group of tinnitus patients. In fact, this is a sub-group that – Tinnitus Hub would argue – is the most important one to involve in CS initiatives, because they are the ones whose lives are most profoundly impacted by the condition.

In addition to the work described above which includes those with lived experience of tinnitus within the research team, the BTA have a well-established practice of including citizens with tinnitus in the work they do. For example, the BTA Consultation Group is made up of citizens who live with tinnitus and have volunteered to advise on work conducted by the BTA, including both research projects and changes made to support services. It is important to recognise that the inclusion of those with lived experience works towards achieving a more representative picture of the experience of those living with tinnitus. However, it is impossible to be representative of the population of those living with tinnitus due to the heterogeneity of the condition.

Misalignment Between Academic and Patient Interests

In general, people with tinnitus want research to be cure-focussed [25]. While some of them see value in strategies that facilitate coping and habituation by reducing tinnitus-associated distress, the prevalent perception among the tinnitus community is that these management strategies have been adequately studied, and efforts now need to focus on discovering treatments that reduce or eliminate the tinnitus percept itself by tackling the underlying causes or mechanisms.

There is further misalignment in how treatment success is defined. In a recent US-based survey patients, most often reported reduction of tinnitus loudness (63%) and complete elimination of tinnitus (57%), whereas audiologists reported decreased awareness (77%), alleviation of stress or anxiety (63%), and increased knowledge of tinnitus (63%) [47]. It is interesting to note that the COMiT International Delphi study that involved patients in the decision-making nominated both tinnitus loudness and tinnitus intrusiveness as core outcomes to be used when assessing whether pharmacological treatments for tinnitus have worked [36]. These approximate to the preferences expressed by patients in the US survey.

Lack of Trust From Either Side

Trust is a key ingredient to productive CS and has to be cultivated carefully [3, 48]. Research can seem like a black box to patients which can make it difficult to understand why, for example, research progresses seemingly slowly. This can, among part of the tinnitus community, foster a perception of researchers "not caring" or "lacking a sense of urgency". On the other hand, researchers might be hesitant to engage with the tinnitus community (even if they acknowledge the value of community involvement) since it could make one vulnerable to criticism or even public attacks on one's work or persona, which can sometimes occur in unmoderated environments such as social media. That said, such attacks do not tend to occur *as a result of* researcher engagement, but rather in the absence of. Hence, an argument could be made that engagement is a prerequisite to bringing both sides closer together. Critical voices, as part of a respectful open debate, are key to bringing both sides closer together. Furthermore, engagement efforts from researchers should ideally extend beyond merely communicating research outcomes through channels like social media. Increased openness and transparency will likely build trust over time.

Lack of Academic Incentives

The greatest incentive to academics can be summarised quite simply as the accessibility of research funding. A study comparing awards for clinical research on hearing disorders with that on diabetes from 2009 to 2011 revealed that hearing research attracted at best only one-fifth of the amount of governmental funding allocated to diabetes research [49]. Instead, tinnitus research tends to be funded by charities, other non-governmental organisations and philanthropists where the size of the awards and the scale of the research programmes are much smaller and arguably also less ambitious. In consequence, this lack of funding and research priority seriously hampers career perspectives for early career researchers committing to the tinnitus topic. In most of the cases, tinnitus research is performed "on the side" at medical or audiological institutes with, for example, small budgets for single PhD projects. This is also true for past or current transnational research consortia like TINNET, ESIT, and TIN-ACT. UNITI is the first research project to offer post-doctoral positions for several years while personal (tenure) career track funding is largely absent. This may be partly due to the inherent multi- or trans-disciplinary nature of the topic which impedes the establishment of a genuine individual profile in any discipline. Furthermore, this could be also explained by missing breakthrough research and respective high-impact publications which are critical ingredients for any successful scientific career. Certainly, this is true for many research fields while in tinnitus research the combination of lacking funding, research priorities, perspectives for mid or late career trajectories, and probably most importantly of a feasible cure or treatment does not provide fertile grounds for such research or publications.

Another incentive to academics perhaps lies in the availability of motivating and enabling factors to engage in a CS approach. The NIHR in the UK is one of the few national government funding bodies that has pioneered a strong policy approach to public involvement [45]. With high-level support from the senior government officials, NIHR has established an organisational infrastructure to support the delivery of meaningful patient involvement including (1) funding schemes dedicated to addressing real-world questions with results that will have a demonstrable impact on the health or healthcare of service users, (2) a national research design service to support researchers in developing high-quality research proposals that are patient focused, and (3) a national advisory group for the promotion and advancement of public involvement. The resulting environment has provided the academic incentive to enable public involvement in tinnitus to flourish in the UK. For example, recent projects funded through the NIHR Research for Patient Benefit scheme include feasibility trials to assess a psychologically informed, audiologist-delivered, manualised intervention for tinnitus [19], and effectiveness of digital hearing aids for tinnitus [15, 16]. Both studies meet our criteria of "genuine" CS projects.

Future Directions and Recommendations

Valuing the Practice of Citizen Science and Practice Standards

The commitment of the NIHR to include the general public in research activity has strengthened over the last decade and the presence and activities of INVOLVE have been important in this achievement. INVOLVE is a national advisory group part of and funded by the NIHR, to support active public involvement in NHS, public health, and social care research. It is one of the few government-funded programmes of its kind in the world.

The NIHR was the first funder of its size and importance globally to review its approach to public involvement [45] and to propose national practice standards. The review comprised a survey, among other data collection methods, and respondents to the NIHR survey felt that the case for the value of public and patient involvement in research had already been made in a compelling way, so that debates about the need for public and patient involvement should now mature into discussions about what forms of involvement work in particular contexts. The authors of the review suggest that their findings and recommendations [45] are transferable to other organisations, countries and individuals.

A set of UK-wide practice standards to improve the consistency and quality of public involvement in research has been developed by INVOLVE through a consultation process and these were publicly launched in 2019 [50]. Standards were proposed for the following themes: (1) Inclusive opportunities, (2) Working together, (3) Support and learning, (4) Communications, (5) Impact, and (6) Governance. Each standard aims to provide clear, concise benchmarks for effective public involvement in health research alongside indicators against which improvement can be monitored. Peer review, performance management, self-regulation, and independent regulation were all suggested as ways the standards could be reached through continuous improvement.

Improved Evaluation and Evidence

The importance of evidence was a recurring theme in the UK NIHR survey [45], particularly in relation to how to best evaluate different methods for public involvement and how to embed the findings into research practice for continuous improvement. To enable this to happen, researchers could be incentivised to collect data on the implementation and impact of their CS methods, and to publish their findings separate from the scientific results addressing the tinnitus research question. For example, the journal *Research Involvement and Engagement* is an interdisciplinary, health and social care journal focussing on patient and wider involvement and engagement in research, at all stages. The journal itself embeds the principles of CS as it is co-produced with patients, academics, policy makers, and service users. We would strongly encourage the tinnitus community to engage with the CS agenda in this way.

Better Involvement of Patient Stakeholders Throughout the Research Process

Many existing tinnitus research projects, networks, consortiums, and other initiatives do in fact involve patients in their activities. For instance, tinnitus organisations may be asked to become a formal partner in a research consortium. This provides a good starting point for CS, since it builds closer connections between the research and patient communities. However, the manner in which patient organisations have been involved to date cannot be considered CS per se, mainly because patient organisations tend to get invited after the research agenda has already been set. Their role therefore becomes limited to public outreach efforts to communicate research results.

We therefore recommend that any new tinnitus research initiative invites patient organisations and other patient representatives early on in the process. In practice, this often means during the early stages of a grant application. At these stages, mutual engagement can still influence the key objectives of the research and the way the research process is designed. Moreover, patient stakeholder organisations should also be included as equal partners in the discussion of research outcomes. This would not only be beneficial for the evaluation of the current research cycle but also inform further research ideas or projects.

Education and Awareness

Education of all stakeholders with respect to CS skills is necessary for any research context and currently largely absent in tinnitus research. We therefore recommend to include CS theory and methodology for any future PhD programme. This inclusion could inform the next generation of researchers early on and may lead to inclusion of CS methodology in research projects. Not all research projects would profit from

CS in the same way but a basic level of understanding of the concepts and methods could be useful in any case. Naturally, it can be more difficult to educate mid to late career academics on CS, but this could be facilitated with postgraduate courses and certificates. The education of patient stakeholders is heavily depending on the educational or occupational status and on the skill set required for the actual CS project. All stakeholders would certainly profit from specific training in moderation, management, and governance of CS processes while further specialisation is driven by requirements of the project.

Education can be considered as a first important step to raise awareness for CS in tinnitus research. Beyond that, we are convinced that dissemination of CS in the academic community would be a further strategy to increase its acceptance and impact. CS should thus be better represented at conferences. Special sessions were already held at two recent TRI conferences, but the last special session was not planned ahead and had to be applied for. We are still far from fixed and dedicated sessions but with current CS-related developments in the tinnitus community, ever-increasing awareness of CS in general, and governmental obligations CS may become an integral part of tinnitus conferences.

Diversity and Inclusion

Diversity and inclusion is a common theme in many contexts of today's society and thus also an issue in CS in tinnitus. This may be especially true for the patient stakeholders with their inherent tinnitus heterogeneity but also social, ethnic, and gender diversity. We propose that diversity should be carefully considered in planning of CS projects with the aim of giving voice to all individuals in an egalitarian fashion. This urge is nicely reflected in the recommendation of the first practice standard of INVOLVE (i.e. inclusive opportunities) and the recently launched BAME project of the BTA. We encourage the use of specialised moderation techniques and methods of collaboration which counteract established social dynamics, mostly expertise and competence asymmetries, by giving voice and safe spaces to non-expert minority stakeholders. Focus groups and Delphi methodology offer good tool sets to these ends (e.g. [14]) although they certainly do not completely remove barriers of social structures and dynamics. Yet, with first experiences gathered in recent CS projects described in this chapter, such methods can be refined and custom-tailored to fit the needs of tinnitus CS. Moreover, the *process character* can be considered essential in any CS project and the co-created establishment of methods and proceedings is a valuable outcome. Looking ahead, it may be feasible to define recommendations with respect to diversity and inclusion which then could act as standards for all CS in tinnitus.

New Technologies, Internet, and Scaling

Due to the COVID-19 restrictions in place for most of 2020, the BTA adjusted the way they worked with many activities being conducted online, instead of face-to face, to maintain social distance and safety. One such event was a webinar which was hosted jointly by the BTA and Tinnitus Hub during Tinnitus Week 2021, which provided research updates and gave those with lived experience the opportunity to ask questions. Questions asked before the event were used to inform the topics of discussion and then there was also the opportunity for discussion about tinnitus research at the end of the panel discussion. This gave all those involved, those with lived experience of tinnitus and researchers, the opportunity to identify and discuss important issues within current tinnitus research.

The above is just one example of how new technologies can be leveraged to reach different, and most importantly wider, audiences. The webinar in question was attended by only about 50 tinnitus patients, but one could easily envisage scaling such events to many hundreds of participants at a time; or alternatively, organising online events with a certain frequency that allows for wide participation. The Tinnitus Talk forum, with over 30,000 registered members, Facebook groups of a similar scale, reddit communities, and other online groups can all be considered fruitful grounds for engaging with a wide audience. Community inputs can be gathered through live video or audio interaction, Q&As, polling, posting comments, rating and sharing of content, and submission of video/audio recordings as input for the research community.

Furthermore, a structured website where users have to log in to engage, like Tinnitus Talk, has the additional advantage of being able to capture data from users. In fact, Tinnitus Hub is seeking funding to integrate a database into the Tinnitus Talk forum, where user data linked to individual accounts can be collected. This or similar efforts could enable large-scale surveys with several time points producing longitudinal data to further study tinnitus natural history as well as treatment journeys. The reach and accessibility of platforms like BTA or Tinnitus Hub would allow for scalability of research which would meet the definition of *big data*. Moreover, such data could represent the general tinnitus population and heterogeneity more validly than more traditionally selected clinical populations [31]. Finally, the application of these technologies could allow for surveys on current topics which could be completed within reasonable time.

Conclusion

In this chapter, we presented completed and on-going CS projects in the field of tinnitus research and introduced the different organisations engaging in these projects. Current challenges identified are the heterogeneity of tinnitus, misalignment between academic and patient interests, dissonance between stakeholders, and lack of academic incentives. In order to improve the status of CS in tinnitus research, we therefore recommend to better value the concept of CS, improve its evidence base and evaluation, further education and awareness, consider more diversity and inclusion, involve patients in all levels of the research projects, and lastly, encourage the use of new technologies including the internet and social media.

Patient involvement in tinnitus research is still in its infancy. A majority of the CS work can currently only be identified in the UK and partly in Europe, while comparable efforts are lacking on an international level. Transnational organisation and harmonisation could be achieved by raising awareness through scientific publishing, conference activities and public dissemination. We hope that this chapter will inspire further CS actions and collaborations to expand our understanding of and treatments for the condition.

Acknowledgments We thank Raj Shekhawat, Jae-Jin Song, Yu-te Lee, Berthold Langguth, and Axel Schiller for helping us to identify CS projects. Furthermore, we are grateful for the Swiss National Fund 'Postdoc Mobility' Grants P400PS_186670, P5R5PS_203068, and to the University Research Priority Program 'Dynamics of Healthy Aging' of the University of Zürich supporting Patrick Neff during the preparation of the manuscript. Maryam Shabbir is funded by the European Union's Horizon 2020 Research and Innovation program under the Marie Sklodowska-Curie grant agreement number 764604.

References

1. Hecker S, Haklay M, Bowser A, Makuch Z, Vogel J, editors. Citizen science: innovation in open science, society and policy. UCL Press; 2018. https://doi.org/10.14324/111.9781787352339.
2. Mahr D, Dickel S. Citizen science beyond invited participation: nineteenth century amateur naturalists, epistemic autonomy, and big data approaches avant la lettre. Hist Philos Life Sci. 2019;41(4):1–9. https://doi.org/10.1007/s40656-019-0280-z.
3. Shirk JL, Ballard HL, Wilderman CC, Phillips T, Wiggins A, Jordan R, McCallie E, Minarchek M, Lewenstein BV, Krasny ME, Bonney R. Public participation in scientific research: a framework for deliberate design. Ecol Soc 2012;17(2). https://doi.org/10.5751/ES-04705-170229.
4. Anderson DP, Cobb J, Korpela E, Lebofsky M, Werthimer D. SETI@home: an experiment in public-resource computing. Commun ACM. 2002;45(11):56–61. https://doi.org/10.1145/581571.581573.
5. Bonney R, Cooper CB, Dickinson J, Kelling S, Phillips T, Rosenberg KV, et al. Citizen science: a developing tool for expanding science knowledge and scientific literacy. Bioscience. 2009;59(11):977–84. https://doi.org/10.1525/bio.2009.59.11.9.
6. Rolfe DE, Ramsden VR, Banner D, Graham ID. Using qualitative Health Research methods to improve patient and public involvement and engagement in research. Res Involv Engagem. 2018;4(1):1–8. https://doi.org/10.1186/s40900-018-0129-8.
7. Heigl F, Kieslinger B, Paul KT, Uhlik J, Dörler D. Opinion: toward an international definition of citizen science. Proc Natl Acad Sci USA; 2019;116(17):8089–8092. doi:https://doi.org/10.1073/pnas.1903393116
8. Eitzel MV, Cappadonna JL, Santos-Lang C, Duerr RE, Virapongse A, West SE, Kyba C, Bowser A, Cooper CB, Sforzi A, Metcalfe AN. Citizen science terminology matters: exploring key terms. Citiz Sci 2017;2(1). https://doi.org/10.5334/cstp.96.s1.
9. Goldman J, Shilton K, Burke J, Estrin D, Hansen M, Ramanathan N, Reddy S, Samanta V, Srivastava M, West R. Participatory sensing: a citizen-powered approach to illuminating the patterns that shape our world. In: Foresight and governance project, white paper; 2009. p. 1–5.
10. Kraft R, Schlee W, Stach M, Reichert M, Langguth B, Baumeister H, et al. Combining mobile crowdsensing and ecological momentary assessments in the healthcare domain. Front Neurosci. 2020;14:145. https://doi.org/10.3389/fnins.2020.00164.
11. Reed MS, Graves A, Dandy N, Posthumus H, Hubacek K, Morris J, Prell C, Quinn CH, Stringer LC. Who's in and why? A typology of stakeholder analysis methods for natural resource management. J Environ Manag. 2009;90(5):1933–49. https://doi.org/10.1016/j.jenvman.2009.01.001.
12. Nowotny H, Scott P, Gibbons M. "Mode 2" revisited: the new production of knowledge. Minerva. 2003;41:179–94. https://doi.org/10.1023/A:1025505528250.
13. Bela G, Peltola T, Young JC, Balázs B, Arpin I, Pataki G, et al. Learning and the transformative potential of citizen science. Conserv Biol. 2016;30(5):990–9. https://doi.org/10.1111/cobi.12762.
14. Fackrell K, Smith H, Colley V, Thacker B, Horobin A, Haider HF, Londero A, Mazurek B, Hall DA. Core Outcome Domains for early phase clinical trials of sound-, psychology-, and pharmacology-based interventions to manage chronic subjective tinnitus in adults: the COMIT'ID study protocol for using a Delphi process and face-to-face meetings to establish consensus. Trials. 2017;18(1):1–1. https://doi.org/10.1186/s13063-017-2123-0.
15. Haines RH, White J, Meakin G, Tan W, Hepburn T, Leighton P, Theriou C, Stockdale D, Almey C, Nicholson R, Hall DA. Protocol for a multi-Centre randomised controlled stand-alone feasibility trial to assess potential effectiveness and cost-effectiveness of digital hearing aids in patients with tinnitus and hearing loss (the HUSH trial). Pilot Feasibility Stud. 2020;6:1–9. https://doi.org/10.1186/s40814-020-00582-5.
16. Smith H, Horobin A, Fackrell K, Colley V, Thacker B, Hall DA. Defining and evaluating novel procedures for involving patients in Core Outcome Set research: creating a meaningful long list of candidate outcome domains. Res Involvem Engage. 2018 Dec;4(1):1–2. https://doi.org/10.1186/s40814-020-00582-5.
17. Adams B, Sereda M, Casey A, Byrom P, Stockdale D, Hoare DJ. A Delphi survey to determine a definition and description of hyperacusis by clinician consensus. Int J Audiol. 2020:1–7. https://doi.org/10.1080/14992027.2020.1855370.
18. Smith H, Fackrell K, Kennedy V, Barry JG, Broomhead E, Hoare DJ. An evaluation of paediatric tinnitus services in UK National Health Service audiology departments. BMC Health Serv Res. 2020;20(1):1–1. https://doi.org/10.1186/s12913-020-5040-y.
19. Taylor JA, Thompson DM, Hall DA, Walker D-M, McMurran M, Casey A, Featherstone D, MacDonald C, Stockdale D, Hoare DJ. The TinMan study: feasibility trial of a psychologically informed, audiologist-delivered, manualised intervention for tinnitus. Int J Audiol. 2020;59(12):905–14. https://doi.org/10.1080/14992027.2020.1788730.
20. Lewis S, Chowdhury E, Stockdale D, Kennedy V. Assessment and management of tinnitus: summary of NICE guidance. BMJ. 2020;368:m976. https://doi.org/10.1136/bmj.m976.
21. Beukes EW, Baguley DM, Jacquemin L, Lourenco MP, Allen PM, Onozuka J, Stockdale D, Kaldo V, Andersson G, Manchaiah V. Changes in tinnitus experiences during the COVID-19 pandemic. Front Public Health. 2020;8:681. https://doi.org/10.3389/fpubh.2020.592878.
22. Phillips JS, Erskine S, Moore T, Nunney I, Wright C. Eye movement desensitization and reprocessing as a treatment for tinnitus. Laryngoscope. 2019;129(10):2384–90. https://doi.org/10.1002/lary.27841.

23. Jackson JG. The cortisol awakening response: a feasibility study investigating the use of the area under the curve with respect to increase as an effective objective measure of tinnitus distress. Am J Audiol. 2019;28(3):583–96. https://doi.org/10.1044/2019_aja-18-0174.
24. Burns-O'Connell G, Stockdale D, Hoare DJ. Soldiering on: a survey on the lived experience of tinnitus in aged military veterans in the UK. Med Humanit. 2019;45(4):408–15. https://doi.org/10.1136/medhum-2019-011671.
25. McFerran DJ, Stockdale D, Holme R, Large CH, Baguley DM. Why is there no cure for tinnitus? Front Neurosci. 2019;13:802. https://doi.org/10.3389/fnins.2019.00802.
26. NIHR Central Commissioning Facility. National standards for public involvement. 2018. https://assets.publishing.service.gov.uk/government/uploads/system/uploads/attachment_data/file/730917/local_action_on_health_inequalities.pdf. Accessed on 02 March 2021.
27. Schlee W, Hall DA, Canlon B, Cima RF, de Kleine E, Hauck F, Huber A, Gallus S, Kleinjung T, Kypraios T, Langguth B. Innovations in doctoral training and research on tinnitus: the European School on Interdisciplinary Tinnitus Research (ESIT) perspective. Front Aging Neurosci. 2018 Jan;12(9):447. https://doi.org/10.3389/fnagi.2017.00447.
28. Hall D, Mohamad N, Firkins L, Fenton M, Stockdale D. Identifying and prioritizing unmet research questions for people with tinnitus: the James Lind Alliance Tinnitus Priority Setting Partnership. Clin Invest. 2013;3(1):21–8. https://doi.org/10.4155/cli.12.129.
29. Ng ZY, Archbold S, Harrigan S, Mulla I. Conspiring together: tinnitus and hearing loss. British Tinnitus Association; 2015. Available from www.tinnitus.org.uk/tef.
30. Schlee W, Schoisswohl S, Staudinger S, Schiller A, Lehner A, Langguth B, Schecklmann S, Simoes J, Neff P, Marcrum S, Spiliopoulou M, et al. Towards a unification of treatments and interventions for tinnitus patients: the EU research and innovation action UNITI. Prog Brain Res. 2021;260:441–51. https://doi.org/10.1016/bs.pbr.2020.12.005.
31. Probst T, Pryss RC, Langguth B, Spiliopoulou M, Landgrebe M, Vesala M, Harrison S, Schobel J, Reichert M, Stach M, Schlee W. Outpatient tinnitus clinic, self-help web platform, or mobile application to recruit tinnitus study samples? Front Aging Neurosci. 2017;9:113. https://doi.org/10.3389/fnagi.2017.00113.
32. Simoes J, Neff P, Schoisswohl S, Bulla J, Schecklmann M, Harrison S, Vesala M, Langguth B, Schlee W. Toward personalized tinnitus treatment: an exploratory study based on internet crowdsensing. Front Public Health. 2019;7:157. https://doi.org/10.3389/fpubh.2019.00157.
33. Hibbert A, Vesala M, Kerr M, Fackrell K, Harrison S, Smith H, Hall DA. Defining symptom concepts in chronic subjective tinnitus: web-based discussion forum study. Interact J Med Res. 2020;9(1):e14446. https://doi.org/10.2196/14446.
34. Hall DA, Hibbert A, Vesala M, Kerr M, Harrison S. Web-based discussion forums reveal the person-centered relevance and importance of tinnitus. Prog Brain Res. 2021;260:205–21. https://doi.org/10.1016/bs.pbr.2020.12.001.
35. Hall DA, Smith H, Hibbert A, Colley V, Haider HF, Horobin A, Londero A, Mazurek B, Thacker B, Fackrell K. Core Outcome Measures in Tinnitus (COMiT) initiative. The COMiT'ID study: developing core outcome domains sets for clinical trials of sound-, psychology-, and pharmacology-based interventions for chronic subjective tinnitus in adults. Trends Hear. 2018;22:2331216518814384. https://doi.org/10.1177/23312165188184.
36. Hall DA, Hibbert A, Smith H, Haider HF, Londero A, Mazurek B, Fackrell K. Core Outcome Measures in Tinnitus (COMiT) initiative. One size does not fit all: developing common standards for outcomes in early-phase clinical trials of sound-, psychology-, and pharmacology-based interventions for chronic subjective tinnitus in adults. Trends Hear. 2019;23:2331216518824827. https://doi.org/10.1177/2331216518824827.
37. Shabbir M, Akeroyd MA, Hall DA. A comprehensive literature search to identify existing measures assessing "concentration" as a core outcome domain for sound-based interventions for chronic subjective tinnitus in adults. Prog Brain Res. 2021;262:209–24.
38. Terwee CB, Prinsen CA, Chiarotto A, Westerman MJ, Patrick DL, Alonso J, Bouter LM, De Vet HC, Mokkink LB. COSMIN methodology for evaluating the content validity of patient-reported outcome measures: a Delphi study. Qual Life Res. 2018;27(5):1159–70. https://doi.org/10.1177/2331216518824827.
39. COMET Initiative. Patients and the public. https://www.comet-initiative.org/Patients. Accessed 02 Mar 2021.
40. Young B, Bagley H. Including patients in core outcome set development: issues to consider based on three workshops with around 100 international delegates. Res Involv Engagem. 2016;2(1):1–3. https://doi.org/10.1186/s40900-016-0039-6.
41. Arnold LM, Crofford LJ, Mease PJ, Burgess SM, Palmer SC, Abetz L, Martin SA. Patient perspectives on the impact of fibromyalgia. Patient Educ Couns. 2008;73(1):114–20. https://doi.org/10.1016/j.pec.2008.06.005.
42. Wolfe F, Smythe HA, Yunus MB, Bennett RM, Bombardier C, Goldenberg DL, Tugwell P, Campbell SM, Abeles M, Clark P, Fam AG. The American College of Rheumatology 1990 criteria for the classification of fibromyalgia. Arthritis Rheum. 1990;33(2):160–72. https://doi.org/10.1002/art.1780330203.
43. Wolfe F, Clauw DJ, Fitzcharles MA, Goldenberg DL, Katz RS, Mease P, Russell AS, Russell IJ, Winfield JB, Yunus MB. The American College of Rheumatology preliminary diagnostic criteria for fibromyalgia and measurement of symptom severity. Arthritis Care Res. 2010;62(5):600–10. https://doi.org/10.1002/acr.20140.
44. Wiggins A, Wilbanks J. The rise of citizen science in health and biomedical research. Am J Bioeth. 2019;19(8):3–14. https://doi.org/10.1080/15265161.2019.1619859.
45. Staniszewska S, Denegri S, Matthews R, Minogue V. Reviewing progress in public involvement in NIHR research: developing and implementing a new vision for the future. BMJ Open. 2018;8(7):e017124. https://doi.org/10.1136/bmjopen-2017-017124.
46. Ocloo J, Matthews R. From tokenism to empowerment: progressing patient and public involvement in healthcare improvement. BMJ Qual Saf. 2016;25(8):626–32. https://doi.org/10.1136/bmjqs-2015-004839.
47. Husain FT, Gander PE, Jansen JN, Shen S. Expectations for tinnitus treatment and outcomes: a survey study of audiologists and patients. J Am Acad Audiol. 2018;29(4):313–36. https://doi.org/10.3766/jaaa.16154.
48. Patel DI, Winkler P, Botello J, Villarreal J, Puga F. The citizen scientist: community-academic partnerships through Translational Advisory Boards. Patient Educ Couns. 2016;99(12):2087–90. https://doi.org/10.1016/j.pec.2016.07.013.
49. Cederroth CR, Canlon B, Langguth B. Hearing loss and tinnitus—are funders and industry listening? Nat Biotechnol. 2013;31(11):972–4. https://doi.org/10.1038/nbt.2736.
50. NIHR Central Commissioning Facility. National standards for public involvement. 2018. http://www.donorhealth-btru.nihr.ac.uk/wp-content/uploads/2018/10/NIHR-Public-Involvement-Standards-2018.pdf. Accessed on 02 Mar 2021.

Mobile Health Solutions for Tinnitus

57

Muntazir Mehdi, Franz J. Hauck, Ruediger Pryss, and Winfried Schlee

Abstract

Modern mobile devices are mainstream and ubiquitous devices. The widespread adoption of mobile devices has resulted in surge of mobile applications (apps) hosted on marketplaces (app stores) of several mobile platforms. Besides other benefits, these apps are also applied in healthcare-related and medical use, for instance, in case of tinnitus, where tinnitus disorder is associated with the perception of ringing sound without external sound source. In particular, for tinnitus, these apps allow provision of tinnitus-related relief, self-help, and general management. The collective aim of this chapter is to foster and report on Mobile Health (mHealth) solutions, in particular mobile apps within the tinnitus context. First, this chapter provides an up-to-date overview of existing mHealth apps available for major mobile platforms. Second, this chapter provides deep insights into quality and effectiveness of said mobile apps for tinnitus treatment and management. Finally, this chapter provides discussions in relation to the tinnitus-related mHealth apps.

M. Mehdi · R. Pryss
Institute of Clinical Epidemiology and Biometry, University of Wuerzburg, Würzburg, Germany
e-mail: ruediger.pryss@uni-wuerzburg.de

F. J. Hauck
Institute of Distributed Systems, Ulm University, Ulm, Germany
e-mail: franz.hauck@uni-ulm.de

W. Schlee (✉)
Institute for Information and Process Management, Eastern Switzerland University of Applied Sciences, St. Gallen, Switzerland
e-mail: winfried.schlee@tinnitusresearch.org

Abbreviations

API	Application programming interface
CBT	Cognitive behavioral therapy
EMA	Ecological momentary assessment
MARS	Mobile application rating scale
MCS	Mobile crowdsensing
mHealth	Mobile health
TRT	Tinnitus retaining therapy

Introduction

State-of-the-art mobile devices entertain a wide array of user base, evident by the fact that approximately 3.6 billion mobile users worldwide existed at the end of year 2020 [1]. Moreover, these mobile devices allow development of new apps using application programming interface (API) provided by device manufacturers and hosting of such apps through respective marketplaces. Consequently, many app developers and publishers from different application domains frequently develop and host new apps to the app marketplaces, thereby, forming an evolving ecosystem of mobile apps. This is evident by the fact that there were around 3.14 million apps in Google's Play Store and nearly 2.10 million apps in Apple's App Store by the end of year 2020 [2]. The extensive development of new apps has caused a wide-spread interest in app consumers for app download and usage; for instance, by the end of year 2020, approximately 218 billion apps were downloaded worldwide by app consumers, increased by nearly 55% since 2016 [3, 4].

Along with others, mHealth has also benefited from rapid growth of mobile apps [5], where mHealth is the application of mobile devices to support healthcare, deliver mobile interventions, or supporting medical and public health practices using mobile devices [6]. Among many, few notable characteristics of mHealth are its potential to support a large volume and variation of users, unrestricted accessibility, and

W. Schlee et al. (eds.), *Textbook of Tinnitus*, https://doi.org/10.1007/978-3-031-35647-6_57

cost-effectiveness. Furthermore, there exist a large number of mHealth apps hosted on all major app stores or marketplaces [7]. At the end of year 2020, around 50 thousand mHealth apps were available on each Google's Play Store and Apples' App Store [8, 9]. To add to the benefits of mHealth apps, recent studies have also reported the helpfulness of mHealth apps in the management of many health problems [10–12]; such is the case with tinnitus, where people who suffer from the tinnitus disorder already use mHealth apps for tinnitus-related relief and management [13, 14].

Tinnitus is defined as "the conscious awareness of a tonal and /or noise sound for which there is no identifiable corresponding external acoustic source," while "tinnitus disorder" is defined as "tinnitus plus tinnitus-associated emotional distress and functional disability" (see Chap. 9). For tinnitus-related relief, a plethora of mHealth apps exist that are easily accessible through several app marketplaces. These mHealth apps are usually designed to reduce tinnitus and have the potential to reach a wide and diverse range of tinnitus patients and thus, these apps could alleviate and sustain workload of [limited] tinnitus-related healthcare providers that are overwhelmed by large numbers of tinnitus patients.

The antecedent benefits of mHealth apps within tinnitus context plus growing interest of research community along with interest in development of tinnitus-related mHealth apps affirms a fast-growing and evolving availability of tinnitus-related apps on app marketplaces. However, presently, the state and availability of these apps for tinnitus can be unknown to most patients and clinicians alike. Therefore, an up-to-date review of app stores and literature to foster and report on tinnitus-related mHealth solutions and apps can contribute significantly to the existing body of knowledge.

Categories of mHealth Solutions

The notable potential of mHealth solutions and apps is embodied in their ability to allow effective management of complex and long-term illnesses as well as chronic disorders like tinnitus. It is noteworthy that many tinnitus patients readily employ mHealth apps for tinnitus-related relief and management [13]. Following are the main categories of mHealth solutions and apps that are currently available on mobile app stores as well as used by tinnitus patients.

Tinnitus Treatment and Management

In the Chaps. 43–59 of this textbook, the currently existing treatment modalities are described in detail. Some of these treatment modalities can be effectively delivered by smartphone apps. As an example, tinnitus masking and sound therapy mHealth apps employ sound manipulation techniques such as, notched sound, acoustic neuromodulation, or amplitude modulation via mobile devices for tinnitus-related relief, while cognitive behavioral treatment (CBT) apps provide necessary information for coping and restructuring cognition and behavior. The development of the CBT apps thereby highly influenced and supported by the research work on Internet-delivered CBT and self-help for effective treatment of tinnitus [15–17], specifically for treatment of psychological comorbidities occurring with tinnitus, such as depression and anxiety [18, 19].

Hearing Protection, Testing, and Enhancement

Tinnitus is known to be confluent with hearing loss in the majority of tinnitus cases [20], where hearing loss has the potential to drastically reduce the overall quality of life of patients [21]. Moreover, it is understood that exposure to increased noise and acoustic trauma can exacerbate and develop tinnitus symptoms [22]. Similarly, variations in hearing loss can result in increased tinnitus-related distress [21, 23]. Nevertheless, in aforementioned cases, on one hand, the use of hearing aids and cochlear implants can reduce tinnitus symptoms [24–26]. While to offset tinnitus-associated predicaments of hearing loss, the hearing protection, enhancement, and testing apps are designed for the users to: (1) assess tinnitus symptoms, (2) reduce tinnitus-related disabilities of hearing processes in daily life, and (3) reduce the likelihood of tinnitus development.

For hearing protection via mobile devices, a variety of apps exist, for example, detection of sound exposure [27], use of smart headphones or earphones [28], and hearing conservation training and education apps [29, 30]. For detection of extreme sound or noise levels, modern mobile devices use the on-chip (embedded) microphone of the mobile device, where accurate detection of sound and noise levels have been reported by some studies [27, 31]. For hearing testing or audiometry, the mHealth apps allow testing of hearing functions on an individual patient level as well as on group levels such that, comparison of testing capabilities can also be carried out with others (such as family members or friends). Moreover, hearing testing mHealth apps allow audiometry on different sound frequencies, pitch, and loudness levels in both silent and noisy environments. The mobile-based audiometry apps allow estimation of pure-tone thresholds [32], and are capable of providing accurate, reliable, and audiologists-quality results [33, 34], even in clinical settings [35, 36], provided that the audio output devices (for instance, headphones) are properly calibrated [37, 38]. For hearing enhancement, mobile devices have the potential to be used as a cheaper alternative to cochlear implants or hearing aids in improving the quality of life of patients suffering from tinnitus [39, 40]. Moreover, hearing enhancement apps offer: (1) auditory education and training programs to improve auditory skills [41, 42], (2) noise removal or reduction [43, 44], 3) audio signal or sound amplification [45], and (4) digital hearing aids using mobile devices [46].

Ecological Momentary Assessment (EMA)

Adding to aforementioned possibilities, one added benefit of mHealth apps is their application in monitoring the health and lifestyle data of patients suffering from complex and long-term illnesses and disorders like tinnitus. These apps therefore not only provide valuable feedback to patients for self-management of their symptoms but also provide clinicians, researchers, and healthcare providers with useful and detailed information relating to health status of patients. Moreover, inclusion of these tracking and monitoring mHealth apps in clinical systems can: (1) rehabilitate and empower patients, (2) enable tailored treatment solutions, and (3) simplify consumption of healthcare resources [47–51]. Ecological momentary assessment (EMA) is a well-established methodological approach to systematically gather assessment data such as, symptomatic, behavioral, cognitive, environmental, psychological, and physiological data from patients or research participants [52, 53]. The EMA methods allow collection of such data in repeated, periodic, and near real-time fashion from participants' native and real-world environment. Furthermore, the patient data are collected in near-experience (close in time to experience) events, thus eliminating the bias caused by retrospective self-reporting approaches [52, 54]. EMA has been widely exploited in psychological research over an extended period of time [55–58], and has been used in context of tinnitus [59–61].

The conventional appropriation of EMA methods can be further enhanced by combining mobile crowdsensing (MCS) approaches. This not only enables swift and convenient collection of assessment data using mobile devices [62–65] but also opens up the opportunities to streamline on-chip (mobile embedded) and auxiliary sensors to contextually enrich the assessment data. Similarly, MCS- based EMA methods can support large-scale assessment data collection in a time and cost-effective way from a variety of [research] participants globally [66–68]. Few existing MCS-based EMA tools have already been reported in literature [51, 69, 70] and have been useful in establishing better insights into understanding tinnitus [49, 61, 71–74].

Mobile Health Apps for Tinnitus

A comprehensive list of commercially available mHealth apps for tinnitus-related treatment and management in Google's Play Store and Apple's App Store are given in Table 57.1 (Sound Therapy and Tinnitus Management) and Table 57.2 (CBT), along with their respective properties. Among the app properties, the "users" property will provide the readers with coverage of the apps' usage; the number of users in case of iOS platform is not provided since the number of users is not publicly available on Apple's App Store. Rating will provide brief insights into app's quality according to the app store's star rating system. Update property gives the last seen update of the app on respective app store. Pricing property gives insights into the costs associated with the apps; herein, the app prices are given in Euros, whereas for free apps, following additional categories exist: Free (I) corresponds to free apps with in-app purchases, and Free (A) corresponds to free apps that are supported by advertisements. The platform property distinguishes between platform-specific user base and signifies their behavior toward the app. Moreover, an asterisk (*) in front of the app name corresponds to the app being reported in literature with technical description about the app development process. Those apps that are evidence based, and whose clinical evaluation is either reported or reviewed in the scientific literature, to the best of our knowledge, are marked with a dagger (†).

The tabulated apps are easily accessible for download for both of the two major mobile platforms (iOS and Android) via their respective marketplaces (Apple's App Store and Google's Play Store). From Tables 57.1 and 57.2, it can be noted that the sound therapy apps for tinnitus masking and distraction using relaxing sounds and sound generators are most widely downloaded and preferred mobile-based solutions for tinnitus treatment and management. Next, the CBT apps for treatment of tinnitus and accompanying conditions (such as, stress, anxiety, and depression) are preferred by the users, with second most number of downloads, where apps of type *CBT chatbots* have higher number of downloads. On the other hand, sound therapy apps, such as *Zen* and *Notch* therapy apps, are the least downloaded mobile apps for tinnitus as of now.

Further from Tables 57.1 and 57.2, it can be noted that most of the mHealth apps for tinnitus treatment and management are freely downloadable through marketplaces with few exceptions, such as tinnitus relief apps like *Stop Tinnitus*, *Tinnitus Therapy lite*, *Tinnitus Help*, *Whist*, *Tinnitus Relief*, and *White Noise lite*, were available at low costs. Even

Table 57.1 Apps providing tinnitus-related relief (Free = royalty free, Free (I) = in-app purchases, Free (A) = ad-supported, Free (I,A) = both). Selection of apps is based on a systematic analysis provided in [75]. App details updated: April 10, 2022. Apps reported and described in the literature are marked with asterisks (*), apps with clinical evaluation are marked with daggers (†) and more details are provided in Table 57.3

App name	Usage	Platform	Users	Rating	Pricing
H&T sound therapy	Tinnitus masking	Android	10 K+	4.2	Free
myNoise*	Tinnitus masking	Android	100 K+	4.2	Free (I)
		iOS		4.6	Free (I)
Oticon ON (Oticon tinnitus sound)	Sound stimulation	Android	500 K+	2.3	Free
		iOS		2.9	Free
Relax melodies	Sound stimulation	Android	10 M+	4.6	Free (I,A)
		iOS		4.8	Free (I)
Relax noise 3*	Tinnitus masking	Android	100 K+	4.2	Free
SimplyNoise*	Tinnitus/stress Control and Management	Android	50 K+	4.1	Free
		iOS		4.3	Free (I)
Starkey relax*	Tinnitus Masking and Management	Android	100 K+	4.3	Free
		iOS		4.0	Free
Stop tinnitus*	Tinnitus masking	Android	100+	2.7	7.95 €
		iOS		1.3	8.03 €
Tinnitracks*	Tinnitus Control and Management	Android	10 K+	4.0	Free (I)
		iOS		3.6	Free (I)
Tinnitus balance app*	Sound stimulation	Android	50 K+	3.7	Free
		iOS		2.3	Free
Tinnitus help*	Tinnitus masking	Android	500+	3.0	9.90 €
		iOS		3.7	15.99 €
Tinnitus notch	Sound stimulation	Android	1 K+	2.7	Free
Tinnitus peace	Sound stimulation	Android	5 K+	3.8	Free
Tinnitus play	Tinnitus masking	iOS		4.2	Free
Tinnitus relief*	Sound stimulation	Android	1 K+	4.0	Free (I,A)
Tinnitus sound therapy	Tinnitus masking	Android	10 K+	4.2	Free (A)
Tinnitus therapy (lite) *†	Tinnitus Therapy and Masking	Android	50 K+	2.7	Free (I)
		iOS		4.3	Free (I)
Tonal tinnitus therapy	Tinnitus therapy	Android	50 K+	3.8	Free (I)
Track your tinnitus	Tinnitus management	Android	1 K+	1.7	Free
		iOS		1.0	Free
Whist – Tinnitus relief*	Sound stimulation	Android	10 K+	4.2	Free (A)
		iOS		3.4	Free
White noise (lite)*	Sound stimulation and tinnitus management	Android	5 M+	4.2	Free
		iOS		4.8	Free (I)
Widex Zen*	Sound stimulation	Android	10 K+	4.0	Free
		iOS		4.4	Free

though many apps are freely downloadable, some of these apps have associated costs in forms of in-app purchases or subscriptions. Similarly, for most of the CBT apps, the apps were freely downloadable; however, the main features of these apps (such as the CBT exercises) are offered as in-app purchases or subscriptions with costs of up to 300 Euros.

In connection to the quality of tinnitus-related apps based on the star ratings (out of five) provided by app users on the respective app store, nearly all tinnitus relief apps scored higher than three (cf. Table 57.1), therefore, indicating at least some level of functionality and quality. The CBT apps (cf. Table 57.2) had better quality as compared to that of tinnitus relief apps since nearly all apps scored higher than 4 (with few exception) for both Android and iOS platforms. It is important to note here that unfortunately, the quality or star ratings provided by the users are highly subjective and reflective of their own opinion. Furthermore, the ratings can be influenced by the provider, or the competitor, of the app

Table 57.2 Apps providing CBT (Free = royalty free, Free (I) = in-app purchases, Free (A) = ad-supported, Free (I,A) = both). Selection of apps is based on a systematic analysis provided in [75]. App details updated: April 10, 2022. Apps reported and described in the literature are marked with asterisks (*), apps with clinical evaluation are marked with daggers (†) and more details are provided in Table 57.3

App name	Usage	Platform	Users	Rating	Pricing
Beltone tinnitus calmer*	CBT and sound therapy	Android	100 K+	4.6	Free (I)
		iOS		4.8	Free
CBT companion	Visual tools for CBT	Android	100 K+	4.5	Free (I)
		iOS		4.7	Free
Diapason for tinnitus*	Game-based tinnitus therapy	Android	50 K+	2.2	Free (I)
		iOS			Free (I)
Mindshift CBT*†	Anxiety control and management	Android	100 K+	4.1	Free
		iOS		4.3	Free
Kalmeda *	Tinnitus therapy	Android	1 K+	3.0	Free (I)
		iOS		3.0	Free (I)
Moodfit—stress and anxiety	Stress and anxiety management and control	Android	50 K+	4.5	Free
Quirk CBT	Self-help CBT	Android	10 K+	3.6	Free (I)
		iOS		4.8	Free (I)
ReSound tinnitus relief*†	CBT, tinnitus and sound therapy	Android	100 K+	4.7	Free (I)
		iOS		4.7	Free (I)
Sanvello—anxiety and depression	Anxiety tracking and management	Android	1 M+	4.3	Free (I)
		iOS		4.8	Free (I)
Stress and anxiety companion	Stress and anxiety management	Android	10 K+	4.2	Free (I)
		iOS		4.2	Free (I)
What's up?	CBT and ACT for stress, anxiety and depression management	Android	500 K+	4.6	Free (I)
		iOS		4.6	Free (I)
Woebot*†	Chatbot for stress and anxiety management	Android	100 K+	4.7	Free
		iOS		4.7	Free
Wysa*†	Chatbot for CBT exercises	Android	1 M+	4.8	Free (I)
		iOS		4.8	Free (I)
Youper*	CBT and ACT based Chatbot	Android	1 M+	4.1	Free (I)
		iOS		4.8	Free (I)

which makes the assessment of app quality unreliable [81]. It is therefore pertinent that alternative measures for quality appraisal of tinnitus-related apps are taken, where the clinical effectiveness of the apps as well as objective quality assessment of the apps using standard tools (such as Mobile Application Rating Scale (MARS) [82] or the multidimensional app-quality assessment tool for health-related apps (AQUA) [83]) can be established.

Effectiveness of Apps

The appstores of Apple and Google are open online platforms allowing everybody to upload a smartphone app as long as the app complies with the regulations of the respective appstore. According to the current regulations, the appstores do not check for empirical evidence of the uploaded mHealth apps. As a result of this policy, a large percentage of health apps in the appstores are available for the users without any proof for clinical efficacy. Thus, there is a fundamental difference between a drug store and an appstore: in a drug store, the client can trust that all the available drugs have gone through a certification process that also involves an empirical validation of the drug—in the appstores such a process for health apps does not exist (yet). This is not necessarily a bad situation, but an important information that should kept in mind when browsing the appstores for health applications. There are several reasons why the majority of health apps have not been empirically testes. One reason is the large cost for a clinical trial. A large percentage of the current health apps have been developed by small start-up companies or private persons that do not have the money to finance a clinical trial. In the current situation, the app provider is not obliged to perform an empirical study. If the app is good and attractive to the users, the provider can make money with the app without investing in a clinical trial. Another reason can also be that the app is currently under clinical evaluation and the study is ongoing. Some providers make the app already available to the users, while the app is being evaluated. Unfortunately, there is no easy way for the user to find out if the mHealth app has been evaluated or not. In Table 57.3, we provide an overview of the apps from Tables 57.1 and 57.2, which have been empirically investigated. The overview is a result of a systematic literature analysis provided in [75]. As can be seen in the table, three out of five apps have not been tested specifically on tinnitus patients. For those apps, that have been tested on tinnitus sufferers, the sample sizes were small. This demonstrates the great need for more scientific studies on the effectiveness of mHealth interventions for tinnitus.

Table 57.3 Apps from Tables 57.1 and 57.2 with empirical studies published in peer-reviewed scientific journals

App name	Study information	Sample	Outcome and results	Additional information	Ref.
Mindshift CBT	Exploratory study, 3 weeks, 5 days/week, minimum 15 min/day	n = 104 Students, not specifically tinnitus sufferers	Outcome measure: PHQ-15, GAD-7, PHQ-9. Results: Significant reduction in somatic anxiety, general anxiety and depression	The app is designed for the cognitive behavioral treatment with a focus on anxiety and depression. Not specifically tested with tinnitus sufferers.	[76]
ReSound relief	Home trial for selected participants, 2 weeks	n = 10 in home trial patients with cochlear implants	Outcome measure: Numeric rating scale. Results: No statistical analysis, descriptive analysis shows large improvements for 3 out of 10 participants		[77]
Tinnitus therapy lite	Convenience sampling, 1 month, 30–45 min / day	n = 5	Outcome measure: Tinnitus handicap inventory (THI) Results: No significant results, small sample size		[78]
Woebot	Randomized controlled trial, experimental group: 2 weeks app usage, control group: Reading a CBT-related book	*n* = 70, college students, not specifically tinnitus sufferers	Outcome measure: PHQ-9, GAD-7, PANAS Results: Significant reduction on depression and anxiety average usage: 12.1 sessions	Not specifically tested with tinnitus sufferers.	[79]
Wysa	Convenience sampling	*n* = 129	Outcome measure: PHQ-9 Results: Significant reduction of depressive symptoms, effect size of 0.63	Not specifically tested with tinnitus sufferers.	[80]

Discussions and Conclusions

The tinnitus-related mHealth apps have the potential to treat, control, and manage tinnitus-related symptoms and distress. The apps for tinnitus treatment and management have the potential to assist patients with self-help and self-management of tinnitus symptoms. The apps for hearing healthcare can assist tinnitus patients in improving their quality of life. The MCS-based EMA and monitoring apps can allow the possibility to acquire tinnitus-related data to better understand this phantom phenomenon. However, in connection to aforementioned mHealth apps, caution is needed by patients and clinicians alike specifically, when it comes to nonregulated and nonclinically validated apps. From patients' perspective, in the process of using such apps for management of tinnitus-related distress, the healthcare providers should be continuously involved. From clinicians' perspective, tinnitus-related apps should be confirmed for suitability and quality prior to recommending to patients such that only effective, nonharmful, and valid apps are used by the patients.

In connection to effective tinnitus-related mHealth apps, although the limited available literature denotes the possibility of using apps for tinnitus control and management; however, there is a certain level of ambiguity due to lack of evidence in connection to the clinical effectiveness of these apps. Further research to identify the clinical effectiveness of these apps in tinnitus context is essential to ascertain the substantial health benefits of tinnitus-related mHealth apps. At present, numerous apps are being used by patients and recommended by healthcare providers without confirmed information in relation to their health benefits. Contemporary quality appraisal methods such as star rating system to gauge objective quality of apps are insufficient and sometimes unreliable, even controlled trials only report on clinical efficacy and overlook certain aspects of the app such as functionality, engagement, elegance, and practicality of apps.

Acknowledgments This publication is a result of research supported by funding from the European Union's Horizon 2020 research and innovation program under the Marie Sklodowska-Curie grant agreement number 722064 (European School for Interdisciplinary Tinnitus Research, ESIT) [84].

References

1. Number of smartphone users worldwide from 2016 to 2023. https://www.statista.com/statistics/330695/number-of-smartphone-users-worldwide/.
2. Number of apps available in leading app stores as of 4th quarter 2020. https://www.statista.com/statistics/276623/number-of-apps-available-in-leading-app-stores/.
3. Mobile app usage-statistics and facts. https://www.statista.com/topics/1002/mobile-app-usage/.
4. Number of mobile app downloads worldwide from 2016 to 2020. https://www.statista.com/statistics/271644/worldwide-free-and-paid-mobile-app-store-downloads/.
5. Kao CK, Liebovitz DM. Consumer mobile health apps: current state, barriers, and future directions. PM&R. 2017;9(5):S106–15.
6. World Health Organization, et al. mhealth: new horizons for health through mobile technologies Geneva: WHO; 2011 (2017). https://www.who.int/goe/publications/goe_mhealth_web.pdf.

7. Carroll JK, Moorhead A, Bond R, LeBlanc WG, Petrella RJ, Fiscella, K. Who uses mobile phone health apps and does use matter? A secondary data analytics approach. J Med Internet Res. 2017;19(4):e125. https://doi.org/10.2196/jmir.5604. http://www.jmir.org/2017/4/e125/
8. Number of mhealth apps available at Google play from 1st quarter 2015 to 4th quarter 2020. https://www.statista.com/statistics/779919/health-apps-available-google-play-worldwide//
9. Number of mhealth apps available in the apple app store from 1st quarter 2015 to 4th quarter 2020. https://www.statista.com/statistics/779910/health-apps-available-ios-worldwide/.
10. Naslund JA, Aschbrenner KA, Barre LK, Bartels SJ. Feasibility of popular m-health technologies for activity tracking among individuals with serious mental illness. Telemed e-Health. 2015;21(3):213–6.
11. Nelson EC, Verhagen T, Noordzij ML. Health empowerment through activity trackers: an empirical smart wristband study. Comput Hum Behav. 2016;62:364–74.
12. Ventola CL. Mobile devices and apps for health care professionals: uses and benefits. Pharm Therapeut. 2014;39(5):356.
13. Deshpande AK, Shimunova T. A comprehensive evaluation of tinnitus apps. Am J Audiol. 2019;28(3):605–16.
14. Smith S, Sereda M. Smartphone apps for tinnitus management. Hear J. 2020;73(2):20–2.
15. Andersson G, Strömgren T, Ström L, Lyttkens L. Randomized controlled trial of internet-based cognitive behavior therapy for distress associated with tinnitus. Psychosom Med. 2002;64(5):810–6.
16. Jun HJ, Park MK. Cognitive behavioral therapy for tinnitus: evidence and efficacy. Korean J Audiol. 2013;17(3):101.
17. Kaldo-Sandstrom V, Larsen HC, Andersson G. Internet-based cognitive—behavioral self-help treatment of tinnitus. Am J Audiol. 2004;13:185.
18. Martinez-Devesa P, Waddell A, Perera R, Theodoulou M. Cognitive behavioural therapy for tinnitus. Cochrane Database Syst Rev. 2007;1:CD012614.
19. Robinson SK, Viirre ES, Bailey KA, Kindermann S, Minassian AL, Goldin PR, Pedrelli P, Harris JP, McQuaid JR. A randomized controlled trial of cognitive-behavior therapy for tinnitus. Int Tinnitus J. 2008;14(2):119–26.
20. Norena A, Micheyl C, Chéry-Croze S, Collet L. Psychoacoustic characterization of the tinnitus spectrum: implications for the underlying mechanisms of tinnitus. Audiol Neurotol. 2002;7(6):358–69.
21. Langguth B, Kreuzer PM, Kleinjung T, De Ridder D. Tinnitus: causes and clinical management. Lancet Neurol. 2013;12(9):920–30.
22. Elgoyhen AB, Langguth B, De Ridder D, Vanneste S. Tinnitus: perspectives from human neuroimaging. Nat Rev Neurosci. 2015;16(10):632–42.
23. Baguley D, McFerran D, Hall D. Tinnitus. Lancet. 2013;382(9904):1600–7.
24. Del Bo L, Ambrosetti U. Hearing aids for the treatment of tinnitus. Prog Brain Res. 2007;166:341–5.
25. Moffat G, Adjout K, Gallego S, Thai-Van H, Collet L, Norena A. Effects of hearing aid fitting on the perceptual characteristics of tinnitus. Hear Res. 2009;254(1–2):82–91.
26. Ruckenstein MJ, Hedgepeth C, Rafter KO, Montes ML, Bigelow DC. Tinnitus suppression in patients with cochlear implants. Otol Neurotol. 2001;22(2):200–4.
27. Sinha S, Kozin ED, Naunheim MR, Barber SR, Wong K, Katz LW, Otero TM, Stefanov-Wagner IJ, Remenschneider AK. Cycling exercise classes may be bad for your (hearing) health. Laryngoscope. 2017;127(8):1873–7.
28. Themann CL, Kardous CA, Beamer BR, Morata TC. 'Internet of ears' and hearables for hearing loss prevention. Hear J. 2019;72(4):32–4.
29. Khan KM, Evans SS, Bielko SL, Rohlman DS. Efficacy of technology-based interventions to increase the use of hearing protections among adolescent farmworkers. Int J Audiol. 2018;57(2):124–34.
30. Watts KL, Welles R, Zurek P. Development of the warfighter's hearing health instructional (whhip) primer app. Mil Med. 2018;183(suppl 1):231–6.
31. Ventura R, Mallet V, Issarny V, Raverdy PG, Rebhi F. Evaluation and calibration of mobile phones for noise monitoring application. J Acoust Soc Am. 2017;142(5):3084–93.
32. Saliba J, Al-Reefi M, Carriere JS, Verma N, Provencal C, Rappaport JM. Accuracy of mobile-based audiometry in the evaluation of hearing loss in quiet and noisy environments. Otolaryngol Head Neck Surg. 2017;156(4):706–11.
33. Bornman ME, et al. Validation of hearTest smartphone application for extended high frequency hearing thresholds. Ph.D. thesis, University of Pretoria, 2017.
34. Chu YC, Cheng YF, Lai YH, Tsao Y, Tu TY, Young ST, Chen TS, Chung YF, Lai F, Liao WH. A mobile phone–based approach for hearing screening of school-age children: cross-sectional validation study. JMIR Mhealth Uhealth. 2019;7(4):e12033. https://doi.org/10.2196/12033. https://mhealth.jmir.org/2019/4/e12033/.
35. Brittz M, Heinze B, Mahomed-Asmail F, Swanepoel DW, Stoltz A. Monitoring hearing in an infectious disease clinic with mhealth technologies. J Am Acad Audiol. 2019;30(6):482–92.
36. Louw C, Eikelboom RH, Myburgh HC, et al. Smartphone-based hearing screening at primary health care clinics. Ear Hear. 2017;38(2):e93–e100.
37. Masalski M, Grysiński T, Krecicki T. Hearing tests based on biologically calibrated mobile devices: comparison with pure-tone audiometry. JMIR Mhealth Uhealth. 2018;6(1):e10. https://doi.org/10.2196/mhealth.7800. https://mhealth.jmir.org/2018/1/e10/.
38. Pickens AW, Robertson LD, Smith ML, Zheng Q, Song S. Headphone evaluation for app-based automated mobile hearing screening. Int Arch Otorhinolaryngol. 2018;22(04):358–63.
39. Kochkin S, Tyler R. Tinnitus treatment and the effectiveness of hearing aids: hearing care professional perceptions. Hear Rev. 2008;15(13):14–8.
40. Trotter M, Donaldson I. Hearing aids and tinnitus therapy: a 25-year experience. J Laryngol Otol. 2008;122(10):1052–6.
41. Lee Y. Mobile application development for improving auditory memory skills of children with hearing impairment. Audiol Speech Res. 2017;13(1):50–61.
42. Olson A, Williams R, Livingston E, Futscher C. Review of auditory training mobile apps for adults with hearing loss. Perspect ASHA Spec Inter Groups. 2018;3(7):12–23.
43. Alamdari N, Yaraganalu S, Kehtarnavaz N. A real-time personalized noise reduction smartphone app for hearing enhancement. In: 2018 IEEE signal processing in medicine and biology symposium (SPMB). IEEE; 2018. p. 1–5.
44. Bhattacharya A, Sehgal A, Kehtarnavaz N. Low-latency smartphone app for real-time noise reduction of noisy speech signals. In: 2017 IEEE 26th international symposium on industrial electronics (ISIE). IEEE; 2017. p. 1280–1284.
45. Chowdhury TA, Sehgal A, Kehtarnavaz N. Integrating signal processing modules of hearing aids into a real-time smartphone app. In: 2018 40th annual international conference of the IEEE engineering in medicine and biology society (EMBC). IEEE; 2018. p. 2837–40.
46. Sharma S, Tiwari N, Pandey PC. Implementation of digital hearing aid as a smartphone application. Proc Interspeech. 2018;2018:1175–9.
47. Badawy SM, Kuhns LM. Economic evaluation of text-messaging and smartphone-based interventions to improve medication adherence in adolescents with chronic health conditions: a systematic review. JMIR Mhealth Uhealth. 2016;4(4):e121.
48. Goldstein BA, Shulman A. Tinnitus outcome profile and tinnitus control. Int Tinnitus J. 2003;9(1):26–31.

49. Muniandi LP, Schlee W, Pryss R, Reichert M, Schobel J, Kraft R, Spiliopoulou M. Finding tinnitus patients with similar evolution of their ecological momentary assessments. In: 2018 IEEE 31st international symposium on computer-based medical systems (CBMS). IEEE; 2018. p. 112–7.
50. Pryss R, Reichert M, Langguth B, Schlee W. Mobile crowd sensing services for tinnitus assessment, therapy, and research. In: 2015 IEEE international conference on Mobile services. IEEE; 2015. p. 352–9.
51. Pryss R, Schlee W, Langguth B, Reichert M. Mobile crowdsensing services for tinnitus assessment and patient feedback. In: 2017 IEEE international conference on AI & Mobile Services (AIMS). IEEE; 2017. p. 22–9.
52. Shiffman S, Stone AA, Hufford MR. Ecological momentary assessment. Annu Rev Clin Psychol. 2008;4:1–32.
53. Stone AA, Shiffman S. Ecological momentary assessment (ema) in behavorial medicine. Ann Behav Med. 1994;16(3):199–202. https://doi.org/10.1093/abm/16.3.199.
54. Walz LC, Nauta MH, Aan Het Rot M. Experience sampling and ecological momentary assessment for studying the daily lives of patients with anxiety disorders: a systematic review. J Anxiety Disord. 2014;28(8):925–37.
55. Ebner-Priemer UW, Trull TJ. Ecological momentary assessment of mood disorders and mood dysregulation. Psychol Assess. 2009;21(4):463.
56. Moore RC, Depp CA, Wetherell JL, Lenze EJ. Ecological momentary assessment versus standard assessment instruments for measuring mindfulness, depressed mood, and anxiety among older adults. J Psychiatr Res. 2016;75:116–23.
57. Shiffman S, Stone AA. Introduction to the special section: ecological momentary assessment in health psychology. Health Psychol. 1998;17(1):3.
58. Trull TJ, Ebner-Priemer UW. Using experience sampling methods/ecological momentary assessment (esm/ema) in clinical assessment and clinical research: introduction to the special section. Psychol Assess. 2009;21(4):457–62. https://doi.org/10.1093/abm/16.3.199.
59. Goldberg RL, Piccirillo ML, Nicklaus J, Skillington A, Lenze E, Rodebaugh TL, Kallogjeri D, Piccirillo JF. Evaluation of ecological momentary assessment for tinnitus severity. JAMA Otolaryngol Head Neck Surg. 2017;143(7):700–6.
60. Henry JA, Galvez G, Turbin MB, Thielman EJ, McMillan GP, Istvan JA. Pilot study to evaluate ecological momentary assessment of tinnitus. Ear Hear. 2012;32(2):179.
61. Probst T, Pryss RC, Langguth B, Rauschecker JP, Schobel J, Reichert M, Spiliopoulou M, Schlee W, Zimmermann J. Does tinnitus depend on time-of-day? An ecological momentary assessment study with the trackyourtinnitus application. Front Aging Neurosci. 2017;9:253.
62. Garcia-Palacios A, Herrero R, Belmonte M, Castilla D, Guixeres J, Molinari G, Baños R, Botella C. Ecological momentary assessment for chronic pain in fibromyalgia using a smartphone: a randomized crossover study. Eur J Pain. 2014;18(6):862–72.
63. Kubiak T, Smyth JM. Connecting domains—ecological momentary assessment in a mobile sensing framework. In: Digital phenotyping and Mobile sensing. Springer; 2019. p. 201–7.
64. Runyan JD, Steenbergh TA, Bainbridge C, Daugherty DA, Oke L, Fry BN. A smartphone ecological momentary assessment/intervention "app" for collecting real-time data and promoting self-awareness. PLoS One. 2013;8(8):e71325.
65. Silk JS, Forbes EE, Whalen DJ, Jakubcak JL, Thompson WK, Ryan ND, Axelson DA, Birmaher B, Dahl RE. Daily emotional dynamics in depressed youth: a cell phone ecological momentary assessment study. J Exp Child Psychol. 2011;110(2):241–57.
66. Probst T, Pryss RC, Langguth B, Spiliopoulou M, Landgrebe M, Vesala M, Harrison S, Schobel J, Reichert M, Stach M, et al. Outpatient tinnitus clinic, self-help web platform, or mobile application to recruit tinnitus study samples? Front Aging Neurosci. 2017;9:113.
67. Rozgonjuk D, Elhai JD, Hall BJ. Studying psychopathology in relation to smartphone use. In: Digital phenotyping and mobile sensing. Springer; 2019. p. 185–99.
68. Vaid SS, Harari GM. Smartphones in personal informatics: a framework for self-tracking research with mobile sensing. In: Digital phenotyping and mobile sensing; 2019. p. 65–92.
69. Kraft R, Schlee W, Stach M, Reichert M, Langguth B, Baumeister H, Probst T, Hannemann R, Pryss R. Combining mobile crowdsensing and ecological momentary assessments in the healthcare domain. Front Neurosci. 2020;14:164.
70. Wilson MB, Kallogjeri D, Joplin CN, Gorman MD, Krings JG, Lenze EJ, Nicklaus JE, Spitznagel EE Jr, Piccirillo JF. Ecological momentary assessment of tinnitus using smartphone technology: a pilot study. Otolaryngol Head Neck Surg. 2015;152(5):897–903.
71. Probst T, Pryss R, Langguth B, Schlee W. Emotion dynamics and tinnitus: daily life data from the "trackyourtinnitus" application. Sci Rep. 2016;6:31166.
72. Probst T, Pryss R, Langguth B, Schlee W. Emotional states as mediators between tinnitus loudness and tinnitus distress in daily life: results from the "TrackYourTinnitus" application. Sci Rep. 2016;6:20382.
73. Pryss R, Probst T, Schlee W, Schobel J, Langguth B, Neff P, Spiliopoulou M, Reichert M. Prospective crowdsensing versus retrospective ratings of tinnitus variability and tinnitus–stress associations based on the trackyourtinnitus mobile platform. Int J Data Sci Analyt. 2019;8(4):327–38.
74. Schlee W, Pryss RC, Probst T, Schobel J, Bachmeier A, Reichert M, Langguth B. Measuring the moment-to-moment variability of tinnitus: the trackyourtinnitus smart phone app. Front Aging Neurosci. 2016;8:294.
75. Mehdi M, Dode A, Pryss R, Schlee W, Reichert M, Hauck FJ. Contemporary review of smartphone apps for tinnitus management and treatment. Brain Sci. 2020;10(11):867. https://doi.org/10.3390/brainsci10110867. https://www.mdpi.com/2076-3425/10/11/867.
76. Paul AM, Fleming CE. Anxiety management on campus: an evaluation of a Mobile health intervention. J Technol Behav Sci. 2019;4:58–61.
77. Tyler RS, Owen RL, Bridges J, Gander PE, Perreau A, Mancini PC. Tinnitus suppression in cochlear implant patients using a sound therapy app. Am J Audiol. 2018;27:316–23.
78. Sabarish, A.; Kruthika, S. Efficacy of sound therapy using android based application in individual with tinnitus. 2019.
79. Fitzpatrick KK, Darcy A, Vierhile M. Delivering cognitive behavior therapy to young adults with symptoms of depression and anxiety using a fully automated conversational agent (Woebot): a randomized controlled trial. JMIR Ment Health. 2017;4:e19.
80. Inkster B, Sarda S, Subramanian V. An empathy-driven, conversational artificial intelligence agent (Wysa) for digital mental Wellbeing: real-world data evaluation mixed-methods study. JMIR Mhealth Uhealth. 2018;6:e12106.
81. Kuehnhausen M, Frost VS. Trusting smartphone apps? to install or not to install, that is the question. In: 2013 IEEE international multi-disciplinary conference on cognitive methods in situation awareness and decision support (CogSIMA). 2013. p. 30–7. https://doi.org/10.1109/CogSIMA.2013.6523820.
82. Stoyanov SR, Hides L, Kavanagh DJ, Wilson H. Development and validation of the user version of the mobile application rating scale (umars). JMIR Mhealth Uhealth. 2016;4(2):e72.
83. O'Rourke T, Pryss R, Schlee W, Probst T. Development of a multidimensional app-quality assessment tool for health-related apps (AQUA). Digit Psychol. 2020;1(2):13–23.
84. Schlee W, Hall DA, Canlon B, Cima RF, de Kleine E, Hauck F, Huber A, Gallus S, Kleinjung T, Kypraios T, et al. Innovations in doctoral training and research on tinnitus: the european school on interdisciplinary tinnitus research (esit) perspective. Front Aging Neurosci. 2018;9:447.

58 Autonomous Tinnitus Management (Self-Help for Tinnitus)

Don J. McFerran and Nic Wray

Abstract

A common refrain heard from people with tinnitus is, "My doctor said there's nothing that can be done." This chapter shows that there are, in fact, are many steps that people can take to help themselves. However, there is no clear signposting through this confusing maze of potential self-treatments and this is of concern as whilst some self-management techniques have been shown to be of benefit, for others the evidence of effectiveness is less conclusive, and for some, there is evidence of no effect or indeed potential harm. It is important for health professionals and patient support organisations to encourage and facilitate evidence-based autonomous interventions such as tinnitus support groups, using reliable information and self-help books, sound therapy and relaxation techniques. People with tinnitus should be discouraged from trying dietary supplements, lasers, and ear-candling. Information from the Internet or social media, and participation in chat-rooms and forums can have benefits, but the quality and reliability of information is variable and could lead to an increase in tinnitus distress.

Rigorous, large-scale studies are called for as a stronger evidence base would help people make better informed decisions about the options they choose to self-manage their tinnitus.

D. J. McFerran (✉) · N. Wray
Tinnitus UK (Formerly the British Tinnitus Association), Sheffield, UK

W. Schlee et al. (eds.), *Textbook of Tinnitus*, https://doi.org/10.1007/978-3-031-35647-6_58

Graphical Abstract

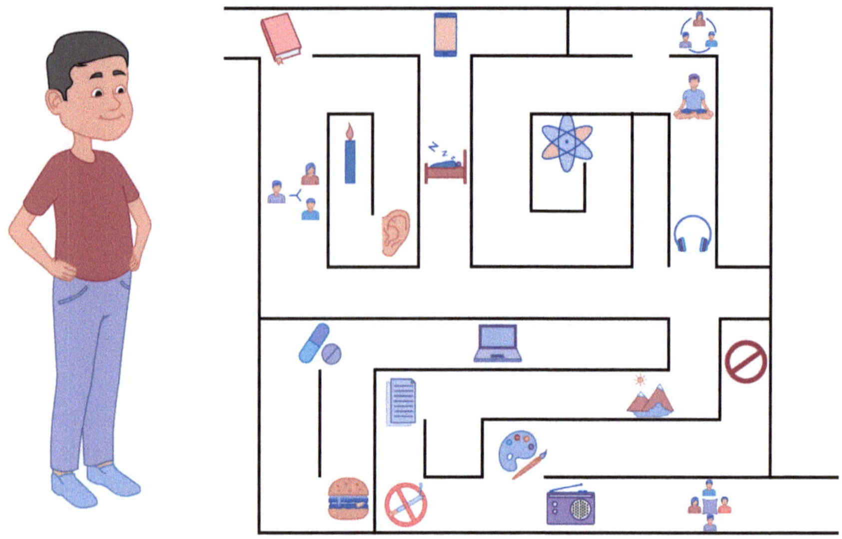

Potentially useful	Use with caution	Avoid!
Self help books	Online information	Home ear wax removal
Apps	Social media	Ear candles
Information leaflets	Chatrooms & forums	Drugs
Sound therapies	Changes to diet	Dietary supplements
Self help groups & befriending	Hearing protection	Lasers
Managing co-morbidities		
Sleep management		
Stopping smoking		
Yoga/Tai chi		
Relaxation		
Hobbies and interests		

Highlights

- Tinnitus information is more widely available than ever before and is recommended as part of a tinnitus management strategy, but not all of it is good quality.
- Peer support can be offered via face-to-face support groups, one to one befriending, or by online resources including online support groups, chatrooms, and forums. The latter offer increased access to tinnitus support. Peer support can help people feel more knowledgeable, more hopeful about their tinnitus, and less isolated and alone.
- Sound therapy (enrichment) is widely used. The evidence base for its use is poor but the safety profile is good.
- General improvements to well-being, fitness, and stress management can be beneficial, but it is unlikely that diet modifications (including reduction of caffeine and alcohol consumption) greatly influence tinnitus.
- In the absence of a known dietary deficiency, there is no evidence that any dietary supplement is effective for tinnitus.
- Hearing protection is underutilised, and appropriate use should be encouraged.

Introduction and Definitions

The original brief for this chapter was that it should describe self-help measures for tinnitus. However, within the healthcare framework there is no clear definition of self-help, and the expression is also used in legal, business, educational, and personal development contexts with varying connotations. In the medical literature, the compound word, self-help, is sometimes qualified in an oxymoronic fashion as guided self-help, minimal guidance self-help or minimal contact self-help. In addition, healthcare writers use other expressions such as self-care, self-directed, and self-management and the choice of terminology often appears arbitrary and overlapping. Self-care and self-management have National Library of Medicine Medical Subject Headings (MeSH). Self-help does not have a MeSH entry and self-directed only has a qualified term "self-directed learning as topic." The MeSH definition for self-care is "Caring for self when ill or positive actions and adopting behaviors to prevent illness" [1]. The MeSH definition for self-management is an "Individual's ability to manage the symptoms, treatment, physical and psychosocial consequences and lifestyle changes inherent in living with a chronic condition. Efficacious self-management encompasses ability to monitor one's condition and to affect the cognitive, behavioral, and emotional responses necessary to maintain a satisfactory quality of life" [2]. Neither of these definitions adequately describe the tinnitus patient's journey to seek a solution to their symptom(s) outside of conventional healthcare pathways.

A further factor to consider is that some measures that are described as self-help have actually had considerable input from experienced healthcare professionals. For example, a patient might use a self-help book or leaflet that has been written by healthcare professionals, who have based the text on the techniques that they use during face-to-face consultations. Healthcare professionals are therefore indirectly involved in the care delivery rather than directly.

For the above reasons, we decided that the current terminology cannot adequately define the boundaries for this chapter, and we altered the title to autonomous tinnitus management. We define this as the measures taken by an individual to address their own medical symptom(s) or condition(s) (in this case tinnitus) without using the direct input of a practitioner of conventional or complementary and alternative medicine.

Using this definition, some modalities such as Internet-delivered cognitive behavioural therapy (ICBT) are excluded because they do generally incorporate some direct contact with healthcare professionals, albeit usually at a distance via phone or email rather than face-to-face. Similarly, some interventions that are partly self-managed such as progressive tinnitus management [3] and Tinnitus Tunes [4] are excluded because an element of contact with healthcare professionals is incorporated. The definition, in contrast, does allow inclusion of the use of a book or information leaflet written by a healthcare professional – as in this case there is no direct contact. Interventions where there is input from trainers who are not healthcare professionals are also acceptable under this definition, allowing interventions such as Qigong and yoga to be considered.

One further complication with this topic is that there is a dearth of good quality evidence: people who are trying to find their own solution to tinnitus do not write articles for peer-reviewed journals regarding their travails. So, rather paradoxically, the majority of the evidence base for a chapter on measures that people use to improve their tinnitus without input from clinicians, comes from clinicians.

Current Usage

A small number of studies have explored the steps that people take to try and improve or eradicate their tinnitus. Most notably, Kutyba et al. [5] collated information from 460 tinnitus patients using an open question about activities they had undertaken, without specialist support, to reduce their tinnitus severity. One hundred eighty-eight participants (40.9%) had undertaken some form of intervention, with acoustic stimulation, distraction techniques, relaxation/meditation/yoga, and physical activity the most popular. Participants were more likely to have undertaken an autonomous intervention if they had higher educational status or more severe tinnitus as determined by the Tinnitus Handicap Inventory (THI) questionnaire [6]. There were limitations to this study: it was retrospective, dependent on people's recall and did not assess the efficacy of the interventions. Also, the study did not address health-information seeking behaviour which is regarded as a coping strategy in its own right [7]. It is therefore likely that the number of self-helping participants in the study is an underestimate.

Simoes et al. [8] undertook a survey of people interacting with Tinnitus Hub, an online self-help platform [9]. Information was obtained from 5017 people, of whom 2916 (58.1%) reported having tried at least one tinnitus treatment previously. The aim of this study was to explore the possibility of personalised tinnitus treatments and consequently did not ask participants whether each intervention was self- or physician-instigated. However, within the results are some interventions that are likely to have been self-instigated: 1562 people reported using "self-sound stimulation"; 1157 had used (dietary) supplements and/or herbal (medicines); 254 had used self-help books.

Beukes et al. [10] explored tinnitus coping strategies among 240 participants who had shown interest in an Internet-based intervention for tinnitus. Among this group, 50 (20.2%) reported using sound enrichment, 43 (17.4%) used techniques to divert their attention, and 13 (5.3%) used relaxation techniques.

Obtaining Information

> Knowledge itself is power - Sir Francis Bacon
> A little learning is a dangerous thing [11]

The first step that most people take when confronted with a new medical condition or symptom is to try and find relevant information, and humanity has been recording information about tinnitus as far back as written records go: text regarding tinnitus has been found on a series of clay tablets discussing medical matters in the library of King Assurbanipal (685–631 BC) in Ninevah in the Neo-Assyrian empire (modern-day Iraq) [12]. Greek and Roman writers also described tinnitus [13], and Hippocrates (460–377 BC) even made the link between tinnitus and hearing loss [14]. Further progress regarding tinnitus emerged with Jean-Marc Itard's work on ear diseases in the eighteenth century, *Traité des maladies de l'oreille et de l'audition* [15]. The first book devoted purely to tinnitus was *Subjective Noises in the Head and Ears: Their Etiology, Diagnosis and Treatment*, by Henry MacNaughton-Jones, published in 1891 [16]. However, most of these writings were aimed at medical professionals and most people at the time they were written will not have had access to the information these scripts contained.

Nowadays, accessibility has dramatically improved: an online search for "tinnitus" returns tens of millions of results and online booksellers list hundreds of English language tinnitus-related books.

The Role of Information in Tinnitus Management

There is a widespread impression among healthcare professionals that information is a key component of tinnitus management. The UK's National Institute for Health and Care Excellence (NICE) state that: "Early provision of relevant information may help the person manage tinnitus better and prevent tinnitus from being intractable and/or distressing" [17], and the authors of the *European Guideline for Tinnitus* state that "having information about tinnitus can be very powerful" [18]. The American Academy of Otolaryngology-Head and Neck Surgery's clinical practice guidelines for tinnitus suggest that clinicians should provide brochures and suggestions for self-help books to their patients experiencing bothersome tinnitus [19]. These recommendations, however, appear to largely be the opinions of their respective committees with scant supportive evidence regarding the therapeutic efficacy of receiving information regarding tinnitus. Such evidence that does exist is presented later in this chapter when considering the various modes of information delivery.

Although people generally want to know more about any health condition they may have, there is some evidence that patients prefer more individualised care and tailored rather than generic information [20].

Types of Information Sought

The evidence review for patient information conducted by NICE [17] suggested that the information people with tinnitus were looking for included:

- Information about changes in tinnitus
- Whether anything can be done to improve the noise
- How tinnitus symptoms can be prevented
- The impact of different management options

However, NICE concluded that the evidence for this recommendation was low quality.

The *European Guideline for Tinnitus* [18] suggested that information topics to be provided to people with tinnitus should include:

- What is tinnitus?
- What causes and maintains it
- Pulsatile tinnitus
- Common misunderstandings and myths
- Hearing loss and hearing aids
- Ear wax removal
- Hyperacusis and tinnitus
- Protecting your hearing
- Habituating to tinnitus
- Relaxation
- Monitoring tinnitus
- Use of sound
- Dealing with sleep problems
- Dealing with the emotional consequences of tinnitus
- Self-help and support groups

This list is more extensive than that suggested in the NICE's *Tinnitus: Assessment and Management*, though no evidence base for this choice was presented.

An in-house study of people accessing the British Tinnitus Association (BTA) website [21] was conducted throughout the month of November 2021 (unpublished data). Firstly, the search term(s) used on the original search engine query was/were considered (Table 58.1).

Secondly, the number of views per webpage was assessed (Table 58.2).

Table 58.1 Terms used to initiate online search that leads to people accessing BTA website

Most common search terms	Explanation (where appropriate)	Clicks through
British Tinnitus Association	An aggregate of two queries: British Tinnitus Association ($n = 1427$) and tinnitus association ($n = 167$)	1594
Pulsatile tinnitus	An aggregate of four queries: Pulsatile tinnitus ($n = 1030$), pulsatile tinnitus NHS ($n = 223$), pulsatile tinnitus in one ear only ($n = 119$) and pulsatile tinnitus changes with head position ($n = 101$)	1473
Tinnitus		1068
Tinnitus after COVID vaccine	An aggregate of five queries: Tinnitus after COVID vaccine ($n = 208$), tinnitus COVID vaccine ($n = 195$), COVID vaccine tinnitus ($n = 175$), tinnitus and COVID vaccine ($n = 143$), COVID vaccine and tinnitus ($n = 118$)	839
TMJ tinnitus	An aggregate of two queries: TMJ tinnitus ($n = 248$) and TMJ and tinnitus ($n = 178$)	426
Silencil	A commercially available supplement claimed to help tinnitus	415
Tinnitus UK		342
Synapse XT	A commercially available supplement claimed to help tinnitus	251
Tinnitus 911	A commercially available supplement claimed to help tinnitus	240
COVID tinnitus	COVID tinnitus ($n = 144$) and tinnitus COVID ($n = 90$)	234
BTA		208
Tinnitus stress	An aggregate of two queries: Tinnitus stress ($n = 100$) and tinnitus and stress ($n = 98$)	198
I hear sounds in my head		148
What causes noises in your head		141
Hyperacusis		135
Hearing music in your head		133
Tinnitus breakthrough 2020		132
Tinnitus society		128
How long does it take for olive oil to clear ear wax		124
Lenire reviews	Lenire is a commercially available device for tinnitus management, available in a few countries through audiology professionals.	115
Musical tinnitus		111
Acouphenol	A commercially available supplement claimed to help tinnitus	106
Misophonia NHS	National Health Service (UK)	102
Eagle hemp CBD gummies tinnitus	CBD or cannabidiol, is the second most prevalent active ingredient in cannabis	91
Tinnitus in children		90

Table 58.2 The number of times individual pages of the BTA website were accessed during a calendar month (November 2021)

Most viewed web page title	Page views
Pulsatile tinnitus	8340
Coronavirus vaccines and tinnitus	7382
Self-help for tinnitus	5405
All about tinnitus	5238
Products for tinnitus (online shop)	4618
Ear wax removal and tinnitus	4502
What does tinnitus sound like?	4046
Musical hallucination (musical tinnitus)	3744
Tinnitus and disorders of the temporomandibular joint (TMJ) and neck	3522
What can I do about it?—Managing your tinnitus	3494
Talk to us (how to access the helpline)	3484
Tinnitus support groups	2734
Tinnitus and stress	2575
Search	2398
I'm hearing noises in my head not my ears!	2191
Sound therapy systems (online shop)	2159
All departments (online shop)	2010
COVID-19 (section)	1973
Sound therapy and tinnitus	1958
Hearing aids and tinnitus	1805
What is tinnitus?	1797
Drugs and tinnitus	1694
Food, drink and tinnitus	1632
Ear plugs (online shop)	1612
Tinnitus and CBD gummies	1590

The findings presented in Tables 58.1 and 58.2 are broadly congruent with the recommendations made in the *European Guideline for Tinnitus* [18] although there were some notable omissions from the latter such as musical tinnitus, the association between temporomandibular joint dysfunction and tinnitus, the role of drugs and the role of foods. The information obtained during the BTA survey may be atypical because the survey was conducted during the COVID-19 pandemic.

Sources of Tinnitus Information

Whilst suggesting that "information is an essential element" [22] of tinnitus management, NICE averred that "On the whole, the general public has poor knowledge of tinnitus" [17]. This statement may seem surprising given the multiple media outlets available to disseminate tinnitus information, and the various parties producing such information. However, although many people turn to the Internet to search for health information, knowledge of specialist sources of help and support may be poor.

In a 2021 survey conducted by international research data and analytics group, YouGov [23], on behalf of the British Tinnitus Association (unpublished data), whilst 43% of respondents said that they or a family member had previously experienced or were currently experiencing tinnitus only 18% claimed to have heard of the British Tinnitus Association [21].

There has been very little research conducted into the information seeking behaviours of people with tinnitus, so our discussion will focus on this behaviour in more general populations.

Methods of obtaining information have changed dramatically over the last quarter of the century with the rise of the Internet and devices capable of accessing it. There are no good resources regarding the information preferences of people with tinnitus, but a recent study examined the health information seeking behaviour of adults in Germany (n = 2151) with one or more chronic illnesses [24]. This showed that most people still prefer to get their health information from a doctor, but the next preferred option was the Internet and smart phones at 39.2%. Paper resources such as books, brochures and magazines were used by 16.5% and self-help groups by only 1.9%.

Online Sources of Information

As mentioned previously, the online world has an abundance of references to tinnitus, and for many people, the Internet is the first place they turn to for health information. In 2009, Pew Research reported that 61% of adult Internet users in the United States had looked online for health information. By 2014, that number had grown to 72% [25], which is broadly in line with usage in Western Europe [26].

Online resources are hosted by a wide variety of organisations including:

- Hospitals and clinics
- Health services, both locally and nationally
- Professional (clinician) organisations
- Open access medical and research journals
- Companies allied to healthcare
- Commercial sites
- Press outlets
- Charities and non-governmental organisations (NGOs)
- Online support groups

Online resources do not have to be text-based which can have advantages in terms of accessibility, responding to personal preference or access requirements. Video, podcasts, webinars, multimedia presentations, and online support groups are often used to provide information, making use of the versatility of digital media.

Online resources are generally accessed through a search engine such as Google or Bing [27]. However, search engines are not impartial. The results they return "are the result of inscrutable and anonymous yet authoritative-seeming processes that can sometimes hide falsity and bias" [28]. Thus, the outcome of an Internet search may depend on multiple factors such as the information-seeker's location, the device being used, the web browser software, the search engine being employed, and previous search history. The most used search engines also prioritise paid advertisements at the top of the search results.

Health information seekers experience varying levels of frustration related to online searching. Frustration with accessing information online is significantly and independently associated with age, race/ethnicity and annual household income [29] and also with lower educational attainment as well as lower income [30], and the authors of both studies highlighted the need for easy access to online health information in diverse populations.

Convenience, coverage, and anonymity are regarded as the main advantages of online information [31], whereas credibility and trustworthiness of health information were noted as limitations by information seekers [32].

Social Media

The definition of social media is broad and constantly evolving but can be defined as "forms of electronic communication (such as websites for social networking and microblogging) through which users create online communities to share information, ideas, personal messages, and other content (such as videos)" [33].

The introduction of online communication services in the 1980s and early 1990s such as CompuServe and AmericaOnline introduced Internet users to bulletin board messaging and real-time online chat. The launch of Six Degrees in 1997, Livejournal in 1999, and Friendster in 2001 kickstarted the development of social media into its current form [34].

Statistics around social media use vary but estimates hover around the 4–4.5 billion mark [35, 36], representing well over half of the global population. Mobile applications make social media platforms easily accessible, with between two-thirds and three-quarters of the world's population estimated to be using a mobile phone [35, 37].

Much of the research on social media and healthcare investigates how health professionals use the platforms, or their potential for disseminating public health information. Relatively few studies focus on the benefits of social media as a self-help management technique.

Researchers have identified several potential benefits to social media use in several long-term conditions, including mental health [38], diabetes [39], and cancer [40]. One study explored tinnitus-related information across three of the most used social media platforms, Facebook, Twitter, and YouTube and concluded that there was considerable tinnitus content [41]. Another study examined the 100 most widely viewed YouTube videos relating to tinnitus [42], finding that most commonly these were produced by people with tinnitus, relating their own story. Relatively few were produced by professionals in the tinnitus field. This highlights one of the caveats of social media, by its very nature it is open to all and there is no quality-check regarding content.

Although other social media platforms have not yet been assessed in the tinnitus scientific press, there is tinnitus content on other sites such as Instagram and TikTok.

Access to online peer support potentially enables people to address issues together, which they have felt to be dealt with unsatisfactorily in traditional settings. This assertion seems to be backed up by four psychological theories and evidence for improved feelings of self-efficacy and group belonging [39].

Table 58.3 presents a summary of potential benefits and challenges relating to social media and their use by people with tinnitus. These are currently hypothetical and have not been subjected to scientific scrutiny.

Trust in social media sources of health information has been shown to be culturally specific [44, 45], whereas expertise-based information from health professionals is universal [44]. However, this trust may be misplaced as others have suggested that social media may disseminate health-related conspiracy beliefs [46].

Sources of Information in Other Formats

Whilst a large majority of people – certainly in high- and middle-income countries – rely on online health information, many online information sources also offer multiple media options, and complement their online offerings with information in more traditional formats. Some organisations, especially hospitals, have been slow to adopt new information technologies and have continued to rely on paper-based information dissemination.

Leaflets

It has long been understood that patients retain only a small proportion of the information relayed to them in a consultation. This was first identified almost half a century ago [47] and although research is scarce, it appears little has changed in patient behaviour in that time [48–50]. In one study, tinnitus patients correctly recalled around one-third of information immediately after a consultation, and this amount dropped one to two weeks later [51]. Recall of information is

Table 58.3 A summary of potential benefits and challenges relating to social media and their use by people with tinnitus. (After Naslund et al. [38]; Reidy et al. [39]; Benetoli et al. [43]; Gentile et al. [40])

Benefits	Example
1. Facilitate social interaction	• Online interaction may be easier for individuals with tinnitus or related hearing problems • Anonymity can help overcome feelings of stigma and embarrassment
2. Access to peer support network	• May reduce feelings of isolation • New relationships can be formed with people who understand tinnitus • Can help to seek information, share experiences and management techniques • Can support friends, family and carers • Validate information
3. Promote engagement and retention in services	• Augment existing interventions to improve engagement • Discredits "nothing can be done" statements • Better understanding of health information
Challenges	
1. Impact on symptoms/ feelings	• Psychosocial comparison • Concentration on tinnitus percept and impact • May reduce in-person interactions and increase feelings of loneliness
2. Facing hostile/ unsupportive interactions	• Cyberbullying is associated with increased anxiety symptoms • Unwanted sharing of self-management techniques • Exposure to advertising for 'cures' and products • Exposure to emotional or non-tinnitus related posts
3. Consequences for daily life	• Risks relating to privacy and confidentiality
4. Inaccurate and unreliable information	• Likely to affect expectations and decision making • Concerns about credibility of information
5. Impact on patient/ healthcare professional relationship	• People may not disclose online activity to healthcare professionals • Could delay seeking help from healthcare professionals

improved if there is additional input in the form of information resources [52]. Written information appears to improve knowledge and satisfaction [53], but may not be enough "to change behaviour and successfully manage the condition for all" [54].

It must be noted that the referenced studies look at leaflets being used in conjunction with a professional intervention, rather than as a pure self-directed action. The caveats regarding accuracy, bias and expertise that apply to online resources similarly apply to leaflets, although the barriers to entry and widespread distribution are much higher.

Among the few studies of information-giving that are available, two have examined the effect of giving leaflets to tinnitus patients. Loumidis, Hallam and Cadge [55] mailed a two-page information leaflet to half of a group of 36 tinnitus patients prior to attending an outpatient appointment. Those who received information were less likely to request professional follow-up care though there was no difference in tinnitus severity as measured by the study's primary outcome measure, the Tinnitus Effects Questionnaire [56]. Hassaan and Trinidade [57] investigated giving patients an information pack comprising six separate leaflets from UK tinnitus charities and a UK tinnitus support group after an initial ENT appointment. Those who received the information packs were much less likely to seek further tinnitus management from the audiology team. Furthermore, among those who did seek audiological tinnitus management, the number failing to attend for that appointment fell from 15.3% to 0.9%. Alteration in tinnitus severity was not assessed in this study. These studies demonstrated the benefits of using information leaflets for the clinical services involved, in terms of resource management, but failed to answer whether such information helped the patients.

Books

A search of online booksellers returns over 600 titles of books with "tinnitus" in the title. These range from scholarly multi-authored textbooks to monographs from pedlars of supplements or those sharing their (self-published) experiences.

Within this range of titles, the array of self-help books ranges from those which are purely informational [58] to those providing a systematic self-help programme [59] or a hybrid approach [60].

There is little information regarding the use of books as a means of disseminating tinnitus information. An Australian study examined the efficacy of bibliotherapy in helping people experiencing tinnitus-related distress [61] and found that, compared to a waiting list control, those who had received a self-help book showed a significant reduction in tinnitus-related distress, which was maintained on 4- and 12-month follow-up. There was, however, considerable dropout from the trial: 35% in the active group failed to complete the study. Another study used bibliotherapy in the form of a cognitive behaviour therapy manual as one arm of a four-arm study [62]. Participants in this arm did not have any therapist contact. There was a high dropout (41.6%) in the bibliotherapy arm, but intention-to-treat analysis showed reduced tinnitus distress compared to the control group.

Press, Television, and Radio

Very little research has examined either the representation of tinnitus in traditional mass media, or the use of these channels by the tinnitus community.

A single study [63] examined coverage of tinnitus in US newspapers by text pattern analysis, and identified five themes: brain stimulation, symptoms, coping, social support, and treatment innovation. These topics differ markedly from the information sought by people with tinnitus.

Studies looking at the media representations of, and information dissemination about, other conditions conclude that such coverage can be misrepresentative, pessimistic, and sensationalised [64–66].

Whilst coverage in mass media could be helpful in raising awareness of a health condition in the general public, coverage may be seen to be "frightening and depressing" to people living with the condition, due to the negative and hyperbolic nature of the stories [65].

Apps for Portable Devices

An app, which is short for application, most frequently refers to a program installed on a smart phone, tablet, or computer. Most apps have a specific and narrow function.

A browse of the common app stores (App Store for Apple, Google Play Store for Android, and Microsoft Store for Windows) returns a long list of free and paid-for apps in response to the search term "tinnitus." Whilst some of these have been developed specifically for tinnitus, others provide sounds for sound therapy, or address problems which are often co-morbid with tinnitus, such as sleep or stress. As recently as 2019, tinnitus apps were only used by a small minority of people living with tinnitus [67].

Tinnitus apps can be classified into four categories based on their purpose: tinnitus education, awareness, and prevention; tinnitus assessment and measurement; tinnitus management; and misinformation [68]. However, only 6% of the content of most popular apps named by survey respondents was information [67]. Respondents in this study mainly were looking to address sleep problems or to mask the tinnitus sound.

Whilst studies have rated apps by quality and feature [68, 69], there is still need for further research, especially in evaluating the efficacy of apps in terms of functions other than sound therapy and cognitive behavioural therapy (CBT) [70, 71].

Evaluation of the Quality of Tinnitus Information

Concern about the quality of online health information has been apparent for more than two decades [72, 73]. "Risky" behaviour in those seeking online information has also been identified [74]. Risky behaviours included not having sufficient knowledge and skills to judge health information quality, tendency to self-medication, not consulting a physician and laxity regarding cyber safety. Further work has confirmed that whilst online health-information seeking is common, few people further consult with a health professional [75].

With social media in particular, the lack of editorial control, the ease of the spread of disinformation, and the tendency for misleading posts to be more popular than those giving accurate, relevant information [76] should be of concern.

Three studies have looked at the quality and readability of tinnitus information, although these have focused on online information [77–79]. All the studies used the DISCERN instrument for rating websites which uses 16 quality indicators, such as clear sources of information, balance, relevance and how up to date the information is [80]. The quality of websites included in the study was considered "fair" [78], "highly variable" but "generally poor" [79] or "limited" [77].

There are very few external accreditation schemes for assessing the quality of health information, and they are not widely used. The Health on the Net Foundation (HON) is an international non-governmental organisation founded to encourage the dissemination of quality health information [81]. In the largest study mentioned above, 18 out of 134 tinnitus websites had obtained HON certification, and these were largely of government origin [79].

The PIF TICK [82] is a UK-wide quality mark for health information which effectively replaced the now-defunct Information Standard [83]. It signifies that an organisation's health information "has been through a professional and robust production process" and has met ten criteria for trustworthy health information.

Whilst consumers may be reassured by accredited sources of information, it should be noted that such accreditation is not a guarantee of quality: both the highest and the lowest ranked websites examined by Fackrell et al. [77] had been accredited by The Information Standard.

Health Literacy

Health literacy refers to a person's ability to understand and use information to make decisions about their health, although definitions and conceptualisations vary. Disadvantaged socioeconomic conditions and, in particular, low educational achievement contribute to low health literacy levels, which in turn leads to low health status and outcomes [84]. However, health literacy is also dependent on the accessibility of healthcare systems, the communication skills of healthcare professionals and the level of complexity of health information [85].

It is generally recommended health information materials be written at a fifth-grade reading level (age 10–11) or lower [86] but more recent guidance urges producers not to use this as a target, nor to rely on readability formulas. Readability formulas ignore the active role of the reader and most factors that contribute to ease of reading and understanding [87].

Low literacy levels are common, even in economically advanced nations. An average of 18.9% of adults in OECD (Organisation for Economic Co-operation and Development) countries are at Level 1 or below (broadly equivalent to primary/elementary school level) [88]. Almost six out of ten Canadians fall into the two lowest literacy categories, a similar proportion of Australians have low literacy skills [89] and in England, 43% of adults aged 18–65 do not have adequate literacy skills to routinely understand health information [90].

Unfortunately, analysis of tinnitus related information showed that much of the information available would be considered "difficult" to read, with mean readability at levels between 10th and 12th grade (age 14–17) [78, 79]. This disparity means that the efficacy of self-help information is likely to be limited.

Peer Support

Peer support involves people taking from shared personal experience to provide knowledge, social interaction, emotional assistance, or practical help to each other, often in a way that is mutually beneficial [91]. Peer support is different from other types of support because the source of support is a similar person with relevant experience.

Peer support can take many forms including online groups, chatrooms and forums, face-to-face support groups or online, telephone or face-to-face befriending on a one-to-one basis.

Peer support has been used by people experiencing a wide range of physical and mental health problems, and a recent survey which compiled information from more than 1000 studies concluded that there is evidence that peer support can help people feel more knowledgeable, confident and happy and less isolated and alone [92].

Face-to-Face Tinnitus Support Groups

There is a long history of tinnitus support groups. The British Tinnitus Association (recently rebranded as Tinnitus UK) [21] was founded in 1979 by people living with tinnitus who had formed support groups in their localities under the aegis of the Royal National Institute for the Deaf [93]. In 1982, the American Tinnitus Association [94] began establishing self-help groups [91], and similar networks exist in many other countries.

Engagement in support groups is low, with estimates ranging from 7% to 20% [95–97]. Barriers to participation include awareness, time constraints and confrontation of negative aspects of the condition [95]. Support groups may have volunteer or professional facilitators, and these may or may not be peers with lived experience of the condition [92, 98]. Most studies have not compared peers alone versus professional or joint peer/professional-led support, but those that do, have found that peers are usually as effective as professionals, particularly when the focus is on emotional or social support [92].

In the first study that comprehensively explored the views of tinnitus support group participants, the most valued features of groups are the knowledge and information provided, the sense of belonging communicated to group members, and the creation and maintenance of a sense of hope towards living with tinnitus [98]. A German study found that quality of life is not associated with tinnitus support group participation [96].

Current guidelines for tinnitus recommend that information about local and national support groups should be given [18, 19, 22].

Online Tinnitus Support Groups

Online tinnitus support groups are a relatively new development, are low cost, and easy to access. The benefits of participation seem to be similar to attending face-to-face support groups [99].

An online American and Canadian study of methods of coping with tinnitus during the COVID-19 pandemic identified a desire for more group online support as one of its key findings [97].

Online Tinnitus Chatrooms and Forums

Online tinnitus chatrooms and forums may be hosted by charities (e.g. Tinnitus UK (formerly British Tinnitus Association) [21], RNID [93]), patient groups (e.g. Tinnitus Hub [9]) or as a sub-section of a wider platform (e.g. Reddit [100]).

A recent analysis of threads from four public online support forums showed that users were able to exchange knowledge and experiences, express complex emotions, gain a network of support, and also engage in non-tinnitus related social conversations [101].

Whilst chatrooms and forums may have moderation policies, it has been noted that lack of control over the quality and reliability of information shared could lead to the propagation of false information. Such information can contribute to increased tinnitus distress, anxiety, purchases of useless products, and delay in seeking appropriate treatment [102].

For people who are particularly vulnerable or prone to psychological stress, it is thought that these groups could be detrimental [101]. As online chatrooms and forums are always available, and not time limited events, there is a risk that by constantly focusing and discussing tinnitus, a person may reinforce their tinnitus by anxiety [99].

Tinnitus Befriending

Befriending can be defined as "a relationship between two or more individuals, initiated, supported and monitored by an agency. The relationship is non-judgmental, mutual, purposeful, and there is a commitment over time" [103].

A wide variety of charitable and voluntary sector organisations offer befriending services across a similarly wide range of physical and mental health conditions. Currently, tinnitus befriending is rare, and no research has yet been undertaken into its effectiveness. A recent systematic review of befriending, however, concluded that there was moderate quality evidence to support the use of befriending for the treatment of individuals with different physical and mental health conditions. Although there was an overall improvement benefit, it is unclear whether befriending does have an impact on outcomes [104], although a previous review did identify that befriending had a modest effect on depressive symptoms and emotional distress in varied patient groups [105].

Sound Therapies

The use of sound in the management of tinnitus has a long pedigree [13] but a poor evidence base. There are many historical references to the use of sound as a tinnitus treatment and Itard, in the second volume of his work, *Traité des maladies de l'oreille et de l'audition* [15], recommended using sounds as close as possible to the sound of the tinnitus: a roaring fire for tinnitus which sounded like wind; burning damp wood for whistling tinnitus; water falling from a vase into a copper bowl for ringing tinnitus.

Sound therapy for tinnitus is typically divided into environmental sound enrichment and wearable sound therapy. The former, as its name suggests, uses a sound source to add sound to the general environment of the tinnitus sufferer. This can be achieved in multiple ways: electronic sound generators produce a range of sounds, often based on nature sounds, such as waves on a beach, wind rustling leaves, the mating call of cicadas or water flowing in a stream. Other non-nature-based sounds are also offered by these devices, such as white or other colours of noise. A study by Handscomb [106] showed that using one manufacturer's environmental sound generator to supply sound therapy at night-time (n = 39) "brook" and "bird" noises were most popular and white noise least so. Relaxing sounds from CDs or MP3 files are also available, and there are anecdotal reports of people deriving benefit from the sound of electric fans, fish tanks' aerators, or wind chimes.

Wearable ear level sound generators (maskers, white noise generators) are generally supplied by healthcare professionals as part of a structured tinnitus management programme. Surprisingly, however, these are also available to buy without any medical or audiological input.

Apps for portable devices (discussed above) can also be used to deliver sound therapy, either as environmental sound enrichment or as wearable sound therapy, using wired or wireless earphones.

People who derive benefit from environmental sound enrichment but share living space with others who prefer quietness, can use headphones, headband earphones or pillows with built-in speakers to restrict the sound experience to themselves – in effect producing a form of wearable sound therapy.

There have been some studies looking at sound therapies provided by healthcare professionals and there have been two Cochrane Reviews of this body of work, one exploring sound therapy (masking) in the management of tinnitus in adults [107] and the other more recent review exploring sound therapy (using amplification devices and/or sound generators) for tinnitus [108]. Both reviews concluded that the available evidence was low quality and was insufficient to support or refute the use of sound therapy for people with tinnitus. However, there were no reports of adverse effects.

There are no studies examining the efficacy of sound therapy devices without involvement of healthcare professionals.

A retrospective study in Poland [5] showed that 188 of 460 participants (40.9%) had used some form of self-help. Among those who had tried to manage their own symptom(s), 116 (61.7%) had used what the authors described as independent acoustic stimulation – they preferred not to use the term sound therapy as it had not been administered by a healthcare professional. This modality was the most frequently administered self-help measure in the study. Simoes et al. performed a questionnaire study of previous treatments used by members of a large UK-based self-help platform for tinnitus patients [8]. This showed that what the authors termed "self-sound stimulation" was the most frequently used modality though it was not clear how often this was a self-instigated measure and how often it had been suggested by a professional. A study of tinnitus coping strategies by Beukes et al. [10] showed that the most commonly used strategy was sound enrichment and interestingly, participants were more likely to report the use of meaningful sound such as using a radio, rather than the non-meaningful sounds usually recommended by healthcare professionals. These observations, together with the widespread availability of environmental sound generators at online retailers, the number of tinnitus-related sound apps and the frequency with which information about sound therapy is accessed (Table 58.2) suggests that sound therapies are acceptable to and widely used by people with tinnitus.

Relaxation

Relaxation techniques are used widely in the management of tinnitus, either as a stand-alone treatment or incorporated into other therapeutic programs. Multiple different techniques have been used. Relaxation is also reported as a frequently used self-help measure among tinnitus patients [5]. It is therefore surprising how little research activity there is regarding stress and relaxation among tinnitus patients. Pupić-Bakrač and Pupić-Bakrač [109] reviewed the available literature and found that when compared to equivalent conditions such as chronic pain, chronic fatigue, and fibromyalgia, stress and its management in tinnitus has attracted much less research interest: there were 16 times more relevant publications for stress in chronic pain; six times more with chronic fatigue; and four times more with fibromyalgia.

Beukes et al. [110] investigated an ICBT intervention and found that the applied relaxation component was rated higher than any other aspect by patients. Beukes et al [111] therefore tried to determine how effective the applied relaxation component was on its own compared to the full ICBT intervention. Unfortunately, the trial suffered from very high dropout rate (possibly due to the COVID-19 pandemic) which compromised interpretation of the results. Nevertheless, among completers, applied relaxation did appear to be an effective intervention. Other studies involving relaxation have given mixed results (e.g. [112, 113]). Relaxation apps are available for smartphones, tablets, and computers, but as yet none have been investigated with respect to effectiveness in tinnitus patients. Similarly, there are no studies addressing relaxation as an autonomous tinnitus management intervention.

Dietary Manipulation

The idea that there is an association between tinnitus and diet is not new. It is almost two millennia since Roman physicians recommended that people with tinnitus should abstain from wine [13]. There have been many reports of food and drink causing tinnitus or exacerbating existing tinnitus and a similarly large number of suggestions of how to manipulate the diet to minimise or eradicate tinnitus.

An Internet search revealed that diet and tinnitus is a common topic for discussion in tinnitus forums and advice regarding food and drink is included in many medical tinnitus websites. The food and drink page of the BTA website is accessed over 54 times a day (Table 58.2), again suggesting that there is considerable public interest. Anecdotally, it is common to hear tinnitus patients reporting that after their own investigations – or sometimes after discussion with healthcare professionals – they have restricted or removed certain items from their diet, most commonly caffeine and alcohol. A comprehensive treatise on this topic is beyond the scope of this chapter but we will investigate some of the more commonly posited associations.

General Diet

There are relatively few studies that have examined the role of the overall diet of people with tinnitus. McCormack et al. [114] using data from the UK Biobank found that persistent tinnitus was less likely among people who had higher fish intake and avoided eggs, whereas it was more common among those with increased intake of fruit and vegetables, increased intake of wholemeal bread and who avoided dairy products. Having bothersome tinnitus, however, was less common among those with increased consumption of wholemeal bread.

Spankovitch et al. [115] used data from the National Health and Nutrition Examination Survey (NHANES). This study used the Healthy Eating Index, a measure of compliance with US dietary recommendations, and found that healthier eating was associated with reduced risk of tinnitus. In particular, lower fat intake and higher fruit intake seemed beneficial.

Tomanic et al. [116] explored tinnitus in a cohort of teenagers and found reduced tinnitus risk with higher consumption of fresh fruit and vegetables. There was an association between increased tinnitus risk and increased consumption of white bread, carbonated drinks, and fast food.

Tang et al. [117] found an increased tinnitus risk among those with lower dietary fibre consumption.

In another study utilising data from the UK Biobank, Dawes et al. [118] reported that a higher intake of vitamin B12 was associated with reduced odds of tinnitus, as was a high-protein intake. By contrast, higher intakes of calcium, iron, and fat were associated with increased odds.

Clearly, there are some contradictory findings among these dietary studies, and this is an area where further research is needed. Association does not imply causality. Furthermore, many of the associations were only associated with minor change in risk so it seems likely that general diet is not a major contributor to tinnitus and changing one's diet may be a disappointing intervention, at least where tinnitus is concerned.

Dietary Supplements

The dietary supplement industry is a huge global business, with an estimated market size of $205 billion in 2021 [119]. There is little global consensus on definitions, taxonomy, and requirements of dietary supplements or herbal medicines [120] and some regions use the term food supplement rather than dietary supplement. In a similar fashion, the regulations around dietary supplements vary from country to country. In many regions, dietary supplements are controlled by food regulating bodies rather than medicine safety agencies.

A study using data from NHANES stated that during 2017–2018, 57.6% of adults, aged 20 and over, reported using at least one dietary supplement in the preceding 30 days [121]. In a study which surveyed 1788 people with tinnitus from 53 countries, 23% of respondents disclosed that they used dietary supplements such as vitamins, minerals, and herbal medicines in an attempt to treat their tinnitus [122]. There were 52 supplements reported in the study, with the most commonly reported being:

- Ginkgo biloba
- Zinc
- Vitamin B12
- Melatonin
- Flavonoids
- Magnesium

The majority (81%) of respondents indicated that taking supplements either had no effect on their tinnitus, or their tinnitus worsened whilst taking the supplement.

Ginkgo Biloba

Ginkgo biloba is a large tree with fan-shaped leaves. Native to China, Japan, and Korea, extracts of Ginkgo leaves have been used medicinally for thousands of years. In several countries, including the United States, Canada, and the UK, Ginkgo extracts are widely available as a food supplement though in parts of Europe the extract is categorised as a drug [123].

Ginkgo has been suggested as a treatment for peripheral vascular disease and cerebral insufficiency, anxiety, dizziness, and tinnitus [122, 123]. Proposed mechanisms by which Ginkgo could improve tinnitus are by increasing inner ear and brain blood circulation and by prevention of cell membrane damage by free radicals [124].

A Cochrane Review, first published in 2004 and most recently updated in 2014, concluded that there is no evidence that Gingko biloba is effective in patients with a primary complaint of tinnitus [123]. However, an earlier review concluded that a specific extract of Ginkgo, EGb761, was superior to placebo [125]. Although generally tolerated well, there are reports of side effects associated with Ginkgo usage and there are reports of Ginkgo interacting with anticoagulants such as warfarin, causing increased bleeding risk [126]. Given the uncertainty about the benefits of Ginkgo biloba as a treatment, and the potential for harm, it is not recommended for use by people with tinnitus [122].

Zinc

Zinc is an important element involved in several physiological functions including neurotransmission.

Prevalence rates of zinc deficiency in people with tinnitus range from 2% to 69%, with elderly people affected more frequently [127]. In 1987, Gersdorff et al. attempted to find a correlation between low blood zinc levels (hypozincaemia) and tinnitus. Such a link was evident only in those with intermittent tinnitus [128]. A population study conducted in South Korea showed no significant difference in blood zinc levels between people with tinnitus and a control group after adjustment for age, sex, and hearing loss [129].

Relatively few studies have looked at zinc as a possible treatment for tinnitus [127, 130, 131]. A Cochrane Review on zinc found no evidence that zinc supplementation improves symptoms in adults with tinnitus [132].

Vitamin B12

Vitamin B12 is an essential vitamin that is synthesised by prokaryotic cells (bacteria and archaea). Eukaryotic cells (animal and plant cells) cannot produce this vitamin, but animals require it for multiple biochemical processes. Different animals use different methods of obtaining vitamin B12: humans derive their B12 from dietary sources. It is present in some foods of animal origin, some fermented foods and some foods of seaweed origin; some foods are fortified with vitamin B12, or it can be obtained as a supplement.

Vitamin B12 deficiency is more common in people who have a plant-based diet and there is some evidence that deficiency is more common among people with tinnitus [133–135]. The results of treating tinnitus patients with vitamin B12 are inconclusive, though there is a weak suggestion of improvement, particularly among those with a pre-existing deficiency [133–135]. This is a topic that merits further, better-controlled research.

Melatonin

Melatonin is a hormone secreted by the pineal gland that is involved in the regulation of the sleep–wake cycle. Melatonin supplements are sold in health food stores, pharmacies, and online in many countries but are not authorised for sale without prescription in the European Union, United Kingdom, Japan, and Australia [136].

Lower plasma levels of melatonin have been found in elderly people with tinnitus compared to those without [137]. Melatonin's properties that could potentially help to alleviate tinnitus include sleep facilitation, free-radical scavenging, antioxidant properties, and its contribution to vasoregulation [19]. A review of studies of melatonin as a tinnitus treatment concluded that melatonin seems to improve sleep disturbance linked to tinnitus, but because of methodological weakness and biases in the evidence base, it could not be assessed whether melatonin is effective for tinnitus itself [138].

Flavonoids

Flavonoids are a large class of phytonutrients found in fruits, vegetables, grains, bark, roots, stems, flowers, tea, and wine. One study has investigated the use of a widely advertisement supplement comprising of a compound of vitamins and flavonoids. Lipoflavinoid Plus® was evaluated alone or when taken with manganese. Neither course of treatment was effective in reducing tinnitus [139].

Magnesium

Magnesium is an abundant element in the body and has been identified as playing a key role in many metabolic functions, including regulation of blood pressure, neurotransmission, and neuromuscular conduction. Low levels of magnesium have been associated with a number of chronic diseases [140], including anxiety [141].

Research studies have shown that serum magnesium levels are lower in people with tinnitus than the general population [142]. Increased susceptibility to noise damage, ototoxicity, and auditory hyperexcitability has also been linked to magnesium deficiency [143]. It has been shown that magnesium supplements can help to prevent or treat some forms of hearing damage [144], and small-scale studies have suggested that they might have a beneficial effect on tinnitus [142, 145].

Proprietary Blends of Dietary Supplements

A wide range of over-the-counter preparations are available and aggressively marketed as tinnitus remedies, particularly through email, online advertising, and social media advertising. All make claims for tinnitus relief, although most add the FDA required disclaimers that "this product is not intended to diagnose, treat, cure or prevent any disease." Most of the products available consist of mixtures of inexpensive and common vitamins, minerals and/or herbal extracts sold at a premium compared to similarly formulated products not directly targeted for tinnitus relief. None have been subjected to rigorous scientific testing on tinnitus populations.

Alcohol

There have been multiple studies into the possible association between tinnitus and alcohol consumption and a recent systematic review considered this subject [146]. The review found 11 relevant cross-sectional studies with significant heterogeneity between studies. After pooled analysis, the authors concluded that there was no relationship between alcohol consumption and the risk of tinnitus.

Caffeine

Avoiding caffeine-containing drinks is one of the most common pieces of tinnitus related advice with various suggested mechanisms by which tinnitus might be associated with caffeine consumption [147]. Biswas et al. [146] reviewed tinnitus studies that had considered caffeine intake and found only three that met their criteria. With this low number of studies, the authors felt unable to draw conclusions but did suggest that it is unlikely that caffeine is a risk factor for tinnitus. Using different study selection criteria, Hofmeister [148] identified seven works that had addressed caffeine consumption and tinnitus, concluding that there was no supporting evidence for restriction of caffeine in tinnitus patients. Subsequent to the publication of these two large reviews, a Brazilian group published a triple blind placebo-controlled trial which concluded that caffeine had no significant effect on psychoacoustic measures, electroacoustic measures, or tinnitus-related degree of discomfort [149].

Cannabidiol

Cannabidiol oils (CBD) are low tetrahydrocannabinol (THC) products extracted from plants of the genus *Cannabis sativa*, which includes marijuana and hemp. Cannabis is the umbrella term for all plants in this genus and CBD is one of over 100 compounds called cannabinoids naturally found in such plants. CBD does not give an intoxicating effect [150]. Whilst cannabis remains illegal in most countries around the world, the status of CBD oil is complex and varied [151].

Cannabinoids have attracted attention as the role of the endocannabinoid system in a wide range of conditions – including mood and anxiety disorders, neuropathic pain, movement disorders, and cardiovascular conditions – has become more understood [152]. Several studies have found cannabinoid receptors in the auditory system [153].

To date, there have been no systematic studies of the effects of cannabinoids on tinnitus in humans [154]. Although cannabinoids have been shown to decrease neuronal hyperactivity in many parts of the brain, the current evidence from animal studies suggests that in the auditory areas of the brain, they may lead to increased neuronal hyperactivity and exacerbate tinnitus [155].

The most recent review evaluating the relationship between cannabis, cannabinoid pathways, and tinnitus concluded that there is no evidence from animal or human studies supporting the use of cannabinoids to relieve tinnitus [156].

Aromatherapy/Essential Oils

Aromatherapy is defined as the "inhalation or bodily application (as by massage) of fragrant essential oils (as from flowers and fruits) for therapeutic purposes" [33]. Essential oils have been used for hundreds of years and are frequently used in food and other products to add flavour or a pleasing scent.

Written in the late tenth or early eleventh century by Persian physician, Avicenna, the Canon of Medicine summarised all the medical knowledge of the time. Lily and spotted orchid oils were mentioned as remedies for tinnitus [157].

In a similar manner to dietary supplements, the use of essential oils may fall under food or drug regulatory programmes, depending on the manner of use. The caveats and exemptions discussed in the dietary supplements section apply here. Although product safety laws apply to essential oils, many plants contain materials that are toxic, irritating, or likely to cause allergic reactions when applied to the skin [158].

There is limited evidence to support the use of aromatherapy to improve sleep quality and reduce stress, anxiety, and depression [159, 160]. There is no evidence to support or refute its use as a treatment for tinnitus.

Smoking

In their systematic review of modifiable lifestyle-related risk factors for tinnitus, Biswas et al. [146] explored the evidence around smoking. They identified 26 studies, 25 cross-sectional and one cohort. Pooled data from the cross-sectional studies showed increased risk of tinnitus in current, ever and former smokers compared to those who had never smoked. The single cohort study showed increased risk in ever and former smokers but not in current smokers.

Physical Therapies and Lifestyle Change

Obesity and Physical Exercise

Biswas et al. [146] conducted a systematic review of tinnitus studies which contained information regarding body mass index (BMI) and tinnitus. They identified 11 studies of which seven provided information regarding tinnitus in individuals who were overweight (BMI $\geq$ 25 kg/m^2) versus normal or underweight (BMI < 25 kg/m^2) and seven studies which provided information on tinnitus in obese (BMI $\geq$ 30 kg/m^2) versus non-obese (BMI < 30 kg/m^2) individuals. Results of the analysis suggested that obesity may be a risk factor for tinnitus but owing to study heterogeneity, further research was recommended.

Online tinnitus support groups contain regular discussions on the topic of high BMI, diet, exercise and tinnitus but there is no evidence regarding this topic and self-help measures: the only evidence comes from medically supervised studies. Özbey-Yücel et al. [161] conducted a randomised controlled trial of 65 obese subjects with tinnitus. Participants were divided into three groups: weight-loss diet and physical activity; weight-loss diet alone; control group with no intervention. Forty-six participants completed the study and at the end of 12 weeks all groups had improved their tinnitus severity as determined by Tinnitus Handicap Inventory [6] questionnaire scores. The active groups fared significantly better than the control group and the greatest change was seen in the diet and physical activity group.

A study by Loprinzi et al. [162] used data from the NHANES study to investigate the association between physical activity and tinnitus. Tinnitus was assessed by self-report; physical activity was assessed by the participants wearing an accelerometer. Among adolescents (12–19 years) increased moderate to vigorous physical activity was associated with significantly fewer reports of tinnitus. Among older adults (72–85 years), a similar but less marked effect was seen with light physical activity.

Qigong and Tai Chi

Qigong and Tai Chi (or T'ai Chi) are forms of Chinese martial art that incorporate exercise in addition to other components. Both have been suggested for use by people with tinnitus. Qigong has been subjected to a randomised controlled trial with 80 patients being randomised to either Qigong training or waiting-list control [112]. Tinnitus severity was assessed by visual analogue scale and Tinnitus-Beeinträchtigungs-Fragebogen (TBF 12) [163] questionnaire scores. The active treatment group showed significant improvement compared to the control group and the effects were particularly marked among participants with somatosensory tinnitus. To date, there are no trials of Tai Chi for tinnitus.

Yoga

Derived from the Sanskrit word yui, "union" yoga is a conglomeration of mental, spiritual, and physical practices. There are several subtypes of yoga and it has long been suggested that practicing yoga can confer multiple health benefits. Several studies have been conducted on the effects of yoga among people with tinnitus, and Gunjawate and Ravi recently collated the available knowledge in a systematic review [164]. Five studies were included in the review: four assessing types of yoga and one assessing relaxation therapy. There was considerable heterogeneity of study design, and the review did not pool results or conduct meta-analysis. Three out of the four studies assessing yoga concluded that it was beneficial. The other study showed that yoga was less helpful than training in coping [165]. Further research was recommended.

Ear and Hearing Care

Ear Wax Removal

Ear wax, or cerumen, is frequently mentioned as a potential cause of tinnitus and wax removal is a common topic for discussion in online tinnitus forums. A visit to a popular online retailer showed a huge array of wax removal products available for sale. Ear drops and sprays included examples containing olive oil, mineral oil, surfactants, sodium bicarbonate, urea hydrogen peroxide, or unspecified plant extracts. Some of these drops were specifically marketed as tinnitus treatments. There were devices for ear canal irrigation including medical style syringes fitted with soft plastic tips, rubber bulb syringes, and spray-bottle irrigation systems. There were plastic and metal instruments for inserting in the ear canal, small endoscopes to allow visualisation of the ear canal, electrically operated suction devices, and cotton buds. There were also many examples of ear candles.

There is no evidence base for many of these products. Most of the ear drops use the same active ingredients as cerumenolytic drops used by physicians and there is an up-to-date Cochrane systematic review of this topic [166]. The authors of the review concluded that there is weak evidence to support the use of ear drops compared to no treatment, but there is no high-quality evidence to suggest which ear drop is most effective or whether such drops are more effective than plain water or normal saline. Reported adverse effects of using cerumenolytic eardrops were generally mild but the evidence was classified as low quality [166].

Cotton buds or cotton tipped swabs are frequently used in attempts at a wax removal: a study of children attending a general paediatric clinic reveal that among 651 patients aged two weeks to 20 years, 401 (61.6%) had used or been subjected to aural cotton tip swabs in the preceding two months [167]. Cerumen impaction of the left ear was worse among those who used cotton tip swabs. Another study [168] found no difference in cerumen impaction among cotton bud users and non-users. A study of 87 children aged 3.5–12 years who presented with otitis externa reported that the majority (61; 70.1%) had their ears cleaned by cotton buds within the 10 days prior to presentation. In conclusion, using cotton buds to clean the ear is common but appears at best ineffective and at worst potentially harmful. There is no good evidence regarding cotton bud usage and tinnitus.

The other ear cleaning intervention for which there is evidence is ear candling and the consensus is that ear candles are ineffective at wax removal and have resulted in significant harm to some patients [169–171]. Their use should be avoided.

Hearing Protection

Noise exposure, both occupational and recreational, is a significant risk factor for tinnitus [172] yet use of appropriate hearing protection remains low. A cross-sectional survey of 10,401 UK adults revealed that 7590 (73.0%) reported exposure to recreational noise in the preceding year but only 158 (2.1%) reported wearing hearing protection for every noisy recreational activity [173]. Kutyba et al. reported that among 188 participants who use some form of self-help measure 1.6% used sound avoidance [5]. Loughran et al. have undertaken a small-scale study to identify targets for interventions to increase earplug usage in noisy recreational settings [174], but this remains an under-researched topic.

Amplification

A range of electronic devices with names such as "sound amplifier," "digital hearing amplifier," "digital hearing enhancer," or "hearing amplifier" are available from online retailers. These devices generally resemble rather crude hearing aids in either behind the ear (BTE) or in the ear (ITE) format. Although these are not specifically marketed for tinnitus, customer reviews of the product show that some purchasers have been buying them for that reason. The number of tinnitus sufferers doing this is unknown as is the outcome of using such devices.

Games and Virtual Reality

There are scattered reports of people using video games to improve their tinnitus, generally a form of distraction [175]. There is also on-going work to investigate whether there is a role for serious games in the management of tinnitus [176–178]. Serious games are games that are designed with the primary purpose other than simple entertainment. Virtual reality is another technique that is being explored regarding a possible tinnitus therapy role [179, 180]. Both these techniques are still at an early stage but if successful, it is not difficult to see both being inducted into the field of autonomous tinnitus management.

Lasers

Low-level laser therapy (LLLT) for tinnitus has been investigated for over 20 years [181]. It has been postulated that LLLT may improve cochlear function and animal studies have found that laser stimulation can induce anatomical and physiological changes in the cochlea [182, 183].

Low-powered lasers are freely available for sale to members of the public, under various brand names and styles, including an over-the-ear device, and a "tinnitus pen."

Studies in humans have investigated the effects of LLLT on both hearing loss and tinnitus, with equivocal results. The risk of bias in studies is high, and the effectiveness of LLLT in the management of tinnitus remains uncertain [184–186]. Deterioration of hearing after laser use has been reported [187].

Hyperbaric Oxygen

Hyperbaric oxygen therapy (HBOT) involves breathing pure oxygen in a specially designed chamber which maintains air pressure two or three times higher than normal. HBOT is a well-established treatment for decompression sickness and has been used in the treatment of sudden sensorineural hearing loss and tinnitus [188].

Hyperbaric oxygen chambers can be accessed by people with tinnitus through referral by a medical practitioner but, perhaps surprisingly, many chambers will also accept self-referral and exploration of tinnitus forums shows that this is a route that some tinnitus patients follow.

A Cochrane Systematic Review evaluating hyperbaric oxygen for idiopathic sudden sensorineural hearing loss (ISSHL) and tinnitus concluded that there is no evidence of a beneficial effect of HBOT on chronic ISSHL or tinnitus [188]. Other workers in the field, however, feel that there is a role for HBOT, at least in the management of sudden sensorineural hearing loss [189].

Comorbidities

Tinnitus has associations with several other conditions including psychological conditions such as anxiety and depression, insomnia, disorders of sound tolerance (hyperacusis), and temporomandibular joint disorders. It is not feasible to assess self-help measures for all these conditions in this chapter, but it is useful to note that there are active online patient support groups and/or non-governmental organisations representing all these disorders. With the exception of hyperacusis the role of self-help or self-care has been scientifically explored for each of these conditions [190–194] and unsurprisingly there is considerable crossover regarding the techniques used. There is some evidence that using self-help measures primarily for one of these conditions can also help comorbidities [192].

Conclusion

A common refrain heard from people with tinnitus is, "My doctor said there's nothing can be done." This chapter shows that there certainly are many things that can at least be tried. However, there is no clear signposting through this confusing maze of potential treatments and there is a risk of those experiencing distressing tinnitus undertaking an eternal search for something to silence their symptom.

This is of concern as whilst some self-management techniques have been shown to be of benefit, for others the evidence of effectiveness is less conclusive, and for some there is evidence of no effect and indeed potential harm.

It is important for health professionals and patient support organisations to encourage and facilitate evidence-based autonomous interventions such as tinnitus support groups, using reliable information and self-help books, sound therapy and relaxation techniques and raise awareness of their availability. People with tinnitus should be strongly discouraged from trying dietary supplements, lasers, and ear-candling. Information from the Internet or social media, and participation in chatrooms and forums can have benefits, but the quality and reliability of information is variable and could lead to an increase in tinnitus distress.

Rigorous, large-scale studies are called for as a stronger evidence base would help people make better informed decisions about the options they choose to self-manage their tinnitus.

References

1. National Library of Medicine Medical Subject Heading (MeSH) for Self-care https://www.ncbi.nlm.nih.gov/mesh/68012648. Accessed 9 Jan 2022.
2. National Library of Medicine Medical Subject Heading (MeSH) for Self- management. https://www.ncbi.nlm.nih.gov/mesh/?term=self+management. Accessed 9 Jan 2022.
3. Myers PJ, Griest S, Kaelin C, Legro MW, Schmidt CJ, Zaugg TL, Henry JA. Development of a progressive audiologic tinnitus management program for Veterans with tinnitus. J Rehabil Res Dev. 2014;51(4):609–22. https://doi.org/10.1682/JRRD.2013.08.0189.
4. Tinnitus tunes. https://www.tinnitustunes.com/. Accessed 9 Jan 2022.
5. Kutyba J, Jedrzejczak WW, Gos E, Bieńkowska K, Raj-Koziak D, Skarżyński PH. Self-help interventions chosen by subjects with chronic tinnitus - a retrospective study of clinical patients. Int J Audiol. 2021;61(8):686–91. https://doi.org/10.1080/14992027.2021.1964040.
6. Newman CW, Jacobson GP, Spitzer JB. Development of the Tinnitus Handicap Inventory. Arch Otolaryngol Head Neck Surg. 1996;122(2):143–8. https://doi.org/10.1001/archotol.1996.01890140029007.
7. Lambert SD, Loiselle CG. Health information seeking behavior. Qual Health Res. 2007;17(8):1006–19. https://doi.org/10.1177/1049732307305199.
8. Simoes J, Neff P, Schoisswohl S, Bulla J, Schecklmann M, Harrison S, Vesala M, Langguth B, Schlee W. Toward personalized tinnitus treatment: an exploratory study based on internet crowdsensing. Front Public Health. 2019;7:157. https://doi.org/10.3389/fpubh.2019.00157.
9. Tinnitus hub. https://www.tinnitushub.com/. Accessed 9 Jan 2022.
10. Beukes EW, Manchaiah V, Andersson G, Allen PM, Terlizzi PM, Baguley DM. Situationally influenced tinnitus coping strategies: a mixed methods approach. Disabil Rehabil. 2018;40(24):2884–94. https://doi.org/10.1080/09638288.2017.1362708.
11. Pope A. A little learning. Essay on Criticism. 1711.
12. Thompson RC. Assyrian prescriptions for diseases of the ears. J R Asiat Soc. 1931:1–25.
13. Stephens SD. The treatment of tinnitus--a historical perspective. J Laryngol Otol. 1984;98(10):963–72. https://doi.org/10.1017/s0022215100147802.
14. Dietrich S. Earliest historic reference of 'tinnitus' is controversial. J Laryngol Otol. 2004;118(7):487–8. https://doi.org/10.1258/0022215041615182.
15. Itard JMG. Traite des maladies de l'oreille et de I'audition. Paris: Mequignon-Marvis; 1821.
16. Mcnaughton-Jones H. Subjective noises in the head and ears: their aetiology, diagnosis and treatment. London: Balliere, Tindall and Cox; 1891.
17. National Guideline Centre (UK). Evidence review for patient information: tinnitus: assessment and management: evidence review B. London: National Institute for Health and Care Excellence (UK); 2020.
18. Cima RFF, Mazurek B, Haider H, Kikidis D, Lapira A, Noreña A, Hoare DJ. A multidisciplinary European guideline for tinnitus: diagnostics, assessment, and treatment. HNO. 2019;67(Suppl 1):10–42. https://doi.org/10.1007/s00106-019-0633-7.
19. Tunkel DE, Bauer CA, Sun GH, Rosenfeld RM, Chandrasekhar SS, Cunningham ER Jr, et al. Clinical practice guideline: tinnitus. Otolaryngol Head Neck Surg. 2014;151(2 Suppl):S1–S40. https://doi.org/10.1177/0194599814545325.
20. Pryce H, Hall A, Shaw R, Culhane BA, Swift S, Straus J, Claesen B. Patient preferences in tinnitus outcomes and treatments: a qualitative study. Int J Audiol. 2018 Oct;57(10):784–90. https://doi.org/10.1080/14992027.2018.1484184.
21. Tinnitus UK (Formerly the British Tinnitus Association). https://www.tinnitus.org.uk/. Accessed 9 Jan 2022.
22. Tinnitus: assessment and management. London: National Institute for Health and Care Excellence (UK); 2020.
23. YouGov. https://yougov.co.uk. Accessed 9 Jan 2022.
24. Gille S, Griese L, Schaeffer D. Preferences and experiences of people with chronic illness in using different sources of health information: results of a mixed-methods study. Int J Environ Res Public Health. 2021;18(24):13185. https://doi.org/10.3390/ijerph182413185.
25. Fox S. Pew Research Center. The social life of health information. 2014. http://www.pewresearch.org/fact-tank/2014/01/15/the-social-life-of-health-information/. Accessed 9 Jan 2022.
26. Eurostat. One in two EU citizens look for health information online. 2021. https://ec.europa.eu/eurostat/web/products-eurostat-news/-/edn-20210406-1. Accessed 9 Jan 2022.
27. Fox S, Duggan M. Pew Research Center. Health online 2013. https://www.pewresearch.org/internet/2013/01/15/health-online-2013/. Accessed 9 Jan 2022.
28. TIME. Search engines may seem all-knowing, but they're not. Here's how to get more trustworthy results. 2018. https://time.com/5318918/search-results-engine-google-bias-trusted-sources/. Accessed 9 Jan 2022.
29. Finney Rutten LJ, Blake KD, Greenberg-Worisek AJ, Allen SV, Moser RP, Hesse BW. Online health information seeking among US adults: measuring progress toward a healthy people 2020 objective. Public Health Reports. 2019;134(6):617–25. https://doi.org/10.1177/0033354919874074.
30. Guo N, Guo Z, Zhao S, Ho SY, Fong DYT, Lai AYW, Chan SS, Wang MP, Lam TH. Digital inequalities in health information seeking behaviors and experiences in the age of web 2.0: a population-based study in Hong Kong. PlosOne. 2021;16(3):e0249400. https://doi.org/10.1371/journal.pone.0249400.
31. Powell J, Inglis N, Ronnie J, Large S. The characteristics and motivations of online health information seekers: cross-sectional survey and qualitative interview study. J Med Internet Res. 2011;13(1):e20. Published 2011 Feb 23. https://doi.org/10.2196/jmir.1600.

32. Chu JT, Wang MP, Shen C, Viswanath K, Lam TH, Chan SSC. How, when and why people seek health information online: qualitative study in Hong Kong. Interact J Med Res. 2017;6(2):e24. https://doi.org/10.2196/ijmr.7000.
33. Dictionary by Merriam-Webster. https://www.merriam-webster.com. Accessed 9 Jan 2022.
34. Shah S. The history of social networking. https://www.digitaltrends.com/features/the-history-of-social-networking/. Accessed 9 Jan 2022
35. Kemp S DataReportal Digital 2021 October Global Statshot report. 2021. https://datareportal.com/reports/digital-2021-october-global-statshot. Accessed 9 Jan 2022.
36. Statista Research Department. Statista. Number of global social network users 2017–2025. https://www.statista.com/statistics/278414/number-of-worldwide-social-network-users/. Accessed 9 Jan 2022
37. O'Dea S. Statista. Number of smartphone users from 2016 to 2021. https://www.statista.com/statistics/330695/number-of-smartphone-users-worldwide/. Accessed 9 Jan. 2022.
38. Naslund JA, Bondre A, Torous J, et al. Social media and mental health: benefits, risks, and opportunities for research and practice. J Technol Behav Sci. 2020;5:245–57. https://doi.org/10.1007/s41347-020-00134-x.
39. Reidy C, Klonoff DC, Barnard-Kelly KD. Supporting good intentions with good evidence: how to increase the benefits of diabetes social media. Journal of Diabetes Science and Technology. 2019;13(5):974–8. https://doi.org/10.1177/1932296819850187.
40. Gentile D, Markham MJ, Eaton T. Patients with cancer and social media: harness benefits, avoid drawbacks. J Oncol Pract. 2018:JOP1800367. https://doi.org/10.1200/JOP.18.00367.
41. Deshpande AK, Deshpande SB, O'Brien C. A study of social media utilization by individuals with tinnitus. Am J Audiol. 2018;27(4):559–69. https://doi.org/10.1044/2018_AJA-18-0033.
42. Basch CH, Yin J, Kollia B, et al. Public online information about tinnitus: a cross-sectional study of YouTube videos. Noise Health. 2018;20(92):1–8. https://doi.org/10.4103/nah.NAH_32_17.
43. Benetoli A, Chen TF, Aslani P. Consumer perceptions of using social media for health purposes: benefits and drawbacks. Health Informatics Journal. 2019:1661–74. https://doi.org/10.1177/1460458218796664.
44. Song H, Omori K, Kim J, Tenzek KE, Hawkins JM, Lin W, Kim Y, Jung J. Trusting social media as a source of health information: online surveys comparing the United States. Korea, and Hong Kong J Med Internet Res. 2016;18(3):e25. https://doi.org/10.2196/jmir.4193.
45. Lin W-Y, Zhang X, Song H, Omori K. Health information seeking in the Web 2.0 age: trust in social media, uncertainty reduction, and self-disclosure. Computers in Human Behavior. 2016;56:289–94. https://doi.org/10.1016/j.chb.2015.11.055.
46. Allington D, Duffy B, Wessely S, Dhavan N, Rubin J. Health-protective behaviour, social media usage and conspiracy belief during the COVID-19 public health emergency. Psychological Medicine. 2021;51(10):1763–9. https://doi.org/10.1017/S003329172000224X.
47. Ley P. Comprehension, memory and success of communications with the patient. J Inst Health Educ. 1972;10:23–9.
48. Kessels RPC. Patients' memory for medical information. Journal of the Royal Society of Medicine. 2003;96:219–22.
49. Richard C, Glaser E, Lussier M-T. Communication and patient participation influencing patient recall of treatment discussions. Health Expect. 2017;20:760–70. https://doi.org/10.1111/hex.12515.
50. Barton Laws M, Lee Y, Taubin T, Rogers WH, Wilson IB. Factors associated with patient recall of key information in ambulatory specialty care visits: results of an innovative methodology. PLoS One. 2018;13(2):e0191940. https://doi.org/10.1371/journal.pone.0191940.
51. Logan K. University of Canterbury. Patient recall of tinnitus information after initial audiological assessment. 2015. https://doi.org/10.26021/5047. Accessed 9 Jan 2022.
52. Gauld VA. Written advice: compliance and recall. J R Coll Gen Pract. 1981;31:553–6.
53. Johnson A, Sandford J, Tyndall J. Written and verbal information versus verbal information only for patients being discharged from acute hospital settings to home. Cochrane Database Syst Rev. 2003;(4):CD003716. https://doi.org/10.1002/14651858.CD003716.
54. Sereda M, Hoare DJ. Self-help interventions for tinnitus. In: Baguley D, Fagelson M, editors. Tinnitus: clinical and research perspectives. San Diego: Plural Publishing; 2016.
55. Loumidis KS, Hallam RS, Cadge B. The effect of written reassuring information on out-patients complaining of tinnitus. Br J Audiol. 1991;25(2):105–9. https://doi.org/10.3109/03005369109079840.
56. Hallam RS, Jakes SC, Hinchcliffe R. Cognitive variables in tinnitus annoyance. Br J Clin Psychol. 1988;27(3):213–22. https://doi.org/10.1111/j.2044-8260.1988.tb00778.x.
57. Hassaan A, Trinidade A. The tinnitus patient information pack: usefulness in intrusive tinnitus. Int J Health Care Qual Assur. 2019;32(2):360–5. https://doi.org/10.1108/IJHCQA-03-2018-0071.
58. Tyler RS, editor. The consumer handbook on tinnitus. 2nd ed. Auricle Ink Publishers. Sedona; 2016.
59. Henry J, Zaugg T, Myers P, Kendall C. How to manage your tinnitus: a step-by-step workbook. San Diego: Plural Publishing Inc.; 2010.
60. McKenna L, Baguley D, McFerran D. Living with tinnitus and hyperacusis, Sheldon Press. London; 2021.
61. Malouff JM, Noble W, Schutte NS, Bhullar N. The effectiveness of bibliotherapy in alleviating tinnitus-related distress. J Psychosom Res. 2010;68(3):245–51. https://doi.org/10.1016/j.jpsychores.2009.07.023.
62. Nyenhuis N, Zastrutzki S, Weise C, Jäger B, Kröner-Herwig B. The efficacy of minimal contact interventions for acute tinnitus: a randomised controlled study. Cogn Behav Ther. 2013;42(2):127–38. https://doi.org/10.1080/16506073.2012.655305.
63. Manchaiah V, Ratinaud P, Andersson G. Representation of tinnitus in the US newspaper media and in Facebook pages: cross-sectional analysis of secondary data. Interact J Med Res. 2018;7(1):e9. https://doi.org/10.2196/ijmr.9065.
64. Bomlitz LJ, Brezis M. Misrepresentation of health risks by mass media. J Public Health (Oxf). 2008;30(2):202–4. https://doi.org/10.1093/pubmed/fdn009.
65. Rees CE, Bath PA. Mass media sources for breast cancer information: their advantages and disadvantages for women with the disease. J Document. 2000;56(3):235–49. https://doi.org/10.1108/EUM0000000007114.
66. Carducci A, Alfani S, Sassi M, Cinini A, Calamusa A. Mass media health information: quantitative and qualitative analysis of daily press coverage and its relation with public perceptions. Patient Educ Couns. 2011;82(3):475–8. https://doi.org/10.1016/j.pec.2010.12.025.
67. Smith S, Sereda M. Smartphone apps for tinnitus management. Hear J. 2020;73(2):20, 22, 23. https://doi.org/10.1097/01.HJ.0000654928.79548.08.
68. Sereda M, Smith S, Newton K, Stockdale D. Mobile apps for management of tinnitus: users' survey, quality assessment, and content analysis. JMIR Mhealth Uhealth. 2019;7(1):e10353. https://doi.org/10.2196/10353. PMID: 30672739; PMCID: PMC6364200.
69. Deshpande AK, Shimunova T. A comprehensive evaluation of tinnitus apps. Am J Audiol. 2019;28(3):605–16. https://doi.org/10.1044/2019_AJA-18-0135.

70. Mehdi M, Riha C, Neff P, Dode A, Pryss R, Schlee W, Reichert M, Hauck FJ. Smartphone apps in the context of tinnitus: systematic review. Sensors. 2020;20:1725. https://doi.org/10.3390/s20061725.
71. Mehdi M, Stach M, Riha C, Neff P, Dode A, Pryss R, Schlee W, Reichert M, Hauck FJ. Smartphone and mobile health apps for tinnitus: systematic identification. Analysis, and Assessment JMIR Mhealth Uhealth. 2020;8(8):e21767. https://doi.org/10.2196/21767.
72. Gottlieb S. Health information on internet is often unreliable. BMJ. 2000;321(7254):136.
73. Cline RJ, Haynes KM. Consumer health information seeking on the Internet: the state of the art. Health Educ Res. 2001;16(6):671–92. https://doi.org/10.1093/her/16.6.671.
74. Zhang D, Zhan W, Zheng C, et al. Online health information-seeking behaviors and skills of Chinese college students. BMC Public Health. 2021;21:736. https://doi.org/10.1186/s12889-021-10801-0.
75. Wong D, Cheung M. Online health information seeking and eHealth literacy among patients attending a primary care clinic in Hong Kong: a cross-sectional survey. J Med Internet Res. 2019;21(3):e10831. https://www.jmir.org/2019/3/e10831
76. Sharma M, Yadav K, Yadav N, Ferdinand KC. Zika virus pandemic-analysis of Facebook as a social media health information platform. Am J Infect Control. 2017;45(3):301–2. https://doi.org/10.1016/j.ajic.2016.08.022.
77. Fackrell K, Hoare DJ, Smith S, et al. An evaluation of the content and quality of tinnitus information on websites preferred by General Practitioners. BMC Med Inform Decis Mak. 2012;12:70. https://doi.org/10.1186/1472-6947-12-70.
78. McKearney R, MacKinnon R, Smith M, Baker R. Tinnitus information online – does it ring true? J Laryngol Otol. 2018;132(11):984–9. https://doi.org/10.1017/S0022215118001792.
79. Manchiah V, Dockens AL, Flagge A, Bellon-Harn M, Azios JH, Kelly-Campbell RJ, Andersson G. Quality and readability of english-language internet information for tinnitus. J Am Acad Audiol. 2019;30(01):031–40. https://doi.org/10.3766/jaaa.17070.
80. Charnock D, Shepperd S, Needham G, Gann R. DISCERN: an instrument for judging the quality of written consumer health information on treatment choices. J Epidemiol Community Health. 1999;53(02):105–11.
81. Health on the Net. https://www.hon.ch. Accessed 9 Jan 2022.
82. PIF TICK. https://piftick.org.uk. Accessed 9 Jan 2022.
83. The Information Standard. https://www.england.nhs.uk/tis. Accessed 9 Jan 2022.
84. Stormacq C, Van den Broucke S, Wosinski J. Does health literacy mediate the relationship between socioeconomic status and health disparities? Integrative review. Health Promot Int. 2019;34(5):e1–e17. https://doi.org/10.1093/heapro/day062.
85. van der Heide I, Poureslami I, Mitic W, Shum J, Rootman I, FitzGerald JM. Health literacy in chronic disease management: a matter of interaction. J Clin Epidemiol. 2018;102:134–8. https://doi.org/10.1016/j.jclinepi.2018.05.010.
86. Stossel LM, Segar N, Gliatto P, Fallar R, Karani R. Readability of patient education materials available at the point of care. J Gen Intern Med. 2012;27(9):1165–70. https://doi.org/10.1007/s11606-012-2046-0.
87. Centers for Medicare and Medicaid Services. Toolkit for making written material clear and effective -toolkit Part 7: using readability formulas. 2021. https://www.cms.gov/Outreach-and-Education/Outreach/WrittenMaterialsToolkit/ToolkitPart07. Accessed 9 Jan 2022.
88. OECD. Skills matter: additional results from the survey of adult skills, OECD Skills Studies.Paris: OECD Publishing; 2019. https://doi.org/10.1787/1f029d8f-en.
89. Oliffe M, Thompson E, Johnston J, et al. Assessing the readability and patient comprehension of rheumatology medicine information sheets: a cross-sectional Health Literacy Study. BMJ Open. 2019;9:e024582. https://doi.org/10.1136/bmjopen-2018-024582.
90. Rowlands G, Protheroe J, Winkley J, Richardson M, Seed PT, Rudd R. A mismatch between population health literacy and the complexity of health information: an observational study. Br J Gen Pract. 2015;65(635):e379–86. https://doi.org/10.3399/bjgp15X685285.
91. McGinnis C. Tinnitus self-help groups. The Hearing Journal. 2001;54(11):50–2. https://doi.org/10.1097/01.HJ.0000293154.16714.ab.
92. National Voices & NESTA. Peer support: what is it and does it work? 2015. Available from https://www.nationalvoices.org.uk/sites/default/files/public/publications/peer_support_-_what_is_it_and_does_it_work.pdf. Accessed 5 Jan 2022.
93. RNID. https://www.rnid.org.uk/. Accessed 9 Jan 2022.
94. American Tinnitus Association (ATA). https://www.ata.org. Accessed 9 Jan 2022.
95. Hu A. Reflections: the value of patient support groups. Otolaryngol Head Neck Surg. 2017;156(4):587–8. https://doi.org/10.1177/0194599817697030.
96. Kofahl C. Associations of collective self-help activity, health literacy and quality of life in patients with tinnitus. Patient Educ Couns. 2018;101(12):2170–8. https://doi.org/10.1016/j.pec.2018.07.001.
97. Beukes EW, Onozuka J, Brazell TP, Manchaiah V. Coping with tinnitus during the COVID-19 pandemic. American Journal of Audiology. 2021;30(2):385–93. https://doi.org/10.1044/2021_AJA-20-00188.
98. Pryce H, Moutela T, Bunker C, Shaw R. Tinnitus groups: a model of social support and social connectedness from peer interaction. Br J Health Psychol. 2019;24(4):913–30. https://doi.org/10.1111/bjhp.12386.
99. Guitton MJ. Telemedicine in tinnitus: feasibility, advantages, limitations, and perspectives. ISRN Otolaryngol. 2013 May;14(2013):218265. https://doi.org/10.1155/2013/218265.
100. Reddit. https://www.reddit.com.
101. Ainscough E, Smith SN, Greenwell K, Hoare DJ. Findings and ethical considerations from a thematic analysis of threads within tinnitus online support groups. Am J Audiol. 2018;27(3S):503–12. https://doi.org/10.1044/2018_AJA-IMIA3-18-0013.
102. American Tinnitus Association 2018. Podcast 10: benefits and pitfalls of an online support community. Available from https://www.ata.org/podcasts/podcast-10-benefits-and-pitfalls-online-support-community. Accessed 5 Jan 2022.
103. Dean J, Goodlad R. Supporting community participation; the role and impact of befriending. Pavilion Publishing and Joseph Rowntree Foundation; 1998.
104. Siette J, Cassidy M, Priebe S. Effectiveness of befriending interventions: a systematic review and meta-analysis. BMJ Open. 2017;7:e014304. https://doi.org/10.1136/bmjopen-2016-014304.
105. Mead N, Lester H, Chew-Graham C, Gask L, Bower P. Effects of befriending on depressive symptoms and distress: systematic review and meta-analysis. 2010. https://www.ncbi.nlm.nih.gov/books/NBK80056/. Accessed 9 Jan 2022.
106. Handscomb L. Use of bedside sound generators by patients with tinnitus-related sleeping difficulty: which sounds are preferred and why? Acta Otolaryngol Suppl. 2006;(556):59–63. https://doi.org/10.1080/03655230600895275.
107. Hobson J, Chisholm E, El Refaie A. Sound therapy (masking) in the management of tinnitus in adults. Cochrane Database Syst Rev. 2012;11(11):CD006371. https://doi.org/10.1002/14651858.CD006371.pub3.
108. Sereda M, Xia J, El Refaie A, Hall DA, Hoare DJ. Sound therapy (using amplification devices and/or sound generators) for tinnitus.

Cochrane Database Syst Rev. 2018;12(12):CD013094. https://doi.org/10.1002/14651858.CD013094.pub2.
109. Pupić-Bakrač J, Pupić-Bakrač A. Comorbidity of chronic tinnitus and psychological stress - which came first, the chicken or the egg? Psychiatr Danub. 2020;32(Suppl 4):412–9.
110. Beukes EW, Manchaiah V, Baguley DM, Allen PM, Andersson G. Process evaluation of Internet-based cognitive behavioural therapy for adults with tinnitus in the context of a randomised control trial. Int J Audiol. 2018;57(2):98–109. https://doi.org/10.1080/14992027.2017.1384858.
111. Beukes EW, Andersson G, Fagelson MA, Manchaiah V. Dismantling internet-based cognitive behavioral therapy for tinnitus. The contribution of applied relaxation: a randomized controlled trial. Internet Interv. 2021;25:100402. https://doi.org/10.1016/j.invent.2021.100402.
112. Biesinger E, Kipman U, Schätz S, Langguth B. Qigong for the treatment of tinnitus: a prospective randomized controlled study. J Psychosom Res. 2010;69(3):299–304. https://doi.org/10.1016/j.jpsychores.2010.04.013.
113. Davies S, McKenna L, Hallam RS. Relaxation and cognitive therapy: a controlled trial in chronic tinnitus. Psychol Health. 1995;10(2):129–43.
114. McCormack A, Edmondson-Jones M, Mellor D, Dawes P, Munro KJ, Moore DR, Fortnum H. Association of dietary factors with presence and severity of tinnitus in a middle-aged UK population. PLoS One. 2014;9(12):e114711. https://doi.org/10.1371/journal.pone.0114711. Erratum in: PLoS One. 2015;10(4):e0123053.
115. Spankovich C, Bishop C, Johnson MF, Elkins A, Su D, Lobarinas E, Le Prell CG. Relationship between dietary quality, tinnitus and hearing level: data from the national health and nutrition examination survey, 1999–2002. Int J Audiol. 2017;56(10):716–22. https://doi.org/10.1080/14992027.2017.1331049.
116. Tomanic M, Belojevic G, Jovanovic A, Vasiljevic N, Davidovic D, Maksimovic K. Dietary factors and tinnitus among adolescents. Nutrients. 2020;12(11):3291. https://doi.org/10.3390/nu12113291.
117. Tang D, Tran Y, Shekhawat GS, Burlutsky G, Mitchell P, Gopinath B. Dietary fibre intake and the 10-year incidence of tinnitus in older adults. Nutrients. 2021;13(11):4126. https://doi.org/10.3390/nu13114126.
118. Dawes P, Cruickshanks KJ, Marsden A, Moore DR, Munro KJ. Relationship between diet, tinnitus, and hearing difficulties. Ear Hear. 2020;41(2):289–99. https://doi.org/10.1097/AUD.0000000000000765.
119. Statista. Total dietary supplements market size worldwide from 2016 to 2028. 2021. Available from https://www.statista.com/statistics/828514/total-dietary-supplements-market-size-globally/. Accessed 29 Dec 2021.
120. Thakkar S, Anklam E, Xu A, Ulberth F, Li J, Li B, et al. Regulatory landscape of dietary supplements and herbal medicines from a global perspective. Regul Toxicol Pharmacol. 2020;114:104647. https://doi.org/10.1016/j.yrtph.2020.104647.
121. Mishra S, Stierman B, Gahche JJ, Potischman N. Dietary supplement use among adults: United States, 2017–2018. NCHS Data Brief, no 399. Hyattsville, MD: National Center for Health Statistics; 2021. https://doi.org/10.15620/cdc:101131.
122. Coelho C, Tyler R, Ji H, Rojas-Roncancio E, Witt S, Tao P, Jun HJ, Wang TC, Hansen MR, Gantz BJ. Survey on the effectiveness of dietary supplements to treat tinnitus. Am J Audiol. 2016;25(3):184–205. https://doi.org/10.1044/2016_AJA-16-0021.
123. Hilton MP, Zimmermann EF, Hunt WT. Ginkgo biloba for tinnitus. Cochrane Database Syst Rev. 2013;(3):CD003852. https://doi.org/10.1002/14651858.CD003852.pub3.
124. Smith GS, Romanelli-Gobbi M, Gray-Karagrigoriou E, Artz GJ. Complementary and integrative treatments: tinnitus. Otolaryngol Clin North Am. 2013;46:389–408.
125. von Boetticher A. Ginkgo biloba extract in the treatment of tinnitus: a systematic review. Neuropsychiatr Dis Treat. 2011;7:441–7. https://doi.org/10.2147/NDT.S22793.
126. Tan CSS, Lee SWH. Warfarin and food, herbal or dietary supplement interactions: a systematic review. Br J Clin Pharmacol. 2021;87(2):352–74. https://doi.org/10.1111/bcp.14404.
127. Coelho CB, Tyler R, Hansen M. Zinc as a possible treatment for tinnitus. Prog Brain Res. 2007;166:279–85. https://doi.org/10.1016/S0079-6123(07)66026-9.
128. Gersdorff M, Robillard T, Stein F, Declaye X, Vanderbemden S. A clinical correlation between hypozincemia and tinnitus. Arch Otorhinolaryngol. 1987;244(3):190–3. https://doi.org/10.1007/BF00464266.
129. Jun HJ, Ok S, Tyler R, Hwang SY, Chae S. Is hypozincemia related to tinnitus?: a population study using data from the Korea National Health and Nutrition Examination Survey. Clin Exp Otorhinolaryngol. 2015;8(4):335–8. https://doi.org/10.3342/ceo.2015.8.4.335.
130. Coelho C, Witt SA, Ji H, Hansen MR, Gantz B, Tyler R. Zinc to treat tinnitus in the elderly: a randomized placebo controlled crossover trial. Otol Neurotol. 2013;34(6):1146–54. https://doi.org/10.1097/MAO.0b013e31827e609e.
131. Yeh CW, Tseng LH, Yang CH, Hwang CF. Effects of oral zinc supplementation on patients with noise-induced hearing loss associated tinnitus: a clinical trial. Biomed J. 2019;42(1):46–52. https://doi.org/10.1016/j.bj.2018.10.009.
132. Person OC, Puga ME, da Silva EM, Torloni MR. Zinc supplementation for tinnitus. Cochrane Database Syst Rev. 2016;11(11):CD009832. https://doi.org/10.1002/14651858.CD009832.pub2.
133. Shemesh Z, Attias J, Ornan M, Shapira N, Shahar A. Vitamin B12 deficiency in patients with chronic-tinnitus and noise-induced hearing loss. Am J Otolaryngol. 1993;14(2):94–9. https://doi.org/10.1016/0196-0709(93)90046-a.
134. Berkiten G, Yildirim G, Topaloglu I, Ugras H. Vitamin B12 levels in patients with tinnitus and effectiveness of vitamin B12 treatment on hearing threshold and tinnitus. B-ENT. 2013;9(2):111–6.
135. Singh C, Kawatra R, Gupta J, Awasthi V, Dungana H. Therapeutic role of Vitamin B12 in patients of chronic tinnitus: a pilot study. Noise Health. 2016;18(81):93–7. https://doi.org/10.4103/1463-1741.178485.
136. Grigg-Damberger MM, Ianakieva D. Poor quality control of over-the-counter melatonin: what they say is often not what you get. J Clin Sleep Med. 2017;13(2):163–5. https://doi.org/10.5664/jcsm.6434.
137. Lasisi AO, Fehintola FA, Lasisi TJ. The role of plasma melatonin and vitamins C and B12 in the development of idiopathic tinnitus in the elderly. Ghana Med J. 2012;46(3):152–7.
138. Miroddi M, Bruno R, Galletti F, Calapai F, Navarra M, Gangemi S, Calapai G. Clinical pharmacology of melatonin in the treatment of tinnitus: a review. Eur J Clin Pharmacol. 2015;71(3):263–70. https://doi.org/10.1007/s00228-015-1805-3.
139. Rojas-Roncancio E, Tyler R, Jun HJ, Wang TC, Ji H, Coelho C, Witt S, Hansen MR, Gantz BJ. Manganese and Lipoflavonoid Plus(®) to treat tinnitus: a randomized controlled trial. J Am Acad Audiol. 2016;27(8):661–8. https://doi.org/10.3766/jaaa.15106.
140. Gröber U, Schmidt J, Kisters K. Magnesium in prevention and therapy. Nutrients. 2015;7(9):8199–226. https://doi.org/10.3390/nu7095388.
141. Boyle NB, Lawton C, Dye L. The effects of magnesium supplementation on subjective anxiety and stress-a systematic review. Nutrients. 2017;9(5):429. https://doi.org/10.3390/nu9050429.
142. Uluyol S, Kılıçaslan S, Yağız Ö. Relationship between serum magnesium levels and subjective tinnitus. Kulak Burun Bogaz Ihtis Derg. 2016;26(4):225–7.

143. Cevette MJ, Vormann J, Franz K. Magnesium and hearing. J Am Acad Audiol. 2003;14(4):202–12.
144. Sendowski I, Holy X, Raffin F, Cazals Y. Magnesium and hearing loss. In: Vink R, Nechifor M, editors. Magnesium in the central nervous system [Internet]. Adelaide, AU: University of Adelaide Press; 2011.
145. Cevette MJ, Barrs DM, Patel A, Conroy KP, Sydlowski S, Noble BN, Nelson GA, Stepanek J. Phase 2 study examining magnesium-dependent tinnitus. Int Tinnitus J. 2011;16(2):168–73.
146. Biswas R, Lugo A, Genitsaridi E, Trpchevska N, Akeroyd MA, Cederroth CR, Liu X, Schlee W, Garavello W, Gallus S, Hall DA. Modifiable lifestyle-related risk factors for tinnitus in the general population: an overview of smoking, alcohol, body mass index and caffeine intake. Prog Brain Res. 2021;263:1–24. https://doi.org/10.1016/bs.pbr.2021.04.005.
147. Trinidade A, Robinson T, Phillips JS. The role of caffeine in otorhinolaryngology: guilty as charged? Eur Arch Otorhinolaryngol. 2014;271(8):2097–102. https://doi.org/10.1007/s00405-013-2648-0.
148. Hofmeister M. Do dietary factors significantly influence tinnitus? Aust J Gen Pract. 2019;48(3):153–7. https://doi.org/10.31128/AJGP-07-18-4643.
149. Ledesma ALL, Leite Rodrigues D, de Castro M, Silva I, Oliveira CA, Bahmad F Jr. The effect of caffeine on tinnitus: randomized triple-blind placebo-controlled clinical trial. PLoS One. 2021;16(9):e0256275. https://doi.org/10.1371/journal.pone.0256275.
150. VanDolah HJ, Bauer BA, Mauck KF. Clinicians' guide to cannabidiol and hemp oils. Mayo Clin Proc. 2019;94(9):1840–51. https://doi.org/10.1016/j.mayocp.2019.01.003.
151. Quinn M. The extract. Is CBD legal worldwide? 2021. https://www.theextract.co.uk/is-cbd-legal-worldwide/?cn-reloaded=1#Difference_between_cannabis_and_CBD. Accessed 9 Jan 2022.
152. Pacher P, Bátkai S, Kunos G. The endocannabinoid system as an emerging target of pharmacotherapy. Pharmacol Rev. 2006;58(3):389–462. https://doi.org/10.1124/pr.58.3.2.
153. Perin P, Mabou Tagne A, Enrico P, Marino F, Cosentino M, Pizzala R, Boselli C. Cannabinoids, inner ear, hearing, and tinnitus: a neuroimmunological perspective. Front Neurol. 2020;11:505995. https://doi.org/10.3389/fneur.2020.505995.
154. Smith PF, Zheng Y. Cannabinoids, cannabinoid receptors and tinnitus. Hearing Research. 2016;332:210–6.
155. Zheng Y, Smith PF. Cannabinoid drugs: will they relieve or exacerbate tinnitus? Curr Opin Neurol. 2019;32(1):131–6. https://doi.org/10.1097/WCO.0000000000000631.
156. Narwani V, Bourdillon A, Nalamada K, Manes RP, Hildrew DM. Does cannabis alleviate tinnitus? A review of the current literature. Laryngoscope Investig Otolaryngol. 2020;5(6):1147–55. https://doi.org/10.1002/lio2.479.
157. Mahdizadeh S, Khaleghi Ghadiri M, Ali Gorji A. Avicenna's canon of medicine: a review of analgesics and anti-inflammatory substances. Avicenna J Phytomed. 2015;5(3):182–202.
158. DiSogra, R. Essential oils for hearing loss, tinnitus, and vertigo. Audiology Today. July/Aug 2019. https://www.audiology.org/news-and-publications/audiology-today/articles/essential-oils-for-hearing-loss-tinnitus-and-vertigo/. Accessed 9 Jan 2022.
159. Cheong MJ, Kim S, Kim JS, Lee H, Lyu YS, Lee YR, Jeon B, Kang HW. A systematic literature review and meta-analysis of the clinical effects of aroma inhalation therapy on sleep problems. Medicine (Baltimore). 2021;100(9):e24652. https://doi.org/10.1097/MD.0000000000024652.
160. Her J, Cho MK. Effect of aromatherapy on sleep quality of adults and elderly people: a systematic literature review and meta-analysis. Complement Ther Med. 2021;60:102739. https://doi.org/10.1016/j.ctim.2021.102739.
161. Özbey-Yücel Ü, Aydoğan Z, Tokgoz-Yilmaz S, Uçar A, Ocak E, Beton S. The effects of diet and physical activity induced weight loss on the severity of tinnitus and quality of life: a randomized controlled trial. Clin Nutr ESPEN. 2021;44:159–65. https://doi.org/10.1016/j.clnesp.2021.05.010.
162. Loprinzi PD, Lee H, Gilham B, Cardinal BJ. Association between accelerometer-assessed physical activity and tinnitus, NHANES 2005–2006. Res Q Exerc Sport. 2013;84(2):177–85. https://doi.org/10.1080/02701367.2013.784840.
163. Zeman F, Koller M, Schecklmann M, Langguth B, Landgrebe M, TRI database study group. Tinnitus assessment by means of standardized self-report questionnaires: psychometric properties of the Tinnitus Questionnaire (TQ), the Tinnitus Handicap Inventory (THI), and their short versions in an international and multi-lingual sample. Health Qual Life Outcomes. 2012;10:128. https://doi.org/10.1186/1477-7525-10-128.
164. Gunjawate DR, Ravi R. Effect of yoga and meditation on tinnitus: a systematic review. J Laryngol Otol. 2021;135(4):284–7. https://doi.org/10.1017/S0022215121000566.
165. Kröner-Herwig B, Hebing G, van Rijn-Kalkmann U, Frenzel A, Schilkowsky G, Esser G. The management of chronic tinnitus--comparison of a cognitive-behavioural group training with yoga. J Psychosom Res. 1995;39(2):153–65. https://doi.org/10.1016/0022-3999(94)00098-p.
166. Aaron K, Cooper TE, Warner L, Burton MJ. Ear drops for the removal of ear wax. Cochrane Database Syst Rev. 2018;7(7):CD012171. https://doi.org/10.1002/14651858.CD012171.pub2.
167. Macknin ML, Talo H, Medendrop SV. Effect of cotton-tipped swab use on ear-wax occlusion. Clin Pediatr (Phila). 1994;33(1):14–8. https://doi.org/10.1177/000992289403300103.
168. Sim DW. Wax plugs and cotton buds. J Laryngol Otol. 1988;102(7):575–6. https://doi.org/10.1017/s0022215100105742.
169. Seely DR, Quigley SM, Langman AW. Ear candles--efficacy and safety. Laryngoscope. 1996;106(10):1226–9. https://doi.org/10.1097/00005537-199,610,000-00010.
170. Ernst E. Ear candles: a triumph of ignorance over science. J Laryngol Otol. 2004;118(1):1–2. https://doi.org/10.1258/002221504322731529.
171. Hornibrook J. Where there's smoke there's fire--ear candling in a 4-year-old girl. N Z Med J. 2012;125(1367):138–40.
172. Bhatt JM, Lin HW, Bhattacharyya N. Prevalence, severity, exposures, and treatment patterns of tinnitus in the United States. JAMA Otolaryngol Head Neck Surg. 2016;142(10):959–65. https://doi.org/10.1001/jamaoto.2016.1700.
173. Armitage CJ, Loughran MT, Munro KJ. Epidemiology of the extent of recreational noise exposure and hearing protection use: cross-sectional survey in a nationally representative UK adult population sample. BMC Public Health. 2020;20(1):1529. https://doi.org/10.1186/s12889-020-09602-8.
174. Loughran MT, Couth S, Plack CJ, Armitage CJ. Identifying targets for interventions to increase earplug use in noisy recreational settings: a qualitative interview study. Int J Environ Res Public Health. 2021;18(24):12879. https://doi.org/10.3390/ijerph182412879.
175. Mail Online. Doctor who got rid of 'incurable' tinnitus: ENT specialist reveals how he retrained his brain to ignore the high-pitched sounds using TV subtitles and video games. 2019. https://www.dailymail.co.uk/femail/article-7036477/Doctor-Tinitusreveals-retraining-brain-ignore-high-pitched-sound.html.
176. Searchfield GD, Sanders PJ, Doborjeh Z, Doborjeh M, Boldu R, Sun K, Barde A. A state-of-art review of digital technologies for the next generation of tinnitus therapeutics. Front Digit Health. 2021;3:724370. https://doi.org/10.3389/fdgth.2021.724370.
177. Wise K, Kobayashi K, Magnusson J, Welch D, Searchfield GD. Randomized controlled trial of a perceptual training game

for tinnitus therapy. Games Health J. 2016;5(2):141–9. https://doi.org/10.1089/g4h.2015.0068.
178. Hoare DJ, Van Labeke N, McCormack A, Sereda M, Smith S, Al Taher H, Kowalkowski VL, Sharples M, Hall DA. Gameplay as a source of intrinsic motivation in a randomized controlled trial of auditory training for tinnitus. PLoS One. 2014;9(9):e107430. https://doi.org/10.1371/journal.pone.0107430.
179. Deshpande AK, Bhatt I, Rojanaworarit C. Virtual reality for tinnitus management: a randomized controlled trial. Int J Audiol. 2021:1–8. https://doi.org/10.1080/14992027.2021.1978568.
180. Malinvaud D, Londero A, Niarra R, Peignard P, Warusfel O, Viaud-Delmon I, Chatellier G, Bonfils P. Auditory and visual 3D virtual reality therapy as a new treatment for chronic subjective tinnitus: results of a randomized controlled trial. Hear Res. 2016;333:127–35. https://doi.org/10.1016/j.heares.2015.12.023.
181. Partheniadis-Stumpf M, Maurer J, Mann W. Softlasertherapie in Kombination mit Tebonin i.v. bei Tinnitus [Soft laser therapy in combination with tebonin i.v. in tinnitus]. Laryngorhinootologie. 1993;72(1):28–31. https://doi.org/10.1055/s-2007-997,848.
182. Wenzel GI, Pikkula B, Choi CH, Anvari B, Oghalai JS. Laser irradiation of the guinea pig basilar membrane. Lasers Surg Med. 2004;35(3):174–80. https://doi.org/10.1002/lsm.20091.
183. Rhee CK, Bahk CW, Kim SH, Ahn JC, Jung JY, Chung PS, Suh MW. Effect of low-level laser treatment on cochlea hair-cell recovery after acute acoustic trauma. J Biomed Opt. 2012;17(6):068002. https://doi.org/10.1117/1.JBO.17.6.068002.
184. Chen CH, Huang CY, Chang CY, Cheng YF. Efficacy of low-level laser therapy for tinnitus: a systematic review with meta-analysis and trial sequential analysis. Brain Sci. 2020;10(12):931. https://doi.org/10.3390/brainsci10120931.
185. Ferreira MC, de Matos IL, de Toledo IP, Honório HM, Mondelli MFCG. Effects of low-level laser therapy as a therapeutic strategy for patients with tinnitus: a systematic review. J Speech Lang Hear Res. 2021;64(1):279–98. https://doi.org/10.1044/2020_JSLHR-20-00066.
186. Talluri S, Palaparthi SM, Michelogiannakis D, Khan J. Efficacy of photobiomodulation in the management of tinnitus: a systematic review of randomized control trials. Eur Ann Otorhinolaryngol Head Neck Dis. 2021:S1879-7296(21)00043-0. https://doi.org/10.1016/j.anorl.2020.10.013.
187. Nakashima T, Ueda H, Misawa H, Suzuki T, Tominaga M, Ito A, Numata S, Kasai S, Asahi K, Vernon JA, Meikle MB. Transmeatal low-power laser irradiation for tinnitus. Otol Neurotol. 2002;23(3):296–300. https://doi.org/10.1097/00129492-200,205,000-00011.
188. Bennett MH, Kertesz T, Perleth M, Yeung P, Lehm JP. Hyperbaric oxygen for idiopathic sudden sensorineural hearing loss and tinnitus. Cochrane Database Syst Rev. 2012;(10):CD004739. https://doi.org/10.1002/14651858.CD004739.pub4.
189. Joshua TG, Ayub A, Wijesinghe P, Nunez DA. Hyperbaric oxygen therapy for patients with sudden sensorineural hearing loss: a systematic review and meta-analysis. JAMA Otolaryngol Head Neck Surg. 2021 Oct;28:e212685. https://doi.org/10.1001/jamaoto.2021.2685.
190. Matcham F, Rayner L, Hutton J, Monk A, Steel C, Hotopf M. Self-help interventions for symptoms of depression, anxiety and psychological distress in patients with physical illnesses: a systematic review and meta-analysis. Clin Psychol Rev. 2014;34(2):141–57. https://doi.org/10.1016/j.cpr.2014.01.005.
191. Ho FY, Chung KF, Yeung WF, Ng TH, Kwan KS, Yung KP, Cheng SK. Self-help cognitive-behavioral therapy for insomnia: a meta-analysis of randomized controlled trials. Sleep Med Rev. 2015;19:17–28. https://doi.org/10.1016/j.smrv.2014.06.010.
192. van Straten A, Cuijpers P. Self-help therapy for insomnia: a meta-analysis. Sleep Med Rev. 2009;13(1):61–71. https://doi.org/10.1016/j.smrv.2008.04.006.
193. Aaron LA, Turner JA, Mancl LA, Sawchuk CN, Huggins KH, Truelove EL. Daily pain coping among patients with chronic temporomandibular disorder pain: an electronic diary study. J Orofac Pain. 2006;20(2):125–37.
194. Albano MG, d'Ivernois JF, de Andrade V, Levy G. Patient education in dental medicine: a review of the literature. Eur J Dent Educ. 2019;23(2):110–8. https://doi.org/10.1111/eje.12409.

Tinnitus Treatment: Evidence and Guidelines

59

Berthold Langguth, Tobias Kleinjung, Winfried Schlee, Sven Vanneste, and Dirk De Ridder

Abstract

It is a hallmark of modern medicine that it claims to be evidence based. This means that clinical decisions are based on research findings. Standardized algorithms have been developed to translate research findings into clinical recommendation. These involve a systematic review of the literature together with meta-analytic aggregation of research findings. The certainty of evidence of the accumulated research findings is evaluated by using methodological criteria. Clinical recommendations are formulated based on the results from research under consideration of the methodological evaluation of how these results were obtained.

In this chapter, we summarize the evidence for efficacy and safety of the various therapeutic interventions for the treatment of tinnitus. We present the most important clinical guidelines and discuss the strength and weaknesses of the evidence-based approach for the management of tinnitus.

B. Langguth (✉)
Department of Psychiatry and Psychotherapy, University of Regensburg, Bezirksklinikum, Regensburg, Germany
e-mail: Berthold.Langguth@medbo.de

T. Kleinjung
Department of Otorhinolaryngology – Head and Neck Surgery, University Hospital of Zurich, University of Zurich, Zürich, Switzerland
e-mail: Tobias.Kleinjung@usz.ch

W. Schlee
Department of Psychiatry and Psychotherapy, Interdisciplinary Tinnitus Clinic, University of Regensburg, Regensburg, Germany

S. Vanneste
School of Psychology, Global Brain Health Institute and Trinity College of Dublin Institute for Neuroscience, Dublin, Ireland
e-mail: sven.vanneste@tcd.ie

D. De Ridder
Section of Neurosurgery, Department of Surgical Sciences, University of Otago, Dunedin, New Zealand
e-mail: dirk.deridder@otago.ac.nz

W. Schlee et al. (eds.), *Textbook of Tinnitus*, https://doi.org/10.1007/978-3-031-35647-6_59

Graphical Abstract

From Evidence to Guidelines

Intervention	Source of evidence	Number of study participants	Efficacy (immediate)	Efficacy (longterm)
Cognitive behavioural therapy	Cochrane Review (Fuller 2020)	2733	Tinnitus severity (SMD): -0.56 THI: -10.91	No evidence due to lack of data
Hearing Aid	Cochrane (Sereda 2018)	590	No significant effects on tinnitus loudness or distress	No data
Cochlear Implant	Meta-Analysis (Oh 2022)	674	Tinnitus score (SMD: -1.32)	Not reported
Auditory Training	Systematic review (Hoare 2010)	269	Available evidence of insufficient quality to make conclusion about efficacy	Not reported
Sound Therapy	Cochrane (Sereda 2018)	590	No significant effects on tinnitus loudness or distress	No data
Tinnitus Retraining Therapy	Meta-analysis (Han 2021)	1345	Significantly increased treatment response	Significantly increased treatment response
Transcranial magnetic stimulation	Meta-Analysis (Lefebvre-Demers 2021)	945	Tinnitus severity (SMD): -0.45	Tinnitus severity (SMD): -0.42
Transcranial direct current stimulation	Meta-analysis (Martins 2022)	1031	Loudness (SMD) -0.35 Distress (SMD): -0.5	Not reported
Ginkgo biloba	Cochrane (Hilton 2013)	1543	No significant effects	Not reported
Antidepressants	Cochrane (Baldo 2012)	610	Insufficient evidence	Not reported
Anticonvulsants	Cochrane (Hoekstra 2011)	453	Insufficient evidence	Not reported
Betahistine	Cochrane (Wegner 2018)	303	No significant effects on tinnitus loudness or distress	Not reported

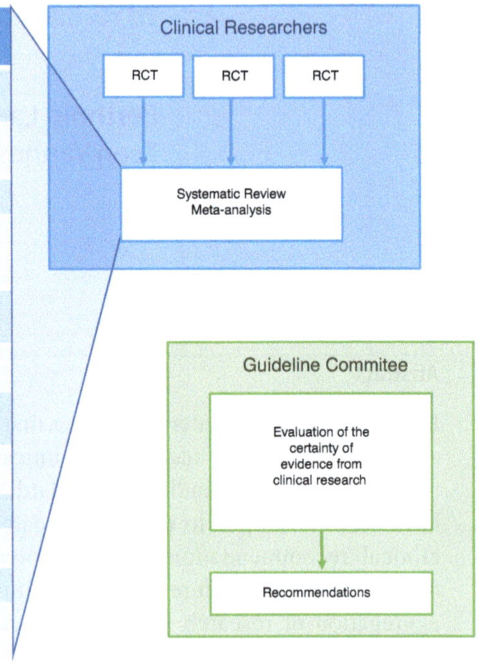

Highlights

- Modern medicine claims that clinical decisions should be based on scientific evidence.
- Clinical guidelines consist of recommendations, which are based on results from research under consideration of the methodological evaluation of how these results were obtained.
- The certainty of evidence in tinnitus research is generally low.
- Relatively good evidence is available for the short-term effectivity of cognitive behavioural therapy on tinnitus severity as assessed by tinnitus questionnaires.
- Good evidence is also available for the treatment of tinnitus with cochlear implants in case of deafness.
- The evidence-based approach has clear strengths but also substantial limitations, especially in a heterogeneous condition such as tinnitus.

Introduction

Tinnitus is treated by a variety of healthcare providers, including audiologists, ENT surgeons, psychologists, neurologists, psychiatrists, neurosurgeons, and others. Large multidisciplinary clinics dedicated to tinnitus are rare, and have some, but usually not all of the abovementioned specialists collaborating to solve the patients' tinnitus. Consequently, a tinnitus patient will be offered very different treatments depending on where patient presents [1, 2]. This indicates that for most patients, the treatment is not based on scientific evidence, but on standard-of-care-practices or recommendations of experts, which are frequently not supported by controlled trials.

This situation shows that the tinnitus field is clearly behind the standards of modern medicine, which are based on the concept of evidence-based medicine. This concept emerged about 50 years ago [3, 4] and since then increasing efforts were made to assess the evidence of effectiveness for therapeutic interventions by performing controlled trials. In the 90s of the last century, several initiatives started to systematically review controlled trials in order to establish an evidence base for clinical guidelines [5, 6].

At the same time, the term "evidence-based medicine" was introduced as "the process of finding, appraising, and using contemporaneous research findings as the basis for medical decisions" [7] or as "the conscientious, explicit and judicious use of current best evidence in making decisions about the care of individual patients" [8].

Evidence-based medicine has two components to it. The first component is the "clinical relevance", which states how good a treatment works. Thus, a treatment that only benefits 20% of all patients may still be very relevant to propose to a

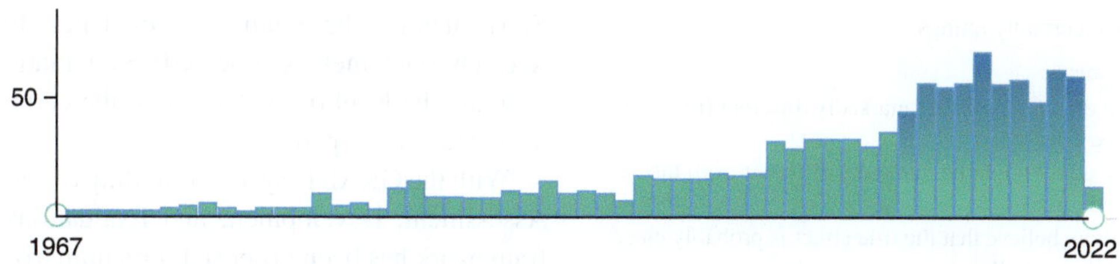

Fig. 59.1 Number of hits for "randomized controlled trials tinnitus" in PubMed (assessed in April 2022)

patient if it has a large effect size, for example, remove the tinnitus sound entirely. The other component is the "statistical significance", which says whether the effect of the treatment differs from a control treatment (in most cases placebo) more than chance level. Whether a difference between a given treatment and the control treatment becomes statistically significant depends on the effect size of the treatment and the sample size of the study. Thus, if you investigate a treatment in a study with a large sample, you may obtain a statistically significant treatment with very little clinical relevance. On the other hand, a treatment with a clinically relevant effect size might not turn statistically significant, if the sample size of the study is not large enough. This dichotomy was nicely expressed by the statistician Altman, who came up with the phrase: "the absence of evidence is not the evidence of absence" [9]. In summary, the absence of scientific proof for a specific tinnitus treatment does not mean the treatment does not work. The treatment may not yet be tested, improperly tested due to biases, or a treatment may be beneficial for a subgroup only. Because of the confusion of statistical significance and clinical relevance, as well as the large amount of trials, not uncommonly with opposite outcomes, guidelines are often developed to help healthcare providers in their clinical practice.

The transition from the results of clinical trials to clinical guidelines is a complex process. The first step is the search of all relevant published reports from clinical trials. The second step is the critical evaluation of the methodological quality of the trials. In a third step, the results must be aggregated. Among other criteria, this involves the evaluation of efficacy, effectiveness, side effects, validity, tolerability, and feasibility. Moreover, inconsistencies in clinical trial results and potential reasons for these inconsistencies (e.g. slight differences in the intervention, differences in study samples, insufficient statistical power, etc.) must be considered. This is further complemented by cost-effectiveness analyses. Finally, there are standardized procedures for guideline committees to integrate all this information to come up with recommendations for the clinical management.

In the field of tinnitus, traditionally many different treatments have been offered to patients, which also reflect the fact that there were no highly effective treatments. With the advent of evidence-based medicine, clinical researchers aimed at evaluating the effectiveness of various treatments by conducting clinical trials. This is far from trivial in the tinnitus field for several reasons [10–12]. First, tinnitus is a heterogeneous condition (see Chap. 7). Second, it is mostly purely subjective, which makes outcome measurement challenging (see Chap. 27), and third, suffering from tinnitus has many facets, which vary from patient to patient. Within the last decades many efforts have been made to establish methodological standards for clinical trials in tinnitus [13–16]. Over the years, more and more clinical trials evaluated the effectiveness of the various tinnitus treatments (see Fig. 59.1, Box 59.1).

These studies enabled systematic reviews and meta-analyses, on which clinical guidelines can be based.

Systematic reviews analyse the literature qualitatively, and can be accompanied by a quantitative meta-analysis if there is a sufficient amount of homogeneous trials to support or permit a quantitative meta-analysis. But even meta-analyses should not be accepted blindly at face value, considering meta-analyses are only as strong as the studies they statistically group. A good meta-analysis cannot correct for poor design or bias in the original source studies. Yet, systematic reviews and meta-analyses based on RCTs are considered the strongest scientific evidence available for creating clinical management guidelines.

In this chapter, we will first discuss the translation of evidence into clinical guidelines and then provide an overview of the available evidence for the various approaches and the recommendations of the various guidelines for tinnitus treatment.

Translating Evidence From Clinical Trials Into Guideline Recommendations

The first step is the definition of the clinical question, including the relevant patient population and the relevant outcomes. Based on a systematic literature search, the appropriate studies and systematic reviews of these will be identified.

Table 59.1 GRADE certainty ratings

Certainty	What it means
Very low	The true effect is probably markedly different from the estimated effect
Low	The true effect might be markedly different from the estimated effect
Moderate	The authors believe that the true effect is probably close to the estimated effect
High	The authors have a lot of confidence that the true effect is similar to the estimated effect

Table 59.2 Levels of evidence for therapeutic studies (from the Centre for Evidence-Based Medicine, http://www.cebm.net)

Level	Type of evidence
1A	Systematic review (with homogeneity) of randomized controlled trials (RCTs)
1B	Individual RCT (with narrow confidence intervals)
1C	All or none study
2A	Systematic review (with homogeneity) of cohort studies
2B	Individual cohort study (including low quality RCT, e.g. <80% follow-up)
2C	"Outcomes" research; ecological studies
3A	Systematic review (with homogeneity) of case-control studies
3B	Individual case-control study
4	Case series (and poor quality cohort and case-control study
5	Expert opinion without explicit critical appraisal or based on physiology bench research or "first principles"

Subsequently, the quality of evidence for all decision-relevant outcomes is assessed. Systematic approaches to evaluate the level of evidence and the certainty of evidence have been developed.

With the GRADE-system (Grading of Recommendations, Assessment, Development and Evaluations), a transparent framework has been proposed for summarizing the evidence and for creating clinical practice recommendations. GRADE has four levels of evidence—also known as certainty in evidence or quality of evidence (Table 59.1).

The certainty of evidence depends on the type of the clinical trials and on the methodological rigor of the trial. An example for a classification system of clinical trials according to the level of evidence is given in Table 59.2. There are also other classification systems that differ slightly in the criteria used.

Evidence from randomized controlled trials starts at high quality and evidence that includes observational data starts at low quality. The certainty in the evidence is increased or decreased by one or two levels according to further study criteria, resulting in a final level of certainty rating (see Fig. 59.2).

Bias occurs when the results of a study do not represent the truth because of inherent limitations in design or conduct of a study [8]. There are several kinds of bias [18]. A first

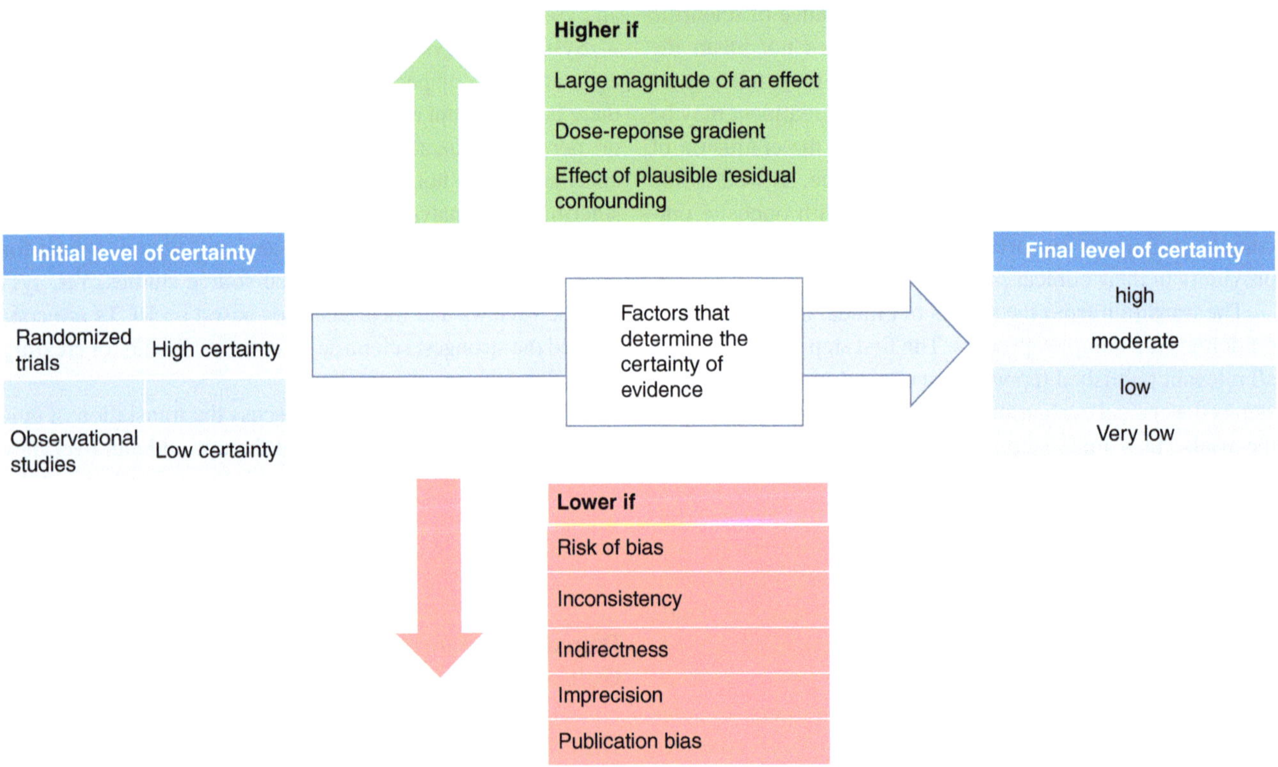

Fig. 59.2 Rating the quality of evidence (from [17]: Source Modified from: J Clin Epidemiol 2011 Apr;64(4):401–6. GRADE guidelines: 3. Rating the quality of evidence Howard Balshem 1, Mark Helfand, Holger J Schünemann, Andrew D Oxman, Regina Kunz, Jan Brozek, Gunn E Vist, Yngve Falck-Ytter, Joerg Meerpohl, Susan Norris, Gordon H Guyatt)

kind is a cognitive bias, in which the way the researchers thinks about the problem at hand is distorted or irrational. A second bias is conflict of interest, in which a person, association, or commercial entity has interests in a specific outcome of the trial. A third bias is statistical bias, which can be related to the way data are selected and sampled, or the statistical technique used. And a fourth type of bias is prejudice, whether conscious or unconscious, for example gender, race, or age-based.

Some of the statistical biases may be controlled for by double-blinding controlled trials.

The GRADE approach to assess *imprecision* focuses on the 95% confidence interval around the best estimate of the absolute effect. Certainty is lower if the clinical decision would likely be different if the true effect were at the upper or lower end of the confidence interval.

Certainty in a body of evidence is highest when there are several studies that show consistent effects. Criteria for *inconsistency* are the similarity of point estimates and the overlap of their confidence intervals, as well as statistical criteria for heterogeneity (e.g. the I2 and chi-squared test).

Indirectness refers to the fact that evidence is most certain when studies directly compare the interventions of interest in the population of interest and report the outcome(s) critical to decision-making. Certainty may be downgraded if the patients studied differ from those to whom the recommendation applies. The same is true, if the setting of a study is different from the real-world condition (e.g. a study of a psychotherapeutic approach by a specialized therapist only indirectly applies to a psychotherapist with less experience).

Publication bias requires inferences about missing evidence. Several statistical and visual methods are helpful in detecting publication bias, despite having serious limitations.

In some circumstances, certainty in the evidence can be rated up (see Fig. 59.2). First, when there is a very large magnitude of effect. Second, when there is a clear dose-response gradient. Third, when residual confounding is likely to decrease rather than increase the magnitude of the effect (in situations where there is an effect).

In GRADE, recommendations can be strong or weak, in favour or against an intervention. Beside the level of evidence and the certainty of evidence, there are also other factors that play a role. Very important is the balance between the desirable consequences and the adverse effects of a given treatment. In addition, variation or uncertainty in patient values and preferences should be considered. In the field of tinnitus, this may be due to the fact that tinnitus patients' expectations of their treatment vary widely. If a patient expects reduction of tinnitus loudness, a treatment, which is effective for reducing tinnitus suffering, might not satisfy the patient. Finally, the resources required for a given treatment recommendation should also be considered.

When integrating all these aspects, it becomes clear that there is a certain margin of discretion in the translating evidence from clinical trials into clinical recommendations. As the weighting of the various aspects is highly subjective, the composition of the guideline committee and their potential conflicts of interest gain relevance. This becomes evident, when recommendations from different guideline teams are compared (see also Table 59.3).

Table 59.3 Evidence for several tinnitus treatments and recommendations of the various guidelines

Intervention	Source of evidence	Number of study participants	Efficacy (immediate)	Efficacy (long term)	Potential harm	US (2014)	Swiss (2019)	European (2019)	NICE (2020)	German (2021)
Cognitive behavioural therapy	Cochrane Review [19]	2733	Tinnitus severity (SMD): −0.56 THI: −10.91	No evidence due to lack of data	Adverse effects are rare	Clinicians should recommend CBT to patients with persistent, bothersome tinnitus. (recommendation)	Efficacy clearly proven	Strong recommendation for cognitive behavioural therapy	If tinnitus is still causing an impact on emotional and social well-being, and day-to-day activities, consider a stepped approach: 1. Digital tinnitus-related cognitive behavioural therapy (CBT) 2. Group-based tinnitus-related psychological interventions including mindfulness-based cognitive therapy, acceptance and commitment therapy or CBT 3. Individual tinnitus-related CBT	Strong recommendation for cognitive behavioural therapy

Intervention	Source of evidence	Number of study participants	Efficacy (immediate)	Efficacy (long term)	Potential harm	US (2014)	Swiss (2019)	European (2019)	NICE (2020)	German (2021)
Hearing aid	Cochrane [20]	590	No significant effects on tinnitus loudness or distress	No data	Not reported	Clinicians should recommend a hearing aid evaluation for patients with hearing loss and persistent, bothersome tinnitus (recommendation)	Patients with a tinnitus pitch below 6 kHz seem to benefit	Weak recommendation for hearing aids	Offer amplification devices to people with tinnitus who have a hearing loss that affects their ability to communicate Consider amplification devices for people with tinnitus who have a hearing loss but do not have difficulties communicating Do not offer amplification devices to people with tinnitus but no hearing loss	Recommendation for hearing aids in case of hearing loss
Cochlear implant	Meta-Analysis [21]	674	Tinnitus score (SMD: −1.32)	Not reported	Not reported	Not mentioned	Not mentioned	No recommendation for cochlear implants	Not mentioned	Strong recommendation for cochlear implants in patients with tinnitus and severe hearing loss/deafness
Auditory training	Systematic review [22]	269	Available evidence of insufficient quality to make conclusion about efficacy	Not reported	Not reported	Not mentioned	Not mentioned	Not mentioned	Not mentioned	Recommendation for auditory training
Sound therapy	Cochrane [20]	590	No significant effects on tinnitus loudness or distress	No data	Not reported	Clinicians may recommend sound therapy to patients with persistent, bothersome tinnitus. (option)	Only limited data from controlled trials	No recommendation	Recommendation for research	Recommendation against sound generators, recommendation against specific sound therapies

(continued)

Table 59.3 (continued)

Intervention	Source of evidence	Number of study participants	Efficacy (immediate)	Efficacy (long term)	Potential harm	US (2014)	Swiss (2019)	European (2019)	NICE (2020)	German (2021)
Tinnitus retraining therapy	Meta-analysis [23]	1345	Significantly increased treatment response	Significantly increased treatment response	Not reported	Not mentioned	Lack of high-quality trials	No recommendation	Not mentioned	Can be considered for long-term treatment
Transcranial magnetic stimulation	Meta-analysis [24]	945	Tinnitus severity (SMD): −0.45	Tinnitus severity (SMD): −0.42	Not reported	Clinicians should not recommend TMS for the routine treatment of patients with persistent, bothersome tinnitus (recommendation against)	Not mentioned	Recommendation against transcranial magnetic stimulation	Recommendation for research	Recommendation against transcranial magnetic stimulation
Transcranial direct current stimulation	Meta-analysis [25]	1031	Loudness (SMD) -0.35 Distress (SMD): −0.5	Not reported	Not reported	Not mentioned	Not mentioned	No recommendation for transcranial electrical stimulation	Recommendation for research	Recommendation against transcranial electrical stimulation
Ginkgo biloba	Cochrane [26]	1543	No significant effects	Not reported	Incidence of side effects low	Clinicians should not recommend Ginkgo biloba, for treating patients with persistent, bothersome tinnitus (recommendation against)	No pharmacological treatment	Weak recommendation against pharmacological treatment	Not mentioned	Strong recommendation against pharmacological treatment
Antidepressants	Cochrane [27]	610	Insufficient evidence	Not reported	Side effects common	Clinicians should not routinely recommend antidepressants, anticonvulsants, anxiolytics, or intratympanic medications for a primary indication of treating persistent, bothersome tinnitus (recommendation against)			Not mentioned	
Anticonvulsants	Cochrane [28]	453	Insufficient evidence	Not reported	Side effects reported in 18% of participants				Not mentioned	
Betahistine	Wegner [29]	303	No significant effects on tinnitus loudness or distress	Not reported	Side effects on placebo level	Not mentioned			Do not offer betahistine to treat tinnitus	

Overview About the Evidence for Therapeutic Interventions in Tinnitus

As mentioned above, many different tinnitus treatments have been evaluated in clinical trials. Box 59.1 provides a (possibly incomplete) overview about therapeutic interventions, which have been investigated in clinical trials.

Box 59.1: Therapeutic Interventions for Tinnitus that Have Been Evaluated with Randomized Controlled Trials

- Pharmacological interventions:
  - Sodium channel blocker
    - Lidocaine
  - Antidepressants
    - Amitriptyline
    - Nortriptyline
    - Paroxetine
    - Sertraline
    - Trimipramine
  - Anticonvulsants
    - Carbamazepine
    - Gabapentin
    - Lamotrigine
    - Selurampanel
  - Benzodiazepines/GABAergic drugs
    - Alprazolam
    - Baclofen
    - Clonazepam
    - Diazepam
  - Glutamatergic drugs
    - Acamprosate
    - Memantine
    - Neremexane
    - Esketamine
  - Muscle relaxants
    - Cyclobenzaprine
    - Orphenadrine
    - Tizanidine
    - Eperisone
  - Others
    - Atorvastatin
    - Betahistine
    - Chinese medicine
    - Cilostazol
    - Cyclandelate
    - Deanxit
    - Ginkgo biloba
    - Melatonin
    - Misoprostol
    - 3,4-Methylenedioxymethamphetamine (MDMA)
    - Naloxone
    - Odansetron
    - Oxytocin
    - Piribedil
    - Pramipexole
    - Vardenafil
    - Vitamin B12
    - Zinc
- Non-pharmacological interventions:
  - Psychotherapy
    - Cognitive behavioural therapy (group setting)
    - Cognitive behavioural therapy (individual setting)
    - Online/Internet-based cognitive behavioural therapy
    - Mindfulness-based therapy
    - Hypnosis
  - Brain/neural stimulation
    - Transcranial magnetic stimulation
    - Transcranial direct current stimulation
    - Direct electrical stimulation
    - Vagus nerve stimulation
    - Transcutaneous electrical neural stimulation
  - Electrical stimulation of the ear/cochlea
  - Bimodal stimulation
    - Vagus nerve stimulation plus sound therapy
    - Electrical skin stimulation plus sound therapy
    - Electrical tongue stimulation plus sound therapy
  - Hearing aids
  - Cochlear implants
  - Sound treatment
    - Noise generator (complete masking)
    - Noise generator (partial masking)
    - Enriched acoustic environment
    - Fractal tones
    - Taylor made notched music training
    - Coordinated reset auditory stimulation
  - Auditory training
  - Music therapy
  - Combination approaches
    - Tinnitus retraining therapy (directive counselling plus sound therapy)
    - Neuromonics (counselling plus acoustic stimulation)
  - Acupuncture
  - Physiotherapy
  - Low-level laser therapy
  - Hyperbaric oxygenation
  - Neurofeedback
  - Virtual reality-based approaches

Among the trials performed, there is a wide variability in the quality of evidence. This does not mean that clinical trials with smaller samples and lower methodological quality are useless. In contrary, these pilot studies may be useful as a first step in a stepwise approach to explore the feasibility of a given treatment, relevant details for the efficacy of an intervention (dose, parameters of the intervention, sensitive outcome parameters, sample characteristics) and provide an estimate of the potential effect size. This is important information for planning randomized controlled trials with a sufficiently large sample size, which then can represent a reliable source for the generation of clinical evidence. Negative results in such exploratory trials can help to sort out certain treatment approaches without the expense of large trials. However, positive results in small exploratory trials without larger confirmatory trials cannot be considered as proof of efficacy.

Some of the interventions mentioned were only investigated in a few studies, others by several studies, which allowed systematic reviews and meta-analyses, so that the conditions for level 1a evidence can be fulfilled (see Table 59.2). Results of these systematic reviews and meta-analyses are summarized in Table 59.3. Cochrane meta-analyses have to follow a high methodological standard and are therefore considered as the "gold standard" [30]. Accordingly, in Table 59.3, we reported the results of the Cochrane meta-analyses, whenever a Cochrane meta-analysis has been performed for a particular intervention in the last 10 years.

In the interpretation of the results, it should be noted that the overall certainty of evidence in the tinnitus field is rather low. Even for cognitive behavioural therapy, the best investigated intervention, which is recommended by all guidelines, both the recent Cochrane meta-analysis [19] and the evidence evaluation of NICE [31], comes to the conclusion that the certainty of most conclusions is "low", meaning that "the true effect might be markedly different from the estimated effect" (Table 59.1).

Table 59.3 only includes interventions for which systematic reviews or meta-analyses are available and which are mentioned in most guidelines. Therefore, we will give a short overview about the evidence of the interventions presented in all chapters of Parts VII and VIII:

Tinnitus Counselling (Chap. 43)

Tinnitus counselling is typically considered as a basic therapeutic approach, which is recommended by all guidelines, even if the evidence for the efficacy from randomized controlled trials is limited. A recent large trial demonstrated the efficacy of a specific form of counselling [32] and additional studies, investigating counselling through specific smartphone apps, are underway [33].

Cognitive Behavioural Therapy for Tinnitus (Chap. 44)

Cognitive behavioural therapy is the best investigated treatment intervention in tinnitus. The main findings from a recent Cochrane meta-analysis [19] are that cognitive behavioural therapy (CBT) may be effective in reducing the score of tinnitus questionnaires at the end of treatment, and that there are few if any adverse effects from receiving CBT (although further research on this is recommended). There is, however, an absence of evidence at 6 or 12 months' follow-up [19].

CBT for tinnitus may have small additional benefit in reducing symptoms of depression although uncertainty remains due to concerns about the quality of the evidence. Overall, there is limited evidence for CBT for tinnitus improving anxiety, health-related quality of life, or negatively biased interpretations of tinnitus.

CBT for tinnitus delivered in person and delivered via the Internet, with some additional email communication from a professional, appear similarly effective, as does CBT delivered individually and group-wise.

Mindfulness and Tinnitus (Chap. 45)

Mindfulness-based treatments are sometimes subsumed under CBT and included in systematic reviews of CBT. A recent systematic review focusing exclusively on mindfulness-based interventions (MBI) [34] concludes that MBI decreases the tinnitus distress scores directly post-therapy based on moderate to high-quality studies. This was found regardless of the heterogeneity of patients, study design, type of MBI, and outcome assessment. Two out of three RCTs found clinically relevant decreases in tinnitus distress scores. No effect of MBIs was observed for depression and anxiety in tinnitus patients. Long-term effects remain uncertain.

Auditory Treatments of Tinnitus (Chap. 46)

Auditory treatments can be divided in four categories: devices for improvement of hearing, sound generators for tinnitus masking, auditory stimulation to induce specific neuroplastic changes in the central auditory system, and auditory training.

Concerning improvement of hearing, there is meta-analytic evidence for the efficacy of cochlear implants on tinnitus in patients with unilateral severe hearing loss or deafness [21, 35]. Even if data come mainly from observational studies and not from RCTs, the effect size of 1.32 is clinically highly relevant. Concerning hearing aids, the evidence from randomized controlled trials is very limited [20]. The relevant question, whether people with tinnitus who have a hearing loss but do not have difficulties communicating, may benefit from hearing aids, has not been addressed in RCTs. The evidence for sound generators is very limited as well [20]. Moreover, concerns were raised that chronic exposition to white noise may have a harmful effect on hearing [36].

Some forms of auditory stimulation such as enriched acoustic environment [37, 38], amplitude modulated tones [39–41], Taylor made notched music training [42, 43], or coordinated reset auditory stimulation [44] aim to reduce tinnitus by the induction of specific neuroplastic changes in the central auditory system. For all these approaches, only data from pilot studies are available, which require confirmation in larger RCTs, before recommendations can be made.

Auditory training approaches encompass various training procedures, e.g. aiming at improving frequency discrimination, sound localization or signal in noise detection. In a systematic review, the quality of the studies investigating auditory training was rated as low and the need for appropriate RCTs was expressed [22].

Tinnitus Retraining Therapy (Chap. 47)

According to a recent meta-analysis [23], TRT as add-on to a standard treatment improved the response rate after 1 month, 3 months, and 6 months. However, the quality of evidence of the available studies has been rated as low with a high risk of bias and the need for appropriate RCTs was expressed.

Tinnitus Pharmacotherapy (Chap. 48)

Various pharmacological agents have been investigated and for several compounds meta-analyses have been performed. Most of these studies were negative. Exceptions are some experimental approaches, which cannot be performed as routine treatments because of side effects (Lidocaine), some positive pilot studies [45–47], which could not yet be replicated by large confirmatory RCTs, and studies that investigated ginkgo biloba in elderly tinnitus patients with dementia [26]. Accordingly, the respective Cochrane meta-analyses for Ginkgo biloba [26], anticonvulsants [28], and antidepressants [27] were negative.

Tinnitus Activities Treatment (Chap. 49)

Tinnitus activities treatment has not been investigated in controlled trials. There exists only one controlled trial, in which tinnitus activities were the basis treatment and patients were randomized to additional sound therapy [48].

Neural Therapy and Botox (Chap. 50)

For neural therapy and botox, only pilot studies are available [49–51], which are far from sufficient for any recommendation.

Neurobiofeedback (Chap. 51)

Different neurobiofeedback paradigms have been investigated in several controlled studies, with promising results [52]. However, large confirmatory studies are needed before recommendations can be made.

Non-Invasive Brain Stimulation (Chap. 52)

Meta-analyses reveal positive effects for both transcranial direct current stimulation (tDCS) [25] and repetitive transcranial magnetic stimulation (rTMS) [24] with a small to medium effect size (between 0.35 and 0.5). For rTMS, an effect size in this range (0.42) has also been observed at follow-up assessments 1 week to 6 months after end of treatment. A recent network meta-analysis investigated the various investigated stimulation protocols of tDCS and rTMS separately, which resulted in effect sizes between −1.89 and 0.11 illustrating the relevance of the specific stimulation protocols [53].

Invasive Brain Stimulation (Chap. 53)

Invasive brain stimulation represents a highly experimental treatment requiring surgical insertion of electrodes under the scull. Epidural, subdural, and deep brain stimulation have shown to be beneficial in case series, but there is far from sufficient data to support their routine clinical use [54].

Bimodal Stimulation for the Treatment of Tinnitus (Chap. 54)

Different forms of bimodal stimulation have been investigated in the last years in randomized controlled trials. One involves the presentation of tones in combination with vagal nerve stimulation via an implanted vagus nerve stimulation device [55], other approaches combined auditory stimulation with electrical stimulation of the face or neck area [56] or the tongue [57]. The approaches differ slightly in the used auditory stimuli and the timing between auditory and electrical stimulation. First studies have shown substantial reductions of tinnitus severity by all three approaches in studies with 20 [56], 30 [55], and 326 [57] participants.

Complementary and Alternative Therapies (Chap. 55)

Of the many complementary and alternative therapies, only a few have been investigated in RCTs. The best-studied among these treatments is probably acupuncture, for which a recent systematic review identified 8 RCTs with 504 participants. Acupuncture had no significant effect on the primary outcome of VAS score compared with control treatment but positive effects on secondary outcomes (THI and TSI score). However, the authors conclude that due to the low quality and small sample size of the included trials, the level of evidence is insufficient to draw any definitive conclusions [58].

E-Health-Based Approach (Chap. 57)

E-Health-based approaches involve online and offline-based treatments including smart phone apps. In particular, the number of smart phone apps for tinnitus management is rapidly growing [59], although the evidence for their efficacy is still very limited.

On the other hand, there is a relative large number of studies investigating Internet-based CBT for tinnitus and revealing that this approach is similarly effective as CBT delivered individually and group-wise [19].

Self-Help Interventions (Chap. 58)

The term "self-help intervention" is used in different contexts with different meanings. Whereas "self-help" means traditionally the mutual exchange of patients in self-help groups, the term "self-help" has been recently also used in the context of online-delivered CBT. A qualitative analysis of the traditional self-help concept revealed that members of self-help group see the importance of their group primarily in social inclusion, psychosocial relief, coping with the disease and new insights in dealing with the disease. A systematic review of the traditional self-help approach concluded that because of the lack of high-quality and homogeneous studies no confident conclusions can be drawn regarding the efficacy of self-help interventions for tinnitus [60].

Guidelines Overview

There exist several guidelines for the management of tinnitus [61]. They vary largely in scope and extent, in their methodological rigor, in their organizational structure, in their actuality and in the composition of the guideline committees. The various guidelines are presented in more detail below.

NICE Guidelines

The NICE guidelines [62] are compiled by the British National Institute for Health and Care Excellence (NICE) according to highest methodological rigor. The guideline development process is highly standardized and transparent [30]. The evidence that was used to develop the recommendations is summarized in 15 evidence reports, which comprise up to 250 pages each [31].

The recommendations of the NICE guidelines differ in several important aspects from other guidelines. One example is the recommendation of hearing aids, where the NICE guideline differentiates between tinnitus patients who have hearing loss that affects their ability to communicate, from those who have hearing loss but no communication difficulties. This differentiation is important, as in the first group, hearing aids are already indicated for improving communication, whereas in the second group, the indication for the hearing aid is primarily its potential to have beneficial effect on tinnitus. This differentiation results in a graded recommendation: amplification devices should be offered to the first group and can be considered in the second group.

Another example is the recommendation for CBT, which considers availability and resources in addition to effectiveness. Thus, the guideline proposes a stepwise approach, starting with digital tinnitus-related CBT, offering group-based psychological interventions (mindfulness based cognitive therapy, acceptance, and commitment therapy or CBT) as the second step and individual CBT as the third step.

In contrast to other guidelines, the NICE guidelines not only make recommendations for or against specific interventions, but also "recommendations for "research". Such a recommendation is given when current evidence for efficacy or safety of a specific intervention is inconclusive or insufficient.

German Guideline

The German guideline has been edited in 2021 by the German Society of Ear-, Nose-, and Throat-medicine as a S3 Guideline [63], which means that the guideline has formally undergone all elements of systematic development (logic, decision and outcome analysis, assessment of clinical relevance of scientific studies and regular review).

The evidence on which the guideline is based is summarized in evidence tables in the appendix of the guideline. Recommendations for and against are provided in three categories each (strong recommendation, recommendation, and no recommendation). For some recommendations, the transition from evidence to recommendation is not entirely comprehensible, especially for recommendations where the German guideline differs from all other guidelines, e.g. in the recommendation for auditory training or in the recommendation against sound therapy (see Table 59.3).

Clinical Practice Guideline: Tinnitus (US)

The US guideline was developed by the American Academy of Otolaryngology—Head and Neck Surgery Foundation (AAO-HNSF) using an explicit and transparent a priori protocol for creating actionable statements based on supporting evidence and the associated balance of benefit and harm and was published in 2014 [64]. Recommendations for and against are provided in four categories each (strong recommendation, recommendation, option, and no recommendation). The US guideline differs from the other guidelines in the case of sound therapy, which is mentioned as a treatment option only in the US guidelines. A major limitation of the US guideline is its compilation date together with the lack of an update.

Swiss Guideline

The Swiss guideline is a very short practice guideline, edited in 2019 by an association of networks of medical practitioners (Medix) [65]. It is neither backed by a medical society nor by experts in the field and there is no information about the methodology of its development. The guideline does not provide recommendations, but a very short summary of the available evidence for various therapeutic interventions.

European Guideline

The European guideline has not been edited by a society, but by a group of clinicians and researchers from different European countries who participated in the EU-funded COST Action TINNET [66]. Neither the procedure for collecting evidence nor the used method for the transition from evidence to clinical recommendations has been described in detail and there is no summary of the evidence, on which the guideline has been based. Recommendations for and against are provided in four categories each (strong recommendation, recommendation, weak recommendation, and no recommendation).

Discussion

The claim of "evidence base" is a hallmark of modern medicine, and this evidence is generated by controlled clinical trials. The results from controlled trials are summarized in systematic reviews and meta-analyses and constitute the basis for the development of clinical guidelines. As mentioned above, the various resulting guidelines differ in several aspects. This has several reasons. First, the guidelines differ in their actuality and thus in the body of evidence on which their conclusions are based. Second, the methodological rigor, the systematics and the transparency, and how evidence was collected from the literature vary largely across guidelines. Third, the transition from evidence to recommendations is a process, which involves subjective evaluations, considerations and balances and thus depends on the constitution of the guideline committee with their individual biases and conflicts of interest. All these factors may explain the variable interpretation of the evidence by different guidelines, which results in a substantial variability across guidelines (see Table 59.3).

This can best be illustrated by, e.g. the optional recommendation of sound treatment only by the US guideline in striking contrast to the recommendation against sound generators, and against specific sound therapies for the German guideline. Some treatments are only recommended by one guideline. For example, auditory training is only recommended by the German guideline.

There is also a considerable difference in the recommendations in case of inconclusive evidence. While most guidelines recommend against in such situations, the NICE guidelines emphasize the need for further research.

An aspect to be considered is also the categorization of recommendations. CBT is strongly recommended by various guidelines, based on an effect size of −0.56 immediately after treatment with low certainty of evidence and an absence of evidence at 6 or 12 months of follow-up [19].

A meta-analysis for transcranial magnetic stimulation reveals the effect size of −0.45 immediately after treatment and −0.42 at follow-up (between 1 week and 6 months after treatment) [24], but is not recommended by any guideline. Thus, a relatively small difference in the evidence results in very different recommendations.

The NICE guidelines provide an explanation for the different assessment of the evidence in this case, by stating "While the committee were able to make recommendations for other reviews based on very limited evidence, they decided that because neuromodulation interventions are currently not offered for tinnitus on the NHS, any recommendation would have a large impact on current practice and there was therefore not enough evidence to support this change" [67]. This implies that the recommendation for new and innovative treatments requires another threshold of evidence as compared to long-standing treatments.

This aspect needs further consideration as it has an impact on the development of innovative treatments, which are urgently needed in the tinnitus field. According to the statement of NICE (which is probably the most innovation friendly guideline, as it provides "recommendations for research" and not "recommendations against" if the evidence for an innovative treatment is not yet sufficient) a new treatment would require a body of evidence for efficacy and safety from several randomized controlled trials together with a convincing meta-analysis of their results, which reveals a higher effect size as compared to the currently recommended treatments. With guideline update cycles of at least 5 years, it would take about 10 years under optimal conditions for a new safe and effective treatment to be recommended in guidelines. As a recommendation in guidelines plays a major role for the implementation in clinical practice, the question arises, whether it can be justified that patients have to wait so long until they can benefit from an innovative therapy. Moreover, a delay of 10+ years from a successfully developed innovative treatment and its clinical implementation will limit the willingness to invest in innovative tinnitus treatments.

There is no doubt that the methodology of evidence-based medicine (EBM) has improved the quality of medical services immensely. But EBM has also its inherent limitations and weaknesses. The methodological gold standard—studying a therapeutic intervention in many multi-centre randomized controlled trials and performing a meta-analysis of their results—aims to focus on the essential aspect of the pathological condition and the therapeutic intervention by removing all patient- and therapist-specific aspects by averaging across many patients and treatment settings.

The more homogeneous the pathophysiology of a given disorder and the more homogeneous the intervention, the more appropriate is this approach. However, if we deal with a heterogeneous condition such as tinnitus (see Chap. 7), this averaging approach has limitations. In this context, it is of utmost importance to identify criteria for meaningful subtypes of tinnitus, as this would allow the investigation of specific interventions for these specific subtypes.

The same applies to the heterogeneity of interventions. In the field of neuromodulation, the investigated interventions vary in many parameters [68]. Pooling all these studies in meta-analyses may not be the most appropriate approach. Recently, the method of network meta-analyses was developed, which enables the aggregated analysis of various interventions. Network meta-analyses for neurostimulation [53, 69] in tinnitus indicate the potential of this approach by demonstrating more promising results as compared to the typical standard meta-analysis. However, these network meta-analyses were not yet considered in the development of guidelines.

A further important aspect is the transferability of results from clinical trials into clinical practice. In case of the administration of a medication, it may be guaranteed that the patients in the real world receive the same treatment as the patients in the clinical trials. However, in case of cognitive behavioural therapy, there might be differences between the treatment provided by the resident psychotherapist with limited tinnitus experience and the specialized therapist in a tertiary referral centre where treatment studies are performed.

Although evidence-based medicine and the development of guidelines have made an important contribution to a scientific approach in medicine, one should be aware of their limitations and the need for further development towards more personalized approaches and an innovation-friendly environment.

Ultimately the goal of the healthcare provider is to help the tinnitus patient. Guidelines are not "laws", merely guidelines, based on as much evidence as we currently have. The clinician treats individual patients and always has a therapeutic freedom to offer off-label treatments, if their use can be justified. This option should not be dismissed, as long as the quality of evidence is low for most if not all current tinnitus treatments. For the individual, case chances of improvement, risks of treatment, alternative options, and the patient's will have to be weighted to come to a reasonable decision.

References

1. Hall DA, Lainez MJ, Newman CW, Sanchez TG, Egler M, Tennigkeit F, et al. Treatment options for subjective tinnitus: self reports from a sample of general practitioners and ENT physicians within Europe and the USA. BMC Health Serv Res. 2011;11:302.
2. Cima RFF, Kikidis D, Mazurek B, Haider H, Cederroth CR, Norena A, et al. Tinnitus healthcare: a survey revealing extensive variation in opinion and practices across Europe. BMJ open. 2020;10(1):e029346.
3. Wennberg J, Gittelsohn. Small area variations in health care delivery. Science. 1973;182(4117):1102–8.
4. Cochrane AL. Effectiveness and efficiency: random reflections on health services. 1972.
5. Davino-Ramaya C, Krause LK, Robbins CW, Harris JS, Koster M, Chan W, et al. Transparency matters: Kaiser Permanente's National Guideline Program methodological processes. Perm J. 2012;16(1):55–62.
6. Smith R. Where is the wisdom...? BMJ. 1991;303(6806):798–9.
7. Rosenberg W, Donald A. Evidence based medicine: an approach to clinical problem-solving. BMJ. 1995;310(6987):1122–6.
8. Sackett DL, Rosenberg WM, Gray JA, Haynes RB, Richardson WS. Evidence based medicine: what it is and what it isn't. BMJ. 1996;312(7023):71–2.
9. Altman DG, Bland JM. Absence of evidence is not evidence of absence. BMJ. 1995;311(7003):485.

10. Langguth B, Kleinjung T, Landgrebe M. Tinnitus: the complexity of standardization. Eval Health Prof. 2011;34(4):429–33.
11. Searchfield G. A commentary on the complexity of tinnitus management: clinical guidelines provide a path through the fog. Eval Health Prof. 2011;34(4):421–8.
12. Hoare DJ, Hall DA. Clinical guidelines and practice: a commentary on the complexity of tinnitus management. Eval Health Prof. 2011;34(4):413–20.
13. Landgrebe M, Azevedo A, Baguley D, Bauer C, Cacace A, Coelho C, et al. Methodological aspects of clinical trials in tinnitus: a proposal for an international standard. J Psychosom Res. 2012;73(2):112–21.
14. Langguth B, Goodey R, Azevedo A, Bjorne A, Cacace A, Crocetti A, et al. Consensus for tinnitus patient assessment and treatment outcome measurement: tinnitus research initiative meeting, Regensburg, July 2006. Prog Brain Res. 2007;166:525–36.
15. Hall DA, Haider H, Szczepek AJ, Lau P, Rabau S, Jones-Diette J, et al. Systematic review of outcome domains and instruments used in clinical trials of tinnitus treatments in adults. Trials. 2016;17(1):270.
16. Hall DA, Smith H, Hibbert A, Colley V, Haider HF, Horobin A, et al. The COMiT'ID study: developing core outcome domains sets for clinical trials of sound-, psychology-, and pharmacology-based interventions for chronic subjective tinnitus in adults. Trends in hearing. 2018;22:2331216518814384.
17. Zhang Y, Akl EA, Schunemann HJ. Using systematic reviews in guideline development: the GRADE approach Res Synth Methods. 2018.
18. Haslam N. Bias in psychopathology research. Curr Opin Psychiatry. 2006;19(6):625–30.
19. Fuller T, Cima R, Langguth B, Mazurek B, Vlaeyen JW, Hoare DJ. Cognitive behavioural therapy for tinnitus. Cochrane Database Syst Rev. 2020;1:CD012614.
20. Sereda M, Xia J, El Refaie A, Hall DA, Hoare DJ. Sound therapy (using amplification devices and/or sound generators) for tinnitus. Cochrane Database Syst Rev. 2018;12:CD013094.
21. Oh SJ, Mavrommatis MA, Fan CJ, DiRisio AC, Villavisanis DF, Berson ER, et al. Cochlear implantation in adults with single-sided deafness: a systematic review and meta-analysis. Otolaryngol Head Neck Surg. 2022:1945998221083283.
22. Hoare DJ, Stacey PC, Hall DA. The efficacy of auditory perceptual training for tinnitus: a systematic review. Ann Behav Med. 2010;40(3):313–24.
23. Han M, Yang X, Lv J. Efficacy of tinnitus retraining therapy in the treatment of tinnitus: a meta-analysis and systematic review. Am J Otolaryngol. 2021;42(6):103151.
24. Lefebvre-Demers M, Doyon N, Fecteau S. Non-invasive neuromodulation for tinnitus: a meta-analysis and modeling studies. Brain Stimul. 2021;14(1):113–28.
25. Martins ML, Souza DDS, Cavalcante M, Barboza HN, de Medeiros JF, Dos Santos Andrade SMM, et al. Effect of transcranial Direct Current Stimulation for tinnitus treatment: a systematic review and meta-analysis. Clin Neurophysiol. 2022;52(1):1–16.
26. Hilton MP, Zimmermann EF, Hunt WT. Ginkgo biloba for tinnitus. Cochrane Database Syst Rev. 2013;(3):CD003852.
27. Baldo P, Doree C, Molin P, McFerran D, Cecco S. Antidepressants for patients with tinnitus. Cochrane Database Syst Rev. 2012;9:CD003853.
28. Hoekstra CE, Rynja SP, van Zanten GA, Rovers MM. Anticonvulsants for tinnitus. Cochrane Database Syst Rev. 2011;(7):CD007960.
29. Wegner I, Hall BA, Smit AL, McFerran D, Stegeman I. Betahistine for tinnitus. Cochrane Database of Systematic Reviews Review. 2018;1–46, https://doi.org/10.1002/14651858.CD013093.pub2.
30. Centre TerwdbtNG. 2020 [updated March 2020]. Available from: https://www.nice.org.uk/guidance/ng155.
31. Centre TerwdbtNG. Tinnitus: assessment and management. Excellence NIfHaC, editor. 2020.
32. Henry JA, McMillan G, Dann S, Bennett K, Griest S, Theodoroff S, et al. Tinnitus management: randomized controlled trial comparing extended-wear hearing aids, conventional hearing aids, and combination instruments. J Am Acad Audiol. 2017;28(6):546–61.
33. Schoisswohl S, Langguth B, Schecklmann M, Bernal-Robledano A, Boecking B, Cederroth CR, et al. Unification of Treatments and Interventions for Tinnitus Patients (UNITI): a study protocol for a multi-center randomized clinical trial. Trials. 2021;22(1):875.
34. Rademaker MM, Stegeman I, Ho-Kang-You KE, Stokroos RJ, Smit AL. The effect of mindfulness-based interventions on tinnitus distress. A systematic review. Front Neurol. 2019;10:1135.
35. Peter N, Liyanage N, Pfiffner F, Huber A, Kleinjung T. The influence of cochlear implantation on tinnitus in patients with single-sided deafness: a systematic review. Otolaryngol Head Neck Surg. 2019;161(4):576–88.
36. Attarha M, Bigelow J, Merzenich MM. Unintended consequences of white noise therapy for tinnitus-otolaryngology's cobra effect: a review. JAMA Otolaryngol Head Neck Surg. 2018;144(10):938–43.
37. Norena AJ, Chery-Croze S. Enriched acoustic environment rescales auditory sensitivity. Neuroreport. 2007;18(12):1251–5.
38. Vanneste S, van Dongen M, De Vree B, Hiseni S, van der Velden E, Strydis C, et al. Does enriched acoustic environment in humans abolish chronic tinnitus clinically and electrophysiologically? A double blind placebo controlled study. Hear Res. 2013;296:141–8.
39. Neff P, Michels J, Meyer M, Schecklmann M, Langguth B, Schlee W. 10 Hz Amplitude Modulated Sounds Induce Short-Term Tinnitus Suppression. Front Aging Neurosci. 2017;9:130.
40. Neff P, Zielonka L, Meyer M, Langguth B, Schecklmann M, Schlee W. Comparison of amplitude modulated sounds and pure tones at the tinnitus frequency: residual tinnitus suppression and stimulus evaluation. Trends Hear. 2019;23:2331216519833841.
41. Schoisswohl S, Arnds J, Schecklmann M, Langguth B, Schlee W, Neff P. Amplitude modulated noise for tinnitus suppression in tonal and noise-like tinnitus. Audiol Neurootol. 2019;24(6):309–21.
42. Okamoto H, Stracke H, Stoll W, Pantev C. Listening to tailor-made notched music reduces tinnitus loudness and tinnitus-related auditory cortex activity. Proc Natl Acad Sci U S A. 2010;107(3):1207–10.
43. Teismann H, Okamoto H, Pantev C. Short and intense tailor-made notched music training against tinnitus: the tinnitus frequency matters. PLoS One. 2011;6(9):e24685.
44. Tass PA, Adamchic I, Freund HJ, von Stackelberg T, Hauptmann C. Counteracting tinnitus by acoustic coordinated reset neuromodulation. Restor Neurol Neurosci. 2012;30(2):137–59.
45. Azevedo AA, Figueiredo RR. Treatment of tinnitus with acamprosate. Prog Brain Res. 2007;166:273–7.
46. Coelho C, Figueiredo R, Frank E, Burger J, Schecklmann M, Landgrebe M, et al. Reduction of tinnitus severity by the centrally acting muscle relaxant cyclobenzaprine: an open-label pilot study. Audiol Neurootol. 2012;17(3):179–88.
47. Kucher K, Johns D, Wagner F, Abd-Elaziz K, Derne C, Sverdlov O, et al. Efficacy and safety of single- and repeated-selurampanel dosing for 2 weeks in patients with chronic subjective tinnitus: results of a randomized, double-blind, placebo-controlled, cross-over, proof-of-concept phase IIa study. Prog Brain Res. 2021;260:423–40.
48. Tyler RS, Stocking C, Ji H, Witt S, Mancini PC. Tinnitus activities treatment with total and partial masking. J Am Acad Audiol. 2021;32(8):501–9.
49. Stidham KR, Solomon PH, Roberson JB. Evaluation of botulinum toxin A in treatment of tinnitus. Otolaryngol Head Neck Surg. 2005;132(6):883–9.
50. Vielsmeier V, Schlee W, Langguth B, Kreuzer PM, Hintschich C, Strohmeyer L, et al. Lidocaine injections to the otic gan-

glion for the treatment of tinnitus-A pilot study. Prog Brain Res. 2021;260:355–66.
51. Sirh SJ, Sirh SW, Mun HY, Sirh HM. Integrative treatment for tinnitus combining repeated facial and auriculotemporal nerve blocks with stimulation of auditory and non-auditory nerves. Front Neurosci. 2022;16:758575.
52. Guntensperger D, Thuring C, Meyer M, Neff P, Kleinjung T. Neurofeedback for tinnitus treatment - review and current concepts. Front Aging Neurosci. 2017;9:386.
53. Chen JJ, Zeng BS, Wu CN, Stubbs B, Carvalho AF, Brunoni AR, et al. Association of central noninvasive brain stimulation interventions with efficacy and safety in tinnitus management: a meta-analysis. JAMA Otolaryngol Head Neck Surg. 2020;146(9):801–9.
54. De Ridder D, Adhia D, Langguth B. Tinnitus and brain stimulation. Curr Top Behav Neurosci. 2021;51:249–93.
55. Tyler R, Cacace A, Stocking C, Tarver B, Engineer N, Martin J, et al. Vagus nerve stimulation paired with tones for the treatment of tinnitus: a prospective randomized double-blind controlled pilot study in humans. Sci Rep. 2017;7(1):11960.
56. Marks KL, Martel DT, Wu C, Basura GJ, Roberts LE, Schvartz-Leyzac KC, et al. Auditory-somatosensory bimodal stimulation desynchronizes brain circuitry to reduce tinnitus in guinea pigs and humans. Sci Translat Med. 2018;10(422):eaal3175.
57. Conlon B, Langguth B, Hamilton C, Hughes S, Meade E, Connor CO, et al. Bimodal neuromodulation combining sound and tongue stimulation reduces tinnitus symptoms in a large randomized clinical study. Sci Translat Med. 2020;12(564):eabb2830.
58. Huang K, Liang S, Chen L, Grellet A. Acupuncture for tinnitus: a systematic review and meta-analysis of randomized controlled trials. Acupunct Med. 2021;39(4):264–71.
59. Mehdi M, Riha C, Neff P, Dode A, Pryss R, Schlee W, et al. Smartphone apps in the context of tinnitus: systematic review. Sensors (Basel). 2020;20(6):1725.
60. Greenwell K, Sereda M, Coulson N, El Refaie A, Hoare DJ. A systematic review of techniques and effects of self-help interventions for tinnitus: application of taxonomies from health psychology. Int J Audiol. 2016;55(Suppl 3):S79–89.
61. Fuller TE, Haider HF, Kikidis D, Lapira A, Mazurek B, Norena A, et al. Different teams, same conclusions? A systematic review of existing clinical guidelines for the assessment and treatment of tinnitus in adults. Front Psychol. 2017;8:206.
62. Lewis S, Chowdhury E, Stockdale D, Kennedy V, Guideline C. Assessment and management of tinnitus: summary of NICE guidance. BMJ. 2020;368:m976.
63. Mazurek B, Hesse G, Dobel C, Kratzsch V, Lahmann C, Sattel H. Clinical practice guideline: chronic tinnitus-diagnosis and treatment. Dtsch Arztebl Int. 2022;119(13):219–25 (Forthcoming).
64. Tunkel DE, Bauer CA, Sun GH, Rosenfeld RM, Chandrasekhar SS, Cunningham ER Jr, et al. Clinical practice guideline: tinnitus. Otolaryngol Head Neck Surg. 2014;151(2 Suppl):S1–S40.
65. Tinnitus. Available from: https://www.medix.ch/wissen/guidelines/augen-und-hno-krankheiten/tinnitus/.
66. Cima RFF, Mazurek B, Haider H, Kikidis D, Lapira A, Norena A, et al. A multidisciplinary European guideline for tinnitus: diagnostics, assessment, and treatment. HNO. 2019;67(Suppl 1):10–42.
67. Centre TerwdbtNG. Tinnitus: assessment and management. 2020.
68. Schoisswohl S, Agrawal K, Simoes J, Neff P, Schlee W, Langguth B, et al. RTMS parameters in tinnitus trials: a systematic review. Sci Rep. 2019;9(1):12190.
69. Chen JJ, Chen YW, Zeng BY, Hung CM, Zeng BS, Stubbs B, et al. Efficacy of pharmacologic treatment in tinnitus patients without specific or treatable origin: a network meta-analysis of randomised controlled trials. EClinicalMedicine. 2021;39:101080.

Part VIII

Future Directions

The Future of Tinnitus Research: "In Crazy We Believe, in Science We Trust"

60

Dirk De Ridder, Sven Vanneste, Aage R. Møller, Tobias Kleinjung, Berthold Langguth, and Winfried Schlee

Abstract

In this chapter, we give an outlook about future research strategies for the tinnitus field. The core question of every scientist, researcher, research team, or research organization is: what do you need to be successful? A literature research reveals characteristics such as multidisciplinarity, open-mindedness, spatial proximity, distributed responsibility, little hierarchy, open communication, trust, innovation, and a common goal. The goal in case of tinnitus research is unambiguously clear, namely finding a cure for tinnitus, to silence the phantom sound.

Success strategies are not domain specific: strategies, which are successful in business and sports, are probably also effective in science. Thus, it is worth to have a look on a highly successful sports team, Emirates Team New Zealand, which won the last editions of the America's Cup, the oldest sports trophy in the world, and which is managed by the founder of the Tinnitus Research Initiative. We will discuss what we can learn from the strategies of the successful sailing team and lay out what is needed in tinnitus research to come closer to our goal, a "cure for tinnitus". The motto is: "in crazy we believe, but in science we trust."

Aage R. Møller has died before the publication of this book.

D. De Ridder (✉)
Section of Neurosurgery, Department of Surgical Sciences, University of Otago, Dunedin, New Zealand
e-mail: Dirk.deridder@otago.ac.nz

S. Vanneste
School of Psychology, Global Brain Health Institute and Trinity College of Dublin Institute for Neuroscience, Dublin, Ireland

A. R. Møller
Neuroscience Program, University of Texas, Dallas School of Brain and Behavioral Sciences, Richardson, TX, USA

T. Kleinjung
Department of Otorhinolaryngology – Head and Neck Surgery, University Hospital of Zurich, University of Zurich, Zürich, Switzerland

B. Langguth
Department of Psychiatry and Psychotherapy, University of Regensburg, Bezirksklinikum, Regensburg, Germany

W. Schlee
Department of Psychiatry and Psychotherapy, Interdisciplinary Tinnitus Clinic, University of Regensburg, Regensburg, Germany

The Future of Tinnitus Research Is Bright, but Why? And Do We Know How to Become Successful in Tinnitus Research?

Entire buildings can be filled with books that describe how one can become successful, especially in business. Only on Amazon.com over 60,000 books are sold with as topic "business" and "success", and 30,000 deal with the "science of success". In PubMed, the most used medical research library, advice can be found on how to build a successful research team [1–3]. The characteristics for success are usually based on the same pillars: (1) Multidisciplinary, (2) Open-mindedness, (3) Common goal and vision, (4) Spatial proximity, (5) Distributed responsibility, (6) Little hierarchy, (7) Open communication, (8) Trust, and (9) Innovation, and a couple more of these managerial buzz words.

Yet, what is success? It could be defined as the state of meeting a predefined prediction or goal. The Tinnitus Research Initiative (TRI) has a predefined goal, which is to cure tinnitus, which it shares with the American Tinnitus Association, the British Tinnitus Association, and many other tinnitus organizations. And thus, success for tinnitus would be when the predictions made by a theory are confirmed by the research experiment, i.e., silence the tinnitus. However, even if a cure is discovered accidentally, by shear serendipity, that would be considered a success. It is

W. Schlee et al. (eds.), *Textbook of Tinnitus*, https://doi.org/10.1007/978-3-031-35647-6_60

assumed that more than 50% of the inventions are actually serendipitous [4]. But luck, and certainly serendipity, can be helped by dedication and hard work. *Thomas Edison*, the wizard of the "invention factory" at Menlo Park, who was elected the greatest inventor of all times, famously stated that "I have not failed 10,000 times, I have just found 10,000 ways that won't work. Our greatest weakness lies in giving up. The most certain way to succeed is always to try just one more time. Genius is 1% inspiration and 99% perspiration". But luck also favors the maniacally dedicated researchers. *Seneca*, Emperor *Nero's famed philosopher-teacher perfectly described this: "luck* is a matter of preparation meeting opportunity". This was translated to science by *Louis Pasteur*, the French microbiologist who invented the germ theory of disease, as follows: "*Dans les champs de l'observation le hasard ne favorise que les esprits prepares*" (In the fields of observation chance favors only the prepared mind). Freely translated to tinnitus this means that when someone is constantly thinking about tinnitus, (s)he will interpret everything in the light of the goal of finding a cure, and signs that may be meaningless for everybody else may be the missing link that serendipitously presents to fill the gap. *August Kekule*, a German theoretical chemist, discovered the chemical structure of benzene, a six-membered ring of carbon atoms with alternating single and double bonds, by interpreting a dream, in which he saw a snake biting its own tail. Needless to say, that if any of us would have the same dream, this would not lead to a discovery.

Furthermore, another aspect of helping luck is taking risks [5]. Indeed, lucky people seem to have a greater tendency than the unlucky to take risks, especially in the social and financial (investment) domains [6]. Thus, taking risks may increase luck to find solutions. This is important, as a computer simulation study has found that even though intelligence/talent has a Gaussian distribution, (financial) success is distributed following a power law or Pareto's 80/20 rule, meaning that 20% of people own 80% of all wealth. The factor explaining this difference according to the computer simulation is randomness, i.e., luck. Thus, the most successful people are not the most talented, but average people who have been lucky [7]. Furthermore, it has been shown that in a mature research field taking risks is more efficient than doing small incremental research for success [8]. Choosing risky experiments may accelerate collective discovery [8].

Thus, from the above, it appears evident that in trying to find a cure for tinnitus, a good team, helped by working hard, delegating work, and taking risks is essential. In a reply to a 12-year-old asking *Richard Branson* what makes success in business, he summarized this eloquently: "*The key enterprising skills I used when first starting out are the very same ones I use today: the art of delegation, risk-taking, surrounding yourself with a great team and working on projects you really believe in*". This applies to business and research in equal terms.

Currently, finding a cure for tinnitus is deemed mostly impossible, and many tinnitus researchers and health-care providers define success as reducing the tinnitus-associated suffering. But that is not the goal of the TRI, nor of the ATA and BTA. The goal is to eliminate the phantom sound. This does not mean that a treatment that reduces tinnitus suffering is worthless. On the contrary, effective treatments for reducing suffering are highly relevant, but for the TRI, they are only milestones on the path toward a cure. And in that sense the TRI does not follow the Olympic Creed which states that "The important thing in life is not the triumph, but the fight; the essential thing is not to have won, but to have fought well".

Apart from the disagreement on the value of the Olympic Creed, we may learn from sports, especially from team sports, as both team sports [9] and health care [10], including tinnitus research, can be regarded as complex adaptive systems [11–14], involving non-linear dynamics and studied by network science. All complex adaptive systems share the same characteristics, irrespective of whether the complex adaptive system is an ant colony, economy, internet, brain, or social group [13, 15]. This also explains how and why *Charles Darwin* and *Alfred Russel Wallace* were both independently inspired by reading the same book on economy (Principle of Population, 1798) by *Thomas Malthus*. Indeed, both adopted the Malthusian economical "*struggle for existence*" as the basis of their biological theory of natural selection in the evolutionary process. This may seem strange but is understandable as the same network science rules that apply to economy also apply to biology within the framework of complex adaptive systems.

The Tinnitus Research Initiative (TRI) was founded by Matteo de Nora with the vision that success in economy, in sports, and in science is based on similar principles.[1] Its founder happens to be also one of the brains behind Emirates Team New Zealand, competing in the America's Cup multiple times but winning the two most recent events in 2017 and 2021. And while everybody in New Zealand and the whole world was thrilled to watch the sailing, or rather flying, of these vessels, one quickly came to the conclusion that Emirates Team New Zealand was destined to win, and that this was very good news for the tinnitus community, for multiple reasons.

First, a little explanation. The America's Cup, affectionally known as the Auld Mug, is the oldest international sporting trophy, dating back to 1851. It is the Formula 1 of sailing, held every 3–4 years, and in 2021 in Auckland, New Zealand, because Emirates Team New Zealand won the previous edi-

[1] We leave it up to the reader to judge to which extent this vision is reflected by the current structure of the academic world.

tion in 2017. And, the winner sets the rules and the design of the boats for the next challenge.

New Zealand is a very beautiful, tiny country, with five million people, very remote, more than 4000 km further than Australia (in a Eurocentric vision). It is known for Lord of the Rings, the Rainbow warrior bombing, its popular prime minister, multiculturalism (Maori and Pacific Islanders, European and Asian), gender equality, the kiwi bird, its stunning landscapes and sports, especially rugby with its famous All Blacks, and…sailing. Pro capita, New Zealand is one of the most successful Olympic medalist winners.

But why is it important that Emirates Team New Zealand won the America's cup? Well it is for multiple reasons.

A first reason, of course, is that the founder of the TRI is one of the two driving forces of this remarkable team, and so we, as TRI, are proud that he and his team won.

A second reason is that New Zealand is a tiny country, and with its lovely people, its commonsense no-nonsense approach beats sailing giants like the UK and USA. Nevertheless, most importantly, because it provides hope for people living with tinnitus, because of the way Matteo de Nora approached this David versus Goliath fight.

First of all is the mind-blowing exceptional design of these boats. They do not sit in the water, they hardly touch the water, and they seem to fly over the water, only in contact with the water by two hydrofoils. These are not sailboats but flyboats (see Fig. 60.1).

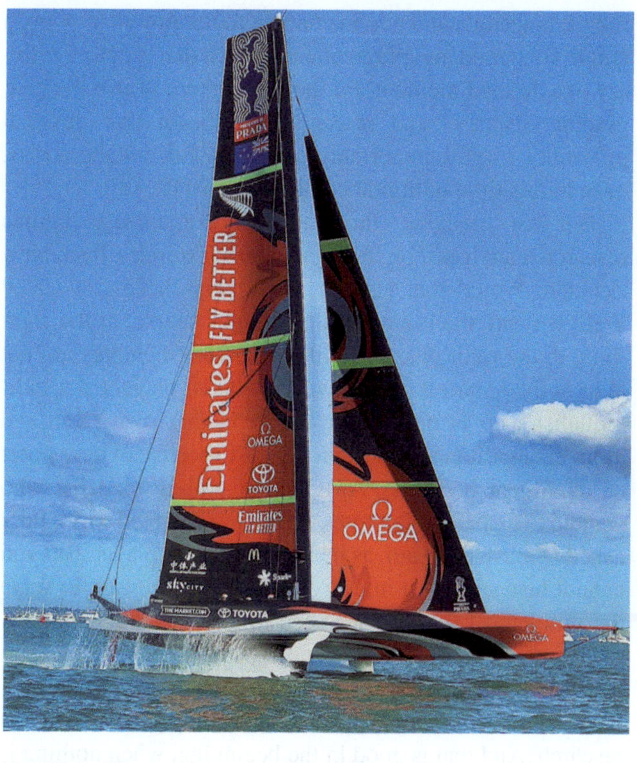

Fig. 60.1 Picture of the exceptional design of the boats that hardly touch the water. Picture taken by Dirk de Ridder

And even more amazing, these sailboats can sail/fly three to four times faster than the speed of the wind. This sounds like magic, something that appears impossible, yet, can be achieved by the right engineering, and not accepting it is impossible, as long as it falls within the laws of physics and biology. Yet, it requires way more than just concocting a sailboat. It requires an extraordinary amount of highly dedicated unrelentless professionalism, rarely seen outside this team, with Grant Dalton taking care of the sailing/flying and Matteo de Nora of the organization, management, politics, and finances. The two form an incredible tandem. According to Wikipedia, the America's Cup "is a test not only of sailing skill and boat and sail design, but also of fundraising and management skills. Competing for the cup is expensive, with modern teams spending more than $100 million each; the 2013 winner was estimated to have spent $300 million on the competition". And Emirates Team New Zealand is probable the team with the lowest budget. Why is this relevant? Because it shows that by being creative even a more restricted budget than the almost unlimited USA and UK budgets does not prevent success. And this is where the tinnitus research world can learn from sailing, as outlined by Grant Searchfield in a talk at the TRI conference in 2018 [16].

So, what can we learn? That success is all about creativity, innovation, team building, dedication, preparation, and professionalism. The fact that a tiny country with a more restricted, albeit still huge budget in most people's counting, can win against very wealthy competitors with almost unlimited financial resources and a selection of a larger number of professional sailors sets the example for tinnitus research. Like Emirates Team New Zealand, tinnitus research is a small community with very limited budgets. But Emirates Team New Zealand proves this is no excuse not to be successful. So, what should we do? Well, we should look at what brought this success about and mimic the story of Emirates Team New Zealand.

What did Emirates Team New Zealand do to win? What is the magic sauce, the secret, and the ingredients of success?

It starts with a motto of one of the sponsors, Toyota, an unlikely motto for a Japanese company: "In crazy we believe" (see Fig. 60.2).

The kiwis, as New Zealanders are called, and call themselves, still embrace risks, and are creative and innovative by necessity. Kiwis have what they call "a number 8 wire mentality" denoting an ability to create or repair anything by using whatever materials are available at hand. They are willing to take chances as a matter of habit, but the risks are calculated, originally based on experience, now aided by artificial intelligence. The kiwis were the first to imagine a catamaran as a foiling yacht. They were the first to put cyclists on a boat. Moreover, they proposed a single hull foil sailboat for the 2021 America's cup. Team New Zealand is also the first to develop a chase boat fueled by hydrogen

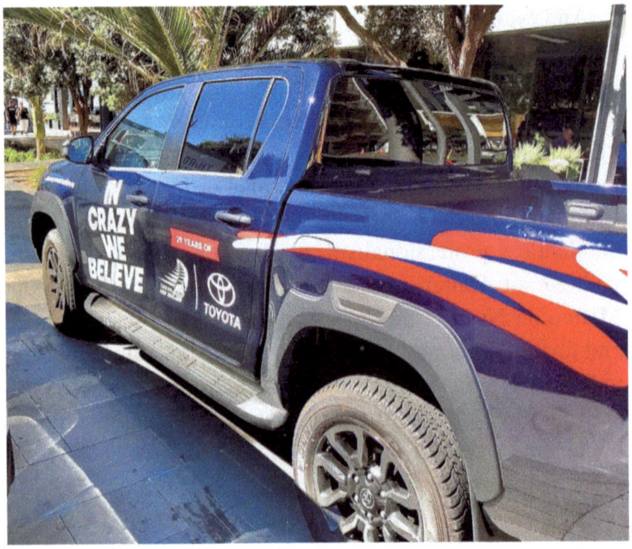

Fig. 60.2 The team motto "in crazy we believe" printed on the team car. Picture taken by Dirk De Ridder

cells, developed in less than a year, which was deemed impossible by specialists. This is what the tinnitus field also must do: embrace crazy ideas, be open-minded to novelty, and follow the Nike logo: Just do it!

So, How Did Emirates Team New Zealand Manage to Win the America's Cup?

The sailboats used in this edition of the America's Cup are actually more akin to airplanes than sailboats. The way these boats fly is based on the same physics that make airplanes fly. Thus, the kiwis realized they needed help from aircraft engineers who design airplane wings, and thus, many young talented aerospace engineers were attracted to help design this boat. But the boat should not take off and leave water, a similar problem encountered by F1 cars. So, Emirates Team New Zealand attracted F1 engineers to help design the boat. Yet, going on uncharted territory comes with a huge amount of new information, and it is critically important to separate signal from noise, to retain valuable information and discard uninteresting data. And that is where artificial intelligence comes in, to help discern relevant patterns in all the new information and use that to perfect the boat. So, a whole new breed of AI people were attracted to help design and perfect the boat. And, oh yes, also some boat designers are needed of course, even if only to design the sails. And as you may guess by now, the sails also are unique. They are double sails, with space between the two leaves, as AI shows this further provides extra speed.

All of this is well, but how do you make this work, specialists from very different domains, all working together? Well, you first need a common language, a "company culture" as marketers tend to call this. And what is this culture? I think it can be summarized by one sentence:

> In crazy we believe, but in science we trust.

So, maybe that should become the philosophy of tinnitus research, promoted, and advocated by the TRI, which was founded by the same person who is co-responsible for Emirates Team New Zealand's exceptional success story.

Matteo de Nora is frustrated he has not been able to create a similar "winning" team within the tinnitus community, when he started funding the TRI. His vision was to do the same thing for tinnitus as what he has done for sailing. And he is right, we have not found a solution for tinnitus at all, even though his contribution has made a landslide of difference, by generating a minimum level of basic knowledge about tinnitus, and by permitting international collaborations, but nothing in comparison to Emirates Team New Zealand.

And there are multiple reasons for that. One reason is that, when Matteo de Nora founded and started funding the TRI, the latter component of the motto "In crazy we believe, in science we trust" was completely absent. There was simply no data about tinnitus, so we did not even know who to put into the team. Consequently, we embraced everybody, creating a very multidisciplinary group, involving psychologists, audiologists, neurologists, ENT surgeons, neurosurgeons, basic scientists, information scientists, etc. This was wonderful, but it came with an equal number of different agendas, different research cultures, individualists afraid of sharing their knowledge, and not, in contrast to the America's Cup, a single concerted and pragmatic approach that requires delivery at a defined moment. Furthermore, there is also the geographic distance, and research has shown that physical proximity is still important for successful collaborations, even in this time of digital connectedness [17, 18].

But just "imagine" that one would organize a tinnitus research team based on the principles of Emirates Team New Zealand. Would that also be an equally successful team? Well, it is all about having all the right people, at the right time, in the right place. And the best team members are not always the smartest, they have to be team players. An individualist who is only interested in his/her own fame and glory cannot fit in a team approach, irrespective of how smart or intelligent he/she is. An Olympic sailing medalist who wanted to be part of Emirates Team New Zealand was kindly asked to leave the team, as he was not a team player. But you cannot be a specialist in everything, and if we want to solve the problem of tinnitus, we need to use the team approach, the Emirates Team New Zealand approach, but with one single vision, not 10 different ones, all going in different directions. And this is what happened in the early years of tinnitus research. And that is good in the beginning, when nothing is known, just like the early explorers of unknown continents, who seem to wander around randomly exploring the unknown. But once the area is charted, a systematic concerted approach is required. And we are still exploring in the tinnitus field, but are at a transition time, when a new approach, an Emirates Team New Zealand approach is needed to bring together what is known into one concerted goal-oriented approach, by a highly dedicated team of creative, innovative specialists who accept to work as a team, to crack the enigmatic code of tinnitus, not for their own fame and glory, but the benefit of the patients and the joy of winning, to understand how the brain and body works.

Even with such an approach, solving the tinnitus problem is not guaranteed, just as you cannot guarantee that Emirates Team New Zealand will win no matter what, but the probability is much higher. Analogous to sailing and other sports you need a little luck, but one can help luck. For example, using artificial intelligence to extract what the wind and currents are like in the area of the races during the last 10 years may help to select the size of the foils. Large foils may be beneficial in low winds, but increase the resistance in the water, so may slow the boat down a little. Small foils have less resistance, and thus can go faster, but cannot lift the boat out of the water when winds are low, so are a little riskier. This targeted, highly professional approach, which also includes calculated risks, is still missing in tinnitus research. We need to consider to really collaborate in the same way Emirates Team New Zealand does.

How Then?

One example of how understanding sailing success can be applied to tinnitus research is neuromodulation as a treatment approach. The basic philosophy is that tinnitus is a phantom sound, characterized by loudness, location, tonality, thoughts, emotions, mood, stress, and other aspects, all integrated in one unified percept for the patient. All the characteristics are likely emergent properties of different, interacting, partially overlapping dynamic networks [19]. Furthermore, the brain communicates with neurotransmitters to the endocrine system and the immune system, and the immune system talks to the brain and endocrine system by cytokines, and the endocrine system communicates with the brain via hormones. But how these systems interact is also determined by one's genetic makeup. In other words, we must accept that trying to find a solution limited to the brain may be insufficient, just as Emirates Team New Zealand had to go beyond building a sailboat with only boatbuilders.

If that is the case, we not only need people specialized in recognizing and extracting patterns of brain activity such as artificial intelligence specialists. We also need geneticists, and people specialized in neuroinflammation, which may be crucially involved in the transition from acute to chronic tinnitus. We need endocrinologists (hormone specialists), as indeed some postmenopausal tinnitus can be improved by hormone replacement therapy, [20, 21] and testosterone has anti-inflammatory effects. [22]. What we can learn from Emirates Team New Zealand is to think further, be creative, have a bold vision, and act accordingly. We need to design innovative brain stimulators that can treat not only one area at the time, like we do now, but simultaneously modulate all the involved networks. And this is not impossible. The stimulators exist [23], but need to be adapted to target tinnitus networks. And we need specialists in advanced functional imaging, so that we can understand how these networks are modified by these novel neuromodulation techniques. These advanced techniques go beyond what we routinely analyze, and may need to incorporate entropy measures to look at information dynamic measures, to look at information transmission, to develop new measures, like aligning brain activity in time, etc.

What is needed is of course funding, not for 1 year, but for 4–10 years, and one single location, or even better two or three locations who compete to find a solution that can silence tinnitus, not only help people to learn and live with the sound. We need an America's Cup for tinnitus research. That requires funding of course, but also a "tinnitus tower", a single place where all these specialists collaborate, developing products that can be tested, fail, tested again,[2] based on specialist insight and artificial intelligence support.

And is all of this impossible? It is just as impossible as admitting it, just like the long-held notion that sailboats cannot go faster than the wind. It takes some craziness to be successful, but craziness is not enough. It requires organized, structured craziness. It requires a highly professional, extremely dedicated, hardworking team of complementary specialists to solve the tinnitus problem. But with the right funding, this Emirates Team New Zealand has shown that what seems impossible can be done.

So, every tinnitus patient should be happy Emirates Team New Zealand won the America's Cup, as it shows the path forward.

Just "imagine" that F1 sponsors, America's Cup sponsors set up a competition, to be held every 4 years, in which the most successful new treatments are tested and compared against each other. Then everyone wants to be a member of the Emirates Team New Zealand Tinnitus team, maybe not the wealthiest, but the most creative, innovative, daring, dedicated, well-organized team, and a low-key team, without arrogance, but all dedicated to win the ultimate trophy: silence tinnitus.

What we can add to Richard Branson's four keys to success (delegate work, take risks, build a good team, and do

[2]According to Samuel Beckett: "Ever failed. No matter. Try again. Fail again. Fail better".

projects you believe in), based on the TRI spirit is that crazy creativity and some Olympic competition could be highly beneficial as well. Does that mean the TRI outlines the only way forward, the only way to success? Of course not, we only outlined one possible way. Variability is the key to evolution, whether in Darwinian biology [24] or Kuhnian science [25], ultimately the fittest will survive. So, it is entirely possible that another strategy than the above proposed by the TRI may be successful in finding a cure, and ultimately whichever way tinnitus is silenced is good.

But, we as tinnitus researchers can learn from Emirates Team New Zealand, we can learn a lot about "winning", based on more than luck or randomness alone, and the same approach could be used for tinnitus, pain, or other pathologies. As long as we believe we can do it, it is possible, on the condition the we embrace the adage "In crazy we believe, in science we trust" [26].

References

1. Gigerenzer G. Simple heuristics to run a research group. Psych J. 2022;11:275.
2. Stanley D, Anderson J. Advice for running a successful research team. Nurse Res. 2015;23(2):36–40.
3. Nguyen E, Xu X, Robinson R. Lessons learned from an academic, interdisciplinary, multi-campus, research collaboration. Innov Pharm. 2020;11(2):13.
4. Kennedy P. Inventology: how we dream up things that change the world. New York: HMH Books; 2016.
5. Stanley TJ. The millionaire mind. Kansas City, MO: Andrews McMeel Publishing; 2000.
6. Maciuszek J, Kolemba M. Perception of risk and risk-taking among the lucky and the luckless. Pol Psychol Bull. 2013;44(3):232–44.
7. Pluchino A, Biondo AE, Rapisarda A. Talent versus luck: the role of randomness in success and failure. Adv Complex Syst. 2018;21(3–4):1850014.
8. Rzhetsky A, Foster JG, Foster IT, Evans JA. Choosing experiments to accelerate collective discovery. Proc Natl Acad Sci U S A. 2015;112(47):14569–74.
9. Chow JY, Davids K, Button C, Shuttleworth R, Renshaw I, Araujo D. Nonlinear pedagogy: a constraints-led framework for understanding emergence of game play and movement skills. Nonlinear Dynamics Psychol Life Sci. 2006;10(1):71–103.
10. Puga F, Stevens KR, Patel DI. Adopting best practices from team science in a healthcare improvement research network: the impact on dissemination and implementation. Nurs Res Pract. 2013;2013:814360.
11. Freeman WJ, Kozma R, Werbos PJ. Biocomplexity: adaptive behavior in complex stochastic dynamical systems. Biosystems. 2001;59(2):109–23.
12. Morowitz H, Singer J, editors. The mind, the brain, and complex adaptive systems. Boulder, CO: Westview Press; 1994.
13. De Ridder D, Maciaczyk J, Vanneste S. The future of neuromodulation: smart neuromodulation. Expert Rev Med Devices. 2021;18(4):307–17.
14. Buckley W. Society as a complex adaptive system. In: Buckley W, editor. Modern systems research for the behavioral scientist. Chicago, IL: Aldine Publishing Company; 1968.
15. Holland J. Complexity. Oxford: Oxford University Press; 2014.
16. Throwing the ball further: what tinnitus research can learn from Team New Zealand's winning of yachting's Americas Cup. Grant Donald Searchfield; Talk at the 11th TRI conference n Regensburg. 2018. https://2018.tri-conf.org/index.php/abstract-book.
17. Salazar Miranda A, Claudel M. Spatial proximity matters: a study on collaboration. PLoS One. 2021;16(12):e0259965.
18. Lee K, Brownstein JS, Mills RG, Kohane IS. Does collocation inform the impact of collaboration? PLoS One. 2010;5(12):e14279.
19. De Ridder D, Vanneste S, Weisz N, et al. An integrative model of auditory phantom perception: tinnitus as a unified percept of interacting separable subnetworks. Neurosci Biobehav Rev. 2014;44:16–32.
20. Chen HC, Chung CH, Chen VCF, Wang YC, Chien WC. Hormone replacement therapy decreases the risk of tinnitus in menopausal women: a nationwide study. Oncotarget. 2018;9(28):19807–16.
21. Lai JT, Liu CL, Liu TC. Hormone replacement therapy for chronic tinnitus in menopausal women: our experience with 13 cases. Clin Otolaryngol. 2017;42(6):1366–9.
22. Bianchi VE. The anti-inflammatory effects of testosterone. J Endocr Soc. 2019;3(1):91–107.
23. Ruffini G, Fox MD, Ripolles O, Miranda PC, Pascual-Leone A. Optimization of multifocal transcranial current stimulation for weighted cortical pattern targeting from realistic modeling of electric fields. NeuroImage. 2014;89:216–25.
24. Darwin C. The origin of species. Ware: Wordsworth; 1998.
25. Kuhn T. The structure of scientific revolutions. 3rd ed. London: University of Chicago Press; 1962.
26. Ridder DD. Why every tinnitus patient should be happy emirates team New Zealand won the America's cup? 2021.

Index

A
Aberrant internal carotid artery, 486, 487
Abnormal neural activity, 695
Acamprosate, 624
Acceptance and commitment therapy (ACT), 263
Acoustic coordinated Reset (CR®) neuromodulation, 579, 583
Acoustic neuroma, *see* Vestibular schwannoma
Acoustic reflex threshold (ART) testing, 358
Acoustic reflexes, 406
Acoustic shock, 30, 31
Acoustic startle reflex, 286
Acoustic stimulation, 657
Active sound avoidance paradigm (ASAP), 289, 290
Activity scheduling, 551
Acupuncture, 708
Acute otitis media (AOM), 388
Acute tinnitus, 619, 620
Adolescents, *see* Childhood tinnitus
Advanced functional imaging, 785
Affective network (AN), 254
Age-related hearing loss, 393
Allergy, 404
Alpha oscillations, 198
Alprazolam, 623
Alzheimer's disease, 303
American Academy of Otolaryngology—Head and Neck Surgery Foundation (AAO-HNSF), 775
American Counselling Association, 531
American Tinnitus Association, 781
America Online, 745
Amino acid metabolism, 708
Amplification, 755
Anterior cingulate cortex (ACC), 225, 226
Anterior inferior cereballar artery (AICA), 369, 428
Anticonvulsants, 619, 624
Antidepressants, 618, 620
Anti-inflammatory effects, 785
Anxiety, 84, 554
  diagnosis and classification, 522
  pathophysiological similarities between *tinnitus*, 522
  screening instruments for, 518
  treatment strategies, 523, 524
Application Programming Interface (API), 731
Arnold-Chiari malformation, 425
Aromatherapy, 711, 712, 753
Arteriosclerotic disease, 440, 441
Arteriovenous fistulas (AVF), 441, 442
Arteriovenous malformations (AVM), 488
Artificial intelligence, 783–785
Ascending pathway, 169–171
Attend, React, Explain, Adapt (AREA), 541, 542
Attentional deficits, 253
Attention-switching model, 254, 255
Audiological assessment
  ABR, 359
  ART testing, 358
  conditions, 353
  LDLs, 356
  OAEs, 358, 359
  otoscopy, 353
  patient history, 353, 355, 359
  psychoacoustic measurement
    clinical protocols, 356
    MML, 357
    residual inhibition, 357
    tinnitus loudness, 357
    tinnitus pitch matching, 356, 357
  PTA and HFA, 353–355
  research assessments, 354, 359
  speech audiometry, 356
  tympanometry, 357, 358
Audiology counselling, 532
Auditory brainstem response (ABR), 61–62, 117, 125, 177, 178, 359
Auditory cortex, 292, 597, 684, 701
  acute noise exposure, 212, 213
  chronic noise exposure, 213
  functional changes, 226–228
  lesion-induced plasticity, 223, 224
  phantom sensation, 223
  structural changes, 225, 226
Auditory hallucination, 20, 21
Auditory nerve fibers, 118
Auditory steady-state responses (ASSR), 177, 178
Auditory system, 234
  anatomy, 103–105
  ascending pathways, 105–108
  bimodal stimulation, 139
  botulinum toxin injection, 138
  clinical manifestations, 138
  cochlear nucleus, 137
  components, 101
  descending pathways, 108, 109
  ear, 102, 103
  electrical stimulation, 138, 139
  extralemniscal and lemniscal auditory pathways, 136, 137
  frequency selectivity, 109–111
  hidden hearing loss, 113
  McGurk illusion, 136
  phantom sensation-based disorders, 112
  physical therapy, 138
  VGLUTS, 137
Auditory treatments
  auditory stimulation, 576–578
  empirical evidence, 580–584
  mechanisms of, 578–580

W. Schlee et al. (eds.), *Textbook of Tinnitus*, https://doi.org/10.1007/978-3-031-35647-6

Auditory-evoked potentials (AEP), 177
  ABRs, 177, 178
  ASSRs, 178
Auditory-limbic dysregulation, 226–228
Auditory-somatosensory stimulation, 701
Autism spectrum disorder (ASD), 288, 289
Autobiographical memory network (AMN), 254, 262
Autoimmune inner ear disease (AIED), 392, 403, 404
Autoinflammatory diseases, 403
Automatic Pilot information processing, 569
Autonomic nervous system, 238, 239, 600
Autonomous tinnitus management
  amplification, 755
  apps for portable devices, 747
  books, 746
  comorbidities, 755
  dietary manipulation, 750–753
  ear wax removal, 754
  games and virtual reality, 755
  health literacy, 748
  hearing protection, 754
  hyperbaric oxygen therapy (HBOT), 755
  information sought, 742–744
  leaflets, 745, 746
  low-level laser therapy (LLLT), 755
  obesity and physical exercise, 753, 754
  online sources, 744, 745
  peer support, 748, 749
  press, television and radio, 747
  Qigong and Tai Chi, 754
  quality of tinnitus information, 747
  relaxation techniques, 750
  role of information, 742
  smoking, 753
  social media, 745
  sound therapies, 749
  sources of information, 745
  sources of tinnitus information, 744
  yoga, 754
Autopilot, 566
Autosomal dominant (AD), 405
Avoidance behaviours, 551
Axonal sprouting, 215

B
Barotrauma, 461
Bayesian brain model, 89
  active perception, 191
  adaptive compensation, 195, 196
  altered predictive process, 199, 200
  auditory information, 196
  belief updating, 193–195
  belief-free and belief-based behaviour, 197
  computational modelling, 200
  free energy, 191, 192
  functional changes, 198
  inference and learning, 191–193
  predictive coding implementation, 192
  prevalence, 195
  self-auditory world interaction, 195
  spontaneous activity, 195, 196
  stress and habituation, 196, 197
  without deafferentation, 199
Behavioural experiments, 551
Behavioural interventions, 549
Benign intracranial hypertension (BIH), 489
Benzodiazepines, 623
Bias, 766
Bilateral Ménière's disease (BMD), 405
Bimodal auditory-somatosensory stimulation, 697, 698
Bimodal stimulation, 773
  bimodal auditory-somatosensory stimulation, 697, 698
  map plasticity changes, 694–697
  mechanism of action, 699–701
  outcomes, 701
  pairing and habituation, 701
  rTMS, 674
  tongue stimulation, 698, 699
  transcranial magnetic stimulation (TMS), 672–674
Blood oxygenation level dependent (BOLD) signals, 168, 659
Botox, 773
Botulinum toxin
  aspect of treatment, 649, 650
  general considerations, 649
  mechanism of action, 645
Botulinum toxin type A injections, 451
Brainstem telangiectasias, 443
British Tinnitus Association, 719, 720, 743, 744, 748, 781

C
Ca^{2+}-binding protein calmodulin (CaM), 118
Caffeine, 752
Calcitonin gene related peptide (CGRP), 649
Caloric tests, 406
Cannabidiol oils (CBD), 753
Cannabinoids, 753
Carotid artery aneurysm, 486
Carotid artery dissection, 486
Carotid dissection (CD), 459
Carotid stenosis, 485, 486
Carotid-cavernous fistula (CCF), 369, 370, 459
Central auditory amplifier, 292
Central auditory system
  amygdala, 129
  auditory cortex, 128, 129
  cingulate cortex, 130
  DCN
    gain, 125
    homeostatic intrinsic plasticity, 125, 126
    homeostatic synaptic plasticity, 126, 127
    overview, 125
  definition, 123
  hippocampus, 129, 130
  inferior colliculus, 127
  nonauditory nuclei, 129
  thalamus, 127, 128
Central gain
  after noise trauma, 208, 209
    auditory cortex, 212, 213
    DCN, 210
    inferior colliculus, 211, 212
    MGB, 212
    VCN, 210, 211
  mechanisms, 215, 216
  sensory deprivation
    axonal sprouting, 215
    excitatory neurotransmission, 214, 215
    GABAergic inhibition, 213, 214
    KCC2 cotransporters, 214
    STDP, 215

Central nucleus of the inferior colliculus (CNIC), 211
Cerebellopontine angle (CPA), 428
Cerebrovascular diseases
    central nervous system, 440
    neuroradiological imaging, 440
    objective tinnitus, 439
    pulsatile tinnitus
        aberrant ICA, 441
        aneurysms, 442, 443
        arterial dissection, 441
        arteriosclerotic disease, 440, 441
        AVF, 441, 442
        brainstem telangiectasias, 443
        causes of, 440
        condylar vein abnormalities, 444
        definition, 439, 440
        fibromuscular dysplasia, 441
        glomus jugulare tumors, 443, 444
        HJB, 443, 444
        internal auditory canal vascular loops, 442, 443
        morphologic abnormalities, 441
        pathophysiologic mechanisms, 440
        persistent trigeminal artery, 442
        proatlantal intersegmental artery, 443
        sigmoid/jugular diverticulum, 444
        sinus thrombosis, 444
        subclavian steal syndrome, 442
        turbulent blood flow, 440
        vascular imaging techniques, 440
        venous angioma of posterior fossa, 444
        vertebrobasilar and carotid dolichoectasia, 442
    subjective tinnitus, 439, 444
Cervical and masticatory somatosensory system
    bimodal stimulation treatment, 451
    cervical collar, 451
    deep neck flexor muscles, 453, 454
    definition, 448
    etiology, 451, 452
    injections, 451
    multidisciplinary treatment, 452
    musculoskeletal treatment, 448–450
    shoulder stabilizing muscles, 454
    TRT, 451
Cervical epidural steroid injection, 451
Cervical spine, 647, 648
C-fiber nociceptor, 649
Child Friendly Tinnitus Model, 478, 479
Childhood tinnitus
    clinical characteristics, 475, 476
    definitions, 467–468
    diagnostics and pathology, 476, 477
    epidemiology, 467
    interviewing, 477
    prevalence, 471–472
    risk factors
        age, 472, 473
        cochlear implants, 473
        co-morbidity, 475
        gender, 473
        hyperacusis, 473
        noise exposure, 474
        ototoxicity, 473, 474
        severity, 475
    study design and populations, 468–470
    treatment
        assessment, 477, 478
        Child Friendly Tinnitus Model, 478, 479
        intervention techniques, 478
        narrative therapy, 478
        outcomes, 480
        reflections and perceptions, 480
        significant improvement, 480
Chronic migraine, 650
Chronic otitis media, 388
Chronic tinnitus, 621–623
Citizen science, 718, 719
Classical conditioning, 240–242, 255, 256
Client Orientated Scale of Improvement in Tinnitus, 533
Clinical otorhinolaryngological assessment
    auscultation, 348
    endoscopy, 348
    ENT, 346, 347
    otoscopy, 347, 348
    supplementary radiological diagnosis, 348
Clinical Outcomes in Routine Evaluation (CORE), 565
Clinically significant tinnitus, 597
Cluster analysis, 707
Cochlea, 124, 125
Cochlear dysfunction, 19
Cochlear implantation, 473, 578, 579, 581, 582
Cochlear nuclei (CN), 137, 213, 292, 701
Cochlear synaptopathy, 124, 125, 178
Cochleovestibular compression syndrome (CVCS), 427
    characteristic features, 427
    classification, 427
    controversy, 428
    diagnostic criteria, 427
    functional anatomy, 428
    meta-analysis, 426
    pathophysiological model, 428–431
    trigeminal neuralgia, 428, 429
Cochrane meta-analyses, 772, 773
Cochrane Risk of Bias 2 tool, 554
Cochrane systematic review, 710, 755
Cognitive ability, 169
Cognitive behaviour therapy (CBT), 28, 508, 509, 521, 618, 619, 772, 776
    activity scheduling, 551
    behavioural activation, 551
    behavioural experiments, 551
    benefits, 558
    cognitive restructuring/reframing, 550
    distress and disability, 546
    exposure therapy, 550
    fear avoidance model, 257, 258, 548, 549
    guided discovery, 550
    habituation model, 256, 257, 546, 548
    history, 255, 256
    journaling and records, 551
    management and meta-analyses, 258
    neurophysiological model, 548
    relaxation and stress reduction techniques, 552
    role-play, 552
    selective attention, 257
    successive approximation, 552
    sympathetic autonomic arousal, 257
    systematic reviews of, 552, 554
    treatment acceptability, 557
Cognitive bias, 767
Cognitive control network (CCN), 254
Cognitive distortions, 549
Cognitive enhancers, 619

Cognitive functioning, 177, 253, 254
Cognitive interventions, 549
Cognitive strategies, 661
Combination hearing aids, 579
COMET approach, 723
COMiT International Delphi study, 725
Co-morbid temporomandibular joint disorders, 646
Complementary alternative medicines (CAM), 706
Compound action potential (CAP), 290
CompuServe, 745
Conditioned response, 255
Conductive hearing loss
  definition, 387
  effect of, 387
  external auditory canal, 387, 388
  middle ear
    AOM, 388
    chronic otitis media, 388
    ETD, 388
    otosclerosis, 389, 390
    stapes surgery, 390, 391
    traumatic lesions, 391
    tumors of, 391
    tympanoplasty, 389
Confidence interval (CI), 61
Congenital rubella/cytomegalovirus infections, 392
Connectome model, 294, 295
Conscious learning, 661
Consciousness, 20
Core hub of the salience network, 29
Core Outcome Measures in Tinnitus (COMiT) initiative, 722
Correlations, 168
Cortex stimulation, 683
Cotton buds, 754
Counselling
  assess patients' counselling needs, 536
  auditory rehabilitation counselling, 532, 533
  counselling content, 535
  counselling styles, 532
  goal setting, 536
  health literacy, 536
  individual experience, 531, 532
  motivation interviewing, 533, 534
  personal adjustment counselling, 533
  role of digital health, 534
  solution focused counselling, 534
Counselling and psychoeducation
  goal setting, 536
  health literacy, 537
  individual experience, 531
COVID-19 infections, 304
COVID-19 pandemic, 744
Critical-period (CP) plasticity, 157
Cross-frequency coupling, 179
Cross-modal plasticity, 153
Cumulative Index to Nursing and Allied Health Literature (CINAHL), 710

D
Daily supplements, 707
Decreased sound tolerance (DST), 235, 594, 595, 602, 603
Deep brain stimulation (DBS), 687
Default mode network, 254
Dehiscent jugular bulb, 372
Delta/theta oscillations, 198
Delusion, 21
Depressed mood, 520
Depression, 84, 179, 554, 673
  diagnosis of, 519
  pathophysiological similarities of, 520
  treatment options for, 521
Descending pathway, 169–171
Diary of Thoughts and Feelings (DTF), 551
Dietary manipulation, 750–753
Dietary supplements, 707, 709, 751
Diffusor Tensor Imaging (DTI), 168
Digital Subtraction Angiography (DSA), 366
Discordant Dysfunction Theory, 243, 602
Distortion product OAE (DPOAE), 358
Distortion product otoacoustic emission (DPOAE), 19, 102, 117
Distress, 179
Diversity and inclusion, 727
Dominant sigmoid sinus with/without dehiscence (DSSD), 490–492
Dopaminergic pathways, 624
Dorsal cochlear nucleus (DCN), 520, 619
  acute noise exposure, 210
  chronic noise exposure, 210
  compensation, 125
  gain, 125
  homeostatic intrinsic plasticity, 125, 126
  homeostatic synaptic plasticity, 126, 127
  overview, 125
Dorsal cortex of the IC (DC), 105
Down's syndrome, 392
DSM-V criteria of major depression, 520
Dural arteriovenous fistulas (DAVF), 442
Dural transverse/sigmoid sinus fistulae, 370, 371
Dysconnectivity disorder, 136

E
Ear, Nose and Throat (ENT), 346, 347
Ecological momentary assessment (EMA), 733
Edge-betweenness centrality, 171
Education, 727
Effectiveness studies, 556
EGb-761 treatment, 304, 305
Electrical stimulation, 701
Electroencephalography (EEG)
  ABRs, 177, 178
  ASSRs, 177, 178
  auditory pathways, 177
  bottom-up and top-down systems, 182
  early cortical electrophysiology, 178
  noise-cancellation/sensory gating model, 182
  predictive coding model, 182
  resting state activity, 179, 180
  signal presentation, 177
  sound stimulation, 177
  subnetworks, 180, 181
  thalamocortical dysrhythmia model, 181
EMBASE, 710
Emirates Team New Zealand, 784–786
Emissary veins function, 372
Emotional strain, 708
Empathy, 533
Endolymphatic hydrops (EH), 373, 401, 402
Endolymphatic sac, 403

ENT Trials Register, 710
Environmental risk
air pollution, 61, 62
chemical exposure, 62, 63
definition, 61, 64
evidence level, 61
noise pollution, 63–65
preventive strategies, 67, 68
radiation exposure, 64–66
urban planning, 66, 67
Epidemiology
heterogeneity, 37
prevalence
any tinnitus (AT), 37–41
severe tinnitus (ST), 38, 42–44
PRISMA guidelines, 37
Etiologic heterogeneity, 73
EU funded COST Action TINNET, 775
European guidelines, 743, 744, 775
European Medicines Agency (EMA) approved drug, 619
Eustachian tube dysfunction (ETD), 388
Eustachian tube function, 347
Evidence for therapeutic studies, 766
Evidence-based medicine, 764, 776
Evolution theory, 12
Exome-based Extreme phenotype (EP) study, 54
Exploding Head Syndrome (EHS), 30
Exposure therapy, 548, 550
External auditory canal, 387, 388
External carotid artery (ECA), 370
External nucleus (ICX), 105
Extra oral approach, 648
Extracranial arteriovenous fistulae, 369
Extradural auditory cortex implant, 685

F
Facial nerve schwannoma, 391
Familial Ménière's disease (FMD), 405, 406
Familial transmission, 52
Fear avoidance model, 548, 549
Fear of Tinnitus Questionnaire (FTQ), 341
Fibromuscular dysplasia (FMD), 366, 367, 441
Fibromyalgia, 147
Flavonoids, 752
Food and Drug Administration (FDA), 619
Fragile X animal model of autism, 288, 289
Fragile X syndrome (FX), 288
Free energy, 191, 192
Functional audiogenic seizure, 31, 32
Functional connectivity, 179
Functional neurological disorders (FND), 31, 32
Functional resonance magnetic imaging (fMRI)
ascending and descending pathway, 169–171
attention system changes, 169
BOLD signals, 168
graph connectivity, 169
independent component analysis, 169
limbic system changes, 169
network-based models, 171
graph theory, 171, 172
triple network model, 172
neural activity, 168
operational interactions, 168
seeding, 168

G
GABAergic drug, 304
Gamma amino butyric type A ($GABA_A$) receptors, 623
Gamma knife surgery, 419
Gamma oscillations, 198
Gap startle reflex model, 129
Gaussian distribution, 782
General diet, 750, 751
Genetic hearing loss, 391, 392
Genetics, 52
adoptees-based studies, 52
candidate gene approaches, 53
characteristics, 51, 52
environmental factors, 52, 53
exome-based extreme phenotype study, 54
familial aggregation, 53
GWAS, 54, 55
homogenous phenotype value, 54
limitations, 56
risk factors, 52, 53
technology improvements, 53
twin studies, 52
variants, 55, 56
Genome-wide association study (GWAS), 54, 55
German guideline, 774
Ginkgo biloba (Chinese Maidenhair), 304, 709, 751
GJB2 gene, 392
Glomus jugulare tumors, 443, 444
Glomus tumors, 391
Glucose metabolism, 708
Glutamate receptor, 118
Glutamate receptor antagonists, 624
Glutamic acid decarboxylase (GAD), 127
Glutathione metabolism, 708
Glycinergic receptor (GlyR), 126
Good counselling, 532
Google's Play Store, 731
GRADE certainty ratings, 766
GRADE-system, 766
Grading of Recommendations Assessment, Development and Evaluation, 554
Graph connectivity, 169
Graph theory, 171, 172, 180, 181

H
Habituation model, 196, 197, 237, 546, 548
Hallucination, definition, 20
Hamilton Rating Scale for Anxiety (HAM-A), 710
Hazards ratio (HR), 61
Head trauma, 391
Health literacy, 748
Health on the Net Foundation (HON), 747
Hearing aids, 579, 580
Hearing impairment, 619, 625
Hearing loss, 597
adaptive compensation, 195, 196
axonal sprouting, 215
conductive hearing loss (*see* Conductive hearing loss)
cortical changes, 213
development, 386
EEG and MEG activity, 179, 180
fMRI, 179
gray and white matter changes, 167
sensorineural hearing loss (*see* Sensorineural hearing loss)

Hearing protection, 754
Hebbian plasticity, 126, 152
Hebbian theory, 239
Herpes simplex virus (HSV), 428
Herpes zoster oticus, 392
Heschl's gyrus (HG), 168
Hidden hearing loss, 19, 113, 125, 178
High frequency audiometry (HFA), 19, 353–356
High jugular bulbs (HJB), 372, 443, 444
Homeopathy, 711
Homogeneous trials, 765
Hormone replacement therapy, 785
Hospital Anxiety and Depression scale (HADS), 305
Human bimodal stimulation clinical studies, 697
Human cytokine synthesis inhibitory factor, 271
Hyperacusis, 216, 243, 244, 522, 594, 625
  acoustic startle reflex, 286
  animal behavioral models, 285, 286
  ASAP, 289, 290
  auditory and pain pathways, 290
  in children, 510
  comorbidities, 27, 285
  definition, 27, 503
  fragile X animal model of autism, 288, 289
  framework, 27
  gain adaptations, 27
  homeostatic model, 27
  human and animal neuroscience studies, 505, 506
  impact/burden, 506, 507
  incidence, 503
  literature review, 503–505
  loudness recruitment, 286–288
  measurement
    audiology-based/psychoacoustic measurement, 507, 508
    questionnaires, 508
  migraine therapy, 27
  prevalence, 27, 285
  recruitment, 28
  residual excitation, 503
  risk factor, 28
  salicylate
    cochlear nuclei, 292
    cochlear output, 290, 291
    high-dose salicylate, 290
    inferior colliculus, medial geniculate body and auditory cortex, 292
    otoacoustic emissions, 290
    reticular formation and cerebellum, 293
    role of stress, 293, 294
    striatum, hippocampus and reticular formation, 292, 293
    suprathreshold amygdala response, 292
    tinnitus-hyperacusis connectome, 294, 295
  somatic manipulation, 503
  tissue-damaging noise, 28
  treatment, 28
    CBT, 508, 509
    multi-modal migraine prophylaxis therapy, 509
    serotonergic medication, 510
    TRT, 509
  ULL, 285
Hyperacusis Questionnaire (HQ), 508
Hyperbaric oxygen chambers, 755
Hyperbaric oxygen therapy (HBOT), 755
Hyperpolarization-activated cationic nucleotide-gated current (H-current), 130
Hypersensitivity to sound, 510

I

ICD 10 criteria, 520
Idiopathic sudden sensorineural hearing loss (ISSHL), 755
Idiopathic tinnitus, 19
Immunogenic labyrinthitis, 392, 393
Independent component analysis, 169
Indirectness, 767
Inferior colliculus (IC), 127, 292, 619, 701
  acute noise exposure, 211
  chronic noise exposure, 211, 212
Influenza, 304
Inner hair cells (IHCs), 117
Internal auditory canal vascular loops, 443
Internal auditory meatus (IAM), 428
Internal carotid artery (ICA) stenosis
  aberrant ICA, 368
  AICA, 369
  aneurysms, 368
  carotid bifurcation, 366
  dissection, 367, 368
  FMD, 366, 367
  persistent stapedial artery, 369
  pseudoaneurysm, 368
International collaborations, 784
Interpeak latency (IPL), 430
Interpretative phenomenological analysis (IPA), 570
Intracranial dural arteriovenous fistula (dAVF), 487, 488
Intracranial hypertension (ICP), 372
Intradural auditory cortex implant, 686
Intradural intracortical implant, 686
Intralabyrinthine schwannomas (ILS), 415
Invasive auditory cortex stimulation, 684, 685, 687
Invasive brain stimulation, 773
  neuromodulation, 683
  pathophysiology of, 681
  symptom generation in the brain, 682
Iowa Tinnitus Handicap Questionnaire, 339
Ischemic stroke, 701

J

James Lind Alliance (JLA), 720, 721
Jugular bulb diverticulum, 372
Jugular vein dominance, 372

K

Kekule, August, 782
Kinesiotape application, 450

L

Labyrinthine concussion, 460
Lamotrigine, 624
L-baclofen, 304
Lenire® System, 699
Lesion-induced plasticity, 223, 224
Levator scapulae, 646
Lidocaine, 646, 647
Limbic system, 225, 226, 238
Local anaesthesics, 649
Local field potential (LFP), 128, 211
Long-term depression (LTD), 126, 127, 215, 673
Long-term potentiation (LTP), 126, 215, 673
LORETA methods, 657
Loudness, 285

Loudness discomfort level (LDL), 356, 595
Loudness intolerance, 288, 289
Loudness recruitment, 286, 287
Low-level laser therapy (LLLT), 755

M
Magnesium, 707, 752
Magnesium supplementation, 710
Magnetic resonance spectroscopy (MRS), 170
Magnetoencephalography (MEG), 583, 686, 697
  ABRs, 177, 178
  ASSRs, 177, 178
  auditory pathways, 177
  bottom-up and top-down systems, 182
  early cortical electrophysiology, 178
  noise-cancellation/sensory gating model, 182
  predictive coding model, 182
  resting state activity, 179, 180
  signal presentation, 177
  sound stimulation, 177
  subnetworks, 180, 181
  thalamocortical dysrhythmia model, 181
Maladaptive coping, 179
Maladaptive plasticity
  hypothesis, 159, 160
  network connectivity, 158, 159
  phantom pain, 160
  structural changes, 158
  tonotopic map changes, 157, 158
Manual therapy, 646
Mastoid emissary vein, 372
McKenna's approach, 548
Medial geniculate body, 292
Medial geniculate body (MGB), 127, 128, 212
Medial prefrontal cortex (mPFC), 225, 226
Medial system, 136
Melatonin, 711, 752
Meniere's disease (MD), 373, 427
  allergy, 404
  audiovestibular examination, 406, 407
  clinical variants
    audio-vestibular symptoms, 405
    BMD, 405
    cluster analysis, 405
    FMD, 405, 406
    UMD, 405
  definition, 401
  diagnosis, 406
  endolymphatic hydrops, 401, 402
  epidemiology, 401
  genetic factors and immune response, 401
  history, 401
  immune response, 403, 404
  magnetic resonance imaging, 407
  migraine, 404
  respiratory and food allergies, 401
  sensory lesions, 402, 403
  symptoms, 401
  tinnitus, 407, 408
  treatment, 408, 409
  vestibular fibrosis, 402
mHealth, 731
Microbiome, 91
Microvascular contacts/compressions (MVC)
  characteristic signs and symptoms, 426
  clinical tinnitus features and electrophysiology, 434
  CVCS, 427
    characteristic features, 427
    classification, 427
    controversy, 428
    diagnostic criteria, 427
    functional anatomy, 428
    meta-analysis, 426
    pathophysiological model, 429–431
    pathophysiology, 428
    trigeminal neuralgia, 428, 429
  definition, 425
  hearing loss
    cochlea-vestibular nerve, 432
    IPL I-III prolongation, 432
    signal transmission, 432
    surgical complications, 433
    treatment, 432
    vascular decompression surgery, 432, 433
  history, 425
  primary and secondary, 425, 426
Migraine, 404
Mindfulness, 772
  evidence for, 564
  in health care and tinnitus management, 564
  impact on tinnitus distress, 564, 565
  loudness, impact of, 566
  non-judgemental attention, 569, 570
  operational definition of, 566
  paying attention, 566–568
  present moment attention, 568, 569
  psychological distress, 565
  risks, 570
Mindfulness based cognitive therapy (MBCT), 549, 564, 570
Mindfulness based stress reduction (MBSR), 564
Mindfulness meditation, 707
MINI International Neuropsychiatric Interview, 518, 519
Minimal clinically important difference (MCID), 333
Minimum masking levels (MML), 357
Mismatch negativity (MMN), 178, 193, 194
Misophonia, 28, 29, 243–245, 594
  complex conditioned stimuli, 607, 608
  protocols for treatment, 608
Mobile Health Apps
  antecedent benefits of, 732
  categories of, 732
  ecological momentary assessment (EMA), 733
  effectiveness of, 735, 736
  hearing Protection, testing, and enhancement, 732, 733
  tinnitus treatment and management, 732
Modified music, 579
Motivation interviewing, 533, 534
MRI-neuronavigation, 674
Muscarinic antagonists, 696
Muscle contraction, 646
Musical hallucinosis, 20, 21
Myofascial trigger point deactivation, 450

N
National Health and Nutrition Examination Survey (NHANES), 750
National Institute for Health and Care Excellence (NICE) guideline, 578
National Institute for Health Research (NIHR) Nottingham Hearing Biomedical Research Unit, 721
National Library of Medicine Medical Subject Headings (MeSH), 741

Natural language processing techniques, 707
Naturecare™, 582
Negative cognitions, 569
Neoplastic disorders, 387
Nerve impulses, 635
Network efficiency, 171
Network resilience, 171
Network-based models
  graph theory, 171, 172
  triple network model, 172
Neural activity, 168, 177
Neural lesions, 403
Neural synchrony, 128
Neural therapy, 645, 773
  clinical importance, 646, 647
  treatment aspects
    cervical spine, 647, 648
    otic ganglion, trigeminal structures and muscles, 648, 649
Neurobiofeedback, 618, 773
Neuroinflammation, 90, 785
  diffusible proinflammatory cytokines, 273, 274
  in animal models, 272, 273
  noise trauma, 271, 272
  noise-induced excitation-inhibition imbalance, 275, 276
  overview, 271
  PV neuron loss, 276, 277
  strain differences, 274, 275
Neuromodulation, 619, 682, 683
Neuromodulators, 170, 171, 619
Neuromodulatory approaches, 662
Neuromonics© treatment, 577
Neuronal excitability, 619
Neuropathic pain, 673
Neurophysiological model, 548
  automatic gain control mechanism, 243
  autonomic nervous system, 238, 239
  brain system, 237, 238
  conditioned reflexes
    principles, 240–242
    role of, 240
  conscious and subconscious function, 236, 237
  decreased neural signal, 242
  discordant dysfunction theory, 243
  habituation, 237
  hyperacusis, 243, 244
  limbic system, 238
  mechanisms, 234–236
  misophonia, 243, 244
  neuronal activity measurements, 243
  pattern recognition, 236
  reverberation, 243
  signal generation, 234
  stimulus, 237
  tensor tympani syndrome, 245
  treatment, 245–247
  two loops, 239, 240
Neuroplasticity
  critical-period plasticity, 157
  developmental plasticity
    cross-modal plasticity, 153
    structural and connectivity changes, 152, 153
  Hebbian plasticity, 152
  homeostatic plasticity, 152
  maladaptive plasticity
    hypothesis, 159, 160
    network connectivity, 158, 159
    phantom pain, 160
    structural changes, 158
    tonotopic map changes, 157, 158
  noise exposure
    assumed safe noise exposure, 155–157
    central, subcortical effects, 154, 155
    peripheral effects, 154
    primary auditory cortex, 155
    traumatic noise, 153, 154
  tonotopic map plasticity
    long-term, 150, 151
    short-term, 150, 151
Neuropsychological model
  attention-switching model, 254, 255
  cognitive behaviour therapy
    fear-avoidance model, 257, 258
    habituation, 256, 257
    history, 255, 256
    management and meta-analyses, 258
    selective attention, 257
    sympathetic autonomic arousal, 257
  cognitive functioning, 253, 254
  development, 261
  frustration-fulfilment hypothesis, 263
  goal-directed behaviour, 262
  mood disorders, 261
  non-auditory factors, 262
  patients' commitment, 261
  primary and secondary care settings, 261
  psychological profiles, 254, 255
  self-focused thinking, 262
  self-perpetuating mechanisms, 262
  suffering in psychology, 263
  tinnitus percept, 262, 263
  tolerance model
    features, 258
    fluctuations of intrusiveness, 258
    helpful attitudes and resources, 258
    need for consideration, 258, 259
    need for self-preservation, 259, 260
    relief through goals, 260
    searching for new self, 260, 261
    sense of identity, 258
    stages, 258
Neuroticism, 27
NICE guidelines, 774, 775
NIHR Research for Patient Benefit scheme, 726
N-methyl-d-aspartic acid (NMDA) receptor pathway, 708
Noise cancellation system, 170, 182, 227
Noise exposure, 474
  assumed safe noise exposure, 155–157
  central, subcortical effects, 154, 155
  peripheral effects, 154
  primary auditory cortex, 155
  traumatic noise, 153, 154
Noise trauma, 208, 209, 461
  auditory cortex, 212, 213
  DCN, 210
  inferior colliculus, 211, 212
  MGB, 212
  VCN, 210, 211
Noise-cancellation/sensory gating model, 182
Noise-induced hearing loss (NIHL)
  measurement, 117, 118
  molecular changes, 119, 120
  OHCs, 118

permanent auditory threshold elevation, 118
stereocilia damage, 118
synapse damage, 118, 119
Noise-related hearing loss, 394
Noise-related trauma, 458
Non-Hebbian plasticity, 126, 127
Non-invasive brain stimulation, 683, 773
transcranial alternating current stimulation (tACS), 670, 671
transcranial random noise stimulation (tRNS), 671
transcutaneous electrical nerve stimulation (TENS), 671
transcutaneous vagus nerve stimulation (tVNS), 671, 672
Non-pulsatile tinnitus, 124, 318, 319, 373, 458
trauma-associated tinnitus
barotrauma, 461
labyrinthine concussion, 460
noise trauma, 461
OChD, 460
perilymphatic fistula, 460
temporal bone fracture, 460
Norepinephrine agonists, 696
Nortriptyline, 623
Nucleus accumbens (NAc), 226–228
Nucleus basalis, 699

O
Obsessive-compulsive disorder (OCD), 29, 516
Obsessive-compulsive personality disorder, 29
Occupational risk
air pollution, 61, 62
chemical exposure, 62, 63
definition, 61, 64
evidence level, 61
multivariate analyses, 64
noise pollution, 63–65
preventive strategies, 67, 68
radiation exposure, 64–66
self-reported tinnitus, 64
stress triggers, 64
Odds ratio (OR), 61
Olympic Creed, 782
OnabotulinumtoxinA (OBTA), 649
Online peer support, 745
Online resources, 744
Online tinnitus chatrooms and forums, 749
Online tinnitus support groups, 753
Operant conditioning, 255, 256, 546
Oral antiarrhythmic drugs, 619
Organic hallucinosis, 20
Oriental medicine, 706
Ossicular chain disruption (OChD), 460
Otic ganglion, 648, 649
Otoacoustic emissions, 102, 290, 406
Otoacoustic emissions (OAE), 358, 359
Otoprotectants, 620
Otosclerosis, 389, 390
Otoscopy, 353
Outer hair cells (OHC), 117, 118, 358, 359
Oxygen therapy, 619

P
Paget's disease, 489
Pain, 138
auditory pathway, 87, 88
C fibers, 86
definition, 84, 85
DSM-5, 85, 86
imbalance
Bayesian brain model, 89
pain input, 88
pain suppression, 88
reward/dysreward system, 89
ipsilateral pathways, 86
lateral pain pathway, 86
mechanism, 84, 85
medial pathway, 86
microbiome, 91
neuroinflammation, 90
pain inhibitory pathway, 86, 87
pathophysiology, 92, 93
PNS, 91
prevalence, 83
risk factors, 84
SNS, 90
treatment, 91
VAS painfulness, 87
Paradoxical lesion, 196
Paragangliomas, 371, 372
Parasympathetic nervous system (PNS), 91
Patient centered multimodal musculoskeletal approach, 450
Patient Centred Outcomes Research Institute (PCORI), 723
Peer support, 748, 749
People and Patient Participation, Involvement and Engagement (PoPPIE), 723
Perception in contrast, 20
Perceptual heterogeneity, 73
Performance intensity (PI) function, 356
Perilymph fistulae, 391
Perilymphatic fistula, 460
Peripheral auditory system, anatomy and physiology, 124, 125
Persistent stapedial artery, 369, 487
Persistent trigeminal artery, 442
Personal adjustment counselling, 533
Phantom auditory perception, 234
Phantom pain, 160
Phantom sensation, 223
Pharmaceutical treatment effects, 621–623
Pharmacotherapy, 618
Phonophobia, 29, 30
Portable devices, 749
Positive allosteric modulators (PAMs), 620
Posterior cingulate cortex (PCC), 658
Posterior semicircular canal dehiscence (PCCD), 373
Post-traumatic stress disorder (PTSD), 29, 516, 521
Prediction error, 182, 191, 192
Predictive coding model, 182
Preferred Reporting Items for Systematic review and Meta-Analyses (PRISMA) guidelines, 37
Prelingual hearing impairment, 392
Proatlantal intersegmental artery, 443
Procaine, 646
Progressive tinnitus management (PTM), 556, 741
Proinflammatory cytokines, 273, 274
Pseudoaneurysm, 368
Pseudomonas aeruginosa infection, 347
Pseudo-pulsatile, 365
Psychiatric co-morbidity
non-psychiatric setting, 517, 518
suicidal patient, 518, 519
Psychiatric treatment, 517

Psychoacoustic measurement of tinnitus
clinical protocols, 356
loudness, 357
MML, 357
pitch matching, 356, 357
residual inhibition, 357
Psychoeducation
and disturbed sleep, 540
interdisciplinary referrals, 541
maintenance and re-emergent tinnitus, 540, 541
psychosocial factors and tinnitus, 537, 538
role of attention-focusing, 539
role of stress, 538, 539
self-efficacy, 540
sound enrichment, 540
thoughts and emotions, 540
Psychological distress, 29
Psychological models, 547
Psychosis, 516
Public and patient involvement
citizen science, 718, 719
British Tinnitus Association, 719, 720
clinical fields, 723
James Lind Alliance (JLA), 720, 721
limitations and challenges, 724, 725
and practice standards, 726, 727
Tinnitus Hub, 721, 722
Publication bias, 767
PubMed, 710, 781
Pulsatile tinnitus (PT), 124, 318, 365, 370, 372, 485
arterial causes
aberrant internal carotid artery, 486, 487
carotid artery aneurysm, 486
carotid artery dissection, 486
carotid stenosis, 485, 486
hyperdynamic state, 487
intrameatal vascular loop, 487
persistent stapedial artery, 487
arteriovenous transition causes
AVM, 488
direct arteriovenous fistula, 488
dural arteriovenous fistula, 487, 488
glomus tympanicum/jugulare, 488, 489
Paget's disease, 489
cerebrovascular diseases
aberrant ICA, 441
aneurysms, 442, 443
arterial dissection, 441
arteriosclerotic disease, 440, 441
AVF, 441, 442
brainstem telangiectasias, 443
causes of, 440
condylar vein abnormalities, 444
definition, 439, 440
fibromuscular dysplasia, 441
glomus jugulare tumors, 443, 444
HJB, 443, 444
internal auditory canal vascular loops, 442, 443
morphologic abnormalities, 441
pathophysiologic mechanisms, 440
persistent trigeminal artery, 442
proatlantal intersegmental artery, 443
sigmoid/jugular diverticulum, 444
sinus thrombosis, 444
subclavian steal syndrome, 442
turbulent blood flow, 440
vascular imaging techniques, 440
venous angioma of posterior fossa, 444
vertebrobasilar and carotid dolichoectasia, 442
physical examination and audiologic evaluation, 493–495
pseudo-pulsatile tinnitus, 492, 493
psychoacoustic characteristics, 493, 494
radiological evaluations, 495
SCDS, 492
trauma-associated tinnitus, 459
venous causes, 489
Arnold-Chiari malformation, 491
BIH, 489
DSSD, 490–492
high jugular bulb, 489, 490
sigmoid sinus diverticulum, 490, 491
Pure tone audiometry, 406
Puretone audiometry (PTA), 353–356
PV neuron loss, 276, 277

Q

Quality of life, 517, 736
Questionnaire data, 548

R

Ramsey Hunt syndrome, 392
Randomized controlled trials (RCTs), 564, 766, 776
Randomized controlled trials tinnitus, 765
Reaction time-intensity function, 286–288
Recruitment, 28
Regular tDCS, 668, 670
Relative risk (RR), 61
Relaxation techniques, 750
Repetititive transcranial magnetic stimulation (rTMS), 773
Research experiment, 781
Residual inhibition (RI), 74, 357
Resting-state fMRI, 168, 169, 171
Rhythmic transcranial magnetic stimulation (rTMS), 657
Ribbon synapses, 117
RNA-sequencing (RNA-seq), 119
Rogerian principles, 533
Role-play, 552
Rostral to dorsal anterior cingulate (rdACC), 170

S

Salicylate
cochlear nuclei, 292
cochlear output, 290, 291
inferior colliculus, medial geniculate body and auditory cortex, 292
otoacoustic emissions, 290
reticular formation and cerebellum, 293
role of stress, 293, 294
striatum, hippocampus and reticular formation, 292, 293
suprathreshold amygdala response, 292
tinnitus-hyperacusis connectome, 294, 295
Salience network (SN), 254
Schwartze's sign, 347
Scientific Committee on Emerging and Newly Identified Hazards and Risk (SCENIHR), 63
Secondary outcomes, 556
Secularization, 10

Seeding, 168
Selective serotonin reuptake inhibitors (SSRI), 623
Self-efficacy, 533, 540
Self-help groups, 259
Self-help interventions, 774
Semicircular canal dehiscence syndrome (SCDS), 492
Sensorineural hearing loss
  age-related hearing loss, 393
  causes of, 391
  definition, 387
  genetic origin, 391, 392
  immunogenic labyrinthitis, 392, 393
  infections, 392
  noise-related hearing loss, 394
  ototoxicity, 393, 394
  SSNHL, 393
  therapy of, 394, 395
Sensory deprivation
  axonal sprouting, 215
  excitatory neurotransmission, 214, 215
  GABAergic inhibition, 213, 214
  KCC2 cotransporters, 214
  STDP, 215
Sensory lesions, 402, 403
Sensory signal, 603
Serenity® System, 696
Serotonergic dysfunction, 521
Sigmoid sinus dehiscence, 372
Sigmoid sinus diverticulum, 372
Signal detection, 233
Signal perception, 233
Signal processing, 659
Single nucleotide variants (SNV), 405
Sinus thrombosis, 444
Sleep deprivation, 253
Small foils, 785
Social isolation, 29
Social media, 745
Solution focused counselling, 534
Solution focused therapy, 533
Somatoform disorder, 516
Somatosensory stimulation, 700
Somatosensory system, 646
  vs. auditory pathways, 378, 379
  bimodal stimulation, 139
  botulinum toxin injection, 138
  clinical manifestations, 138
  cochlear nucleus, 137
  electrical stimulation, 138, 139
  extralemniscal and lemniscal auditory pathways, 136, 137
  McGurk illusion, 136
  physical therapy, 138
  somatosensory tinnitus
    characteristics, 379
    health professionals, 379
    patient's medical history, 379
    pre-test probability, 379–381
    symptoms, 379
    types of, 379
  stimulus, 381, 382
  VGLUTS, 137
Somatosensory tinnitus (SST), 646
Somatostatin (SOM)-expressing inhibitory neurons, 276
Sound deprivation
  frequency tuning, 146
  inhibition and excitation, 146, 147
  neural plasticity, 147
Sound generating devices, 582
Sound generators, 579
Sound loudness, 179
Sound maskers, 618
Sound therapy, 749
  general principles, 603, 604
  hearing loss, 606, 607
  instrumentation, 604
  issue of the "mixing point", 605
  rule of sound therapy, 604
  and sleep, 604
  specific recommendations for, 605
  stochastic resonance, 605, 606
Sound-evoked response, 292, 293
Speech audiometry, 356, 406
Speech discrimination scores (SDS), 649
Speech recognition thresholds (SRT), 356
Speech-in-noise tests, 119
Spike-time dependent plasticity (STDP), 126, 127, 215
Spontaneous discharge rate (SR), 119
Spontaneous firing rate (SFR), 210
Spontaneous otoacoustic emission (SOAE), 102
St John's Wort (SJW), 710
Standardized psychometric tools, 661
Stapes surgery, 390, 391
Statistics, 745
Stereotactic radiosurgery (SRS), 416
Stimulation frequency, 674
Stress, 196, 197
Stress accumulation, 260
Stress is synonymous, 552
Stress reduction techniques, 552
Stroop test, 169, 253
Structural imaging, 167, 168
Subclavian steal syndrome, 442
Subjective tinnitus, 346, 646
Subjective Tinnitus Severity Scale (STSS), 340
Sudden deafness, 393
Sudden sensorineural hearing loss (SSNHL), 393
Suicide, 323
Sulpiride, 624
Superior canal dehiscence, 29
Superior cervical sympathetic ganglion, 648
Superior semi-circular canal dehiscence (SCCD), 373, 510
Swiss guideline, 775
Sympathetic nervous system (SNS), 90
Synaptic genes, 54
Syndromic hearing loss (SHL), 392
Systematic reviews, 552

T
Talking therapy, 257
Task-based fMRI, 168, 169
Temporal coherence, 146
Temporary threshold shifts (TTS), 124, 154, 155
Temporomandibular joint, 648
Temporomandibular joint disorder, 29
Tensor tympani nerve, 648
Tensor Tympani Syndrome, 245
Thalamocortical dysrhythmia, 128, 181, 198
Theta frequency synchronization, 696
Threshold equalizing in noise (TEN) testing, 19

Tinnitus, 594, 635
  acute and chronic tinnitus, 21
  affective component, 19
  and anxiety, 521–524
  and depression, 519–521
  animal models, types of, 303
  audiological assessment (*see* Audiological assessment)
  auditory hallucination, 20, 21
  auditory treatments of, 772, 773
  biomarkers, 19
  brain stimulation techniques, 684, 685, 687
  challenges, 307, 308
  classification and etiology, 123, 124
  clinical neuroimaging
    advantages and disadvantages, 365
    arterial vascular abnormalities, 366–369
    arteriovenous pathologies, 369–372
    colour duplex sonography, 366
    computed tomography, 366
    contrast enhanced MR angiography, 366
    definitions, 365
    Digital Subtraction Angiography, 366
    limiting factors, 366
    magnetic resonance imaging, 366
    non-invasive identification, 365
    plane of acquisition, 366
    pre- imaging assessment, 365
    pre-imaging assessment, 365
    pulsatile tinnitus, 366
    TOF MRA, 366
    venous causes, 372, 373
  clinical observations, 316
  cochlear dysfunction, 19
  cognitive behavioural therapy, 302, 772
  complementary and alternative therapies, 773
  definition, 19, 20, 22, 233, 234
  diagnostic assessment
    challenging, 317
    clinical characteristics, 317, 318
    features, 318
    history, 318
    indication, 318
    life-threatening emergency, 318
    non-pulsatile tinnitus, 318, 319
    pulsatile tinnitus, 318
    stepwise decision-tree approach, 317
    subforms, 316
    symptomatic treatment, 319
  diagnostic criteria, 20, 22
  E-Health based approaches, 774
  history
    classical antiquity, 5–7
    clinical intake interview, 325
    clinical practice, 324
    cognitive behavioral therapy, 325
    demographic data, 324
    depression and anxiety, 323
    diagnostic and therapeutic management, 324
    early middle ages, 8, 9
    enlightenment, 11
    follow-up assessments, 323
    health disorders, 325
    high middle ages, 9
    intake interview, 323
    items list, 324
    late antiquity, 7, 8
    late middle ages, 9, 10
    loudness, 325
    modern times, 11–14
    otologic and audiologic assessment, 322
    psychological and psychiatric assessment, 323
    psychological and social factors, 322
    renaissance, 10
    scientific revolution, 11
    severity, 323
    sound characteristics, 324, 325
    structured interviews, 323
    suicide, 323
    time course, 322
    tinnitus diary, 327
    tinnitus-related impairment, 325–327
    worsen tinnitus, 325
  mindfulness and, 772
  musical hallucinosis, 20, 21
  neural correlates (*see* Electroencephalography (EEG)) (*see* Magnetoencephalography (MEG))
  neurofeedback studies in, 656
  objective and subjective tinnitus, 21
  pathophysiology, 19
  pharmacological treatments
    Alzheimer's disease, 303
    brain stimulation therapies, 305–307
    EGb-761, 304, 305
    GABAergic drug, 304
    gabapentin, 304
    glutamatergic neurotransmission, 303
    medications, 303
    memantine, 303
    N-methyl-d-aspartate receptor, 303
  symptoms, 19
  therapeutic interventions, 771, 772
  tinnitus activities treatment, 773
  tinnitus pharmacotherapy, 773
  tinnitus retraining therapy, 773
Tinnitus activities treatment (TAT)
  clinician, role of, 633
  components of
    concentration, 639, 640
    evidence for, 641
    hearing, 636, 637
    sleep disturbances, 637, 638
    thoughts and emotions, 635, 636
  history, 632, 633
Tinnitus Beeinträchtigungs Fragebogen (TBF-12), 340
Tinnitus Cognitions Questionnaire (TCQ), 340, 341
Tinnitus Coping Style Questionnaire (TCSQ), 341
Tinnitus counseling, 772
Tinnitus distress, 556, 648
Tinnitus drug discovery, 625, 626
Tinnitus Effects Questionnaire, 746
Tinnitus extreme phenotype (TEP), 407
Tinnitus Functional Index (TFI), 338, 450, 564
Tinnitus Functional Inventory, 552
Tinnitus grading, 517
Tinnitus Handicap Index (THI), 564
Tinnitus Handicap Inventory (THI), 305, 337, 340, 516, 552, 649, 742
Tinnitus Handicap Inventory score, 624
Tinnitus Handicap Questionnaire (THQ), 339
Tinnitus Handicap/Support Scale (TH/SS), 340
Tinnitus heterogeneity
  clinical subtypes, 76
  in comorbidities, 73, 74

etiologic factors, 73
gender aspects
in auditory processing, 75
in sound processing, 74, 75
neuronal mechanisms, 75
genetic variants, 76, 77
implications, 77
interference, 74
patient databases, 76
perceptual characteristics, 73
severity, 74
treatment response, 74, 76
Tinnitus Hub, 721, 722
Tinnitus index (TI), 211
Tinnitus loudness, 357
Tinnitus masking, 234
Tinnitus pharmacotherapy, 773
Tinnitus pitch matching, 356, 357
Tinnitus questionnaires, 552, 553
clinical assessment, 331
correlations, 338
definition, 330
development, 338
factor analysis, 338
FTQ, 341
limitations, 342
loudness, 330
psychometric and methodological aspects
cultural and language bias, 334
feasibility, 333
minimal clinical important improvement, 333
outcome domains, 334, 335
reliability, 333
responsiveness, 333
severity, 334
standardization and norming, 333
translation, 334
validity, 331
quantification, 330
quantitative assessment, 335, 336
rating scales, 341, 342
responses, 338
self-report measurement, 336
severity, 331
STSS, 340
TCQ, 340, 341
TCSQ, 341
TFI, 338
TH/SS, 340
THI, 337, 340
THQ, 339
Tinnitus Activities Questionnaire, 339
Tinnitus Severity Index, 340
treatment, 338
TRQ, 338, 339
TSS, 339
Tinnitus Reaction Questionnaire (TRQ), 338, 339
Tinnitus Research Initiative (TRI), 781, 782
Tinnitus retraining therapy (TRT), 28, 247, 451, 509, 599, 600
audiological evaluation, 595, 596
changes in implementation of, 610
clinical goals of, 593, 594
conditioned reflexes, 600–602
diagnosis, 596, 597
hyperacusis, 597
long term evaluation of, 609
patients' categorization and main features of, 598
prolonged exacerbation, 597, 598
result of, 608, 609
structures interview and questionnaires, 594, 595
Tinnitus Sample Case History Questionnaire (TSCHQ), 326, 353
Tinnitus Severity Index (TSI), 340
Tinnitus Severity Scale (TSS), 339
Tinnitus signal, 592
Tinnitus treatment
clinical trials, 765–767
EEG neurofeedback for
auditory α and δ band power, 657, 658
chronic tinnitus, 656, 657
differential EEG neurofeedback protocol, 658
early attempts, 655, 656
fMRI approaches, 659, 660
protocols, 658, 659
and recommendations, 768–770
Tomographic approaches, 659
Tongue stimulation, 698, 699
Tortuous carotid artery, 486
Traditional Chinese Medicine (TCM)
acupuncture, 708
aromatherapy, 711, 712
clinical practice guidelines and CAM, 712
dietary supplements, 709
Ginkgo biloba (Chinese Maidenhair), 709
homeopathy, 711
melatonin, 711
Placebo effect, 713
St John's Wort (SJW), 710
Transcranial alternating current stimulation (tACS), 670, 671
Transcranial direct current (tDCS)
high-definition tDCS, 670
regular tDCS, 668, 670
stimulation (tDCS), 357, 669, 773
Transcranial electrical stimulation, 669
Transcranial magnetic stimulation (TMS), 672, 673, 685
Transcranial random noise stimulation (tRNS), 671
Transcutaneous electrical nerve stimulation (TENS), 671
Transcutaneous vagus nerve stimulation (tVNS), 671, 672
Transduction process, 124
Transient-evoked otoacoustic emission (TEOAE), 102, 359
Translabyrinthine resection, 418, 419
Trauma-associated stress disorder (PTSD), 462
Trauma-associated tinnitus
cervical, 461, 462
head and neck injuries, 458
medicolegal aspects, 462
noise-related trauma, 458
non-pulsatile tinnitus
barotrauma, 461
labyrinthine concussion, 460
noise trauma, 461
OChD, 460
perilymphatic fistula, 460
temporal bone fracture, 460
PTSD, 462
pulsatile tinnitus, 459
symptoms, 458, 459
Traumatic brain injury (TBI), 273
sound tolerance, 31
Traumatic life events, 516
Traumatic noise, 153, 154
Trigeminal nerve, 648
Trigeminal neuralgia, 428, 429

Triple network model, 172
Tympanometry, 357, 358
Tympanoplasty, 389
Typical high-frequency hearing loss, 596

U
UK National Institute for Health and Care Excellence's (NICE) guidelines, 564
UK's National Institute for Health and Care Excellence (NICE), 742
Uncomfortable loudness levels (ULL), 285
Unilateral Ménière's disease (UMD), 405

V
Vagus Nerve Stimulation (VNS), 687, 688, 694, 695, 700, 701
Variability, 786
Varicella zoster virus, 392
Ventral Cochlear Nucleus (VCN)
  acute noise exposure, 210
  chronic noise exposure, 210, 211
Ventromedial prefrontal cortex (vmPFC), 167
Vertebrobasilar and carotid dolichoectasia, 442
Vesicular glutamate transporters (VGLUT-2), 126
Vesicular glutamate transporters (VGLUTS), 137
Vestibular aqueduct, 403
Vestibular evoked myogenic potentials (VEMPs), 406
Vestibular fibrosis, 402
Vestibular schwannomas (VS)
  brainstem and cerebellum, 416
  diagnosis, 416
  disequilibrium, 415
  dizziness and headache, 416
  growth, 416
  ILS, 415
  incidence, 415
  symptoms and signs, 415
  tinnitus
    conservative treatment, 417
    gamma knife surgery, 419
    microsurgery, 417, 418
    retrosigmoid/suboccipital resection, 418, 419
    symptoms, 417
    translabyrinthine resection, 418, 419
    translabyrinthine surgery, 419
    tumor size, 417
  treatment, 416, 417
Video head impulse test, 407
Virtual reality, 755
Visual analogue scores (VAS) painfulness, 87
Visual snow (VS), 21
Visual snow syndrome (VSS), 199
Vitamin B12 deficiency, 752
Vitamin d supplements, 707
Vitamins, 707
Voltage-gated channel acting compounds, 619
Voxel-based morphometry (VBM), 167

W
Wearable ear level sound generators, 749
Western medicine, 707
Williams syndrome, 289

Y
Yoga, 754
YouTube videos, 745

Z
Zinc, 751